Surgery of Cranial Base Tumors

Surgery of Cranial Base Tumors

Editors

Laligam N. Sekhar, M.D., F.A.C.S.
Professor
Department of Neurosurgery
University of Pittsburgh School of Medicine
and
Co-Director
Center for Cranial Base Surgery
Presbyterian University Hospital
Pittsburgh, Pennsylvania

Ivo P. Janecka, M.D., F.A.C.S.
Associate Professor
Department of Otolaryngology
Eye and Ear Institute
University of Pittsburgh School of Medicine
and
Co-Director
Center for Cranial Base Surgery
Presbyterian University Hospital
Pittsburgh, Pennsylvania

RAVEN PRESS ♦ NEW YORK

Raven Press, Ltd., 1185 Avenue of the Americas, New York, New York 10036

© 1993 by Raven Press, Ltd. All rights reserved. This book is protected by copyright. No part of it may be reproduced, stored in a retrieval system, or transmitted, in any form or by any means, electronic, mechanical, photocopying, recording, or otherwise, without prior written permission of the publisher.

Made and Bound in Hong Kong

Library of Congress Cataloging-in-Publication Data

Surgery of cranial base tumors/editors, Laligam N. Sekhar, Ivo P. Janecka.
    p. cm.
    Includes bibliographical references and index.
    ISBN 0-88167-877-5
    1. Skull base—Tumors—Surgery—Atlases. I. Sekhar, Laligam N.
II. Janecka, Ivo P.
    [DNLM: 1. Brain Neoplasms—surgery—atlases. 2. Skull Neoplasms—surgery—atlases. WE 17 S961]
RD662.5.S88 1993
616.99'481059—dc20
DNLM/DLC
for Library of Congress   92-6787
                                                                                            CIP

    The material contained in this volume was submitted as previously unpublished material, except in the instances in which some of the illustrative material was derived.
    Great care has been taken to maintain the accuracy of the information contained in the volume. However, neither Raven Press nor the editors can be held responsible for errors or for any consequences arising from the use of the information contained herein.
    Materials appearing in this book prepared by individuals as part of their official duties as U.S. Government employees are not covered by the above-mentioned copyright.

9 8 7 6 5 4 3 2 1

This book is dedicated to our teachers, colleagues, and our patients.

Our families, and especially our wives, Barbara Sekhar and Cheryl Janecka, provided invaluable support for all our professional activities and development. Our children and our students continue to be an inspiration to seek better solutions now and for the future.

Contents

Contributing Authors	xi
Foreword *by Peter J. Jannetta*	xv
Foreword *by Eugene N. Myers*	xvii
Preface	xix

General Principles/Diagnostic Evaluations

1. Introduction: General Neurosurgical Operative Techniques and Instrumentation in Cranial Base Surgery ... 1
   Laligam N. Sekhar, Atul Goel, and Chandranath Sen

2. Introduction: General Otolaryngologic/Plastic Surgery Operative Techniques and Instrumentation in Cranial Base Surgery ... 11
   Ivo P. Janecka

3. MRI and CT in the Evaluation of Skull Base Masses ... 15
   William L. Hirsch, Jr. and Hugh D. Curtin

4. Balloon Test Occlusion ... 33
   Joseph A. Horton, Charles A. Jungreis, and Frank Pistoia

5. Interventional Neuroradiology: Embolization ... 37
   Charles A. Jungreis and Joseph A. Horton

6. Cerebral Revascularization in Cranial Base Surgery ... 45
   Mark E. Linskey, Laligam N. Sekhar, and Chandranath Sen

7. Special Anesthetic Considerations in Cranial Base Tumor Surgery ... 69
   Rene M. Gonzalez

8. Methods of Neurophysiological Monitoring During Cranial Base Tumor Resection ... 83
   Robert J. Sclabassi, Donald N. Krieger, Donald J. Weisz, and John Durrant

Surgical Anatomy

9. The Anterior and Middle Cranial Fossae Including the Cavernous Sinus and Orbit ... 99
   Johannes Lang

10. Anatomy of the Paranasal Sinuses ... 123
    Johannes Lang

11. Anatomy of the Posterior Cranial Fossa 131
    Johannes Lang

Operative Techniques

12. Anterior and Anterolateral Craniofacial Resection 147
    Ivo P. Janecka and Laligam N. Sekhar

13. Anterior, Anterolateral, and Lateral Approaches to Extradural
    Petroclival Tumors 157
    *Laligam N. Sekhar, Chandranath Sen, Carl H. Snyderman,
    and Ivo P. Janecka*

14. Transoral Approach to Intra/Extradural Tumors 225
    H. Alan Crockard

15. The Transmaxillary Approach to the Clivus 235
    H. Alan Crockard

16. Facial Translocation Approach to Nasopharynx, Clivus, and
    Infratemporal Fossa 245
    *Ivo P. Janecka, Chandranath Sen, Laligam N. Sekhar, and
    Daniel W. Nuss*

17. The Transmandibular–Transcervical Approach to the Skull Base 261
    Yosef P. Krespi and Gady Har-El

18. Transtemporal and Infratemporal Approach for Benign Tumors
    of the Jugular Foramen and Temporal Bone 267
    *Barry E. Hirsch, Laligam N. Sekhar, and
    Donald B. Kamerer*

19. Surgical Excision of Petrous Apex Lesions 291
    *Ricardo Ramina, Joao J. Maniglia, and
    Carlos E. Barrionuevo*

20. Petrosal Approach to Clival Tumors 307
    Ossama Al-Mefty

21. Classification, Technique, and Results of Surgical Resection of
    Petrous Bone Tumors 317
    *Shlomo Pomeranz, Laligam N. Sekhar, Ivo P. Janecka,
    Barry E. Hirsch, and Sai S. Ramasastry*

22. The Transsphenoidal Approach to Invasive Sellar and Clival Lesions 337
    Rudolf Fahlbusch and Michael Buchfelder

23. Translabyrinthine/Transcochlear Approaches 351
    Derald E. Brackmann

24. The Middle Fossa Approach 367
    Derald E. Brackmann

25. Surgical Strategy for Jugular Foramen Tumors 379
    Madjid Samii and Walter Bini

26. Extreme Lateral Transcondylar and Transjugular Approaches 389
    Chandranath Sen and Laligam N. Sekhar

Reconstruction

27. Regional Flaps and Craniofacial Skeleton 413
    Ivo P. Janecka and Carl H. Snyderman

28. Microvascular Reconstruction of the Cranial Base 427
    *Kenneth C. Shestak, Neil Ford Jones, and
    Sai S. Ramasastry*

29. Facial Nerve Management and Reconstructive Techniques 435
    Ivo P. Janecka, Laligam N. Sekhar, and Erick Stephanian

30. Reanimation of the Paralyzed Face Without the Facial Nerve 449
    Mark May and Steven M. Sobol

31. Alloplastic Materials in Skull Base Reconstruction 461
    Jan Helms and Götz Geyer

Treatment of Specific Tumors

32. Esthesioneuroblastoma 471
    Robert W. Cantrell

33. Transzygomatic and Transpalatal Excision of Juvenile Nasopharyngeal
    Angiofibroma with Intracranial Extension: The Surgical Procedure ... 477
    Stephen J. Haines and Arndt J. Duvall III

34. Juvenile Angiofibroma 485
    Wolfgang Draf

35. Nasal/Paranasal Sinus Carcinoma 497
    Ivo P. Janecka, Laligam N. Sekhar, and Eugene N. Myers

36. Tuberculum Sella and Olfactory Groove Meningiomas 507
    Ossama Al-Mefty

37. Cavernous Sinus and Sphenocavernous Neoplasms: Anatomy and
    Surgery 521
    Laligam N. Sekhar, Donald A. Ross, and Chandranath Sen

38. Petroclival Meningiomas 605
    Laligam N. Sekhar, Tariq Javed, and Peter J. Jannetta

39. Combined Supra- and Infra-Parapetrosal Approach for Petroclival
    Lesions 661
    Takanori Fukushima

40. Transcondyle Approach for Foramen Magnum Meningiomas 671
    Akira Hakuba and Takeshi Tsujimoto

41. Clivus Chordomas 679
    Edward R. Laws, Jr.

42. Microsurgical Anatomy of Acoustic Neuromas 687
    Albert L. Rhoton, Jr.

43. Acoustic Neurilemoma: Otological Approaches 715
    Jean-Marc Sterkers

44. Facial Nerve Neurilemomas 725
    Ivo P. Janecka and Laligam N. Sekhar

45. Jugular Foramen Neurilemoma 731
    Sam E. Kinney

46. Trigeminal Neurilemoma 737
    Ian F. Pollack and Laligam N. Sekhar

47. Glomus Jugulare Tumors 747
    C. Gary Jackson, Charles I. Woods, and Philip N. Chironis

48. Glomus Vagale Tumors 763
    Eugen J. Dolan and Patrick Gullane

49. Orbital Surgery 769
    Jack Rootman and Felix Durity

50. Surgical Management of Craniopharyngioma 787
    Dachling Pang

51. Osseous Lesions of Anterior and Middle Base 809
    Patrick J. Derome and A. Visot

Rehabilitation/Complications

52. Rehabilitation of Swallowing 819
    Carl H. Snyderman and Jonas T. Johnson

53. The Central Electroauditory Prosthesis 825
    *William F. House, William E. Hitselberger,
    Jed A. Kwartler, and Derald E. Brackmann*

54. Complications of Skull Base Operations 831
    *Chandranath Sen, Carl H. Snyderman, and
    Laligam N. Sekhar*

Subject Index 841

Contributing Authors

Ossama Al-Mefty, M.D., *Professor, Division of Neurological Surgery, Loyola University Medical Center, 2160 South First Avenue, Maywood, Illinois 60153*

Carlos E. Barrionuevo, M.D., *Associate Professor, Department of Otology, Hospital de Clinicas, University Federal of Paraná, Bispo Don José 2505, Curitiba, Paraná, Brazil 80420*

Walter Bini, M.D., *Neurosurgical Clinic, Nordstadt Hospital, Haltenhoffstr 41, 3000 Hannover, Germany*

Derald E. Brackmann, M.D., *Clinical Professor, Department of Otolaryngology, University of Southern California, Los Angeles, House Ear Clinic and Institute, 2100 West Third Street, First floor, Los Angeles, California 90057*

Michael Buchfelder, M.D., *Universitat Erlangen Nurnberg, Schwabashaslage 6, D 8520 Erlangen, Germany*

Robert W. Cantrell, M.D., *Fitz-Hugh Professor and Chairman, Department of Otolaryngology and Head and Neck Surgery, University of Virginia, Box 430, University of Virginia Medical Center, Charlottesville, Virginia 22908*

Philip Chironis, M.D., *Otolaryngology, Head and Neck Surgery, 951 South Beach Boulevard, La Habra, California 90631*

H. Alan Crockard, F.R.C.S., *Consultant Neurosurgeon, Department of Surgical Neurology, The National Hospital for Neurology and Neurosurgery, Maida Vale, London, W9 1TL, United Kingdom*

Hugh D. Curtin, M.D., *Professor, Department of Radiology, University of Pittsburgh, 230 Lothrop Street, Pittsburgh, Pennsylvania 15213*

Patrick J. Derome, M.D., *Professor, Department of Neurosurgery, Hopital Foch, 40 rue Worth, 92151 Suresnes, France*

Eugen J. Dolan, M.D., F.R.C.S.(C), *Department of Neurosurgery, The Billings Clinic, 2825 Eighth Avenue North, P.O. Box 35100, Billings, Montana 59107-5100*

Wolfgang Draf, M.D., PhD., *Professor of Medicine, Department of Ear, Nose, and Throat Diseases, Head, Neck, and Facial Plastic Surgery, Communication Disorders, Klinikum Fulda Teaching Hospital, University of Marburg, Pacelliallee 4, D6400 Fulda, West Germany*

Felix Durity, M.D., *Associate Professor, Division of Neurosurgery, University of British Columbia, 700 West Tenth Avenue, Vancouver, British Columbia, Canada V57 4E9*

John Durrant, M.D., *Center for Clinical Audiology, Department of Otolaryngology, University of Pittsburgh School of Medicine and Montefiore University Hospital, Pittsburgh, Pennsylvania 15213*

Arndt J. Duvall, III, M.D., *Department of Otolaryngology, University of Minnesota, Center for Craniofacial and Skull Base Surgery, Box 96 UMHC, B590 Mayo Memorial Building, 420 Delaware Street South East, Minneapolis, Minnesota 55455*

Rudolf Fahlbusch, M.D., *Professor and Chairman, Department of Neurosurgery, University of Erlangen-Nürnberg, Kopfklinikum, Schwabachanlage, 852 Erlangen, Germany*

Takanori Fukushima, M.D., D.M.Sc., *Professor, Department of Neurosurgery, Co-Director, USC-Skull Base Center, University of Southern California, 1200 North State Street, Los Angeles, California 90033*

Götz Geyer, M.D., *Universitats Hals-Nasen-Ohren Klinik, Josef-Schneider-Str. 11, 8700 Würzberg, Germany*

Atul Goel, M.D., *Lecturer, Department of Neurosurgery, KEM Hospital, 400 012 Bombay, India*

René M. Gonzalez, M.D., *Clinical Associate Professor, Department of Anesthesiology and Critical Care Medicine, Eye and Ear Hospital of the University of Pittsburgh Medical Center, 230 Lothrop Street, Pittsburgh, Pennsylvania, 15213*

Patrick Gullane, M.B., Bch., F.R.C.S.(C), *Professor, Department of Otolaryngology, University of Toronto, Toronto General Hospital, Eaton Wing, North 7, 200 Elizabeth Street, Toronto, Ontario, M5G 1L7, Canada*

Stephen J. Haines, M.D., *Associate Professor, Departments of Neurosurgery and Otolaryngology, University Hospital, University of Minnesota, 420 Delaware Street South East, Minneapolis, Minnesota 55455*

Akira Hakuba, M.D., D.M.S., *Professor and Chairman, Department of Neurosurgery, Osaka City University Medical School, 1-5-7, Asahi-machi, Aveno-ku, Osaka 545, Japan*

Gady Har-El, M.D., *Department of Otolaryngology, SUNY-Health Sciences Center at Brooklyn, and the Long Island College Hospital, Brooklyn, New York 11201*

Jan Helms, M.D., *Professor, Universitats Hals-Nasen Ohren-Klinik, Josef-Schneider-Str. 11, 8700 Wurzburg, Germany*

Barry E. Hirsch, M.D., *Assistant Professor, Department of Otolaryngology, Eye and Ear Institute Pavilion, University of Pittsburgh, 203 Lothrop Street, Pittsburgh, Pennsylvania 15213*

William L. Hirsch, Jr., M.D., *Department of Radiology, Presbyterian University Hospital, 230 Lothrop Street, Pittsburgh, Pennsylvania 15213*

William E. Hitselberger, M.D., *2222 Ocean View Avenue, Suite 119, Los Angeles, California 90057*

Joseph A. Horton, M.D., *Department of Radiology, Presbyterian University Hospital, 230 Lothrop Street, Pittsburgh, Pennsylvania 15213*

William F. House, M.D., *Hoog Memorial Hospital, 361 Hospital, Newport Beach, California 92663*

C. Gary Jackson, M.D., F.A.C.S., *The Otology Group, 1811 State Street, Nashville, Tennessee 37203*

Ivo P. Janecka, M.D., F.A.C.S., *Associate Professor, Department of Otolaryngology, Eye and Ear Institute, Suite 500, and Co-Director, Center for Cranial Base Surgery, University of Pittsburgh School of Medicine, Presbyterian University Hospital, 203 Lothrop Street, Pittsburgh, Pennsylvania 15213*

Peter J. Jannetta, M.D., *Professor and Chairman, Department of Neurosurgery, Presbyterian University Hospital, 230 Lothrop Street, Room 9402, Pittsburgh, Pennsylvania 15213*

Tariq Javed, M.D., *Department of Neurosurgery, Presbyterian University Hospital, 230 Lothrop Street, Pittsburgh, Pennsylvania 15213*

Jonas T. Johnson, M.D., F.A.C.S., *Division of Head and Neck Oncology and Immunology, Department of Otolaryngology, University of Pittsburgh School of Medicine, and Eye and Ear Institute, Suite 500, 230 Lothrop Street, Pittsburgh, Pennsylvania 15213*

Neil Ford Jones, M.D., *Associate Professor, Department of Plastic Surgery, University of Pittsburgh, 6B Scaife Hall, Pittsburgh, Pennsylvania 15261*

Charles A. Jungreis, M.D., *Associate Professor, Department of Radiology and Neurological Surgery, University of Pittsburgh School of Medicine, Presbyterian University Hospital, Pittsburgh, Pennsylvania 15213*

Donald B. Kamerer, M.D., *Professor, Department of Otolaryngology, Montefiore University Hospital, Eye and Ear Institute Pavilion, Suite 500, 203 Lothrop Street, Pittsburgh, Pennsylvania 15213*

Sam E. Kinney, M.D., *Department of Otolaryngology, Cleveland Clinic Foundation, 9500 Euclid Avenue, Cleveland, Ohio 44106-5034*

Yosef P. Krespi, M.D., *Director, Department of Otolaryngology, Head and Neck Surgery, St. Luke's/Roosevelt Hospital Center, and Professor of Otolaryngology, Columbia University College of Physicians and Surgeons, 425 West 59th Street, New York, New York 10019*

Donald N. Krieger, Ph.D., *Assistant Professor, Department of Neurological Surgery, University of Pittsburgh, University Health Center, Children's Hospital, One Children's Place, Pittsburgh, Pennsylvania 15213*

Jed A. Kwartler, M.D., *Assistant Professor, Department of Surgery, Section of Otolaryngology, University of Medicine and Dentistry, New Jersey Medical School, 185 South Orange Avenue, Newark, New Jersey 07103*

Johannes Lang, M.D., *Professor, Institute of Anatomy, University of Würzburg, Koellikerstrasse 6, W-8700 Würzburg, Germany*

Edward R. Laws, Jr., M.D., *Professor and Chairman, Department of Neurological Surgery, George Washington University Medical Center, 2150 Pennsylvania Avenue, North West, Washington, D.C., 20037*

Mark E. Linskey, M.D., *Senior Resident, Department of Neurosurgery, University of Pittsburgh, 230 Lothrop Street, Pittsburgh, Pennsylvania, 15213*

Joao J. Maniglia, M.D., *Associate Professor, Department of Otorhinolaryngology, Hospital de Clinicas-University Federal of Paraná, Bispo Don José 2502, Curitiba, Paraná, Brazil 80420*

Mark May, M.D., F.A.C.S., *Clinical Professor, Department of Otolaryngology, Head and Neck Surgery, University of Pittsburgh, 510 South Aiken Avenue, Pittsburgh, Pennsylvania 15232*

Eugene N. Myers, M.D., F.A.C.S., *Professor and Chairman, Department of Otolaryngology, University of Pittsburgh School of Medicine, and Eye and Ear Institute, 203 Lothrop Street, Pittsburgh, Pennsylvania 15213*

Dachling Pang, M.D., F.R.C.S.(C), F.A.C.S., *Associate Professor, Department of Neurosurgery, Chief, Pediatric Neurosurgery, Children's Hospital of Pittsburgh, University of Pittsburgh School of Medicine, 3705 Fifth Avenue, Pittsburgh, Pennsylvania 15213*

Frank Pistoia, M.D., *Department of Radiology, Presbyterian University Hospital, Room 9402, 230 Lothrop Street, Pittsburgh, Pennsylvania 15213*

Ian F. Pollack, M.D., *Assistant Professor, Department of Neurosurgery, University of Pittsburgh, Presbyterian-University Hospital, 9402 DeSoto at O'Hara Streets, Pittsburgh, Pennsylvania 15213*

Shlomo Pomeranz, M.D., *Lecturer, Department of Neurosurgery, Hadassah University Hospital, Hebrew University, Ein Karem, P.O. Box, 12000, Jerusalem, Israel 91120*

Sai S. Ramasastry, M.D., *Associate Professor, Department of Plastic Surgery, University of Pittsburgh, 6B Scaife Hall, Pittsburgh, Pennsylvania 15261*

Ricardo Ramina, M.D., *Neurosurgeon, Curitiba Skull Base Foundation, Hospital Das Nacóes, R. Goncalves Dias 713, 80420, Curitiba, Brazil*

Albert L. Rhoton, Jr., M.D., R. D. Keene Family Professor and Chairman, Department of Neurological Surgery, University of Florida Medical Center, 1600 South West Archer Road, Room M-219, P.O. Box 100265, Gainesville, Florida 32610

Jack Rootman, M.D., F.R.C.S., Professor, Department of Ophthalmology and Pathology, University of British Columbia and Vancouver General Hospital, 2550 Willow Street, Vancouver, British Columbia V5Z 3N9

Donald A. Ross, M.D., Assistant Professor, Section of Neurological Surgery, University of Michigan, 1500 East Medical Center Drive, Ann Arbor, Michigan 48109

Madjio Samii, M.D., Professor, Department of Neurosurgery, Hannover Medical School, Director of Neurosurgical Clinic, Nordstadt Hospital, Haltenhoff Str. 41, 3000 Hannover, Germany

Robert J. Sclabassi, M.D., Ph.D., Professor, Department of Neurological Surgery, Electrical Engineering, and Behavioral Neuroscience, University of Pittsburgh, University Health Center, Children's Hospital, Pittsburgh, Pennsylvania 15213

Laligam N. Sekhar, M.D., F.A.C.S., Professor, Department of Neurosurgery, Co-Director, Center for Cranial Base Surgery, University of Pittsburgh School of Medicine, Presbyterian University Hospital, Room 9402, 230 Lothrop Street, Pittsburgh, Pennsylvania 15213

Chandranath Sen, M.D., Associate Professor, Department of Neurosurgery, Mount Sinai Medical Center, Box 1136, 5 East 98 Street, New York, New York 10029

Kenneth C. Shestak, M.D., Assistant Professor, Department of Plastic Surgery, University of Pittsburgh, 6B Scaife Hall, Pittsburgh, Pennsylvania 15261

Carl H. Snyderman, M.D., Assistant Professor, Center for Cranial Base Surgery, University of Pittsburgh School of Medicine, and Department of Neurosurgery, Eye and Ear Institute, Suite 500, 203 Lothrop Street, Pittsburgh, Pennsylvania 15213

Steven M. Sobol, M.D., Head and Neck Surgery, 2 Memorial Drive, Suite 300, Decatur, Illinois 62526

Erick Stephanian, M.D., Department of Neurosurgery, Presbyterian University Hospital, Room 9402, 230 Lothrop Street, Pittsburgh, Pennsylvania 15213

Jean-Marc Sterkers, M.D., Professor, Department of Otorhinolaryngology, Paris Hospital, 4 rue Michel Ange, 75016 Paris, France

Takeshi Tsujimoto, M.D., Department of Neurosurgery, Osaka City University Medical School, 1-5-7, Asaki-machi Abeno-ku, Osaka 545, Japan

A. Visot, M.D., Department of Neurosurgery, Hospital Foch, 40 Rue Worth, 92151 Suresnes, France

Donald J. Weisz, Ph.D., Associate Professor, Department of Neurological Surgery and Behavioral Neuroscience, University of Pittsburgh, University Health Center, Children's Hospital, One Children's Place, Pittsburgh, Pennsylvania 15213

Charles I. Woods, M.D., Assistant Professor, State University of New York Health Sciences Center, Syracuse, New York 13204

Foreword

How dependent we are upon the wide spectrum of recently developed diagnostic techniques in the practice of contemporary surgery. How dependent we are upon recently developed technical advances for the formulation of new operative areas of expertise. In an interesting reversal of fortune, these dependencies have given surgeons some basic freedoms: freedom from morbidity, freedom from mortality, freedom from blood loss, freedom from neurological deficits, freedom from worry about our patients.

This interesting dichotomy, dependency with freedom, plus a third ingredient, academic collegiality, has enabled astute, contemporary leaders in neurosurgery and otolaryngology to develop new approaches to old, previously insurmountable problems. It is almost as if this wondrous tripartite impaction of attitude has actually *caused* these many good things to happen.

Included among the many good things that have been happening and will continue to happen even more profoundly is the development of the surgery of cranial base tumors. By working together collegially, by collaborating with diagnostic experts in an active way, and by laboring together with other experts therapeutically, the insurmountable problems of yesteryear have not always remained so. As we learn to utilize the newer techniques, as we learn to work together efficiently and not as the starkly solo practitioner of yore, we revise old standards, we set new standards, and we develop new areas of expertise. Part of this development is that of sharing this expertise with our colleagues. As new ideas, new techniques, and new applications are shared, a snowball of further new ideas, new techniques, and new applications develops almost geometrically. Many surgeons in many institutions are now working together, carefully evaluating these previously untreatable, often recurrent tumors, applying new techniques, and further evaluating results carefully and independently. A critical mass of skull base tumor surgeons now exists.

Although several recent and excellent textbooks are in our libraries and are frequently used when we approach cranial base tumors, no surgical atlas has been published until now, despite a real need for such. This atlas, edited by Sekhar and Janecka, is authored by multiple contributors who have created much that is state-of-the-art in the area of surgical techniques. The book is organized so that it can be utilized easily and effectively by surgeons working in the area. The first section deals with diagnostic testing, both imaging and physiologic. This is followed by lessons from the neurosurgical/anatomical master of surgical anatomy of the cranial base, Johannes Lang of Würzburg. Then specific operative approaches, which comprise our "brain-saving" techniques, are presented in an orderly fashion. Description of techniques of reconstruction are followed by descriptions of specific techniques for various tumor resections. The important areas of rehabilitation and complications are then lucidly addressed.

The superb art work by Jon Coulter is an important part of the atlas. This book fills a great need in an admirable way and should be in the library of every surgeon interested in and working in the surgery of cranial base tumors, no matter what vantage point the surgeon comes from. In this atlas, we have a synthesis of the best that can be done in our evaluation and treatment of these devastating lesions.

Peter J. Jannetta, M.D.

Foreword

The first venture for surgery of the cranial base was carried out at the University of Pittsburgh in 1974 for a patient suffering intractable pain from a primary carcinoma of the palate involving the ethmoids, which had failed 17 operative procedures and two courses of radiation therapy. Being familiar with the work of Ketcham, members of the Department of Otolaryngology and Neurological Surgery carried out a craniofacial resection. Since then, the two departments have had a commitment to improvement of the diagnosis and management of these tumors and the Center for Cranial Base Surgery, which is the essence of multidisciplinary activity, was developed.

It's been thrilling over these last several decades to witness the proliferation of diagnostic, therapeutic, and reconstructive techniques in this area. This book, *Surgery of Cranial Base Tumors,* is an exceptionally comprehensive book which will give the reader a great deal of information as to the most contemporary forms of diagnosis and patient evaluation, such as CT and MR scanning, balloon test occlusion, and interventional neuroradiology. Contemporary anesthetic techniques and electrophysiological monitoring have made this type of surgery quite safe and are detailed in several chapters. The complex surgical anatomy is very well outlined in the early chapters and specific operative approaches are then detailed by anatomical area. Many of these operative approaches, such as the facial translocation approach to the nasopharynx, clivus, and infratemporal fossa, the anterior, anterolateral, and lateral approaches to extradural petroclival tumors, are innovative, contemporary, and provide the reader with an idea of the creative instincts which are being brought to bear on the management of tumors of the cranial base.

These areas are amplified in the section on specific tumor types and much is to be gained by reading these chapters, each one written by experts in the field whose names are indelibly linked with management of these tumors. Appropriate emphasis is placed on reconstruction, particularly with microvascular free flaps, which are the most contemporary and versatile means of reconstruction, as well as rehabilitation of certain aspects of the patient's function, which is often hampered by the tumor and/or the surgery. Ample space is provided for clear discussion of the management of complications of these procedures.

This book is one which, in my opinion, will be an excellent addition to the literature now building on contemporary management of cranial base tumors. Much is to be admired about the selection of topics and authors and the book is a tribute to its co-editors, Dr. Laligam Sekhar and Dr. Ivo Janecka, and to the current contemporary surgery requiring multimodality treatment and the utmost of multidisciplinary action.

Eugene N. Myers, M.D.

Preface

Cranial base surgery is one of the most exciting and challenging frontiers for neurosurgeons and otolaryngologists alike. Although "cranial base surgery" or "skull base surgery" usually refers to the removal of tumors that occur at the base of the brain and/or involve the basicranium, other types of lesions are also encompassed by this discipline. Developmental lesions such as basal encephaloceles and craniosynostosis are treated using the principles of cranial base surgery. Complex traumatic lesions of the basicranium are better treated because of the advances in cranial base surgery. Finally, complex vascular lesions at the base of the brain, such as aneurysms and arteriovenous malformations, can be better managed by the advanced cranial base exposures developed for tumor surgery. This book deals predominantly with tumor surgery, but the techniques presented here can be applied to the other lesions as well.

This book is the first comprehensive color atlas that details the important new surgical techniques in this field. The chapters discuss the indication for the procedure, illustrate operative techniques by means of drawings, radiographs, and operative photographs, and discuss complications and results. The majority of the illustrations are by Jon Coulter, and in combination with the photographs, make the learning of this complex surgery easier.

The book is organized into six sections. The first section provides the general principles of cranial base operations, operative instrumentation, and microsurgical operative technique. Preoperative patient evaluation with computed tomography, magnetic resonance imaging, and arteriography are discussed. Balloon occlusion testing of the internal carotid artery and embolization techniques of tumors are illustrated. Principles of anesthesia for cranial base operations, cerebral revascularization, and neurophysiological monitoring are discussed.

The second section on surgical anatomy consists of three chapters written by one of the greatest neuroanatomists of our time, Professor Johannes Lang. Further information about cavernous sinus anatomy, posterior fossa anatomy, and other pertinent surgical anatomy can also be found in the relevant chapters.

The third section deals with specific operative approaches, such as the subtemporal and infratemporal approach, extended frontal approach, transoral approach, transmaxillary approach, facial translocation approach, and the extreme lateral transcondylear approach.

In the fourth section, cranial base reconstruction is discussed in detail. This includes regional flaps, the facial skeleton, microvascular flaps, facial nerve reconstruction, facial reanimation techniques, and the use of alloplastic material.

The fifth section is the largest and contains details regarding operative excision of specific tumor types or anatomic sites. Examples include cavernous sinus tumors, petroclival lesions, esthesioneuroblastoma, glomus tumors, and orbital lesions.

The last section includes chapters on rehabilitation of swallowing, and of anacusis using a central electroauditory prosthesis. Complications and their management are also discussed in this section.

Neurosurgeons and otolaryngologists will be particularly interested in this book. However, all physicians, nurses, and other health care professionals who care for patients with skull base lesions will also find it interesting and a valuable source of information.

Surgeons who are interested in learning cranial base surgery must realize that reading a book such as this is only a part of the learning process. Rigorous training in basic microsurgery, an exquisite knowledge of skull base anatomy gained by repeated anatomic dissections, and observations of and training with individuals who are experienced in cranial base surgery are essential ingredients of the training process.

Laligam N. Sekhar
Ivo P. Janecka

Surgery of Cranial Base Tumors

CHAPTER 1

Introduction

General Neurosurgical Operative Techniques and Instrumentation in Cranial Base Surgery

Laligam N. Sekhar, Atul Goel, and Chandranath Sen

The emergence of skull base surgery as a separate neurosurgical subspecialty has been a rapid ascendancy occurring within the last decade. It is encouraging to note that many young and talented surgeons are getting interested in this field of neurosurgery. This augurs well for the future of this specialty.

Tumors of the cranial base are defined as those that arise at the base of the brain, with a tendency to invade the basicranium, those arising from the cranial bones themselves, or those originating just below the cranium, often involving the paranasal sinuses, the infratemporal fossa, or the parapharyngeal space. Such lesions may arise in the neural, vascular, or meningeal structures of the nervous system or in bone or cartilage of the skull base, or they may originate in the extracranial tissues and invade the skull base secondarily. Although the term "cranial base tumors" groups together a variety of neoplasms, they share certain common features and problems because of the complex anatomical region that they occupy. Figures 1 and 2 show the benign and malignant tumors operated by LNS or CNS during the last 7 years.

The cranial base is conveniently classified into anterior, middle, and posterior parts that correspond to the respective cranial fossae. Some authors have divided the middle and posterior cranial base into three compartments: the sphenoid base, the petrous temporal base, and the clivus.

The skull base, with its complex collection of blood vessels and nerves and irregular bony topography, is an anatomically complex region. It is essential to have a three-dimensional image of these structures and to be able to decipher the relationships from all angles. The skull base surgeon must therefore have an exact understanding of the anatomy of this region gained by repeated cadaveric dissections. Laboratory training with vascular and neural anastomosis and microdissection is also important. Advanced training with experienced surgeons in this field is necessary to grasp the subtleties of technique as well as nuances of preoperative and postoperative care. Ability to work for long hours under a microscope is a prerequisite. A high degree of technical competence, patience, and courage to successfully tackle the problems that are likely to be encountered are essential for the skull base surgeon.

Even though many neoplasms involving the cranial base are benign or locally confined malignant lesions, radical resection of extensive lesions remains difficult. The reasons for this include: the necessity to retract the brain to achieve tumor exposure, with the possibility of retraction-related cerebral injury; the involvement by the tumor of basal blood vessels, injury to which may lead to stroke and/or death; the involvement of the cranial nerves, injury to which may result in significant functional deficits; and the potential for a postoperative cerebrospinal fluid (CSF) leakage through the skin, paranasal sinuses, or nasopharynx, which may be fol-

---

L. N. Sekhar: Department of Neurosurgery, Center for Cranial Base Surgery, University of Pittsburgh School of Medicine, Presbyterian University Hospital, Pittsburgh, Pennsylvania 15213.
A. Goel: 9, Type IV Flats, Seminary Hills, Nagpur, 440006 India.
C. Sen: Department of Neurosurgery, Mt. Sinai Medical Center, New York, New York 10029.

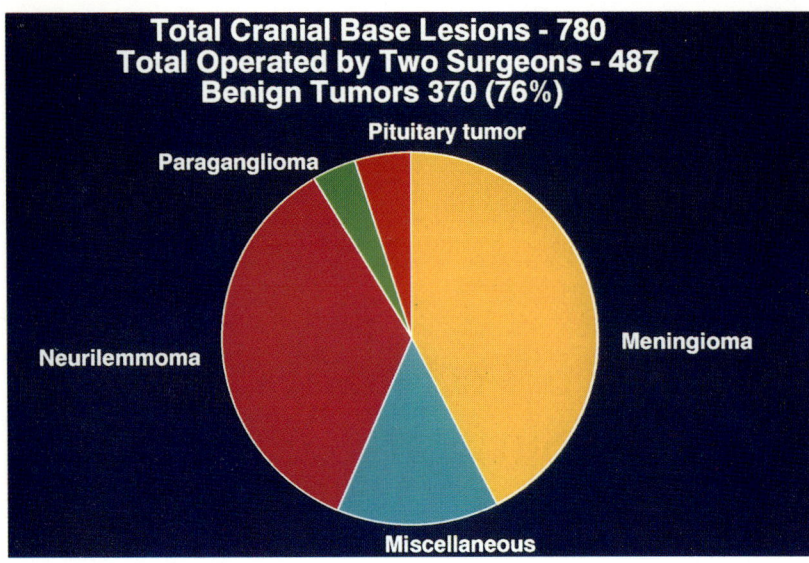

FIG. 1. Chart showing the number of benign tumors operated by the two senior authors (LNS and CNS).

lowed by meningitis and death. However, several advances have occurred during the past decade that permit a total or near total resection of many such neoplasms with low morbidity. These advances include an improved understanding of cranial base anatomy, resulting in the introduction of new operative approaches; the improved management of the petrous and cavernous internal carotid artery; surgery within the cavernous sinus; the preservation and/or reconstruction of cranial nerves involved by the tumor; and improved cranial base reconstruction techniques, using regional and distant vascularized flaps. Advancements in neuroanesthetic techniques and in neurophysiological monitoring methods, the introduction of balloon occlusion tests to monitor the adequacy of collateral circulation, and the preoperative embolization of vascular tumors have also contributed to the refinements in skull base surgery. The friendly collaboration of specialists from different disciplines, and surgeons from the same discipline, has been a very important stimulus for the growth of this discipline.

The keys to the success of operations for cranial base lesions include the avoidance of brain, vascular, or cranial nerve injury; the avoidance of postoperative cerebrospinal fluid fistula or infection; and the use of an operative approach that allows good visualization of all essential anatomical structures to enable total tumor resection.

Successful skull base surgery is a team effort. Apart from the neurosurgeon, the team includes otolaryngologists, plastic and reconstructive surgeons, radiologists, anesthesiologists, critical care and rehabilitation experts, and nurses. A weak link anywhere in this chain can adversely affect the success of these major operations. A large part of the skull base lies adjacent to the structures of the ear, nose, throat, and paranasal sinuses, and an otolaryngologist with special training in skull base proce-

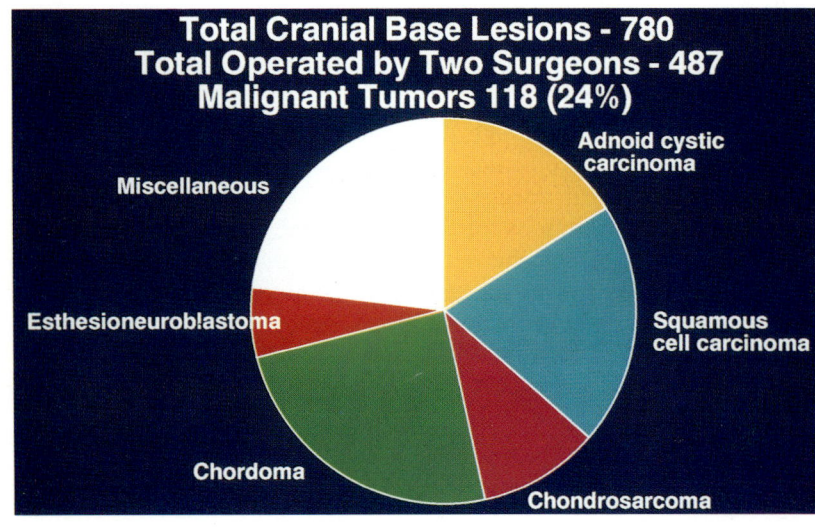

FIG. 2. Chart showing the number of malignant tumors operated by the two senior authors (LNS and CNS).

dures is an important partner in most of the surgical procedures. The teamwork helps not only in bringing together expertise from different specialties but also provides an opportunity for intermittent relaxation during a prolonged surgery and better involvement of the various groups in the postoperative phase. However, it is essential for each member of the team to know their exact role during the operation, and for one person to be ultimately responsible for the patient. In long operations, the presence of another neurosurgeon who works synergistically is of great assistance. Apart from other things, a good communication and relationship with teammates is vital.

In order to justify extensive operative procedures to remove cranial base neoplasms, one must show that the procedure can be performed safely and that the outcome is better than it would be if the disease progressed naturally, or if other treatment modalities such as irradiation or chemotherapy were used. The efficacy of such extensive surgical resection in providing long-term control or cure of benign and malignant lesions of the cranial base has been documented for some lesions; for others, it requires further study and documentation.

PATIENT EVALUATION

The patient who has been referred to a neurological surgeon for a specialized cranial base surgery operation has in most cases already been seen by an internist, a neurologist, or an otolaryngological surgeon. Even then, most patients have a poor understanding of the exact nature of their problem. It is mandatory for the patients and their relatives to know the long-term outlook of the tumor itself, as well as to understand what is involved in the surgery and, in particular, what complications may occur. Preoperative evaluation includes careful physical and neurological examinations. These data should carefully be recorded because they serve as the baseline for all further follow-up studies. The progression of the signs and symptoms and the physiological age of the patient significantly influence the decision concerning whether to operate. The specific requirements of a patient's job activity are collectively important factors in this delicate tabulation of the pros and cons of the surgical intervention. Preoperative studies useful in the evaluation of these patients include computed tomography (CT), especially bone algorithms, magnetic resonance imaging (MRI), cerebral angiography, and a balloon occlusion test of the internal carotid artery (ICA) with clinical and cerebral blood flow measurements. Interventional neuroradiological embolization procedures often help in reducing the blood supply of vascular tumors.

In addition to the extensive radiographic workup, preoperative evoked potential studies are often useful. They provide both a measure of the existence of subclinical neurologic compromise and a baseline for comparison of intraoperative evoked potential measurements. Other preoperative testing may be necessary. Audiometric and visual field testing are important adjunctive studies in some cases. A full endocrinologic evaluation may be necessary for tumors in suprasellar or parasellar locations. For patients with suspected malignant neoplasms, a complete metastatic workup is important.

Some patients undergoing cranial base surgery have concomitant medical illnesses. Because these illnesses may impact on the intraoperative and postoperative care of the patient, it is important that they be well defined and properly controlled prior to surgery. Therefore preoperative consultation with a specialist in general internal medicine or the appropriate medical subspecialty is advisable, whenever the history or physical examination reveals a systemic illness. A *cranial base nurse coordinator* is an important member of the skull base team. The job of the coordinator is to make sure that the patient and the relatives understand the nature of the problems and to support them psychologically in both the preoperative and postoperative periods. The nurse coordinator makes daily rounds to the patients on the ward and provides a direct link between them and the surgeon. The link continues when the patients are discharged home. This person proves to be very important for follow-up of patients on an outpatient basis.

ANESTHESIA

The special requirements for cranial base anesthetic management are to maintain perioperative hemodynamic stability, reduce intracranial pressure, protect the brain in the event of vascular occlusion, and allow neurophysiological monitoring of cranial nerve and brain function. Anesthesia is induced with sodium thiopental and short-acting muscle relaxants. After endotracheal intubation, an inhalation agent such as isoflurane is used to maintain anesthesia along with nitrous oxide and oxygen. A constant intravenous infusion of low-dose sodium thiopental (2 mg/kg/hr) may be used to reduce the requirement for inhalation agents and to relax the brain. Long-acting muscle relaxants are avoided to permit electrophysiological monitoring of the muscle activity. Tracheostomy is employed when it is anticipated that the patient may have postoperative difficulty with airway protection.

Intermittent pneumatic compression of the lower limbs is used during the operation to reduce the incidence of deep vein thrombosis. To maintain a normothermic state, the patient lies on a foam mattress covered with a heating blanket. Moderate hypothermia (32–34°C) and barbiturate coma may be used for brain protection. During the operation, the blood lost is replaced as much as possible with colloid solutions rather than crystalloids. Overinfusion of crystalloids should be avoided because it may cause excessive postoperative edema. The prothrombin time and platelet count must be checked intraoperatively when blood loss exceeds 1 liter, and appropriate blood component therapy should be undertaken.

A skull base operation consists of three phases: the first is the exposure of the lesion; the second is the removal of the tumor with reconstruction of cranial arteries and nerves if necessary; and the third is the reconstruction of the cranial base.

SURGICAL EXPOSURE

The exposure of skull base lesions usually involves extensive bone work. The exposure must be adequate and yet should not be excessive. The wide exposure helps in reducing the operating distance of the deep lesions from the surgeon, reduces the need for brain retraction, and provides space for maneuvering. An adequately planned incision should take into account any previously existing incisions, the vascularity of the flap, cosmesis, and the course of the facial nerve. The exposure should take into consideration proximal and distal control blood vessels, and any additional surgery that may be required in the future. Restricted exposures may sometimes lead to difficulties in handling complex problems.

Electrophysiological monitoring of the cranial nerves that may be subjected to surgical manipulation can help to avoid injury to those nerves. Such monitoring can also aid the surgeon in identification of the nerves when the anatomy is distorted. Monitoring may include that of facial muscle activity, extraocular muscle activity, and visual evoked responses. Monitoring of appropriate brain electrical activities such as the brain stem evoked response (BSER), somatosensory evoked response (SSER), and electroencephalogram (EEG) is equally important.

INSTRUMENTATION

The surgeon should be in a comfortable working position during the prolonged surgery. A specially designed surgical chair (Fig. 3) helps in providing adequate hand and back rest. A Zeiss–Contraves microscope is an essential part of the instrumentation. The addition of a 35 mm camera and high-quality television equipment enables both the anesthesiologist, the scrub nurse, and others to observe the proceedings of the operation. Recordings can also be used for teaching purposes. A reciprocating saw and various types of power driven burrs and drills are essential (Fig. 4). Bipolar cautery is the most important tool for dissection and tumor removal (Fig. 5). While working to remove tumors rapidly, a different type of bipolar is used (Aesculap) from the instrument used to perform delicate dissection (Malis irrigation bipolar). Microinstruments necessary for vessel and nerve repair should always be available (Fig. 6). A good and flexible retractor system is essential. But the surgeon should learn to apply minimal or no brain retraction most of the time. The use of osteotomies of facial bones is very helpful to reduce brain retraction. Resection of small areas of noneloquent brain can also help to eliminate severe brain retraction. Instruments required for a routine skull base case are shown in Figs. 7–10. Instruments helpful in transoral surgery are shown in Fig. 11. In cases of deep seated firm tumors, a CO_2 laser is occasionally useful. Different types of contact lasers currently

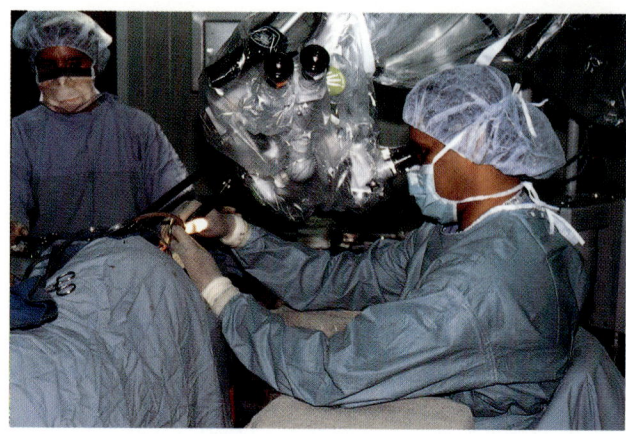

FIG. 3. Picture showing the specially designed chair and the surgeon working in the comfortable operating position.

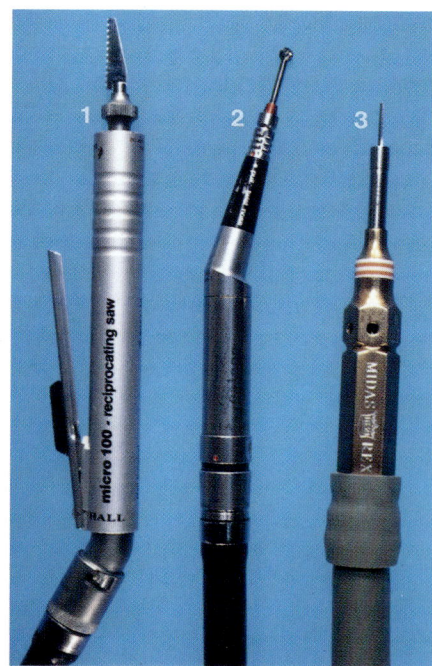

FIG. 4. (1) Hall Micro 100 reciprocating saw (Zimmer). (2) Osteon drill (Zimmer). (3) Midas Rex drill system.

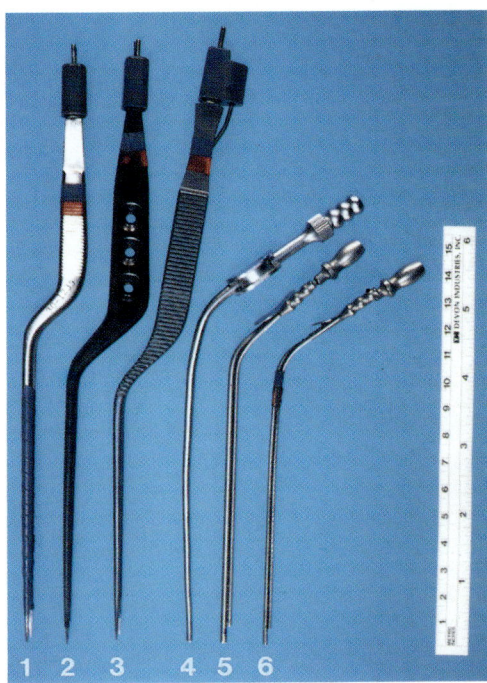

FIG. 5. (1) Hardy bipolar forceps, bayonet $8\frac{1}{4}$ in. (Codman). (2) Bipolar forceps, bayonet, insulated $8\frac{2}{4}$ in. (Aesculap). (3) Malis irrigation bipolar (Codman). (4) Fukushima suction (PMT). (5) William House suction irrigation 6-8 French (Storz). (6) William House suction irrigation 5-7 French (Storz).

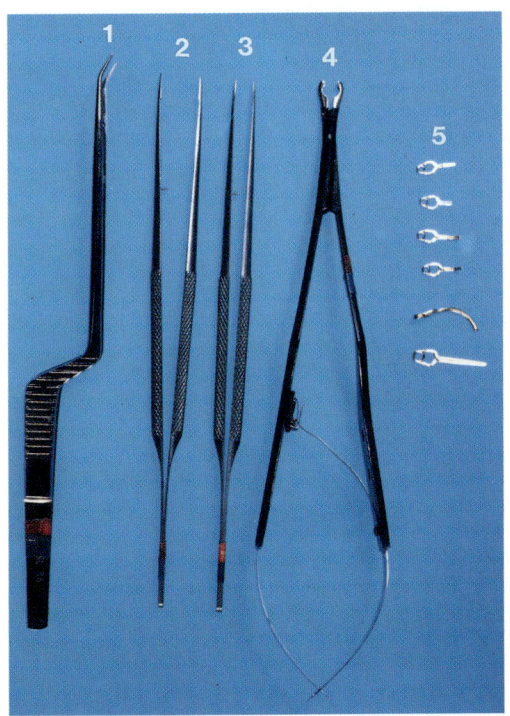
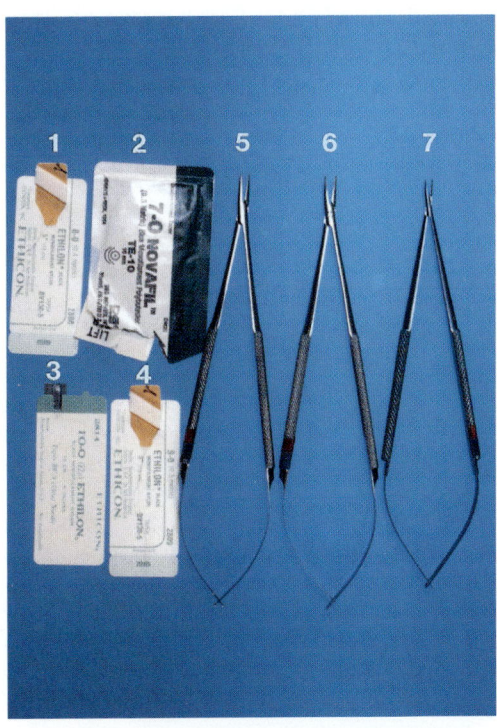

FIG. 6. A: (1) Angled microbayonet forceps, Neurofed (Weck). (2) Microvascular tying forceps, titanium straight 7 in. (Codman). (3) Microvascular tying forceps, curved 7 in. (4) Yasargil aneurysm clip applier (Aesculap). (5) Small and large temporary clips (Aesculap). **B:** (1) 8-0 Nylon, BV 130-5 (Ethicon). (2) 7-0 Novafil +E-10 (Davis and Geck). (3) 10-0 Nylon, BV-6 needle (Ethicon). (4) 9-0 Nylon, BV-3 needle (Ethicon). (5, 6) Jacobsen microneedle holders (Scanlan). (7) Microvascular needle holder, titanium, curved tip (Codman).

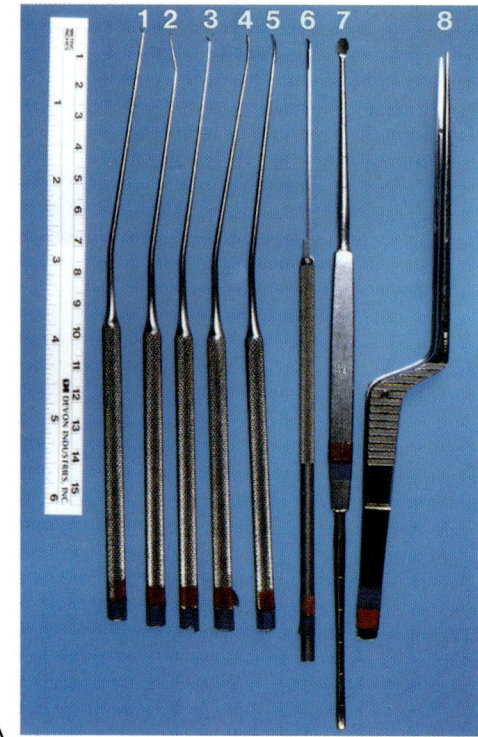
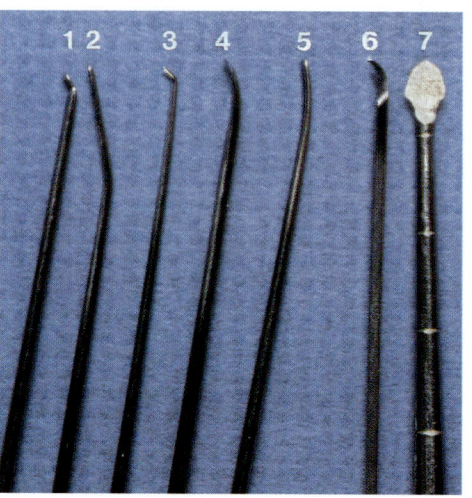

FIG. 7. A: (1) Rosen dissector, Jannetta (V. Mueller). (2) Angled dissector, Jannetta (V. Mueller). (3) A 45 degree hook, Jannetta (V. Mueller). (4) Sacks dissector, Jannetta (V. Mueller). (5) Duckbill dissector, Jannetta (V. Mueller). (6) Beaver knife handle and blade (Alpin Surgical). (7) Cottle elevator (Edward Weck). (8) Straight microbayonet forceps (Edward Weck). **B:** (Tips of the instruments in part **A**). (1) Rosen dissector, Jannetta (V. Mueller). (2) Angled dissector, Jannetta (V. Mueller). (3) A 45 degree hook, Jannetta (V. Mueller). (4) Sacks dissector, Jannetta (V. Mueller). (5) Duckbill dissector, Jannetta (V. Mueller). (6) Beaver knife handle and blade (Alpin Surgical). (7) Cottle elevator (Edward Weck).

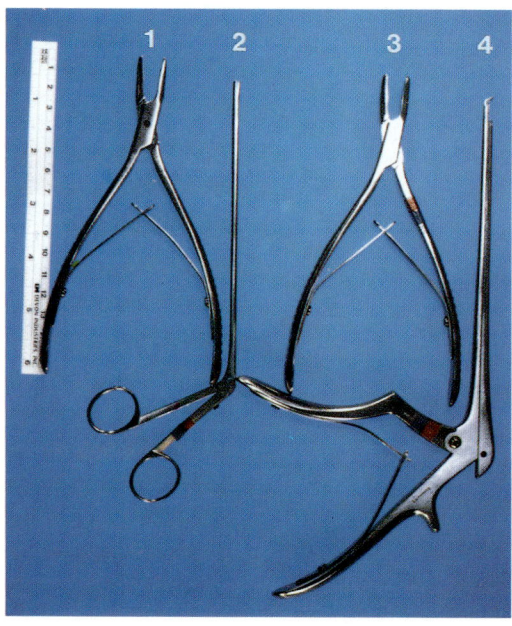

FIG. 8. (1) Lempert Rongeur, straight (Codman). (2) Micropituitary forceps (Codman). (3) Beyer–Lempert Rongeur, curved (Codman). (4) A 1-mm Hardy sella punch, 7 in. (Codman).

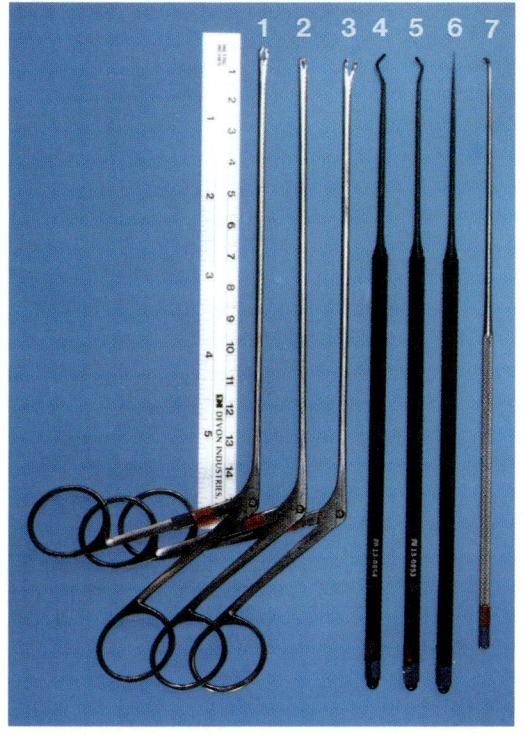
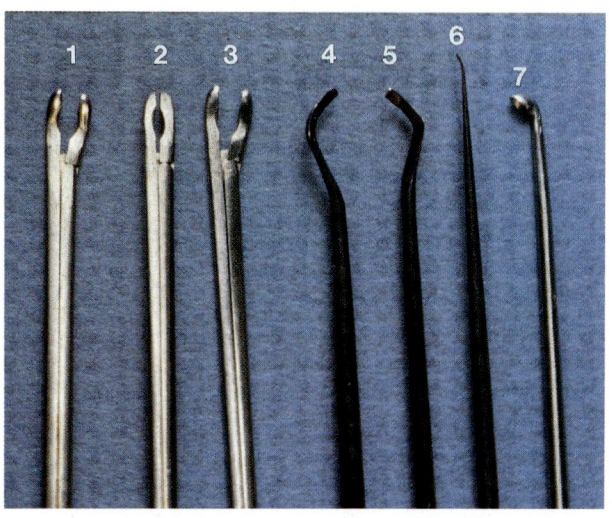

FIG. 9. A: (1) Rhoton microcup forceps, straight (Richards). (2) Rhoton microcup forceps, right (Richards). (3) Rhoton microcup forceps, left (Richards). (4) Shea Robertson excavator, left (Richards). (5) Shea Robertson excavator, right (Richards). (6) Shea Robertson 45 degree pick, sharp (Richards). (7) Rhoton microcurette, angled (V. Mueller). **B:** (Tips of the instruments in part **A**). (1) Rhoton microcup forceps, straight (Richards). (2) Rhoton microcup forceps, right (Richards). (3) Rhoton microcup forceps, left (Richards). (4) Shea Robertson excavator, left (Richards). (5) Shea Robertson excavator, right (Richards). (6) Shea Robertson 45 degree pick, sharp (Richards). (7) Rhoton microcurette, angled (V. Mueller).

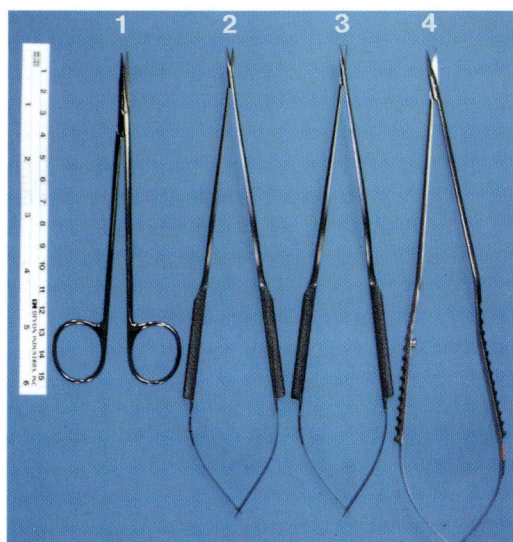

FIG. 10. (1) Tenotomy scissors (Weck). (2) Rhoton titanium straight scissors (Codman). (3) Malis titanium curved scissors (Codman). (4) Serrated straight scissors (Connell Neurosurgical, Redmond).

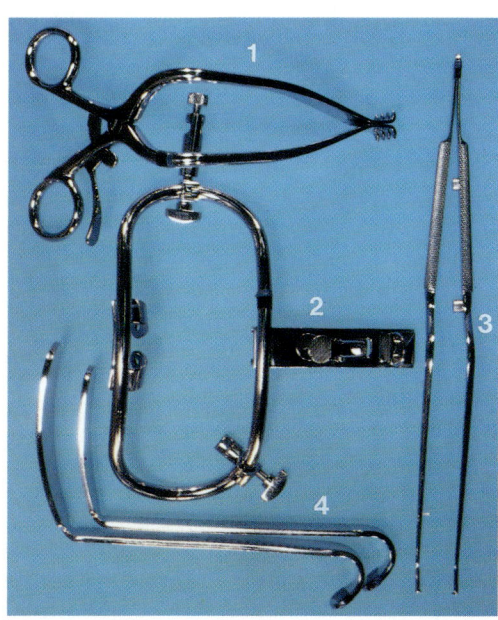

FIG. 11. Crockard transoral instrumentation (Codman). (1) Large pharyngeal retractor. (2) Transoral retractor body with blade connectors. (3) Large and small retractor blades. (4) Ligament grasping forceps.

under development may prove to be very useful. A Cavitron ultrasonic aspiratory (CUSA) is helpful when the tumor is moderate in terms of consistency and vascularity.

PERIOPERATIVE MANAGEMENT

If there is a significant dural repair made during the operation, spinal fluid drainage, strictly regulated by volume, is continued for 1 or 2 days. Other wound drains are removed usually within 3–4 days. Broad spectrum antibiotic coverage is started preoperatively and continued postoperatively until the drains are removed. The patient should be ambulated as early as possible. If the patient remains confined to bed, subcutaneous heparin prophylaxis is employed. Sequential compression stockings should be continued in the postoperative stage until the patient is ambulated.

TUMOR OPERATION

It is important for the surgeon to formulate a clear plan for tumor excision preoperatively, based on the anatomical location of the tumor, the extent of neurovascular involvement, and experience of the surgeon. The surgeon must decide whether the tumor can be removed by a single approach or combination of approaches, and if staged resection is necessary. Once tumor exposure has been obtained, it is important to become oriented to the distorted anatomy. All dissections must be carried out under direct vision. Use of a monopolar nerve stimulator can be very helpful in the identification of cranial nerves, some of which may be very thin and splayed over the tumor capsule.

The removal of the tumor is dependent on whether the tumor is benign or of a low- or high-grade malignancy. In those tumors that are high-grade malignancies, the resection is done in an *en bloc* fashion, that is, without entering the substance of the tumor itself. This is to avoid spillage of the tumor contents. After the *en bloc* resection, frozen sections are performed to check the tumor margins. If any tumor remnants are found, further piecemeal tumor resection will then be performed to complete the tumor resection.

Despite the use of extensive osteotomies or other basal approaches, some amount of brain retraction is inevitable. Recording of BSER from the contralateral ear has been a useful means of monitoring distortion of the upper brain stem that may result from such retraction. Tactics available for relaxing the brain depend on whether the majority of the operation is to be performed extradurally or intradurally. In *extradural operations,* removal of CSF via a lumbar subarachnoid drainage can effectively provide brain relaxation. Lumbar drainage should be avoided when there is a large intracranial mass with pressure differential across the various compartments. Ventricular puncture for drainage of CSF or opening of the basal cisterns intradurally is an available option if there is no distortion of the ventricles from the tumor mass. Osmotic agents and diuretics are also useful. Proper positioning of the head of the patient relative to the neck and heart to permit unimpeded venous drainage is very important during lengthy operations. Proper neuroanesthetic management can greatly help to reduce brain retraction. In *intradural operations* when a large intradural mass is present, steroids are administered 2–3 days in advance. Both cisternal drainage and tumor debulking prior to dissection will reduce the requirements for brain retraction. Whenever possible, the retractors are removed entirely, such that the duration of retraction is minimized. All exposed brain surfaces must be kept covered and moist since drying makes the tissues very friable and prone to contusions and abrasions from the slightest manipulation. Wet Biocol sponge should be placed over the exposed convexity and rubber dams and cottonoid strips under the retractor blades. The actual tumor removal depends on the consistency and vascularity of these tumors. For the most part, meningiomas and neurilemomas are removed with the help of suction, suction irrigation, and bipolar cautery, as well as sharp and blunt microsurgical instrumentation. In cases of large and giant-sized tumors, arachnoidal planes may be missing and all efforts are made to preserve the pial plane. When critical vessels and nerves are encountered, dissection is done from the normal to abnormal area, parallel to the direction of the encased structure. Sharp dissection is preferable in the proximity of blood vessels and nerves. The surgeon should be prepared to temporarily occlude the vessel and to provide alternate circulation with the help of a graft as and when necessary. In situations where vascular injury is anticipated, the case is discussed with the anesthesiologist in advance and plans are made to institute a combination of barbiturate or etimodate-induced electroencephalographic burst suppression. Temporary hypertension and moderate hypothermia are also helpful in situations where temporary vascular occlusion is necessary. Dissection of the small perforators may be most tedious and difficult in this regard. Occasionally, it is necessary to leave some tumor behind, as when dissection from the perforators is not possible. Whenever injury to the cranial nerves occurs during surgery, a surgeon should be prepared to perform reconstruction either by direct suture or by graft.

RECONSTRUCTION

A good reconstruction is essential to avoid postoperative complications. Reconstruction is crucial to avoid postoperative infection by sealing potential sites of cerebrospinal fluid leakage. The open paranasal sinuses must be obliterated and the continuity of the lateral and posterior pharyngeal walls must be restored at the end of the surgical procedure. Any dural lacerations must be closed meticulously, either by primary suture or with the use of a graft of the parietal pericranium or fascia lata. The closure does not have to be watertight but an attempt must be made to suture and to plug any holes with the aid of small pieces of fat (fat plugs). Sutures must be placed around the entire circumference of the defect under magnification. Autologous fibrin glue is a useful adjunct to seal small holes. However, too much reliance on fibrin glue may prove deceptive. The paranasal sinuses are usually not inhabited by virulent flora. They should be completely denuded of mucosa. A vascularized flap such as a galeal or a pericranial flap is laid into the sinus, and the sinus is packed with autogenous fat. This will become vascularized in time. When the operative defect is large, when a large communication exists with the sinuses or the oronasopharynx or the exterior surface, and in patients who have had prior extensive surgery or radiation therapy, a vascularized flap reconstruction is essential. Such a flap may be a regional, such as a temporalis flap, or a trapezius flap. In patients where these flaps are not suitable, a rectus abdominis or latissimus dorsi free flap transfer is necessary.

COMPLICATIONS

Meticulous attention to every detail from preoperative planning to postoperative care and follow-up is essential for a favorable outcome. Complications are related to several factors. The histology of the lesion, whether benign or malignant, will indicate the extent and nature of involvement of various neural and vascular structures as well as the feasibility of dissection of these structures from the tumor. The size of the lesion and the extent of involvement of the basal dura, bone, and neurovascular structures—that is, whether there is unilateral or bilateral involvement of the cavernous sinuses, petrous apices, jugular foramina, and internal carotid or vertebral arteries—may predict an increased probability of developing complications. Location of the lesion will dictate the extent of brain retraction or resection that may be needed to expose it. A history of previous operations will indicate that scarring may obscure the dissection planes. Previous irradiation will predispose to wound-related problems, which may present as cerebrospinal fluid leakage and infection. CSF leakage in the postoperative period is one of the most frustrating problems faced by the skull base surgeon. As with other complications, it is best prevented. Prevention requires a meticulous reconstruction of the cranial base after removal of the tumor. It is this stage of the operation that is prone to errors as the surgical team is usually exhausted and shortcuts and oversights are more likely. The amount of CSF leakage depends on the site of the leak and the size of the fistula. Increasing volume of subdural and intraventricular air usually indicates a persistent communication of the subarachnoid space with the exterior and hence a likelihood of CSF leak. Elevated CSF pressure can be managed by lumbar spinal drainage. However, if the fistula is large or if CSF dynamics are normal, reoperation is essential. Increase in intracranial air and recurrence of leak after cessation of CSF drainage are indications for surgical repair. It must be carefully planned so that it is performed only once. Hydrocephalus may develop as a late complication of cranial base surgery, especially after multiple operations and/or radiation therapy, and may manifest as CSF leak. Insertion of a ventriculoperitoneal shunt usually controls the CSF leak in such cases.

Infections remain the most dreaded complication. Despite the frequent communication of the intradural contents with the paranasal sinuses and pharynx and also lengthy operative procedures, the incidence of serious infections is surprisingly low. Precautions to prevent desiccation and ischemia of tissues and gross contamination are crucial for prevention of infection. One must be very aggressive with the closure of the oropharynx and the nasopharynx. If these structures are exposed, they should be sealed meticulously by primary closure if possible, supplemented by a good local or distant vascularized flap. When infection does occur, drainage of the abscess, treatment with appropriate antibiotics, and the provision of adequate vascularized tissue such as regional flaps often lead to a dramatic improvement.

The surgical approach used may result in obligatory loss of certain cranial nerve function and must be thoughtfully selected for maximum exposure and safe removal of the tumor. Cranial nerve palsies constitute long-term morbidity. Recovery often occurs with time. An aggressive attempt must always be made to reconstruct them whenever their continuity is disrupted. Thus many of the postoperative problems can be anticipated on the basis of a detailed preoperative clinical as well as radiological evaluation. A surgeon must always anticipate complications in order to prevent morbidity and to manage complications effectively when they arise.

POSTOPERATIVE FOLLOW-UP

Immediately after surgery, the patient should be nursed in an intensive care unit with facilities for acute respiratory care for 48 hr or longer if necessary. The presence of a neurointensivist skilled in the management of these kinds of patients is very essential. Usually a CT scan is performed on the first postoperative day to evaluate the patient in cases where there has been a major cranial base operation even if there is no neurological problem. This CT scan serves both to prepare the surgeon for any impending problems and also to facilitate in the decision-making process as to when the patient can be taken out of the intensive care unit. If the patient has had vascular grafting or suturing during the operation, a postoperative angiogram is mandatory to serve as a baseline. Patients who spend the longest time in the intensive care unit are those with lower cranial nerve palsies with tracheostomies and gastrostomies, who require critical care nursing because of difficulty with their cough reflex. Patients undergoing prolonged operative procedures should have a nasogastric tube placed for early gastric decompression and for subsequent feeding. When tracheostomy has been utilized, the tracheostomy tube should be left in place for 24–48 hr or until the patient demonstrates a satisfactory upper airway. Wide fluctuations in the blood pressure should be avoided in the postoperative phase. Fluid and electrolyte deficits must be replaced in sufficient quantities to allow hemodynamic stability. Back and limb care should be vigorously pursued in patients who will need prolonged bed nursing.

In-house rehabilitation of patients is very crucial when there are major neurological deficits and cranial nerve palsies. Prolonged neurological deficits and cranial nerve palsies will require outpatient rehabilitation. The social and financial situation of the patient may affect the rehabilitation of the patient.

The referring specialist should be closely and constantly kept aware of the progress of the patient in the hospital. The specialist can actively take part in the management of the patient after discharge from the hospital. Careful and long-term follow-up by neurological examination and MRI or CT scanning are essential. The frequency of follow-up will depend on the nature of the operation and the neurological problems with the patient. The patients are usually seen 2–3 weeks after their discharge from the hospital. They may, however, be contacted on telephone by the nurse coordinator at frequent intervals. The next follow-up is between 3 months and 1 year when a MRI or a CT scan is repeated to assess the tumor residue or recurrence.

A skull base surgeon often deals with patients who are critically ill. The surgeon realizes that these unfortunate people need specialized services, care, and love. The surgeon uses every available tool but is always aware of the Great Natural Force that makes the human body work in health and heals it in disease.

Based on the management of many patients with difficult skull base lesions, the senior author has developed a motto that is very useful to surgeons working in this field. The first part is borrowed from the Boy Scouts of America:

Be Prepared; Do Not Despair.

The surgeon should be prepared for many problems that may arise during operations. However, when serious complications arise, do not despair; many of them can be managed effectively with a good result.

CHAPTER 2

Introduction

General Otolaryngologic/Plastic Surgery Operative Techniques and Instrumentation in Cranial Base Surgery

Ivo P. Janecka

The history of medicine is full of examples of sudden discoveries leading to new advances in understanding or implementation of treatment modalities. This usually follows a pattern of knowledge transfer from basic to clinical science (e.g., immunology to transplantation) or "skill transfer" from one clinical field to another (microsurgery from otology to plastic surgery and neurosurgery).

The establishment of cranial base surgery as a new field of surgical oncology, however, exemplifies the "convergent evolution" of several disciplines exhibiting "critical maturation" in specific areas. New skills, critical judgment, and symbiotic surgeons' interaction came into play. The development of cranial base surgery crossed the boundaries of neurosurgery–otolaryngology–plastic surgery in a way never witnessed before. The sudden appearance of cranial base surgery as a surgical reality was facilitated by the precision of new CT/MR imaging and recognition that single specialty limitation at the cranial base can be translated into multispeciality surgical feasibility. A new field was born.

An important aspect of "survival" of any new field of medicine is its acceptance as a practical alternative to historic standards. This goal is best achieved, I think, through education and true understanding of the benefits, risks, and the invariable present-day limitations.

It is to this goal that this textbook is dedicated. As with any written communication, it will not be all encompassing to all readers. This textbook represents an expression of "current" practices in surgical techniques and management of cranial base neoplasms. As the first color textbook on the subject of cranial base surgery, it provides a framework and background for future, undoubtedly more advanced publications.

Since the 1950s, there have been sporadic attempts to surgically treat malignant lesions of the cranial base as a last therapeutic effort by a few daring clinicians. The oncological success was limited and the complications were many. The surgical approaches used were technically restrictive in their exposure of key anatomic structures and tumor margins as well as the surgeon's options for reconstruction (1,2).

The first breakthrough came in the late 1960s when Tessier (3) reported on his successful experience in treating children with congenital craniofacial deformities. His work put forth the foundation for *craniofacial surgery,* demonstrating in principle the feasibility of mobilizing and repositioning craniofacial skeletal units with an acceptable rate of complications. It is this accomplishment that opened the door to the current plethora of surgical approaches to the cranial base. These approaches can be broadly categorized as techniques of craniofacial disassembly and range from the subtemporal–infratemporal approach to an expanded facial translocation technique.

Oncologic understanding of the behavior of various tumors has permitted the anticipation of true tumor extent so essential to our ability to secure clear surgical

---

I. P. Janecka: Center for Cranial Base Surgery, University of Pittsburgh School of Medicine, Presbyterian University Hospital, and Department of Otolaryngology, Eye and Ear Institute, Pittsburgh, Pennsylvania 15213

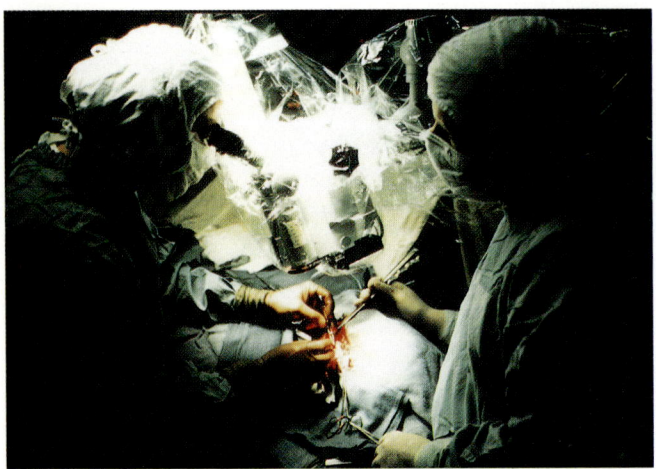 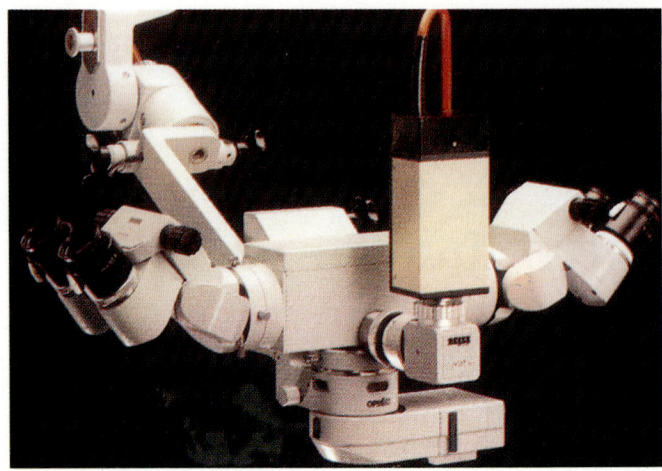

FIG. 1. A: Use of operating microscope in skull base surgery. **B:** Zeiss operating microscope with optical systems for two surgeons as well as video attachment.

margins. "Standard" histologic evaluation of neoplastic tissue has been augmented by immunohistochemistry, which permits the pathologist to define the tumor cell of origin with much greater precision.

The introduction of a *microscope* into surgery dates back to the 1920s when Nylen (4) used a single lens scope for ear surgery. It took over 40 years before the microsurgical era began on a broader front. House (5) popularized it with otolaryngologists, Olivecrona with neurosurgeons (6,7), and Harii (8) with plastic surgeons. Each specialty benefitted enormously from magnified binocular surgical visualization, and as the optics improved the visualization, concentrated training refined surgeons' dexterity.

Today, the operating microscope is indispensable in cranial base surgery (Fig. 1). The precision of surgical intervention lessens the surgical morbidity and also opens new technical territories. Microsurgery of cranial nerves and microvascular surgery are two major examples (9,10).

Reconstruction is an indispensable phase of any complex surgical procedure. The greater the involvement of critical anatomic structures during surgery, the greater the demand on the integrity of reconstruction. The primary usage of autologous vascularized tissue, which respects the regional neurovasculature, is the hallmark of sound reconstruction. The concerted effort of microvas-

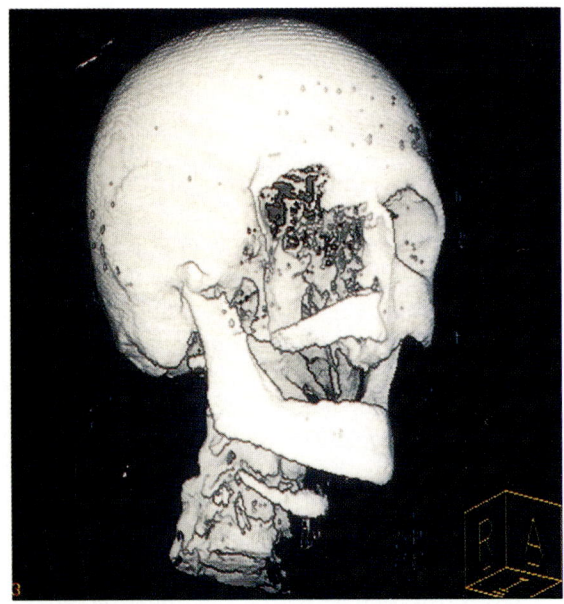 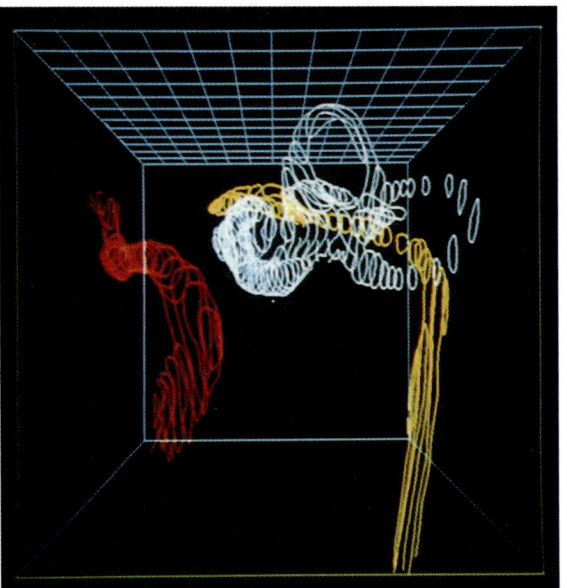

FIG. 2. A: Simulation of an approach to cranial base (via facial translocation) on an ISG work station. **B:** Computer-generated images of left temporal bone anatomic structures: internal carotid artery (*red*), facial nerve (*yellow*), and labyrinth (*white*).

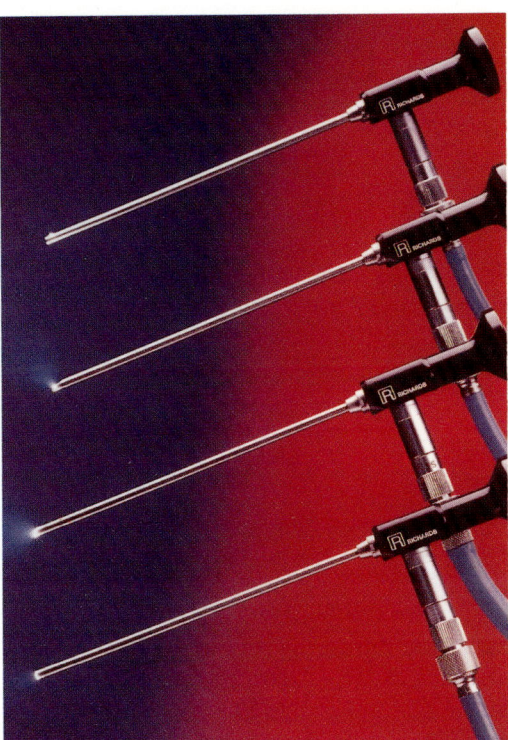

FIG. 3. Fibro-optic endoscopes with angled view (note direction of light beams).

numerous regional as well as microvascular flaps attest to this, offering valid reconstructive options to most of our patients.

Success of cranial base surgery is proportional to our ability to match cranial base approaches with cranial base neoplasms. In general, the more of the tumor periphery that can be reached without tumor manipulation, the better the approach. Such surgical access provides the maximum safety for a procedure, gives us the best chance to secure clear oncologic tissue margins, and sets the stage for primary reconstruction. Surgical simulation can be performed on CT/MR work stations (e.g., ISG System) (Fig. 2A) or computer-generated images of anatomic structures (Fig. 2B).

In a significant way, advancing *instrumentation* has also contributed to the progress of cranial base surgery. It has permeated all phases of our clinical practice; from the diagnostic workup through intraoperative monitoring to the postoperative follow-up.

In spite of ever advancing quality of diagnostic imaging, the diagnosis is still only a probability (even if at times an extremely high one). The progress in fibro-optic research has resulted in the design of precision endoscopic instrumentation (Fig. 3). From the "macro" rigid endoscopes have evolved micro and flexible endoscopes. These tools permit access, for direct visualization and biopsy, to previously unreachable or difficult to reach segments of cranial base anatomy. Miniaturization seems to have no fundamental limits. A 1-mm (in diameter) flexible endoscope with photographic capabilities (currently available) is only one example.

cular surgeons to find new flaps feasible for transfer by microvascular methodology enhanced our knowledge of vascular territories of skin and muscle, as well as the bone. The richness of reconstructive methods available today for cranial base surgery came out of this effort. The

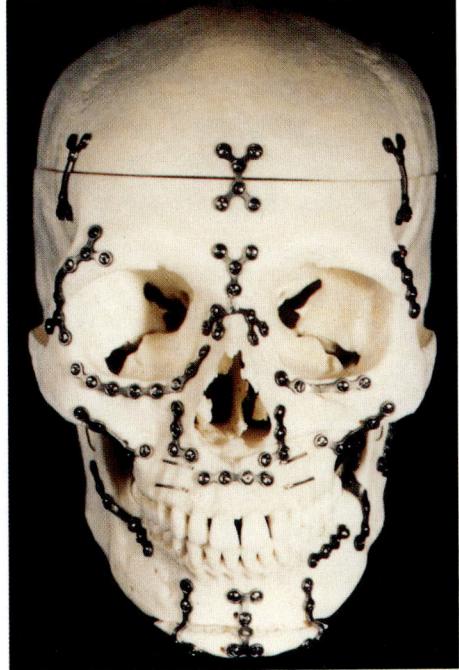
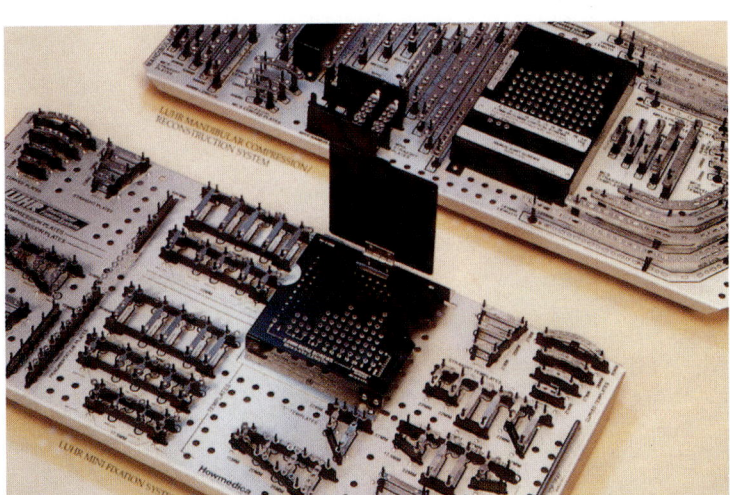

FIG. 4. A: Example of the use of miniplate fixation on a dry skull (by Stortz). **B:** One of several miniplate craniofacial sets available today.

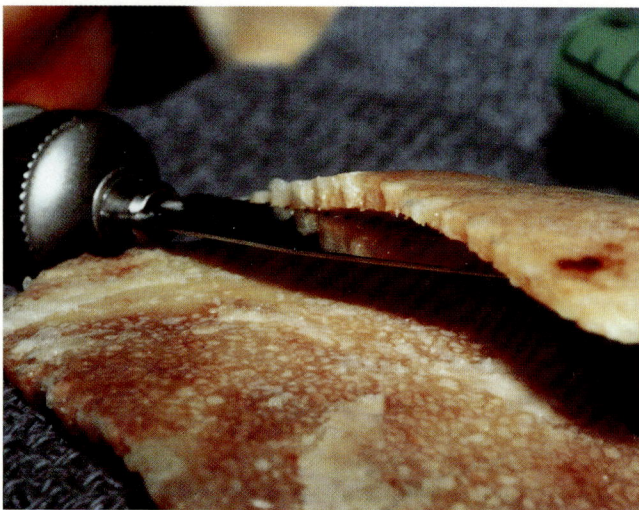

FIG. 5. Reciprocating blade of Micro 100 saw splitting calvarial bone.

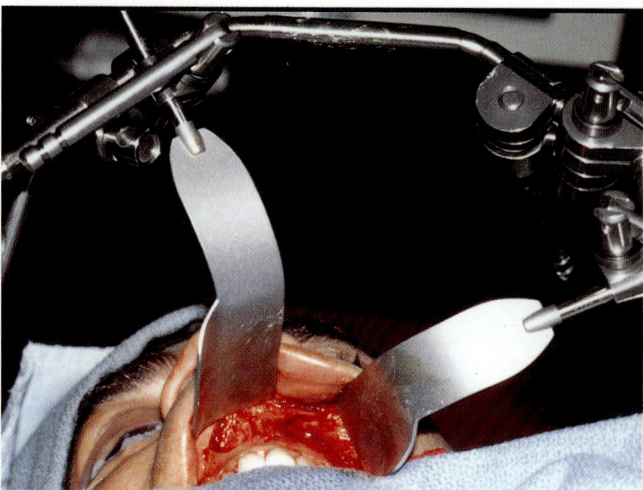

FIG. 7. Omni Tract retractor used in "degloving" approach to skull base.

Another preoperative option for securing tissue for diagnosis from the depth of the cranial base is with the use of CT/MR-guided needle biopsy.

The operating room for cranial base surgery displays state-of-the-art instrumentation. From magnetically operated microscope stands (e.g., Cotraves) allowing instantaneous optical adjustments, to mini or microplating systems (Fig. 4A) of internal bone fixation used for reassembly of craniofacial skeleton (e.g., Synthes and Howmedica craniofacial sets) (Fig. 4B). Various oscillating or reciprocating minisaws are available, allowing us to perform thin osteotomies (e.g., Hall Micro 100) (Fig. 5).

Craniotomes and drills may reach up to 80,000 rpm (e.g., Midas Rex system). An array of attachments and bits (Fig. 6), ranging from micro to macro sizes, from cutting edge to diamond surfaces, and straight as well as angulated hand pieces, are available with many systems.

The full use of the achieved surgical exposure requires adequate retraction—either manual or mechanical. For long microsurgery (e.g., temporal bone) or unusual approaches (e.g., "degloving"), mechanical retraction is preferred. The often encountered inflexibility of previous systems has been overcome by the Omni Tract retractor offering three-dimensional multiblade adjustments (Fig. 7).

Cranial base surgery involves complex procedures. Each participating surgical discipline can offer specific knowledge and expertise, as well as instrumentation. Members of the Cranial Base Team must learn to participate in the available educational cross-fertilization. Our patients will be the greatest benefactors of this collaboration rich in intellect and dexterity.

REFERENCES

1. Smith RR, Klopp CT, Williams JM. Surgical treatment of cancer of the frontal sinus and adjacent areas. *Cancer* 1954;7:991–994.
2. Ketcham AS, Wilkins RH, Van Buren JM, et al. Combined intracranial facial approach to the paranasal sinuses. *Am J Surg* 1963;106:698–703.
3. Tessier P. Osteotomies totales de la face: syndrome de Crouzon, syndrome d'Apert, oxycephalies, scaphocephalies, turricephalies. *Annales de Chirurgie Plastique* 1967;12:273–286.
4. Nylen CO. The otomicroscope and microsurgery 1921–1971. *Acta Otolaryngol* 1972;73:453.
5. House WF. Surgical exposure of the internal auditory canal and its content through the middle cranial fossa. *Laryngoscope* 1961;71:1363–1385.
6. Kurze T, Doyle JB Jr. Extradural intracranial (middle fossa) approach to the internal auditory canal. *J Neurosurg* 1962;19:1033–1037.
7. Kurze R. Microtechniques in neurological surgery. In: Shillito J Jr, Mosberg WH, eds. *Clinical neurosurgery.* Baltimore: Williams & Wilkins, 1964;128–137.
8. Harii K, Ohmori K, Ohmori S. Hair transplantation with free scalp flaps. *Plast Reconstr Surg* 1974;53:410.
9. McCraw J, Dibbell D, Carraway J. Clinical definition of independent myocutaneous vascular territories. *Plast Reconstr Surg* 1977;60:341.
10. Janecka IP. Microvascular reconstruction in head and neck surgery. *Adv Otolaryngol Head Neck Surg* 1988;2:205–226.

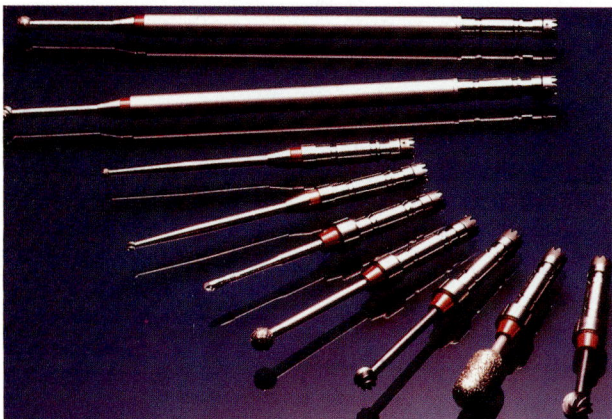

FIG. 6. Range of drill bits available for macro and micro drilling of skull (Hall Osteon).

CHAPTER 3

MRI and CT in the Evaluation of Skull Base Masses

William L. Hirsch, Jr. and Hugh D. Curtin

In the evaluation of skull base lesions two primary issues must be addressed: first, the identity of the tumor, and second, the precise extent of the lesion.

W. L. Hirsch, Jr. and H. D. Curtin: Department of Radiology, University of Pittsburgh, Pittsburgh, Pennsylvania 15213.

CT AND MRI TECHNIQUES

Magnetic resonance imaging (MRI) and computed tomography (CT) are complementary not competitive tools in the initial evaluation of skull base lesions.

CT is better at detecting calcification (Fig. 1) and at evaluating the effect of the lesion on the bone of the skull base (Fig. 2). CT examination of the skull base requires

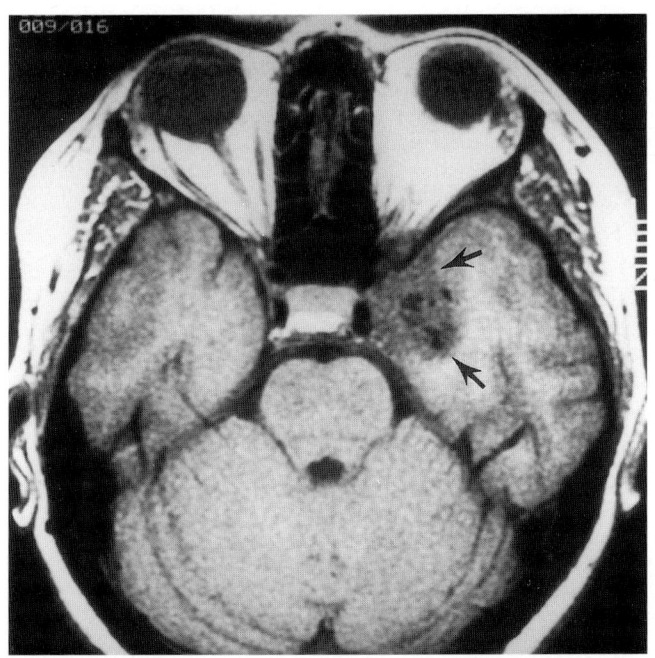 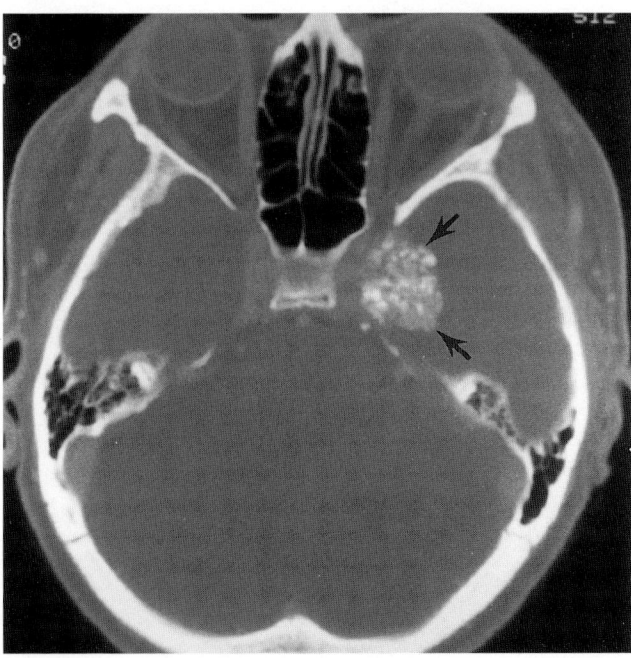

FIG. 1. Calcified meningioma.* **A:** Axial spin echo (SE) (600/20) (TR/TE) MRI. There is a left parasellar mass with intermediate signal intensity (arrows). The low signal (dark) spots within the mass may be vascular flow voids or calcifications. **B:** Axial CT (bone algorithm) shows dense calcification within this meningioma (arrows).

* All the magnetic resonance (MR) images used in this chapter are obtained using a spin echo (SE) technique. If the TR is less than 1000, the image is T1 weighted. If the TR is 2000–3000, the image is T2 weighted.

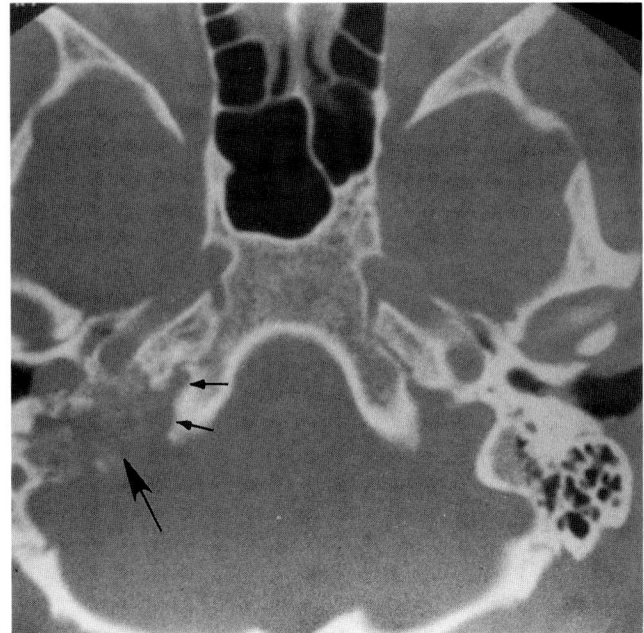
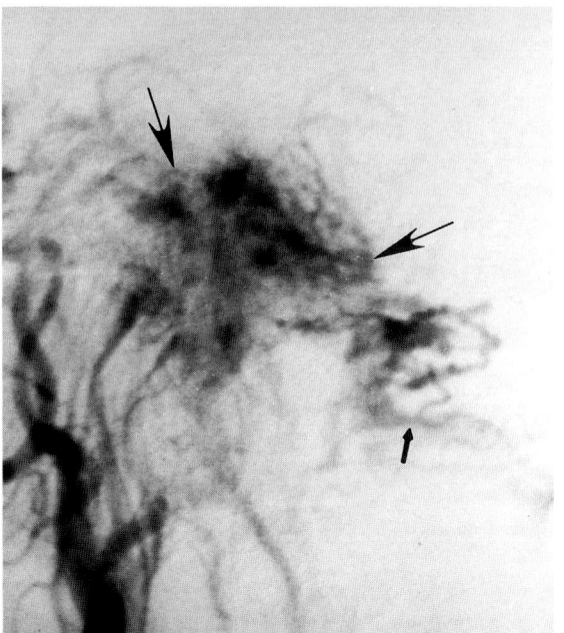
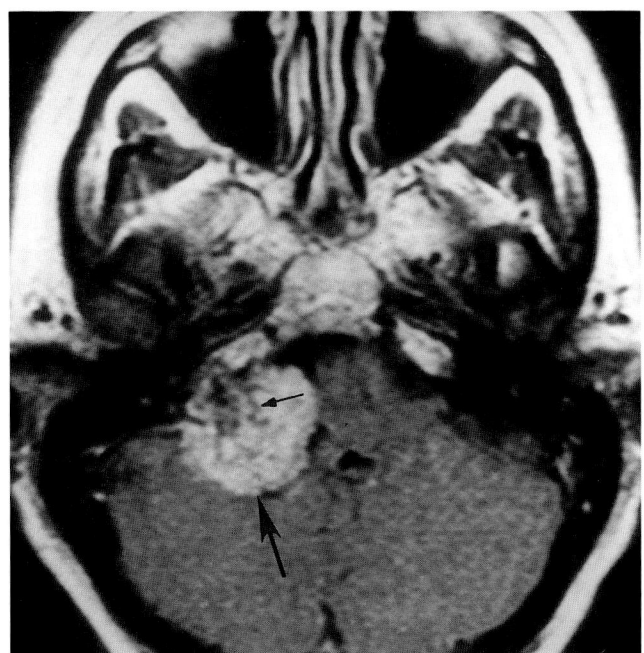

FIG. 2. Paraganglioma (glomus jugulare). **A:** Axial CT (bone algorithm). There is erosion of the lateral wall of the right jugular fossa (*large arrow*). The medial wall (*small arrows*) is normal and not eroded. Compare this with the normal left jugular fossa. **B:** Lateral external carotid angiogram: glomus jugulare tumors are very vascular (*large arrows*). They often have early draining veins (*small arrow*). They are supplied by branches of the external carotid. In particular, the ascending pharyngeal artery almost always makes a significant contribution. Preoperative embolization is used in some institutions to reduce lesion vascularity. **C:** Axial SE (650/30) postcontrast MRI. Paragangliomas are typically densely enhancing (*large arrow*). Serpentine flow voids (*small arrow*) within the mass indicate that it is a highly vascular lesion. The presence of flow voids within a densely enhancing mass in the jugular fossa is highly suggestive of a glomus jugulare tumor. However, in small paragangliomas, vascular flow voids are often not visualized.

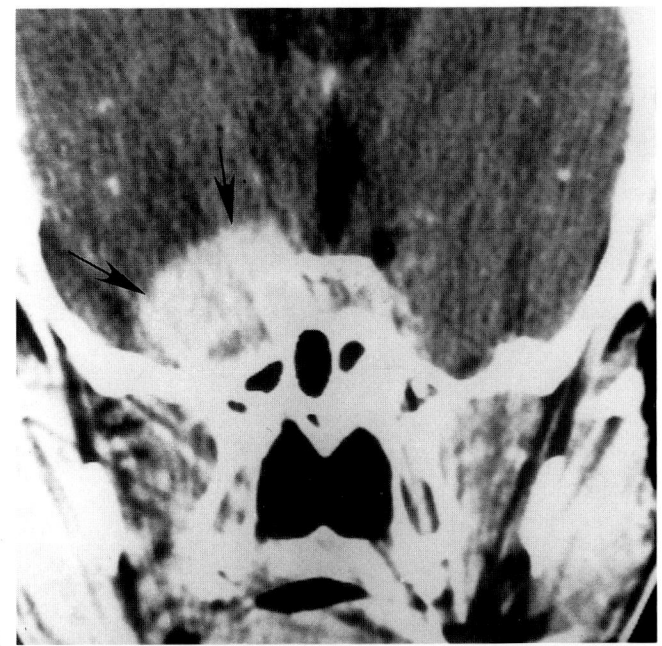
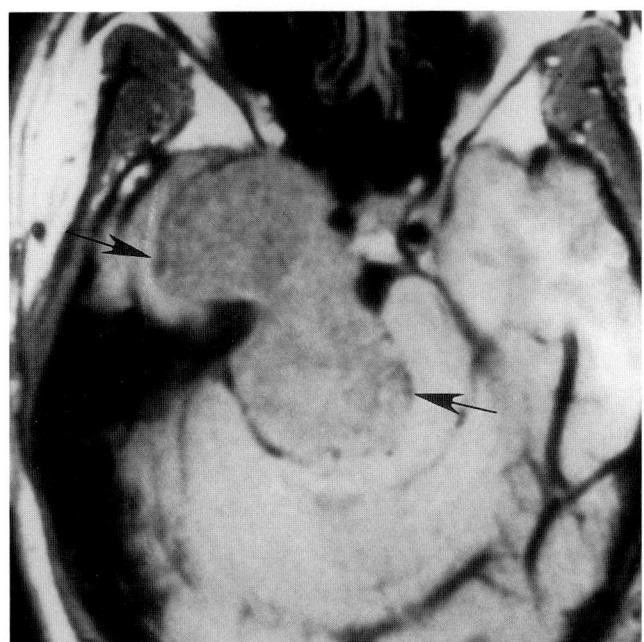
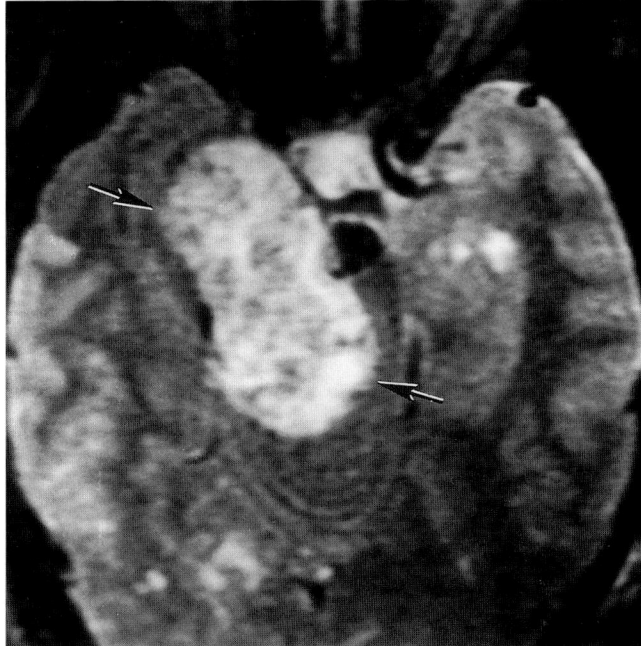

FIG. 3. Trigeminal nerve sheath tumor. **A:** Coronal postcontrast CT. There is a large enhancing tumor (*arrows*) in the right parasellar region. **B:** Axial SE (800/20) MRI. The mass (*arrows*) is intermediate in signal on this T1-weighted image. The right carotid is displaced but not surrounded by tumor. The relationship of the tumor to the carotid artery is better demonstrated by MRI than by CT. **C:** Axial SE (2500/100) MRI. The mass (*arrows*) has primarily high T2 signal, although there are mottled areas of lower signal. Nerve sheath tumors typically have intermediate signal on T1-weighted images and high signal on T2-weighted images. They may displace the carotid but almost never narrow it the way meningiomas do. Also unlike meningiomas, calcification is very rare in nerve sheath tumors.

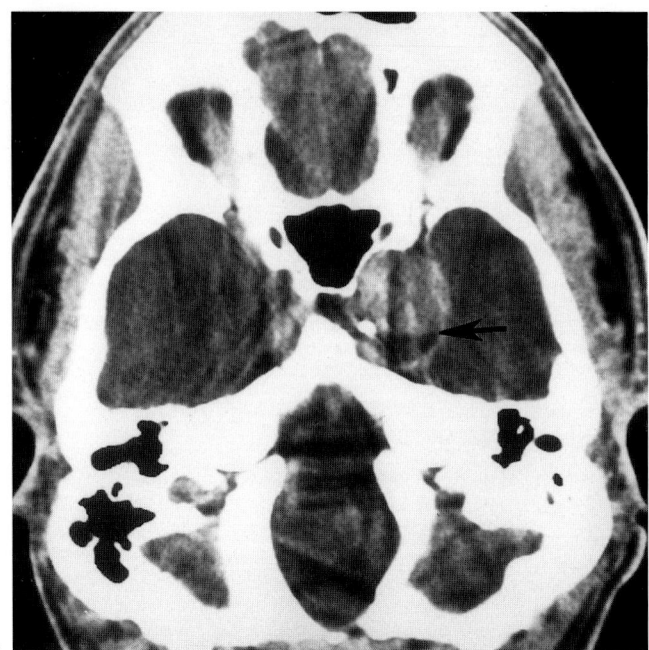 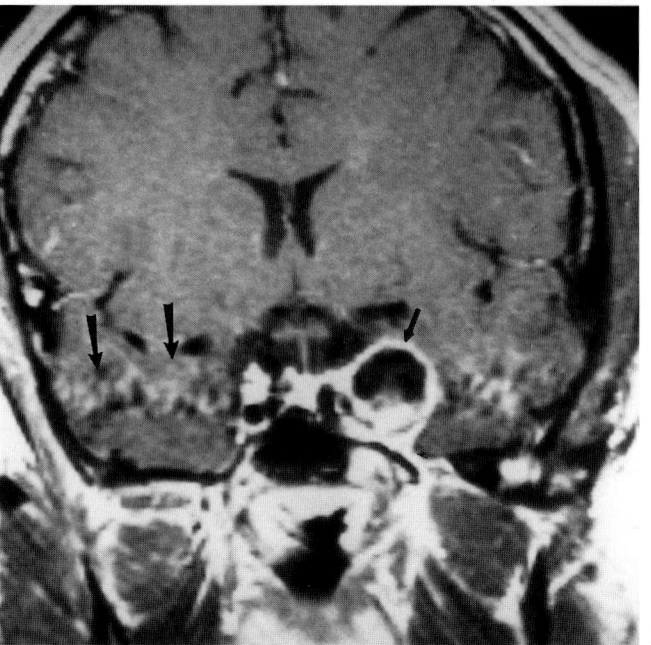

FIG. 4. Parasellar aneurysm. **A:** Axial postcontrast CT shows a round enhancing mass in the left parasellar region. The posterior nonenhancing region (*arrow*) represents mural thrombus. If this thrombus is soft, it can be extruded from the aneurysm during intra-aneurysmal balloon embolization. It may be safer to sacrifice the parent vessel in such cases. **B:** Coronal MRI following contrast (Gd-DTPA). The wall of the aneurysm enhances (*small arrow*). Phase encoding artifact (*large arrows*) is evidence of flow within the aneurysmal lumen.

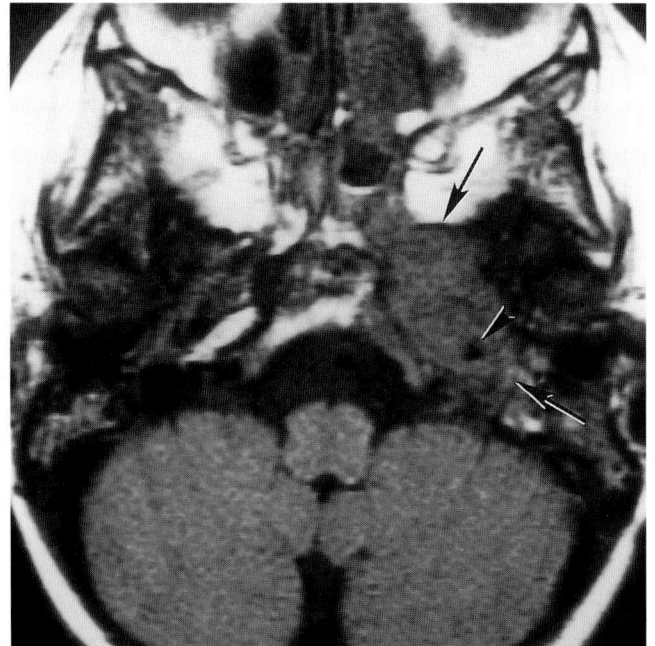 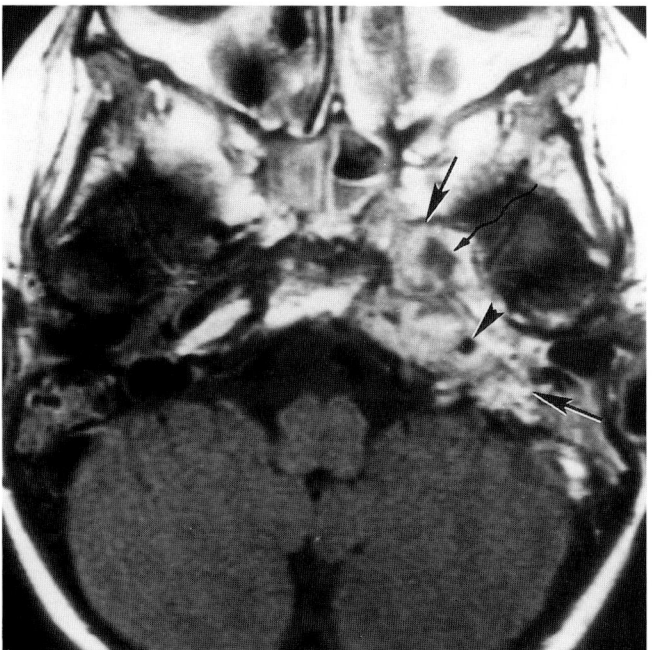

FIG. 5. Treated rhabdomyosarcoma. **A:** Axial SE (600/20) MRI. This nasopharyngeal rhabdomyosarcoma (*arrows*) extends superiorly into the left petrous apex. It has replaced marrow fat and has surrounded the left carotid artery (*arrowhead*). **B:** Postgadolinium MRI shows generalized enhancement of the mass (*arrows*). A central nonenhancing area (*wavy arrow*) may represent necrosis. The signal difference between the neoplasm and the surrounding fat is less than on the precontrast study (compare with **A**). The carotid artery still appears as a flow void on this enhanced scan (*arrowhead*).

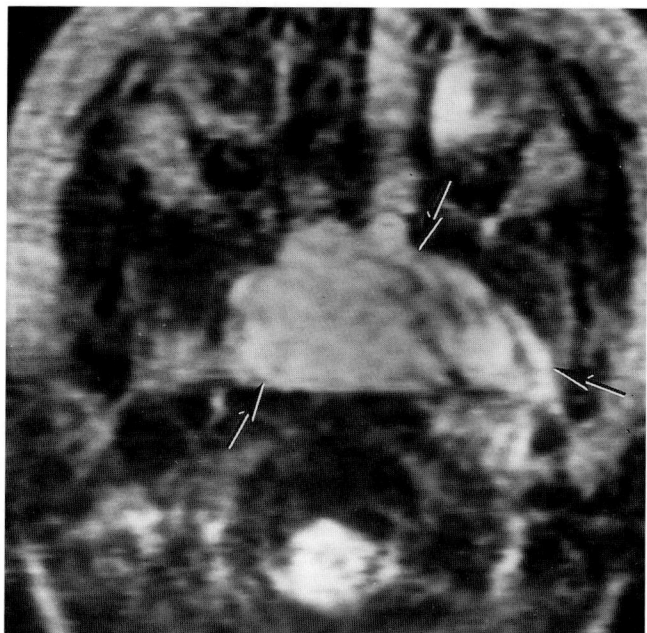 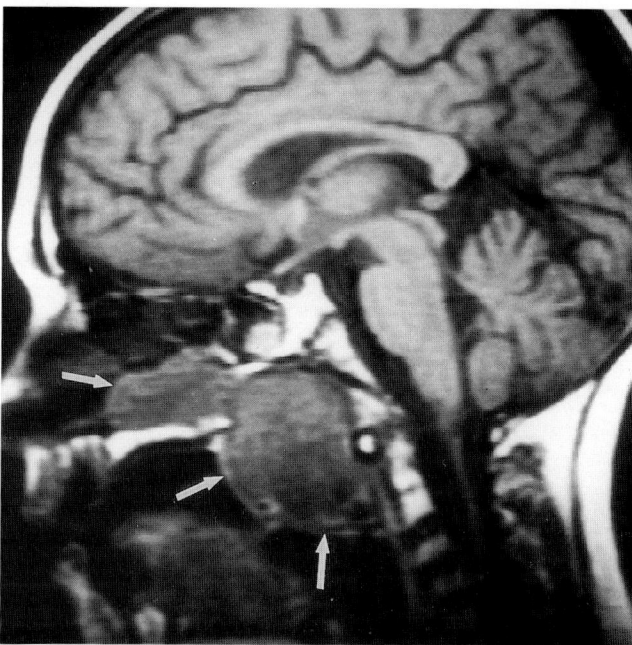

FIG. 5. *Continued.* **C:** Axial SE (3000/100) MRI. This rhabdomyosarcoma has high T2 signal (*arrows*). Most rhabdomyosarcomas have intermediate or low T2 signal. The high signal in this case may be an effect of the chemotherapy and radiation therapy this patient received. **D:** Sagittal SE (600/20) MRI without contrast shows the mass protruding into the nasopharynx and the posterior nasal cavity (*arrows*).

thin sections (3 mm or less), a small field of view (16–18 cm), soft tissue and bone algorithms, and enhancement with iodinated contrast. We perform both axial and direct coronal CT in most cases.

MRI is superior in demonstrating the relationship of a skull base mass to soft tissue structures (including cranial nerves), the carotid artery, the jugular vein, and the brain (Fig. 3). MRI is also better than CT in excluding aneurysm (Fig. 4). This is particularly important in the evaluation of parasellar masses. As with CT, MRI of the skull base is time consuming. T1-weighted spin echo (SE) images are particularly helpful because they show good contrast between skull base neoplasms (which are usually intermediate in signal intensity) and surrounding fat (which has high T1 signal intensity) (Fig. 5A). We perform thin section (3-mm) axial and coronal T1-weighted images both before and after contrast. Both sequences are performed because on postcontrast images the margins between enhancing neoplasm and fat may be obscured since both enhancing tumor and fat have T1 high signal (Fig. 5B). We also perform axial T2-weighted images. These pulsing sequences require 60–90 min of scanner time. Volume acquisitions and fat nulling techniques may play a greater role in the future and hopefully will shorten the length of the exam.

TUMOR IDENTIFICATION

Final determination of tumor type almost always requires biopsy. Predictions can be made based on the apparent site of origin of the tumor. Some tumors can arise anywhere in the skull base. These include meningiomas, bone or soft tissue sarcomas, and metastasis (Fig. 6). Other tumors have a predilection for the anterior, middle, or posterolateral aspects of the skull base.

Preferred sites of various tumors are summarized in Fig. 7. Some lesions almost always occur in a specific location. Examples include juvenile angiofibromas, which occur in the pterygopalatine fossa (Fig. 8); esthesioneuroblastomas (olfactory neuroblastomas), which arise from olfactory epithelium (Fig. 9); cholesterol granulomas, which arise at the petrous apex (Fig. 10); paragangliomas, which arise in the carotid sheath, jugular bulb, or middle ear (Fig. 2); and chordomas, which usually arise in the basisphenoid, basiocciput, or along the endocranial surface of the clivus.

In addition to location, some tumors have characteristic imaging features that suggest a specific diagnosis. Such features include hyperostosis in meningiomas; calcification in some chondrosarcomas (Figs. 11 and 12) and meningiomas (Fig. 1) (1,2); vascular flow voids apparent on MRI scans of juvenile angiofibromas (Fig. 8) (3) and paragangliomas (Fig. 2) (4); and high T1 signal, which can be present in a few chordomas and more characteristically in lesions with obstructed air cells such as cholesterol granuloma (Fig. 10) and mucocele (Fig. 13) (5). Air cells obstructed by sinus tumors may vary widely in signal characteristics. The variability reflects differences in protein content of the mucoid material within the obstructed sinuses. The imaging characteristics of various tumor types are summarized in Table 1.

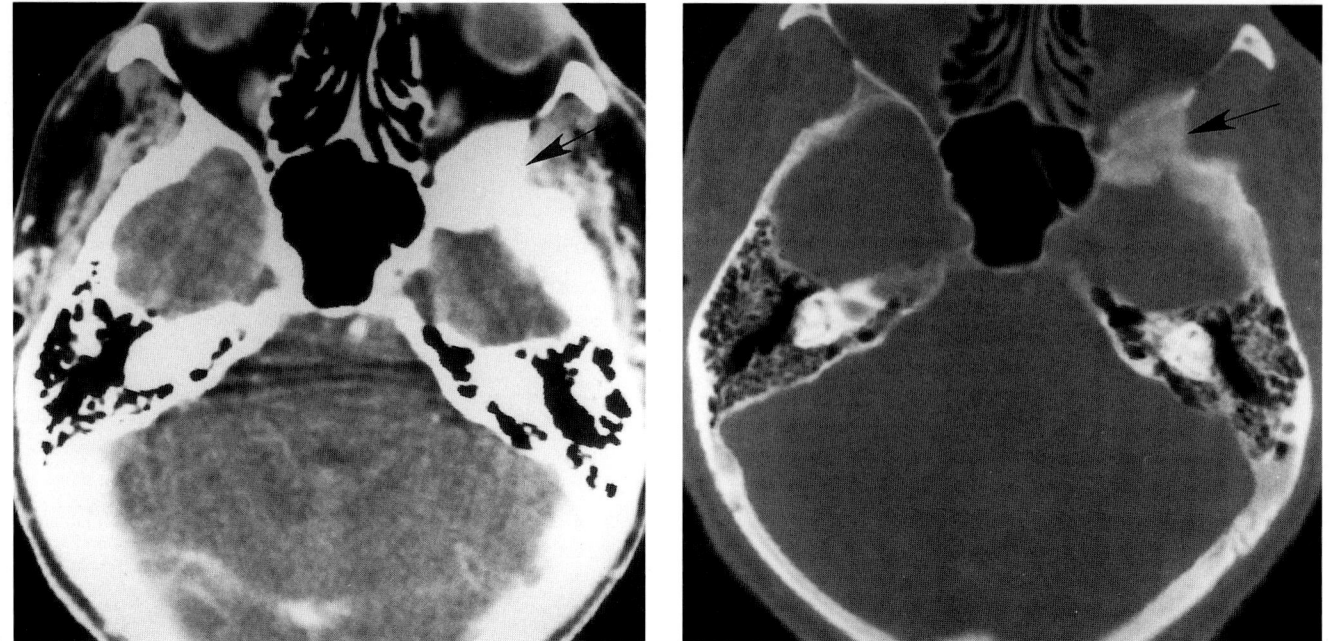

FIG. 6. Metastatic prostrate cancer. **A, B:** The lateral wall of the left orbit is expanded (*arrows*). This lesion would be hard to differentiate from an en plaque meningioma.

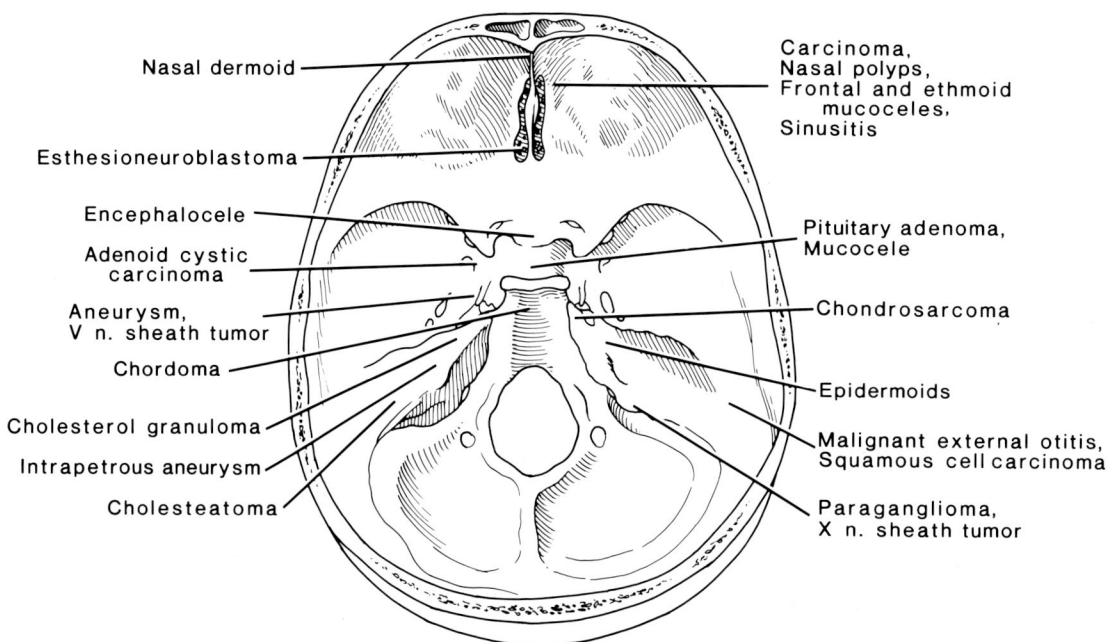

FIG. 7. Sites of origin of skull base tumors. **A:** Intracranial surface in the skull base. Some tumors may arise anywhere within the skull base including meningiomas, metastases, and sarcomas. Most tumors have a predilection to arise in a certain region of the skull base as outlined in the figure.

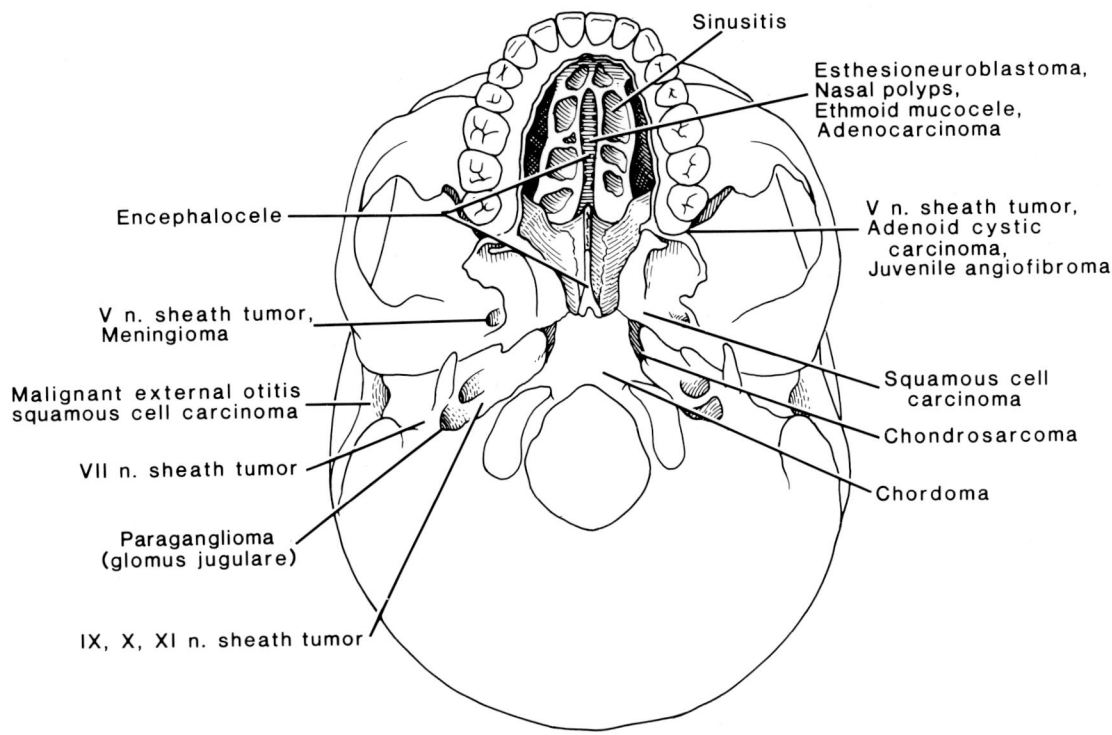

FIG. 7. *Continued.* **B:** Extracranial surface of the skull base (maxilla removed).

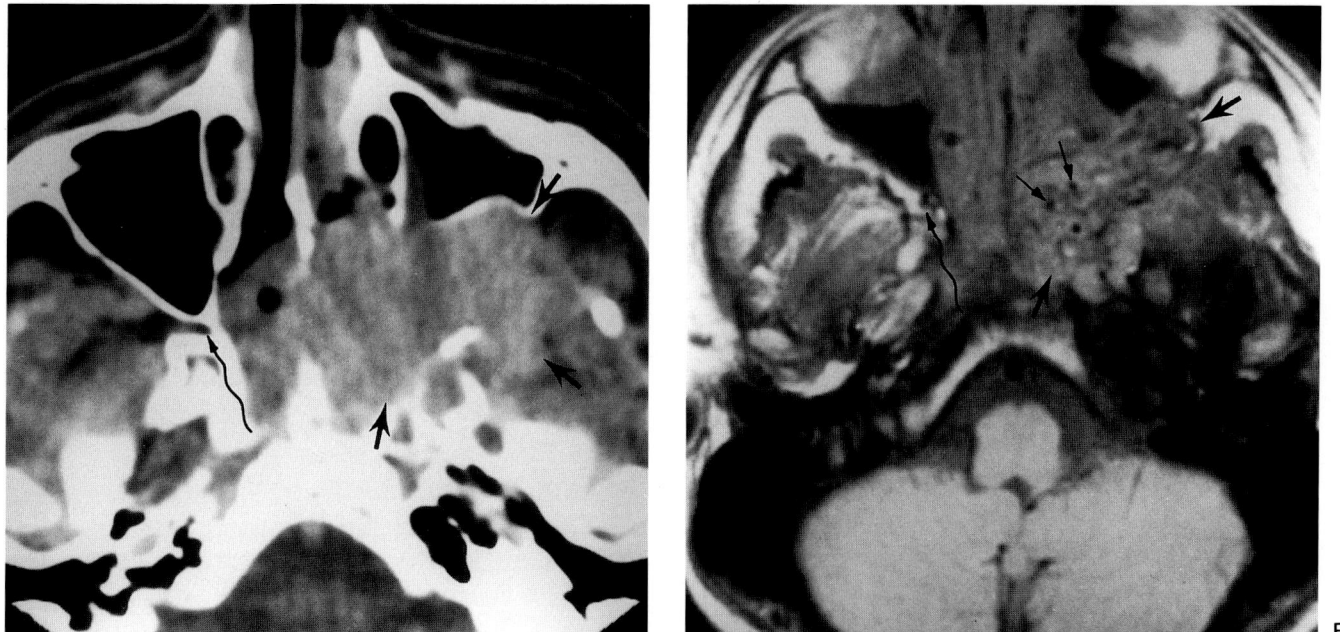

FIG. 8. Juvenile angiofibroma. **A:** Postcontrast axial CT shows a mass expanding the left pterygopalatine fossa (*arrows*). All juvenile angiofibromas arise in this region. This mass extends medially into the nasopharynx and laterally into the infratemporal fossa through the pterygomaxillary fissure. The normal right pterygopalatine fossa contains fat and is not expanded (*wavy arrow*). **B:** Axial SE (800/20) MRI. The lobulated mass (*large arrows*) is of intermediate T1 signal intensity. There are low signal flow voids within the mass (*small arrows*) that represent vessels and are characteristic of this very vascular tumor. The normal fat in the right pterygopalatine fossa is bright (high signal) on this T1-weighted image (*wavy arrow*).

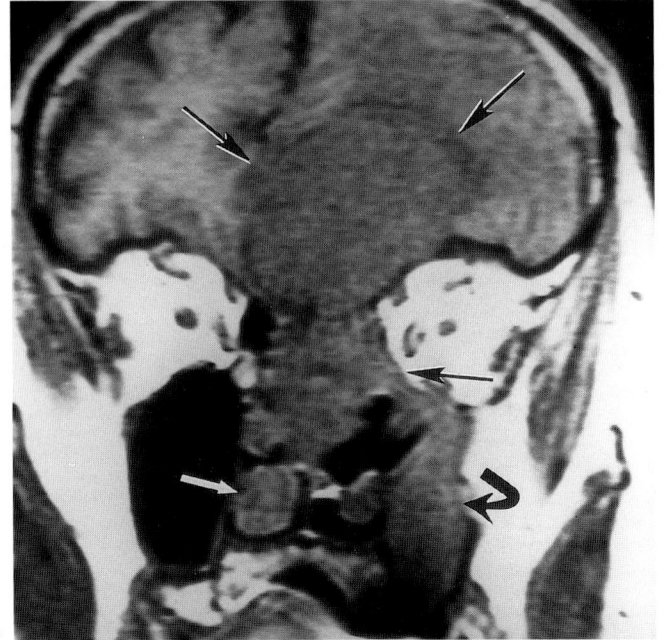
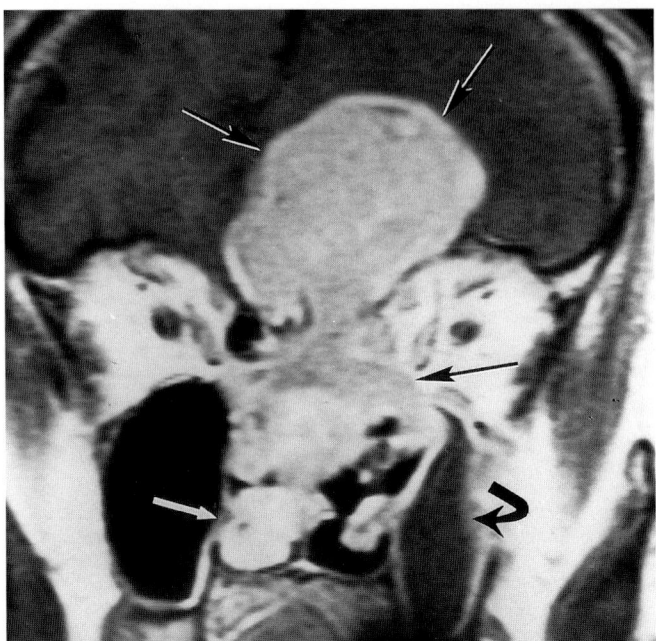
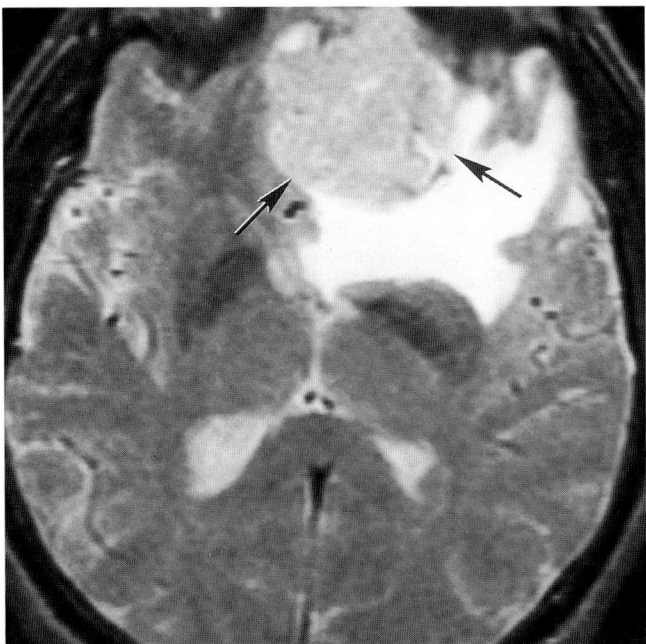

FIG. 9. Esthesioneuroblastoma (olfactory neuroblastoma). **A:** Coronal SE MRI (600/20). There is a large mass in the nasal cavity extending into the anterior cranial fossa (*black arrows*). The mass has intermediate signal characteristics similar to gray matter. The signal of the mass is indistinguishable from the signal within the obstructed left maxillary sinus (*curved arrow*) and from the inferior right nasal turbinate (*white arrow*). **B:** Postcontrast MRI at the same level. There is intense enhancement of the tumor (*black arrows*). The neoplastic tissue can now be differentiated from the obstructed maxillary sinus (*curved arrow*) where only the mucosa surrounding the obstructed secretions enhances. The neoplasm can also be differentiated from the right inferior turbinate (*white arrow*), which enhances more intensely than the tumor. **C:** Axial SE MRI (2500/80). The neoplastic tissue is of intermediate signal intensity, more intense than gray or white matter, but less intense than CSF (*arrows*). The high T2 signal surrounding the tumor represents edema in the adjacent frontal and temporal lobes.

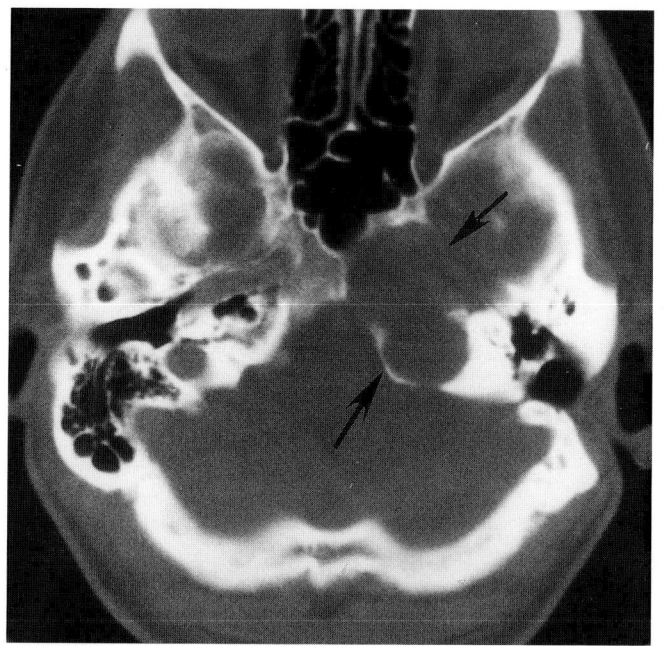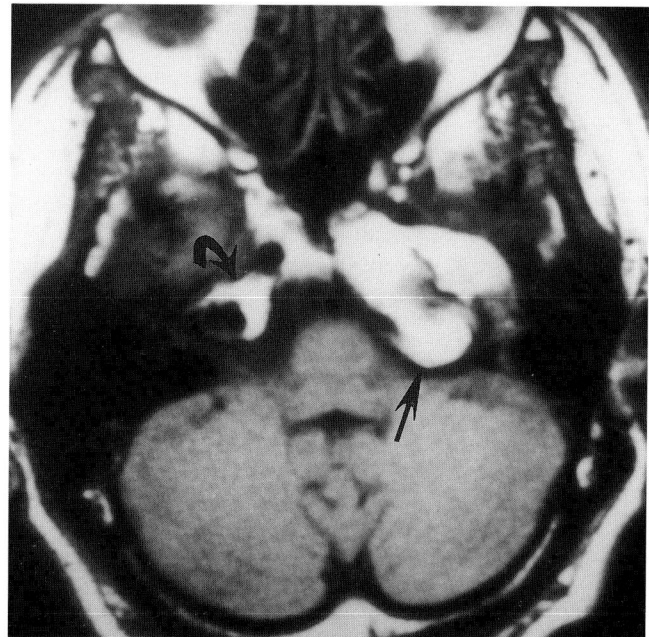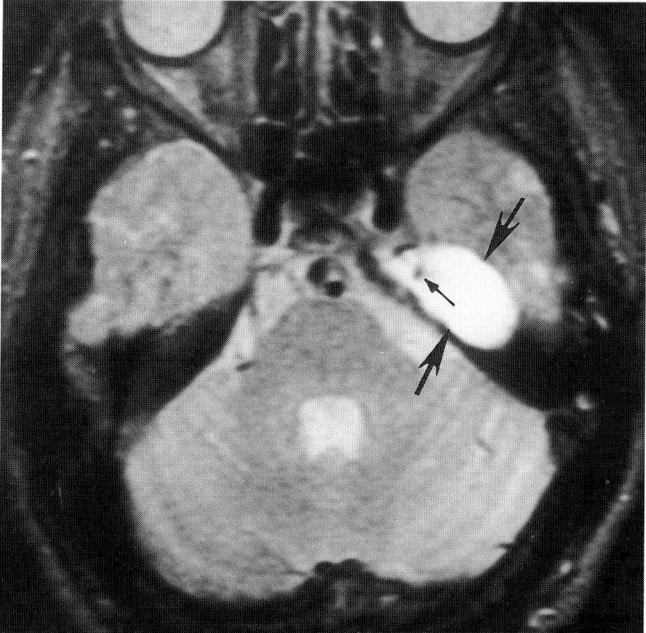

FIG. 10. Cholesterol granuloma. **A:** Axial CT (bone algorithm). Typically, cholesterol granulomas are expanding smooth walled lesions of the petrous apex (*arrows*). On soft tissue windows, they are intermediate in density between cerebral spinal fluid (CSF) and brain. **B:** Axial SE (600/20) MRI. On T1-weighted images cholesterol granulomas typically appear bright (*straight arrow*). These lesions are similar in signal intensity to the normal fat in the contralateral petrous apex (*curved arrow*) but can be differentiated because they are expansile and because fat is low in signal (dark) on T2-weighted images. **C:** Axial SE (2500/75) MRI. On T2-weighted images cholesterol granulomas (*large arrows*) are predominantly bright (high signal) although they may contain some areas of lower signal (*small arrow*). The characteristic high signal on T1-weighted images distinguishes cholesterol granulomas from other masses in this area.

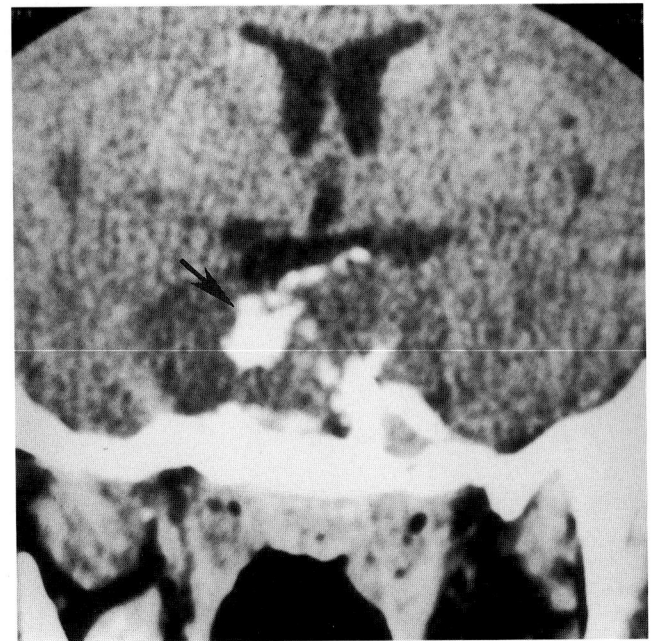
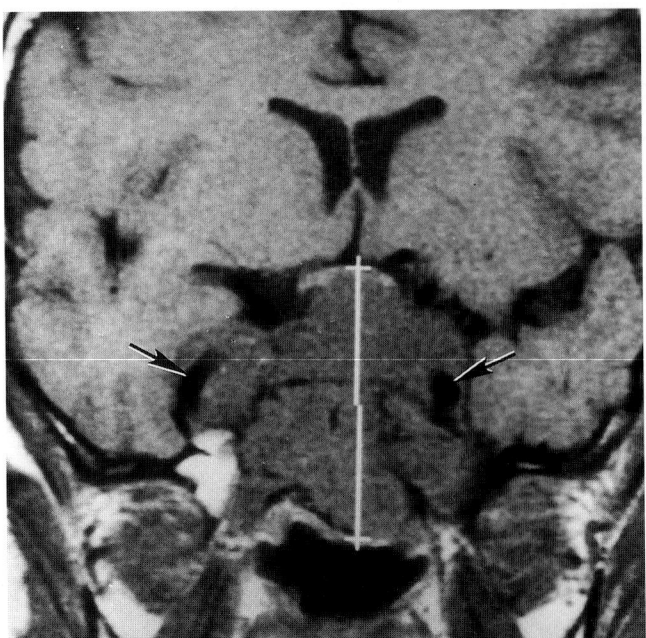
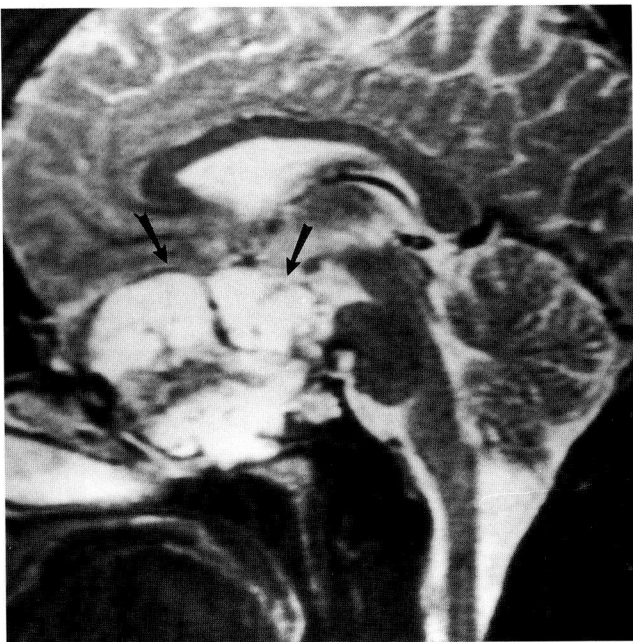

FIG. 11. Chondrosarcoma. **A:** Coronal noncontrast CT. There are areas of dense calcification within the mass (*arrow*). **B:** Coronal SE (800/20) MRI. A large mass of intermediate T1 signal replaces the clivus and sella and involves both cavernous sinuses. Both carotid arteries (*arrows*) are engulfed by the neoplasm. **C:** Sagittal SE (2500/100) MRI. The mass is high signal on a T2 basis (*arrows*). Chordomas and chondrosarcomas both typically have high signal on T2-weighted images and therefore may be hard to differentiate on the basis of imaging. A few chordomas have high signal on a T1 basis, which may provide a clue to the correct diagnosis. Chondrosarcomas usually arise at sutures lateral or anterior to the clivus and this may help differentiate them from chordomas that are typically more central. However, with large lesions such as this, the site of origin is hard to determine.

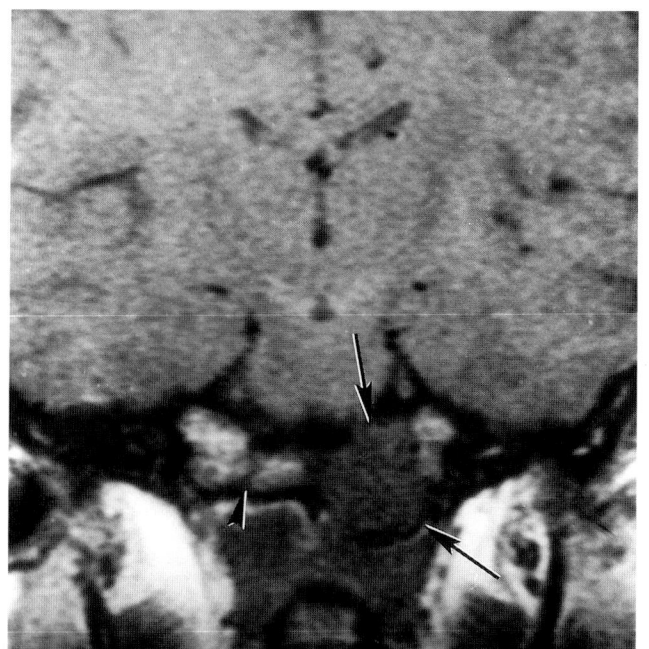
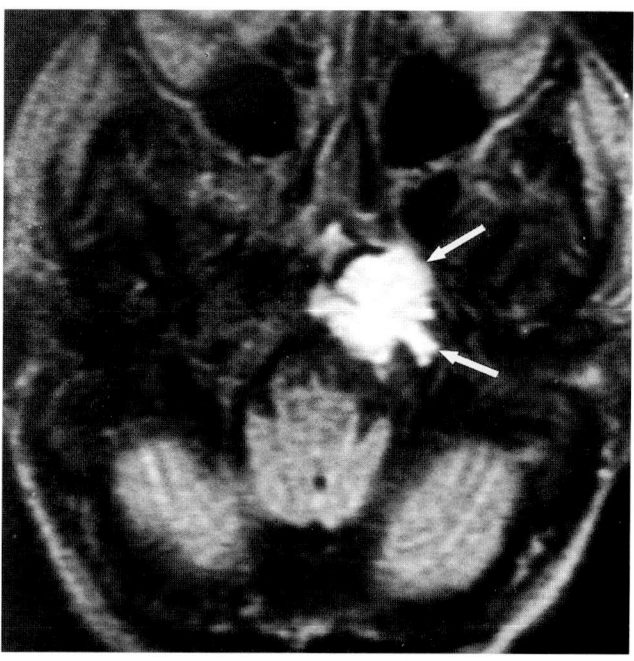

FIG. 12. Chondrosarcoma. **A:** Coronal SE (600/20) MRI. There is an intermediate signal mass (*arrows*) replacing the normal marrow fat in the skull base. The center of the tumor is the petro-occipital synchondrosis. Note the normal right petro-occipital synchondrosis (*arrowhead*). **B:** Axial SE (2500/100) MRI. The mass is high signal on a T2 basis (*arrows*). Skull base chondrosarcomas frequently arise at sutures such as the petro-occipital synchondrosis or in the region of the nasal cavity and paranasal sinuses. They are usually intermediate in signal on a T1 basis and high signal on a T2 basis.

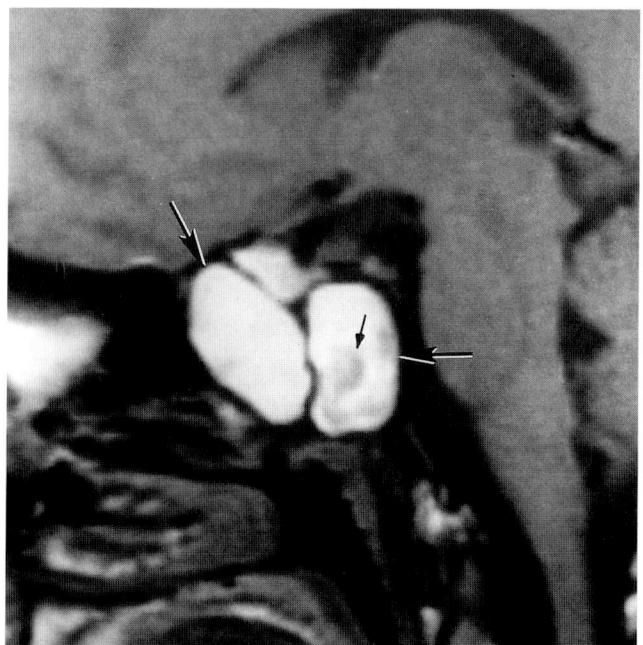
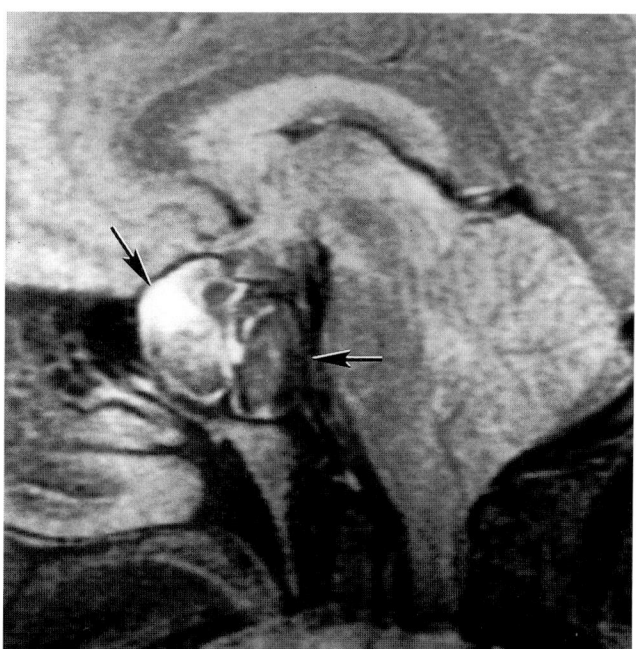

FIG. 13. Mucocele. **A:** Sagittal SE (600/20) MRI. There is expansion of the sphenoid air cells (*large arrows*). The sinus contents are primarily high signal although within the posterior sphenoid air cell there is lower signal material (*small arrow*). **B:** Sagittal SE (3000/75) MRI. On a T2 basis the contents of the obstructed air cells vary in intensity: anteriorly they are high signal; posteriorly they are of lower signal. The mucus within obstructed air cells (*arrows*) may have extremely varied signal characteristics, depending on the length of obstruction, viscosity of the mucus, and water content. Very inspissated secretions can appear dark on all pulsing sequences and can even look like an aerated cell. In ambiguous cases, CT may be needed to differentiate obstructed from aerated air cells.

TABLE 1. Imaging characteristics of tumors[a]

Neoplasm	T1 signal	T2 signal	Location	Special features
Adenoidcystic carcinoma	Intermediate	Intermediate	Middle	Perineural spread often involves pterygopalatine fossa
Aneurysm	Variable	Variable	Middle	Flow void or laminated clot
Bacterial sinusitus	Low	High	All	Sclerosis of sinus wall if chronic
Cholesteatoma	Intermediate	Intermediate or high	Posterolateral	Erosion of scutum or ossicles, may enhance peripherally
Cholesterol granuloma	High	High	Posterolateral	Almost always at petrous apex, rare in middle ear, high T1 signal suggests diagnosis
Chondrosarcoma	Intermediate	High	All	Arises at sutures, large dense "popcorn-like" calcification
Chordoma	Intermediate, occasionally high	High	Middle	Clivus involved in almost all cases, may have areas of high T1 signal, may have matrix calcifications
Dermoid	Variable	Variable	Anterior	Bridge of nose and cribriform region, bony canal may connect intra- and extracranial components
Encephalocele	Low	High	All	
Epidermoids	Low	High	Middle/posterolateral	Usually similar to CSF in MRI signal and CT density, may have internal echoes that distinguish it from CSF
Esthesioneuroblastoma	Intermediate	Intermediate	Anterior	Involves cribriform plate, occasional hyperostosis
Fibrous dysplasia	Intermediate	Variable	Anterior/middle	Characteristic amorphous high density bone on CT, enhancement of dysplastic bone best seen on MRI
Fungal sinusitus	Low	Low	Anterior/middle	Foci of increased density within sinus on CT, marked hypointensity on T2-weighted images
Juvenile angiofibroma	Intermediate	Intermediate or high	Middle	Vascular flow voids on MRI
Lymphoma	Intermediate	Intermediate	Anterior/middle	
Malignant external otitis	Intermediate	Intermediate or high	Posterolateral	*Pseudomonas* infection in elderly diabetics, may mimic carcinoma of external canal on imaging
Meningioma	Intermediate	Intermediate or high	All	Vascular on angiography, hyperostosis of adjacent bone is a frequent finding
Mucocele	Variable	Variable	Anterior/middle	Signal varies with viscosity of contents, the peripheral mucosa may enhance
Nerve sheath tumor	Intermediate	High	Middle/posterolateral	Usually high T2 signal; almost never calcifies
Paragangliomas (glomus tumors)	Intermediate	Intermediate or high	Posterolateral	Middle ear or lateral jugular foramen (pars vascularis), vascular flow voids on MRI
Pituitary adenoma	Intermediate	Intermediate	Middle	Intramural cysts or hemorrhage may have variable signal
Polyps	Variable	High	Anterior	
Sarcomas	Intermediate	Intermediate or high	All	
Squamous cell carcinoma	Intermediate	Intermediate	Anterior/middle	

[a] Table based on refs. 1–5, 7, 8, and 12–18.

AVENUES OF SPREAD

Many tumors involve the skull base by direct extension. These include malignant lesions such as esthesioneuroblastoma (Fig. 13), lymphoma, and squamous cell carcinoma (6,7).

Other tumors, particularly adenoid cystic carcinoma and nerve sheath tumors, spread along nerves (Fig. 14). This can result in enlargement of the neural foramina, which can be detected by CT or MRI. More subtle perineural spread that does not enlarge the foramen can be detected at the point where the cranial nerves exit the skull base. Perineural spread should be suspected if the fat around the exiting nerve is replaced with soft tissue (8–10). Cranial nerves III, IV, V_1, and VI are surrounded by fat in the superior orbital fissure, V_2 by fat in the pterygopalatine fossa, V_3 by fat just inferior to the foramen ovale, and VII by fat surrounding the extracranial opening of the stylomastoid foramen. Cranial nerves IX, X, XI, and XII emerge beneath the skull base close to the carotid artery and jugular vein. A mass close to these vessels may represent perineural extension.

Meningiomas seldom grow along nerves; instead, they spread along the dural coverings lining the intracranial surface of the skull base. Dural spread is best detected on enhanced MRI scans. There is often a "dural tail" of enhancing meninges around meningiomas (Fig. 15). This dural tail is rarely seen in other tumors and can only be detected on enhanced MRI scans; it is not visible on CT because of the overlying bone. The histopathologic

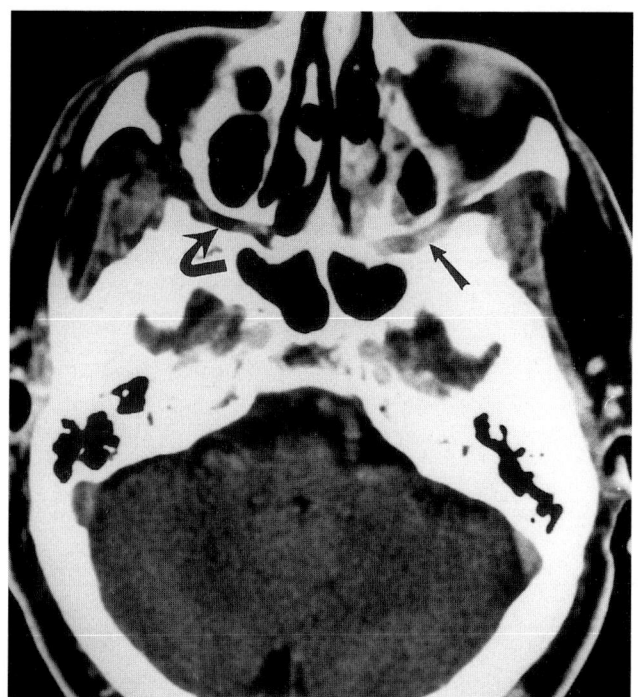

FIG. 14. Adenoidcystic carcinoma. Axial enhanced CT shows obliteration of the fat in the left pterygopalatine fossa (*straight arrow*). Compare this with a normal hypodense fat in the right pterygopalatine fossa (*curved arrow*). Perineural extension is characteristic of adenoidcystic carcinoma. It spreads centrally along the branches of the trigeminal nerve. Once in the pterygopalatine fossa it can spread along branches supplying the lacrimal gland through the inferior orbital fissure and into the orbit. It can also spread intracranially along V_2 through foramen rotundum into the cavernous sinus. Involvement of the pterygopalatine fossa is recognized on CT as abnormal increased density, whereas on T1-weighted MR images it is recognized as abnormal decreased signal intensity on unenhanced T1-weighted images.

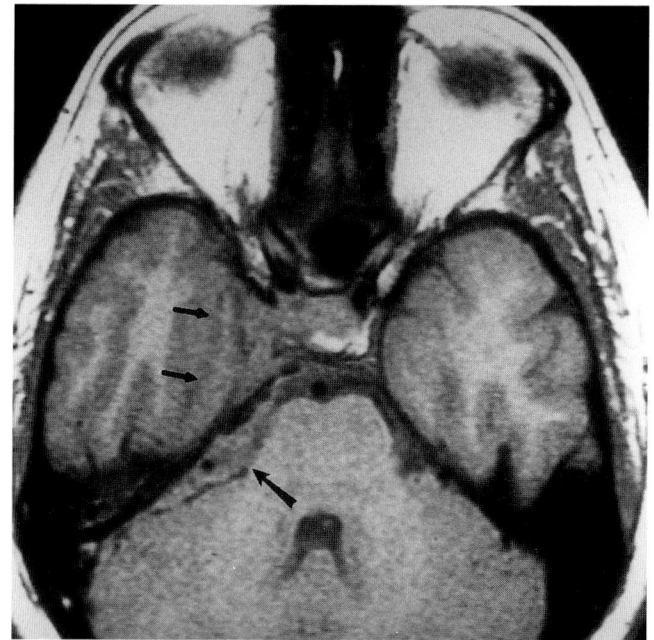
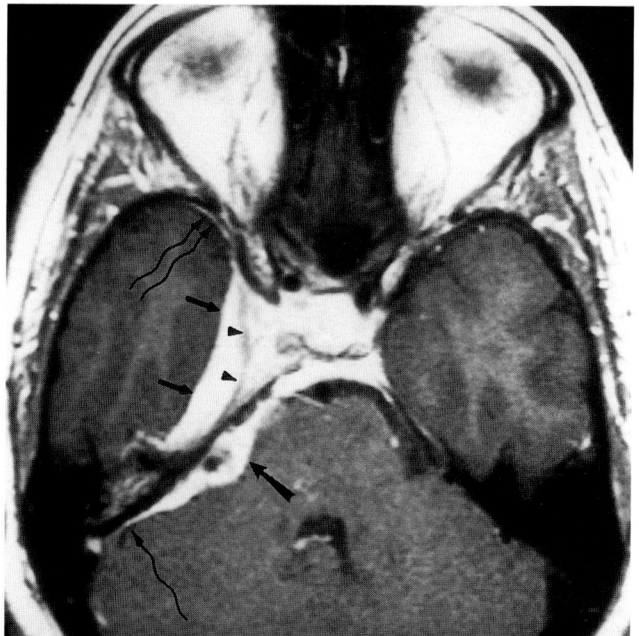

FIG. 15. Meningioma. **A:** Axial SE (500/20) MRI. On unenhanced images there is some fullness in the right cavernous region (*small arrows*). In addition, tumor is growing along the posterior surface of the petrous bone (*large arrow*). **B:** Postcontrast MRI shows the lesion much more clearly. The lateral wall of the cavernous sinus (*arrowheads*) is highlighted by the tumor growing medial and lateral (*small arrows*) to it. The tumor extends along the posterior surface of the petrous bone and along the dorsum sella (*large arrow*). Note the enhancing "dural tail" (*wavy arrow*) extending along the posterior aspect of the petrous bone and also along the greater wing of the right sphenoid bone (*paired wavy arrows*). The histopathologic significance of the dural tail remains to be established (see text).

features of the dural tail are not fully known: some contend that it represents hyperemic meninges with congested veins while others suggest that dual tails harbor microscopic and macroscopic islands of meningioma cells. If the latter proves true, it may explain the recurrence of some meningiomas (11).

IMAGING AS A GUIDE TO SURGICAL MANAGEMENT

Many skull base tumors have a high recurrence rate. Chordomas are a prime example (Fig. 16). Recurrences may be so common in part because these tumors are so

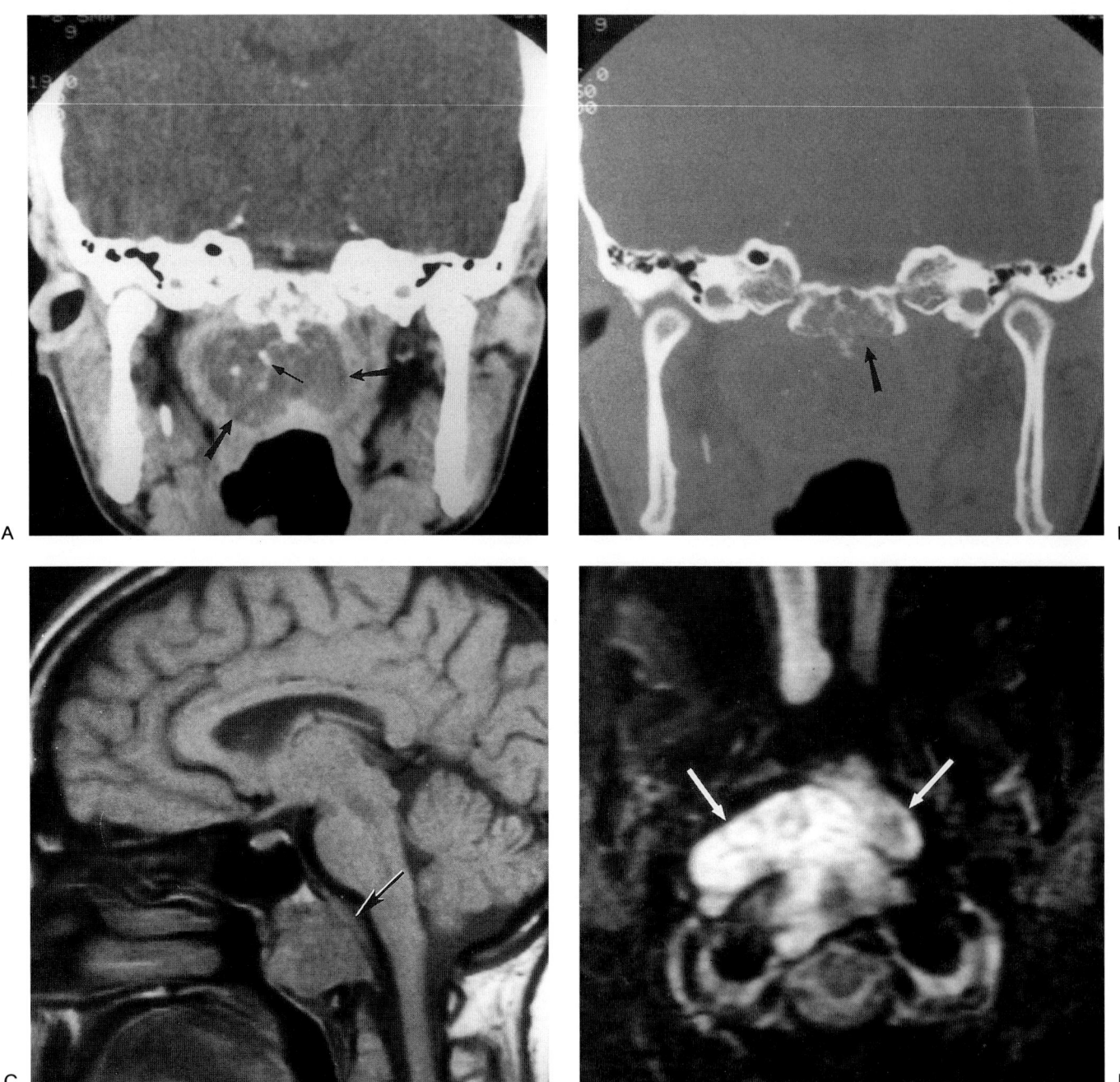

FIG. 16. Chordoma. **A:** Coronal CT shows a low dense mass (*large arrows*) protruding into the nasopharynx. There are small calcifications or fragments of partly destroyed bone within the mass (*small arrow*). **B:** Bone algorithm of the same slice shows irregular erosion of the nasopharyngeal cortex of the clivus (*arrow*). **C:** Sagittal SE (600/25) MRI. The mass bulges into the nasopharynx and extends inferiorly to the level of C1. The mass has broken through the intracranial cortex of the clivus (*arrow*). Most chordomas, like this one, are intermediate in signal on T1-weighted images. Chordomas may have foci of high T1 signal, which, when present, are highly suggestive of chordoma. **D:** Axial SE (2500/100) MRI. Chordomas almost always are high signal on T2-weighted images (*arrows*).

difficult to remove completely. Carefully performed and analyzed imaging can fairly precisely define the location and extent of skull base lesions preoperatively. This foreknowledge allows precise planning of the operation, which may increase the chance for long-term control or cure of the tumor.

There are several "problem areas" in the imaging of skull base masses, which deserve special mention. In tumors involving the paranasal sinuses, it can be difficult on CT to differentiate between neoplastic tissue and adjacent obstructed air cells. However, MRI is usually able to make this distinction because of its greater ability to characterize soft tissues. Multiple pulsing sequences and images with contrast may be necessary (12–14) (Fig. 9).

Another problem area is the relationship of skull base lesions to vascular structures, particularly the carotid artery and jugular vein. By CT these enhancing structures are often very similar in density to enhancing tumor (Fig. 3A). Dynamic bolus contrast CT can help differentiate vessel from tumor but this procedure is time consuming and may require multiple injections of contrast to trace the vessel. Differentiation of tumor from vessel is easier by MRI (Fig. 3B). The carotid artery appears as a signal void, easily contrasted from surrounding tumor. Evaluation of the jugular vein is more difficult because the blood flow within it is slower and more variable. Flow rate variations result in a myriad of possible MRI signal characteristics. In this situation, it is important to perform special flow-sensitive sequences (such as gradient echo or flow saturation images) to differentiate tumor from slowly flowing blood in the jugular fossa or vein. MRI angiography, which is able to demonstrate large vessels such as the parasellar carotid artery and jugular vein, may help in difficult cases. In some cases, conventional angiography is still needed.

POSTOPERATIVE EVALUATION

The purpose of imaging studies in the immediate postoperative period is to define complications of surgery, such as cerebral edema, bleeding, or infection. CT is ideal for this purpose because it is easy to perform, readily available, and rapid. At the soft tissue window and level settings, air, fat packing, and gelfoam can appear to have similar low density (Fig. 17). A wide window setting is needed to differentiate fat from air. At the bone window and level settings these different densities are easy to distinguish. Edema and blood at the surgical bed usually preclude accurate assessment for residual tumor on scans done shortly after surgery. Early postoperative CT and angiography can also be useful in confirming the patency of carotid artery bypass grafts (Fig. 18).

Baseline postoperative scans are obtained at 3 months

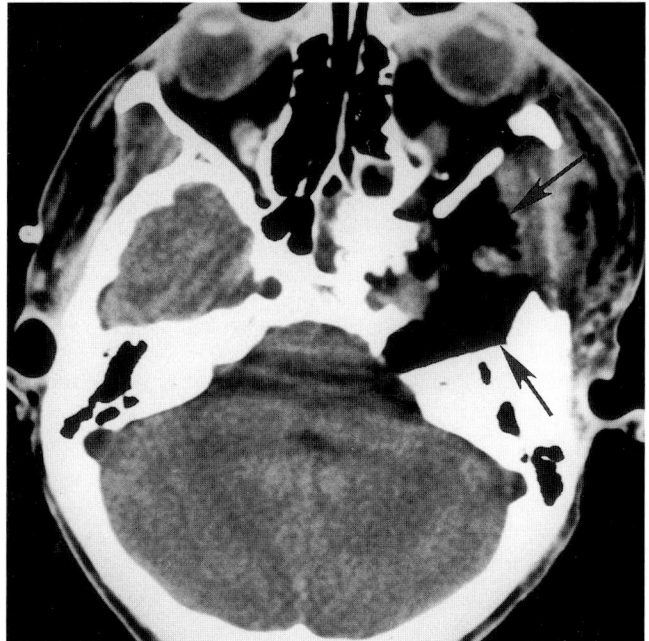
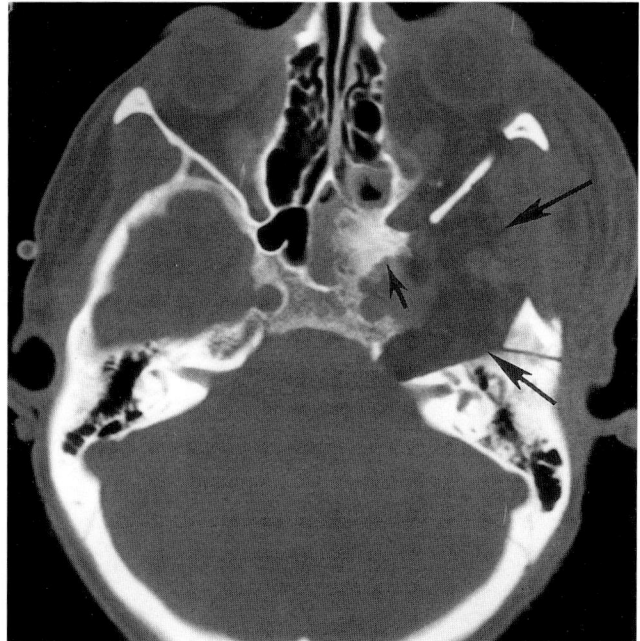

FIG. 17. Meningioma, immediate postoperative scan. **A:** Axial unenhanced CT. There is a large low density area in the operative bed (*arrows*). At these window and level settings it is impossible to tell if this low density represents air, gelfoam, or fat packing. **B:** Axial CT at the same level as **A** but at a wider window setting. The low density material (*large arrows*) represents fat packing. It is the same density as the fat in the orbits but is much higher in density than the air in the ethmoid and sphenoid sinuses. There is still some hyperostotic bone on the left lateral wall on the sphenoid sinus (*small arrow*). Hyperostotic bone frequently contains viable neoplastic cells.

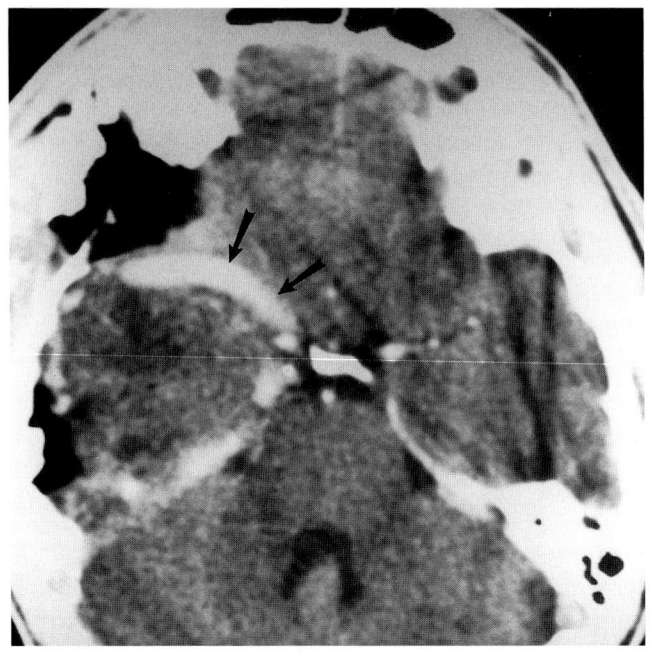
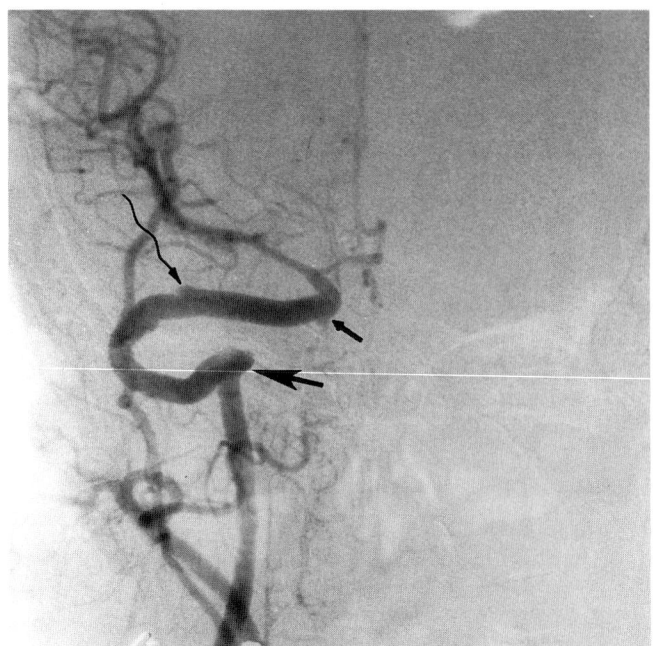
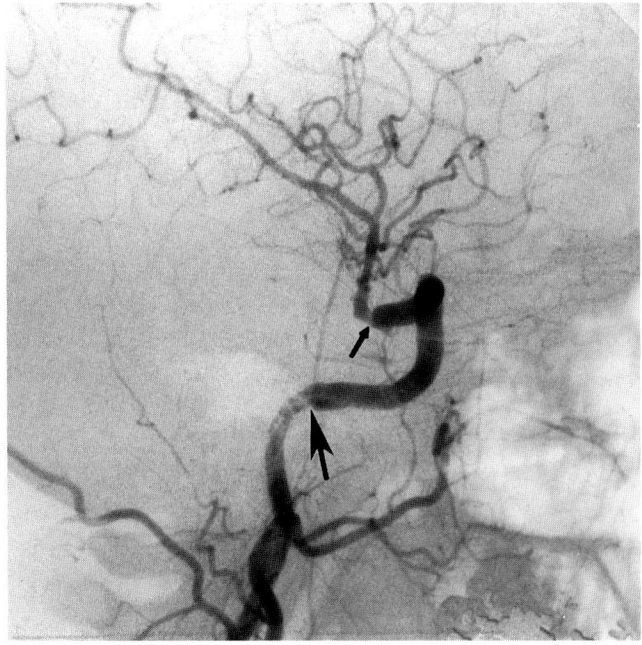

FIG. 18. Carotid bypass graft. **A:** Axial enhanced CT shows the vein graft (*arrows*) densely opacified with contrast. There is no evidence of thrombosis of the graft. **B, C:** AP and lateral angiogram. Proximally there is an end-to-end anastomosis between the vein graft and the native carotid (*large arrows*). Distally there is an end-to-side anastomosis between the vein graft and the supraclinoid carotid artery (*small arrows*). Mild irregularities of the graft (*wavy arrow*) can represent valves or branching veins that have been ligated prior to graft insertion.

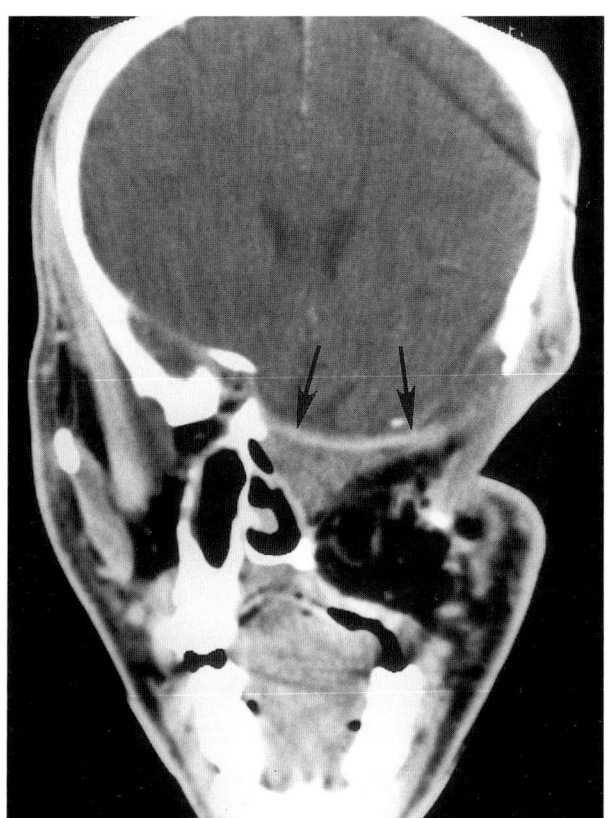 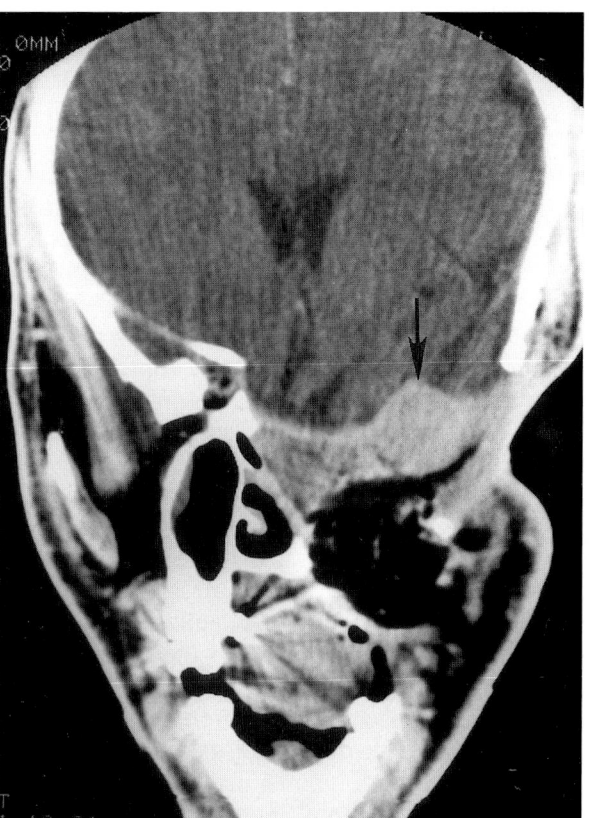

FIG. 19. Recurrent chordoma. **A:** Coronal enhanced CT 3 months after surgery. A temporalis muscle flap (arrows) separates the nasal cavity from the intracranial contents. The flap enhances following contrast. **B:** Coronal enhanced CT at the same level as **A**, but 9 months after surgery. There is marked expansion of the lateral aspect of muscle flap (arrow). This indicates tumor recurrence. Normally, one would expect further contraction of the muscle flap. Any expansion of the flap after the 3-month postoperative scan is highly suggestive of tumor recurrence.

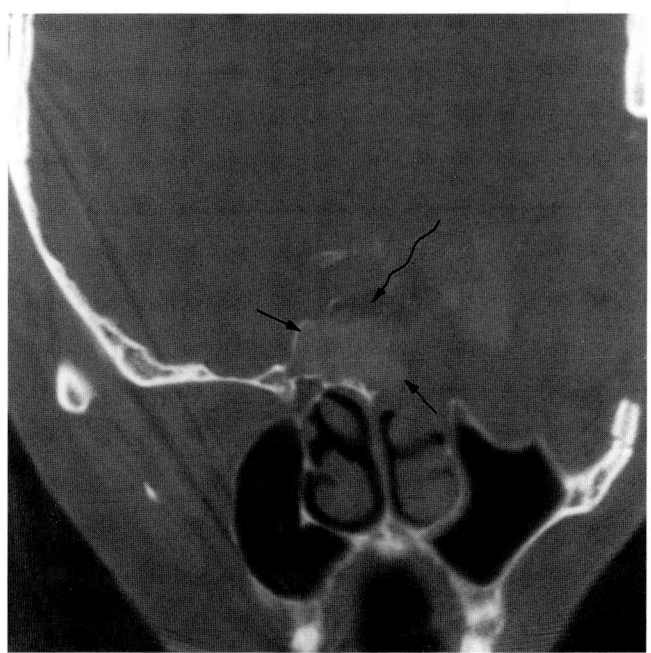 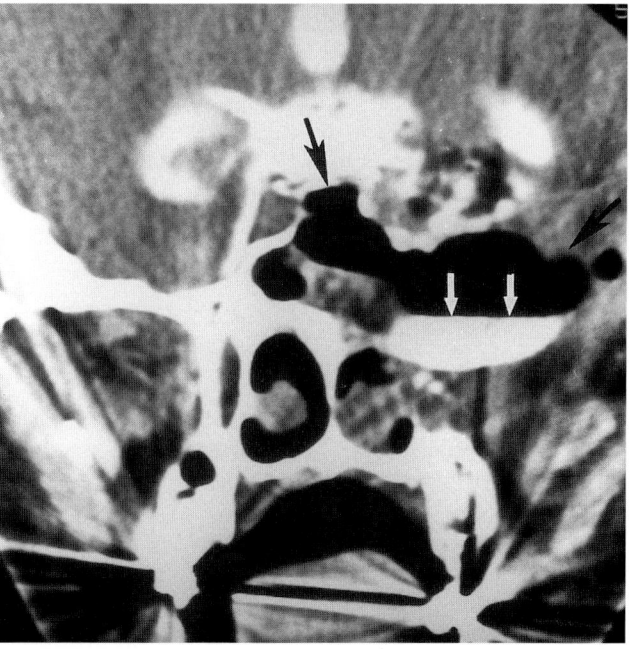

FIG. 20. CSF leak. **A:** Coronal CT (bone algorithm) following intrathecal contrast. There is surgical absence of the floor of the left middle cranial fossa and left lateral wall of the sphenoid sinus. The subarachnoid contrast opacified the sphenoid sinus (arrows). The sinus is partially packed with fat (wavy arrow). **B:** The patient did not respond to lumbar drainage and after 2 weeks a repeat cisternogram shows a large cavity in the left infratemporal region (black arrows), which is contiguous with the sphenoid sinus and contains an air-contrast level (white arrows).

following surgery. This is done because often tumor recurrence can only be recognized on serial studies. The distortion of normal fat planes by the surgery itself as well as the variable enhancement characteristics of muscle flaps make tumor recurrence very difficult to detect on a single study. Changes induced by adjuvant chemotherapy and radiation therapy can further complicate the postoperative appearance of the surgical site. Usually recurrence can only be definitely defined by changes (usually mass effect), which can only be appreciated by comparison with earlier studies (Fig. 19). We are unsure if MRI has a distinct advantage over CT in follow-up scanning.

CSF leak is a frequent postoperative complication. Often the leaks will seal spontaneously or following measures (such as a lumbar drain) that lower CSF pressure. In cases of persistent leak, CT with intrathecal contrast and radionuclide cisternography are still the mainstays in diagnosis. Contrast is injected into the lumbar subarachnoid space and the patient is positioned head down. The patient is usually placed prone with the neck extended, and coronal 3-mm cuts through the surgical bed with bone algorithms are obtained (Fig. 20). In spite of strong clinical evidence of CSF leak, these studies are frequently negative.

REFERENCES

1. Oot RF, Melville GE, New PFJ, et al. The role of MR and CT in evaluating clival chondroma and chondrosarcomas. *AJNR* 1988;9:715–723.
2. Lee Y, Tassel PV. Craniofacial chondrosarcomas: imaging findings in 15 untreated cases. *AJNR* 1989;10:165–170.
3. Lloyd GAS, Phelps PD. Juvenile angiofibroma: imaging by magnetic resonance, CT and conventional techniques. *Clin Otolaryngol* 1986;11:247–259.
4. Olsen WL, Dillon WP, Kelly WM, Norman D, Brant-Zawadzki M, Newton TH. MR imaging of paragangliomas. *AJNR* 1986;7:1039–1042.
5. Press GA, Hesselink J. MR imaging of cerebellopontine angle and internal auditory canal lesions at 1.5 T. *AJNR* 1988;9:241–251.
6. Mills SE, Frierson HF. Olfactory neuroblastoma: a clinicopathologic study of 21 cases. *Am J Surg Pathol* 1985;9:317–327.
7. Som PM, Dillion WP, Sze G, Lidov M, Biller HF, Lawson W. Benign and malignant sinonasal lesions with intracranial extension: differentiation with MR imaging. *Radiology* 1989;172:763–766.
8. Laine FJ, Braun IF, Jensen ME, Nadel L, Som PD. Perineural tumor extension through the foramen ovale: evaluation with MR imaging. *Radiology* 1990;174:65–71.
9. Curtin HD, Williams R, Johnson J. CT of the perineural tumor extension: pterygopalatine fossa. *AJR* 1985;144:163–169.
10. Curtin HD, Wolfe P, Snyderman N. Facial nerve between the stylomastoid foramen and the parotid: computed tomographic imaging. *Radiology* 1983;149:165.
11. Goldsher D, Litt A, Pinto R, Bannon RK, Kricheff I. Dural "tail" associated with meningiomas on Gd-DTPA-enhanced MR images: characteristics, differential diagnostic value, and possible implications for treatment. *Radiology* 1990;176:447–450.
12. Som PM, Shapiro MD, Biller HF, Sasaki C, Lawson W. Sinonasal tumors and inflammatory tissues: differentiation with MR imaging. *Radiology* 1988;167:803–808.
13. Dillon WP, Som PM, Fullerton GD. Hypointense MR signal in chronically inspissated sinonasal secretions. *Radiology* 1990;174:73–78.
14. Som PM, Dillon WP, Fullerton GD, Zimmerman RA, Rajagopalan B, Marom Z. Chronically obstructed sinonasal secretions: observations on T1 and T2 shortening. *Radiology* 1989;172:515–520.
15. Zinreich SJ, Kennedy DW, Malat J, et al. Fungal sinusitis: diagnosis with CT and MR imaging. *Radiology* 1988;169:439–444.
16. Som PM, Shugar JM, Troy K, et al. The use of magnetic resonance and computed tomography in the management of a patient with intrasinus hemorrhage. *Arch Otolaryngol Head Neck Surg* 1988;114:200–202.
17. Elster AD, Challa VR, Gilbert TH, Richardson DN, Contento JC. Meningiomas: MR and histopathologic features. *Radiology* 1989;170:857–862.
18. Watabe T, Azuma T. T1 and T2 measurements of meningiomas and neuromas before and after Gd-DTPA. *AJNR* 1989;10:463–470.

CHAPTER 4

Balloon Test Occlusion

Joseph A. Horton, Charles A. Jungreis, and Frank Pistoia

The routine Matas test (manual compression of the cervical carotid artery for 15 min with neurological testing), the so-called balloon Matas test (BMT—same as the traditional Matas test, but rather than using manual compression a balloon is used to occlude the internal carotid artery—ICA), and the BMT with stump pressure measurement were successively developed to determine whether it would be safe to occlude a carotid artery. All fail to detect a group of patients who are at risk for developing a delayed stroke if the carotid artery is permanently occluded. In fact, in a large series of each of these, the delayed stroke rate is a surprisingly constant 10–15%.

We have used the stable xenon/CT technique for measurement of cerebral blood flow (CBF) *during* balloon occlusion of the internal carotid artery to identify patients at risk for delayed stroke. First, we anticoagulate the patient with 7000 units of heparin and introduce a double lumen, 100-cm Swan–Ganz balloon catheter into the internal carotid artery. We then test the patient's neurological status continuously for 15 min. If the patient develops a neurological deficit, the balloon is immediately deflated, the heparin reversed with protamine, and the test concluded: the patient will definitely not tolerate permanent carotid occlusion. This would place the patient in (our category) group IV (clinical failure with balloon occlusion).

Group IV comprises only about 5% of the patients we have examined. The remaining 95% do not develop a neurological deficit with temporary carotid occlusion. In these patients, we deflate the balloon but leave it in place in the ICA, move the patient to the CT scanner where the CBF study will be done, reinflate the balloon, and do a CBF study. After this has been completed, we deflate and remove the balloon catheter, wait about 20 min for the xenon to be exhaled, and repeat the CBF study. In this way, we are able to obtain the "occluded" study and have an "unoccluded" study with which to compare it.

CBF data comparing occluded and unoccluded studies have shown that patients fall into three groups. Group I patients show no difference in hemispheric CBF (hCBF) whether the balloon is inflated or deflated. Group II patients display a mild but symmetric decrease in hCBF with ICA occlusion. Patients in both these groups (I and II) are at minimal risk for delayed stroke following permanent ICA occlusion (Figs. 1 and 2). In over 40 patients at our institution in groups I and II whose ICAs were ligated at surgery through necessity, only one (<2.5%) had a delayed stroke; that stroke occurred some days after surgery and was likely the result of thromboembolism rather than cryptic hemodynamic insufficiency. Generally, patients in groups I and II have hCBF values greater than 30 cc/100 g per minute.

Group III patients show a more pronounced and almost always asymmetric decrease in hCBF, more on the occluded side. These patients are at greatly increased risk for delayed stroke with permanent carotid occlusion. We are aware of 11 group III patients in the United States who had permanent ICA occlusion. Ten of these patients (>90%) had perioperative stroke. Although the number of patients in this group is not large, there can be little doubt of the significance of identifying the group. Group III patients represent 14% of the over 300 patients in whom we have done the balloon test/CBF study. It is important to emphasize that this group has a normal clinical evaluation with temporary balloon occlusion and is not identified by neurological examination alone.

J. A. Horton and C. A. Jungreis: Department of Radiology, University of Pittsburgh School of Medicine, and Presbyterian University Hospital, Pittsburgh, Pennsylvania 15213.

F. Pistoia: Department of Neuroradiology, St. Vincents Hospital, Indianapolis, Indiana, 46240.

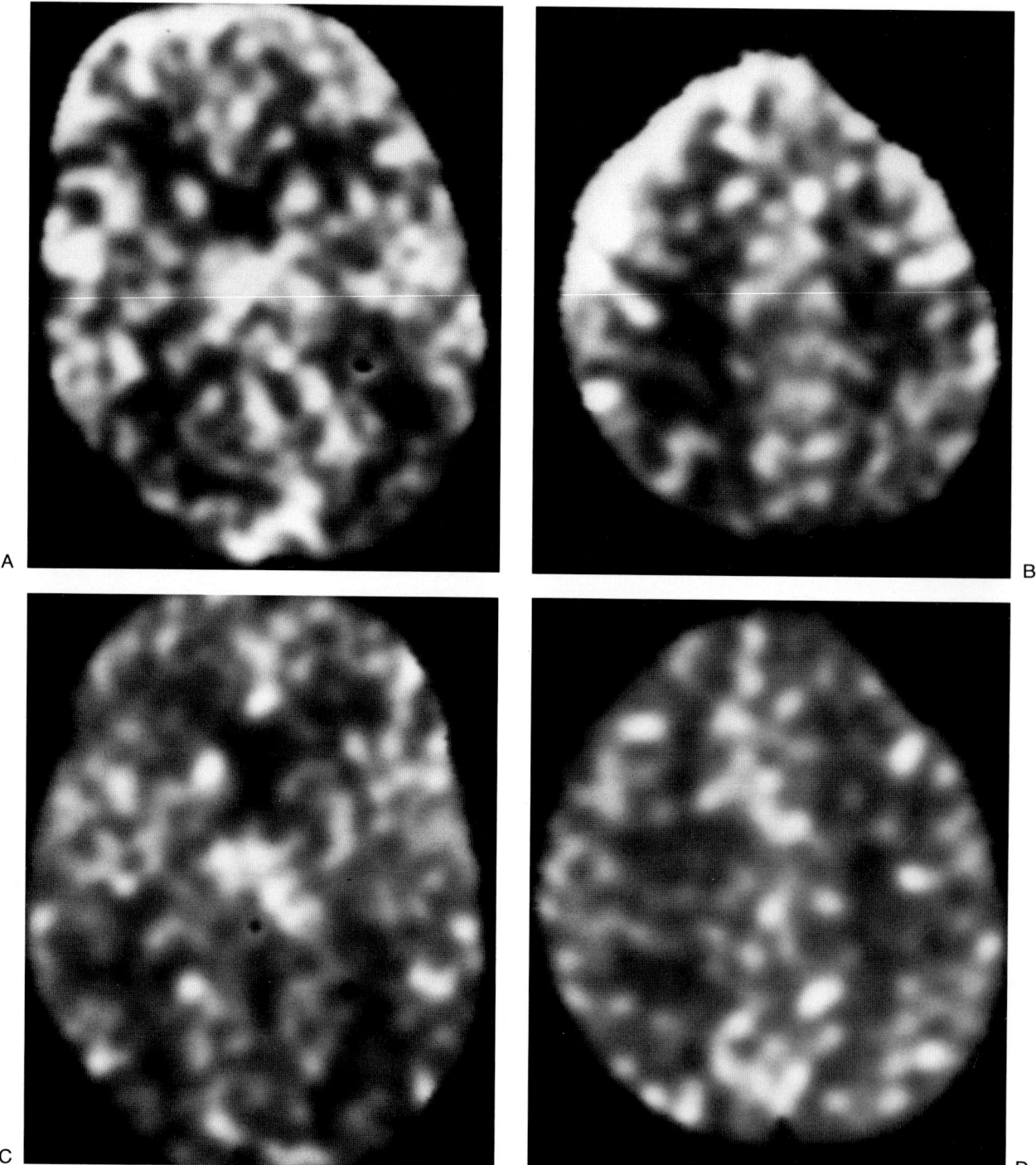

FIG. 1. A,B: Xenon-enhanced CT/CBF study with balloon deflated in the "unoccluded" study. There is symmetric CBF. **C,D:** The "occluded" study shows a mild symmetric decrease in hCBF. This patient exhibits criteria for group II: mild, symmetric decrease in hCBF.

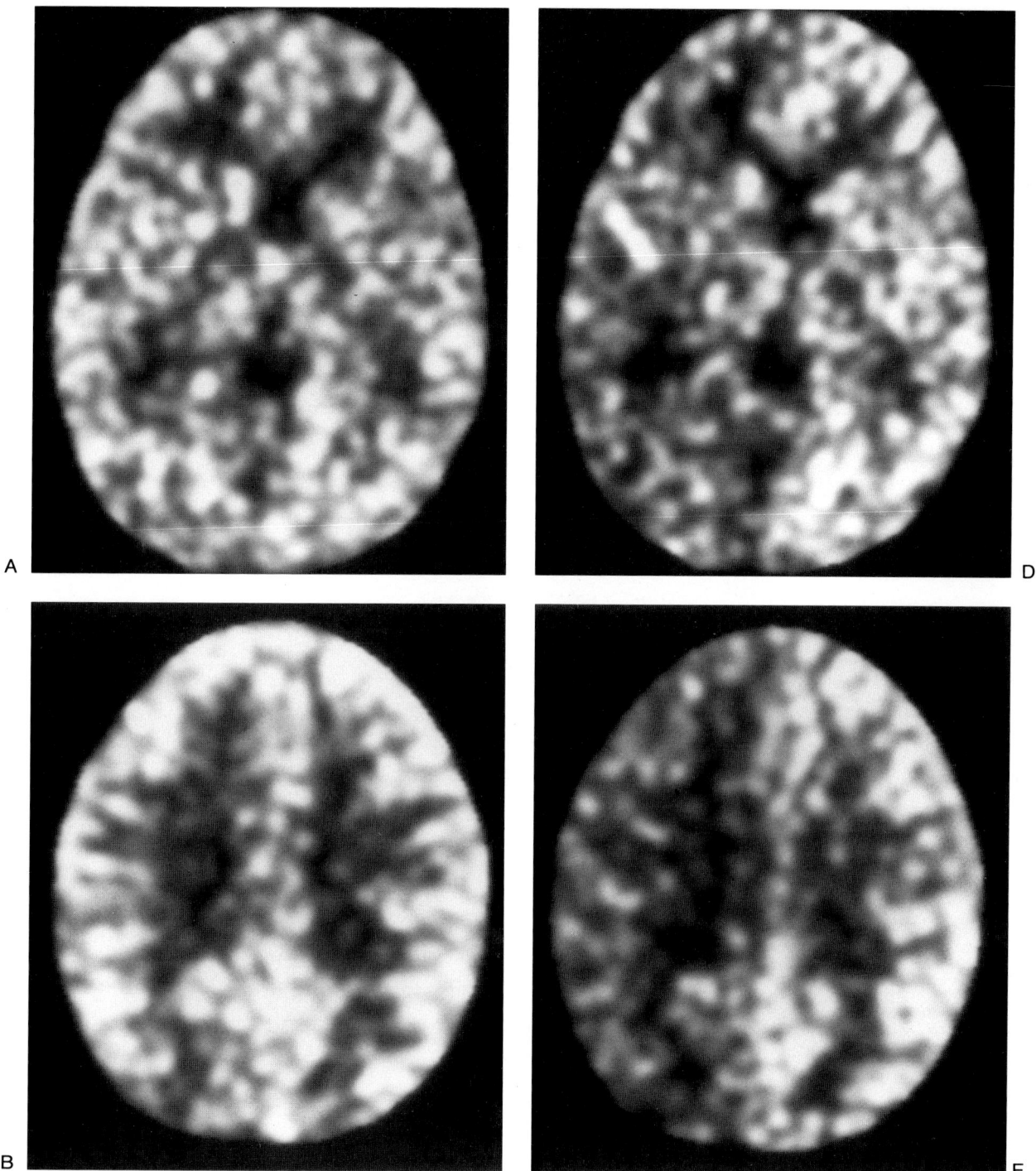

FIG. 2. A–C: This three-level study shows symmetric CBF with the balloon deflated. **D–F:** Inflating the balloon causes a *marked* decrease in right hCBF. Note that during this period the patient was clinically asymptomatic. This patient exhibits criteria for inclusion in group III: markedly asymmetric decrease in hCBF.

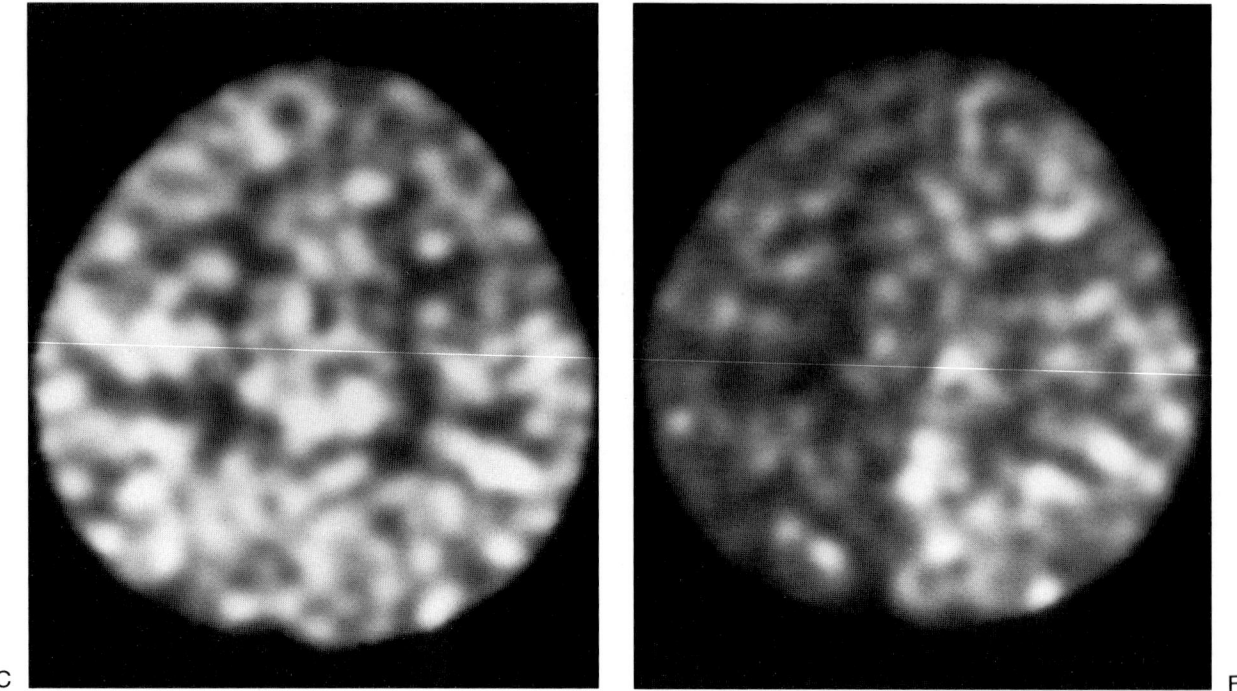

FIG. 2. *Continued.*

CHAPTER 5

Interventional Neuroradiology: Embolization

Charles A. Jungreis and Joseph A. Horton

BASIC CONSIDERATIONS

Skull base tumors often have rich vascular supplies. Prior to surgical resection, it may be desirable to devascularize a tumor using endovascular techniques (embolization) (Fig. 1). Many factors are involved in deciding whether or not a patient is a candidate for preoperative embolization. These include the vascular anatomy, the planned surgical objective, and the neurologic status of the patient.

To evaluate the vascular anatomy, a thorough angiogram must be performed (Fig. 2). Superselective angiography rather than subselective angiography is often required for two reasons. The first is that the angioarchitecture of the tumor may not be apparent on less selective injections. That is, the feeding vessels and the tumor blush might only be clearly demonstrated with superselective angiography (Fig. 3).

The second reason to perform highly selective angiography is that small "dangerous" anastomoses are plentiful in the skull base but not easily visualized angiographically (1). For example, the middle meningeal artery frequently has small anastomoses with the ophthalmic artery in the orbit or with the cavernous portion of the internal carotid artery. Embolization in the presence of such anastomoses would put the normal territories at risk. With superselective angiography, these dangerous anastomoses are more likely to be apparent and are therefore more likely to be avoided (Fig. 4). The relative ease and safety with which embolization versus surgical occlusion can be performed must also be balanced (Figs. 5 and 6).

Once catheter position has been attained and immediately before embolization, angiography is performed. If dangerous anastomoses are opacified, then the catheter might require repositioning. When the angiogram appears "safe," we proceed with provocative testing using sodium amytal (for central nervous system evaluation) and/or lidocaine (for retinal and cranial nerve evaluation) (2–4). We advocate provocative testing because even superselective angiography may not see important small vessels. Dosages of sodium amytal and lidocaine vary depending on the size of the vessel but range between 10 and 100 mg.

For example, if one were embolizing a middle meningeal artery that was supplying a cavernous sinus meningioma, 20 mg of lidocaine would be injected into the vessel just before injecting any emboli even if the vessel appeared to fill only the tumor. If neurologic testing remained unchanged, then embolization would be performed. If, on the other hand, the lidocaine had induced an ipsilateral monocular blindness, one would be obliged to modify the procedure. The modification might entail changing the position of the catheter and

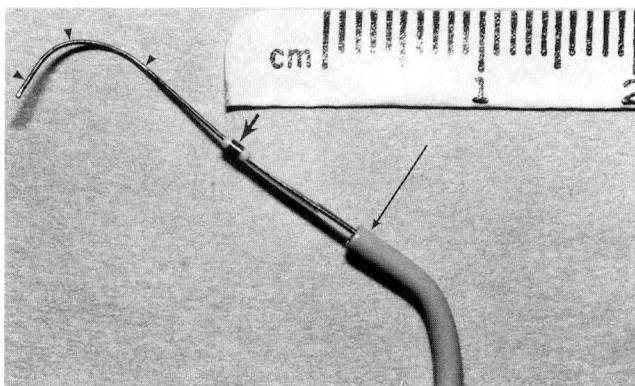

FIG. 1. Catheters. The coaxial assembly consists of a standard cerebral catheter through which a microcatheter and microguidewire are advanced. *Long arrow,* 5 French catheter; *short arrow,* tip of microcatheter; *arrowheads,* microguidewire.

C. A. Jungreis and J. A. Horton: Department of Radiology, University of Pittsburgh School of Medicine, and Presbyterian University Hospital, Pittsburgh, Pennsylvania 15213.

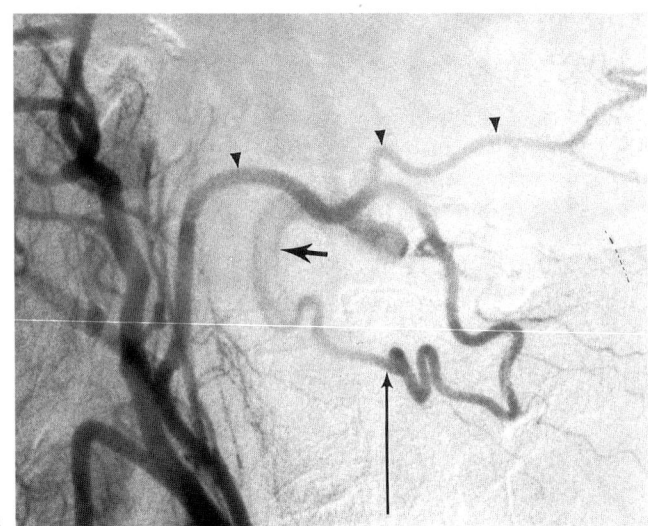 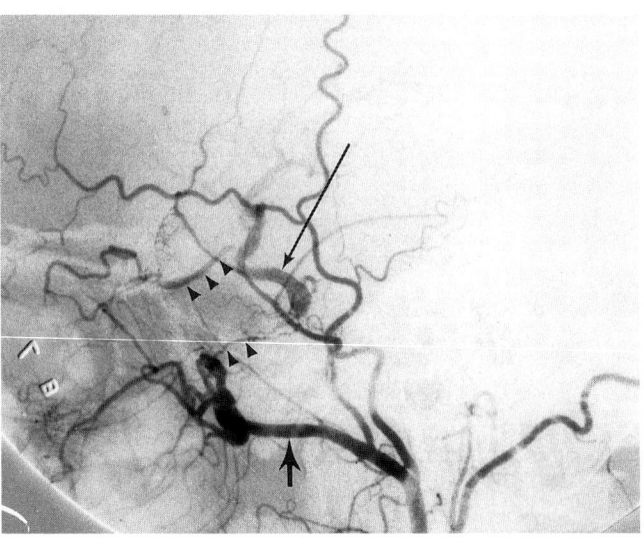

FIG. 2. Dangerous anastomoses. **A:** Occipital–vertebral anastomosis. Lateral view of external carotid artery angiogram. The occipital artery has a branch at C2 that fills the vertebral artery. An occipital artery embolization would place the vertebral–basilar territory at risk. *Long arrow,* C2 anastomosis; *short arrow,* vertebral artery; *arrowheads,* occipital artery. **B:** Internal maxillary–internal carotid anastomosis. Lateral view of external carotid artery angiogram. Branches of the internal maxillary artery opacify the internal carotid. *Long arrow,* internal carotid artery; *short arrow,* internal maxillary artery; *double arrowheads,* vidian artery filling cavernous portion of the internal carotid artery; *triple arrowheads,* ophthalmic artery filled via orbital collaterals that in turn fill the internal carotid.

FIG. 3. Skull base meningioma. **A:** Contrast-enhanced CT. The superior extent of the tumor deforms the inferior right frontal lobe. *Arrows,* meningioma. **B:** Lateral view of distal external carotid artery angiogram. The middle meningeal artery is large, but no definite tumor blush is apparent. *Long arrow,* middle meningeal artery in floor of middle cranial fossa; *short arrow,* position eventually attained with microcatheter. **C:** Lateral view of superselective middle meningeal artery angiogram. The microcatheter is intracranial. The tumor is extremely vascular, demonstrating a large blush, a finding not appreciated on the less selective external carotid angiogram (compare with **B**). *Arrow,* tip of the microcatheter and the same point identified in **B**; *arrowheads,* microcatheter as it courses through the middle meningeal artery. **D:** Lateral scout view showing the microcatheter in the position from which the superselective angiogram and the embolization were performed. *Arrow,* tip of the microcatheter. **E:** Postembolization angiogram. The tip of the microcatheter remains in the same position. The tumor blush is decreased (compare with **C**). Normal branches are preserved. *Arrow,* tip of the microcatheter.

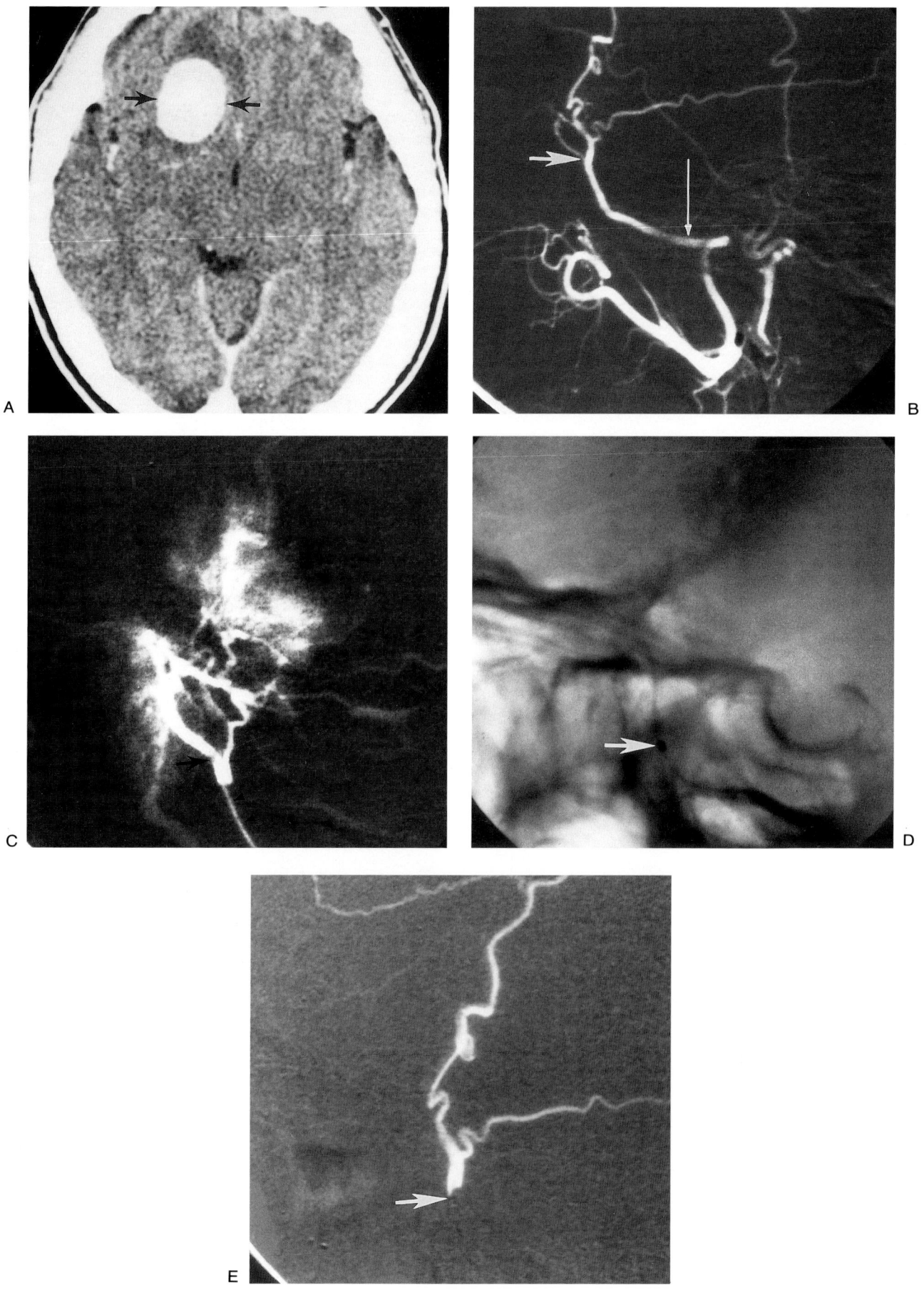

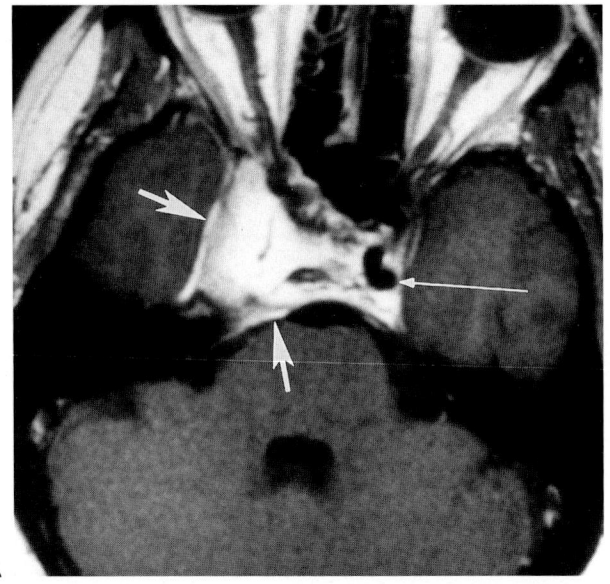

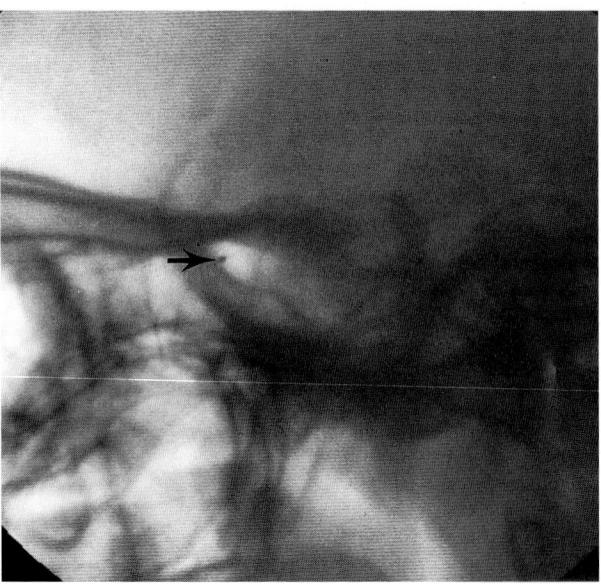

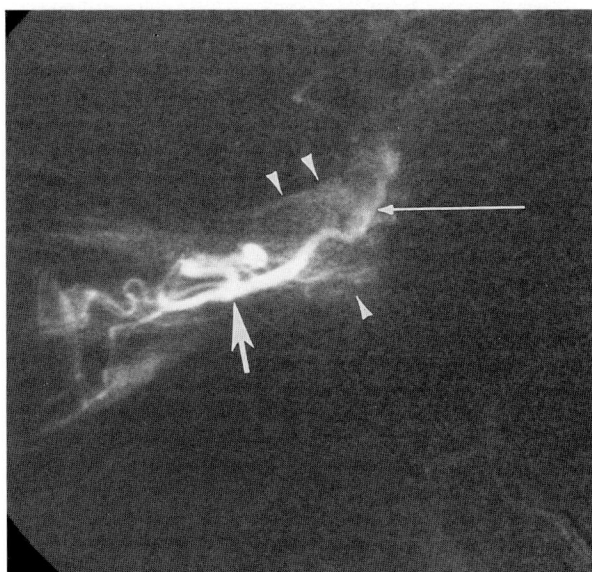

FIG. 4. Cavernous meningioma. **A:** Gadolinium-enhanced MRI demonstrates a right cavernous mass that is almost totally occluding the right internal carotid artery. The left internal carotid artery is normal with the flow, causing it to appear black on MRI. *Long arrow,* left internal carotid artery; *short arrows,* mass. **B:** Lateral scout view with microcatheter in the intracranial middle meningeal artery. The situation appears similar to the previous case (Fig. 3). *Arrow,* tip of microcatheter. **C:** Superselective angiogram of middle meningeal artery. In this case, however, not only does the tumor opacify, but so do the ophthalmic, internal carotid, and middle cerebral arteries. Embolization in this position would jeopardize important normal territories. While the catheter position is similar in Figs. 3 and 4, the angiograms are quite different. The patient in Fig. 3 was embolized successfully. The patient in Fig. 4 was not embolized. *Long arrow,* supraclinoid internal carotid artery; *short arrow,* ophthalmic artery; *arrowheads,* tumor blush.

FIG. 5. Angiofibroma in a 20-year-old male. **A:** MRI postgadolinium demonstrates an enhancing mass centered in the pterygopalatine fossa. *Arrows,* mass. **B:** Lateral angiogram of internal maxillary artery. The tumor vascularity is demonstrated. *Broad arrow,* internal maxillary artery; *long arrow,* middle meningeal artery; *short arrow,* accessory meningeal artery. **C:** Superselective angiogram of the middle meningeal artery demonstrates that this vessel contributes little to the tumor. Such information is difficult to extract from the less selective angiogram. *Long arrow,* middle meningeal artery. **D:** Angiogram of the distal internal maxillary artery. The tumor blush is substantial. *Broad arrow,* distal internal maxillary artery. **E:** Angiogram of accessory meningeal artery. This vessel also supplies the tumor. *Short arrow,* accessory meningeal artery. **F:** Postembolization angiogram of the internal maxillary artery. Only the distal internal maxillary artery and the accessory meningeal artery were embolized. The tumor blush is decreased (compare with **B**). The middle deep temporal artery is preserved, as is the middle meningeal artery. The middle deep temporal artery is particularly important to preserve since it contributes to the supply of the temporalis muscle, which in turn must remain vascularized in case it is required for reconstruction. *Broad arrow,* internal maxillary artery; *long arrow,* middle meningeal artery; *short arrow,* accessory meningeal artery; *broken arrow,* middle deep temporal artery.

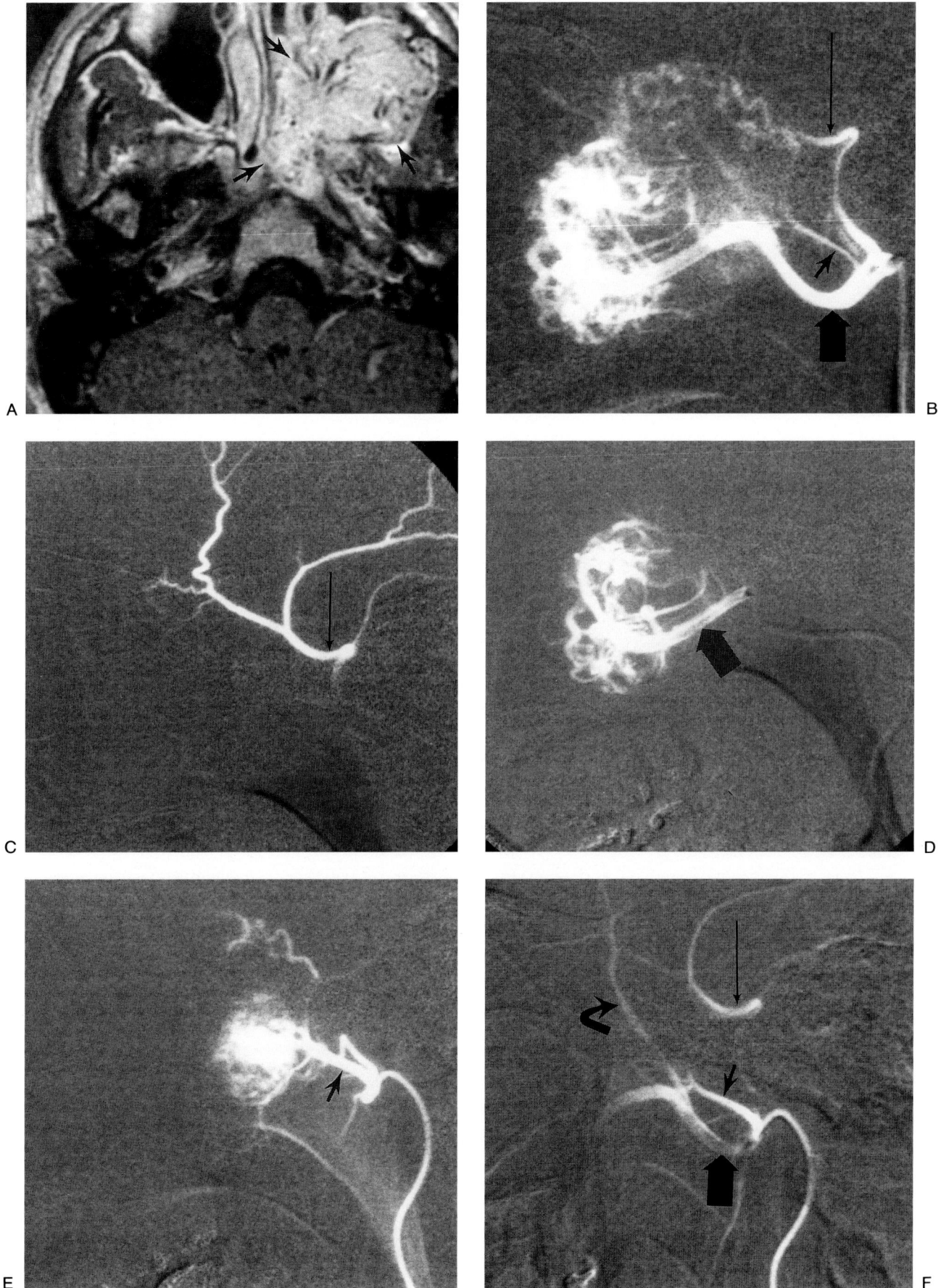

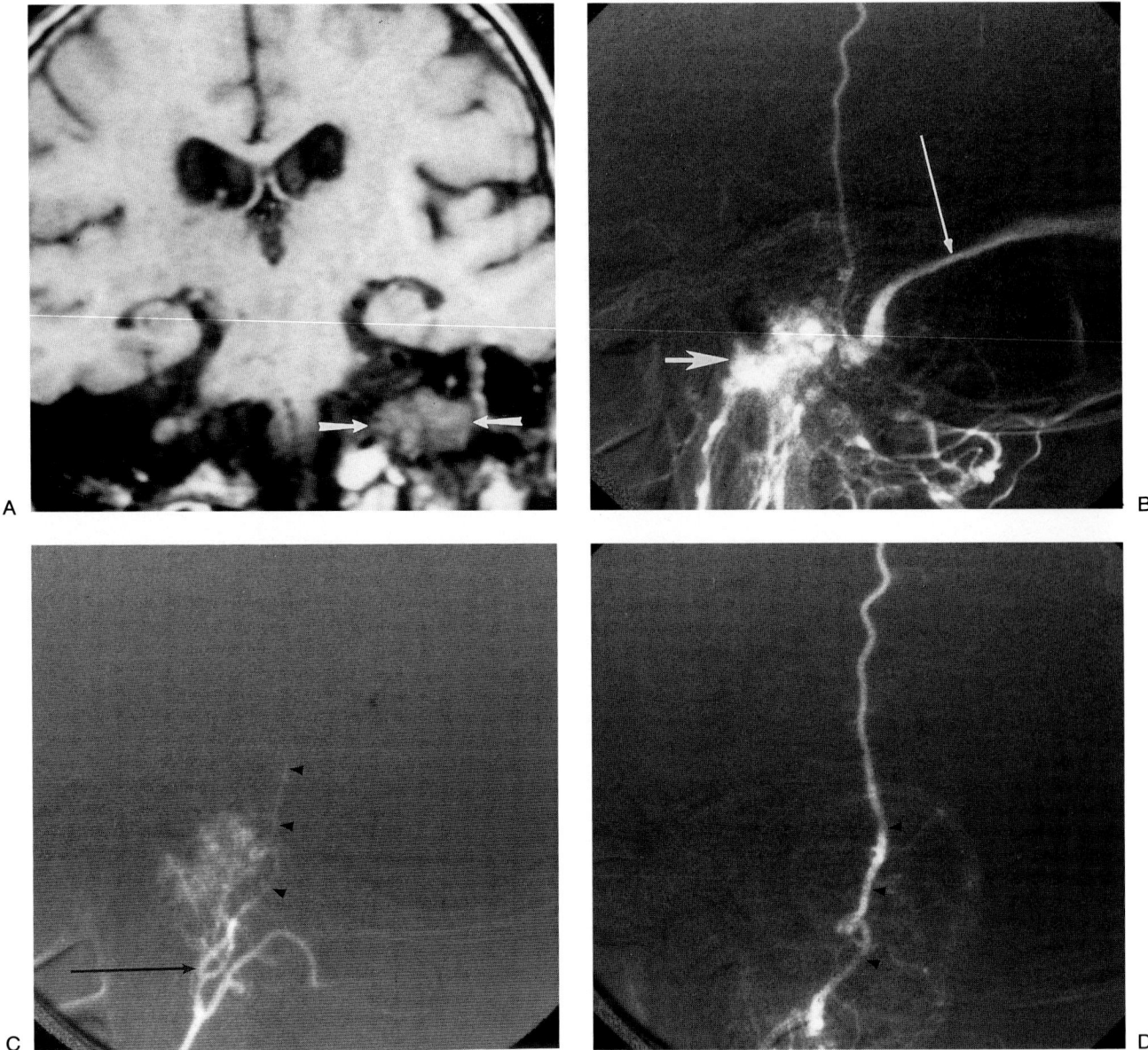

FIG. 6. Jugular paraganglioma. **A:** Coronal MRI shows the tumor in the jugular foramen. *Arrows,* tumor. **B:** Lateral external carotid artery angiogram. The tumor is vascular and demonstrates arteriovenous shunting. *Long arrow,* transverse sinus; *short arrow,* tumor. **C:** Selective angiogram of the distal external carotid. A fine pattern of neovascularity is seen. *Arrow,* the point to which the catheter was advanced for the embolization; *arrowheads,* distal superficial artery. **D:** Postembolization angiogram. The tumor blush is reduced. The superficial artery is preserved. *Arrowheads,* superficial artery.

TABLE 1. Data on four exemplary cases

Case	Diagnosis	Age/sex	Feeding arteries[a]	Embolic agent
Figure 3	Meningioma	50/F	Branches of MMA	PVA[b]
Figure 4	Meningioma	28/F	ICA	None
			MMA	+Lidocaine, no embo
			Ophthalmic	None
Figure 5	Angiofibroma	20/M	Ophthalmic	None
			Distal IMA	Gelfoam powder/PVA
			Accessory meningeal artery	Gelfoam powder/PVA
Figure 6	Paraganglioma	56/M	Petrosal branch MMA,	+Lidocaine, no embo
			Posterior auricular	Gelfoam powder/PVA
			Ascending pharyngeal	Gelfoam powder/PVA

[a] MMA, middle meningeal artery; ICA, internal carotid artery; IMA, internal maxillary artery.
[b] PVA, polyvinyl alcohol.

retesting in the new position, using particulate emboli larger than the presumed size of the dangerous anastomoses, or aborting the procedure. In addition, as an embolization progresses, repeat angiograms and repeat testing are performed periodically because the hemodynamics of the vascular bed are changed by the embolization. Vascular channels that were not filled initially may subsequently become perfused as the distal runoff decreases. The changed hemodynamics potentially put new territories at risk (see Table 1).

TECHNICAL CONSIDERATIONS

Many catheter systems have been developed (5,6) (Fig. 1). In general, a larger caliber catheter is usually an advantage since if large particles are required, they can easily be passed. However, microcatheters or open ended guide wires offer an advantage since a more selective position can be attained, which means there is less chance of unintentional embolization of normal territories (7). We usually start a case with standard cerebral catheters ranging between 5 and 7 French so that if a microcatheter is required, it can be inserted coaxially without changing the base catheter.

Many embolic agents are available. Since this type of embolization is performed as a preoperative procedure, permanent agents such as acrylics (cyanoacrylates) are not usually required. Small particles appear to be the agents of choice and include polyvinyl alcohol (PVA) foam, absorbable gelatin powder (Gelfoam Powder, The Upjohn Company, Kalamazoo, MI 49001), and combinations thereof. Roadmapping capabilities and live subtraction angiography are indispensable fluoroscopic tools that must be available before these procedures are attempted.

PATIENT PREPARATION

Preoperative care includes clear liquids the morning of the procedure, appropriate laboratory values, and informed consent. The risks of embolization will vary depending on the territory to be embolized and include stroke, death, blindness, cranial nerve deficits, and skin necrosis. During the procedure cardiac monitoring and blood pressure monitoring are always performed. Intravenous sedation may be used, but we prefer not to use general anesthesia so that neurologic testing can be performed when necessary. If embolization involves external carotid artery vessels, we administer 2–5 in. of nitropaste (nitroglycerin ointment) at the beginning of the procedure to prevent vasospasm in these particularly reactive vessels (8).

Following embolization, the patient is kept at bed rest with close neurological monitoring. Most procedures are performed via the femoral artery and frequent checks of the puncture site are required. The patient is not permitted to bend the ipsilateral hip for 8 hr. This means that the patient may not sit up or bend the involved leg for that length of time. Bleeding and/or hematoma formation are controlled by direct pressure to the puncture site. A normal diet can be resumed, but intravenous fluids are continued until the patient is tolerating oral feedings. Ischemic territories from the embolization may cause significant pain and analgesics are used as required. The use of steroids is controversial and they are not used routinely. If the patient was receiving steroids prior to the embolization, then they are continued postprocedure. In general, we suggest an interval of approximately 5–7 days between the embolization and the surgery to allow the initial edema to subside and the necrosis to "soften" the mass.

REFERENCES

1. Lasjaunias P, Berenstein A. *Surgical neuroangiography, vol 1: Functional anatomy of craniofacial arteries.* New York: Springer-Verlag, 1987;242.
2. Wada J, Rasmussen T. Intracarotid injection of sodium amytal for the lateralization of cerebral speech dominance. *J Neurosurg* 1960;17:266–282.
3. Horton JA, Kerber CW. Lidocaine injection into external carotid

branches: provocative test to preserve cranial nerve function in therapeutic embolization. *AJNR* 1986;7:105–108.
4. Horton JA, Dawson RC. Retinal Wada test. *AJNR* 1988;9:1167–1168.
5. Berenstein A, Kricheff II. Catheter and material selection for transarterial embolization: technical considerations. Part I. *Radiology* 1979;132(3):619–630.
6. Berenstein A, Kricheff II. Catheter and material selection for transarterial embolization: technical considerations. Part II. *Radiology* 1979;132(3):631–639.
7. Jungreis CA, Berenstein A, Choi IS. Use of an open-ended guidewire: steerable microguidewire assembly system in surgical neuroangiographic procedures. *AJNR* 1987;8:237–241.
8. Erba M, Jungreis CA, Horton JA. Nitropaste for prevention and relief of vascular spasm. *AJNR* 1989;10:155–156.

CHAPTER 6

Cerebral Revascularization in Cranial Base Surgery

Mark E. Linskey, Laligam N. Sekhar, and Chandranath Sen

All the major vessels supplying blood to the brain must traverse the cranial base en route to their destinations. Cranial base surgical approaches usually involve the visualization, manipulation, and displacement, while direct neoplastic involvement may necessitate the temporary occlusion or resection of these vessels. While postoperative cranial nerve dysfunction can be debilitating to patients, the major morbidity and mortality associated with cranial base surgery arise from cerebral ischemia related to the management of the major blood vessels supplying the brain. The purpose of this chapter is to describe the various techniques available for cerebral revascularization for cranial base surgery, to outline how one decides whether revascularization will be necessary in any given patient, and to suggest the most suitable settings for each technique.

ASSESSING THE NEED FOR REVASCULARIZATION

As long as the planned operative approach for a patient involves the exposure and manipulation of the great vessels supplying the brain, that patient should undergo a pretreatment evaluation of the risk of vessel occlusion. Even if temporary or permanent vessel occlusion is not anticipated preoperatively, unforeseen technical difficulties might require their use. Pretreatment evaluation of the risk of temporary or permanent internal carotid artery (ICA) or vertebral artery (VA) occlusion thus becomes one of the cornerstones of the therapeutic decision-making process.

In our institution, the risk of ICA occlusion is assessed with a 15-min clinical balloon test occlusion (BTO) followed by an ICA-occluded stable xenon/CT scan cerebral blood flow (XeCBF) study (19,26). The details of these studies are outlined in the chapter by Horton et al., and the three patient risk categories defined by these studies are outlined in Fig. 1.

Patients who fail the clinical BTO are at high risk for stroke even with temporary occlusion. These patients may require a prophylactic bypass procedure if the need for temporary occlusion is anticipated and should not undergo ICA sacrifice without revascularization. Patients who pass the BTO but have an ICA-occlusion CBF less than or equal to 30 ml/100 g/min are at low risk for stroke with short temporary occlusion but are at moderate risk for stroke with long temporary or permanent ICA occlusion. Temporary occlusion in these patients should be accompanied by induced hypertension and pharmacological brain protection, and a revascularization procedure should probably be performed if permanent ICA sacrifice is required. Patients who pass both parts of the pretreatment evaluation are at low risk for stroke with ICA sacrifice and thus do not require cerebral revascularization. Three exceptions to this principle would be patients who are very young, since ICA sacrifice may lead to an increased risk of delayed ipsilateral ischemic deficits (8,31,32,50,51) or *de novo* aneurysm formation (23) over the course of their lifetime, patients who have a contralateral berry aneurysm, which has been shown to grow and/or rupture after contralateral ICA sacrifice (10,18,27,46,56,68), and patients who may be expected to have tumor involvement of the contralateral ICA some time in the future.

The posterior circulation is more difficult to evaluate.

M. E. Linskey and L. N. Sekhar: Department of Neurosurgery, Center for Cranial Base Surgery, University of Pittsburgh School of Medicine, and Presbyterian University Hospital, Pittsburgh, Pennsylvania 15213.
C. Sen: Department of Neurosurgery, Mt. Sinai Medical Center, New York, New York 10029.

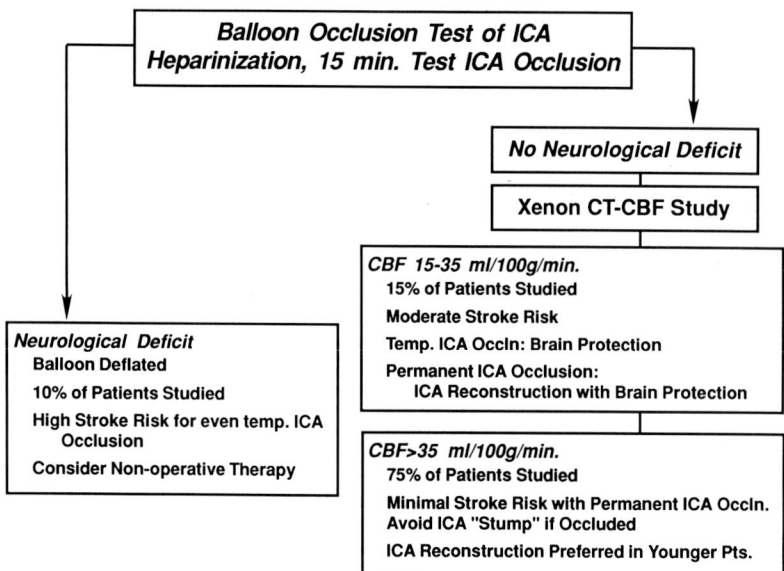

FIG. 1. Algorithm dividing patients into one of three categories for risk of stroke based on the results of a preoperative 15-min clinical ICA BTO followed by an ICA-occluded Xe/CT CBF study.

A 15-min clinical BTO of the cervical VA is significant if positive but provides little information about the effects of occlusion distal to the vertebrobasilar junction. Performing a BTO distal to the take-off of the posterior inferior cerebellar artery (PICA) is dangerous since the balloon occludes a large segment of artery and has led to brain stem and cerebellar strokes from perforator occlusion. A four-vessel cerebral angiogram evaluating the competency of both posterior communicating arteries, the presence or absence of VA dominance, and the presence or absence of significant atherosclerotic occlusive disease in the cervical VAs or the basilar artery (BA) is still the mainstay for estimating the adequacy of posterior circulation collateral flow distal to the PICA.

ANESTHESIA AND MONITORING

A detailed discussion of anesthesia techniques and intraoperative electrophysiological monitoring can be found in the chapter by Gonzalez and Sclabassi et al. This section serves to amplify certain points that are particularly important during cerebral revascularization.

Cerebral hemispheric function is monitored continuously intraoperatively with somatosensory evoked potentials (SSEPs) and limited channel electroencephalography (EEG). Brain stem function is monitored using contralateral brain stem auditory evoked potentials (BSAEPs) and SSEPs. Monitoring evoked potentials provides assurance that the patient is tolerating vessel occlusion intraoperatively and provide a warning if graft thrombosis or distal embolization occurs.

There are several ways that the anesthesia team can help prevent both ischemia during temporary vessel occlusion and hyperperfusion once revascularization has been completed. Raising the blood pressure approximately 20 mm Hg during temporary occlusion helps improve collateral blood flow (11) while moderate hypothermia (32–34°C) and barbiturate- or etomidate- (Abbot Laboratories, North Chicago, IL) induced coma to the point of burst suppression on EEG may provide some brain protection during ischemia in high and moderate risk patients (9,34,78). Finally, autoregulation of CBF may be impaired or absent in patients who have been revascularized with high-flow vein grafts at the base of the brain. Thus systemic hypotension or hypertension must be avoided at all costs once the graft has been completed. It is particularly important not to use large volumes of crystalloid or colloid to compensate for the loss of peripheral vascular resistance during general anesthesia since this can lead to relative volume overload, which usually leads to hypertension at the time of emergence (12).

SAPHENOUS VEIN HARVESTING AND PREPARATION

Autologous saphenous vein provides the best substrate for performing high-flow interposition or bypass grafts and for patch graft repair of damaged large diameter vessels. A great deal has been written about the best solutions and temperature for the irrigation and storage of vein grafts and the dangers of graft distention under pressure. For an excellent review, the reader is referred to the article by Sundt and Sundt (73) as well as the related letter-to-the-editor response (52).

We routinely use the great saphenous vein from the upper thigh since we most often deal with large diameter arteries in the cranial base and since the vein in this location is usually large enough to avoid the need for hydrostatic graft distention. Graft lengths of 25–30 cm can be

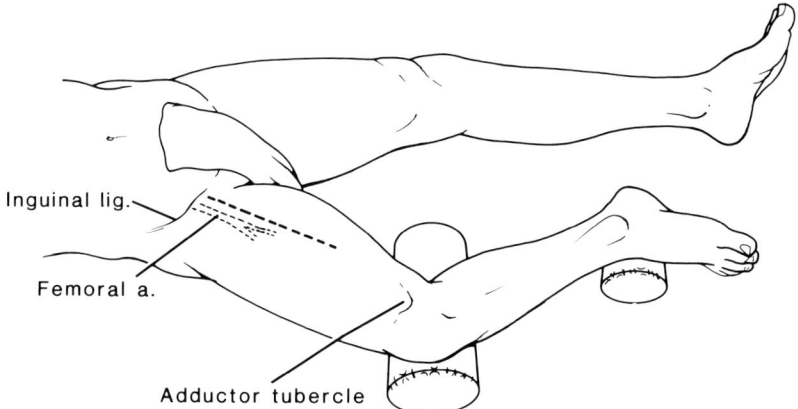

FIG. 2. This drawing shows the positioning of the patient's lower extremity for harvesting proximal saphenous vein. The incision is shown with a *dashed line* and is begun medial to the femoral pulse just below the inguinal ligament and is directed toward the adductor tubercle.

obtained in this manner, although for short interposition grafts, only the proximal 8–10 cm are routinely harvested. If a smaller diameter vein is necessary for a bypass graft to cortical or posterior fossa arteries, then saphenous vein from the lower leg is used and the reader is referred to several good references for descriptions and diagrams of the operative dissection (41,71,73).

The upper thigh is prepped and draped in the standard fashion, being careful to extend the prep 5 cm above the inguinal ligament and to support the knee slightly flexed on a padded roll with the hip everted (Figs. 2–4). The femoral pulse is palpated at the inguinal ligament and a longitudinal incision made approximately 1 cm medial to the pulse. The greater saphenous vein is identified where it penetrates the cribriform fascia and is followed distally into the medial thigh. A readily identifiable venous trifurcation or quadrification is invariably present just prior to entrance of the vein through the cribriform fascia. Care is taken not to touch or manipulate the vein during sharp dissection. Once a sufficient length is exposed, the adventitia of the vein is injected with a dilute solution of papaverine (2.4 mg/ml) using a 26-gauge needle. Vein tributaries are tied off at least 1 mm away from the main vein segment with 4-0 silk sutures. The vein is stored *in situ* by packing the wound with sponges soaked in dilute papaverine, which are not removed until necessary.

Once a decision is made that saphenous vein will be needed, the packing is removed from the wound and the appropriate length of vein is harvested after marking the proximal end of the vein graft and double tying the proximal and distal vein stumps with 2-0 silk ties. The vein graft is gently irrigated without overdistention with room temperature dilute heparinized saline. The graft is stored in the same solution for a few minutes during transfer to the cranial operative field.

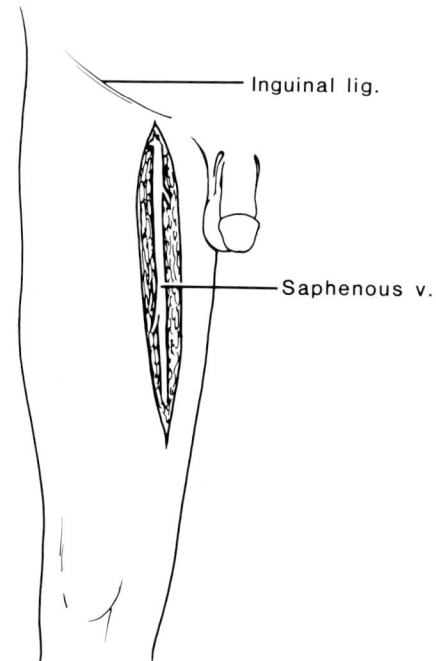

FIG. 3. Drawing of the exposed greater saphenous vein.

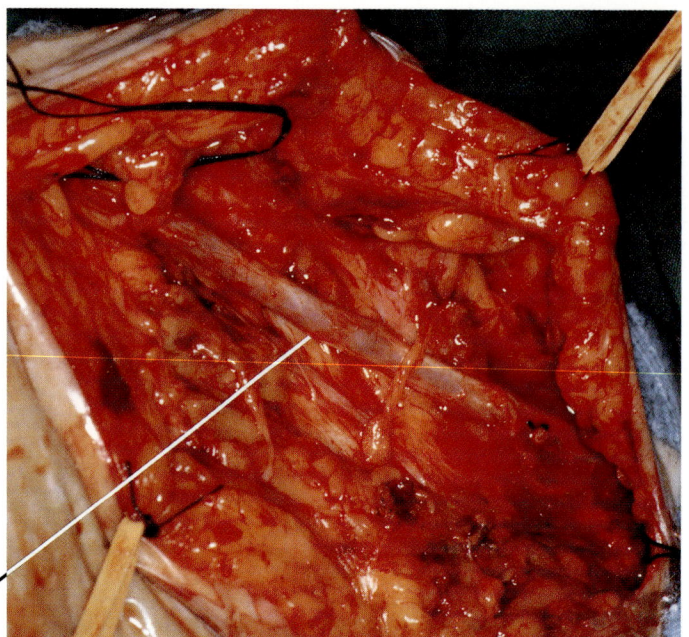

Saphenous vein

FIG. 4. An intraoperative photograph of the greater saphenous vein properly exposed *in situ*.

ARTERY-TO-ARTERY MICROANASTOMOSIS

The microanastomosis of small arteries is required when performing a superficial temporal artery (STA) or occipital artery (OA) bypass to a cortical artery or to a recipient artery in the posterior fossa. The techniques are also applicable to reimplantation of small arteries if they become severed during the course of cranial base exposure or tumor dissection. This anastomosis is performed under the microscope with a magnification of 20–40× (Fig. 5).

The donor artery should be at least 1 mm in diameter; preferably 1.5–2 mm in diameter. The recipient vessel should be at least 1.5 mm in diameter. A 1.0–1.5-cm segment of recipient artery is chosen with the smallest number of collaterals. The arachnoid around the recipient artery is opened with microscissors and any minute penetrating branches are coagulated with bipolar cautery. A rubber dam is inserted beneath the free segment of recipient artery (Fig. 5A). The adventitia is peeled off the distal 1–2 mm of donor artery, and the donor artery lumen is irrigated with heparinized saline. A microclip is placed at either end of the isolated segment of recipient artery. A longitudinal arteriotomy is made in the middle of the isolated segment with microscissors. The lumen is irrigated with heparinized saline. The end of the donor

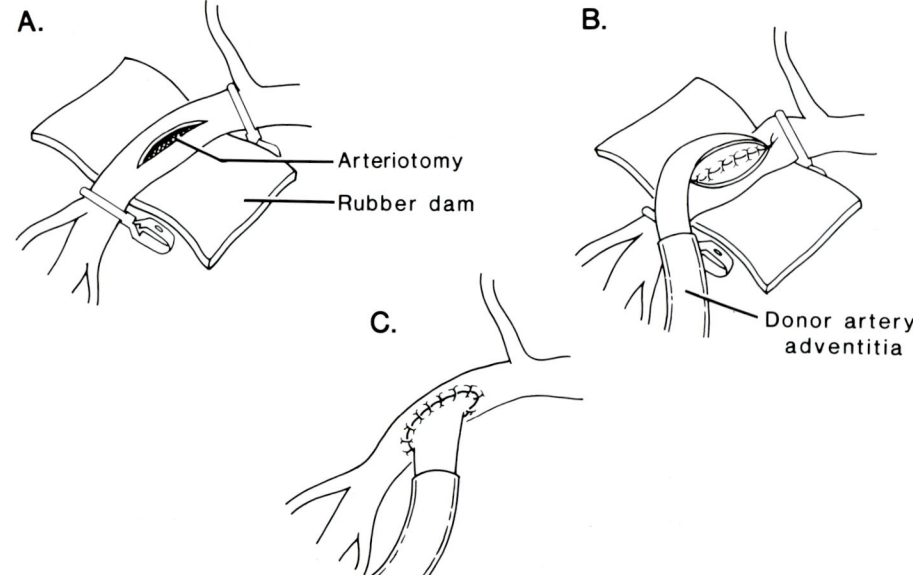

FIG. 5. The steps involved in performing an artery-to-artery microanastomosis (20–40×). See the text for a detailed description of the technique.

artery is cut obliquely to correspond to the size of the arteriotomy. The anastomosis is performed using approximately 10–12, interrupted 10-0 monofilament nylon sutures beginning with the back wall of the anastomosis (Fig. 5B). If the OA is used as the donor artery, then 9-0 sutures may be necessary. Prior to placing the last stitch, the clip on the donor artery is released, clearing any air or debris from the anastomosis. All clips are then removed (Fig. 5C). Any bleeding from the suture line is usually self-limiting but may occasionally require a small amount of Surgicel (Johnson & Johnson, Inc., New Brunswick, NJ), Gelfoam (Upjohn, Kalamazoo, MI), or an additional suture to stop.

VEIN-TO-ARTERY MICROANASTOMOSIS

This section describes the anastomosis of a large vein graft (4–6-cm diameter) to a large artery at the base of the brain (Fig. 6). If a smaller diameter vein graft is used to anastomose with a cortical or posterior fossa artery, the procedure is technically similar to that described for artery-to-artery microanastomosis with the exception of the use of 8-0 monofilament nylon sutures for the anastomosis and the need for a slightly longer longitudinal arteriotomy on the recipient artery.

Under the microscope, the end of the vein is denuded of adventitia for a distance of 2 mm. For an end-to-end anastomosis, the recipient artery is divided after application of a proximal temporary aneurysm clip. The ends of the artery and vein are bevelled and spatulated if necessary, and two 7-0 or 8-0 monofilament nylon sutures are placed at diametrically opposed points to attach the vein to the artery (Fig. 6A). Heparinized saline is used intermittently to irrigate both vessel lumina. The rest of the anastomosis is completed with interrupted 7-0 or 8-0 sutures, beginning with the back wall (Fig. 6B).

For an end-to-side anastomosis, the recipient artery segment is isolated between temporary aneurysm clips. A linear arteriotomy is made in the isolated artery segment. The vein graft is cut on an angle and the end is spatulated to fit the length of the arteriotomy. Heparinized saline is used intermittently to irrigate both vessel lumina. Two apical tacking stitches are placed with 7-0 or 8-0 monofilament nylon (Fig. 6C). The back wall of the anastomosis is finished with interrupted sutures (Fig. 6D), followed by the front wall.

Once the final anastomosis is near completion, the clips are removed, and any air is evacuated from the graft. The entire graft is again irrigated with heparinized saline. The last stitch is then placed (Fig. 6E). Most bleeding from the suture line stops spontaneously, but occasionally a small amount of Surgical or Gelfoam or an additional suture may be required. Occasionally, the recipient artery at the base of the brain may be involved with atherosclerosis. In this case, an endarterectomy

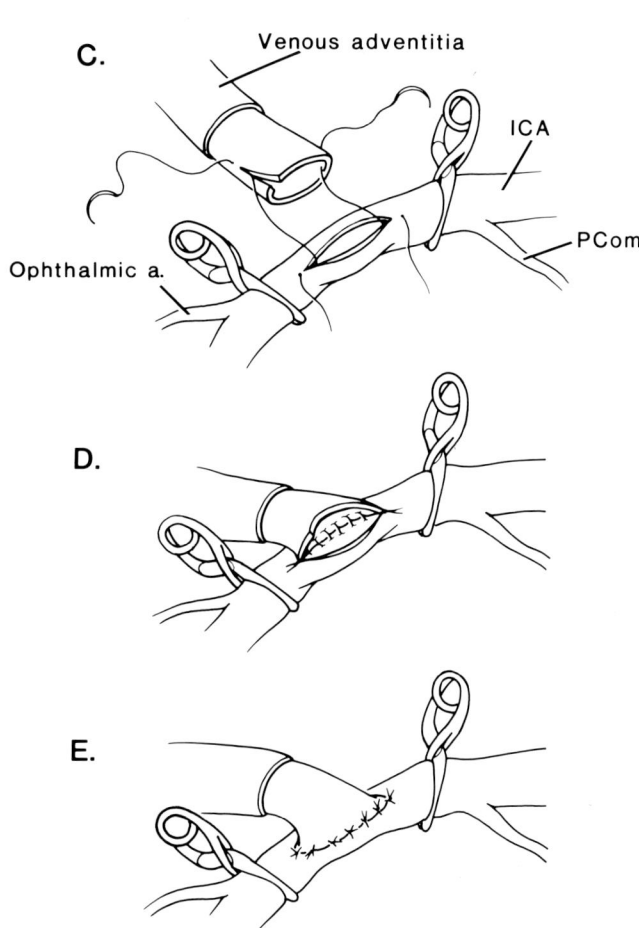

FIG. 6. The steps involved in performing an end-to-end (**A, B**) and an end-to-side (**C–E**) anastomosis of a large vein graft (4–6-cm diameter) to a large artery at the base of the brain. See the text for a detailed description of the technique.

must be performed prior to anastomosis, taking care to tack down any distal intimal flap. A low dose intravenous heparin infusion is used during the graft anastomosis in older patients, patients with malignant tumors, and patients who have hypercoagulability for any reason.

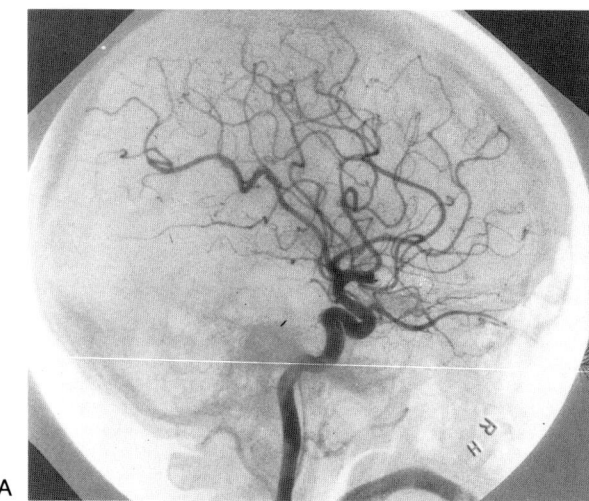 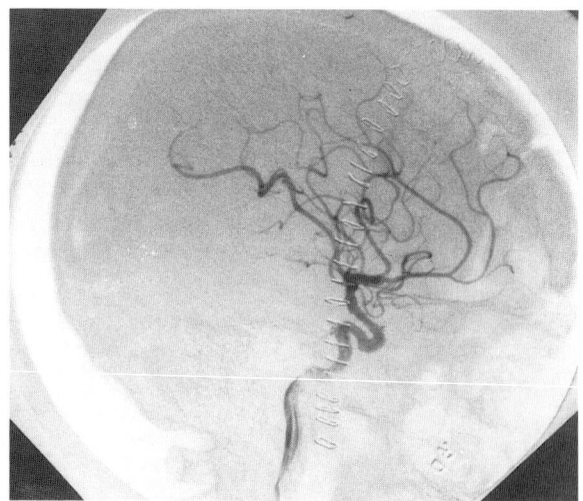

FIG. 7. Lateral views of a preoperative (**A**) and postoperative (**B**) right ICA angiogram of a 32-year-old woman with neurofibromatosis and a grade III right cavernous sinus meningioma. Operative dissection led to a tear in the supraclinoid segment of the right ICA without arterial tissue loss. The tear was repaired primarily with preservation of flow through the ICA.

VESSEL REPAIR IN SERIES

Venous Patch Grafting

Occasionally, during operative exposure or during dissection of neoplasm from an encased cranial base artery, a hole will result in the artery. If actual tissue loss has not occurred, the tear is best repaired primarily (Figs. 7 and 8). However, if significant tissue loss has occurred, then primary repair could lead to stenosis of the artery. In this setting, the best form of repair is with a venous patch graft (Figs. 9–12). The edge of the hole in the artery is trimmed smoothly into a diamond shape. A patch of saphenous vein is cut into a diamond, slightly larger than the defect. It is lowered into place using 2–4 apical 7-0 or 8-0 monofilament nylon tacking sutures (Fig. 9A). The lumen of the isolated artery is intermittently irrigated with heparinized saline. The rest of the patch is sealed with interrupted 7-0 or 8-0 sutures (Fig. 9B). Prior to the placement of the last stitch, the temporary clips are removed to evacuate any air and irrigated with heparinized saline.

Petrosal to Upper Cervical ICA Interposition Grafting

Saphenous vein interposition grafting of the upper cervical or petrosal ICA has been successfully performed by several surgeons (28,39,48,61,62,76). Our approach

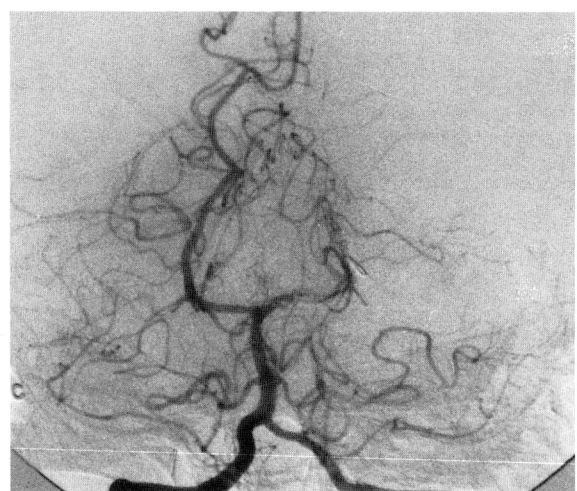 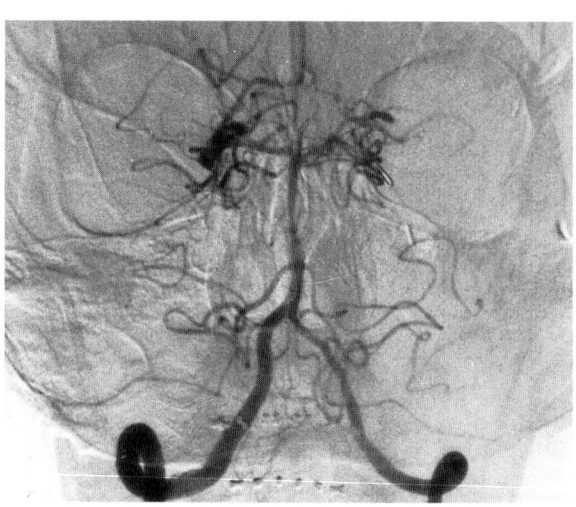

FIG. 8. Anteroposterior views of a preoperative (**A**) and postoperative (**B**) right vertebral angiogram of a 47-year-old woman with a grade IV right cavernous sinus meningioma. Operative dissection led to a tear in the mid-basilar artery without arterial tissue loss. The tear was repaired primarily with preservation of flow through the basilar artery.

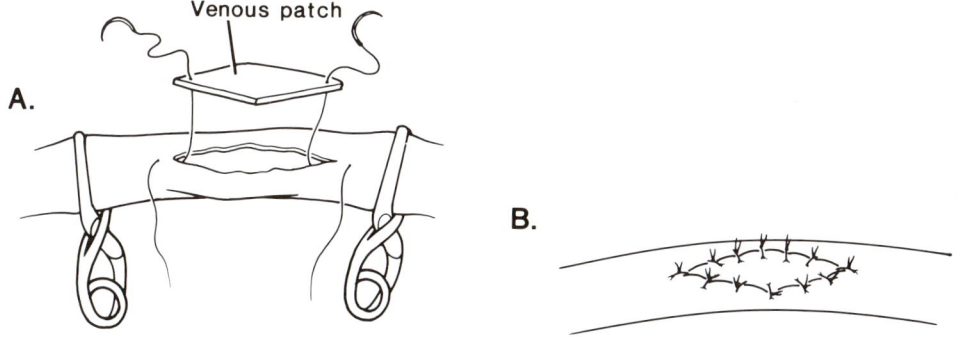

FIG. 9. The steps involved in performing a venous patch graft of a damaged artery are shown: tacking the patch in place (**A**) and the completed patch graft (**B**). See the text for a detailed description of the technique.

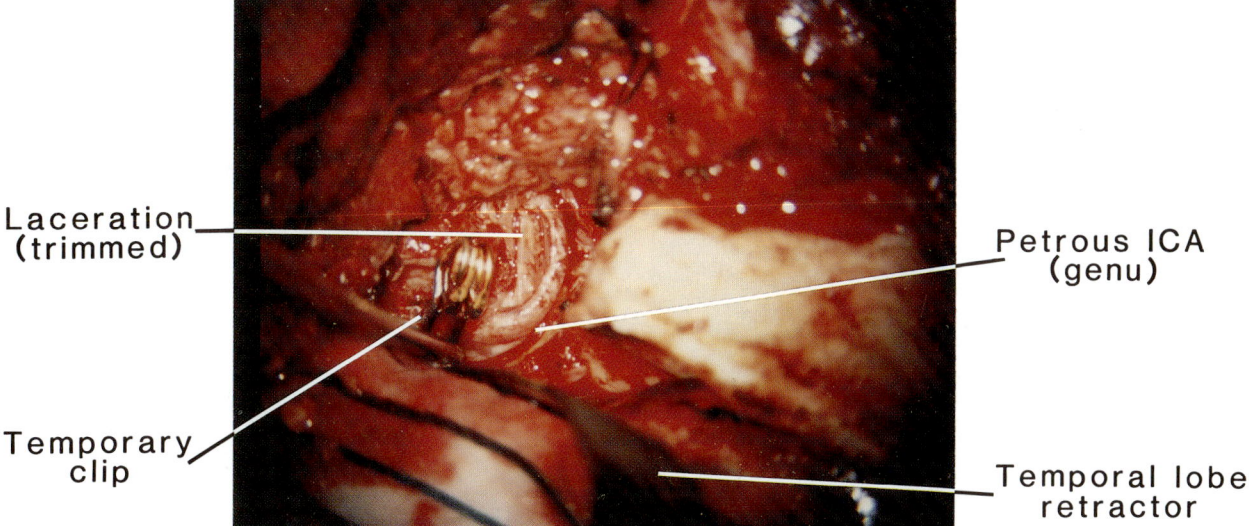

FIG. 10. Intraoperative photograph of a tear in the petrous ICA, which occurred during operative exposure. The photograph was taken after trimming the defect to accept a venous patch graft. A temporary clip is visible proximal to the tear and a distal clip is present on the supraclinoid ICA (not shown).

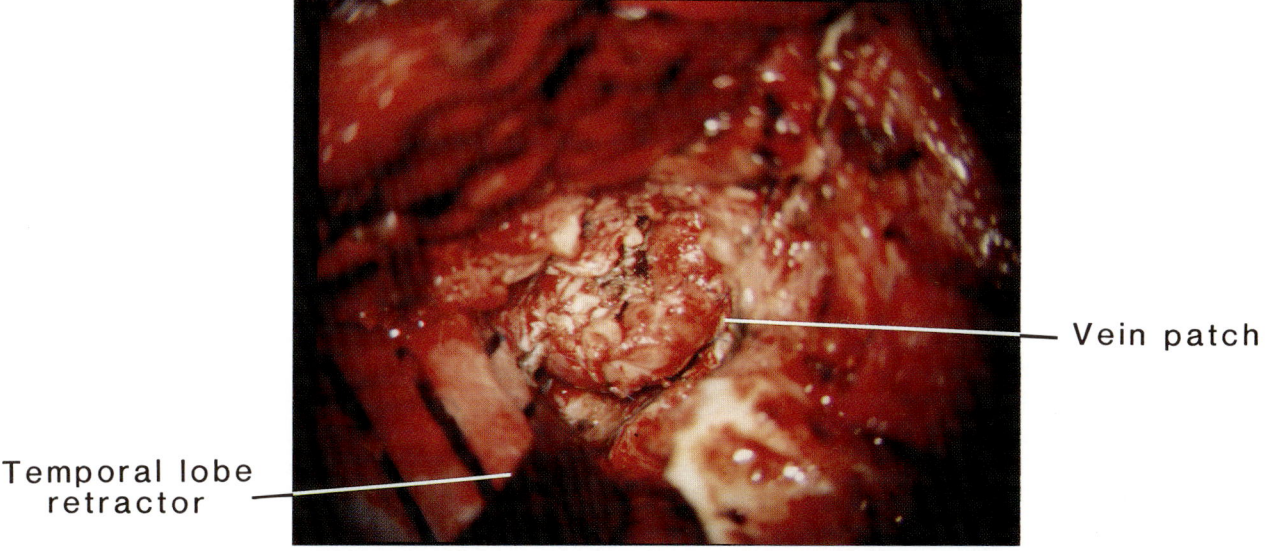

FIG. 11. Intraoperative photograph of the petrous ICA tear seen in Fig. 10 after completion of the venous patch graft and removal of both temporary clips. Excellent pulsation of the petrous ICA was present.

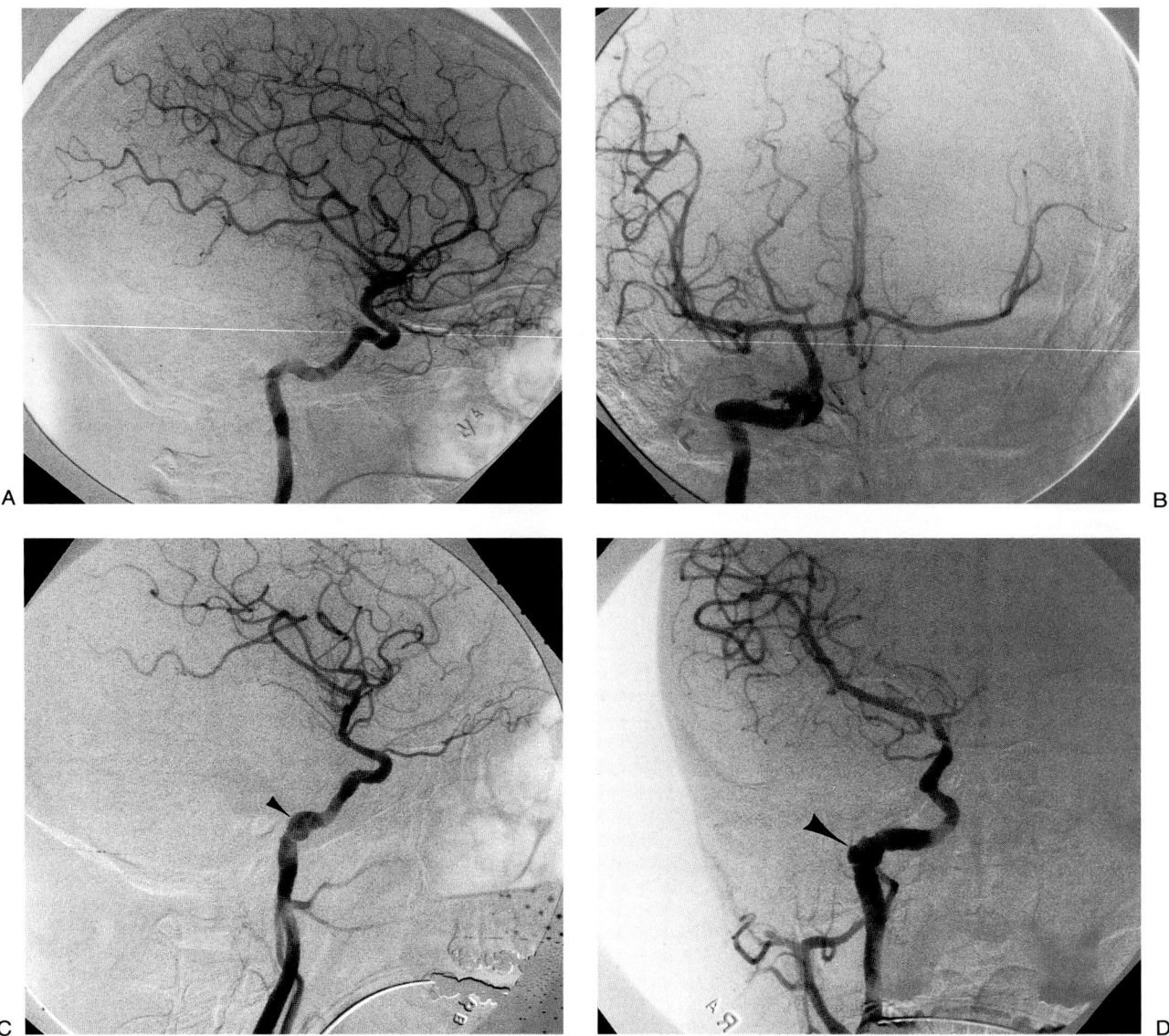

FIG. 12. Preoperative lateral (**A**) and anteroposterior (**B**) views of a right ICA cerebral angiogram from the patient in Figs. 10 and 11 showing displacement of the petrous ICA from a giant trigeminal neurilemoma. The venous patch graft site is visible on the postoperative angiogram (*arrows*) (**C, D**) along with excellent filling of the petrous ICA.

to the petrous and upper cervical ICA has previously been published (61) and involves a subtemporal–infratemporal fossa approach as outlined in the chapter by Sekhar et al. ("Anterior, Anterolateral, and Lateral Approaches to Extradural Petroclival Tumors"). The exposure provided with this approach is demonstrated in Fig. 13 and representative examples are presented in Figs. 14–16. An end-to-end saphenous vein-to-ICA anastomosis is performed across the involved segment. The graft length is tailored to the length of ICA resected. Intraluminal shunting is not performed.

Petrosal to Supraclinoid ICA Cavernous Sinus Bypass

The feasibility of a petrosal to supraclinoid ICA cavernous sinus bypass (P-S bypass) using saphenous vein was first described in cadavers by Sekhar et al. (60). Since then, the procedure has been used clinically by our group (62), as well as by Spetzler et al. (64), and studied in cadavers by Al-Mefty et al. (1). The operative approach to the cavernous sinus is outlined in the chapter by Sekhar et al. ("Cavernous Sinus and Sphenocavernous Neoplasms: Anatomy and Surgery"). The operative expo-

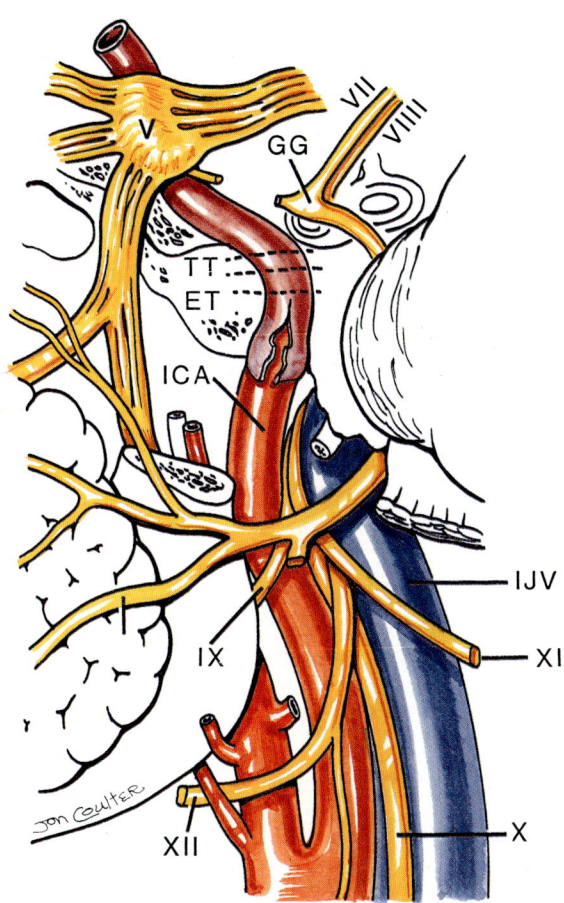

FIG. 13. These figures illustrate the exposure of the upper cervical ICA and of the petrous ICA by a subtemporal and preauricular infratemporal fossa approach. Note the relationship of the eustachian tube (ET), tensor tympani muscle (TT), cochlea, and geniculate ganglion (GG) to the genu of the petrous ICA. Cranial nerves, roman numerals; internal jugular vein, IJV.

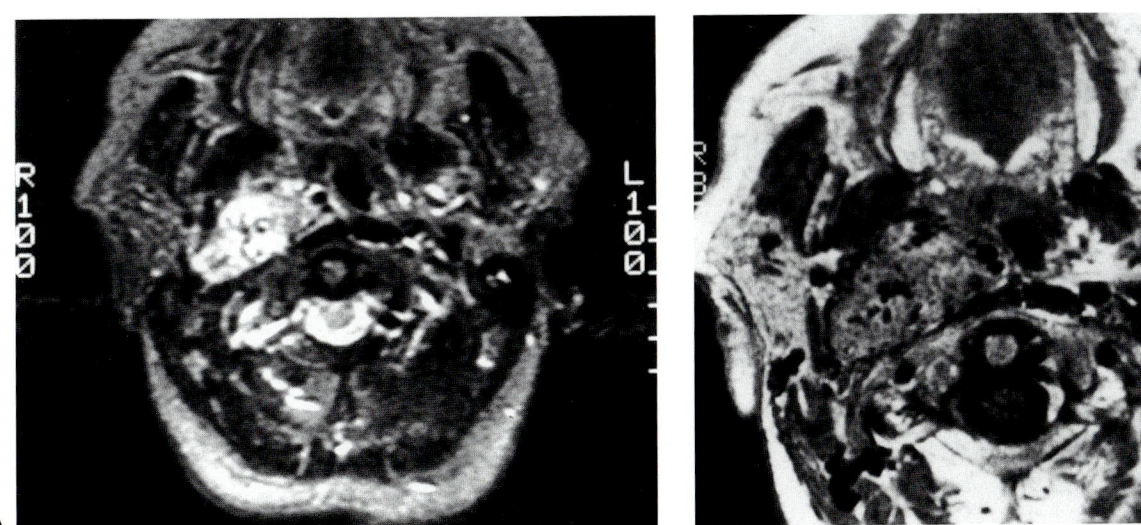

FIG. 14. Preoperative axial MRI scans of a 64-year-old woman with a right cervical glomus tumor intimately involving the upper cervical segment of the ICA. The upper cervical ICA was resected with the tumor and an upper cervical-to-petrous ICA vein graft was performed (cf. Fig. 15). **A:** TR 2867, TE 80; **B:** gadolinium enhanced; TR 600, TE 20.

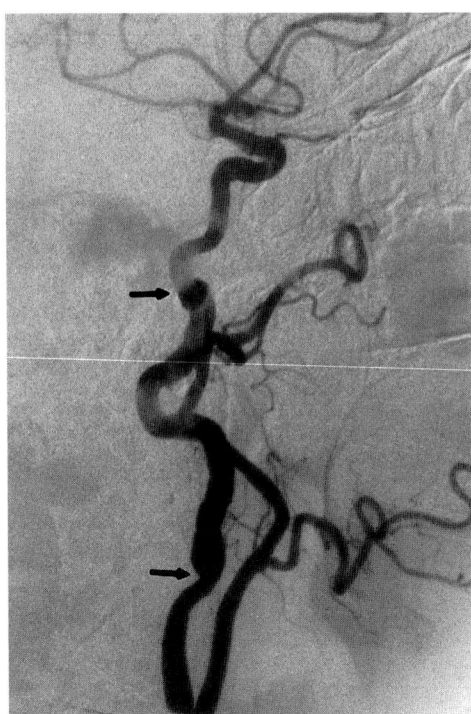

FIG. 15. Postoperative lateral vein of a right CCA angiogram from the patient in Fig. 14, demonstrating a functioning upper cervical-to-petrous ICA saphenous vein graft. The proximal and distal anastomoses are indicated by *arrows*.

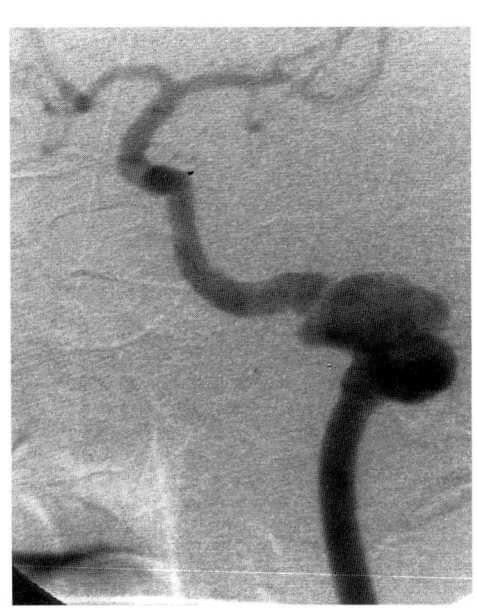 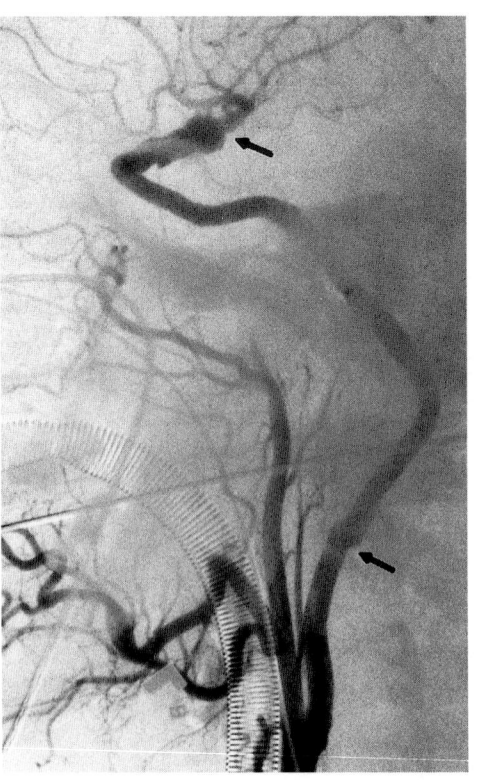

FIG. 16. A preoperative oblique view of a left ICA angiogram of a 34-year-old man with an aneurysm of the left petrous ICA (**A**). The aneurysm was resected with placement of a long cervical-to-petrous ICA saphenous vein graft. The postoperative lateral angiogram (**B**) shows excellent filling of the graft and the distal ICA territories as well as the proximal and distal anastomoses (*arrows*).

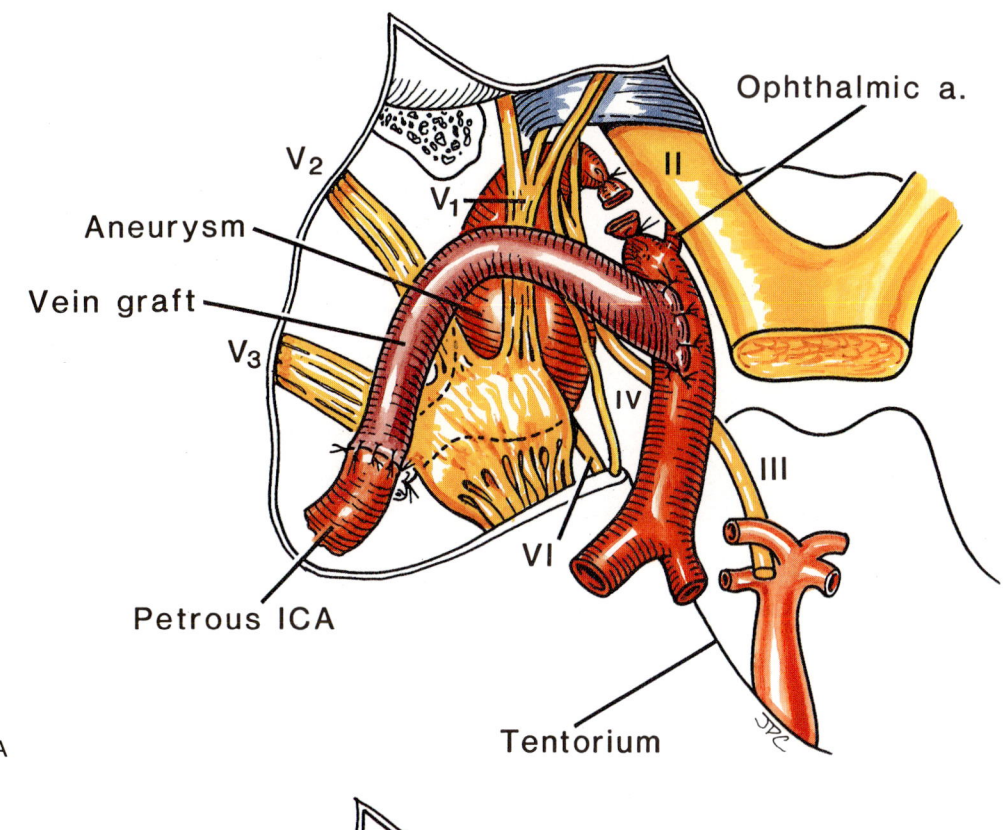
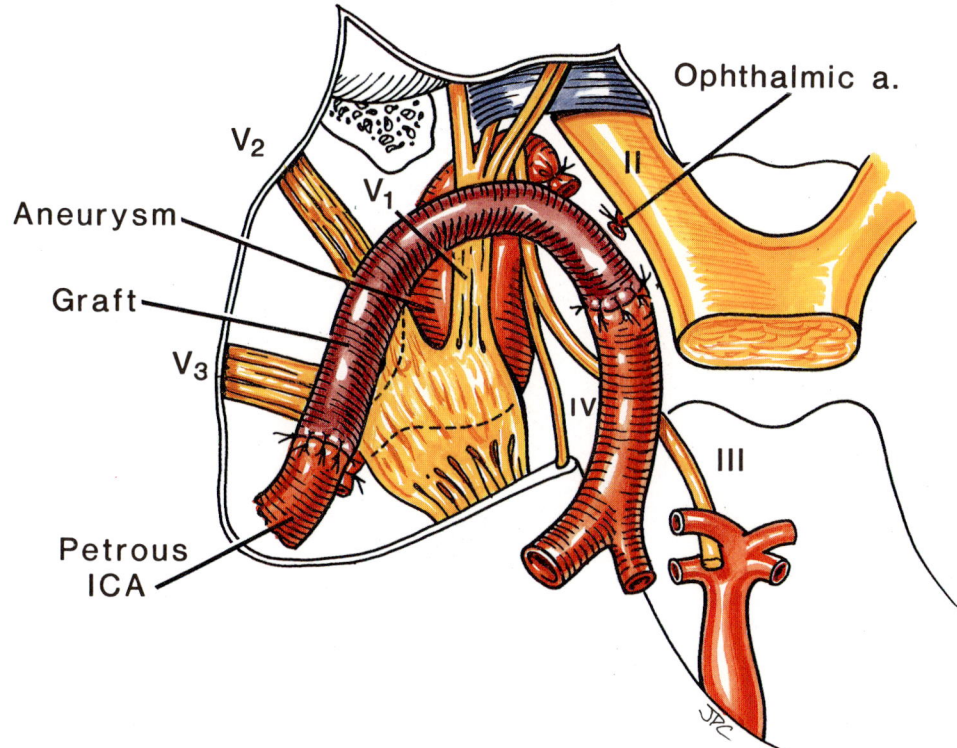

FIG. 17. Drawings depicting the operative exposure for performing a saphenous vein bypass of the intracavernous ICA using an end-to-side distal anastomosis (**A**) or an end-to-end distal anastomosis (**B**). The end-to-end anastomosis can occasionally be performed infraclinoid, sparing the ophthalmic artery, when sufficient healthy ICA is present (cf. Fig. 18). The end-to-side anastomosis is designed to spare the ophthalmic artery when sufficient healthy infraclinoid ICA is not present. Roman numbers depict cranial nerves.

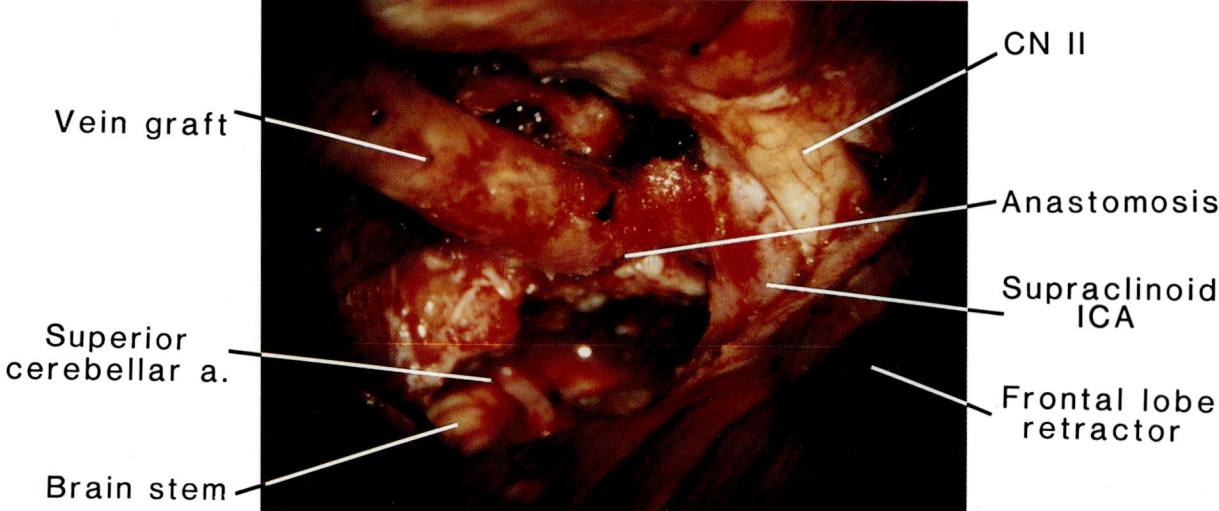

FIG. 18. Intraoperative photograph demonstrating an infraclinoid, end-to-end distal anastomosis in a P-S bypass placed in a 51-year-old woman with a grade III left cavernous sinus meningioma.

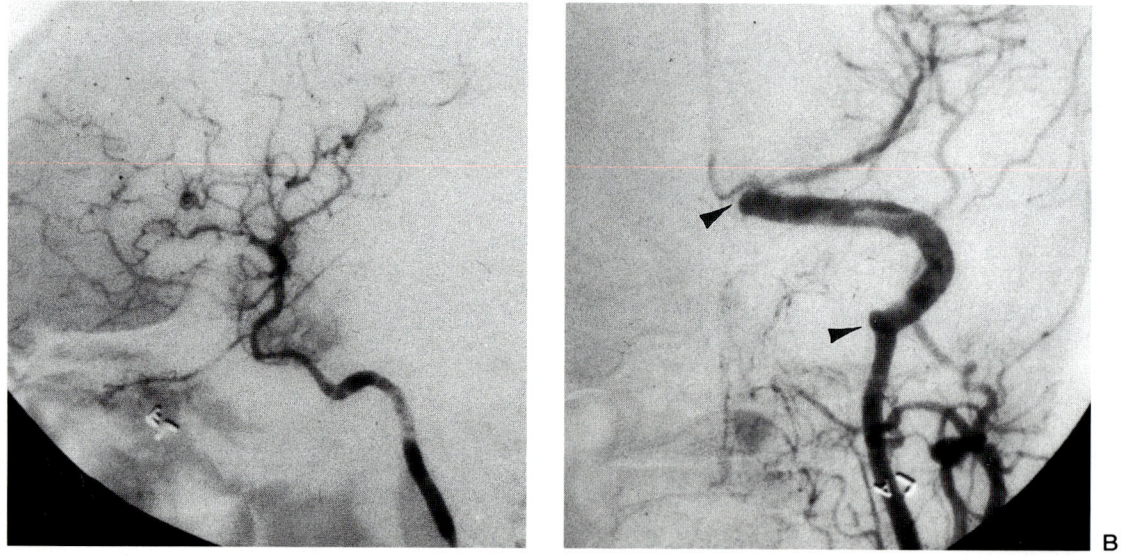

FIG. 19. Preoperative left lateral (**A**) and postoperative anteroposterior (**B**) angiograms of a 24-year-old woman with a grade IV left cavernous sinus meningioma where the cavernous ICA was resected along with the tumor with placement of a P-S bypass using an end-to-end distal anastomosis. The proximal and distal anastomoses are clearly seen (*arrows*) as is filling of the ipsilateral ACA and MCA via a patent graft.

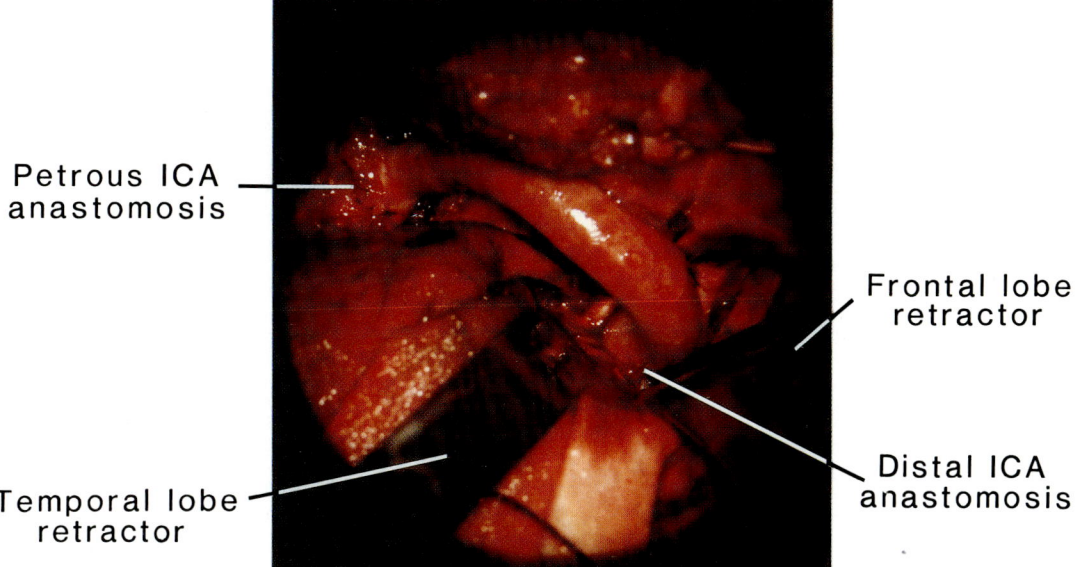

FIG. 20. Intraoperative photograph of a 39-year-old woman with a traumatic left intracavernous carotid artery aneurysm with life-threatening epistaxis, who was treated with surgical trapping of the left cavernous sinus ICA and placement of a P-S bypass with an end-to-side distal anastomosis (cf. Fig. 21).

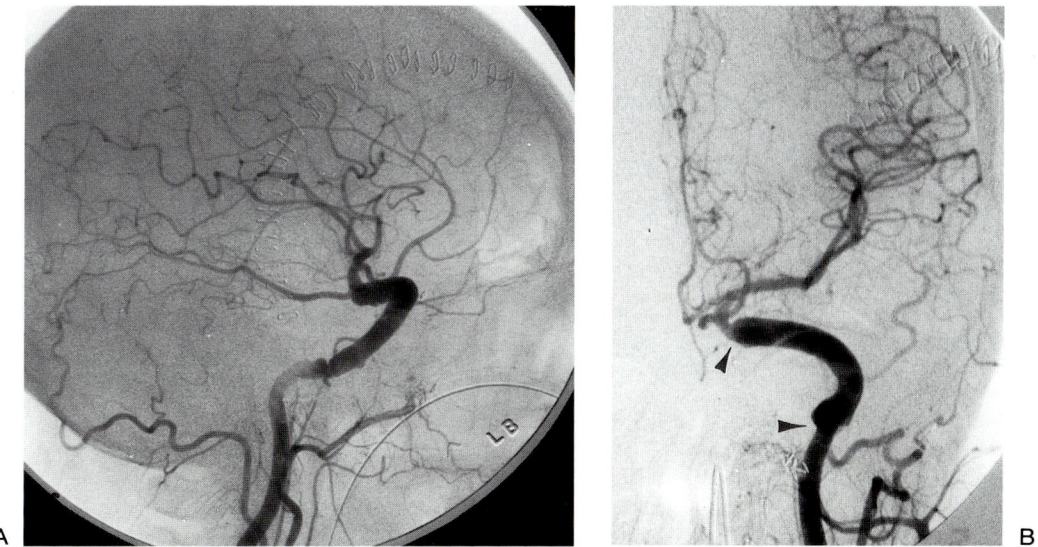

FIG. 21. Postoperative lateral (**A**) and anteroposterior (**B**) views of a left ICA angiogram from the patient in Fig. 20. The graft is patent with filling of the ipsilateral ACA, MCA, and PCA. The proximal and distal anastomoses are visible (*arrows*).

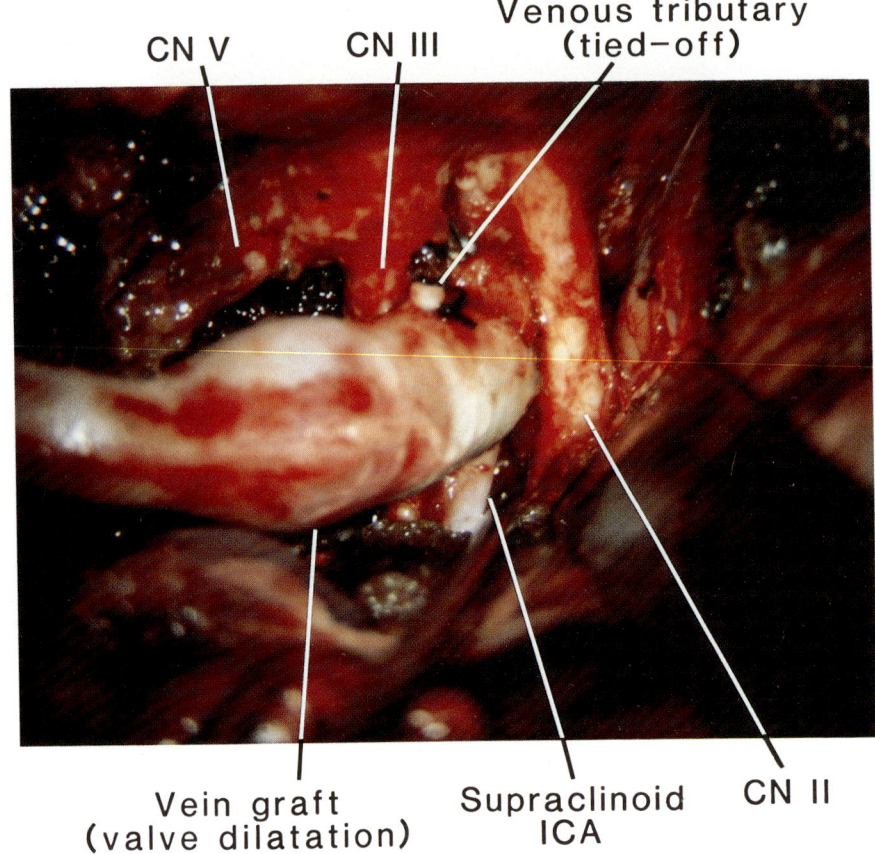

FIG. 22. Intraoperative photograph demonstrating a supraclinoid, end-to-side distal anastomosis is a P-S bypass placed in a 50-year-old man with a grade V left cavernous sinus meningioma. The dilatation from a venous valve and a tied-off venous tributary are clearly seen.

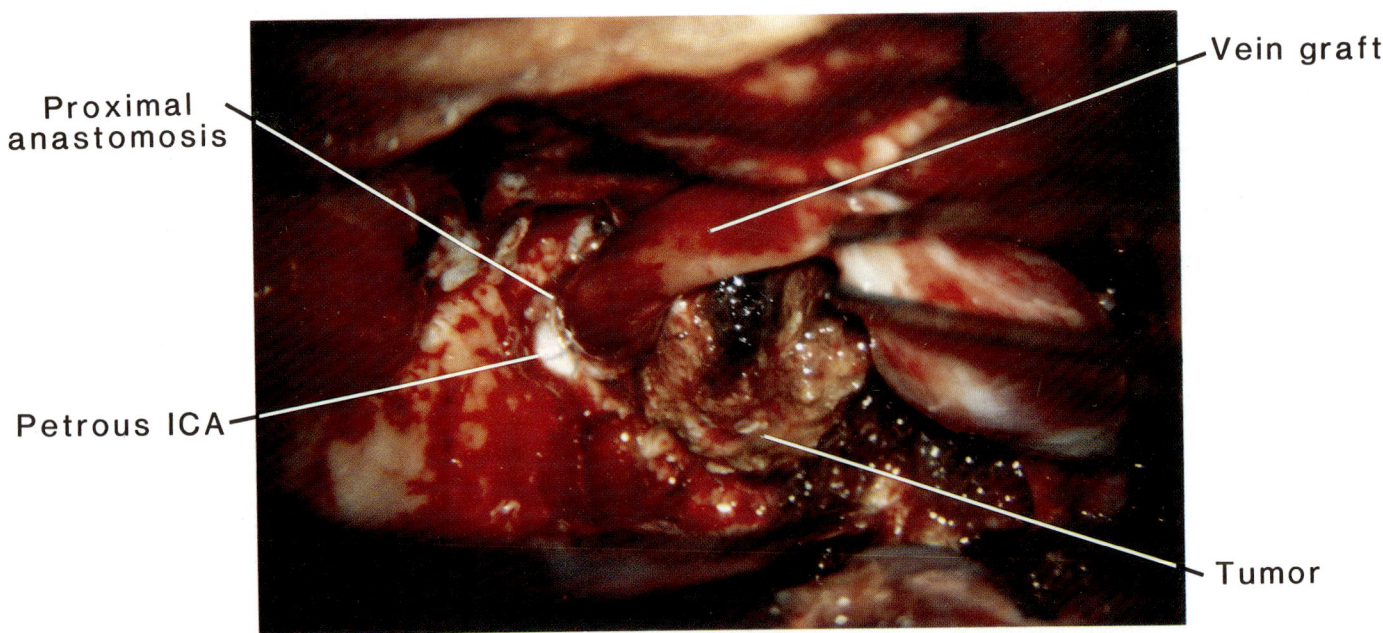

FIG. 23. Intraoperative photograph of the same patient as Fig. 22, demonstrating the petrous ICA end-to-end proximal anastomosis.

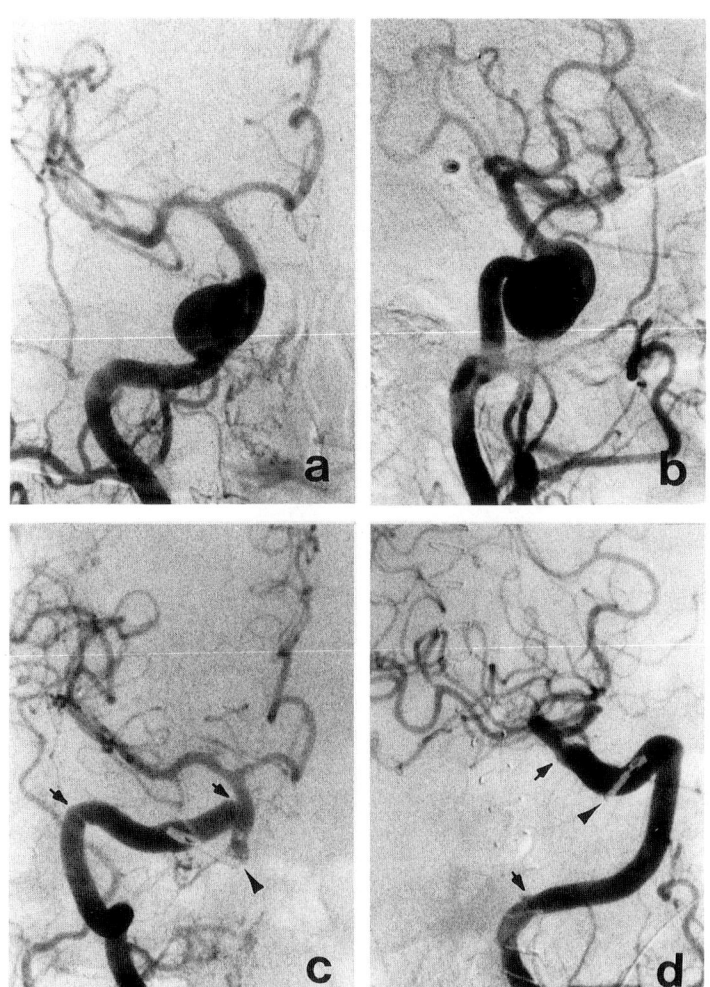

FIG. 24. Preoperative (**A, B**) and postoperative (**C, D**) anteroposterior and lateral ICA angiograms of a 68-year-old woman with a large right intracavernous carotid artery aneurysm treated by surgical trapping with placement of a P-S bypass using an end-to-side distal anastomosis. Postoperatively the graft is patent with excellent filling of the ipsilateral ACA and MCA. Both anastomoses are visible (*arrows*) as is an aneurysm clip placed on the ICA just proximal to the ophthalmic artery (*arrowhead*).

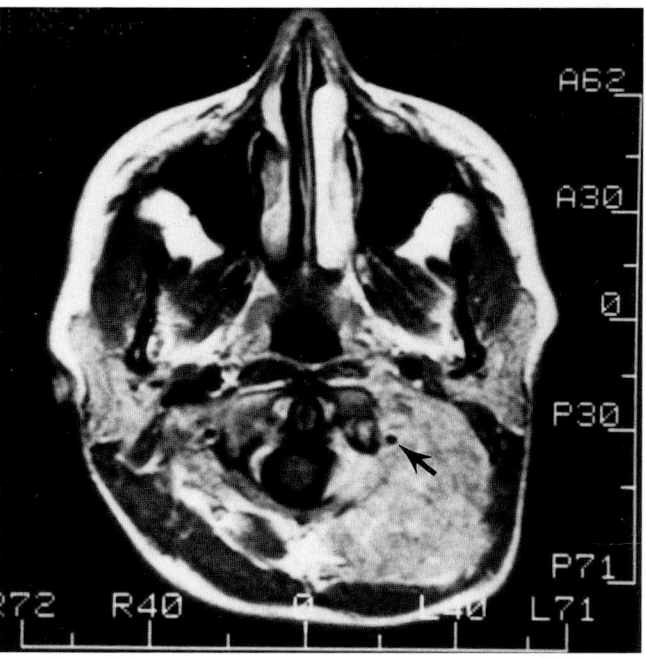

FIG. 25. Preoperative axial MRI (TR 550, TE 20) of a 27-year-old woman with a meningioma by C1 and the left cranial–vertebral junction intimately involving the upper left VA (*arrow*) (cf. Figs. 24–26).

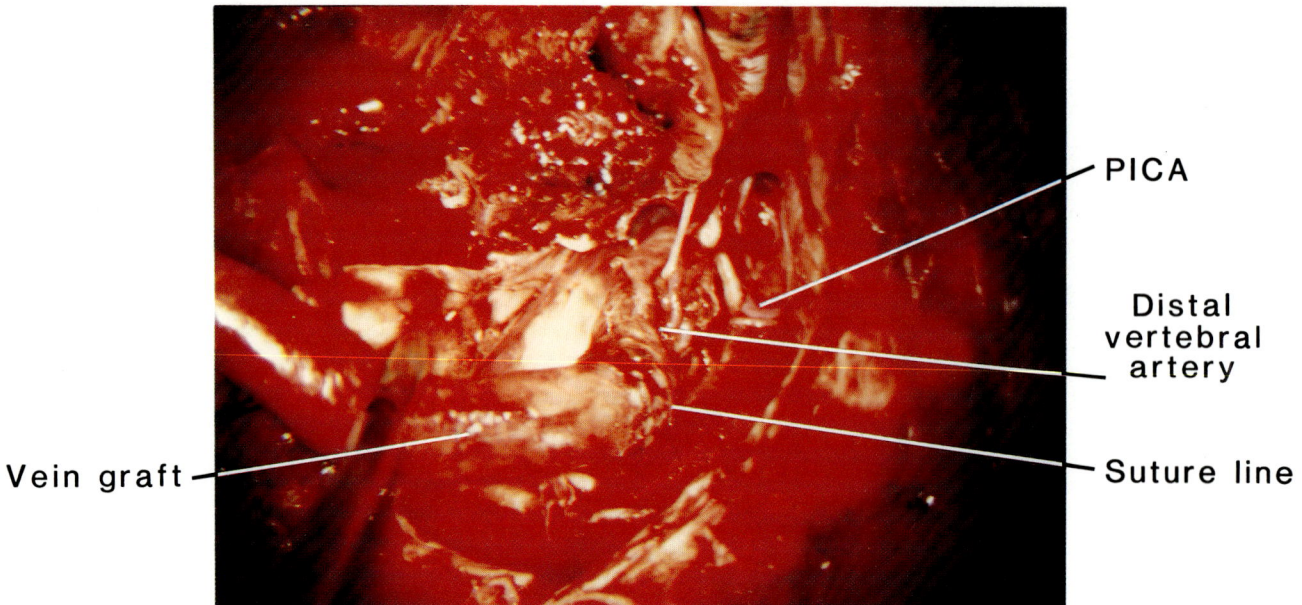

FIG. 26. Intraoperative photograph of the patient in Fig. 23 after resection of the upper left VA along with the tumor and placement of a saphenous vein interposition graft. The distal intradural anastomosis is made just proximal to the PICA.

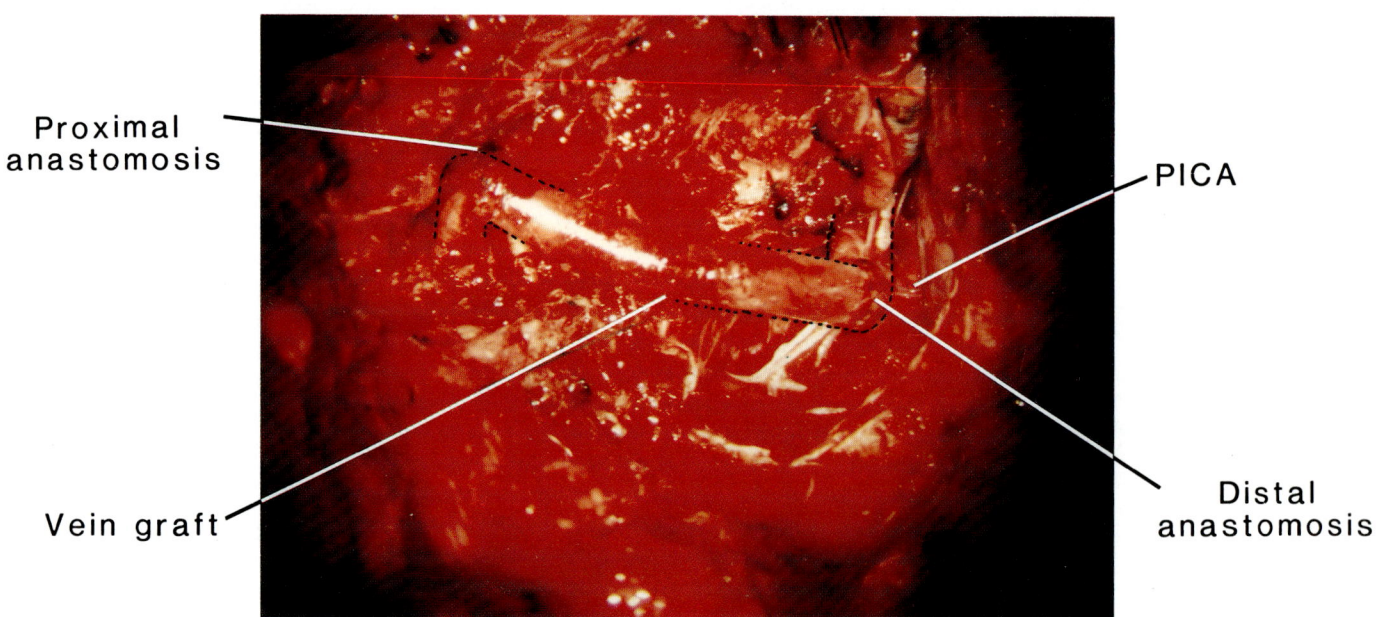

FIG. 27. Intraoperative photograph of the same patient from Figs. 23 and 24, showing the whole interposition graft with both anastomoses.

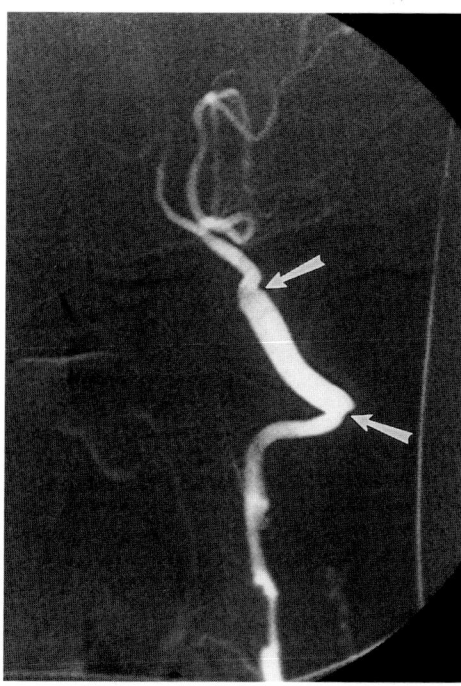

FIG. 28. A postoperative left lateral vertebral angiogram of the patient in Figs. 23–25, showing a patent graft with good filling of the basilar artery as well as the location of both anastomoses (arrows).

sure provided and the two types of P-S bypass employed are demonstrated in Fig. 17. The proximal anastomosis is end-to-end while the distal anastomosis can be end-to-end or end-to-side, depending on the status of the ophthalmic artery and the length of healthy ICA present proximal to the ophthalmic artery. Representative examples are presented in Figs. 18–24.

An additional temporary clip must be placed on the ophthalmic artery if an end-to-side distal anastomosis is chosen. The distal anastomosis is performed prior to the proximal anastomosis. Back-bleeding from the intracavernous ICA from anastomotic intracavernous branches is stopped by packing the cavernous ICA lumen with Surgical. The length of the saphenous vein graft is 5–6 cm. Intraluminal shunting is not used.

TABLE 1. *University of Pittsburgh Center for Cranial Base Surgery vein graft revascularization procedures 1985–1990*

Types of procedure	Number
P-S bypass (supraophthalmic end-to-side)	16
P-S bypass (infraophthalmic end-to-end)	2
Cervical to supraophthalmic carotid (end-to-side)	1
Cervical to petrous carotid (end-to-end)	7
Extradural to intradural vertebral artery (end-to-end)	1
Petrous carotid venous patch graft	2
Total	29

TABLE 2. *University of Pittsburgh Center for Cranial Base Surgery vein graft revascularization procedures 1985–1990*

Type of lesion	Number
Benign	
Meningioma	16
Chemodectoma	1
Craniopharyngioma	1
Malignant	
Malignant meningioma	1
Squamous cell carcinoma	1
Rhabdomyosarcoma	1
Mucoepidermoid carcinoma	1
Vascular	
Petrous carotid aneurysm	1
Cavernous sinus aneurysm	2
Cervical carotid aneurysm	2
Iatrogenic laceration of the petrous carotid	2
Total	29

Vertebral Artery Interposition Grafting

The VA proximal to the origin of the PICA may sometimes have to be resected with a foramen magnum or craniovertebral junction tumor. If the patient does not tolerate a clinical BTO of that VA, then a saphenous vein interposition graft may need to be performed (Figs. 25–28). The principles and techniques involved are the same as those described for the petrosal or high cervical ICA interposition grafting and our operative approach to the VA at the craniovertebral junction is described in the chapter by Sen and Sekhar ("Extreme Lateral Transcondylar and Transjugular Approaches").

Reimplantation

Occasionally during dissection for exposure, or in the process of removing tumor from one of the major arteries at the base of the brain, that artery may be avulsed from its parent artery [e.g., superior cerebral artery (SCA), anterior inferior cerebellar artery (AICA), or PICA]. Since these are end arteries with little collateral flow, the patient should be immediately placed in barbiturate- or etomidate-induced coma until burst suppression is achieved by EEG and an attempt made to reimplant the avulsed artery onto the parent artery using the artery-to-artery microanastomosis technique already described. If reimplantation is not technically possible, then an attempt must be made to perform an extracranial-to-intracranial (EC-IC) bypass to the avulsed artery as described in the following sections.

Vein Graft Results

Over the period from 1985 to 1990, we have performed 29 vein graft revascularization procedures dur-

TABLE 3. University of Pittsburgh Center for Cranial Base Surgery vein graft revascularization graft occlusions, N = 4 (14%)

Case	Graft type	Time of occlusion	Cause	Course
1	Cervical to petrous carotid (end-to-end)	Less than 24 hr after surgery	Compressing neck wound hematoma	Fogarty embolectomy unsuccessful; new graft placed; graft patent
2	P-S bypass (supraophthalmic end-to-side)	Intraoperative	Undersized vein graft (<3 mm diameter)	Patient was in the low-risk category, so the graft was not revised
3	P-S bypass (supraophthalmic end-to-side)	Intraoperative	Atheroma of the supraclinoid ICA led to ICA dissection and occlusion distal to the distal ICA anastomosis	The ICA occluded up to the carotid bifurcation, leading to massive infarction and death
4	P-S bypass (supraophthalmic end-to-side)	Intraoperative	The vein used as a graft had previously been exposed in situ during the first stage of resection (? endothelial injury)	Patient was in the low-risk category so the graft was not revised

ing cranial base surgery. Twenty-one patients were female and eight were male. Patient age ranged from 13 to 81 years. The types of vein graft revascularization procedures are listed in Table 1. The types of lesions requiring revascularization during cranial base surgery are outlined in Table 2. Acute graft occlusions occurred in four patients (14%) either intraoperatively or within 24 hr of surgery (Table 3). All acute occlusions resulted from technical problems that are potentially avoidable. One acute occlusion led to the only death in the series (3% mortality rate). This patient was in the low-risk category by preoperative assessment but sustained a distal ICA dissection with occlusion all the way up to the carotid bifurcation, eliminating all posterior communicating artery collateral circulation and isolating the MCA territory. The long-term clinical and neuroimaging outcomes are described in Table 4. Hemispheric deficits and infarctions on neuroimaging in the absence of graft occlusion are most likely caused by temporary ICA occlusion during graft placement. The majority occurred early in the series, before the institution of moderate hyperthermia, induced hypertension, and etomidate- or barbiturate-induced coma during temporary occlusion in moderate and high-risk patients. All 25 vein graft revascularizations that were patent 24 hr after surgery remain patent and without evidence of delayed pathology by angiogram 2–60 months after graft placement (mean 1.5 years).

TABLE 4. University of Pittsburgh Center for Cranial Base Surgery vein graft revascularization procedures 1985–1990, preoperative stroke risk and outcome

Risk category[a]	Immediate postoperative hemispheric deficit	Persistent clinical hemispheric deficits	Neuroimaging evidence of infarction
Low risk N = 13	1 (8%)	1 (8%)	1 (8%)
Moderate risk N = 8	5 (63%)	1 (13%)	1 (13%)
High risk N = 2	2 (100%)	2 (100%)	2 (100%)
Passed clinical BTO, but Xe CT/CBF not done[b] N = 5	0	0	0
Vertebral artery interposition graft N = 1	0	0	0

[a] Low risk, passed a 15-min clinical BTO and had an ICA-occluded CBF > 30 cc/100 g/min. Moderate risk, passed a 15-min clinical BTO but had an ICA-occluded CBF ≤ 30 cc/100 g/min. High-risk, failed the 15-min clinical BTO.

[b] These five patients were assessed early in our experience, prior to the addition of the Xe CT/CBF study to preoperative evaluation.

EC-IC BYPASS GRAFTING

Extracranial-to-Distal Middle Cerebral Artery Bypass

The use of the EC–distal MCA bypass was shown to be ineffective for the prevention of strokes from atherosclerotic cerebrovascular disease by the EC-IC cooperative study (24). However, the EC–distal middle cerebral artery (MCA) bypass has a definite role in providing immediate flow to the MCA territory in the face of acute reduction or elimination of proximal MCA blood supply. EC–distal MCA bypass in cranial base surgery has several roles. First, an EC–distal MCA bypass may allow a high-risk patient who failed the BTO to later pass the BTO, moving that patient into the moderate- or low-risk category and thus reducing the subsequent risk of cranial base surgery (29,49). Second, an EC–distal MCA at the beginning of cranial base surgery in high-risk patients may provide enough collateral flow to allow for safe temporary ICA occlusion during the definitive procedure. Third, an EC–distal MCA bypass may supply enough flow to revascularize the MCA territory in patients where the cranial base tumor is large enough to involve the M1 segment of the MCA, placing this segment at risk for sacrifice at surgery. In high-risk patients, an EC=distal MCA bypass may not supply enough flow to supply the whole hemisphere should the ICA require sacrifice (59). In these patients, we prefer the higher flow P-S bypass or a petrosal or high cervical ICA interposition vein graft for permanent revascularization.

In order to be adequate for an EC–distal MCA bypass, the donor artery must be at least 1 mm in diameter. The most common artery used is either the parietal or frontal branch of the STA; however, the STA has been found to be unsuitable (<1 mm diameter, <70 mm length) in 8% of cadaver specimens studied (44). When the STA is inadequate or was sacrificed during prior surgery, then the OA can sometimes be used (66,80). If neither artery is adequate, then a short vein graft (<10 cm) from the larger, more proximal STA can be used to supply the distal MCA (40,58,74).

Advantages of using a scalp artery as the donor vessel include a higher patency rate than EC–distal MCA venous grafts, and the need to perform only one anastomosis. Disadvantages are a lower initial flow rate than EC–distal MCA venous grafts (42 ± 21 ml/min versus 67 ± 36 ml/min) (25) and a higher incidence of donor vessel spasm.

The incisions used for STA-MCA and OA-MCA bypasses are demonstrated in Fig. 29. In each case, the scalp artery is traced prior to incision with a Doppler probe. The artery is isolated with sharp dissection, leaving a cuff of connective tissue and adventitia attached. Small branches are coagulated with bipolar cautery and large ones are divided between 6-0 ligatures. The artery is traced as proximal as possible to provide maximum length. The artery is then occluded proximally with a temporary clip and the lumen irrigated with heparinized saline as the clip is opened and closed. It is covered with gauze soaked in dilute papaverine until needed. A small craniotomy is performed 6 cm above the external auditory meatus and, after locating a suitable recipient artery near the angular gyrus, an end-to-side anastomosis is performed as previously described, using 10-0 monofila-

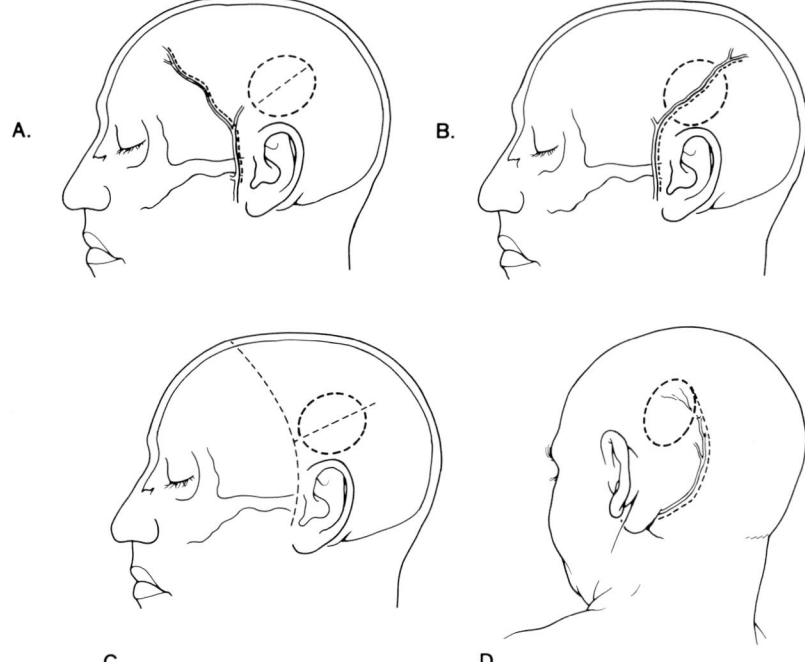

FIG. 29. Drawings showing the craniotomy location (*heavy dotted line*) and incisions used for performing a STA-to-MCA bypass (**A–C**) and an OA-to-MCA bypass (**D**). Drawing (**C**) demonstrates the incision combining a bicoronal craniotomy incision with an incision for a STA-to-MCA bypass.

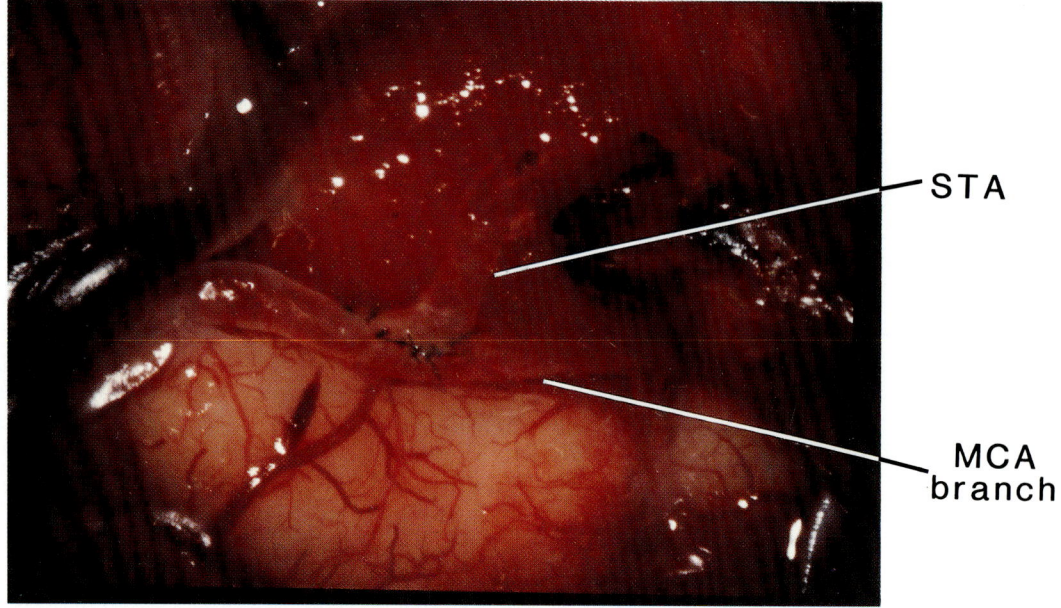

FIG. 30. Intraoperative photograph of a completed left STA-to-MCA bypass in a 58-year-old with bilateral cavernous sinus aneurysms who presented with spontaneous ipsilateral ICA thrombosis and reversible, blood pressure-dependent, left hemisphere ischemic deficits.

ment nylon and end-to-side suturing. The dura is closed around the donor artery and a hole is fashioned in the bone flap to allow access for the donor artery without compression. The overlying muscle and scalp are then tightly reapproximated. Representative cases are presented in Figs. 30–32.

Extracranial-to-Proximal Anterior Circulation Arteries

Diaz et al. (21) were the first to describe an STA-to-proximal MCA bypass in 1985. Since then, others have described or performed long (>10 cm) saphenous vein bypasses from the external carotid artery (ECA) or CCA

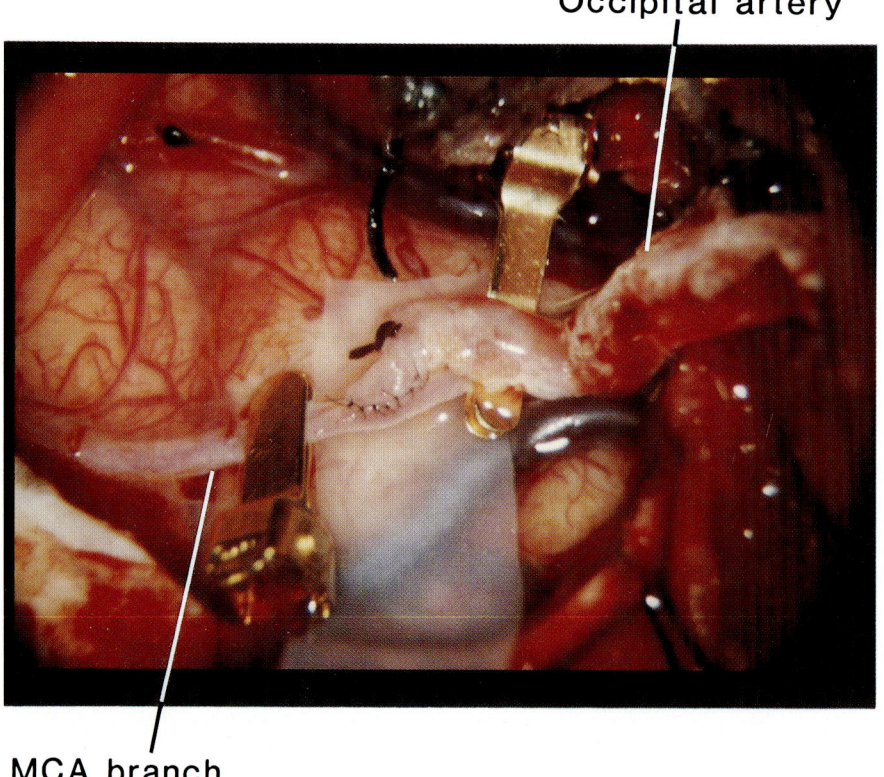

FIG. 31. Intraoperative photograph of a completed right OA-to-MCA bypass in a 27-year-old woman with a giant craniopharyngioma intimately involving the M1 segment of the right MCA. The bypass was placed prior to an attempt at tumor resection. Her ipsilateral STA had been sacrificed during surgery at another institution years ago.

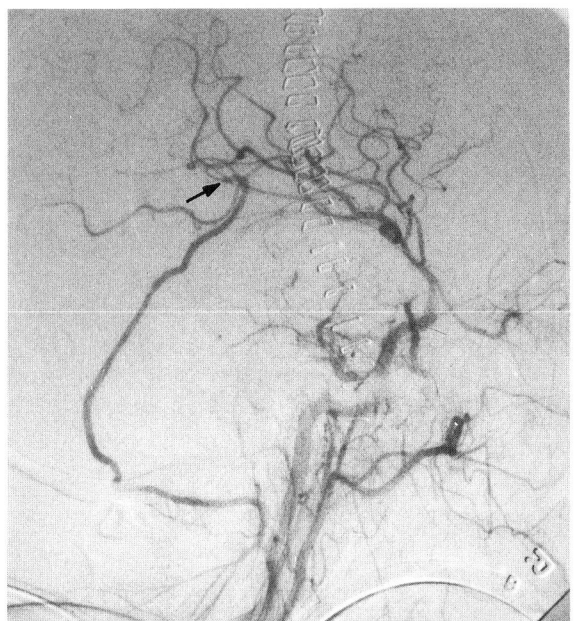

FIG. 32. Postoperative lateral right CCA angiogram from the patient in Fig. 29, showing a patent bypass with good filling of the right MCA. The microanastomosis is labeled with an *arrow*.

to the proximal MCA (21,71). There have also been reports of long saphenous vein bypass grafts from the CCA to the supraclinoid ICA (38,43). The advantage of long vein bypasses are that they provide a higher volume of flow than distal MCA bypasses and that this flow is anterograde and thus more physiologic. The disadvantages are that they are technically more difficult than distal MCA bypasses to perform and run a higher risk of occlusion than short grafts. These proximal bypass grafts have a limited role in cranial base surgery where short interposition proximal vein grafts, which provide the same volume of anterograde flow and run less risk of thrombosing, can be performed more easily during cranial base exposure.

Posterior Circulation Bypass Grafting

The role of posterior circulation bypass grafting in cranial base surgery has yet to be defined. In patients with poor anterior-to-posterior circulation collaterals who require temporary or permanent occlusion of their dominant artery or only VA, an OA-PICA bypass (3-5,33,36,37,57,69) could theoretically provide the necessary collateral blood flow. Likewise, in patients with poor anterior-to-posterior circulation collaterals who require temporary or permanent occlusion of the midbasilar artery or of the dominant or only VA distal to the PICA, an STA-SCA bypass (2,5,6) or an ECA-posterior cerebral artery (PCA) saphenous vein bypass (70,71) could theoretically provide the necessary collateral blood flow. An anatomic study in cadavers (63) has shown that the best sites for posterior circulation bypass anastomosis are the pretonsilar segment of the PICA, the perimesencephalic segment of the SCA, and the perimesencephalic segment of the PCA. The OA-PICA bypass is performed through a unilateral suboccipital craniectomy with resection of the ipsilateral arch of C1 (7,33,36,57,69) and the STA-SCA and ECA-PCA saphenous vein bypasses are performed via a subtemporal approach with splitting of the tentorium near the fourth cranial nerve (2,6,70,71).

POSTOPERATIVE MEDICAL MANAGEMENT

If a saphenous vein graft is used for revascularization, the patient is given 1000 mg of intravenous methyl prednisolone intravenously to reduce the inflammatory graft response that has been reported within vein grafts (53,54). Steroids are continued postoperatively (40 mg intravenously every 6 hr) for 48 hr and then tapered. Strict blood pressure control is imperative postoperatively in patients with saphenous vein grafts to try and limit the incidence of intracerebral hemorrhage and hyperperfusion edema, which have occasionally been reported with vein graft revascularization (12,16,30,35,69). In patients with arterial EC–distal MCA bypass grafts in place, isovolemic hemodilution has been shown to increase the immediate postoperative regional blood flow provided by these relatively low flow grafts, which take time to mature and increase flow (79).

All patients who undergo cerebral revascularization are placed on subcutaneous heparin 5000 units every 8 hr, beginning 24 hr postoperatively and continued for 10 days. Since there is some evidence to suggest that antiplatelet therapy can reduce the development of "accelerated atherosclerosis" in bypass grafts (15,47), all patients are started on aspirin 325 mg/day beginning 1 week after operation. There is also some evidence to suggest that long-term control of VLDL and LDL levels postoperatively may assist in slowing the development of atherosclerotic lesions (14).

COMPLICATIONS

Complications of cerebral revascularization include ischemia, hyperperfusion hemorrhage or edema, pseudoaneurysm formation, subdural hematomas, and subdural hygromas. Ischemia can result from graft thrombosis, dissection of the recipient artery, or distal embolization. Acute bypass thrombosis is most often related to undersized vein grafts or narrowed anastomoses (12,62), inadequate flow through the vein graft (12,17,45,55), technical errors leading to graft torsion or kinking (21,22,53), and external graft compression by bone or fascial edges (20,21,53), as well as endothelial damage caused by poor graft harvesting and preparation techniques or vascular clamps (21,22,53). Delayed bypass thrombosis is most often related to internal fibrous thickening with "accelerated atherosclerosis" (13,53,67,77). Dissection of the recipient artery most often occurs when that artery segment is involved with atherosclerotic placque. To prevent this, a limited endarterectomy should be performed, being careful to tack down any distal intimal flap. Distal embolization can result from either a thrombosed graft or occasionally just from temporary clamping. Intraoperative SSEPs are very useful in warning when embolization has occurred, allowing a search for the embolus with subsequent embolectomy.

Hyperperfusion hemorrhage or edema seems to be a rare problem most often associated with saphenous vein grafts, presumably related to the impairment or loss of CBF autoregulation through the high-flow graft (12,15,30,35,71). For this reason, strict postoperative blood pressure control is essential. Postbypass intracerebral hemorrhage has also been reported with STA-MCA bypass, but this is usually associated with reperfusion of an area of developing infarction (24). Pseudoaneurysm formation is most often related to technical errors with poor anastomotic technique (22) or arterial weakening due to adjacent infection (61).

Rarely, a distal cortical artery bypass may be complicated by subdural hematoma formation secondary to poor anastomotic technique (58). Subdural hygroma formation can also occur with distal cortical artery bypasses (72) but is much more common with the subtemporal approach for ECA-PCA saphenous vein bypass (71). Sundt et al. (71) now routinely place a subdural-atrial shunt during ECA-PICA bypass. Other complications unique to posterior circulation bypass include occasional homonymous hemianopia from temporary occlusion of the PCA (70), occasional persistent ataxia after bypass to the PICA or SCA (69,71), and a small incidence of temporal lobe hematoma as a result of either retraction or venous infarction using the subtemporal approach to the SCA or PCA (70,71).

LONG-TERM OUTCOME

Nothing is known about the 10- and 20-year patency rates of cerebral revascularization grafts. We do know that STA-MCA patency rates are about 96% at 4.5 years (24) and that the short-term patency rates of OA-PICA bypasses run between 92 and 94% (33,69). The more lengthy cardiothoracic experience with coronary artery bypass grafts suggests that saphenous vein grafts have a lower long-term patency rate than arterial grafts (42,75). This observation appears to hold true for cerebral revascularization grafts with short-term patency rates reported between 71 and 94% for long vein grafts (25,30,53,58,71) and between 90 and 100% for short vein grafts (40,53). One observation from the femoral artery-to-popliteal artery experience is that long-term saphenous vein graft patency is inversely related to graft length (20), and this appears to hold true for cerebral revascularization vein grafts as well (53). P-S bypasses are usually performed in patients without significant atherosclerotic disease, are short, and go from a large vessel to another large vessel. Of the 15 P-S bypass grafts that were patent 24 hr after operation, all are still patent without evidence of late pathology 2–60 months after placement (mean 18 months). Long-term follow-up data for cerebral revascularization grafts will only come from meticulous patient follow-up, including periodic cerebral angiography.

REFERENCES

1. Al-Mefty O, Khalil N, Elwany MN, Smith RR. Shunt for bypass graft of the cavernous carotid artery: an anatomical and technical study. *Neurosurgery* 1990;27:721–728.
2. Ausman JA, Diaz FG, de los Reyes RA. Posterior circulation revascularization: superficial temporal artery to superior cerebellar artery anastomosis. *J Neurosurg* 1982;56:766–776.
3. Ausman JI, Diaz FG, de los Reyes RA. Extracranial–intracranial anastomoses in the posterior circulation. In: Berguer R, Bauer B, eds. *Vertebrobasilar arterial occlusive disease.* New York: Raven Press, 1984;313–319.
4. Ausman JI, Diaz FG, Dujovny M. Posterior circulation revascularization. *Clin Neursurg* 1986;33:331–343.
5. Ausman JI, Diaz FG, Vacca DF, et al. Superficial temporal and occipital artery bypass pedicles to superior, anterior inferior, and posterior inferior cerebellar arteries for vertebrobasilar insufficiency. *J Neurosurg* 1990;72:554–558.
6. Ausman JI, Lee MC, Chater N, et al. Superficial temporal artery to superior cerebellar artery anastomosis for distal basilar artery stenosis. *Surg Neurol* 1979;12:277–282.
7. Ausman JI, Lee MC, Klassen AC, et al. Stroke: what's new? *Minn Med* 1976;59:223–227.
8. Barnett HJ. Delayed cerebral ischemic episodes distal to occlusion of major cerebral arteries. *Neurology* 1978;28:769–774.
9. Batjer HH, Frankfurt AL, Purdy PD, et al. Use of etomidate, temporary arterial occlusion, and intraoperative angiography in surgical treatment of large and giant cerebral aneurysms. *J Neurosurg* 1988;68:234–240.
10. Batjer H, Mickey B, Samson D. Enlargement and rupture of a distal basilar artery aneurysm after iatrogenic carotid occlusion. *Neurosurgery* 1987;20:624–628.
11. Boysen G, Engell HC, Henriksen H. The effect of induced hypertension of internal carotid artery pressure and regional cerebral blood flow during temporary carotid clamping for endarterectomy. *Neurology* 1972;22:1133–1144.
12. Brown WE, Ansell LV, Story JL. The technique of saphenous vein bypass graft from the common carotid artery to the middle cerebral artery. In: Erickson DL, ed. *Revascularization for the ischemic brain.* Mount Kisco, NY: Futura Publishing, 1988;167–199.
13. Buckley BH, Hutchins GM. Accelerated "atherosclerosis." A morphological study of 97 saphenous vein coronary artery bypass grafts. *Circulation* 1977;55:163–169.
14. Campeau L, Enjalbert M, Lesperance J, et al. The relation of risk factors to the development of atherosclerosis in the saphenous-vein bypass grafts and the progression of disease in the native circulation. A study 10 years after coronary bypass surgery. *N Engl J Med* 1982;307:73–78.
15. Chesebro JH, Clements IP, Fuster V, et al. A platelet-inhibitor-drug trial in coronary bypass operations. Benefit of perioperative dipridamole and aspirin therapy on early postoperative vein-graft patency. *N Engl J Med* 1982;307:73–78.

16. Collice M, Arena O, Riva M. Complications after subclavian–cortical middle cerebral artery bypass. *Neurosurgery* 1986;18:483–486.
17. Dean RH, Yao JS, Stanton PE, et al. Prognostic indicators in femoral popliteal reconstructions. *Arch Surg* 1975;110:1287–1293.
18. DeMorais JY, Lana-Peixoto MA. Bilateral intracavernous carotid aneurysms: treatment by bilateral carotid ligation. *Surg Neurol* 1978;9:379–381.
19. deVries EJ, Sekhar LN, Horton JA, et al. A new method to predict safe resection of the internal carotid artery. *Laryngoscope* 1990;100:85–88.
20. DeWeese JA, Rob CG. Autogenous venous grafts ten years later. *Surgery* 1977;82:775–784.
21. Diaz FG, Umansky F, Mehta B, et al. Cerebral revascularization to a main limb of the middle cerebral artery in the sylvian fissure. An alternative approach to conventional anastomosis. *J Neurosurg* 1985;63:21–29.
22. Diaz FG, Pearce J, Ausman JI. Complications of cerebral revascularization with autogenous vein grafts. *Neurosurgery* 1985;17:271–276.
23. Dyste GN, Beck DW. De novo aneurysm formation following carotid ligation: case report and review of the literature. *Neurosurgery* 1989;24:88–92.
24. The EC/IC Bypass Study Group. Failure of extracranial–intracranial arterial bypass to reduce the risk of ischemic stroke. Results of an international randomized trial. *N Engl J Med* 1985;313:1191–1200.
25. Eguchi T. Results of EC-IC bypass with and without long vein graft. In: Spetzler RF, Carter LP, Selman WR, et al, eds. *Cerebral revascularization for stroke.* New York: Thieme-Stratton, 1985.
26. Erba SM, Horton JA, Latchaw RE, et al. Balloon test occlusion of the internal carotid artery with stable xenon/CT cerebral blood flow imaging. *AJNR* 1988;9:533–538.
27. Faria MA, Fleischer AS, Spector RH. Bilateral giant intracavernous carotid aneurysms treated by bilateral carotid ligation. *Surg Neurol* 1980;14:207–210.
28. Fish U, Oldring DJ, Senning A. Surgical therapy of internal carotid artery lesions of the skull base and temporal bone. *Otolaryngol Head Neck Surg* 1980;88:548–554.
29. Fox AJ, Vinuela F, Pelz DM, et al. Use of detachable balloon for proximal artery occlusion in the treatment of unclippable cerebral aneurysms. *J Neurosurg* 1987;66:40–46.
30. Friedrich H, Laas J, Walterbusch G, et al. Extra-cranial bypass procedure with saphenous vein grafts. *J Thorac Cardiovasc Surg* 1986;34:57–62.
31. German WJ, Black SP. Cervical ligation for internal carotid aneurysms: an extended follow-up. *J Neurosurg* 1965;23:572–577.
32. Gomensoro JB, Maslenikov V, Azambuga N, et al. Joint study of extracranial arterial occlusion. *JAMA* 1973;244:985–991.
33. Hopkins LN, Martin NA, Hadley MN, et al. Vertebrobasilar insufficiency. Part 2: microsurgical treatment of intracranial vertebrobasilar disease. *J Neurosurg* 1987;66:662–674.
34. Hossman KA. Barbiturate protection of cerebral ischemia. In: Carlson LA, Paoletti R, Sirtori CR, et al, eds. *International conference on atherosclerosis, Milan, 1977.* New York: Raven Press, 1978;251–256.
35. Iwabuchi T, Kudo T, Hatanaka M, et al. Vein graft bypass in the treatment of giant aneurysm. *Surg Neurol* 1979;12:463–466.
36. Khodad G. Occipital artery–posterior inferior cerebellar artery anastomosis. *Surg Neurol* 1979;12:463–466.
37. Khodad G. Atherosclerotic occlusive disease of the vertebrobasilar system in young adults and its surgical consideration. *Acta Neurochir (Wien)* 1978;45:147–154.
38. Lazar ML, Clark K. Microsurgical cerebral revascularization: concepts and practice. *Surg Neurol* 1973;1:355–359.
39. Lesoin F, Autricove A, Villette L, et al. The antero-external approach to the internal carotid artery at the base of the skull and intrapetrously. In: Dolenc VV, ed. *The cavernous sinus.* New York: Springer-Verlag, 1987;311–319.
40. Little JR, Furlan AJ, Bryerton B. Short vein grafts for cerebral revascularization. *J Neurosurg* 1983;59:384–388.
41. LoGerfo FW, Haudenschild CC, Quist WC. A clinical technique for prevention of spasm and preservation of endothelium in saphenous vein grafts. *Arch Surg* 1984;119:1212–1214.
42. Loop FD, Cosgrove DM, Lytle BW, et al. An 11-year evolution of coronary arterial surgery (1967–1978). *Ann Surg* 1979;190:444–455.
43. Lougheed WM, Marshall BM, Hunter M, et al. Common carotid to intracranial internal carotid bypass venous graft. Technical note. *J Neurosurg* 1971;34:114–118.
44. Marano SR, Fischer DW, Gaines C, et al. Anatomical study of the superficial temporal artery. *Neurosurgery* 1985;16:786–790.
45. Marko JD, Barner HB, Kaiser GC, et al. Operative flow measurements and coronary artery bypass graft patency. *J Thorac Cardiovasc Surg* 1976;71:545–547.
46. Matsuda M, Handa J, Saito A, et al. Ruptured cerebral aneurysm associated with arterial occlusion. *Surg Neurol* 1983;20:4–12.
47. Metke MP, Lie JT, Fuster V, et al. Reduction of intimal thickening in canine coronary bypass vein grafts with dipyridamole and aspirin. *Am J Cardiol* 1979;43:1144–1148.
48. Miyazaki S, Fukushima T, Fujimaki T. Resection of high-cervical paraganglioma with cervical-to-petrous internal carotid artery saphenous vein bypass. Report of two cases. *J Neurosurg* 1990;73:141–146.
49. Morioka TM, Matsushima T, Fujii, et al. Balloon test occlusion of the internal carotid artery with monitoring of compressed spectral arrays (CSAs) of electroencephalogram. *Acta Neurochir (Wien)* 1989;101:29–34.
50. Nishioka H. Report on the cooperative study of intracranial aneurysms and subarachnoid hemorrhage. Section VIII, Part 1. Results of the treatment of intracranial aneurysms by occlusion of the carotid artery in the neck. *J Neurosurg* 1966;25:660–682.
51. Oldershaw JB, Voris HC. Internal carotid artery ligation, a follow-up study. *Neurology* 1966;16:937–938.
52. Paniszyn CC. Preparation of vein bypass grafts. *J Neurosurg* 1987;67:788–789.
53. Pearce J, Diaz FG, Ausman JI, et al. Saphenous vein grafts in neurovascular surgery, their value and limitations. In: Spetzler RF, Carter LP, Selman WR, et al., eds. *Cerebral revascularization for stroke.* New York: Thieme-Stratton, 1985;372–378.
54. Pearce JE, Dujovny M, Ho KL, et al. Acute inflammation and endothelial injury in vein grafts. *Neurosurgery* 1985;17:626–634.
55. Pereira BM, Weinstein PR, Zea-Longa E, et al. Effect of blood flow rate and donor vessel diameter on the patency of carotid venous bypass grafts in dogs. *Surg Neurol* 1989;31:195–199.
56. Poppen JL. Specific treatment of intracranial aneurysms. Experiences with 143 surgically treated patients. *J Neurosurg* 1951;8:75–102.
57. Roski RA, Spetzler RF, Hopkins LN. Occipital artery to posterior inferior cerebellar artery bypass for vertebrobasilar ischemia. *Neurosurgery* 1982;10:44–49.
58. Samson DS, Gewertz BL, Beyer CW, et al. Saphenous vein interposition grafts in the microsurgical treatment of cerebral ischemia. *Arch Surg* 1981;116:1578–1582.
59. Samson DS, Neuwelt EA, Beyer CW, et al. Failure of extracranial–intracranial arterial bypass in acute middle cerebral artery occlusion: case report. *Neurosurgery* 1980;6:185–188.
60. Sekhar LN, Burgess J, Akin O. Anatomical study of the cavernous sinus emphasizing operative approaches and related vascular and neural reconstruction. *Neurosurgery* 1987;21:806–816.
61. Sekhar LN, Schramm VL Jr, Jones NF. Operative exposure and management of the petrous and upper cervical carotid artery. *Neurosurgery* 1986;19:967–982.
62. Sekhar LN, Sen CN, Jho HD. Saphenous vein graft bypass of the cavernous internal carotid artery. *J Neurosurg* 1990;72:35–41.
63. Shrontz C, Dujovny M, Ausman JI, et al. Surgical anatomy of the arteries of the posterior fossa. *J Neurosurg* 1986;65:540–544.
64. Spetzler RF, Fukushima T, Martin N, Zabramski JM. Petrous carotid-to-intradural carotid saphenous vein graft for intracavernous giant aneurysm, tumor, and occlusive cerebrovascular disease. *J Neurosurg* 1990;73:496–501.
65. Spetzler R, Rhodes RS, Roski RA, et al. Subclavian to middle cerebral artery saphenous vein bypass graft. *J Neurosurg* 1980;53:465–469.
66. Spetzler RF, Schuster H, Roski RA. Elective extracranial–intracranial arterial bypass in the treatment of inoperable giant aneurysms of the internal carotid artery. *J Neurosurg* 1980;53:22–27.

67. Spray TL, Roberts WC. Changes in saphenous veins used as aorto-coronary bypass grafts. *Am Heart J* 1977;94:500–516.
68. Stuntz TJ, Ojemann GA, Alword EC. Radiographic and histologic demonstration of an aneurysm developing on the infundibulum of the posterior communicating artery. *J Neurosurg* 1970;33:591–596.
69. Sundt TM Jr, Piepgrass DG. Occipital to posterior inferior cerebellar artery bypass surgery. *J Neurosurg* 1978;48:916–928.
70. Sundt TM Jr, Piepgrass DG, Houser OW, et al. Interposition saphenous vein grafts for advanced occlusive disease and large aneurysms in the posterior circulation. *J Neurosurg* 1982;56:205–215.
71. Sundt TM Jr, Piepgrass DG, Marsh R, et al. Saphenous vein bypass grafts for giant aneurysms and intracranial occlusive disease. *J Neurosurg* 1986;65:439–450.
72. Sundt TM Jr, Whisnant JP, Foda NC, et al. Results, complications, and follow-up of 415 bypass operations for occlusive disease of the carotid system. *Mayo Clin Proc* 1985;60:230–240.
73. Sundt TM III, Sundt TM Jr. Principles of preparation of vein bypass grafts to maximize patency. *J Neurosurg* 1987;66:172–180.
74. Tew JM Jr. Reconstructive intracranial vascular surgery for prevention of stroke. *Clin Neurosurg* 1987;66:172–180.
75. Tyras DH, Codd JE, Willman VL. Bypass grafts to the left anterior descending coronary artery. Saphenous vein versus internal mammary artery. *J Thorac Cardiovasc Surg* 1980;80:327–333.
76. Urken ML, Biller HF, Hainoy M. Infratemporal carotid artery bypass in resection of a skull base tumor. *Laryngoscope* 1985;95:1472–1477.
77. Vlodaver Z, Edwards JE. Pathologic changes in aortic–coronary arterial saphenous vein grafts. *Circulation* 1971;44:719–728.
78. Wilkinson E, Spetzler RF, Carter LP, et al. Intraoperative barbiturate therapy during temporary vessel occlusion in man. In: Spetzler RF, Carter LP, Selmen WR, et al., eds. *Cerebral revascularization for stroke.* New York: Thieme-Stratton, 1985;397–402.
79. Wood JH, Polyzoidis KS, Kee DB Jr, et al. Augmentation of cerebral blood flow induced by hemodilution in stroke patients after superficial temporal–middle cerebral arterial bypass operation. *Neurosurgery* 1984;15:535–539.
80. Yonekawa Y, Yasargil MG. Extra-intracranial arterial anastomosis: clinical and technical aspects. Results. In: Karyenbuhl H, Brihaye J, Loew F, et al., eds. *Advances and technical standards in neurosurgery,* vol 3. New York: Springer-Verlag, 1976;48–78.

CHAPTER 7

Special Anesthetic Considerations in Cranial Base Tumor Surgery

Rene M. Gonzalez

Major advances in pharmacology, technology, and the subspecialty of neurosurgical anesthesiology in the last decade have given neuroanesthesiologists an unprecedented amount of understanding and control of many physiologic processes that ultimately affect the functioning of the central nervous system (CNS). It has become increasingly clear that the drugs we administer and the things we do—or do not do—behind the surgical drapes can have significant impact on the ultimate neurologic outcome. The ten major goals of anesthetic management of the skull base surgery patient can be summarized as follows:

1. Tight maintenance of hemodynamic stability.
2. Prevention of increases in intracranial pressure.
3. Maintenance of cerebral perfusion and oxygenation.
4. Maintenance of a still surgical field.
5. Facilitating surgical exposure of the tumor.
6. Facilitating appropriate electrophysiologic monitoring of the brain and cranial nerves.
7. Replacing blood loss and preventing and treating coagulopathies.
8. Providing a smooth, safe, and rapid emergence from general anesthesia so that a "postoperative baseline" neurologic exam may be performed shortly after the operation.
9. Continuation of all of the above considerations in the recovery room/intensive care unit postoperatively.
10. Postoperative airway management.

R. M. Gonzalez: Eye and Ear Institute, and Department of Anesthesiology and Critical Care Medicine, University of Pittsburgh School of Medicine, Pittsburgh, Pennsylvania 15213.

In addition to the above, the anesthesiologist must also take into account each patient's individual medical problems and must consider how each organ system might affect or be affected by the choice of anesthetic agents and technique. Unfortunately, there is no perfect drug available for neurosurgical anesthesia; all drugs have their limitations. Instead, what is available is a large armamentarium of drugs and techniques, and a large body of knowledge of pharmacokinetics and drug interactions—both in healthy patients and in patients with specific organ dysfunctions—that enable us to predict fairly well how an individual patient will respond to a given dose of a certain drug. Also available are increasingly sophisticated monitors to provide feedback for our predictions. In an average cranial base tumor operation, we administer 10–20 different drugs and use approximately 15 different monitoring devices.

The goal of this chapter is to relate the techniques, drugs, philosophy, and approaches we have been using at the University of Pittsburgh to provide anesthesia for the patient undergoing surgical removal of cranial base tumors. In addition, we try to convey some major perianesthetic concerns and challenges as well as the limitations in our knowledge and techniques.

SOME ANESTHETIC AGENTS AND THEIR EFFECTS ON INTRACRANIAL CONTENTS

All the inhalational and intravenous anesthetic agents in clinical use have significant effects on the intracranial contents, either directly or indirectly (1–4). A brief general discussion of our current knowledge of the subject follows and is summarized in detail in Table 1.

Most sedatives, analgesics, and anesthetic agents de-

TABLE 1. *Effects of anesthetic agents on systemic hemodynamics, cerebral circulation, and intracranial contents*

Anesthetic	MAP	CMRO$_2$	CBF	Cerebrovascular autoregulation	CO$_2$ responsiveness	CSF production	Resistance to CSF absorption	ICP	ICP if hyperventilated	Seizures
Inhalation										
Halothane	↓↓	↓	↑↑	Abolished	Yes	↓	↑	↑↑	—	No
Enflurane	↓↓	↓	↑	Abolished	Yes	↑↑	↑	↑↑	—	Yes (in high doses and with hypocapnia)
Isoflurane	↓↓	↓↓	↑	Maintained unless high dose	Yes	—	↓	↑	—	No
N$_2$O	—	?↓	?↓	? Maintained	? Yes	?	?	?	?	No
Intravenous										
Thiopental	↓↓	↓↓	↓	Maintained	Yes	—	—	↓↓	↓	No
Etomidate	↓	↓↓	↓	Maintained	Yes	?	?	↓↓	↓	?
Fentanyl	↓	— or ↓ (dose-dependent)	— or ↓	Maintained	Yes	—	↓	—	↓	In very high doses

Source: From ref. 41, with permission.
Abbreviations: MAP, mean arterial pressure; CMRO$_2$, cerebral metabolic oxygen consumption rate; CBF, cerebral blood flow; ICP, intracranial pressure; CSF, cerebrospinal fluid.

press EEG activity and decrease the cerebral metabolic oxygen consumption rate ($CMRO_2$). In clinically useful doses, the decrease in $CMRO_2$ is most profound with barbiturates and isoflurane. This decrease in the brain's metabolic demand may be viewed as a favorable property of anesthetics on the CNS. Possible exceptions include ketamine, enflurane (at very high concentrations under conditions of hypocapnia), laudanosine (a metabolite of the neuromuscular blocker atracurium), and nitrous oxide. These agents have been reported in large doses to produce either increases in $CMRO_2$ or seizure-like activity on EEG. This would be an undesirable effect during neurosurgery. Much controversy exists, however, regarding nitrous oxide; many investigators report that, like other inhaled anesthetics, it lowers $CMRO_2$.

All anesthetic agents are cardiovascular depressants to varying degrees (Table 1). Great care must be taken to avoid systemic hypotension with its attendant risk for cerebral hypoperfusion, particularly in the patient with intracranial hypertension who requires a high cerebral perfusion pressure. The blood pressure-lowering effects of the anesthetics can, however, serve a useful purpose in the patient with impaired cerebral autoregulation or a damaged blood–brain barrier, by blunting the hypertensive response to surgical stimulation, which carries the risk of hypertensive cerebral edema or hemorrhage.

All sedatives, analgesics, and anesthetics are respiratory depressants. Because of the risks of hypercarbia-induced increases in ICP, cranial base surgery patients should be mechanically hyperventilated intraoperatively. To facilitate mechanical ventilation and to help assure a perfectly still surgical field, neuromuscular blockers ("muscle relaxants") are frequently employed. Some of the neuromuscular blockers have cardiovascular side effects, such as tachycardia or histamine-mediated hypotension, which must be taken into account.

All currently used potent inhalation anesthetics (halothane, enflurane, and isoflurane) can significantly increase ICP and produce intraoperative brain protrusion, probably by a variety of mechanisms, including cerebral vasodilation and an imbalance of CSF production and absorption. This effect on cerebral vasodilation and ICP is probably most prominent with halothane and enflurane and least significant with isoflurane. Fortunately, it has been demonstrated that the increases in ICP induced by the potent inhalation anesthetics in patients with intracranial masses can be minimized by hyperventilation. For the above reasons, isoflurane (with hyperventilation) enjoys the most popularity of all the inhalational anesthetics for neurosurgical procedures. However, significant increases in ICP may still occur in patients with very high baseline ICP when isoflurane is administered, in spite of moderate levels of hyperventilation.

An ideal neuroanesthetic agent would possess all the following properties: perservation of hemodynamic stability and cerebral perfusion, no increase in ICP, decrease in cerebral metabolic demands, cerebral protective effect in ischemia, and short duration of action or at least instant reversibility with an antidote. As can be gleaned from the above discussion and from Table 1, no such agent currently exists. Although several agents possess many desirable qualities, all possess some undesirable side effects. As a result, modern neurosurgical anesthetic management usually consists of a blend or balance of many different pharmaceuticals, intravenous and inhalational.

CLINICAL ANESTHETIC MANAGEMENT

Preoperative Preparation

An important goal of the preoperative visit is to gather data on the patient's neurologic and general medical condition (5). A physical exam, with particularly careful evaluation of the upper airway, must be performed. All efforts must be made to optimize the patient's general medical condition prior to surgery. Close communication with medical consultants is essential.

In addition to obtaining a list of allergies, current drug therapy must be reviewed during the preoperative evaluation, since adverse interactions of these drugs with drugs used as part of the anesthetic management must be considered. Many of the patient's drugs (e.g., antianginals, antihypertensives, digitalis, anticonvulsants, steroids, hormone replacements) may, and should, be continued on the morning of surgery either parenterally or with a small sip of water.

Preoperative sedatives and narcotics should be used sparingly if at all. In general, premedicants leading to hypoventilation and CO_2 retention should be avoided in patients with reduced intracranial compliance. It is also our belief that patients having lengthy neurosurgical procedures are exquisitely sensitive to sedatives, which may contribute to delayed awakening and impaired neurologic assessment at the end of the procedure. A thorough preoperative explanation of the anticipated perioperative events by the anesthesiologist to the patient serves as a nonpharmacologic antidote to anxiety.

Monitoring

Major advances in monitoring technology now permit tight control of physiologic parameters and early detection of physiologic derangements and end-organ dysfunction.

Our list of "routine" monitors for *all* cranial base procedures is rather extensive and is illustrated in Fig. 1. A few brief comments are in order.

In general, the antecubital approach is our route of choice for placement of the CVP or Swan–Ganz cath-

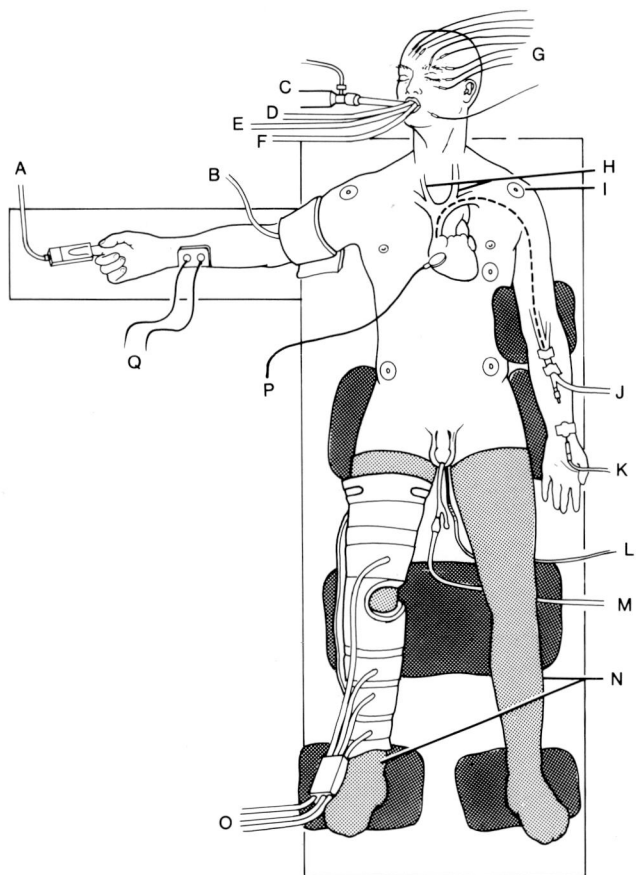

FIG. 1. Monitoring and equipment setup for cranial base surgery. A, pulse oximeter; B, blood pressure cuff; C, capnograph and mass spectrometer; D, esophageal stethoscope; E, pharyngeal temperature probe; F, orogastric suction tube; G, EEG, EMG, and EP; H, alternate route for central line (external or internal jugular vein); I, ECG; J, central venous line (basilic vein); K, arterial line; L, rectal temperature probe; M, urinary catheter; N, antiembolism stockings; O, sequential leg compression device; P, precordial Doppler; Q, peripheral nerve stimulator. (From ref. 41, with permission.)

eter. If this proves technically impossible, we then proceed to cannulate the external or internal jugular vein (preferably contralateral to the surgical site) or, finally, the subclavian vein. When the subclavian route is used, a chest x-ray should be obtained to rule out pneumothorax, since positive pressure ventilation can quickly convert a small pneumothorax into a tension pneumothorax, which could be catastrophic in a neurosurgical patient.

Our neuroanesthesiologists have been increasingly using a relatively new technology, computer-processed two-channel electroencephalography (EEG), for monitoring cerebral electrical function intraoperatively, especially during induction of anesthesia and during vascular cross-clamping. These user-friendly EEG monitors require only five small scalp electrodes and thus can sometimes be used even if the surgical area requires a wide sterile prep. They continuously display right versus left cerebral hemispheric activity and may be useful for detection of seizure activity, unilateral ischemia, or guidance in dosage when barbiturate infusions are used.

Monitoring for intraoperative venous air embolism is discussed in another section.

In our institution, electrophysiologic monitoring of the neuraxis and appropriate cranial nerves is performed during all cranial base tumor resections. This monitoring is performed by a separate, dedicated team, whose approach is discussed by Sclabassi et al. Close cooperation is required between the anesthesia team and the electrophysiology team to avoid interfering with each other (e.g., not dislodging electrodes or endotracheal tubes, not administering neuromuscular blockers when cranial nerve EMGs are being monitored).

Almost all intraoperative monitoring should be continued during transport to the recovery room using portable monitors. Intensive monitoring should be continued throughout the recovery room stay until the patient has (a) completely recovered from the anesthetic drugs and (b) demonstrated stability of all vital physiologic parameters and absence of neurosurgical complications.

Induction and Maintenance of Anesthesia

After the establishment of appropriate monitoring and intravenous access, the patient is nearly ready for general anesthesia (6–9).

The next important issue to be addressed is the adequacy of the patient's airway. The anesthesiologist must make a critical judgment. Might the anatomy of this individual patient's airway lead to difficulty with (a) mask ventilation or (b) endotracheal intubation after induction of general anesthesia? This is an especially important question in patients with intracranial lesions, in which even a few moments of hypoxia or hypercarbia could have devastating CNS effects. It is also a particularly pertinent question for patients with invasive skull base tumors or previous skull base surgery, in which there may be anatomical compromise of the upper airway or temporomandibular joint. A systematic, meticulous examination of each individual feature of the patient's upper airway anatomy, as well as consultation with the neurosurgeons and otorhinolaryngologists, and a "high index of suspicion" for potential airway problems is mandatory.

If there is any question regarding a difficult airway, general anesthesia should *not* be induced first. A safe, rational approach is to topically anesthetize the upper airway and perform an awake examination or intubation with either a conventional direct laryngoscope or a fiberoptic scope. In our experience, with adequate explanation and with meticulous, sequential application of local anesthetic solutions to the upper airway, patients reliably tolerate awake laryngoscopy and intubation very well, with little or no need for sedation (with its attendant risk of hypercarbia and increased ICP) and with minimal change in vital signs. Supplemental oxygen via nasal cannula is recommended during awake intubation.

If the patient's airway anatomy and mobility are assessed to be within normal limits, then intravenous induction with "asleep" laryngoscopy and tracheal intubation are planned. "Preoxygenation" with 100% O_2 for 2–3 min prior to induction has been shown to protect against the arterial oxygen desaturation that can take place during laryngoscopy and tracheal intubation. During preoxygenation, "voluntary hyperventilation" is initiated by asking the patient to take deep, rapid breaths. This is done in order to lower the ICP and to protect against the CO_2 retention, which is always a possibility during laryngoscopy, especially if the airway turns out to be difficult to manage.

After preoxygenation and voluntary hyperventilation, general anesthesia may be induced. This is usually accomplished using fast-onset intravenous agents, such as thiopental or etomidate. The goal is rapid but smooth induction of the unconscious state so that rapid control of the airway and hyperventilation may be quickly reestablished using bag and mask. More intravenous agents (thiopental, etomidate, fentanyl, lidocaine) are titrated in prior to laryngoscopy and intubation. The goal is to administer enough of these anesthetic agents to blunt the hypertensive response to tracheal intubation without excessively depressing the blood pressure prior to intubation.

Constant attention to the arterial line pressure during induction is thus critical. Everything possible is done to avoid blood pressure changes. Hypotension and hypertension are quickly but carefully treated with vasopressors or depressors, fluids, and table position.

A neuromuscular blocker is administered to facilitate laryngoscopy, since coughing, straining, or bucking can increase ICP. Of note, the fast-onset, short-acting neuromuscular blocker succinylcholine has been reported to increase ICP in animals and humans. The increase in ICP, however, appears to be reliably prevented in both animals and humans by "defasciculation" (administration of a small subparalyzing dose of a nondepolarizing neuromuscular blocker a few minutes prior to the administration of succinylcholine). The slower acting, nondepolarizing neuromuscular blockers (curare, pancuronium, metacurine, vecuronium, atracurium) do not appear to have any significant direct effect on ICP, but histamine-mediated systemic hypotension may be seen with rapid administration of large doses of curare and possibly atracurium.

As soon as the trachea is intubated and tube position confirmed by auscultation, the tube is carefully secured either with adhesive tape or by suturing around the jaw or teeth (Fig. 2). Hyperventilation is then resumed, and an arterial blood gas determination is made.

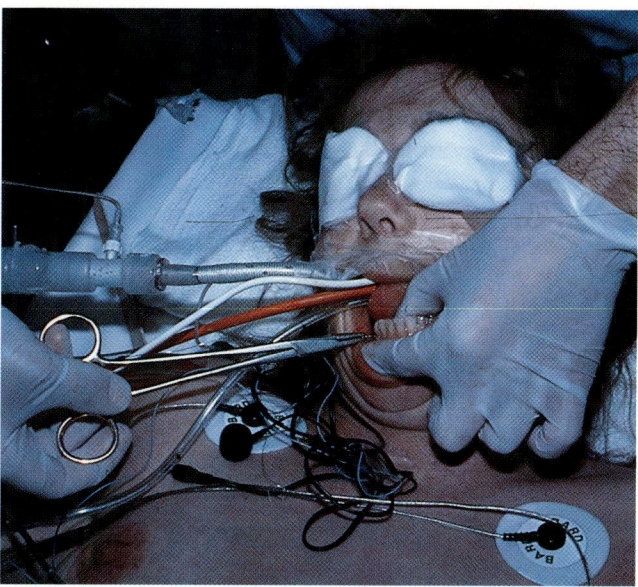

FIG. 2. Careful securing of the endotracheal tube by means of adhesive tape and wire suturing around the teeth or the jaw.

General anesthesia is maintained with a combination of drugs (component anesthesia). Agents are selected that lack undesirable effects on $CMRO_2$ and intracranial dynamics and that are compatible with the individual patient's medical condition (e.g., cardiovascular disease).

A narcotic-based technique is frequently employed for several reasons: hemodynamic stability; decrease in $CMRO_2$; effective blunting of the hypertensive response to surgical stimulation; lack of increase in ICP; and availability of antagonists (Narcan) that make reversal possible at the end of the case. Our narcotic agent of choice is usually fentanyl, because it is shorter acting and produces less blood pressure depression than morphine. Based on the pharmacokinetics of fentanyl in normal patients, I prefer to build up a fentanyl base of approximately 8–10 μ/kg during induction and prior to incision, and to supplement with 1–2 $\mu g/kg/hr$ as needed throughout the case. We attempt to discontinue all narcotics in the last 1–2 hr of the procedure in order to achieve rapid awakening. Sufentanil shares these properties with fentanyl; however, sufentanil was recently reported to produce significant cerebral vasodilation and increase in ICP in dogs.

We frequently employ a low-dose (1–2 mg/kg/hr) infusion of pentothal as one component of our anesthetic, because barbiturates can reduce ICP and may afford some brain protection during cerebral ischemia. However, even the ultra-short-acting barbiturate pentothal can accumulate and produce hypotension or delayed awakening. Since there is no available antidote for barbiturates, we discontinue pentothal infusions routinely 1–2 hr prior to the anticipated end of the case (or even earlier for cases of very long duration or patients who are elderly, debilitated, or have hepatic dysfunction).

Neuromuscular blockers are frequently used in neurosurgical anesthesia because they help ensure a still surgical field while permitting a "light" anesthetic, facilitate mechanical hyperventilation, and are reversible with available antagonists at the end of the case. One notable situation in which neuromuscular blockers are undesirable is during EMG monitoring for identification of cranial nerves. In these cases, a deeper level of general anesthesia, with its attendant risk for profound cardiovascular depression, must be maintained to keep the patient from moving.

The inhalational agent isoflurane may be used to help maintain general anesthesia, prevent intraoperative awareness, and decrease $CMRO_2$. The cerebral vasodilation and increased ICP induced by the inhalational agents can be minimized by hyperventilation and use of low concentrations. The use of inhalational agents is often necessary when intraoperative EMG monitoring is required, since this precludes the use of neuromuscular blockers.

Application of the skull-pin head-holder and surgical incision are potent stimuli that can produce acute hypertension. Infiltration of these sites with local anesthetic solution helps blunt this acute hypertensive response.

A "light" anesthetic technique is usually desirable for intracranial surgery, so that the patient awakens quickly after the conclusion of the surgical procedure. This permits an early baseline postoperative neurological exam and thus allows early detection of neurosurgical complications, and hopefully earlier intervention. It is our belief that intracranial surgery renders the CNS exquisitely sensitive to all CNS depressants. This may result from the multiple mechanical, thermal, and chemical insults sustained by the brain during surgery. Exposure of the brain to cold, dry air, electrocautery, retraction ischemia, and irrigation with antibiotic-containing solutions must disturb the normally finely tuned milieu of the CNS. As a result, prolonged and more profound sedation and respiratory depression seem to result from doses of drugs that do not excessively sedate patients undergoing noncraniotomy procedures.

Thus, in order to reliably achieve the goal of prompt emergence, several steps may be taken. First, all anesthetic agents need to be given in lower, titrated doses. Second, agents that are short-acting, or easily washed out, or for which there are available antagonists or "reversal agents" should be used. Long-acting sedatives should be avoided. Third, a thorough knowledge and skillful application of the pharmacokinetics of each drug, both in healthy patients and in patients with impaired drug metabolism (renal or hepatic insufficiency, abnormal blood chemistries), are necessary. Fourth, anesthetic agents should be discontinued or withheld for enough in advance of the end of the case to facilitate prompt emergence. Adequate neuromuscular blockade keeps lightly anesthetized patients from moving during the closure. As can be seen, planning for the emergence from anesthesia begins prior to the selection of premedication and induction agents.

Fluid Management

Many cranial base tumor patients are hypovolemic on the day of surgery due to a variety of reasons, including poor oral intake, administration of diuretics and radiocontrast dyes, and supine diuresis (10–13). Excessive fluid deficits may lead to electrolyte disorders, such as hypokalemia, which can predispose to intraoperative arrhythmias. Significant hypovolemia can also be particularly dangerous during the induction of general anesthesia and positive pressure ventilation, because it may lead to profound hypotension and compromised cerebral perfusion. Hypovolemia with low CVP may also predispose to venous air embolism.

Preoperative fluid deficits and intraoperative fluid losses must therefore be replaced judiciously to prevent excessive hypotension and organ ischemia on induction and during maintenance of general anesthesia. Efforts should also be made to avoid profound hypovolemia secondary to excessive intraoperative administration of diuretics. In our experience, overdiuresis almost invariably results in the need to replace large amounts of fluid just to maintain acceptable blood pressures under general anesthesia; aggressive diuresis is thus felt by us to be of questionable value.

On the other hand, excessive fluid administration may produce increased cerebral edema and intracranial pressure, particularly in the presence of a disrupted blood–brain barrier. Thus our general philosophy is to maintain the patient's volume status near the "dry" side of normovolemia, just sufficient to maintain adequate blood pressures under general anesthesia. This is accomplished by continuous monitoring of arterial and central venous or pulmonary artery pressure and urine output.

Cerebral edema is especially a concern with transfusion of hypotonic solutions (such as half-normal saline), which behave like free water and rapidly cross the blood–brain barrier. Since glucose is rapidly metabolized, the administration of solutions that contain only glucose (such as D5W) is physiologically nearly equivalent to administering distilled water. For these reasons, hypotonic solutions are avoided in intracranial surgery, and isotonic electrolyte solutions (normal saline, lactated Ringer's, Plasmalyte-A, and Normosol) are preferred. Of the isotonic crystalloid solutions, we prefer to use Plasmalyte or Normosol because their compositions, particularly pH and osmolality, so closely resemble that of normal serum.

Replacement of fluid deficits with colloid solutions

(5% albumin, plasma protein fraction, or hetastarch) may be helpful in minimizing cerebral edema. These solutions are effective volume expanders. In the presence of an intact blood–brain barrier, these molecules remain in the intravascular space longer than isotonic crystalloid solutions. Studies in normal rabbits suggest that increases in brain water and ICP are reduced when colloids are used for hemodilution instead of crystalloid solutions. We therefore use 5% albumin and plasma protein fraction (PPF) fairly liberally for volume replacement in neurosurgical patients. Both of these products are derived from human plasma but both are heat treated and are felt to be free of infectious risk. It should be noted that disruptions of the blood–brain barrier in an experimental model using cold thermal injury produced a marked increase in albumin permeability in cats. The starch-derived colloid solution hetastarch (Hespan) should probably be administered with caution in neurosurgical patients because of its potential, when administered in large doses (e.g., greater than 1.5 liters in an average-sized patient), to produce a heparin-like coagulopathy.

There is now evidence suggesting that hyperglycemia (even blood glucose levels as low as 160–180 mg/dl) may worsen neurologic outcome in ischemic cerebral injuries. The reason for this phenomenon is unclear. It is therefore prudent to avoid glucose-containing solutions in neurosurgical patients, because of the risk of cerebral ischemia. Intraoperative blood glucose levels should be checked periodically.

Positioning

Special attention must be given to proper positioning of skull base surgery patients. Close cooperation and planning between the anesthesiologist and surgeon are important.

For cranial base tumors that involve the anterior and middle cranial base, most of our patients are placed in the supine position with the head turned and secured by either the Mayfield skull clamp or horseshoe headrest. Posterior fossa procedures are usually performed in the lateral or prone positions. The sitting position is rarely, if ever, used at the University of Pittsburgh.

Frequently in neurosurgery, the head is deliberately elevated in order to improve venous drainage from the wound and to facilitate surgical exposure. Head elevation, however, may have adverse effects, with the greatest risk associated with the full-sitting position. Complications may include orthostatic hypotension and decreased cerebral perfusion pressure, endotracheal tube and atrial catheter tip migration, tension pneumocephalus, and venous air embolism.

Careful protection of pressure points is necessary to prevent injury to weight-bearing areas such as the scapulae, elbows, sacrum, calves, and heels. We advocate the routine use of an egg crate foam mattress. Additionally, care is taken to pad all joints and to place all joints in an anatomically neutral position to prevent joint and nerve injury. In the awake patient, ligaments and muscles limit the motion of joints. Since muscle tone is obtunded by anesthesia, excessive joint extension or flexion may occur when a patient is lifted or turned. Damage to joints and adjacent structures is a distinct possibility.

Special care must be taken to protect the "down" ear from folding and bearing weight during long cases in the lateral position. A dedicated stretcher *must* be kept immediately outside the operating room during cases in the lateral or prone positions. Should CPR become necessary, the patient can be flipped onto the stretcher and resuscitated in the supine position.

Finally, steps are taken to minimize the tendency for venous stasis and consequent thrombosis in the legs. Thigh-high antiembolism stockings are used in addition to encircling pneumatic wraps (TED Sequential Compression Device) that are intermittently inflated from distal to proximal to compress and massage the legs.

Facilitating Surgical Exposure

Surgical exposure of the brain can be enhanced by the administration of diuretics, hyperventilation to lower arterial Pco_2, reduction of cerebral venous pressure, control of arterial blood pressure, and removal of CSF (14–16).

Mannitol is the osmotherapeutic agent of choice for ICP reduction, either alone or in combination with furosemide. Mannitol causes withdrawal of brain water into the intravascular compartment, thereby decreasing brain bulk. Although doses between 0.5 and 2.0 g/kg were used in the past, lower doses (0.25 g/kg) have proved to be as effective. Beneficial effects can be seen as soon as 15 min after administration. Mannitol must be used cautiously in patients with congestive heart failure, as transient intravascular hypervolemia ensues, which may increase CVP, blood pressure, and ICP. A small (5–10 mg) dose of furosemide may be given prior to mannitol to avoid this problem. The ability of loop diuretics (furosemide) to lower ICP without raising intravascular volume or blood osmolality is theoretically an advantage over the osmotic diuretics. Furosemide has been shown to potentiate the brain bulk-reducing effects of mannitol. Reports of the effectiveness of furosemide alone in the treatment of intracranial hypertension have been conflicting. Small doses (5–10 mg) of furosemide may induce a large diuresis under general anesthesia. Therefore, to avoid unnecessary fluid shifts and electrolyte losses, it is best to start with low doses of diuretics.

Hyperventilation to lower arterial Pco_2 reduces cerebral blood volume, thereby reducing brain bulk and ICP.

In cooperative individuals, voluntary hyperventilation starts prior to anesthesia induction. When this is not possible, airway control is obtained as early as possible following induction, and hyperventilation is rapidly initiated. In previously normocapnic patients, acute hyperventilation to a P_{CO_2} range of 25–30 mm Hg probably provides maximum intracranial decompression with minimal risk of cerebral ischemia. Acute reductions in P_{CO_2} to 20 mm Hg or less are avoided since this may reduce cerebral blood flow to the point of ischemia and may produce alkalosis, which can decrease the release of oxygen from hemoglobin to tissues.

Surgical exposure can also be facilitated by reduction of cerebral venous pressure with a slight head-elevated position. Application of positive end-expiratory pressure (PEEP) or other ventilatory patterns that increase mean intrathoracic pressure have a potential to increase cerebral venous pressure and ICP in patients on mechanical ventilation. Muscle relaxants help reduce elevated ICP in patients by decreasing resistance to mechanical ventilation.

Careful control of blood pressure can help improve surgical exposure. Systemic blood pressure is usually maintained at low-normal levels during most of the surgical dissection, except in the case where carotid artery clamping is required. Deliberate hypotension reduces blood loss and the number of transfusions and the clear surgical field can improve surgical conditions and reduce surgical time. However, the neurosurgeons at the University of Pittsburgh rarely request deliberate hypotension. The blood pressure is maintained in the high-normal range during carotid cross-clamping.

Withdrawal of CSF through a lumbar subarachnoid catheter may improve surgical exposure (Fig. 3). We commonly place the catheters into the lumbar subarachnoid space at L3–L4 in the lateral position following induction of anesthesia, after adequate neuromuscular blockade to assure patient immobility and after the patient is being hyperventilated. Since CSF is formed at a rate of 0.35–0.40 ml/min, with a total CSF volume of 150 ml, slow withdrawal of 20–60 ml of CSF usually results in excellent relaxation of intracranial contents. Drainage is usually initiated at the request of the surgeon.

POTENTIAL COMPLICATIONS

Cranial Nerve Cardiovascular Reflexes

Abrupt reflex cardiovascular alterations frequently occur during cranial base surgery because of surgical manipulations near the eye, the carotid body in the neck, the dura, the brain stem, or the cranial nerves in the posterior cranial fossa (17–19). The trigeminal and vagus nerves are commonly involved. The acute alterations include severe hypotension or hypertension, severe brady- and tachy-dysrhythmias, cardiac conduction abnormalities, and other ECG changes. The surgeon should be immediately notified of any arrhythmia or hemodynamic aberration so that the offending stimulation (retraction, traction, irrigation) of the brain stem or cranial nerve can quickly be discontinued. In most cases, the cardiovascular change is transient and disappears shortly after the surgical stimulus is removed. Treatment with antiarrhythmic drugs is rarely necessary unless the arrhythmia is life-threatening and sustained.

Venous Air Embolism

Air bubbles can enter or be drawn into the circulation during craniotomy, particularly when the surgical field is above the level of the heart and when the CVP is low (34–40). The site of entry is frequently felt to be noncollapsible venous channels such as diploic veins and dural sinuses. Although air embolism is most commonly associated with sitting craniotomies, an 8% incidence (as detected by precordial Doppler) has been reported with craniotomies in the lateral position. Entrainment of air may be slow and continuous. Air bubbles that embolize the pulmonary vasculature may increase pulmonary dead space and thus reduce the expired end-tidal carbon dioxide concentration measured on capnography, impair gas exchange, and produce hypercarbia, hypoxia, and pulmonary vasoconstriction. Large air emboli may form an "air lock" (right ventricular filling pressures and cardiac output), resulting in hypotension, arrhythmias, and cardiovascular collapse. In addition, venous air bubbles may occasionally cross into the left side of the heart via

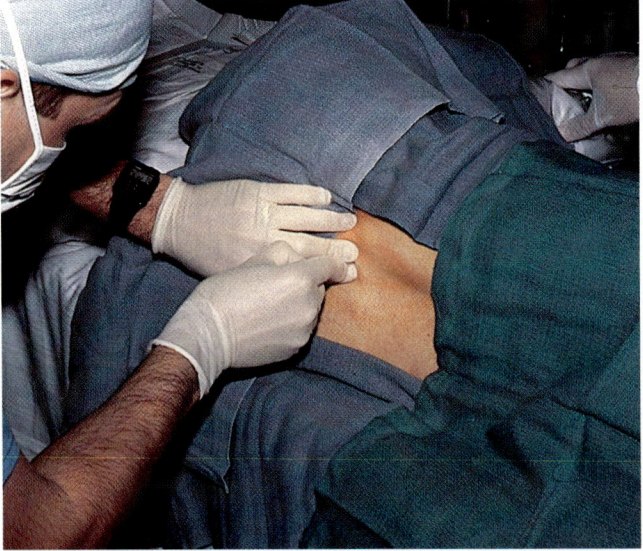

FIG. 3. Insertion of lumbar CSF drain in the lateral decubitus position.

an intracardiac defect or pulmonary shunt and become arterial or "paradoxical" air emboli. It is noteworthy that 27% of patients with no known heart disease have a probe patent foramen ovale and thus are at risk for paradoxical air embolism in the presence of venous air embolism.

Prevention, early detection, and rapid treatment of venous air embolism are thus very important. Preventative measures include avoiding "head-up" positions as much as possible, as well as avoiding sever hypovolemia (i.e., low CVP).

Several monitoring modalities assist in detection of air in the circulation. The most sensitive widely used modality is the precordial Doppler ultrasound transducer, which can detect as little as 0.1 ml of air and even microbubbles in a saline flush. Larger air emboli may be detected by an acute decrease in end-tidal CO_2, acute appearance of an increase in end-tidal nitrogen (N_2) gas, or increase in pulmonary artery pressure. Late occurring manifestations of large air emboli include "millwheel" murmur detectable via the esophageal stethoscope, hypotension, cardiac arrhythmias, or ECG changes suggestive of right heart strain. Transesophageal echocardiography, a relatively new technology still not in widespread clinical use, may be the most sensitive method for detecting air emboli in the circulation.

The first step in managing an air embolism should be to notify the surgeon of its occurrence so that the source of air entry can be identified and closed with bone wax or sutures. Flooding the surgical field with irrigation solution can transiently halt the entrainment of air and be a very useful temporizing measure.

The patient should be immediately placed in the headdown position to raise the CVP and to diminish the negative pressure gradient between the surgical field and the heart. If possible, the table is rotated so that the patient is in the "left side down" position. This may help prevent a large air bubble in the right atrium or ventricle from moving into the pulmonary outflow tract and forming an "air lock."

Nitrous oxide, if being used, should be discontinued since nitrous oxide dissolved in the blood will difuse into and thus expand air bubbles, and since 100% inspired oxygen may be desirable should cardiovascular or respiratory compromise ensue.

The CVP catheter should be aspirated to withdraw some of the air bubbles from the central circulation. Special CVP catheters and pulmonary artery catheter introducer sheaths with multiple side holes have been designed to enhance the efficacy of air aspiration.

Elevation of the CVP and maintenance of hemodynamic stability by volume infusion and vasopressors may be desirable or necessary. In addition, jugular venous compression or a positive pressure Valsalva maneuver may aid the surgeon in detecting the open vessel responsible for the air entry. The use of positive end-expiratory pressure (PEEP) to elevate intrathoracic pressure to prevent further emboli is controversial. The concern is that PEEP might differentially increase right atrial pressure, resulting in a right-to-left shunt, and thus possibly paradoxical air embolism, in patients with a patent foramen ovale. Experiments to test this hypothesis have been inconclusive.

Blood Transfusion and Coagulopathy

Blood loss may be extensive in skull base surgery, especially with highly vascular tumors and extensive reconstruction of the cranium. Transfusion-related coagulopathies (31–33) can occur after infusion of multiple units (usually 10 or more) of stored blood. Coagulopathy can be a devastating problem in neurosurgery, since even a small intracranial hematoma can produce significant mass effect in the rigid cranial vault. Coagulopathy may manifest as oozing into the surgical field, hematuria, gingival bleeding, or bleeding from venous puncture sites. When such bleeding occurs in a patient who did not have a coagulopathy preoperatively, the differential diagnosis is either dilutional thrombocytopenia, deficiencies of clotting factors (V, VIII), disseminated intravascular coagulation (DIC), or hemolytic transfusion reaction. There have also been reports suggesting that surgical disruption of brain tissue itself can produce a coagulopathy.

Therefore "STAT" intraoperative coagulation studies should be obtained at the earliest suspicion of coagulopathy, in order to guide rational management. The studies we feel are most useful are the prothrombin time (PT), partial thromboplastin time (PTT), platelet count, Ivy bleeding time, and the thromboelastogram (TEG). The first three are sent by special courier to the coagulation lab and labeled "STAT for OR"; the latter two are performed in the OR. We do not hesitate to obtain "STAT" intraoperative hematology consults for more complex coagulopathies not responsive to platelets or fresh frozen plasma (FFP). Anticipation of ongoing need for blood products and close communication with the blood bank are important.

Statistically, dilutional thrombocytopenia is the most common cause of a hemorrhage problem in a patient who has received multiple units of blood. Transfusion of 8–10 units of platelet concentrate is indicated when this is documented or highly suspected.

Protein clotting factors, particularly V and VIII, are labile in stored whole blood. They are even more scarce in packed red blood cells, where much of the plasma (and therefore the clotting factors) has been removed in the blood banking process. Therefore clotting factor deficiency or dilution may occur when large amounts of whole blood older than a few days or packed red blood cells are given to a patient. The treatment is fresh frozen plasma (FFP) or specific factor concentrates. A useful clinical guideline is that 2 units of FFP and 8–10 units of platelet concentrate may be needed after every 5–10 units of blood transfused to restore diluted clotting elements.

Other complications of blood transfusions include hypothermia, transfusion reactions (hemolytic, febrile, and allergic), disease transmission (viral hepatitis in 7% of transfused patients, AIDS), citrate intoxication causing hypocalcemia, and infusion of microaggregates.

As a general rule, we try to keep the hemoglobin level at or above approximately 10 g/dl in patients who had normal preoperative levels. We feel this is a reasonable compromise between minimizing blood transfusion with its attendant risks and yet assuring a reasonable blood oxygen carrying capacity. It is advisable to continue supplemental oxygen for several days into the postoperative period if the patient's hemoglobin is allowed to drop intraoperatively.

Predeposit of autologous blood (autodonation) is becoming a more routine procedure at the University of Pittsburgh. Predonation is suitable for many patients scheduled for elective surgical procedures in which the need for transfusion is anticipated. Donations may be scheduled as frequently as every 72 hr, with the last phlebotomy performed at least 72 hr prior to surgery to permit restoration of plasma volume. Withdrawal of four or more units is possible if oral iron therapy is administered. Autologous red blood cell products have a shelf life of 35–42 days, depending on the preservative employed.

We also employ a device that salvages and reinfuses blood ("cell saver") from extradural sites when skull base tumors are contained within the dura. Such blood has the advantages of being completely compatible, warm, and immediately available. Contraindication includes tumor cell contamination of the salvaged blood, and thus the surgeon and anesthesiologist must determine whether or not autotransfusion is appropriate prior to each operation.

Carotid Artery Cross-Clamping

It is sometimes necessary to temporarily cross-clamp or permanently sacrifice the carotid artery during resection of tumors near the cavernous sinus (1,20–24). Preoperative assessment of the adequacy of collateral cerebral blood flow is made by a carotid balloon test occlusion during arteriography in patients in whom carotid clamping is a consideration. It is important intraoperatively during carotid cross-clamping to maintain the systemic arterial pressure at or slightly above the upper level of the patient's normal blood pressure in order to maintain adequate collateral blood flow; careful infusion of volume or vasopressors may be necessary.

Cerebral ischemia and seizures are the two major concerns during carotid cross-clamping. Both of these conditions can be detected on electroencephalogram (EEG). Patients in whom carotid clamping is a possibility are started on phenytoin anticonvulsant therapy preoperatively. Serum phenytoin levels are checked to confirm therapeutic levels.

The ideal level of P_{CO_2} during cerebral ischemia is controversial. There is theoretical concern that hyperventilation could actually reduce collateral blood flow to ischemic areas, since hypocarbia produces cerebral vasoconstriction in normal cerebral arterioles. However, local accumulation of acid metabolites in ischemic areas causes cerebral vessels to dilate, a situation known as vasomotor paralysis. It has thus been proposed that if blood pressure is maintained during focal cerebral ischemia, hyperventilation-induced vasoconstriction may shunt blood away from normal areas of brain and toward the ischemic but vasodilated areas, a potentially favorable phenomenon. This has been referred to as "inverse steal" or "Robin Hood" syndrome (taking from the rich to give to the poor). Since there is no practical way of knowing what will actually happen to regional CBF in a given patient, most anesthesiologists maintain *normo*carbia for patients undergoing carotid surgery (e.g., endarterectomy). Thus the advantages of hyperventilation to reduce brain bulk must be weighed against the potential benefits of normocapnia during regional cerebral ischemia. Hypercarbia is most likely detrimental in both of these respects and therefore undesirable.

The subject of cerebral protection from ischemia has deservedly received much attention. Since most anesthetic agents reduce cerebral metabolic rate and thus demand, in theory they could protect the brain during ischemia. Barbiturates, in doses that produce burst suppression on the EEG, have been fairly convincingly demonstrated to improve neurologic and neuropathologic outcome in acute focal ischemia in animal models. This protective effect has been demonstrated when barbiturates were administered before, or as long as 30 min after, the ischemic insult. The mechanism for this protection may be a reduction in cerebral metabolic demand or vasoconstriction of normal vessels, which may improve the distribution of CBF to ischemic areas. Because of these studies, we feel that administration of pentothal prior to carotid cross-clamping is rational. This must be done cautiously because a large dose of pentothal may depress the blood pressure. There is some evidence in animals that isoflurane may also have cerebral protective effects against ischemia. Many other drugs (anticonvulsants, corticosteroids, local anesthetics, calcium channel blockers, anti-inflammatory agents, free radical scavengers) are being studied for possible protection against cellular injury in different scenarios of cerebral ischemia. To date, results have been insufficient to warrant routine clinical use of these agents.

Tension Pneumocephalus

Air frequently collects in the intracranial spaces during neurosurgery (25-31). In fact, small subdural pneumocephalus is frequently detected on postcraniotomy CT scan or skull film and is generally felt to be of little clinical significance. However, if present in sufficient volume and under pressure, subdural intracranial gas may produce mass effect and severe postoperative focal or global neurologic pneumocephalus.

Pneumocephali as large as several hundred milliliters have been reported. Subdural air probably begins to accumulate intraoperatively when the dura is opened. Air presumably is drawn in as CSF leaks out and as the brain shrinks due to hyperventilation, steroids, and diuretics. The most dramatic cases of large postcraniotomy pneumocephalus have been reported in patient whose operations were performed in the sitting position and in patients with CSF drainage devices in whom excessive CSF drainage occurred inadvertently. With closure of the dura, air loculates intracranially and usually dissects to the frontal portion of the cranial vault due to the usual supine position of the patient following surgery. As the brain expands postoperatively (due to surgical edema and cessation of hyperventilation and reaccumulation of CSF), the presence of a large pneumocephalus can increase ICP and produce cerebral compression.

An interesting link may exist between tension pneumocephalus and venous air embolism. The arachnoid granulations of the cerebral venous sinuses act as one-way valves to allow CSF to flow into the superior sagittal sinus when a critical opening pressure is reached. Saidman and Eger (28) have postulated that gas under pressure in the intracranial CSF space might escape via the arachnoid granulations into the venous blood as venous air emboli. Luce (30) has demonstrated that intracranial gas under pressure can produce venous gas emboli (which could be misdiagnosed as neurogenic pulmonary edema).

Nitrous oxide dissolved in the blood can diffuse from the bloodstream into gas-containing spaces in the body and produce an increase in volume or pressure. There has thus been concern that nitrous oxide might enter an intracranial air pocket and enlarge the size of a pneumocephalus. It has therefore been suggested by some authors that nitrous oxide be discontinued (or its inspired concentration diminished) just prior to dural closure.

Other reasonable practices to help reduce the risk of pneumocephalus include filling the surgically created cavity with fluid before closure of the dura and diminishing the degree of hyperventilation a bit to reexpand the brain prior to dural closure.

The risk of postoperative tension pneumocephalus is one more indication for attempting to tailor an anesthetic plan that will allow rapid awakening and early postoperative neurologic evaluation. The presence of unexpected postoperative neurologic deficit not easily attributable to the surgery or anesthetic should signal the possibility of tension pneumocephalus in the differential diagnosis. Definitive diagnosis can be made with an emergency CT scan and frequently even with lateral plain skull films. The treatment consists of emergency decompression of the gas pocket via twist drill holes into the cranium overlying the pneumocephalus.

Hypothermia

Heat loss and hypothermia are common intraoperative complications in surgical patients under general anesthesia. A number of factors contribute to this phenomenon, including: cold ambient operating room temperatures; heat loss via the respiratory tract due to the cold, dry inspired anesthetic gases; heat loss due to evaporation of the skin prep and via the surgical incision; decreased metabolic rate under general anesthesia; impairment of homeothermic mechanisms (such as cutaneous vasoconstriction and shivering) by general anesthetics; and administration of cold irrigation and intravenous fluids, especially refrigerated blood products.

Because it lowers cerebral metabolic rate, deliberate profound hypothermia was popular 15-20 years ago for cerebral protection against ischemia. Profound hypothermia has since fallen into disfavor for several reasons: it can depress myocardial contractility, increase myocardial irritability and the risk of life-threatening arrhythmias, shift the oxyhemoglobin dissociation curve toward decreased oxygen release, increase blood viscosity and compromise microcirculatory flow, and delay emergence from general anesthesia. For all these reasons, it is our practice to attempt to avoid large, rapid decreases in body temperature. Several modalities are employed, including heating and humidification of inspired anesthetic gases, use of both a water-heated blanket and a reflective "space blanket," and administration of all blood products through a warming device. In spite of these efforts, we usually observe a mild degree of hypothermia (34.5-35.5°C rectal) in our skull base tumor resections. This degree of mild to moderate hypothermia may actually afford some of the cerebral protective effects of more profound levels of hypothermia without some of the risks. Patients should be gradually rewarmed toward normothermia toward the end of the case to facilitate a rapid awakening from anesthesia.

Postoperative Airway Management

Intraoperative trauma to respiratory centers or to cranial nerves IX, X, and XII, direct surgical trauma to the upper airway, and placement of surgical pharyngeal packs are common during cranial base surgery and can have important airway management implications. Injury to cranial nerves IX, X, and XII may be associated with impaired upper airway sensation, swallowing dis-

TABLE 2. *Factors that affect postoperative airway management (extubate versus tracheostomy versus leave intubated) in cranial base surgery patients*

Difficult intubation preoperatively?
Pulmonary dysfunction preoperatively or intraoperatively?
Prolonged emergence from anesthesia and surgery? (obtunded patient?)
Hypothermia?
Preoperative or suspected intraoperative CN IX or X deficit?
Surgical involvement (hematoma, edema, TMJ dysfunction) of upper airway?

coordination, and vocal cord paralysis. We keep our patients intubated in the immediate postoperative period if there is any concern that trauma to the pharyngeal or laryngeal nerve supplies has occurred. This critical decision is always made in conjunction with the surgeons. If the patient's airway was difficult to manage on induction, even more caution is warranted postoperatively. See Table 2.

Nausea and Vomiting

Nausea and vomiting are frequently seen in the recovery room. Surgical manipulation of the middle ear, vestibular nerve, and posterior fossa, as well as drainage of blood into the stomach, may increase the incidence of nausea in some cranial base tumor patients. The increase in ICP that accompanies vomiting may be particularly detrimental in these patients.

It is therefore our practice to pass an oro- or nasogastric tube after the induction of anesthesia for decompression of gastric contents. Prophylactic administration of antiemetics intraoperatively may prolong emergence from general anesthesia because of sedative side effects. However, if the awake recovery room patient shows evidence of nausea, we quickly treat with intravenous droperidol, a butyrophenone, which in low doses (1.25 mg) is effective for antiemesis but does not produce significant sedation.

CONCLUSION

An operation for a lesion near the base of the brain is a complex endeavor, combining the unique challenges of anesthesia for neurosurgery, head and neck cancer surgery, and surgical procedures of long duration. Attention to details and close communication among all members of the health care team are key ingredients for success.

REFERENCES

1. Messick JM, Newberg LA, Nugent M, Faust RJ. Principles of neuroanesthesia for the non-neurosurgical patient with CNS pathology. *Anesth Analg* 1985;64:143.
2. Adams RW, Gronert GA, Sundt TM, Michenfelder JD. Halothane, hypocapnia and cerebrospinal fluid pressure in neurosurgery. *Anesthesiology* 1972;37:510.
3. Adams RW, Chucchiara RF, Gronert GA, Messick JM, Michenfelder JD. Isoflurane and cerebrospinal fluid pressure in neurosurgical patients. *Anesthesiology* 1981;54:97.
4. Grosslight K, Foster R, Colohan A, Bedford R. Isoflurane for neuroanesthesia: risk factors for increases in intracranial pressure. *Anesthesiology* 1985;63:533.
5. Egbert LD, Battit GE, Turndorf H, Beecher HK. The value of the preoperative visit by an anesthetist. *JAMA* 1963;185:553.
6. Berthoud M. Pre-oxygenation—how long? *Anaesthesia* 1983;38:96.
7. Haigh J, Nemoto E, DeWolf A, Bleyaert A. Comparison of the effects of succinylcholine and atracurium on intracranial pressure in monkeys with intracranial hypertension. *Can Anaesth Soc J* 1986;33:421.
8. Milde L, Milde J. The cerebral hemodynamic and metabolic effects of sufentanil in dogs (abstract). *Anesthesiol Rev* 1987;14:25.
9. Domino K. Anesthesia for cranial base tumor operations. In: Sekhar L, Schramm V, eds. *Tumors of the cranial base: diagnosis and treatment*. Mount Kisco, New York: Futura Publishing Company, 1987.
10. Smith DS. Fluid management of the neurosurgical patient. 37th Annual ASA Refresher Course Lectures, 1986.
11. Todd MM, Tommasino C. The effects of acute isovolemic hemodilution on the brain: a comparison of crystalloid and colloid solutions (abstract). *Anesthesiology* 1984;61:A122.
12. Gazendam J. Composition of isolated edema fluid in cold-induced edema. *J Neurosurg* 1979;51:70.
13. Lanier WL, Stangland KJ. The effects of dextrose infusion and head position on neurologic outcome after complete cerebral ischemia in primates. *Anesthesiology* 1987;66:39.
14. Marshall LF, Smith RW, Ranscher LA, Shapiro HM. Mannitol dose requirements in brain-injured patients. *J Neurosurg* 1978;48:169.
15. Schettin A, Stahurski B, Young HF. Osmostic and loop diuresis in brain surgery: effects on plasma and CSF electrolytes and ion excretion. *J Neurosurg* 1982;56:679.
16. Wilkinson HA, Rosenfeld S. Furosemide and mannitol in the treatment of acute experimental intracranial hypertension. *Neurosurgery* 1983;12:405.
17. Lall NG, Jain AP. Circulatory and respiratory disturbances during posterior cranial fossa surgery. *Br J Anaesth* 1969;41:447.
18. Drummond JC, Todd MM. Acute sinus arryhthmia during surgery in the fourth ventricle: an indication of brainstem irritation. *Anesthesiology* 1984;60:232.
19. Nagashima C. Cardiovascular complication on upper vagal rootlet section for glossopharyngeal neuralgia. *J Neurosurg* 1976;44:248.
20. Hoff JT, Smith AL, Hankinson HL, Nielsen SL. Barbiturate protection from cerebral infarction in primates. *Stroke* 1975;6:28.
21. Michenfelder JD, Milde JH. Influence of anesthetics on metabolic, functional and pathologic responses to regional cerebral ischemia. *Stroke* 1985;6:405.
22. Moseley JL, Lavrent JP, Molinary GF. Barbiturates attenuation of the clinical course and pathologic lesions in a primate stroke model. *Neurology* 1975;25:870.
23. Smith AL, Hoff JT, Nielsen SL, Larson CP. Barbiturate protection in acute focal cerebral ischemia. *Stroke* 1974;5:1.
24. Michenfelder JD, Milde JH, Sundt TM. Cerebral protection by barbiturate anesthesia. *Arch Neurol* 1976;33:345.
25. Lunsford LD, Maroon JC, Sheptak PE, Albin MS. Subdural tension pneumocephalus. *J Neurosurg* 1979;50:525.
26. Grundy BL, Spetzler RF. Subdural pneumocephalus resulting from drainage of cerebrospinal fluid during craniotomy. *Anesthesiology* 1980;52:269.
27. Toung T, Donham RT. Tension pneumocephalus after posterior fossa craniotomy. *Neurosurgery* 1983;12:164.
28. Saidman LF, Eger EI. Change in cerebrospinal fluid pressure during pneumoencephalograph under nitrous oxide anesthesia. *Anesthesiology* 1965;26:67.
29. Artru AA. Nitrous oxide plays a direct role in the development of tension pneumocephalus intraoperatively. *Anesthesiology* 1982;57:59.
30. Luce HM. Increasing intracranial pressure with air causes air em-

bolism, not neurogenic pulmonary edema. *J Appl Physiol* 1981;50:967.

31. Reed RL, Ciavarella D, Heimback DM, et al. Prophylactic platelet administration during massive transfusion. *Ann Surg* 1986; 203:40.
32. Miller RD, Brzica SM. Blood, blood component, colloid and autotransfusion therapy. In: Miller RD, ed. *Anesthesia.* New York: Churchill Livingstone, 1981;885.
33. Curran JW, Lawrence ON, Jaffe H, et al. Acquired immunodeficiency syndrome (AIDS) associated with transfusion, *N Engl J Med* 1984;310:69.
34. Albin MS, Carroll RG, Maroon JC. Clinical considerations concerning the detection of venous air embolism. *Neurosurgery* 1978;3:380.
35. Gronert GA, Messick JM, Cucchiara RF. Paradoxical air embolism from a patent foramen ovale. *Anesthesiology* 1979;50:548.
36. Gildenberg PL, O'Brien RP, Britt WJ. The efficacy of Doppler monitoring for the detection of venous air embolism. *J Neurosurg* 1981;54:75.
37. Matjasko J, Petrozza P, Mackenzie CF. Sensitivity of end-tidal nitrogen in venous air embolism detection in dogs. *Anesthesiology* 1985;63:418.
38. Cucchiara RF, Nugent M, Seward JB. Air embolism in upright neurosurgical patients: detection and localization by two-dimensional transesophageal echocardiography. *Anesthesiology* 1984; 60:353.
39. Bowdle TA, Artru AA. Treatment of air embolism with a special pulmonary artery catheter introducer sheath in sitting dogs. *Anesthesiol Rev* 1987;14:20.
40. Oliver S, Cucchiara R, Nishimura R, Michenfelder J. Parameters affecting the occurrences of paradoxical air embolism. *Anesthesiol Rev* 1987;14:22.
41. Gonzales RM, Khalouf FK. Special anesthetic challenges in skull base tumor surgery. In: Jackson CG, ed. *Surgery of skull base tumors.* New York: Churchill Livingstone, 1991.

CHAPTER 8

Methods of Neurophysiological Monitoring During Cranial Base Tumor Resection

Robert J. Sclabassi, Donald N. Krieger, Donald Weisz, and John Durrant

Surgical treatment of tumors at the base of the skull carries significant risk to the functioning of the cranial nerves, the brain stem, and the cerebral hemispheres. This risk is due both to problems associated with maintaining adequate blood supply to the brain stem and cerebral hemispheres and to the effect of various operative maneuvers aimed at adequately exposing the tumor and removing it. These risks may be reduced if appropriate information concerning the relationships between surgical manipulations and their impact on the functioning of the patient's central nervous system is available to the surgeon. In order to provide information of this type, aimed at reducing both the probability and severity of injury to the neural tissue, there have been developed and are being used methodologies for obtaining and evaluating multimodal neurophysiological measures in real-time, during surgery to the cranial base.

Intraoperative neurophysiological monitoring provides a real-time control loop around a system composed of the surgeon and the patient. The goals of this control loop are both the reduction of morbidity and a dynamic assessment of structure–function relationships of the patient's nervous system. This is accomplished by making specific and sensitive measurements that reflect the interactions between the surgeon's intraoperative manipulations and the functioning of the patient's central nervous system (CNS). These goals require obtaining real-time measurements of CNS function that can be closely correlated with operative manipulations. To achieve these goals within a time frame that is of value to the progress of the operation, multiple channels of data need to be acquired, processed, and displayed rapidly. At the University of Pittsburgh, these measurements are made using a distributed computer system (NeuroNet), developed specifically for this purpose. NeuroNet provides extensive multidimensional computing and data display capabilities in the operating room and remote sites.

This chapter reviews the intraoperative monitoring approach used by our group to provide multimodality, neurophysiological monitoring during cranial base tumor resection. In particular, we present a detailed description of our overall approach to this complex monitoring problem and of the system developed to implement this approach. The technical approaches to the acquisition and interpretation of these neurophysiological measures are then presented. Finally, we discuss the implications of this approach to the successful performance of cranial base surgery.

THE PITTSBURGH APPROACH

The surgeon needs information about the functional status of the nervous system, during surgery, in order to adapt the surgical strategy in such a way as to minimize morbidity. Immediate knowledge of the physiological effect of each surgical manipulation is an irreplaceable help in the pursuit of aggressive surgical techniques, such as those involved in operating at the cranial base (36). Thus the objective of intraoperative monitoring during cranial base tumor cases is to help the surgeon produce minimum morbidity; and when it is necessary to produce morbidity, to do so in a controlled fashion, that is,

---

R. J. Sclabassi, D. N. Krieger, and D. Weisz: Center for Clinical Neurophysiology, Department of Neurological Surgery, University of Pittsburgh School of Medicine, and Children's Hospital, Pittsburgh, Pennsylvania 15213.

J. Durrant: Center for Clinical Audiology, Department of Otolaryngology, University of Pittsburgh School of Medicine, and Montefiore University Hospital, Pittsburgh, Pennsylvania 15213.

to provide information about what is being done and what are its consequences.

It has long been appreciated that the patient's physiological status is dynamic, and that during surgery rapid and life-threatening changes may occur. This realization has led to the sophisticated patient monitoring by anesthesiologists where extensive physiological monitoring is routinely used to maintain the homeostatic status of the patient (10). This monitoring may be thought of as putting a control loop around the anesthesiologist and the patient for the purposes of life support. Some information is available from these procedures that also reflect the stress on the central nervous system, for example, changes in heart rate related to both brain stem and vagal stimulation. However, the comparative ability to evaluate the nervous system by either clinical means or by the commonly used physiological monitoring tools available to the anesthesiologists is limited during anesthesia.

These limitations in the ability to assess nervous system function have led to the development of neurophysiological intraoperative monitoring techniques. The various neurophysiological measures described in this chapter provide objective measures of nervous system function and have significant potential of providing ongoing and relevant information about the status of the central nervous system. Neurophysiological measures have value in many types of operative procedures (6,19,22); however, the ones described in this chapter are most useful in cranial base surgery, which requires particularly complex and lengthy surgical procedures.

Depending on the surgical procedure, we routinely measure electrical activity dependent on the functioning of the brain stem (brain stem auditory evoked potentials and brain stem somatosensory evoked potentials), the cortex (the electroencephalogram, somatosensory evoked potentials, and visual evoked potentials), and cranial nerves II, III, IV, V, VI, VII, VIII, X, XI, and XII. It is imperative that the measures utilized are both specific to the neural tissue being manipulated and sensitive to changes in the functioning of the neural tissue produced by the surgical manipulations. Many of these measures are obtained, displayed, and interpreted simultaneously, permitting a multidimensional assessment of the integrity of the neural structures at risk. In addition, many of these measures provide information not only about function itself but also about variables that indirectly affect function, such as blood flow, hypoxia, and hypotension.

An additional important aspect necessary for successful intraoperative monitoring is the planning and execution of surgical procedures in such a way that the neurophysiologists are in close communication with all other members of the surgical team, including surgeons, neuroanesthesiologists, and neuroradiologists. This preoperative and intraoperative communication between the members of the surgical team ensures that the appropriate neurophysiological measures are used during the case, that the neuroanesthesiologist is prepared to switch anesthetic technique in support of the requirements imposed by each technique, and that the significance of observed changes are appreciated by all members of the operative team.

Our conceptual approach requires that the neurophysiologist understand the nature of the patient's pathology, the operative strategy of the surgeon, and the anesthesiologist's approach to the management of that particular patient. It requires that the surgeon understand the level of information that the neurophysiologist can provide as the operative procedure is evolving, and it requires that the neuroanesthesiologist understand the effects of the pharmacological manipulations on the monitoring tools available to the neurophysiologist. Thus the keystone of the Pittsburgh approach to intraoperative monitoring is the close and continuous interchange of information between all the members of the surgical team.

Attention to detail begins prior to the patient being taken to the operating room. It is our policy that all patients for whom intraoperative monitoring is ordered undergo preoperative neurophysiological studies to determine baseline responses (see Figs. 6A and 7A). The reasons for this are many: these include introducing the neurophysiology monitoring concept to the patient, ensuring that the neurophysiologist understands the nature of the case to be monitored, ensuring that the peculiarities of the patient's responses be understood prior to arrival in the operating room, and determining the existence of unsuspected second lesions. This approach has the support of the surgeons, who write specific orders for every patient who is to be evaluated and monitored.

The neurophysiologists participate in preoperative discussions concerning patient management and also attend and participate in the surgical complications conferences. Thus the neurophysiologist has a detailed understanding of each patient and his or her unique monitoring requirements prior to the case, as well as an appreciation for the outcome of the case and for the role that intraoperative monitoring may have played in that outcome. This close coordination between the neurophysiologist and the surgeon not only ensures the most appropriate and highest quality intraoperative monitoring, but facilitates the evolution of improved monitoring techniques to better provide the types of information the surgeons need and desire.

The neurophysiologists must communicate with the surgeon and the anesthesiologist concerning the anesthetic requirements prior to the start of the case to ensure that no conflicts exist over the required anesthetic approach. For example, when will the use of paralytic or potent inhalation agents interfere with neurophysiological monitoring? Many of the monitoring procedures desired by the surgeons place competing and complex demands on the anesthesiologists. Thus a variety of anesthesia techniques may be used at different times during a single operative procedure to enable the appropriate neurophysiological measurements when needed.

Based on this information and on anticipation of what may happen, the appropriate subset of monitoring tools from the total armamentarium must be selected prior to the beginning of the case. For example, if an injury to a carotid artery occurs during tumor resection and it is desired to place the patient under pentobarbital protection, the neurophysiologists must be prepared to provide a measure of burst suppression from both ongoing electroencephalographic activity and median nerve evoked potentials. Thus the need for EEGs must have been anticipated prior to the draping of the patient. Finally, at some point prior to the actual beginning of surgery, the surgical team must be informed about the quality of the recordings, that is, how consistent or variable they are.

Pertinent information during the case is entered into the computer record and is appended to the operative data (see notes in Figs. 6B and 7B). These notes provide a permanent record of the case and alert the neurophysiologist observing the case across the network of any significant changes. In addition, a continuous log sheet with the time of each saved response, stimulating sites, and any additional information relevant to the operation is maintained.

THE MONITORING SYSTEM

The Center for Clinical Neurophysiology at the University of Pittsburgh has developed an intraoperative monitoring system, NeuroNet, specifically designed to implement the approach to intraoperative monitoring described in this chapter. NeuroNet is a distributed computing system based on work station and local area network technology, which provides user-transparent, shared file systems and powerful interprocess communication protocols to facilitate sharing and consulting on real-time neurophysiological data (16,17,28). This system is described in detail because it has allowed us to support as many as three cranial base tumor cases at the University Health Center of Pittsburgh while at the same time monitoring six or more other cases and three diagnostic laboratories.

Computer Network Architecture

The standard configuration of NeuroNet uses a 10-Mbit/sec Ethernet (IEEE 802.3) as its backbone, with functionally organized subnetworks implemented using 12-Mbit/sec token-passing rings (Fig. 1). The subnets are organized around functionally distinct activities to minimize the bandwidth required to support the transmission of data across the Ethernet. There are two advantages to this arrangement. First, data transmission rates for token-passing rings are greater, under high-demand loading, than for Ethernet, and the functional organization of the rings allows us to take advantage of this. Second, the subnets function as independent networks with the Ethernet serving as a link between them, providing robust local ring function; that is, if the Ethernet backbone fails, the subnets are not directly affected. Neu-

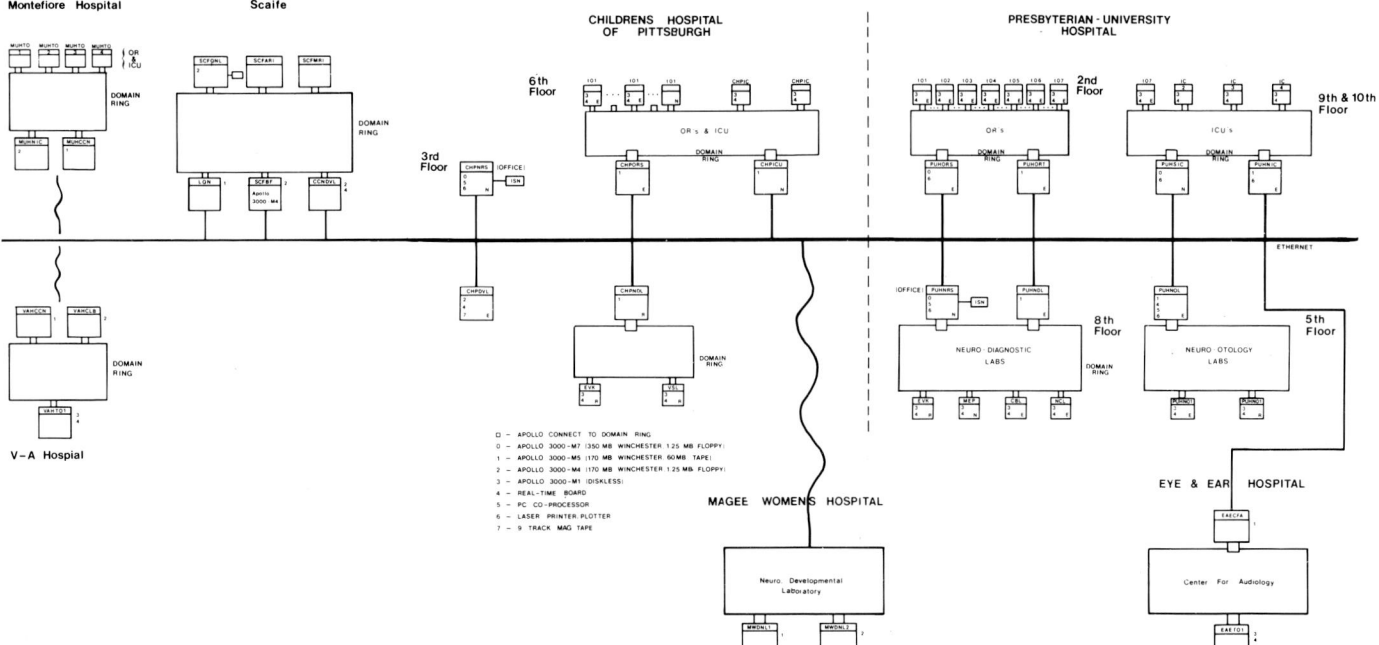

FIG. 1. NeuroNet configuration installed at the Center for Clinical Neurophysiology at the University of Pittsburgh. By using this distributed computer system, as many as three cranial base tumor and ten other surgical procedures have been monitored simultaneously.

roNet is supported by a set of decentralized file servers, a minimum of one to a subnet. On critical subnetworks, servers are placed in pairs to provide redundancy in case of hardware failure. In addition, the entire tree structured file system, available on the servers, is transparently accessible from any node on the network.

Instrumentation Systems

Diskless work stations are mounted in instrumentation racks and configured with appropriate electronics to support various data acquisition tasks including EEGs and EPs (Fig. 2A) and EMGs (Fig. 2B). The instrumentation racks are taken to whichever operating room the procedure is being performed in and booted, across the network, from the closest available server. Multiple racks may be used in parallel on the same case if the number of variables to be monitored is greater than the capacity of a single rack. The data being acquired on these systems are transparently accessible, in real-time, across the network for both review and analysis.

These instrumentation racks perform a number of functions, including stimulus control and generation, data acquisition, signal processing, and data display. Controllers for all peripheral devices sit on either a SCSI or AT-compatible bus that is interfaced to the 32-bit central bus. Each work station has a high-resolution (1024 by 1280 pixel), either black-and-white or 8-bit color monitor.

Data acquisition is accomplished through analog interface hardware on a single board: either the DT 2821 (Data Translation, Marlboro, MA) or the DAP 2400 (Microstar Laboratories, Redmond, WA). These boards include a 12-bit A/D converter with a 16-channel multiplexer, a two-channel 12-bit D/A converter, a 16-bit TTL I/O word, and a 1-MHz real-time programmable clock. On the DT board, interrupt-driven DMA block-mode transfers are supported for both A/D and D/A converter operation; while the Microstar board has a DSP chip and individual programmable control for both sampling rate and gain for each channel. All data manipulations are handled by calls to the NDF (Neuro Data File) library.

The EPs and EEGs are obtained simultaneously on the same instrumentation rack (Fig. 2A). This rack, besides a work station as described previously, includes a Grass Model 12-4 amplifier, a Grass Model S10DSCM somatosensory stimulator, and a Grass Model A10CTCM auditory stimulator. If visual evoked potentials are required, a Grass Model P22 stimulator configured to be used with fiber optics stimulating cables is used. In addition, the rack contains a four-channel oscilloscope for visually examining all data as they are obtained from the patient.

The EMGs are obtained from up to eight channels on an instrumentation rack specifically configured for this purpose (Fig. 2B). This rack may also be used for EEGs and EPs, as may the rack configured for EPs and EEGs be used for EMGs. This rack contains a Grass Model

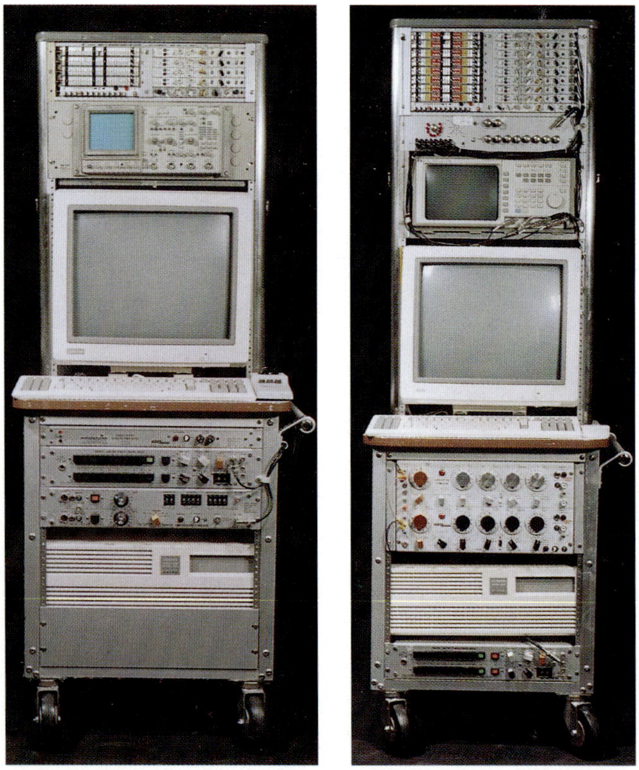

FIG. 2. A: EP and EEG instrumentation racks used in the operating room as part of the NeuroNet system. **B:** EMG instrumentation rack also used in support of these cases.

12-8 amplifier for recording the signals, and an eight-channel switchable auditory monitor for listening to the myogenic action potential activity on either all eight channels simultaneously or any one of the eight channels individually. The rack also contains a modified Grass Model 88 somatosensory stimulator used for direct stimulation of the cranial nerves. Finally, the rack also contains a four-channel oscilloscope for observing the unprocessed signals.

Signal Processing Algorithms

Real-time signal processing algorithms may be executed on the data acquired on any data acquisition node either on that node or on any other work station on the network. The algorithms implemented include a wide and constantly expanding set of signal processing capabilities including artifact rejection, averaging, moving averaging, digital filtering, integration, differentiation, differencing, peak detection and tracking, noise estimation, and various spectral estimators including discrete Fourier transforms, autoregressive procedures, and maximum likelihood procedures. Figure 3 shows an example of an averaged square wave, its moving average, digitally filtered version, and the estimated noise all acquired and displayed simultaneously.

Other signal processing capabilities, which have been integrated into the system and which are useful in monitoring cranial base tumor cases, include discrete Fourier transforms in parts (31), discrete Wigner–Ville distributions (32), complex demodulation (27,29), and instantaneous frequency (30).

In addition to signal processing, different display options are provided depending on the processing algorithm used. In the local display routines, whenever a signal processing function is invoked, the raw signal may also be displayed. This not only assists in recognition of any distortion, which may be introduced by the signal processing technique, but also facilities recognition of important signal features. Facilities are provided for display calculations in the same window or in separate windows, and for displaying subsegments of the results in separate windows (Fig. 4). Feature identification and tracking facilities are provided, which allow specific data components of interest to be identified, followed, and compared to baseline data in multiple windows simultaneously.

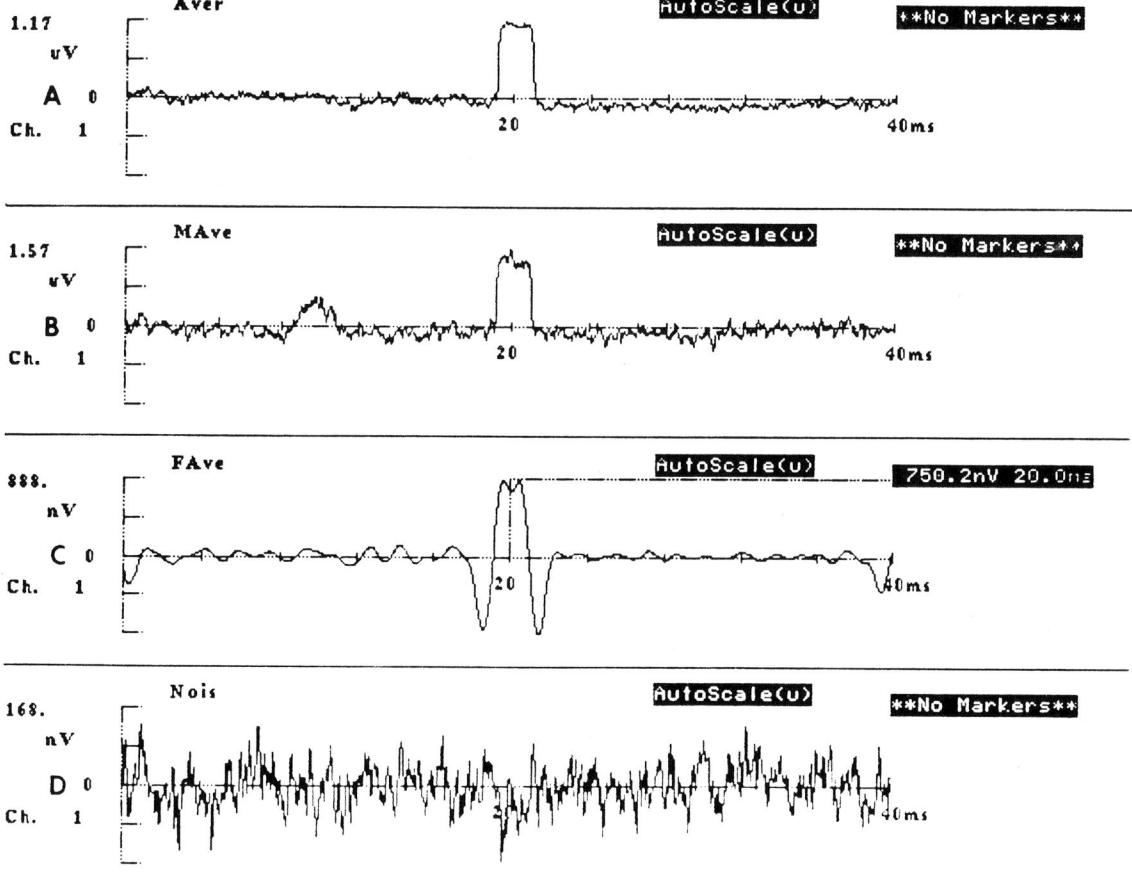

FIG. 3. Example of (**A**) averaged, (**B**) moving averaged, (**C**) digitally filtered average, and (**D**) noise signals displayed in one window of an instrumentation rack.

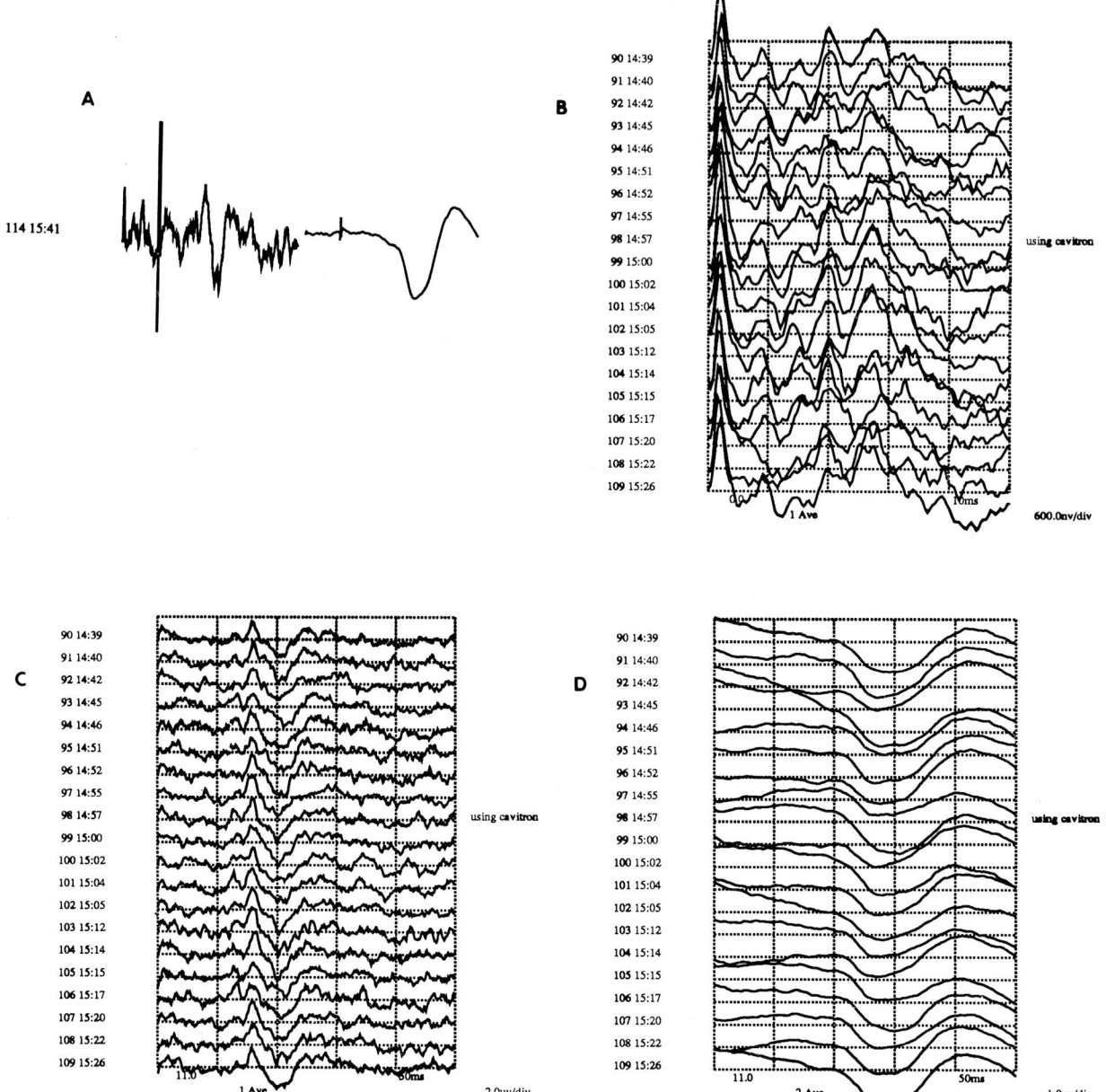

FIG. 4. Display of multimodality data from cranial base surgery. **A:** Combined data including BAEP, BSEP, and MSPs. Segmented waterfall display of **(B)** BAEPs, **(C)** BSEPs, and **(D)** MSPs.

NEUROPHYSIOLOGICAL MEASURES

The neurophysiological measures routinely used in this center provide a functional map of much of the entire neuraxis. These include: the electroencephalogram (EEG), an unstimulated measure of cortical function suitable for providing information concerning the degree of cortical activation related to either metabolic process (e.g., hypoxia) or to pharmacological manipulation (e.g., pentobarbital-induced burst suppression to protect the patient's cortical function) (21); the somatosensory and visual cortical potentials (SEPs and VEPs), which provide additional measures of cortical function specific to certain pathways and vasculature; the auditory and somatosensory brain stem potentials (BAEPs and BSEPs), which provide information about the functioning of the brain stem again specific to certain pathways (24); and finally, EMGs produced by muscles innervated by the various cranial nerves, which provide information about both the cranial nerves themselves and their underlying brain stem nuclei (14).

General Procedures

Neurophysiological recording during cranial base procedures can rapidly become quite complex. It is not unusual to monitor as many as nine different neurophysiological variables simultaneously; for example, EEG, BAEPs, and BSEPs, SEPs, and EMGs relating to five different cranial nerves (III, IV, V, VI, and VII). This requires a well organized and theoretically parsimonious approach to monitoring.

Where possible, all scalp electrodes are placed according to the International 10/20 system of electrode placement (33). Recording electrodes are placed symmetrically to provide for control recordings from the side contralateral to the surgery, even when electrodes may not be positioned in the standard recording sites. The patient is prepared for monitoring by measuring the head according to the 10/20 system and marking it appropriately for the desired electrode placement. If possible, this is accomplished in the operating room holding area, since this permits more accurate and rapid placement of electrodes in the operating room.

All recordings are performed using subdermal needle electrodes. Electrodes that are not in the operative field, but that are on the scalp and not accessible during surgery, are either sutured or stapled in place. Electrodes on the face, which are placed for recording EMG activity, are taped in place. Electrodes in the operative field are placed by the surgeons using sterile technique, usually early in the procedure. The electrodes are checked for impedance values and are accepted if the impedance is less than 10,000 ohms. If electrodes fail the impedance test and all connections are intact, the faulty electrodes are identified and replaced. In all cases, every effort is made to reduce noise and artifact to obtain a robust and consistent potential.

Baseline responses are obtained before draping the patient and compared to the preoperative evaluation. Significant differences must be accounted for, since signal deterioration may be due to patient positioning. The baseline responses are displayed as a background display on the computer monitor so that differences may be automatically calculated and displayed. A waterfall display window is used to follow the patterns of the change over a period of time during the case. New responses are automatically updated to this display as they are saved from the current data display. Thus the waterfall display provides a comparative record of the patient's data and facilitates the process of identifying significant changes in activity.

Neuroanesthetic Considerations

It is well known that the type of anesthesia, the patient's blood pressure, cerebral blood flow, body temperature, hematocrit, and blood gas tensions all affect the functioning of the patient's central nervous system and thus the intraoperatively observed neurophysiological measures (12).

The cranial base tumor cases are typically performed using isoflurane or a modified balanced narcotic procedure (7). However, muscle relaxants are rarely used, as the monitoring of the EMGs related to cranial nerve function is a major factor in the successful outcome of these cases.

The anesthesiologist typically uses constant infusion techniques to minimize the use of inhalation agents and to maintain as constant as possible a baseline level of functioning. The neurophysiologist notes whenever a medication bolus is given in anticipation of decrements in response quality.

Throughout the surgical procedures, close communication is maintained with the anesthesiologists regarding any changes in blood pressure, temperature, heart rate, or muscle tone, since changes in any of these variables may alter the responses.

Electroencephalogram

The functioning of the cerebral cortex is extremely sensitive to changes in arterial oxygenation and insufficient cerebral blood flow or an inadequate partial pressure of oxygen; this sensitivity is rapidly reflected in the EEG (18). Oxidative metabolism supplies the energy for maintainance of the membrane potential of nerve cells and the EEG is directly dependent on the transmembrane potentials of neurons; thus it reflects disturbances of cerebral metabolism such as hypoxia. Some factors that may contribute to ischemic events in cranial base tumor patients are decreased oxygen-carrying capacity due to hypovolemia or decreased cerebral perfusion pressure due to factors associated with decreased systemic arterial pressure, increased intracranial pressure, or mechanical obstruction of cerebral vessels (8).

The major use that we have seen in monitoring EEG during cranial base cases has been related to clamping and bypassing of the internal carotid artery in patients who have failed a preoperative blood flow study. This is usually related to the repair of a tear to the internal carotid artery, which can be associated with the removal of tumor from the cavernous sinus. To control the bleeding during a repair of this type, proximal and distal control of the internal artery is required, potentially reducing blood flow to the brain. Associated with this decreased availability of blood may be hypoxia caused by an inability of the remaining members of the vasculature to adequately perfuse the brain. The second most useful application of EEG monitoring in these cases has been to help define the occurrence of embolic phenomena, which is again represented by decreased blood flow and therefore potentially an ischemic event. In both of these situations EEG monitoring can be useful both to identify the presence of an insult and to define the degree of burst suppression if barbiturate brain protection is instituted.

We routinely provide two channels of continuous EEG monitoring during cranial base cases. This minimal configuration is felt to be adequate, since the problems we are, in general, concerned with are not related to precise focality but rather are of global or hemispheric importance. The electrode configuration utilized is P_3/F_3 and P_4/F_4, which provides two parasagittal planes, one on the operative side and the other contralateral to the operative side, providing a continuous comparative control. This electrode configuration may be simplified to P_3/F_z and P_4/F_z, if the desired frontal sites are not available. These same electrodes are also used to obtain cortical somatosensory evoked potentials; the dual function served permits a reduction in the number of electrodes used during the procedure. Because we routinely use these same electrodes to monitor the median nerve SEPs, we set the bandpass of the amplifiers to that which is appropriate for these measures; specifically, the high-pass filter is set at 1 Hz and the low-pass filter is set at 1000 Hz. The gain is set between 10,000 and 50,000 depending on the level of cerebral activity demonstrated by the anesthetized patient.

The EEG is observed both as the ongoing unprocessed signal and in a Fourier transformed representation (Fig. 5). The raw EEG is observed continuously on an oscilloscope, provided on each rack, and may also be observed on the work station screen. The oscilloscope is set to provide a 0.1-sec/div sweep speed to provide a rapid visual estimate of the continuous frequency. The Fourier transformed data may be displayed as either a compressed spectral array (CSA) or as a density spectral array (DSA), depending on the preference of the neurophysiologist. In either case, both the instantaneous frequency and the spectral edge may be estimated and overlaid on the displays. Because the signals, on which the spectra are being computed, have significantly higher frequency content than that normally of interest in the EEG, the spectral coefficients above an arbitrary value, typically 30 Hz, may be suppressed. Figure 5A presents an example of the EEG obtained during the repair of a torn internal carotid artery; while Figs. 5B and 5C show the corresponding CSAs and DSAs, respectively.

The typical pattern seen in these measures during cerebral hypoperfusion is a reduction or loss in high-frequency activity and the appearance of large-amplitude slow waves in the Δ range (1–4 Hz). We have even seen decreases in cerebral blood flow produced by radiographically verified cerebral emboli. The EEG appearances of any ischemic or hypoxic events are similar and differentiation between the various putative causative factors is made by being particularly attentive to the clinical situation; for example, blood pressure, ECG, oxygen saturation, administered drugs, and surgical manipulations may all have an observable effect. Other concurrent factors that may alter the EEG are changes in depth of anesthesia, temperature changes, and changes in CO_2 content. These factors may be recognized by their relatively slow onset, lasting for several minutes, in contrast to the changes of ischemia, which generally occur within seconds. One must keep in mind that there are situations where the EEG may be acutely depressed upon injection of an anesthetic that rapidly passes the blood–brain barrier. Such situations may be found in high-dose opioid anesthesia, where fentanyl induces an immediate

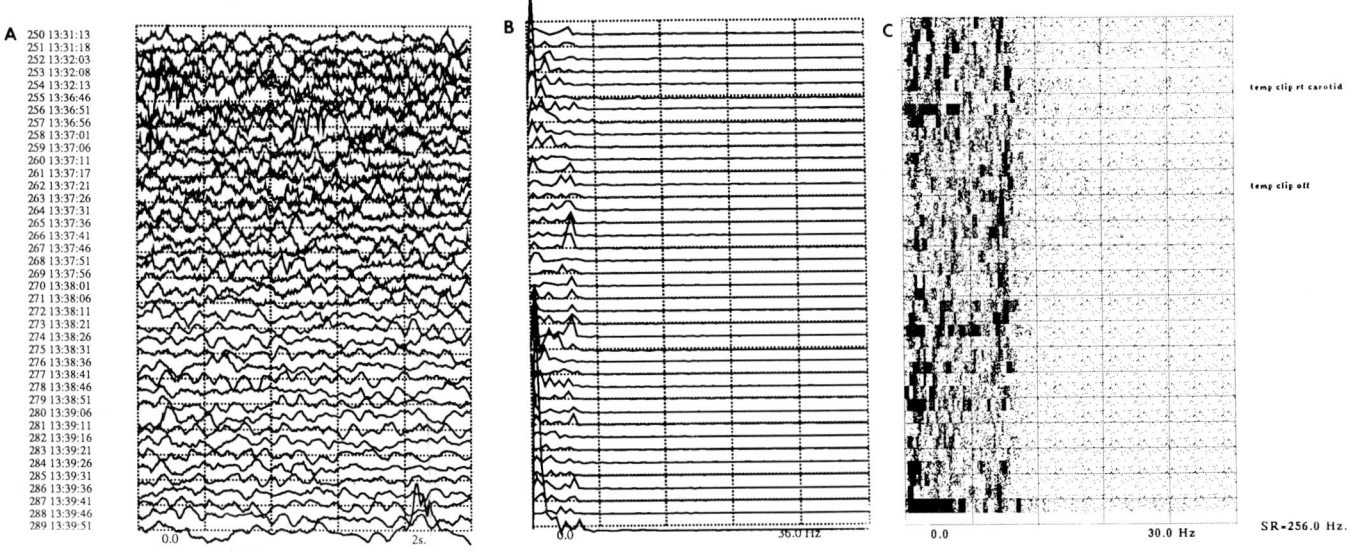

FIG. 5. A: One channel of raw EEG obtained during repair of internal carotid artery damaged during tumor resection. **B:** Compressed spectral array (CSA) presentation of the power spectra computed on the EEG in (**A**). **C:** Density spectral array (DSA) presentation of the same data showing an alternative method available for presenting the EEG data.

and marked reduction of fast frequency activity in the EEG, with an increase in low-frequency, high-amplitude activity in the Δ range (8).

A simple but useful summary of possible changes is that decreased frequency with increased amplitude (34) implies an ischemic event to the cortex, widespread frequency slowing and decreased amplitude usually imply brain stem ischemia (25), while ischemic events affecting the thalamus and the internal capsule produce unremarkable changes in the EEG (34) but possible significant changes in the somatosensory evoked potential.

Somatosensory System

Median nerve somatosensory evoked potentials (MSPs) are used to aid in determining the functional integrity of the somatosensory cortex and the ascending somatosensory system primarily in the region of the brain stem and forebrain. These potentials are useful both in preventing or reducing surgical morbidity during procedures that pose potential harm to the upper cervical cord and in assessing the level of hypoxia in cortical tissue (9).

Stimulation of the median nerve elicits a series of potentials that ascend from the stimulus site to the somatosensory cortex (Fig. 6A). Typically, the most peripheral recording site is Erb's point, which is above the clavicle, lateral to the insertion of the sternocleidomastoid muscle. A negative potential with a latency of 9–10 msec can be recorded at Erb's point and is probably generated by the branches of the brachial plexus. An electrode at cervical C_7 records a complex wave at 11–14 msec that consists of a small negative peak at 11 msec, a larger negative peak at 12–13 msec, and a positive peak at approximately 14 msec. The N_{11}, $N_{12/13}$, and P_{14}-msec peaks are probably generated at the dorsal root entry of the cervical spinal cord (N_{11}), the uppermost region of cervical spinal cord ($N_{12/13}$), and in the medial lemniscus of the brain stem (P_{14}) (5). Two negative peaks at 18 and 20 msec are easily seen at P_3 and P_4 parietal recording sites. These two negative peaks may appear as one negative

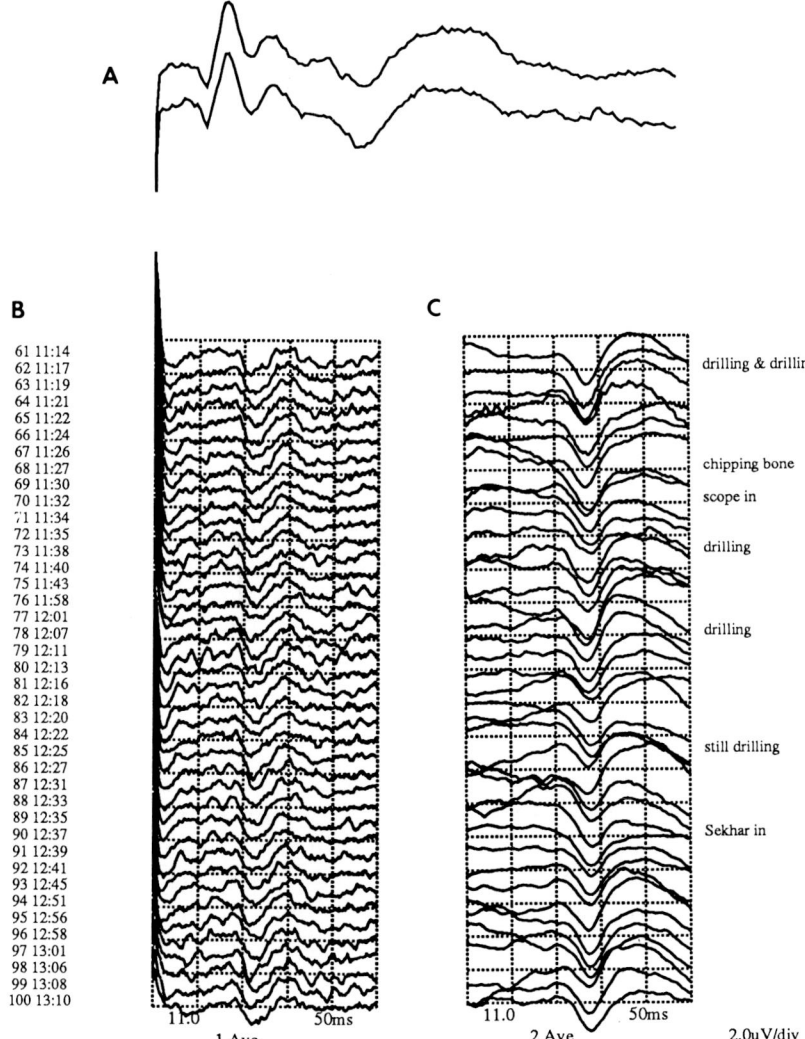

FIG. 6. A: Preoperative evaluation of median nerve somatosensory evoked potentials obtained from cranial base tumor patient. B: Intraoperative BSEPs obtained from median nerve stimulation followed and displayed in a waterfall display. C: MSPs obtained simultaneously with BSEPs to median nerve stimulation. Note sequence number, time, data, and comments appended to data.

complex in the operating room. The N_{20} wave is generated in the primary somatosensory cortex along the posterior bank of the central fissure (1). At longer latencies (approximately 25–100 msec), additional positive (P_{30}) and negative peaks are seen. These waves are generated by secondary somatosensory areas in the parietal lobe and by cortical association areas (11). We normally monitor the P_{14} (medial lemniscal activity) and the cortical N_{20} activity to assess conduction and P_{30} to assess cortical perfusion.

The recording and stimulating electrodes are applied following the patient's intubation, but prior to final positioning. The stimulating electrodes are needle electrodes and are applied subdermally, above the median nerve at the wrist, with the leads firmly taped to the patient's extremities to secure them during positioning. Following final positioning, a forehead ground electrode and P_3, P_4, F_3, and F_4 recording electrodes are applied in their nominal positions, if possible. The P_3 and P_4 recording electrodes should be placed 2 cm posterior and 7 cm lateral to C_z on the left (P_3) and right (P_4) scalp, respectively. The F_3 and F_4 recording electrodes are placed 3 cm anterior and 7 cm lateral to C_z. Again, these positions are optimal; however, many times the planned incision does not allow these positions to be used. In those cases, we attempt to place the electrodes as close as possible to recording sites. In some cases, these electrodes are placed using sterile technique by the surgeon, in the operative field, after the incision is completed.

The stimulus intensity is usually preset at 30 volts and adjusted as necessary to maximize the response, while producing minimal patient movement. The occurrence of the stimulus pulse is delayed by 10 msec when monitoring concurrently with the brain stem auditory evoked potential (Fig. 4A). If right and left median nerve responses are being observed concurrently, then the two stimuli are separated by 100 msec. If BAEP and SEPs are being monitored concurrently, a stimulation rate of 9.3 Hz is used; if bilateral SEPs are being monitored a stimulus rate of 3.3 Hz is used. In either case a pulse width of 0.1 μsec is used.

Ideally, baseline responses are obtained individually for each recording condition, prior to the draping of the patient, in order to alleviate any technical difficulties prior to the beginning of surgery. If MSPs are acquired by themselves, usually 128 stimuli are used to elicit each averaged response; however, on some patients stable responses are seen with numbers of stimuli as low as 32. These data are compared with the preoperative evaluation and used as baseline data throughout the case. When somatosensory and auditory data are being gathered simultaneously, usually 512 stimuli are used; however, when the BAEPs are of excellent quality the number of stimuli presented may be decreased to as low as 256.

In the operating room, we usually record and display the P_{14} brain stem responses (BSEPs) on Channel 1, using the same vertex to mastoid electrodes utilized to obtained the BAEPs (Fig. 6B). This allows the BSEPs to be recorded simultaneously with the BAEPs, and the cortical somatosensory evoked potentials (MSPs) (Fig. 4). The MSPs are recorded from parietal to frontal electrodes and are displayed on Channel 2, simultaneously with the farfield data (Fig. 6B). The gains used are between 100,000 and 500,000 on Channel 1 and between 20,000 and 50,000 on Channel 2. However, these values can be adjusted for the individual patient's response amplitude, with the usual value being 200,000 on Channel 1 and 20,000 on Channel 2. The bandwidths used are 100–3000 Hz on Channel 1 and 1–1000 Hz on Channel 2.

The N_{20} and P_{30} waves are sensitive to certain types of anesthetics. Barbiturates and inhalation anesthetics (e.g., isoflurane, ethrane, and halothane) will markedly decrease the amplitude of the cortically generated activity, including N_{20}, in a dose-dependent, but individualized, manner. Of the inhalation anesthetics, isoflurane produces the weakest effects on cortical activity. Thus in those cases where a balanced narcotic technique may not be used, due to the need to measure EMG activity, isoflurane is used as the anesthetic. The balanced anesthetic (a combination of nitrous oxide, a muscle relaxant, and a minor tranquilizer) is the much preferred method for recording SEPs by themselves. In cases in which isoflurane is used to supplement another form of anesthesia, a concentration of under 0.4% should produce minimal effects on the cortical somatosensory activity in adults; however, these effects are very individualized and even low levels of inhalation agents may reduce the amplitudes of cortically generated activity in some patients (26). The somatosensory short latency potentials behave similarly to those from the auditory system and are unaffected by most anesthetic manipulation. Temperature changes significantly influence the SEP latency. For each degree Celsius of local cooling, the nerve conduction velocity decreases by about 2.5 m/sec. During long operations, of this type, a drop in temperature around the nerve being stimulated can result in a progressive increase in N_{20} latency, unrelated to surgical intervention. Also latencies may be transiently affected when the surgeon irrigates with physiological solution at cooler temperatures; thus it is recommended that warm saline be used for irrigation.

For the cortical responses, the amplitude and latency of the N_{20}/P_{30} complex are of primary concern. In general, a decrease of more than 50% in amplitude or an increase of more than 10% in latency is communicated to the surgeon. Another response is taken as soon as possible to confirm the stability of the change. The neurophysiologist consults with the anesthesiologist to determine if a change in blood pressure, level of anesthesia, or type of anesthesia could have contributed to the observed changes in the amplitude and/or latency of the evoked potential. In the case when the potentials are completely lost, the neurophysiologist immediately reports the loss and then checks to ensure that all electrodes and their connections are intact.

Auditory System

Monitoring the function of cranial nerve VIII is used to aid in preserving hearing, locating CN VIII, and determining if the overall function of the brain stem is altered.

The classic BAEP consists of a minimum of five and a maximum of seven peaks (Fig. 7A). The first five peaks, Jewett Waves I through V, are the principal peaks used in clinical practice. All occur with 10 msec of a brief click or tone presentation. Wave I is generated in the auditory portion of CN VIII. Its latency is approximately 1.5–2.1 msec in a normal adult. Wave I is present on the ipsilateral side to the stimulus but is not usually seen on the contralateral side. Wave II is generated bilaterally at or in the proximity of the cochlear nucleus. The latency between Waves I and II is approximately 0.8–1.0 msec. The amplitude of Wave II on the contralateral side may be greater than on the ipsilateral side. Wave III is generated bilaterally from the lower pons near the superior olive and trapezoid body. The latency between Waves I and III is approximately 2.0–2.3 msec in a normal adult. Wave III may be smaller on the contralateral side than on the ipsilateral side. Waves IV and V are probably generated in the upper pons or lower midbrain, near the lateral lemniscus or possibly near the inferior colliculus (2). In ipsilateral recordings, Waves IV and V may fuse into a complex that can vary between two identifiable components with a common base to a single wave with a tall wide peak. On the contralateral side the peaks tend to be more easily identified. Wave V tends to be the most robust peak and is typically the last to disappear when stimulus intensity is reduced. In addition, there tends to be a large negative-going wave following Wave V, which aids the neurophysiologist in identifying Wave V. Wave V is most closely followed during these cases.

The BAEP is stimulated using one of several techniques, depending on the surgical procedure involved—and thus whether or not the auricle is retracted—and other considerations. Most often, we use miniature open-air high-fidelity earphones (i.e., commonly used

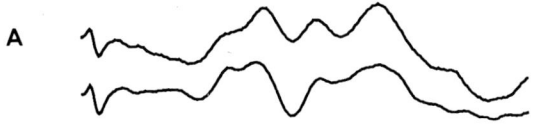

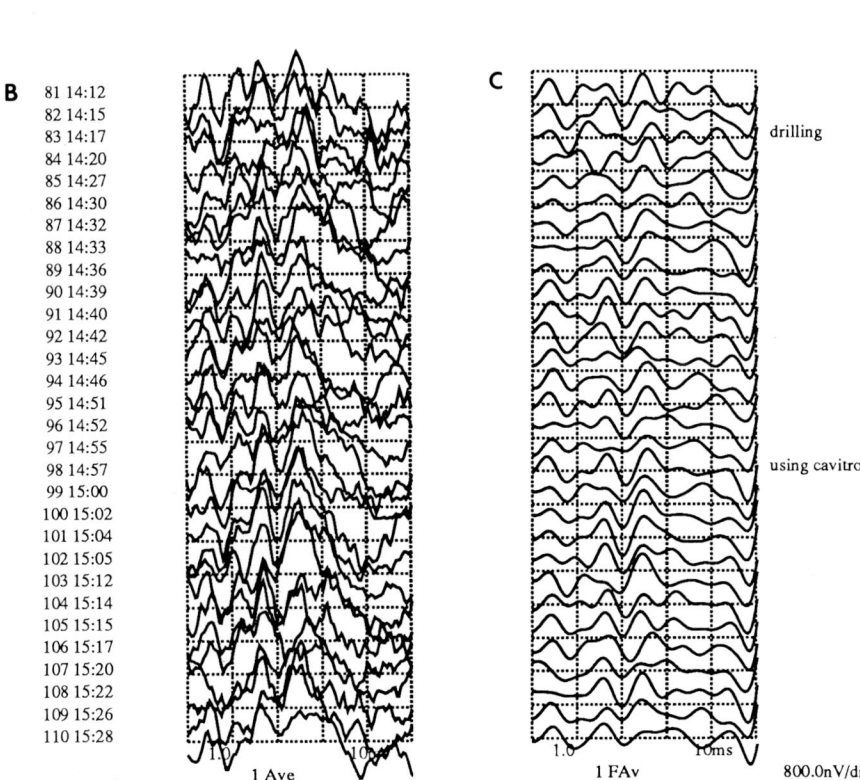

FIG. 7. A: Preoperative evaluation of BAEPs. **B:** Intraoperative BAEPs. **C:** Digitally filtered BAEPs obtained simultaneously with the data displayed in (**B**).

with personal tape players or radios), which rest in the concha of the ear. The earphones, along with the recording electrodes, are applied following the patient's intubation, prior to final positioning of the patient. After verifying that the earphones are working, they are securely taped in the ears with transparent tape, so that they may remain visible. At the same time, the taping must be adequate to prevent fluids from getting to the earphones and into the ear canal, which might cause device failure or a conductive hearing loss, respectively. Following final patient positioning, the vertex (C_z) and ear recording electrodes are placed. The contralateral ear electrode is placed over the mastoid (M_n) and the electrode for the operative side is placed in the pinna of the earlobe (A_m). In some cases, it is not possible to place an ipsilateral stimulating earphone and recording electrode because of the planned surgical incision. In those cases, we monitor only the contralateral responses, which still provide valuable information concerning the status of the brain stem.

For a wide variety of cranial base tumors monitored, the intensity level of the click is set to approximately 70 dB nHL. However, when the patient is known to have a hearing loss and/or a given patient's responses are not well defined, higher intensity levels may be required. In such cases an intensity level of 85 dB nHL is typical. Rarefaction and compression clicks are applied in an alternating fashion to minimize the apparent stimulus artifact. The stimulus rate is usually set between 9.3 and 19.3 Hz, because of the well known effects of higher stimulus rates on response latencies (35). The interstimulus intervals may be randomized to minimize contamination with phase-locked or quasi-periodic noise.

Baseline responses, for each ear, are acquired prior to the beginning of surgery. Usually 1024 stimulus presentations are used for the baseline data; however, the number of stimuli may be adjusted to as few as 256 depending on the quality of the responses. These data are compared with the preoperative evaluation and used as baselines throughout the case. If auditory responses are being obtained concurrently with either somatosensory or visual responses, the auditory stimulus is always presented first in the stimulus sequence. Usually, the second stimulus in the sequence is presented 10 msec after the auditory stimulus is presented, allowing the BAEP to fully develop prior to the activation of the second system being monitored.

In the operating room, we usually record and display the BAEP responses on Channel 1, using vertex to mastoid or earlobe electrodes (Fig. 7B). This permits these farfield auditory responses to be observed sequentially with the farfield somatosensory responses on the same channel.

Waves I to V are relatively resistant to sedative medication and general anesthetics. Thus these responses place no constraints on the anesthesiologist. However, they are sensitive to temperature changes, with absolute and interpeak latencies increasing by approximately 0.20 msec/°C.

The latency of Wave V is the primary concern in intraoperative monitoring of the BAEPs, since this is the most robust and easily identifiable of the waves in this response (Fig. 7B). In general, any repeatable or systematic change in the latency of Wave V that exceeds 0.3 msec is reported to the surgeon. However, clear changes in the waveshape, even with latency shifts less than 0.3 msec, are noted. The next sample is taken as soon as possible in order to confirm the stability of the change. In the case where the potentials are completely lost, the neurophysiologist reports the loss and then immediately checks to ensure that both the stimulating system and the recording electrodes are intact.

Visual System

Visual evoked potentials (VEPs) are used to aid in determining the functional integrity of the visual system, primarily in the region of the optic nerves, chiasm, and optic radiations. The recorded activity is generated either at the retina (electroretinogram) or at the cortex.

Stimulation of the visual system using a bright flash is not recommended for diagnostic purposes due to intersubject variability (3), except in selected situations; however, in the operating room this is a very helpful and effective technique. Four waves are typically seen in the visual evoked potential: P_{60}, which is thought to be generated in subcortical structures; and N_{70}, P_{100}, and N_{120}, which are all thought to be generated in the primary visual cortex (15).

For stimulation of the visual system, we use a fiber optics system, which is positioned directly under the eye, but not on the globe, and securely taped in place. This fiber optics stimulator is designed to be mounted on the flash stimulator driven by a Grass photic stimulator (P22), and this stimulator is then set at maximum intensity. Recording electrodes are placed at O_1 and O_2, both referenced to C_z.

The stimulus rate used for the visual data is 1.3 Hz and the observation window is 200 msec. A bandwidth of 1–100 Hz and a gain of 20,000 are used. Usually we record only one channel of visual data along with simultaneous somatosensory data or interspersed with auditory data. If the visual data are obtained in conjunction with somatosensory data, the visual stimulus is delayed to occur 98 msec after the somatosensory data, and at least three channels of data are collected: one for the BSEPs, the second for the MSPs, and the third for the VEPs.

Baseline responses are obtained individually for each recording condition during the surgical preparation period, so that any technical difficulties can be alleviated prior to the beginning of surgery. If the VEPs are acquired by themselves, usually 128 stimuli are used to elicit each averaged potential. These data are compared with the preoperative data and used as baseline data throughout the case.

In the operating room, we usually record and display visual activity in conjunction with either somatosensory or auditory data, depending on the system of interest.

Electromyographic Evaluation of Cranial Nerve Function

Cranial nerve function is monitored continuously during skull base surgery for two reasons: first, to establish the location and orientation of the cranial nerves in the operative field; and second, to preserve functioning in the cranial nerves and their related brain stem nuclei (20).

The major observed variables are the electromyograms (EMGs) from the appropriate muscle group innervated by the cranial nerves of interest. The cranial nerves, along with the associated muscle groups, that are usually monitored using EMG techniques are: the facial nerve (VII), and the orbicularis oculi, oricularis oris, and the mentalis muscles innervated by the zygomatic branch, the buccal branch, and the mandibular branch, respectively; the abducens nerve (VI) and the lateral rectus muscle; the trigeminal nerve (V) and the masseter muscle; the trochlear nerve (IV) and the superior oblique muscle; and the oculomotor nerve (III) and the medial and inferior rectus, and inferior oblique muscles of the eye. When appropriate, the functioning of the glossopharyngeal (IX), vagus (X), the spinal accessory (XI), and the hypoglossal (XII) cranial nerves are monitored by placing electrodes in the stylopharyngeus, the cricothyroid, the trapezius, and the intrinsic muscles of the tongue, respectively. In general, the cranial nerves ipsilateral to the operative side are monitored; however, when appropriate, bilateral activity is monitored.

Three different types of electrodes are used to record the EMGs. These are: fine wire electrodes, which have the highest impedance and the narrowest field of view; subdermal needles, which have an intermediate impedance and a larger field of view; and disk surface electrodes, which have the lowest impedance and the largest field of view (by field of view is meant the integrated level of electrical activity). Our recording techniques are essentially the same for all cranial nerves and all muscle groups. Subdermal platinum needle electrodes are utilized in bipolar recording configurations; that is, all recordings are done between a pair of electrodes inserted into the same muscle group. There is one exception to the bipolar recording technique: we occasionally record transfacially between the orbicularis oculi and the mentalis muscles to reduce the number of channels allocated to monitoring CN VII. Bipolar recordings are used to minimize confusion regarding which cranial nerve or branch of a cranial nerve is producing the observed EMG. The electrodes are normally placed prior to the start of the procedure; however, occasionally electrodes are placed in a sterile field by the surgeons. The EMG electrodes are held in place with tape and benzoine. We favor the needle electrodes over the fine wire and disk electrodes, because of the signal characteristics that they provide and their ease of application and maintenance.

The amplifier bandpass is set from 10 to 1000 Hz, and a gain of 5000–20,000 is routinely used. The unstimulated EMG activity from up to eight channels is monitored continuously throughout the case. This ongoing activity is continuously monitored on an oscilloscope and periodic episodes of interesting activity may be saved into a computer file.

Most importantly, the sound from all channels of activity is monitored continuously. Our system has the capability of amplifying the activity on eight channels simultaneously and driving an audio system with this amplified signal. This system has gauges that measure the relative amounts of activity on each channel, allowing the channel with the most activity to be isolated and listened to by itself if so desired. In addition, the system has suppressor circuits, which suppress the artifactual sounds related to bipolaring and stimulating. The importance of the audio system in identifying the level of activity in the muscle groups cannot be stressed too much. These signals are listened to continuously for evaluation of nerve function both by the neurophysiologists and by the surgeons. Four categories of EMG activity are observed: (a) no activity, which in an intact nerve is the best situation, but which may also be the case in a nerve that has been sharply dissected; (b) irritation activity, which sounds like soft intermittent flutter and is consistent with working near the nerve; (c) injury activity, which sound like a continuous, nonaccelerating tapping and which can be an indicator of permanent injury to the cranial nerve; and (d) a "killed-end" response, which sounds like an accelerating firing pattern and is an unequivocal indicator of nerve injury (23). It is important to note that a sharply cut nerve may produce only a brief burst of activity; thus monitoring cannot be expected to replace extreme caution when working near the cranial nerves.

Besides these signals of interest, various electrical artifacts must be identified and ignored. These include high-frequency electrode pops, activity related to electrode manipulation, static from surgical instruments, and activity produced by irrigation.

In addition to monitoring the ongoing EMG activity related to the various cranial nerves, the various cranial nerves may also be electrically stimulated. This is usually done to determine the location of the nerve in the operative field, since many times the nerve is enveloped by tumor and may not be directly observable, or to determine the functional integrity of the nerve (4). The most common example of this procedure is the direct stimulation of CN VII. We use Grass S44 or S88 stimulators to control the stimulus rate, pulse duration, stimulus intensity, and switching of the sound system. A stimulus isolation transformer is utilized to drive a monopolar stimulating electrode. The stimulating electrode is a low impedance (≤1000 ohms) electrode, with the shaft insulated to, but not including, the tip. These devices are capable of producing currents as high as 150 mA, requiring care in their use. The return path for the stimulating current is provided by a metal electrode inserted into the adjacent muscle mass. The stimulus used is a constant voltage, with a pulse frequency of 10 Hz, and a pulse width of 100 μsec. The voltage amplitude is typically varied between 0.1 and 1 volt. In some situations, where very precise localization of the nerve is required, bipolar stimulating electrodes are used. However, the great majority of the time, the question being asked is: Is the nerve there?

When CN VII is stimulated, usually all three branches are observed on the oscilloscope. The parameters typically measured for the stimulated VIIth nerve EMGs are the voltage threshold required to produce the evoked response of 0.3–0.5 volts, the latency to onset of 8–10 msec, and a peak-to-peak voltage of 1.0–2.0 mV (Fig. 8) (13). These parameters are measured at the beginning and end of the case, and whenever appropriate during the case. In addition, we have the capability to integrate the evoked EMG and use the area of the evoked EMG response as a criteria of change. Other cranial nerves may be stimulated as needed, and the same parameters are measured if appropriate.

SUMMARY

This chapter reviews our approach to the intraoperative monitoring of neurophysiologic function during cranial base surgery. The commonly accepted principal goal of intraoperative monitoring is to prevent morbidity, and at a certain level this is true; however, the more fundamental goal of intraoperative monitoring is to provide the surgical team with information that allows them to accomplish the desired operative objective with as optimal a surgical strategy as possible, while having a clear idea of what surgical morbidity is being induced along the way. This latter goal is particularly important in cases where the degree of difficulty is high and it is virtually impossible to prevent morbidity.

Essentially, we place a real-time feedback control loop around the dynamic, changing, system comprised of the surgeon and the patient. This requires a strong commitment to the concept that the central nervous system of the patient is highly sensitive to the operative manipulations of the surgeon and that appropriately observed variables may predict lesions about to develop. This information permits the surgeon to dynamically modify the approach to the operation and thereby minimize the degree of morbidity induced in the patient.

Based on these considerations and viewpoints, the neurophysiologists, who support the intraoperative monitoring service for the Cranial Base Tumor Center at the University of Pittsburgh Medical Center, have evolved an integrated approach to the problem of assessing the dynamic functional status of the patient's nervous system and of providing this information to the rest of the surgical team in as relevant and clear fashion as is possible. This approach is based on the combined experience of monitoring more than 300 cranial base surgeries to date.

Neurophysiological monitoring differs from that provided by the anesthesiologist in fundamental ways, and it is important to recognize and appreciate the distinctions. The monitoring performed by the anesthesiologists is aimed at maintaining the patient's homeostasis. That is, the anesthesiologist wishes to preserve the life of the patient and is focused on those measures that provide information concerning this most fundamental issue.

The use of evoked potentials in the evaluation and monitoring of patients with neurological or potential neurological deficits provides a set of objective measures of nervous system function, which are more specific and reliable than previously used methods of nervous system monitoring (36). EMG measures are highly specific and reliable. The EEG measures are also highly reliable; how-

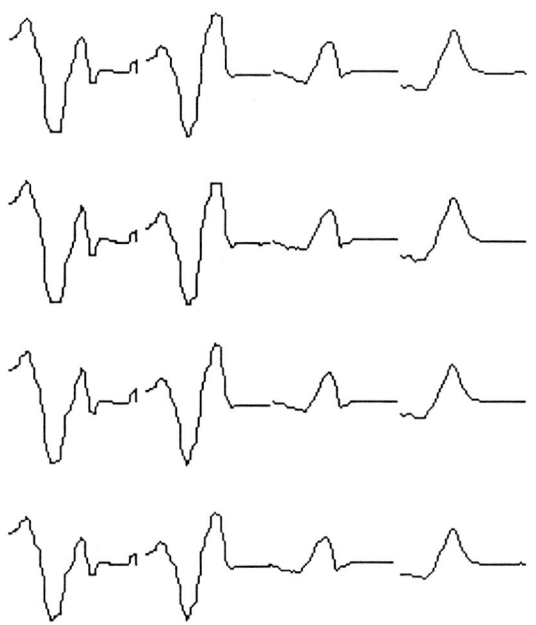

FIG. 8. Intraoperative EMG evoked by stimulation of CN VII and recorded from the orbicularis oculi, the orbicularis oris, the mentalis muscles, and between the orbicularis oculi and the mentalis muscles simultaneously.

ever, they are routinely used to assess more global factors than the EMGs.

Many apparently benign surgical manipulations may have significant effects on the neural responses and resultant clinical condition. For example, retraction of structures that are close to, or within, the pathway being monitored, noise and vibration from drilling, and heat diffusion from lasers, all affect the underlying neural tissue and the neurophysiological responses.

Stringent time constraints exist in intraoperative monitoring of neurophysiological function, and damage to the central nervous system may occur rapidly, over seconds. This constraint has inspired the development of methods for extracting and analyzing evoked potential, EMG, and EEG waveforms rapidly and efficiently. A corollary of the increased sensitivity required to decrease the monitoring time is a higher rate of individually false positive measures. These are usually rapidly identified as such and produce no disruption in the flow of the case.

In support of the intraoperative monitoring of these measures we have developed a distributed computer system, NeuroNet, specifically configured to support the considerations discussed in this chapter. This system provides both off-line and real-time signal processing and data review capabilities, and it addresses many of the problems associated with the acquisition, processing, and display of multivariate neurophysiologic data in these complex cases.

Monitoring of these measures in the operating room uses computationally based techniques and presents a significant step forward in reducing patient morbidity due to surgery. Previously, the integrity of the central nervous system could only be examined clinically when the patient recovered from anesthesia; however, the measures described in this chapter provide an immediate assessment of the effects of surgery on the nervous system with implications for modifying surgical techniques.

ACKNOWLEDGMENTS

The authors wish to acknowledge the collaboration of our surgical and neuroanesthetic colleagues; in particular, Laligam Sekhar, Chandra Sen, Ivo Janecka, Carl Snyderman, Barry Hirsch, Andrew Kofke, Mark Bloom, and James Krugh.

REFERENCES

1. Allison T. Developmental and aging changes in human evoked potentials. In: Barber C, Blum T, Nodar R, eds. *Evoked potentials III.* Boston: Butterworth, 1987;72–90.
2. Buchwald JS, Haung CM. Far-field acoustic responses: origins in the cat. *Science* 1975;189:382–384.
3. Ciganek L. The EEG response to light stimulus in man. *Electroencephalogr Clin Neurophysiol* 1961;13:165–172.
4. Daube JR, Harper CM. Surgical monitoring of cranial and peripheral nerves. In: Desmedt JE, ed. *Neuromonitoring in surgery.* Amsterdam: Elsevier, 1989;115–138.
5. Desmedt JE, Cheron G. Central somatosensory conduction in man: neural generators and interpeak latencies in the far-field components recorded from neck and right or left scalp and earlobes. *Electroencephalogr Clin Neurophysiol* 1980;50:382–403.
6. Desmedt JE. *Neuromonitoring in surgery.* New York: Elsevier, 1989.
7. Domino KB. Anesthesia for cranial base tumor operations. In: Sekhar LN, Schramm VL, eds. *Tumors of the cranial base: diagnosis and treatment.* Mount Kisko, NY: Futura Publishing Company, 1987.
8. Freye E. *Cerebral monitoring in the operating room and the intensive care unit.* Boston: Kluwer Academic Publishers, 1990.
9. Gentili F, Lougheed WM, Yamashiro K, Corrado C. Monitoring of sensory evoked potentials during surgery of skull base tumors. *Can J Neurol Sci* 1985;12:336–340.
10. Gerson GR. Monitoring during anesthesia. Boston: Little, Brown, 1981.
11. Goff WR, Williamson PD, Vangilder JC, Allison T, Fisher TC. Neural origins of long latency evoked potentials recorded from the depths and from the cortical surface of the brain in man. In: Desmedt JE, ed. *Progress in clinical neurophysiology,* vol 2. Basel: Karger, 1980;126–145.
12. Grundy BL. Intraoperative monitoring of sensory-evoked potentials. *Anesthesiology* 1983;58:72–87.
13. Harner SG, Daube JR, Beatty CW, Ebersold MJ. Intraoperative monitoring of the facial nerve. *Laryngoscope* 1988;98:209–212.
14. Kamura J. *Electrodiagnosis in diseases of nerve and muscle.* Philadelphia: FA Davis, 1983.
15. Kraut MA, Arezzo JC, Vaughan HG. Intracortical generators of the flash VEP in monkeys. *Electroencephalogr Clin Neurophysiol* 1985;62:300–312.
16. Krieger DN, Lofink RM, Doyle EL, Burk G, Sclabassi RJ. NeuroNet: implementation of an integrated clinical neurophysiology system. *Med Instrum* 1987;21(6):296–303.
17. Krieger DN, Burk G, Sclabassi RJ. NeuroNet: a distributed real-time system for monitoring neurophysiological function in the medical environment. *Computer* 1991;24(3):45–55.
18. Meyer JS, Marx PW. The pathogenesis of EEG changes during cerebral anoxia. In: Van der Drift JHA, ed. *Cardiac and vascular diseases/Handbook of electroencephalography and clinical neurophysiology,* vol 14A. Amsterdam: Elsevier, 1972;5–11.
19. Moller AR. Evoked potentials in intraoperative monitoring. Baltimore: Williams & Wilkins, 1987.
20. Moller AR. Electrophysiological monitoring of cranial nerves in operations in the skull base. In: Sekhar LN, Schramm VL, eds. *Tumors of the cranial base: diagnosis and treatment.* Mount Kisko, NY: Futura Publishing Company, 1987.
21. Niedermeyer E, Lopes da Silva F. *Electroencephalography.* Baltimore: Urban and Schwarzenberg, 1987.
22. Nuwer MR. *Evoked potential monitoring in the operating room.* New York: Raven Press, 1986.
23. Prass RL, Kinney SE, Hardy RW, Hahn JF, Luders H. Acoustic (loud-speaker) facial EMG monitoring: II, Use of evoked EMG activity during acoustic neuroma resection. *Otolaryngol Head Neck Surg* 1987;97(6):541–551.
24. Regan D. *Human brain electrophysiology: evoked potentials and evoked magnetic fields in science and medicine.* New York: Elsevier, 1989.
25. Roger J, Roger A, Gastaut H. Electro-clinical correlation in 36 cases of vascular syndromes of brainstem. *Electroencephalogr Clin Neurophysiol* 1954;6:164(abstract).
26. Samra SK. Effect of isoforane on human median nerve evoked potentials. In: Ducker TB, Brown RH, eds. *Neurophysiology and standards of spinal cord monitoring.* New York: Springer-Verlag, 1988.
27. Sclabassi RJ, Harper RM. Laboratory computers in neurophysiology. *Proceed IEEE* 1973;61(11):1602–1614.
28. Sclabassi RJ, Lofink RM, Doyle EL. NeuroNet: a distributed microprocessor network for clinical neurophysiology. In: Geisow MJ, Barret AN, eds. *Microcomputers in medicine.* New York: Elsevier, 1987.

29. Sclabassi RJ, Sun M, Krieger DN, Scher MS. Time-frequency analysis of the EEG signal. *Proc ISSPA* 1990;935–938.
30. Sclabassi RJ, Sun M, Krieger DN, Jasiukaitis P, Scher M. Time-frequency domain problems in the neurosciences. In: Boashash B, ed. *Methods and applications of time frequency signal analysis,* chapter 23. Longman Cheshire, Melbourne, Australia, 1992.
31. Sun M, Li CC, Sekhar LN, Sclabassi RJ. Efficient computation of the discrete pseudo Wigner distribution. *IEEE Trans Acoustics, Speech, Signal Processing* 1989;37(11):1735–1742.
32. Sun M, Li CC, Sekhar LN, Sclabassi RJ. A Wigner frequency analyser for nonstationary signals. *IEEE Trans Instrum Measurement* 1989;38(5):961–966.
33. Tyner FS, Knott JR, Mayer WB. *Fundamentals of EEG technology: vol I, basic concepts and methods.* New York: Raven Press, 1983.
34. Van der Drift JHA. The EEG in cerebro-vascular disease. In: Vinken PJ, Bruyn GW, eds. *Handbook of clinical neurology,* vol 11. Amsterdam: North-Holland, 1972;267–291.
35. van Olphen AF, Rodenberg M, Verwey C. Influence of stimulus repetition rate on brainstem evoked responses in man. *Audiology* 1979;18:388–394.
36. Villani RM. Forward. In: Grundy BL, Villani RM, eds. *Evoked potentials: intraoperative and ICU monitoring.* New York: Springer-Verlag, 1989.

CHAPTER 9

The Anterior and Middle Cranial Fossae Including the Cavernous Sinus and Orbit

Johannes Lang

ORBIT

The *superior wall of the orbit* is formed primarily by the frontal bone. The lesser wing of the sphenoid bone forms its most posterior segment and transmits the optic nerve. The medial aspect of the superior wall may be split by extensions of the frontal or ethmoid sinuses. Medially, the anterior and posterior ethmoidal foramina lie at the junction (or on the superior wall) of the superior wall with the lamina papyracea. In about 50% of skulls, there may be up to five foramina. The locations of these foramina are quite variable, and the posterior ethmoidal foramen may be as close as 1–2 mm to the orbital opening of the optic canal in some cases. The lateral orbital wall is formed by the greater wing of the sphenoid bone posteriorly and by the zygomatic bone anteriorly.

At about the middle of the lateral orbital rim but behind the attachment of the orbital septum, about 80% of adults have a small bulge called the marginal tubercle of the zygomatic bone. Near this tubercle, and about 11 mm below the frontozygomatic suture, the lateral bulbar retinaculum, which is the lateral part of the aponeurosis of the levator palpebrae muscle, and the lateral canthal ligament are attached. The lateral bulbar retinaculum is the strongest attachment of the ocular bulb. This is important, since the four rectus muscles tend to pull the ocular bulb backward, and the oblique muscles exert tension on the bulb anteriorly and medially.

Like the other orbital walls, the borders of the *medial orbital wall* are not clearly marked. Superiorly, the frontal bone curves into the wall formed by the ethmoid bone. Below this area, most of this wall borders on the maxilla posteriorly and superiorly the lesser wing of the sphenoid bone; the orbital lamina of the palatine bone; and in front, the lacrimal bone. The orbital lamina of the ethmoid bone is paper thin (lamina papyracea) and is supported by the walls of the ethmoidal cells. These cells vary in number and orientation.

Portals of the Orbit

The largest portals of the orbit are the superior and inferior orbital fissures. The superior border of the *superior orbital fissure* is formed by the lesser wing of the sphenoid bone, and sometimes the frontal bone also forms a part of the lateral border. The inferior border is formed by the superior rim of the greater wing of the sphenoid bone. The medial wall is formed by the body of the sphenoid bone. The superior orbital fissure connects the middle cranial fossa with the orbit. At the orbital face of the posterior part of the greater wing of the sphenoid bone, a small bony tongue is present from which originates part of the lateral rectus muscle. In the region of the middle of the superior border of the superior orbital fissure, a small bony spine may be present.

The *inferior orbital fissure* is bordered by the greater wing of the sphenoid bone superiorly, by the zygomatic bone anteriorly, and by the maxilla inferiorly. From the middle of the inferior orbital fissure, a shallow bony sulcus (rarely, a canal) runs anteriorly and slightly medially and forms the infraorbital canal. This sulcus lodges the infraorbital nerve and artery. The upper wall of the infraorbital canal usually has gaps or small canals, through which one or more small twigs of the infraorbital artery pass to supply the contents of the orbit.

Optic Canal

Via the optic canal, the optic nerve with its integuments and the ophthalmic artery run to the orbit. Occa-

---

J. Lang: Institute of Anatomy, University of Würzburg, W-8700, Würzburg, Germany.

sionally, a bony canal transmitting the ophthalmic artery may be present (in 1% of our specimens), 1–2 mm below the optic nerve canal (39). Figure 1 shows the optic canal in newborns and adults at the intracranial and the orbital openings and the middle segment.

The medial wall of the optic canal can be seen from the sphenoid sinus in approximately 80% of specimens. In these specimens the sphenoid sinus bordered the canal of the optic nerve, from which it is separated by only a thin bony lamella. The upper and lower walls of the optic canal may also be pneumatized. In about 13% of specimens, the posterior ethmoidal cells border totally the medial wall of the canal of the optic nerve and the ophthalmic artery.

Contents of the Orbit

The periosteal layer of the dura lines the inner surface of the optic canal at its cranial end. At the orbital end, the two layers of the dura appear to diverge. The outer layer extends as the periorbital layer and the deeper layer of the dura accompanies the arachnoid (and a subarachnoidal space) and the pia of the optic nerve to the sclera of the eyeball.

Hayreh and Dass (19,20) noted that the ophthalmic artery usually arises at the medial circumference of the internal carotid artery. The origin may be higher and rarely lateral to the optic nerve (Figs. 2 and 3). In our study it was observed that the artery usually entered the optic canal medial to the optic nerve to exit lateral to it at the orbital end of the canal (12).

The inferior orbital fissure is occupied by the orbitalis muscle; its size usually is underestimated. At the orbital side, this muscle is also covered by periorbita. In the area of the infraorbital sulcus, the periorbita runs into the periosteal layer of the infraorbital sulcus and canal. The same relationships are found at the ethmoidal, orbitofacial, and orbitotemporal canals, as well as in the region of the meningo-orbital foramina. Because the periorbital vessels connect the orbital contents and the orbital bones

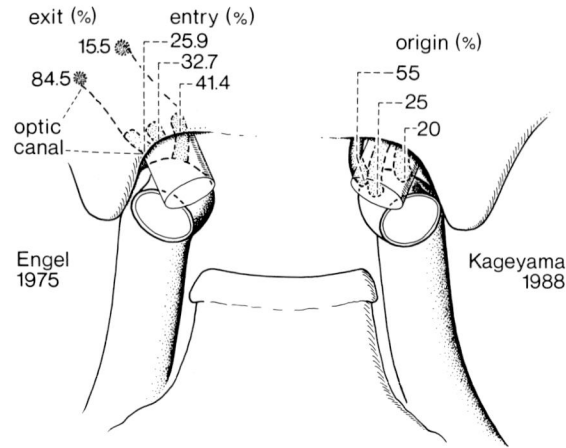

FIG. 2. Ophthalmic artery and its relationships with the optic canal.

with the neighboring paranasal sinuses, they can carry infections to the orbit.

The recti and the levator palpebrae superioris muscles arise from the common tendinous ring situated at the apex of the orbit (Fig. 4). The superior and medial portal

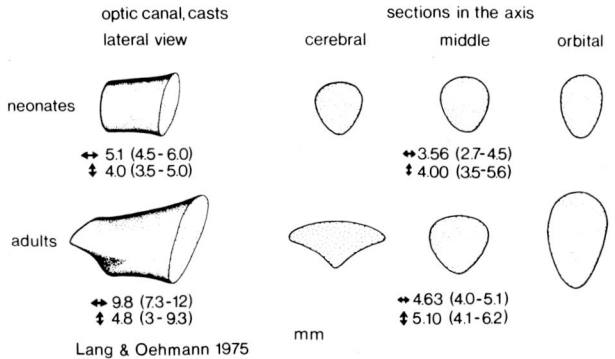

FIG. 1. Optic canal shape and measurements in neonates and adults.

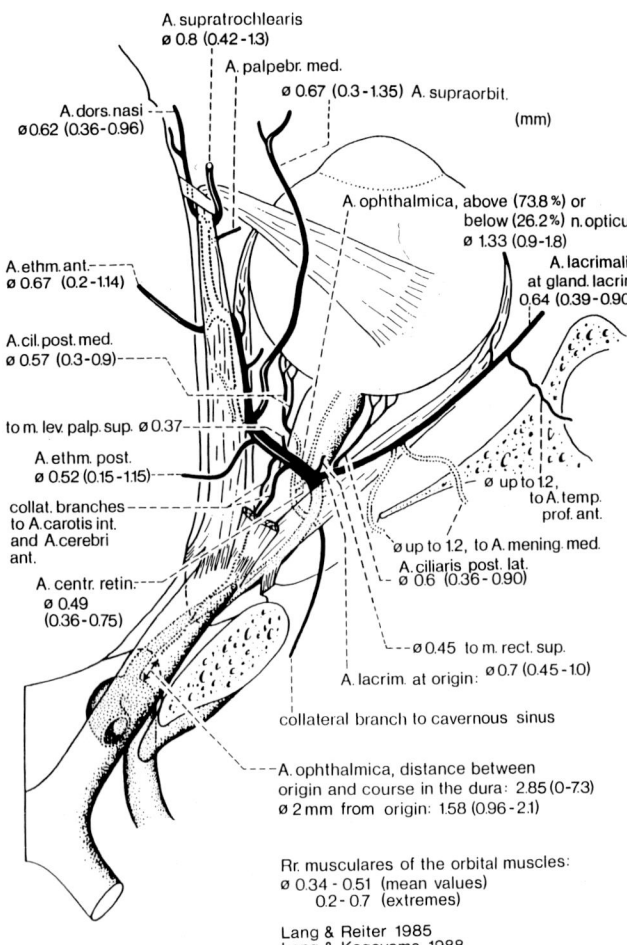

FIG. 3. Common course of the ophthalmic artery.

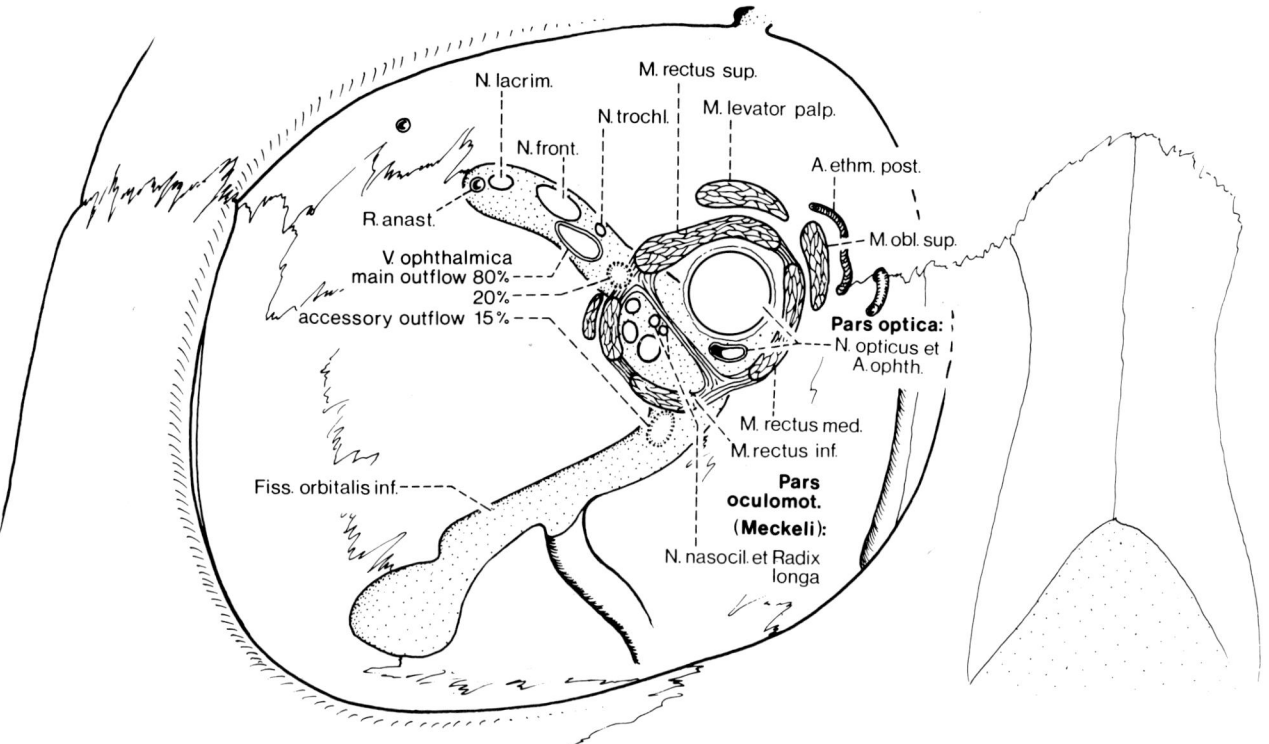

FIG. 4. Area of origin of extraocular muscles at the apex of the orbit.

of the superior orbital fissure is called the pars optica, while the inferior and lateral portal is called the pars oculomotoria. The oculomotor nerve (usually divided into a superior and an inferior ramus), abducent, and nasociliary nerves run through the ring's lateral and inferior portal. The tendinous ring embraces the medial part of the superior orbital fissure as well as the orbital end of the optic canal. Lateral to the tendinous ring, the lacrimal nerve, often accompanied by a twig of the middle meningeal artery, runs through the superior orbital fissure. The ophthalmic vein, frontal, and trochlear nerves traverse in the compartment lateral to the ring, medial to the lacrimal nerve. Numerous variations of the course of the ophthalmic vein have been described (40,46).

After the removal of the orbital roof, the twigs of the ophthalmic and the trochlear nerve may be seen through the periorbita. In some cases, flat layers of fat lie between the periorbita and nerves (38). The frontal and the lacrimal nerves separate off from the ophthalmic nerve in the cavernous sinus. In the anterior part of the cavernous sinus, the trochlear nerve crosses the oculomotor nerve from laterally to superomedially, to lie on the superior aspect of the superior oblique muscle. From the superior aspect, after the frontal nerve is mobilized and further fatty tissue is removed, the levator palpebrae superioris muscle can be seen.

During the operative approaches to the orbital cone, the nerve to the levator palpebrae superioris muscle should be preserved. In 85%, the nerve embraces the medial border of the superior rectus muscle and reaches the levator palpebrae superioris muscle from below. In the remainder, the nerve runs through the superior rectus muscle at different zones. The approach between the lateral rectus muscle and the levator palpebrae superioris and the superior rectus muscle is dorsally broader than that between superior oblique muscle and the superior rectus and levator palpebrae superioris muscles. The connective tissue fasciae of the eye muscles are closely woven in the anterior portion of the bulb (cingulum bulbi). They are relatively thin behind it, in the region of the orbital apex.

Connective Tissue in the Orbit

The orbital volume is occupied by the eyeball and its moving apparatus, as well as vessels, nerves, and fatty tissue. The orbital apex is well suited to provide little friction for the movements of the optic nerve and the muscles as well as for the ball and socket joint of the eyeball. In 54 orbits, Hugo and Stone (24) found that the weight of the intraorbital fatty tissue ranged from 5 g to more than 10 g. According to Rohen (70), the septa of the connective tissue between the fatty lobules are oriented in an equatorial–transverse direction in the frontal parts of the orbit and more sagittally in the posterior region. In addition to cingulum bulbi, Koornneef (31) observed the presence of circular arrangements of the connective tissue septa between periorbita and vagina bulbi in the posterior one-third of the bulb in frontal sections. We could not confirm the presence of such an arrangement at this level (53). Several investigators have distinguished five intraorbital fat compartments (25,67). Two are accessible through the upper eyelid and three through the lower eyelid. However, others believe that special parts of fat cannot be differentiated.

After the lateral orbital wall is removed, the periorbita is seen. Frequently, in the superior part, the lacrimal nerve and artery shimmer through the periorbita as does a part of the posterior aspect of the lacrimal gland and, laterally, the lateral rectus muscle. The anterior part of the lateral rectus muscle is covered by connective tissue and therefore (in anatomical preparations) is not visible. Woven into the periorbita or below it, a ramus communicans of the lacrimal nerve runs, supplying the gland with secretory fibers from the pterygopalatine ganglion. Arterial anastomoses also often occur between branches of the infraorbital artery below and the lacrimal artery above. After the periorbita is cut, a thin fatty tissue is seen covering most of the lateral rectus muscle, which is supplied by the abducent nerve. Schurmann (72) found that the lateral orbitotomy offers a favorable approach to this area, particularly for laterally lying tumors that do not reach the orbital apex. Other ophthalmic surgeons believe, however, that it is possible to reach the orbital apex via this approach (5,60).

The slant of the lateral orbital wall should be kept in mind. The orbital apex is deep and far medial in the operative area, and the greater wing of the sphenoid bone must be removed during this approach. However, this wing also forms part of the base of the middle cranial fossa. Berke (3a) noted that, depending on the position of the tumor, the lateral rectus muscle can be moved up or down. A view of the important structures in the retrobulbar region is possible after the lateral rectus muscle is removed (Fig. 5).

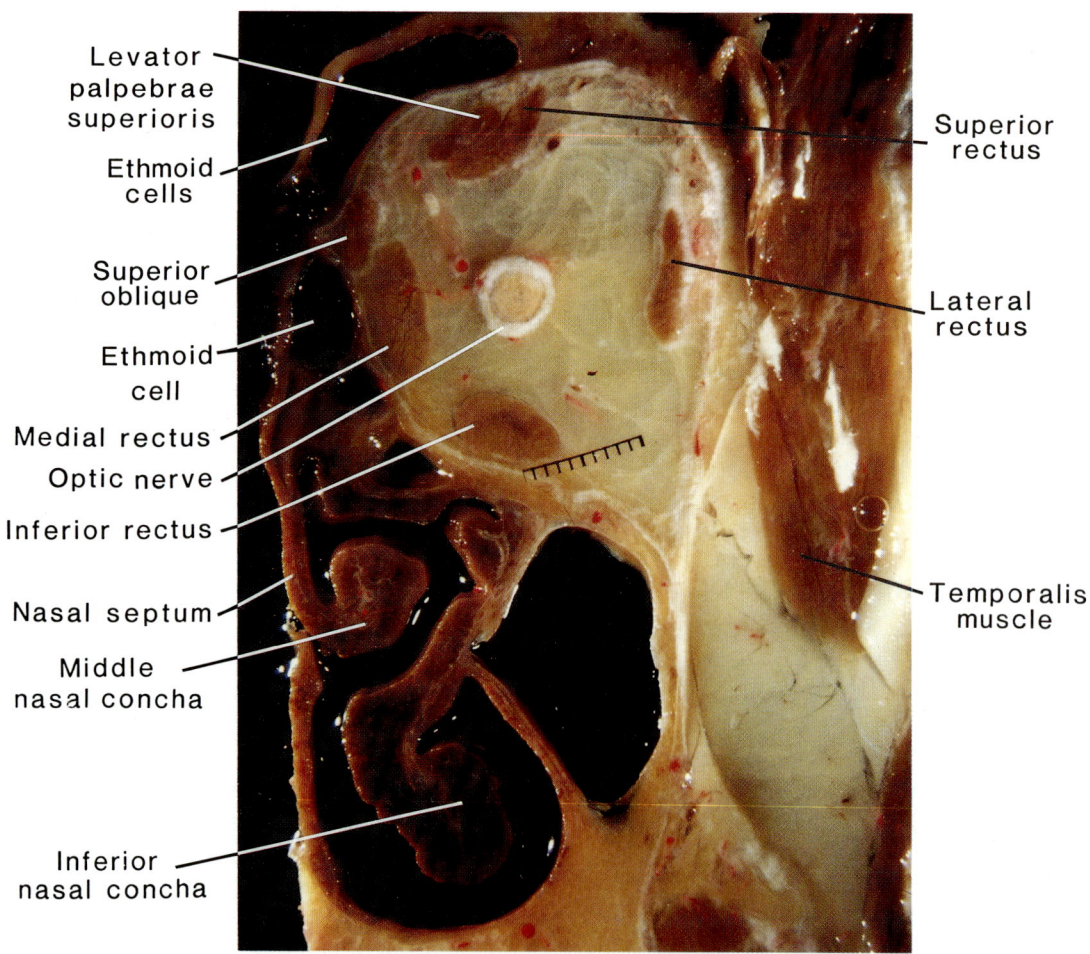

FIG. 5. Coronal section posterior to the eyeball.

ANTERIOR CRANIAL FOSSA

The anterior cranial base is deeper medially than it is laterally. The floor of the anterior cranial fossa is formed by the frontal, ethmoid, and sphenoid bones (anterior superior part of the body and the lesser wing). The foramen cecum lies in front of the crista galli. Usually, this foramen is filled with a small extension of dura that is traversed by small blood vessels. Rarely, and only in young children, veins connecting the superior sagittal sinus with nasal veins may be seen traversing the foramen cecum. Encephaloceles occasionally pass through the area of the foramen cecum (78).

The cribriform plate on each side contains about 44 foramina and anterolaterally includes the cribroethmoid foramen. The olfactory fila pass through the cribriform plate, along with small dural and arachnoidal extensions and branches of the posterior and anterior ethmoid arteries. The largest nasal branch of the anterior ethmoid artery and the anterior ethmoid nerve leave the cranial cavity through the cribroethmoid foramen. We have also seen a vein that was connected to an inferior vein of the forebrain passing through the lamina cribrosa.

Meningo-orbital foramina are sometimes present in the orbital roof and branches of the ophthalmic or middle meningeal artery may pass through these foramina. The planum sphenoidale is located behind the lamina cribrosa. The average distance between the foramen cecum and the tuberculum sellae was seen to be 42.5 mm (range 28–50 mm).

Dura Mater

The dura of the anterior cranial fossa consists of collagen fibers oriented in different directions. Thick dural zones are seen above the planum sphenoidale and behind the lesser wing of the sphenoid bone. In the area of the olfactory fossa, the dura mater is relatively thin.

The dura and floor of the anterior cranial fossa are supplied by the ethmoidal arteries, the frontal branch of the middle meningeal artery, and the internal carotid artery (ICA). Twigs of the ethmoidal arteries pierce the lamina cribrosa to reach the medial and lateral walls of the nasal cavity. One of the branches that is normally large and well developed is the anterior falceal artery supplying the falx cerebri. The frontal branch of the middle meningeal artery supplies the lateral floor of the anterior cranial fossa and usually reaches the orbit through meningo-orbital foramina.

Brain and Blood Vessels Related to the Anterior Cranial Fossa

The orbital surface of the frontal lobe has a variable pattern of sulci and gyri, but the presence of the olfactory sulcus is a constant feature. The olfactory tract is located near the posterior part of the olfactory sulcus, in a small olfactory cistern. Medial parts of the orbital surface and the olfactory bulb and tract are supplied by the medial frontobasal artery, which is a branch of the anterior cerebral artery, and usually also by branches of the recurrent artery of Heubner. The lateral part of the brain in this area is supplied by the lateral frontobasal artery, a branch of the middle cerebral artery.

In our specimens, venous drainage of the posteromedial areas of the orbital surface was via the medial orbital vein, the vein of the olfactory gyrus, and the anterior cerebral veins. These veins drain the blood to the basal vein of Rosenthal (48). From the anterior parts of the orbital surface, some veins drain to the superior and inferior sagittal sinus.

MIDDLE CRANIAL BASE ANATOMY

Skull

The middle cranial base comprises the bony floor of the middle cranial fossa and the sella turcica region. The bony floor of the middle cranial fossa is bounded anteriorly by the posterior border of the lesser wing of the sphenoid bone and its lateral extension, the crista alaris (Sylvi). The frontal bone, the parietal bone, the squama of the temporal bone, and the great wing of the sphenoid bone meet here, usually in an H-shaped suture zone called the pterion. In this normally thick, bony area, in about 40% a bony canal for the frontal branch of the middle meningeal artery or a meningeal sinus is present (6). A little below the crista alaris, we found (in 21%) a communication between the middle cranial fossa and orbit, called the posterior meningo-orbital foramina. Through these canals run vessels that anastomose with the middle meningeal artery and branches of the ophthalmic artery, most commonly the lacrimal artery. The greater wing of the sphenoid bone forms most of the floor and part of the lateral wall of the middle cranial fossa. Laterally, this wing connects to the squamous portion of the temporal bone, which also constitutes the lateral bony floor of the middle cranial fossa. Medially and posteriorly, the greater wing abuts the petrous part of the temporal bone and the bony carotid canal.

Rostral to the petrous part of the temporal bone, the thickest part of the middle cranial fossa is usually the area of the mandibular eminence, anterior to the fossa mandibularis. The deepest area of the middle cranial fossa is at the upper border of the zygomatic process of the temporal bone near its articular tubercle.

Middle Cranial Fossa Portals

The medial part of the *superior orbital fissure* is wide; laterally, it narrows and turns superiorly and anteriorly.

Its superior border is formed by the inferior surface of the lesser wing, and its medial boundary by the inferior root of the lesser wing and a part of the body of the sphenoid bone. The inferior border of the superior orbital fissure is the superior margin of the greater wing of the sphenoid bone. The fissure is always widest medial to the spine of the lateral rectus muscle and narrowest at about 5 mm medial to its lateral end.

In adults, the *foramen rotundum* is a canal about 4 mm long. Its internal aperture lies below the inferior medial border of the superior orbital fissure. Postnatal enlargement of the foramina rotundum, ovale, and spinosum and their topographical changes have been described (49).

The *maxillary nerve* runs through the middle cranial fossa to the pterygopalatine fossa. Its average intracranial length between the trigeminal ganglion and the foramen rotundum was found to be 10.33 mm (range 4.5–15.1 mm). Within the foramen rotundum, the nerve contains an average of 14 (1–30) fascicles and two arteries (47). In one case with agenesis of the ICA, a large branch of the maxillary artery was found traversing the foramen rotundum and another coursing through the foramen ovale united rostral to the trigeminal ganglion (13). The branches supplied one hemisphere of the brain. In about 10% of cases studied, Sondheimer (74) found veins in the foramen rotundum with diameters of 1–3 mm; these veins were on the medial circumference of the foramen rotundum and came from the pterygoid process of the sphenoid bone.

The *mandibular nerve* exits the middle cranial fossa through the foramen ovale. Its average intracranial length between the trigeminal ganglion and the foramen ovale measured 6.63 mm (range 2.9–11.1 mm) (75). This foramen also occasionally carries the accessory meningeal branch from the middle meningeal artery and the meningeal branch of the mandibular nerve. Also within the foramen ovale is a large caliber venous plexus that connects to the cavernous sinus, usually to the middle meningeal vein, and less commonly to a paracavernous sinus. The plexus ascends as far as the trigeminal ganglion in 68% of cases and always reaches the proximal maxillary nerve and the anterior upper half of the intracranial mandibular nerve (73). Below the skull, this plexus is connected to the pterygoid venous plexus.

About 98% of the time, the *foramen spinosum* is posterior and lateral to the foramen ovale (6). Like the foramen rotundum, it is a short bony canal, usually shortest on the medial side. Between the perinatal period and adult life, the canal approximately doubles in length (18). Duplicate foramina spinosa have been found in dried skulls and in roentgenograms (58). Sondheimer (74) believes that duplication of the foramen spinosum is not associated with early bifurcation of the middle meningeal artery outside the skull. Lindblom (58) found that the foramen spinosum was absent in 0.4% of cases and that the middle meningeal artery arose from the ophthalmic artery instead of entering the skull through the foramen spinosum. This vessel is surrounded by the middle meningeal veins, which are in the form of sinuses.

On the right side, we found the foramina rotundum, ovale, and spinosum situated more medially than on the left, whereas on the left side, the foramina lie slightly more rostrally than on the right (56).

The foramen of Vesalius carries the basal emissary vein from the cavernous sinus and was present on the right side in 49% of our specimens and on the left in 36%. It lies dorsal (mediodorsal more often than laterodorsal) to the foramen rotundum. A small nerve also may pass through this foramen into the cavernous sinus (nervulus sphenoidalis lateralis). Rarely, this foramen is incomplete dorsally (42).

The anterior surface of the petrous part of the temporal bone has a trigeminal impression. It extends down and forward to the foramen lacerum internum and the sulcus of the greater and lesser superficial petrosal nerves.

Below the impression for the triangular part of the trigeminal nerve runs the canal for the ICA. Its superior and anterior surfaces were dehiscent in 96% of our cases. This dehiscence, which was closed by connective tissue and which we called the inferior petrosphenoid ligament, varied in size and shape. Lateral to the trigeminal impression, the openings for the greater and lesser petrosal nerve sulci can be identified. The genu of the facial nerve canal normally is covered by a bony lamella but in about 15% of specimens there was no bone covering it.

The greater (GSPN) and lesser petrosal (LSPN) nerves run forward, medially, and inferiorly, embedded in dura close to the bone. Below the trigeminal ganglion, the GSPN pierces the transverse part of the inferior petrosphenoid ligament and is joined by sympathetic fibers (deep petrosal nerve). Together with these fibers, it then enters the pterygoid canal, where it forms the nerve of the pterygoid canal. Below or at the level of the sphenoid sinus, this nerve runs forward to the pterygopalatine ganglion in the pterygopalatine fossa. The lesser petrosal nerve passes into the middle cranial fossa a little inferior and more rostrally to the GSPN. It is embedded in the external layer of dura and pierces the transverse part of the inferior petrosphenoid ligament to end in the otic ganglion. In about 15% of cases, however, the lesser petrosal nerve pierces the great wing (usually lateral and dorsal to the foramen spinosum) to reach the inferior surface of the skull (Arnold's canal).

The GSPN is usually accompanied by an arterial branch from the middle meningeal artery, called the petrosal artery, and less frequently by a branch from one of the caroticocavernous branches. This branch runs to the geniculate ganglion and to parts of the labyrinthine and tympanic segments of the facial nerve. The lesser petrosal nerve is also accompanied by a branch of the middle

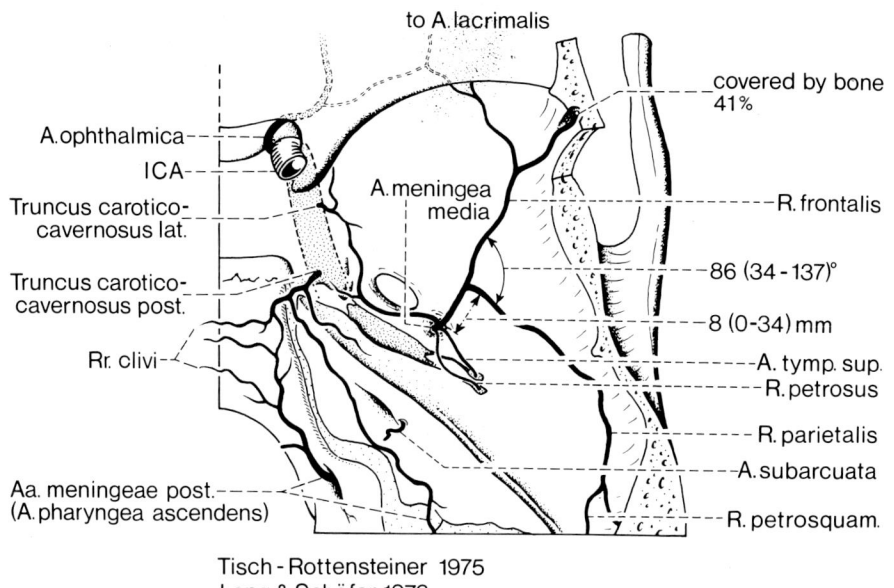

FIG. 6. Arteries to the bottom of the middle cranial fossa and their anastomoses.

meningeal artery, the superior tympanic artery, which supplies the tensor tympani muscle and an area of the mucosa of the tympanic cavity.

The arcuate eminences of newborns and young children are always visible. In later childhood, bony tubercles (juga cerebralia) sometimes develop in this area, and the eminence is clearly visible in only 50% of adults (49). Under the arcuate eminence lies the superior semicircular canal.

The superior border of the petrous temporal bone forms a variable angle with the midsagittal plane. Lateral to the arcuate eminence lies the often very thin tegmen tympani, which sometimes has dehiscences. Slightly inferior and lateral to the tegmen is the internal petrosquamosal suture, visible in most skulls of young children and sometimes in adults.

The superior petrosal sinus is found along the upper crest of the petrous bone, embedded in dura of the tentorium cerebelli posteriorly.

The arteries supplying the floor of the middle cranial fossa are mainly branches of the middle meningeal artery, whereas numerous anastomoses with branches of the caroticocavernous branches are found in the medial parts of the fossa (Fig. 6).

HYPOPHYSEAL AREA AND THE CAVERNOUS SINUSES

Osteology

The hypophyseal fossa is located in the middle of the skull base. The many variations in the bony surroundings of the pituitary gland are due partly to the complex embryology of the sphenoid bone. This bone arises in the middle of the cartilaginous basin of the skull, in which there are 18–19 ossification centers. Between the anterior and posterior parts of the sphenoid is a layer of cartilage (intrasphenoidal synchondrosis), which occasionally persists until the end of the first year of life (sometimes up to the fourth year), although its upper end is already ossified at birth. Ossification of the dorsum sellae is usually in progress at birth.

The middle part of the anterior boundary of the sella turcica is formed by the tuberculum sellae, a structure that varies in shape. The dorsum sellae forms its posterior boundary and its lateral extensions are the posterior clinoid processes. The floor of the sella is part of the sphenoid body. On either side of the pituitary, it slopes down and laterally toward the floor of the middle cranial fossa. The clinoid processes are important sites of dural attachment.

In the pituitary fossa, a depression at the site of the pituitary gland was seen in only about half of our specimens. Instead of a fossa, there is frequently a plateau, which is flat in approximately 20%. Various other combinations make up the remainder (56).

The anterior wall of the pituitary fossa usually is separated from the prechiasmal sulcus by a rounded transverse ridge, which extends from side to side between the inferior borders of the two optic canals. This ridge is known as the tuberculum sellae and can be seen roentgenographically. Less frequently, there is a rounded transition from the anterior wall of the pituitary fossa into the prechiasmal sulcus. The ridge at the anterior border of the prechiasmal sulcus is the limbus sphenoidalis. The tuberculum sellae is situated about 3 mm (1–5 mm) deeper than the limbus. We found the angle between the planum sphenoidale and the tuberculum to be on average 25° (9–43°) (32).

The floor of the pituitary fossa has in rare cases a median craniopharyngeal canal and in children contains a foramen or a vascular channel (lateral craniopharyngeal canal) in the area of the superior orbital fissure.

Variations of the Sella Turcica

Sellar Bridges

Sellar bridges are bone structures running between the anterior and posterior clinoid process. When present, they are usually bilateral, though they may be incomplete. Platzer (68) found sellar bridges in 5.9% of 220 half skulls. Our own investigations indicate that sellar bridges are laid down in cartilage at an early stage of development and ossify in early childhood.

Bony bridges between the lateral border of the pituitary fossa and the apex of the anterior clinoid process demarcate an orifice known as the *caroticoclinoid foramen* or carotid foramen, as the ICA runs out of the cavernous sinus through this closed and usually circular ring of bone. An accessory bony bridge also may arise from the middle clinoid process, which occasionally fails to fuse completely with an extension of the anterior clinoid process, thus producing an almost closed ring. Completely closed caroticoclinoid foramina were present in about 10% of specimens, and the numbers in children and adults were roughly equal.

Sellar Spine

This variation was first examined in a 23-year-old Caucasian man (39). The osseous spine protruded from the dorsal side of the pituitary fossa into the fossa itself. A spine protruding into the pituitary fossa was seen anatomically and radiographically in five living patients (10). It appears that this spine is a remnant of the anterior end of the notochord.

Cavernous Sinus

The transverse dural plate of the pituitary region varies in length and breadth. The middle part, which spans the sella turcica and is perforated for the pituitary stalk, is the diaphragma sellae. Lateral and dorsal to the diaphragma, the transverse plate merges into a basin of varying depth. The lateral boundary of the basin is the anterior petroclinoid fold, the anterolateral extension of the tentorium cerebelli. Posteromedially, the basin is bounded by the posterior petroclinoid fold, which represents the posteromedial extension of the tentorial notch. Near the anterior clinoid process, the medial fibers radiate above the optic nerve canal and unite with the transverse fibers of the dura on the planum sphenoidale (36).

The lateral fibers run along the posterior margin of the lesser wing of the sphenoid and contribute to the relatively thick dural layer at this site. The fibers in the basin region of the transverse plate are likewise largely derived from the anterior radiation of the tentorium. The entry portal for the oculomotor nerve is formed by a concave border, sharp rostrally and rounded dorsally. Behind the oculomotor nerve, the basin consists of fibers that originate from the ramification zone of both petroclinoid folds and form dense bundles dorsally. Anteriorly, these fibers diverge into a relatively thin roof for the cavernous sinus. The entry portal of the oculomotor nerve is usually located at the anterior border of the basin.

Dura Mater

The diaphragma sellae stretches from the tuberculum sellae to the upper border of the dorsum sellae and the posterior clinoid processes (Fig. 7). In most specimens in one study, its width exceeded its length, but in 16%, it was approximately square.

Near the diaphragmatic foramen, the dural covering of the pituitary is usually very thin and consists of circular fibers. At the exit portal for the ICA and the posterior clinoid process, the diaphragma becomes thicker.

Medial to the anterior clinoid process, the ICA crosses the transverse plate. This part of the vessel has a curve that is convex forward and medially, where it passes from the cavernous to the subarachnoid part.

With advancing age, the diaphragmatic foramen seems to enlarge. In addition to the infundibulum, the superior hypophyseal arteries often pass through this foramen to reach the anterior lobe. Occasionally, one of these arteries penetrates the diaphragma.

Pituitary Cisterns

The arachnoid invariably extends through the diaphragmatic foramen and spreads out on the upper surface of the anterior lobe of the pituitary (Fig. 8). Adults have a fluid-filled space within this arachnoid tissue, known as the pituitary cistern, which usually enlarges with advancing age. The cistern can extend for a variable distance forward and laterally and occasionally even overlaps the posterior lobe.

There are usually two superior *hypophyseal arteries* (Fig. 9) but there may be one to four in number. They branch off from the medial and undersurface of the subarachnoid part or where the ICA briefly runs through the diaphragma sellae. These arteries run back and up toward the infundibulum, reaching it at various levels. On their way to the pituitary stalk, some small twigs branch off to the undersurface of the optic chiasma and optic nerve and to the tuber cinereum. At the pituitary stalk, they usually form an arterial circle, from which the real

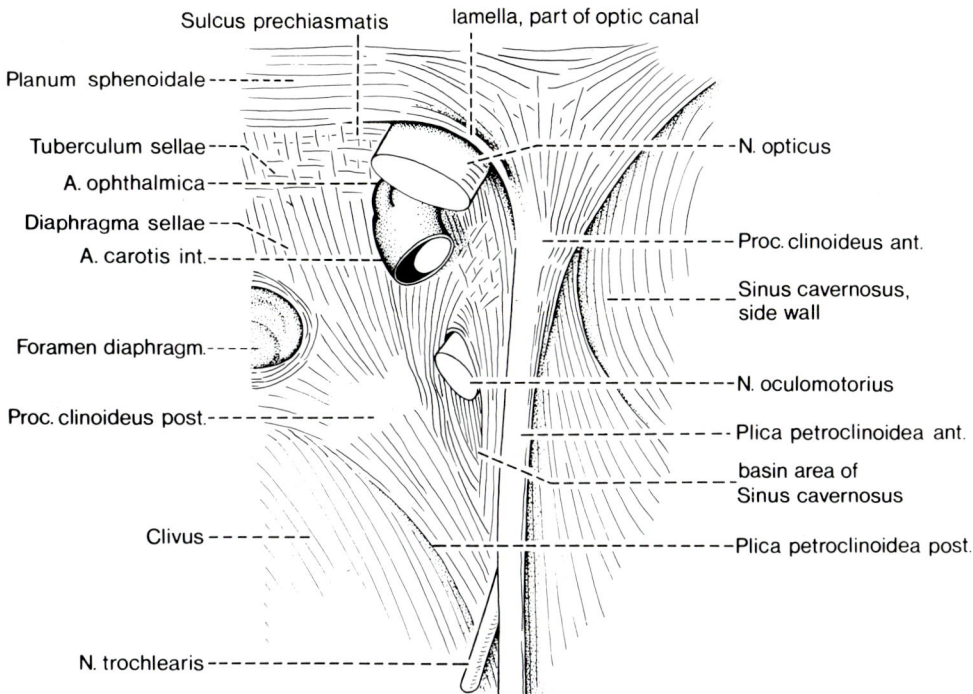

FIG. 7. Course of the dural fibers in the hypophyseal area.

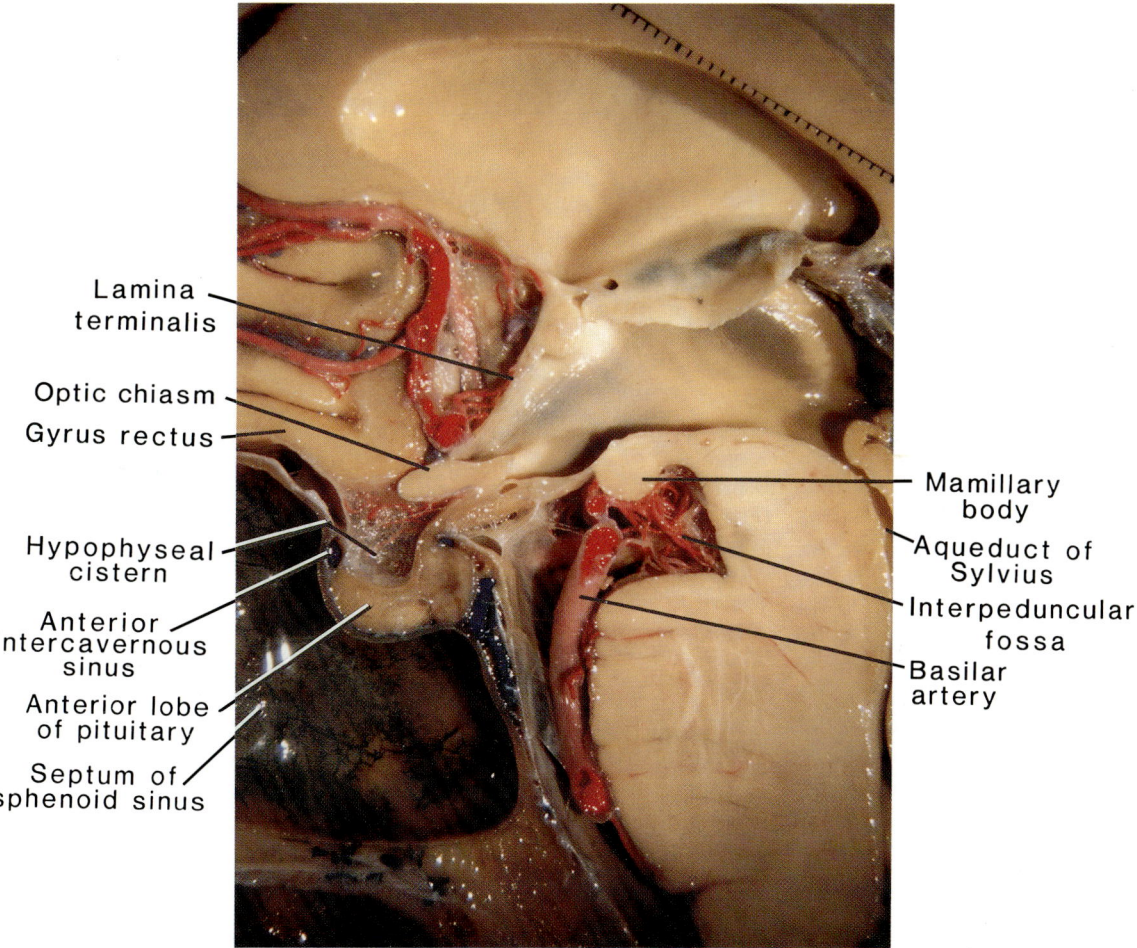

FIG. 8. Median sagittal section showing pituitary cisterns.

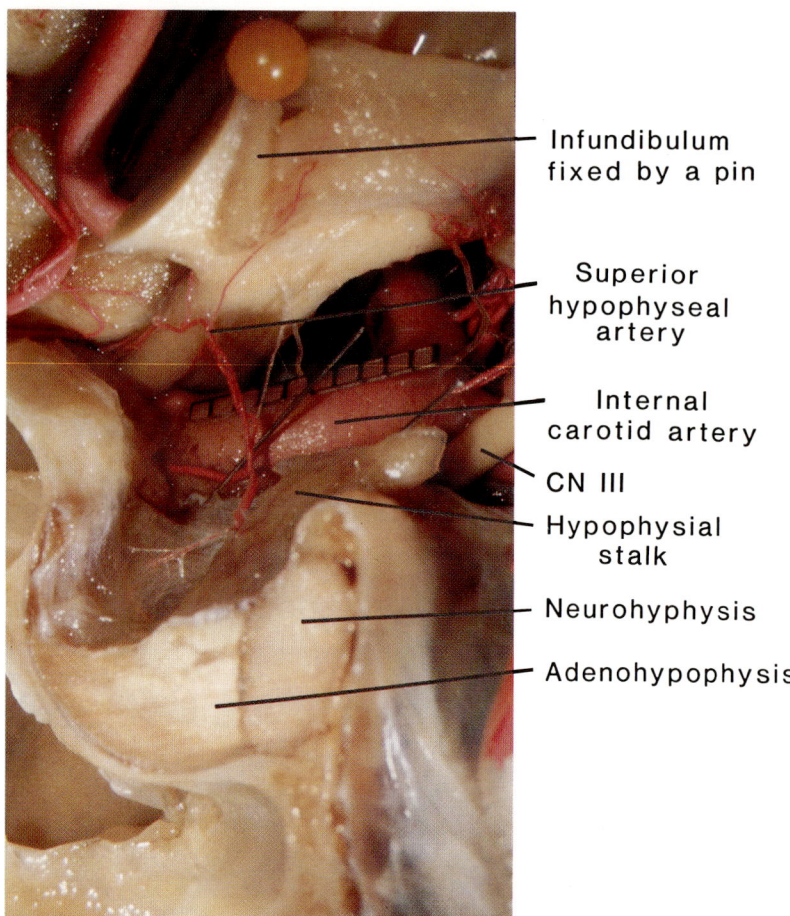

FIG. 9. Dissection showing the origin of the superior hypophyseal artery.

superior hypophyseal arteries originate; they commonly run downward on the anterior and lateral sides of the pituitary stalk.

Accessory Hypophyseal Arteries

Small branches from the posterior communicating artery are often found, which run to the tuber cinereum and contribute to the supply of the infundibulum. They also anastomose with the superior hypophyseal artery.

Caroticocavernous Arteries

Two to six small arteries arise from the cavernous part of the ICA (54). Usually, there are two main trunks, which we call the posterior and lateral caroticocavernous trunks. The posterior caroticocavernous trunk branches off near the posterior curve of the ICA and is commonly known as the meningohypophyseal trunk. It runs first dorsally inside the cavernous sinus, then it divides into two or three branches. The inferior hypophyseal artery usually runs medially and forward. It commonly pursues a tortuous course between the ICA and the dorsum sellae, running medially to the basal part of the posterior pituitary lobe, where it frequently divides into two branches embracing the posterior lobe. The remaining branches supply the tentorium and the clival dura. For variations and twigs see Lang (41). *Capsular arteries* generally arise from the cavernous ICA or from the posterior caroticocavernous trunk. They run through the medial blood space of the cavernous sinus in the cleft between the pituitary capsule and the periosteum. The lower branches enter the bone through nutrient foramina and supply the floor of the pituitary fossa, also contributing to the blood supply of the mucosa of the sphenoidal sinus. The upper branches of this vessel may pierce the pituitary capsule and contribute to the supply of the pituitary (middle inferior and anterior hypophyseal arteries). There are usually left–right anastomoses between these pituitary vessels and also between the capsular arteries. The *inferolateral trunk* usually arises from the inferior or lateral segment of the midportion of the intracavernous carotid artery and often courses lateral to the adjacent nerve. The artery probably supplies the dura and cranial nerves in this area.

Hypophyseal Veins

Blood from the sinusoids of the distal adenohypophysis drains by various routes into the cavernous sinus. Some of the blood may run up into the anterior intracavernous sinus (developed in about 80%), whereas some runs down to a posterior intercavernous sinus. Blood drainage from the neurohypophysis runs into the posterior superior intercavernous sinus or directly into the cavernous sinus itself. Blood from the pituitary stalk region also drains into the upper intercavernous sinuses and the network of pial vessels.

At operation, the anterior lobe of the pituitary looks yellowish and feels relatively firm, whereas the posterior lobe appears gelatinous and gray. Hardy (17) stated that the anterior lobe is surrounded by a potential cleft in which venous capillaries run between the pituitary capsule and the periosteum of the sella turcica. The posterior lobe, on the other hand, usually is attached firmly to the posterior wall of the pituitary fossa.

Pituitary Capsule

Ciric (7) studied the pituitary capsule with an operating microscope in 150 patients undergoing transsphenoidal hypophysectomy. He believes that the anterior and posterior lobes and the pituitary stalk are surrounded by a common layer of connective tissue of simple structure, which he called the hypophyseal capsule.

Lateral Wall of the Cavernous Sinus and the Nerves in It

We have noted that the lateral wall (sagittal plate) of the right cavernous sinus (Fig. 10) is usually closer to the vertical plane than the corresponding wall of the left cavernous sinus (40). Furthermore, the right-sided foramina rotundum and ovale lie closer to the median plane than those on the left. The lateral wall of the cavernous sinus is formed from the dura of the middle cranial fossa and can be separated into a superficial layer (adjacent to the brain) and a deep layer. After the superficial layer (lamina propria) is dissected away, the ophthalmic, maxillary, and trochlear nerves come into view together with the oculomotor nerve and outer wall of the cavum trigeminale. The ophthalmic nerve runs from the upper edge of the trigeminal ganglion forward and up to the superior orbital fissure, passing through it above the third nerve. At the level of the posterior clinoid process, the nerve usually sends out the dural branch, which runs backward into the sagittal plate of the cavernous sinus. This branch continues, usually accompanied by the tentorial branch, into the tentorium cerebelli (Arnold's nerve).

Within the foramen rotundum, the *maxillary nerve* contains an average of 14 fascicles, although there can be anywhere from 1 to 30 fascicles (47).

The *mandibular nerve* is embedded in the lateral wall of the cavernous sinus. Within the lateral wall of the cavernous sinus, *the trochlear nerve* is enveloped by an arachnoid sheath, on which there also may be arachnoid granulations. In our specimens it was found that the *trochlear nerve* entered the inferior surface of the tentorium cerebelli in only 21% of cases. In the remainder, its entry was in the angle between the diverging anterior and posterior clinoid folds. In about 20%, the trochlear nerve is seen in two or more branches.

The *oculomotor nerve* enters the transverse plate of the cavernous sinus at its "pore." The anterolateral margin of the pore is sharp. A pocket of dura and arachnoid accompanies the nerve for 6–8 mm into the cavernous sinus (37). In its intracisternal portion, the nerve is

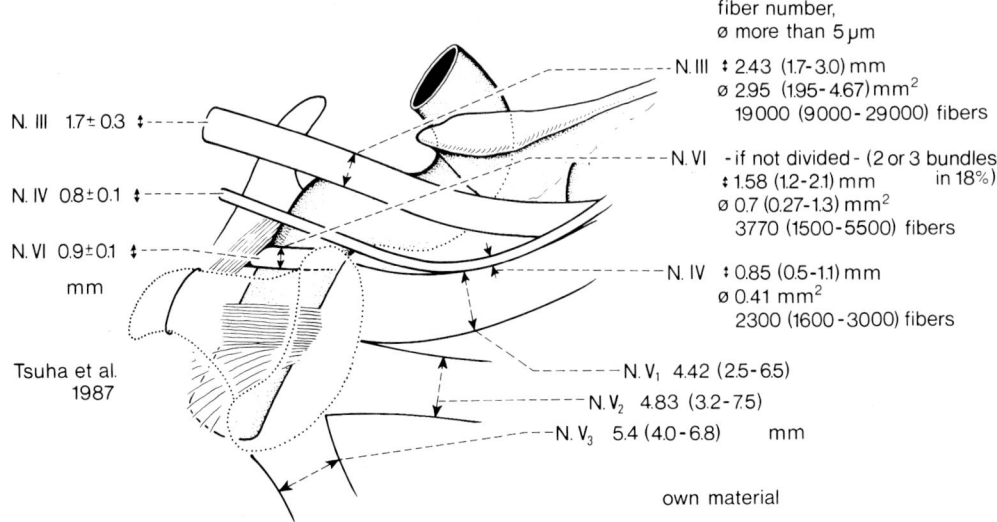

FIG. 10. Nerves in the lateral wall of the cavernous sinus.

usually oval but tends to flatten as it runs into the cavernous sinus.

The *abducens nerve* (Fig. 11) first runs anteriorly and laterally within the cisterna pontis to its opening in the dura, which lies in the lateral region of the clivus. Sheaths of dura and arachnoid accompany the nerve through its portal into the basilar plexus. The portal of entry for the abducent nerve in the cavernous sinus is posteroinferior to the posterior clinoid process. It then proceeds rostrally lying lateral to the ICA, enveloped in its sheaths of dura, arachnoid, and connective tissue (37). It is the only nerve to the orbital muscles that runs within the cavernous sinus. Near the posterior curvature of the ICA, the nerve normally broadens and flattens and, in 18%, breaks into two and, rarely, three bundles.

The attachment zones of *the superior sphenopetrosal ligament* (*abducent bridge*) present small bony spurs. Gruber divided them into the posterior petrosal process of the sphenoid bone, arising from the lateral margin of the backrest of the Turkish saddle, and the posterior (sphenoid) process of the petrosal part, arising from the apex of the petrosal part. If the two bony spurs are close or fused, they form a bony bridge arching over the beginning of the groove for the inferior petrosal sinus. The abducent nerve (and the inferior petrosal sinus) runs beneath this bridge. The space below it is known as Dorello's canal. Sometimes the nerve is divided into two segments, part above and below the ligament.

The *abducens nerve* ran below the upper border of the *trigeminal ganglion* in 84% on the right and in 77.3% on the left in our specimens. In the remainder, it first ran above the ganglion, turning only in its subsequent course downward and medially toward the ophthalmic nerve.

Internal Carotid Artery

The course of the ICA in the cavernous sinus is shown in Figs. 11–13. Inside the cavernous sinus, the two internal carotid arteries are separated by an average distance of 12 mm (4–18 mm) between their medial walls. About half the time, the ICA follows an S-shaped course within the cavernous sinus. The artery ascends deeply into the sinus, almost as far as the posterior clinoid process, then bends at a right angle. In about one-third of specimens, the S-shape was even more pronounced, and in the remainder it followed an almost straight course (52,75).

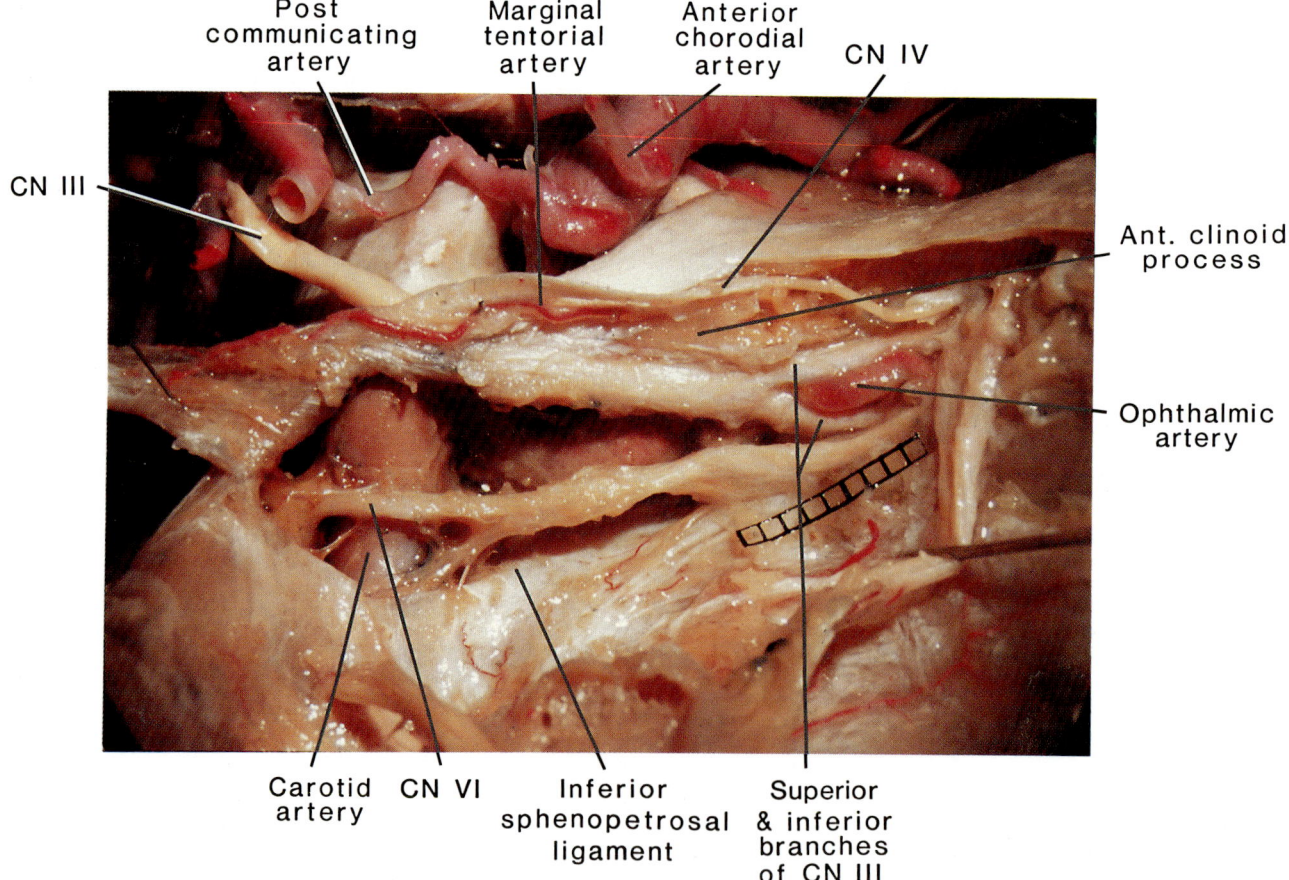

FIG. 11. Abducens, oculomotor, and trochlear nerves: their course in the cavernous sinus and in the apex of the orbit.

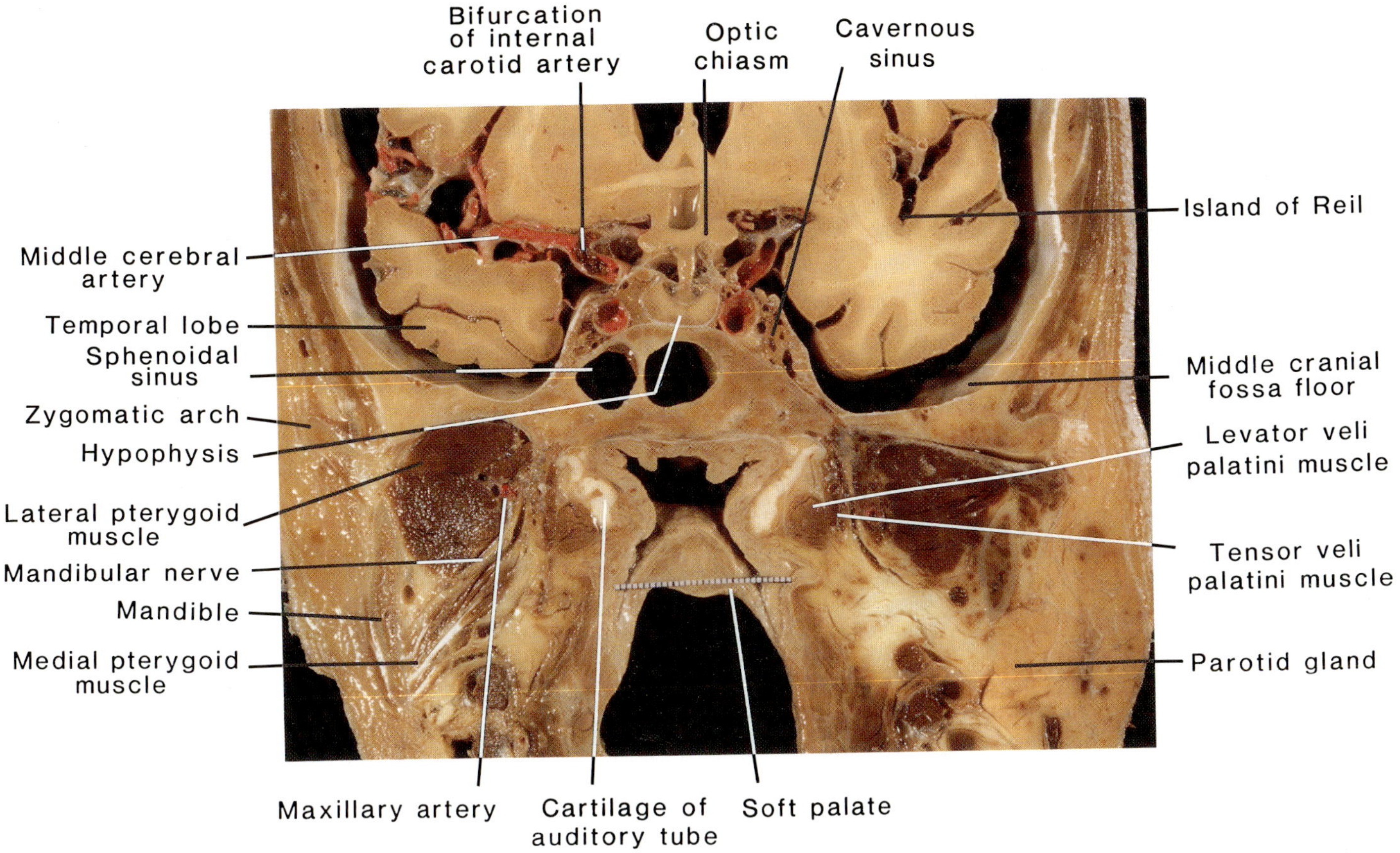

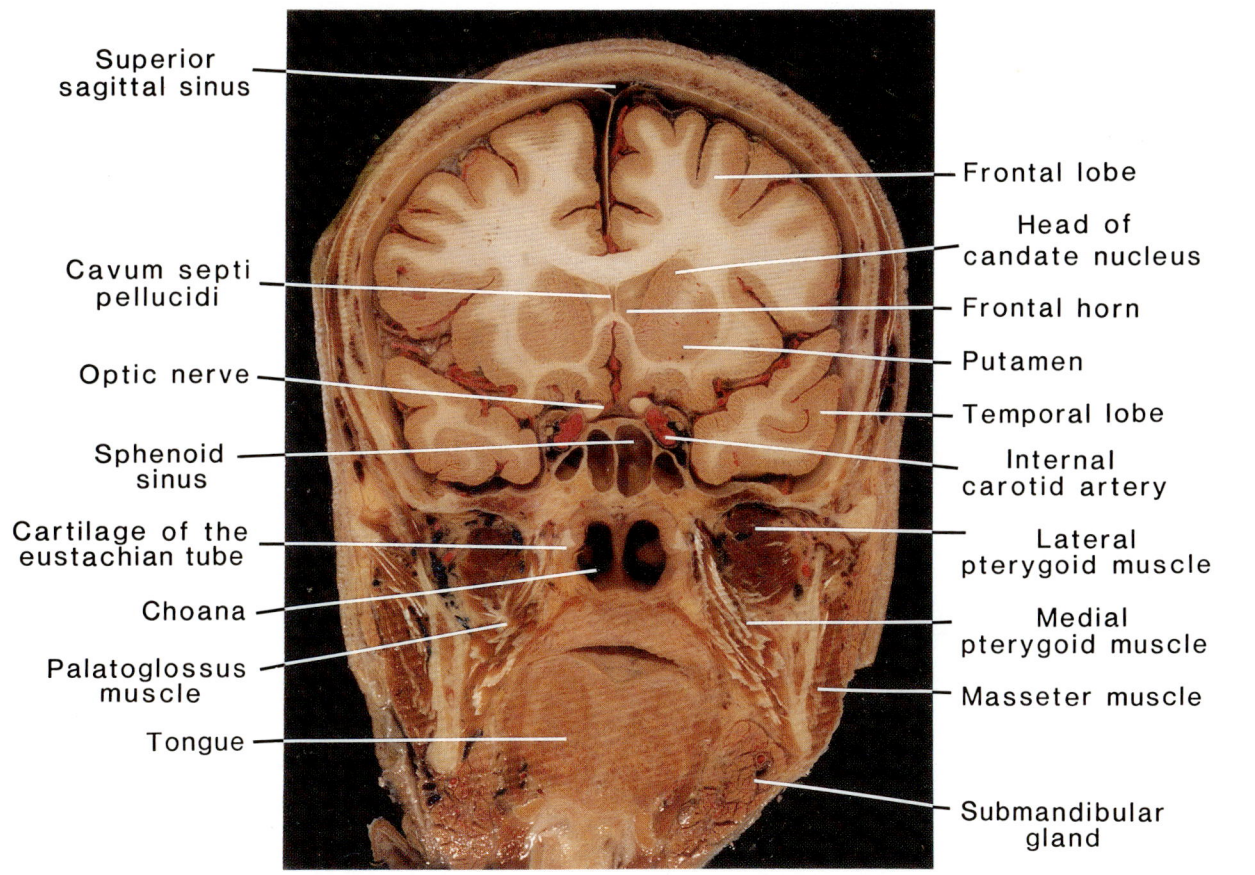

FIG. 12. Coronal section of the head—posterior view.

FIG. 13. Coronal section of the head.

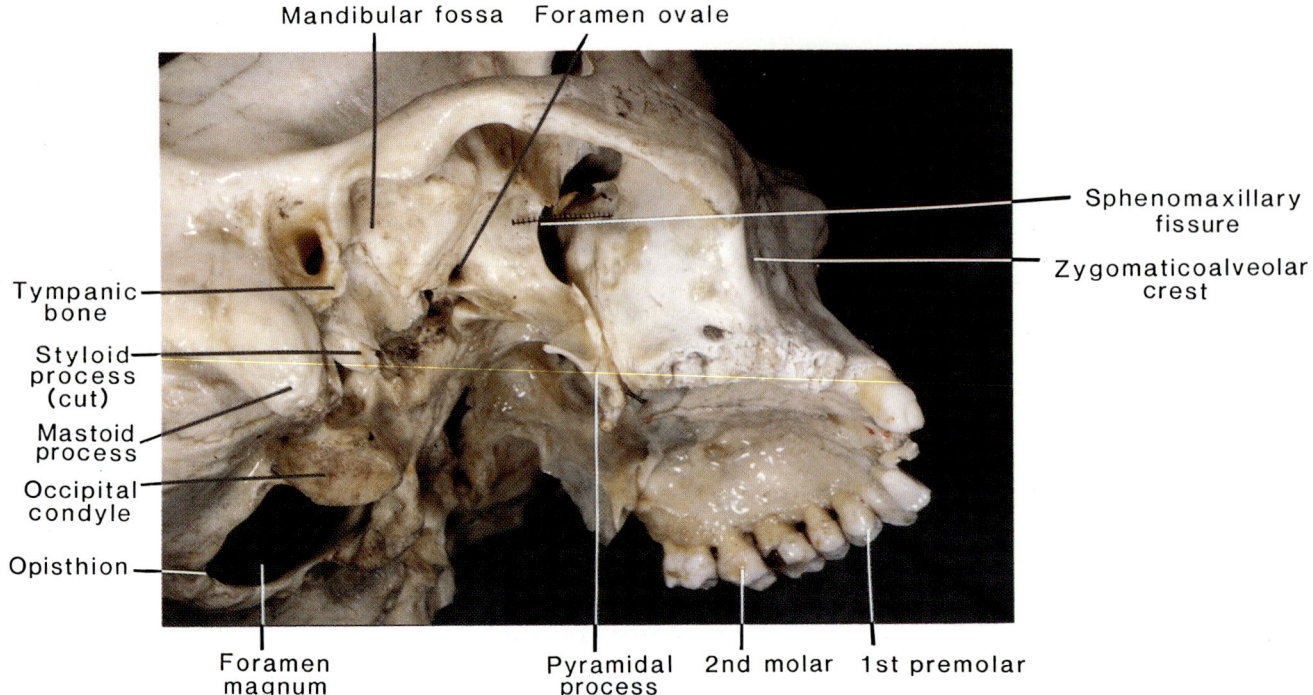

FIG. 14. View of the infratemporal fossa.

Inferior Skull Base Anatomy

The anterior border of the inferior orbital fissure (Figs. 14 and 15) is the maxillary tuber, which increases in size postnatally, especially between the fifth and eighth years of life. The pterygopalatine fossa is posterior to the posteromedial part of the tuber maxillae. The inferior orbital fissure is narrower medially and wider laterally and is bordered above by the great wing of the sphenoid bone and below by the maxillary tuber. In about half the population, the anterior lateral border is formed by the zygomatic bone, and in the other half, by the sphenoid and maxillary bones. Rarely (mainly in older people), this part of the fissure is thinned, and orbital fat may project

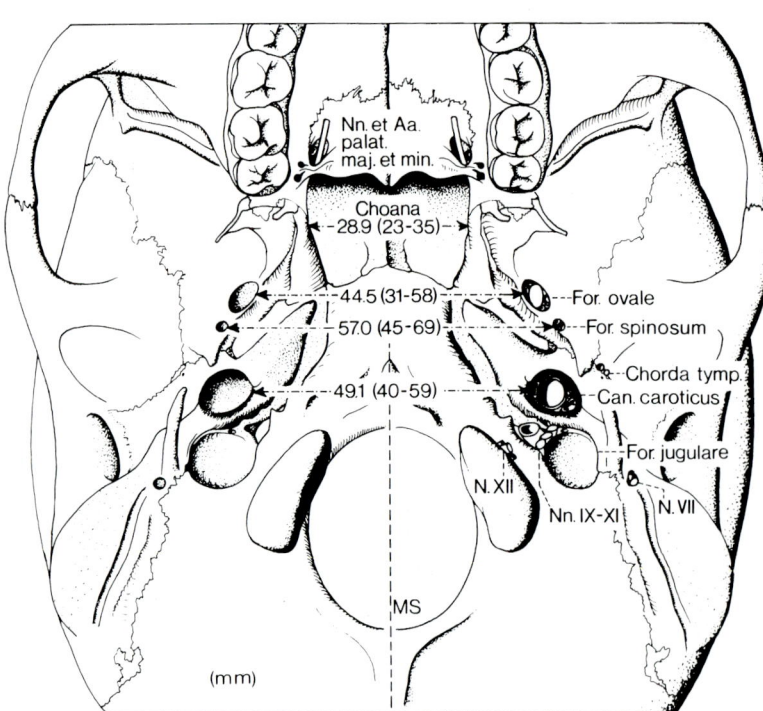

FIG. 15. Important portals of the inferior skull base.

into the temporal fossa as a "fat hernia" (55). Below the inferior orbital fissure are the alveolar foramina, through which the superior posterior alveolar branches of the maxillary nerve are transmitted to the lateral wall of the maxillary sinus (50). These nerves and the accompanying vessels supply the mucous membrane of the maxillary sinus, the molars and premolars of the upper jaw, and parts of the gingiva.

Behind the infraorbital fissure is the *infratemporal fossa*, which lies mainly below the great wing of the sphenoid bone. Dorsolaterally, the squama of the temporal bone forms the temporomandibular joint. A groove usually is found immediately behind the inferior orbital fissure, and behind this groove is the sphenomaxillary crest (21). Behind this crest, in the lateral part of the infratemporal fossa, is the infratemporal spine, which is shaped like a three-sided pyramid. The infratemporal spine connects with the sphenomaxillary crest anteriorly and the infratemporal crest laterally and posteriorly (79).

Medial to the infratemporal fossa, the lateral plate of the pterygoid process projects downward. Postnatally, like the maxillary bone, the pterygoid process grows inferiorly (45). The lateral plate of the pterygoid process is oriented dorsally and laterally. The pterygospinal ligament extends between the lateral lamina of the pterygoid process and the spine of the ala. Sometimes this ligament is ossified in both children and adults. These bony bridges are called *laminae pterygospinosae* and are found medial to, below, or lateral to the foramen ovale. In the last case, thermocoagulation of the trigeminal ganglion may be difficult or impossible. The so-called spinous processes of the lateral pterygoid lamina have different shapes, are sometimes duplicated, and may lie in the upper or lower part of the lateral lamina. The medial lamina of the pterygoid process is shorter than the lateral lamina.

The superior and anterior parts of the pterygoid process lie slightly posterior to the maxillary tuber. The space between these two bony structures is called the *sphenomaxillary fissure* and forms the lateral opening of the pterygopalatine fossa. Within this fossa are the pterygopalatine ganglion, the pterygopalatine part of the maxillary artery, veins, and fatty tissue.

The *anterior wall of the pterygopalatine fossa* is the tuber of the maxilla; the *medial wall* is composed of the vertical lamina of the palatine bone, and the *posterior wall* is the pterygoid process.

The posterior and lateral parts of the infratemporal fossa are bounded by the squamous temporal bone. This part is triangular. Behind the squama are the tympanic part of the temporal bone and the inferior process of the tegmen tympani. The lateral ligament of the temporomandibular joint originates in the *articular tubercle* (Figs. 16 and 17).

Medial to this is the articular fossa, which can be transverse or oblique, and fibrous cartilage covers part of the joint between the articulate disc and the squamous part of the temporal bone. The *articular eminence* is medial to the articular tubercle. Like the articular fossa, it is covered by thin fibrous cartilage.

The *mandibular fossa* is usually the thinnest zone of the middle cranial fossa. It should be remembered that the gonial angle of the mandible prevents direct transmission of forces from the corpus mandibulae to the ramus.

Between the retroarticular process and a small zone medial to it, the tympanic part of the petrous bone connects with the squamous part via the tympanosquamous suture. The *petrotympanic fissure* lies more medially. The inferior process of the tegmen tympani grows downward shortly before and after birth; later, between this process and the tympanic part of the temporal bone, one or two foramina may be found, through which run the chorda tympani nerve and the inferior tympanic artery.

The *tympanic part of the temporal bone* is posterior to the tympanosquamous and tympanopetrous suture and fissure. A horseshoe-shaped annulus tympanicus has been identified in newborns, situated nearly horizontally. The pars tensa of the tympanic membrane is embedded in this ring-shaped bone. In the superior part the annulus is absent, in the incisura Rivini. The pars flaccida of the eardrum is situated in this area and is loosely attached at the squama. During childhood, tympanic bone grows laterally, medially, and anteriorly to form the solum tympani and the lower wall of the musculotubal canal. Posterior to and against the carotid canal and the jugular fossa, the vagina of the styloid process grows inferiorly.

The *styloid process* develops from the second branchial arch (as do the stylohyoid ligament and the lesser horn of the hyoid bone). In newborns, the styloid process is directed anteriorly and medially; later in life it lies more vertically. Rarely, the styloid process can reach up to the hyoid bone. Bony and cartilaginous chips are sometimes found in the stylohyoid ligament. In these cases, and when the styloid process reaches the hyoid bone, the blood vessels of the neck and of cranial nerves V, VII, IX, and X may be compressed, especially with extension of the head. Attacks of unconsciousness and/or lesions of the phrenic, glossopharyngeal, and superior laryngeal nerves have been described (57). Posterolateral to the styloid process is the opening of the facial canal, the stylomastoid foramen.

Postnatally, the mastoid process develops behind the pars tympanica or the annulus tympanicus. The intermastoid line (line between the apices of the two mastoid processes) usually crosses the area of the occipital condyle. Medial to the mastoid process is a groove called the digastric sulcus. In 93% of specimens, its medial border has a ridge, called the paramastoid crest (8). The posterior belly of the digastric muscle arises in the digastric

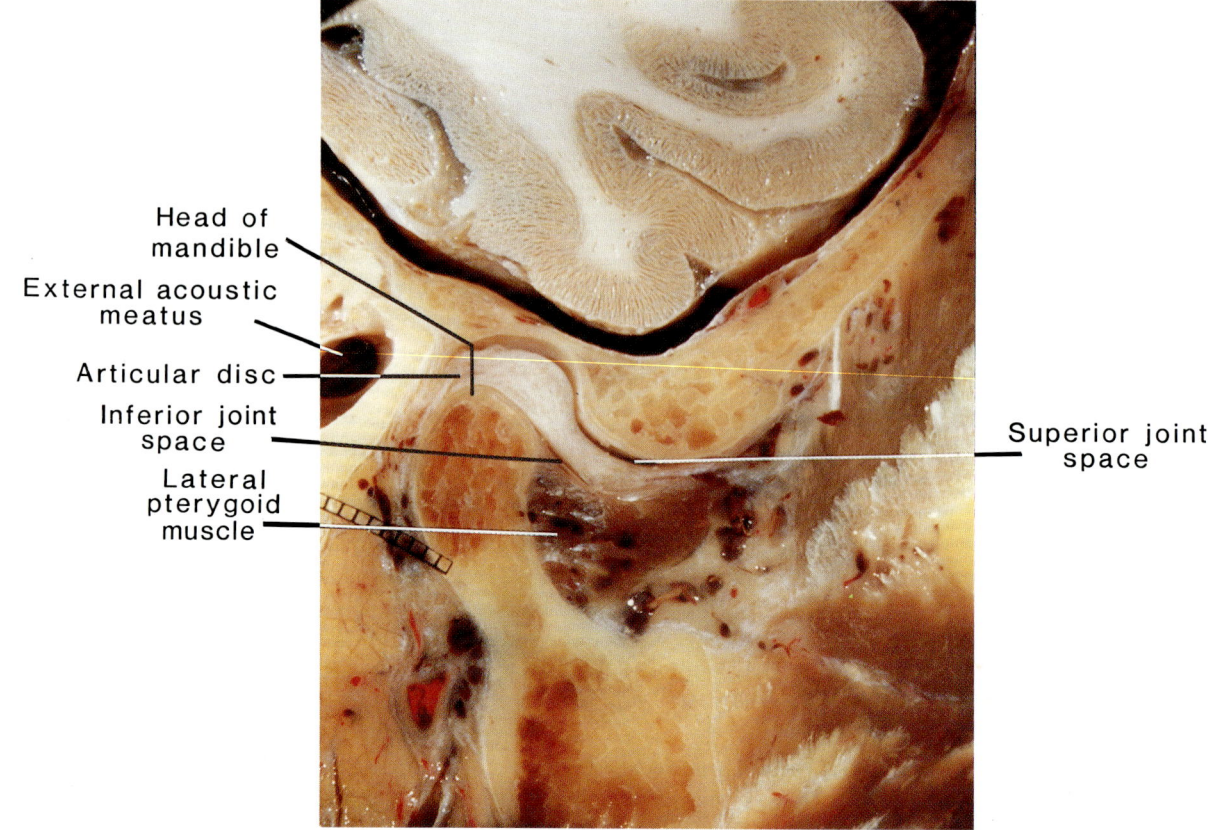

FIG. 16. Temporomandibular joint.

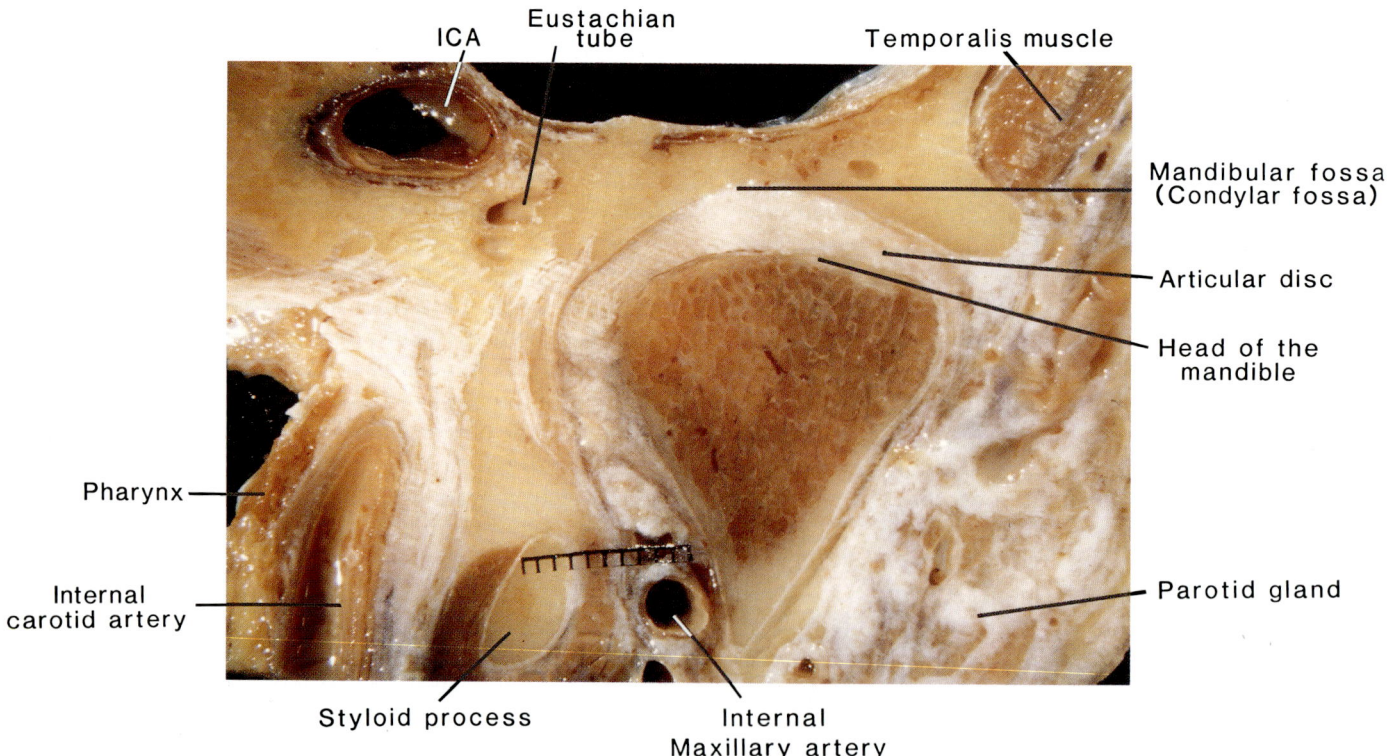

FIG. 17. Coronal section through the temporomandibular joint.

sulcus and the paramastoid crest. In well-pneumatized mastoid processes, this sulcus is visible from inside the mastoid process, and the surgeon can follow it to the mastoid part of the facial canal. A groove of the occipital artery can usually be found medial to the paramastoid crest, and the artery runs in or below this groove.

Portals for Nerves and Vessels

The maxillary nerve runs through the *foramen rotundum* (Fig. 15) into the pterygopalatine fossa. Within the foramen rotundum, the nerve has an average of 14 fascicles (range 1–30) and is usually accompanied by two small arteries.

The mandibular nerve exits through the *foramen ovale*. A venous plexus surrounds the mandibular nerve and connects veins and sinuses of the inner skull base with veins on the outer skull base. The middle meningeal artery, surrounded by a venous plexus of the middle meningeal veins, runs through the foramen spinosum. In about 40% of specimens, a foramen of Vesalius transmitting a sphenoid emissary vein was seen.

The opening of the eustachian tube is dorsal and medial to the foramen spinosum. The pars ossea of the auditory tube is the inferior part of the musculotubal canal; and the groove for the tensor tympani muscle, the upper part. The two grooves are divided by a bony bridge of variable thickness. The bony part of the eustachian tube in adults is 11–12 mm long. The cartilaginous portion of the eustachian tube is 20–25 mm long together 36, 2 (31–42) mm (65a) and runs obliquely from lateral to medial and inferiorly, with an angle to the horizontal plane.

The external opening of the *carotid canal* (Fig. 15) is usually oval in shape. This canal carries the ICA, the venous plexus and veins around the artery, and the sympathetic nerves.

Muscles of the Inferior Cranial Base

The *lateral pterygoid muscle* (Fig. 16) has two parts, a flat superior portion—the infratemporal head—and the inferior belly—the pterygoid head. These are separated by horizontal septa of connective tissue (23). The proximal portions of each part of the muscle are surrounded by fascia, and the two fasciae meet about 10 mm in front of the temporomandibular joint.

The origin of the *infratemporal head of the lateral pterygoid muscle* lies on the infratemporal planum and the infratemporal spine of the lower surface of the great sphenoidal wing, medial to the infratemporal crest. The pterygoid muscle is bordered laterally by the temporal muscle. It runs nearly horizontally and dorsolaterally and merges with the pterygoid head a short distance anterior to the temporomandibular joint. The infratemporal head of the pterygoid muscle inserts on the medial half of the mandibular neck, slightly superior to the insertion of the pterygoid head. A portion of its tendon runs in the capsule of the temporomandibular joint and its disc (23,66), and the axis of the muscle forms an approximately 20° angle with the zygomatic arch. It was once thought that the articular disc and the condyle were extensions of the pterygoid muscle. Several investigators have stated that the superior head of the lateral pterygoid muscle serves to close and/or stabilize the temporomandibular joint, probably directing the forces of mastication to the articular eminence (29).

The *inferior head of the lateral pterygoid muscle* originates on the outer surface of the lateral lamina of the pterygoid process. The muscle fibers run dorsally and superiorly. The belly of the muscle contracts to effect opening of the mouth by pulling the condylar process of the mandible and the articular disc forward, while the head of the mandible rotates on the articular disc.

Origin of the Temporal Muscle

Figure 18 shows the origin of the temporalis muscle on the lateral surface of the skull, the temporal fossa, and the posterior border of the frontal process of the zygomatic bone. The deep portion of the temporal muscle originates from the infratemporal spine and crest, connective tissue of the inferior orbital fissure, and from the external opening of the foramen rotundum (79).

Origin of the Masseter Muscle

The *superficial part* of the masseter muscle originates on the inferior surface of the zygomatic bone or on the zygomatic process of the maxilla. A small portion of this muscle arises on the outer surface of the zygomatic bone.

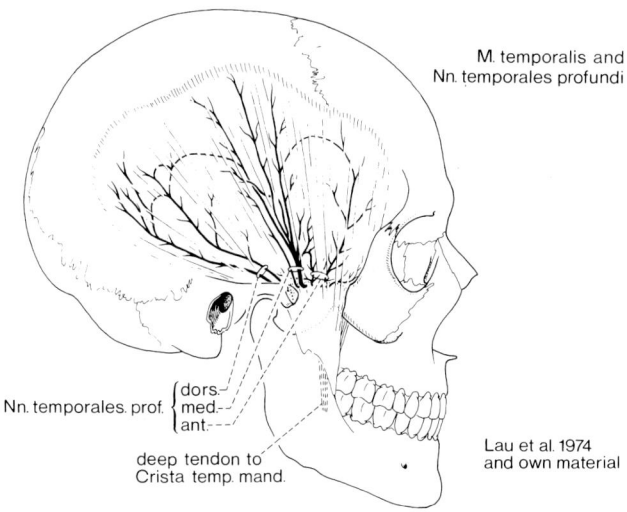

FIG. 18. Temporalis muscle and its nerves.

The *deep part* of the masseter muscle originates in the inferior and medial surface of the zygomatic arch. It extends dorsally to the capsule of the temporomandibular articulation.

Medial Pterygoid Muscle

We divide the muscle into two portions. The main portion arises in the pterygoid fossa, including the pyramidal process of the palatine bone. The smaller, accessory portion arises from the posterior surface of the maxillary tuber.

The uvular muscle arises from the inferior surface of the horizontal lamina of the palatine bone, immediately medial to the insertion of the tensor veli palatini muscle.

The levator veli palatini muscle originates from tuberosities that lie anterior to the external aperture of the carotid canal, in an area bordered by the inferior surface of the apex of the petrous bone. Part of this area is formed by the tympanic portion of the temporal bone. Other fibers of this muscle arise on the medial lamina of the cartilaginous portion of the auditory tube.

The deep portion of the *tensor veli palatini* muscle originates in the salpingopharyngeal fascia; other fibers are connected loosely with the lower border of the lateral or anterior lamellae of the auditory tube. Fibers also arise in the semicanal of the tensor tympani and the scaphoid fovea.

Styloid Process and Origin of Muscles

The stylopharyngeal muscle originates in the superomedial border of the styloid process. At the lateral surface of the styloid process is the origin of the stylohyoid muscle, and at the superior portion or along its anterior border is the origin of the styloglossus muscle (Fig. 17).

Nerves of the Inferior Skull Base

The *sympathetic trunk* is interwoven in the prevertebral cervical fascia. The superior cervical ganglion is located between the first and third cervical vertebrae (2). In 62.3% of cases (40% bilaterally and 22% unilaterally), a sympathetic ganglion is found, anterior to the sixth cervical vertebra (although it may lie anywhere between the third and seventh cervical vertebrae).

The superior cervical sympathetic ganglion is supplied mainly by branches of the ascending pharyngeal artery (44). Lateral to the sympathetic trunk, the ventral rami of the cervical nerves pierce the lamina profunda of the cervical fascia.

Rami of C1 and C2 are connected with the hypoglossal nerve and the sympathetic trunk. It has been noted that these branches supply infrahyoidal muscles. The sympathetic trunk also has connections to the superior laryngeal nerve. As a rule, one or two branches of the superior cervical ganglion of the sympathetic trunk run to the ICA, and one branch goes to the internal jugular vein.

The *glossopharyngeal nerve* leaves the skull through the anterosuperior medial portion of the jugular foramen. Its inferior ganglion lies at the outer skull base, where a small fossa, the fossula petrosa, sometimes is seen between the external aperture of the carotid channel and the jugular fossa.

The tympanic nerve, a small branch of the ninth cranial nerve, courses with a branch of the ascending pharyngeal artery through the canaliculus tympanicus to the middle ear cavity. Two to six glomera, from which chemodectomas can arise, are present in the course of this nerve (15). After the glossopharyngeal nerve sends out another branch to anastomose with the vagus nerve, it courses along the outer surface of the ICA and turns medial to the internal jugular vein. The nerve then runs inferiorly and anteriorly to the ICA. The landmark for the nerve here is the stylopharyngeal muscle, which it also supplies; the nerve has been seen piercing this muscle in about 12% of cases (62).

The nerve then runs in the stylopharyngeal fascia to the margin between the superior and middle pharyngeal constrictor muscles. Rarely, the nerve pierces the superior constrictor muscle, but it always anastomoses with the auricular branch of the vagus nerve, the sympathetic trunk, and the facial nerve. The anastomosis with the facial nerve may be with its extracranial portion or digastric branch. These anastomoses provide a means for the sensory fibers from the pinna to reach the ninth cranial nerve.

Inferior to the inferior ganglion of the glossopharyngeal nerve, one or two branches (the rami sinus carotici), which anastomose with branches of the tenth cranial nerve and the sympathetic trunk, run to the pressoreceptive zone of the carotid sinus and carotid glomus. In addition, three to four pharyngeal branches of the ninth cranial nerve run to the posterior surface of the pharynx, tonsillar branches extend to the tonsillar capsule, and lingual branches run to the pharyngeal part of the tongue: the vallate and foliate papillae, the vallecula glossoepiglottica, and the upper surface of the epiglottis.

Motor branches of the ninth nerve (together with the tenth nerve) supply the stylopharyngeal muscle and the upper constrictors of the pharynx. The ninth nerve also provides sensory innervation of the posterior third of the tongue (taste fibers to the vallate papillae) and dorsal parts of the mouth cavity, the isthmus faucium, and the pharynx. Sensory areas innervated by this nerve include the isthmus faucium, the palatine tonsil, the pharyngeal surface of the tongue, the posterior and lateral walls of the pharynx, the tympanic cavity, the auditory tube, and a small area posterior to the ear.

Vagus Nerve

Vagus nerve bundles run to the ovoid dural pore in the area of the jugular foramen, where the superior ganglion of the tenth cranial nerve is located. One to three anastomoses with the glossopharyngeal nerve were found in this area and in more inferior parts. The internal branch of the accessory nerve branches off below the margo terminalis sigmoidea of the jugular foramen and intersects the vagus nerve.

The auricular branch of the vagus nerve branches off from the lower circumference of the superior ganglion of the nerve and usually contains fibers from the glossopharyngeal nerve. This branch courses through the jugular fossa and then runs in a small channel through the petrous part of the temporal bone on the posterior or anterior circumference of the mastoid portion of the facial nerve and also contains glomera. Anastomoses between the ninth and seventh cranial nerves also occur in this area. The auricular branch of the vagus nerve then courses through the temporal bone to the tympanomastoid fissure, in rare cases along with the facial nerve branch to the stylomastoid foramen, and provides part of the innervation of the lateral surface of the tympanic membrane and the external auditory canal. A small branch of the superior ganglion of the vagus nerve is thought to course posteriorly in the posterior fossa, in particular around the occipital sinus.

The inferior ganglion of the tenth nerve is anterior to the transverse processes of the first and second cervical vertebrae. In more than 50% of our specimens, we found large veins running through the ganglion area.

The motor fibers of the vagus nerves are axons of the ambiguous nucleus in the medulla oblongata and (along with the fibers of the glossopharyngeal nerve) supply the constrictor muscles of the pharynx and the stylopharyngeal, levator veli palatini, palatoglossus, palatopharyngeal, and laryngeal muscles.

The sensory fibers of the mucous membrane of the pharynx, the thyroid gland, and the parathyroid gland run centrally in the pharyngeal branches of the vagus nerve. Glomera laryngea have been found on the superior laryngeal nerve (77) and on the inferior laryngeal nerve (30). These findings are important in understanding the origins of glomus tumors.

Accessory Nerve

From 6 to 16 (average 10.66) cranial root fiber bundles of the accessory nerve are found to anastomose with the spinal part of the nerve. These fibers are composed of axons of the inferior portion of the ambiguous nucleus and run in the pharyngeal branches of the vagus nerve and in the recurrent laryngeal nerve. The spinal portion of the accessory nerve is composed of fiber bundles that leave the spinal cord between the anterior and posterior root fiber bundles, sometimes as far inferior as the seventh cervical segment.

The nucleus of the accessory nerve in the spinal cord extends from the caudal third of the inferior olive to between the fourth and seventh (although usually between the fourth and sixth) cervical segments, slightly dorsal to the ventral column. The spinal roots of the accessory nerve emerge from the lateral portion of the spinal cord or, occasionally, in line with the dorsal nerve roots. The most inferior fibers may come from the sixth or the seventh cervical segment.

The roots of the accessory nerve unite to ascend between the dentate ligament and the dorsal rootlets of the spinal nerve and then pass through the foramen magnum posterior to the vertebral artery. We found one to three fibers from the dorsal rootlets of the first dorsal cervical root and occasionally fibers of second or third cervical root anastomose with the spinal root of the accessory nerve.

In the area of the anastomoses between the first cervical nerve and the spinal roots of the accessory nerve, a ganglion was visible macroscopically on the right side in 41% of specimens and on the left in 43% (42). It is possible that sensory fibers of the first cervical nerve also go to the deeper portions of the spinal cord via the eleventh cranial nerve and its descending roots. In addition, proprioceptive fibers from the muscles supplied by the accessory nerve (sternocleidomastoid and trapezius muscles) may enter the spinal cord via the dorsal rootlets.

In the jugular foramen area, the accessory nerve runs immediately posterior to the vagus nerve, embedded in the nerve guide plate. Tandler (76) found that this nerve then runs posterior to the internal jugular vein in 33% of cases and anterior to the vein in 66%. In 85% of our specimens, the eleventh nerve traversed anterior to the jugular vein, and in the other 15% posterior to the jugular vein, to the sternocleidomastoid muscle and anastomosed with branches of the cervical plexus. The sternocleidomastoid branch of the occipital artery runs a short distance with the accessory nerve. This nerve (and the cervical plexus) supply the sternocleidomastoid and trapezius muscles.

Hypoglossal Nerve

An average of 13.6 root fiber bundles leave the sulcus between the pyramid and the olive of the medulla oblongata. The hypoglossal canal was divided into two canals in 12.7% of our specimens on the right and in 25% on the left. The dural pores were duplicated in 65% of specimens. The nerve fiber bundles (and their sheaths) always united inside the hypoglossal canal.

The canal for the hypoglossal nerve made a 45° (average) angle to the midsagittal plane (71). The nerve (and sometimes also the posterior fossa meningeal branch) is surrounded by a venous plexus, a dural sheath, and an arachnoidal sheath.

On the outer skull base, the hypoglossal nerve runs on the medial surface of the internal jugular vein and on the lateral surface of the vagus nerve in 92% of cases. Then the twelfth nerve curves around the occipital artery or its first branch to the sternocleidomastoid muscle to course first to the lateral, and then to the anterior, surface of the external carotid artery (ECA). In about 8% of cases, the nerve curves around the ECA distal to the origin of the occipital artery, then takes a lateral course on the outer surface of the ECA and posterior to the internal jugular vein (59). The hypoglossal nerve connects with the ventral rami of C1 and C2: ventral ansa between them.

The descending branch of the nerve leaves the main trunk $14.3\bar{x}$ mm distal to the ansa. A communicating branch with the lingual nerve always was present on the outer surface of the hyoglossus muscle (14,61).

It is important to note that the fibers of the first and second cervical nerves supply the longus capitis, rectus capitis anterior, and the infrahyoid muscles. The lingual twigs of the hypoglossal nerve supply the genioglossus, hyoglossus, styloglossus, and intrinsic muscles of the tongue. When a lesion is present on the side of the hypoglossal nerve, the tongue (especially the genioglossus) points to the side of the lesion. When bilateral lesions of the hypoglossal nerve are present, it is impossible to move the tongue at all, and disturbances in swallowing and speech also occur. Occasionally, glossospasm and fibrillation of the tongue are seen when such lesions are small.

Vessels of the Parapharyngeal Space

Binswanger (3) first showed that the *carotid sinus* was not always located on the origin of the ICA but might be found at the termination of the common carotid artery or its location might include both the origin of the ICA and the termination of the common carotid artery.

The *internal carotid artery* most often bifurcates between the third and fourth cervical vertebrae. The left-sided bifurcation was slightly inferior than that on the right. For a description of the variations possible in the origin of the common carotid artery and the twigs of the external carotid artery see Lang (43). The ICA ascends in the lateral parapharyngeal space to the external opening of the carotid canal in the temporal bone. Herrschaft (22) noted that the ICA can elongate, coil, or kink in 10–20% of cases (this was seen in only 10% of our specimens). Tortuosities generally develop only when arteriosclerosis is present; whereas coiling of the artery may be a congenital condition due to lack of stretching of the internal carotid arteries during descent of the carotids (4).

Proximal kinking of this vessel is most often directed dorsally; and distal kinking is directed ventrally (43).

The *ascending pharyngeal artery* originated directly as a branch of the ECA in 55.6% of 63 half heads (44). In 11.1% of cases, it was a branch of another artery that left the ECA and in 12.7% of cases, it originated near the bifurcation of the common carotid artery. In 8%, the ascending pharyngeal artery was a branch of the occipital artery, and in about 5%, a branch of the ICA.

The ascending pharyngeal artery usually runs in an almost straight course. In 39% of cases it ran medial, and in 35%, anteromedial to the ICA. In about 9%, the proximal two-thirds of the ascending pharyngeal artery ran rostral to the ICA. In approximately 80% of our cases, the ascending pharyngeal artery divided into branches that ran to the muscles of the pharynx, to the tenth and twelfth cranial nerves, to the sympathetic trunk, and to lymph nodes in the parapharyngeal and retropharyngeal spaces. Other branches may extend to the pharyngeal tonsil, auditory tube, cranial base, and foramina of the posterior cranial fossa. The longus capitis, longus colli, and anterior rectus muscles also are supplied by this vessel. Other branches may run medial to the styloglossus, stylopharyngeal, and stylohyoid muscles.

One branch of the ascending pharyngeal artery to the jugular foramen was seen in 50% of cases, two branches in 37.5%, and three branches in 10.5%. These represent meningeal branches to the posterior cranial fossa (dura and bone). Most originated in the infracranial portion of the artery, although in 30%, the vessels were from the middle; and in 8%, the vessels were from the proximal distribution. In about 4% of specimens, the branch to the jugular foramen was a twig of the occipital artery. Two branches of the ascending pharyngeal artery ran to the inferior cranial base in about 33% of cases, one branch in 19%, and four branches in 5.4%. Branches of the distal ascending pharyngeal artery usually ran to the epipharynx, pharyngeal tonsil, and auditory tube. In the last case, the vessel anastomosed with the ascending palatine artery, the sphenopalatine artery, and the arterial network in the tympanic cavity.

The *ascending palatine artery* was found to originate on the facial artery in 71% of cases and on the ECA in 29% (51). Its most important branch is the tonsillar branch, but the palatine branch is important during transpalatine approaches to the clivus in the upper cervical column.

Infratemporal Fossa: Masticatory Space, Vessels, and Nerves

The main vessel of the infratemporal fossa is the *maxillary artery,* which is an end branch of the ECA and which takes a variable course to the lateral pterygoid muscle. In 50% of our specimens, the pterygoid part of the maxillary artery ran parallel to the Frankfort plane or within 5° upwards.

The first part of the maxillary artery is the retromandibular portion, which courses behind the mandible and sends one or two small branches to the tympanic membrane and one branch each to the deep auricular, anterior tympanic, and the middle meningeal arteries. The accessory middle meningeal artery usually branches off from this twig but also may arise directly from the maxillary artery. The middle meningeal artery supplies part of the pterygoid muscles and the tensor veli palatini muscle.

The second part of the maxillary artery, the pterygoid part, extends obliquely anteromedially and was found by different investigators to run medial or lateral to the inferior head of the lateral pterygoid muscle. The middle meningeal artery branches off proximal to the inferior alveolar artery when this artery takes a lateral course and vice versa when it takes a medial course (33,34). Branches of the pterygoid part of the maxillary artery run to the pterygoid muscles, the masseter muscle, and as deep temporal arteries. These last branches course superiorly and then run in small grooves of the temporal squama.

The pterygopalatine part of the maxillary artery courses through the sphenopalatine fissure in the pterygopalatine fossa and anteriorly to the pterygopalatine ganglion and veins. The branches of this vessel are the anterior deep temporal, posterior superior alveolar, infraorbital (the infraorbital and the superior and posterior alveolar arteries often have a common trunk), greater palatine, and sphenopalatine arteries. One group of researchers twice found a sphenopalatine vein running from the sphenopalatine foramen to the inferior border of the sphenomaxillary fissure, immediately posterior to the periosteal layer of the maxillary sinus (65). In the other cases they examined, the veins were very small.

Tumors in the infratemporal fossa cause deafness, auditory canal pain, and anesthesia of the mandibular nerve distribution, as well as asymmetry of the soft palate, trismus (when the pterygoid muscles are involved), and swelling in the area of the zygomatic arch. Aneurysms of the maxillary artery are very rare; only four cases had been described prior to 1966, and all were diagnosed when the aneurysm ruptured. In one report, a 53-year-old woman presented with pain anterior to the left ear; a congenital saccular aneurysm of the maxillary artery was found intraoperatively in the area of the lateral pterygoid muscle (69).

The course of the maxillary artery to the lingual and inferior alveolar nerves varies greatly.

The *mandibular nerve* is lateral and anterior to the eustachian tube and tensor veli palatini muscle, inferior to the foramen ovale, and medial to the lateral pterygoid muscle. It is surrounded by the venous plexus of the foramen ovale and is near the accessory middle meningeal artery and the meningeal branch of the mandibular nerve. The otic ganglion is located medial to the mandibular nerve.

The posterior branch of the mandibular nerve is the auriculotemporal nerve, two branches of which surround the middle meningeal artery and later unite to form the nerve that extends posterior to the temporomandibular joint in the parotid region.

The chorda tympani nerve lies medial to the lateral pterygoid muscle. It courses between the petrotympanic fissure or the spine of the ala major and the lingual nerve. Other medial and superior branches of the mandibular nerve send twigs to the pterygoid, tensor tympani, and tensor veli palatini muscles. The deep temporal nerves course on the superior margin of the infratemporal head of the lateral pterygoid muscle and enter the temporal muscle from the medial side. The masseter nerve runs through the mandibular incisura to the masseter muscle; the buccal nerve runs between the two heads of the lateral pterygoid muscle to the outer surface of the buccinator muscle, supplying the skin and the mucous membrane of the neck. The lingual and inferior alveolar nerves run through the pterygoid hiatus to the lateral border of the medial pterygoid muscle and its fascial sheath. This hiatus is bordered by the inferior limit of the pterygoid head of the lateral pterygoid muscle, the superior and posterior borders of the medial pterygoid muscle, and the neck of the mandible. The lingual nerve may originate as one to three roots. It may receive a branch from the inferior alveolar nerve, the sympathetic plexus, and the otic ganglion.

Veins of the Inferior Skull Base

The most important vein in the parapharyngeal space is the internal jugular vein. The bulb of this vein is located anteriorly, lateral to the margo terminalis sigmoidea of the jugular foramen. From this landmark, the bulb extends superiorly. When an extremely high jugular bulb is located more medially, it can be found immediately lateral to the inferior area of the internal auditory meatus. More laterally located high jugular bulbs bulge into the floor of the middle ear cavity. This has implications for cranial base surgery. A high jugular bulb may be inadvertently entered while opening the internal auditory canal by retrosigmoid–transmeatal approach. Such a bulb may restrict the exposure afforded by a translabyrinthine approach. A laterally placed high jugular bulb may be mistaken for a glomus tumor upon otoscopy.

In one study of 257 temporal bones, the jugular bulb was elevated (superior to the lower perimeter of the tympanic annulus) in 6% (64). The internal jugular vein normally takes a lateral course in the parapharyngeal space, slightly posterior to the ICA.

Vertebral Artery and Veins

The *prevertebral segment of the vertebral artery* (the first segment) is that segment between the artery's origin and the transverse foramen, which this artery enters. This segment was first approached surgically by Crawford et al. (9) to manage lesions causing osteal stenosis.

The *transverse segment* (the second segment) is the portion between the transverse foramen and the C2–C3 intercervical space. Kuttner (35) and Oljenick (63) were the first to surgically approach this segment. Elkin and Harris (11), Hardin et al. (16), and Jung (26) used this approach to treat traumatic vertebral arteriovenous aneurysms and neurovascular complications secondary to spondylosis.

The *third segment* lies between the C2 transverse foramen and the posterior fossa dura. The *fourth segment* extends from the dural entrance to the vertebrobasilar junction.

Jung and Kehr (27) defined arterial hypoplasia as an arterial diameter of less than 2 mm, measured radiographically, and by incomplete or retarded filling with contrast material on serial roentgenograms. A "single" vertebral artery refers to the total absence of one artery or presence of a nonfunctional (hypoplastic) artery as identified roentgenographically by retarded filling with contrast material (1). Jung (28) found complete absence of the vertebral artery in 2.5% of cases and functional aplasia of one artery in 6%. Argenson et al. (1) noted unilateral hypoplasia of the vertebral artery in 9.3% of cases on the right and 3.7% on the left. Jung (28) found that hypoplasia occurred three times as often on the left as on the right. Bilateral hypoplasia of the vertebral arteries was found in 3.7% of Africans.

In the transverse foramina, the vertebral artery is surrounded by the vertebral venous system and the sympathetic elements and lies anteromedially in the canal, in contact with the anterior root of the transverse process, more or less in the region of the uncus. Normally, the artery has an undulating course from one transverse process to the other. As it passes between the periosteum of the uncus and the vertebral body, one or more small veins may be interposed. The largest vertebral vein ran between the artery and the periosteum of the anterior bony root of the transverse process in two cases.

REFERENCES

1. Argenson C, Francke JP, Sylla S, Dintimille H, Papasian S, di Marino V. The vertebral arteries (segments V_1 and V_2). *Anat Clin* 1980;2:29–41.
2. Becker RF, Grunt JA. The cervical sympathetic ganglia. *Anat Rec* 1957;127:1–14.
3. Binswanger. Anatomische Untersuchungen uber die Ursprungsstelle und den Anfangsteil der Carotis interna. *Arch Psychiatry* 1879;9:351.
3a. Berke RN. A modified Kronlein operation. *Arch Ophthalmol* 1954;51:609–632.
4. Brosig HJ, Vollmar J. Chirurgische Korrektur der Knickstenosen der A. carotis interna. *Munch Med Wochenschr* 1974;116:19.
5. Buschmann W, Linnert D. Wandel der Indikation und der Technik in der Chirurgie retrobulbarer Orbitatumoren. *Klin Monatsbl Augenheilkd* 1978;171:1–12.
6. Chandler SB, Derezinski CF. The variations of the middle meningeal artery within the middle cranial fossa. *Anat Rec* 1935;62:309–319.
7. Ciric I. On the origin and nature of the pituitary gland capsule. *J Neurosurg* 1977;46:596–600.
8. Corner EM. On the temporal fossa. *J Anat Physiol* 1896;30:377–385.
9. Crawford E, de Baker M, Fields W. Roetgenographic diagnosis and surgical treatment of the basilar artery insufficiency. *JAMA* 1958;168:509–514.
10. Dietemann JL, Lang J, Francke JP, Bonneville JF, Clarisse J, Wackenheim A. Anatomy and radiology of the sellar spine. *Neuroradiology* 1981;21:5–7.
11. Elkin DC, Harris MH. Arteriovenous aneurysm of the vertebral vessels. Report of 10 cases. *Ann Surg* 1946;124:934–951.
12. Engel A. *Ursprungs- und Verlaufsvariationen der ersten Ophthalmica-Strecke.* Medical Dissertation, Wurzburg, 1975.
13. Fisher AG. Case of complete absence of both internal carotid arteries with a preliminary note on development of stapedial artery. *J Anat Physiol* 1914;48:37–46.
14. Fitzgerald MJT, Law ME. The peripheral connexions between the lingual and hypoglossal nerves. *J Anat* 1958;92:178–199.
15. Guild SR. A hitherto unrecognized structure, the glomus jugularis, in man. *Anat Rec* 1941;79:29.
16. Hardin C, Wilimason W, Steegmann A. Vertebral artery insufficiency produced by cervical osteoarthritic spurs. *Neurology* 1960;10:855–858.
17. Hardy J. Transsphenoidal microsurgery of the normal and pathological pituitary. *Clin Neurosurg* 1969;16:185–217.
18. Hassmann H. *Form, MaBe und Verlaufe der Schadelkanale: des Canalis infraorbitalis, Canalis incisivus, Canalis palatinus major, Foramen spinosum und Meatus acusticus internus.* Medical Dissertation, Wurzburg, 1975.
19. Hayreh SS, Dass R. The ophthalmic artery. I. Origin and intracranial and intra-canalicular course. *Br J Ophthalmol* 1962;46:65–98.
20. Hayreh SS, Dass R. The ophthalmic artery. II. Intraorbital course. *Br J Ophthalmol* 1962;46:165–185.
21. Henle J. *Handbuch der Nervenlehre des Menschen.* Braunschweig: Vieweg & Sohn, 1871.
22. Herrschaft H. Cerebrale Durchblutungsstorungen bei extremer Schlingenbildung der A. carotis interna. *Munch Med Wochenschr* 1968;46:2694–2702.
23. Honee GLJM. The anatomy of the lateral pterygoid muscle. *Acta Morphol Neerl Scand* 1972;10:331–340.
24. Hugo NE, Stone E. Anatomy for a blepharoplasty. *Plast Reconstr Surg* 1974;53:381–383.
25. Johnson JB, Hadley RC. The aging face. In: Converse JM, ed. *Reconstructive plastic surgery.* Philadelphia: Saunders, 1964.
26. Jung A. Resection de l'articulation uncovertebrale et ouverture de trou de conjugaison par voie anterieure dans le traitement de la nevrealgie cervico-brachiale. Technique operatoire. *Mem Acad Chir* 1963;89:361–367.
27. Jung A, Kehr P. *Pathologie de l'artere vertebrale et des racines nerveuses dans les arthroses et les traumatismes du rachis cervical.* Paris: Masson, 1972.
28. Jung FM. *Les traumatismes du rachis cervical avec lesions de l'artere vertebral.* Thesis in Medicine, Strasbourg, 1974.
29. Juniper RP. The superior pterygoid muscle. *Br J Oral Surg* 1981;19:121–128.
30. Kleinsasser O. Das Glomus laryngicum inferior. Ein bisher unbekanntes, nicht chromaffines Paraganglion vom Bau der sog. Carotisdruse im menschlichen Kehlkopf. *Arch Ohr-, Nas-Kehlk-Heilkd* 1964;184:214–224.
31. Koornneef L. New insights in the human orbital connective tissue. *Arch Ophthalmol* 1977;95:1269–1273.
32. Krauss J. *Messungen zur cranio-cerebralen Topographie.* Medical Dissertation, Wurzburg, 1987.

33. Krizan Z. Beitrage zur keskriptiven und topographischen Anatomie der A. maxillaris. *Acta Anat* 1960;41:319–333.
34. Krizan Z. Uber die fraglichen Korrelationen und uber die Entwicklung einiger Typen der A. Maxillaris. *Acta Anat* 1960;42:71–87.
35. Kuttner H. Die Verletzungen und traumatischen Aneurysmen der Vertebralgefabe am Halse und ihre operative Behandlung. *Beitr Klinis Chir* 1917;108:1–60.
36. Lang J. Zur Vascularisation der Dura mater cerebri. II. Vascularisierte Durazotten am Eingang in den Canalis opticus. *Z Anat Entwicklungsgesch* 1973;141:223–236.
37. Lang J. Eintritt und Verlauf der Hirnnerven (III, IV, VI) "im" Sinus cavernosus. *Z Anat Entwicklungsgesch* 1974;145:87–99.
38. Lang J. Uber die Vascularisation der Periorbita. *Gegenbaurs Morphol Jahrb* 1975;121:174–191.
39. Lang J. Structure and postnatal organization of heretofore uninvestigated and infrequent ossifications of the sella turcica region. *Acta Anat* 1977;99:121–139.
40. Lang J. Praktische Anatomie. Begr v R von Lanz, W Wachsmuth. *Fortgef u hrsg v.* J Lang, W Wachsmuth. Vol 1, part 1B. Berlin: Springer 1979.
41. Lang J. Uber die Pteriongegend und deren klinisch wichtigem Abstand zum Nervus opticus. 1. Pteriongegend. *Neurochirurgia (Stuttg)* 1983;26:161–163.
42. Lang J. *Clinical anatomy of the head. Neurocranium–orbit–craniocervical regions.* New York: Springer, 1983.
43. Lang J. *Clinical anatomy of the posterior cranial fossa and its foramina.* New York: Thieme, 1991.
44. Lang J, Heilek E. Anatomische-klinische Befunde zur A. pharyngeal ascendens. *Anat Anz* 1984;156:177–207.
45. Lang J, Hetterich A. Beitrag zur postnatalen Entwicklung des Processus pterygoideus. *Anat Anz* 1983;154:1–31.
46. Lang J, Kageyama I. Clinical anatomy of the ophthalmic artery and cavernous sinus. In: Samii M, ed. *Surgery of the sellar region,* vol 2. Springer, 1991;145–148.
47. Lang J, Keller H. Uber die hintere Pfortenregion der Fossa pterygopalatina und die Lage des Ganglion pterygopalatinum. *Gegenbaurs Morphol Jahrb* 1978;124:207–214.
48. Lang J, Koth R, Reiss G. Uber die Bildung, die Zuflusse und den Verlauf der V. basalis und der V. cerebri interna. *Anat Anz* 1981;150:385–423.
49. Lang J, Maier R, Schafhauser O. On the postnatal magnification of the foramina rotundum, ovale and spinosum and their topographical changes. *Anat Anz* 1984;156:351–387.
49a. Lang J, Oehmann G. Formentwicklung des Canalis opticus, seine Maße und Einstellung zu den Schädelebenen. *Verh Anat Ges* 1976;70:567–574.
50. Lang J, Papke J. Uber die klinische Anatomie des Paries inferior orbitae und dessen Nachbarstrukturen. *Gegenbaurs Morphol Jahrb* 1984;130:1–47.
51. Lang J, Preis K-H. A. palatina ascendens, Ursprung, Verlauf und Zweige. *HNO* 1981;29:391–396.
52. Lang J, Reiter U. Uber den Verlauf der Hirnnerven in der Seitenwand des Sinus cavernosus. *Neurochirurgia (Stuttg)* 1984;27:93–97.
53. Lang J, Reiter U, Reiter W. Topographie des Orbitainhaltes. Teil II: Uber die Kammerung des Corpus adiposum orbitae. *Neurochirurgia (Stuttg)* 1991;34:1–5.
54. Lang J, Schafer K. Uber Ursprung und Versorgungsgebiete der intracavernosen Strecke der A. carotis interna. *Gegenbaurs Morphol Jahrb* 1976;122:182–202.
55. Lang J, Schlehahn FA. Uber die postnatale Entwicklung der Fissurae orbitales. *Gegenbaurs Morphol Jahrb* 1981;127:849–859.
56. Lang J, Tisch-Rottensteiner KF. Uber Form und Formvarianten der Sella turcica. *Verh Anat Ges* 1977;71:1279–1282.
57. Lesoine W. Das Stylo-Kerato-Hyoidale Syndrom. *DA Heft* 1976;38:2381.
58. Lindblom K. A roentgenographic study of the vascular channels of the skull. *Acta Radiol* 1936;30:146.
59. Lowy R: Ueber das topographische Verhalten des Nervus hypoglossus zur Vena jugularis interna. *Anat Anz* 1910;37:10–12.
60. Maroon JC, Kennerdell JS. Lateral microsurgical approach to intraorbital tumors. *J Neurosurg* 1976;44:556–561.
61. Mizuno N, Akimoto C, Mochizuki K, Matsuschima R. Experimental studies of efferent fibers in the hypoglossal nerve in the cat: a scanning electron microscopic observation in the lingual mucosa following transsection of the nerve, and a degeneration study with silver impregnation methods. *Arch Histol Jpn* 1973;35:99–113.
62. Muller T. *Uber die Verbreitung des N. glossopharyngeus im Bereich des Gaumens und die Anastomosen des N. hypoglossus im Spatium parapharyngeum.* Medical Dissertation, Wurzburg, 1985.
63. Oljenick I. Uber die Unterbindung der Arteria vertebralis. *Zentralbl Chir* 1917;44:1067–1069.
64. Overton SB, Ritter FN. A high placed jugular bulb in the middle ear: a clinical and temporal bone study. *Laryngoscope* 1973;83:1986–1991.
65. Pearson BW, MacKenzie RG, Goodman WS. The anatomical basis of the transantral ligation of the maxillary artery in severe epistaxis. *Laryngoscope* 1969;79:969–984.
65a. Pahnke JW. Beiträge zur klinischen *Anatomie der Tuba auditiva.* Habilitationsschrift Würzburg 1991.
66. Petersen H. Braus' Lehrbuch der Anatomie. *Roux' Arch Entwicklungsmechanik Organismen* 1925;106:26–32.
67. Pickrell KL. Reconstructive plastic surgery of the face. In: Walton JH, ed. *Clinical symposia,* vol 20. Canada: Ciba, 1968.
68. Platzer W. Zur Anatomie der "Sellabrucke" und ihrer Beziehung zur A. carotis interna. *ROFO* 1957;87:613–616.
69. Rankow RM. Congenital aneurysm of the maxillary artery. *Plast Reconstr Surg* 1966;37:291–294.
70. Rohen J. Morphologische Studien zur Funktion des Lidapparates beim Menschen. *Gegenbaurs Morphol Jahrb* 1953;93:43–97.
71. Schmidt HM. Uber die postnatale Entwicklung der Vertikalabstande zwischen der Lamina cribrosa und kraniometrischen Messpunkten und Schaedelebenen. *Verh Anat Ges* 1975;69:799–805.
72. Schurmann K. Neurochirurgische Aufgaben in der Orbita. *Arch Otorhinolaryngol* 1974;207:253–282.
73. Simoes S. Relacoes anatomicas do seio emisario do forame ovale suas implicacoes clinico-chirurgicas. *Arq Neuropsiquiatr* 1973;31:1–9.
74. Sondheimer FK. Basal foramina and canals. In: Newton TH, Pott DG, eds. *Radiology of the skull and brain. The skull.* St Louis: CV Mosby, 1971;287–347.
75. Strobel FJ. *Uber Lagebeziehungen des Ganglion trigeminale.* Medical Dissertation, Wurzburg, 1980.
76. Tandler J. Die Entwicklung der Lagebeziehung zwischen N. accessorius und V. jugularis interna beim Menschen. *Anat Anz* 1907;31:473–480.
77. Watzka M. Uber Paraganglien in der Plica ventricularis des menschlichen Kehlkopfes. *Dtsch Med Forsch* 1963;1:19–20.
78. Whitaker SR, Sprinkle PM, Chou SM. Nasal glioma. *Arch Otolaryngol* 1981;107:550–554.
79. Zenker W. Das "Spatium buccotemporale" und die anderen Fascienraume der tiefen seitlichen Gesichtsregion. *Z Anat Entwicklungsgesch* 1955;118:371–390.

CHAPTER 10

Anatomy of the Paranasal Sinuses

Johannes Lang

The paranasal sinuses include the *maxillary, sphenoid, frontal,* and *ethmoid* sinuses (18). The ethmoid sinuses are subdivided into the anterior, middle, and posterior sinuses or cells. The walls of the paranasal sinuses do not correspond to the bony walls suggested by their names, that is, maxillary, sphenoid, and frontal sinuses.

MIDDLE NASAL MEATUS AND PARANASAL SINUSES

The *middle nasal meatus* (Fig. 1) is bounded above by the attachment of the middle nasal concha, below by the attachment of the inferior nasal concha, below by the attachment of the inferior nasal concha, and medially by the middle turbinate. The *middle nasal concha* is part of the ethmoid bone. Its anterior part is attached at the agger nasi and at the skull base lateral to the cribriform plate, and posterior to the lateral nasal wall at the ethmoid bone and perpendicular plate of the palatine bone. The sphenopalatine foramen lies immediately posterior or above to the posterior attachment of the middle concha (11).

SEMILUNAR HIATUS

The semilunar hiatus (Fig. 2) is bordered above by the ethmoidal bulla and below by the uncinate process of the ethmoid bone. Its anterosuperior end is usually covered by the middle nasal concha. In one series of 111 specimens, the anterior end of the hiatus was in front of the anterior end of the middle nasal concha in 2% of cases; in these cases the middle nasal concha was underdeveloped. In 5% it was at the same level as the anterior attachment of the middle concha, in 43% between 1 and 10 mm behind the attachment, and in 47% of cases 11–20 mm behind it. In one case (0.9%) the anterior end of the semilunar hiatus was 23 mm posterior to the anterior attachment of the turbinate. The length of the semilunar hiatus was between 14 and 22 mm and its medial–lateral extent was between 0.5 and 3.0 mm (17).

ETHMOIDAL BULLA

The term *ethmoidal bulla* (Fig. 2) was first used by Zuckerkandl (27) and it indicates that this part of the bone is pneumatized. In the specimens studied the ethmoidal bulla was 18 mm (range 9–28 mm) long, and 5.4 mm (range 2–13 mm) high. Zuckerkandl (27) recorded lengths between 20 and 26 mm. Soemmering (23) and Grünwald (5) termed the bulla, if it is nonpneumatized, the lateral torus. In our material the bulla was pneumatized in 70% of cases; in the rest a lateral torus extended to the junction of the medial and inferior orbital walls.

Frontal Recess

Initially, a *frontal recess* arises from the superior part of the middle meatus. The frontal recess may extend widely and grow into the frontal bone (direct formation of the frontal sinus) (8,19). Other anterior ethmoidal cells also sprout from the recess; they too can grow into the frontal bone (indirect formation of the frontal sinus).

J. Lang: Institute of Anatomy, University of Würzburg, W-8700 Würzburg, Germany.

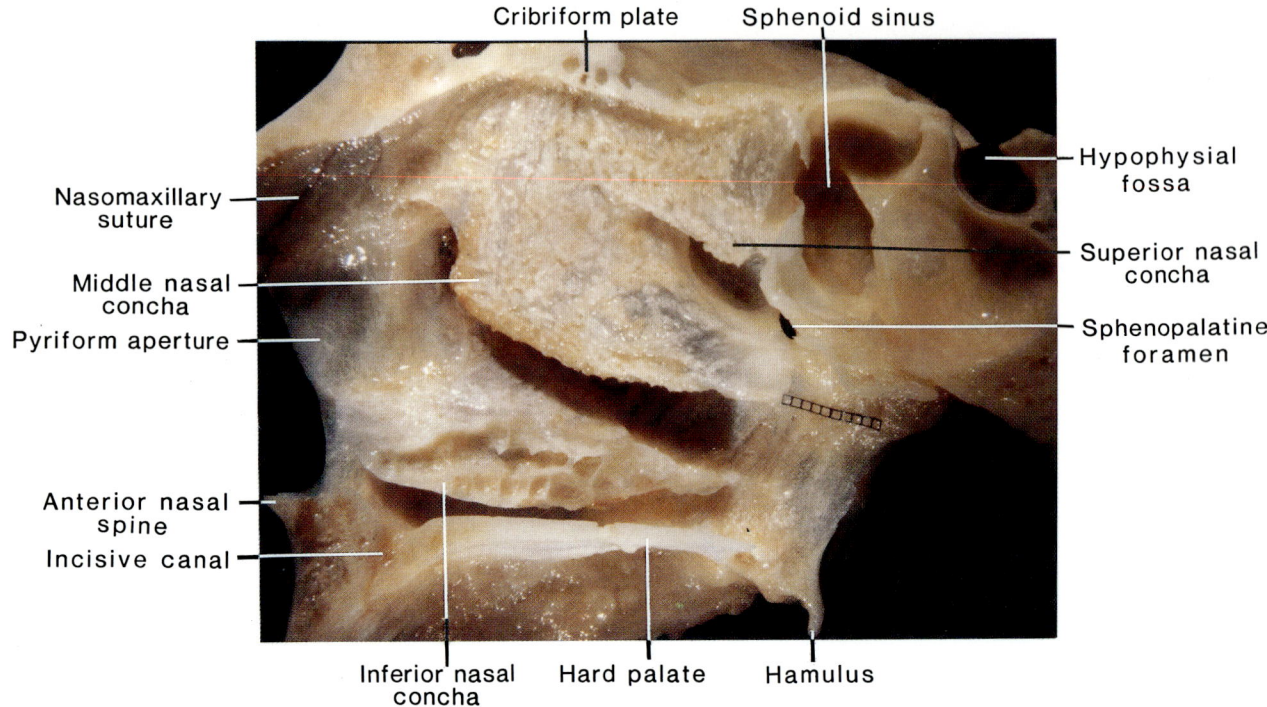

FIG. 1. Lateral wall of the nose.

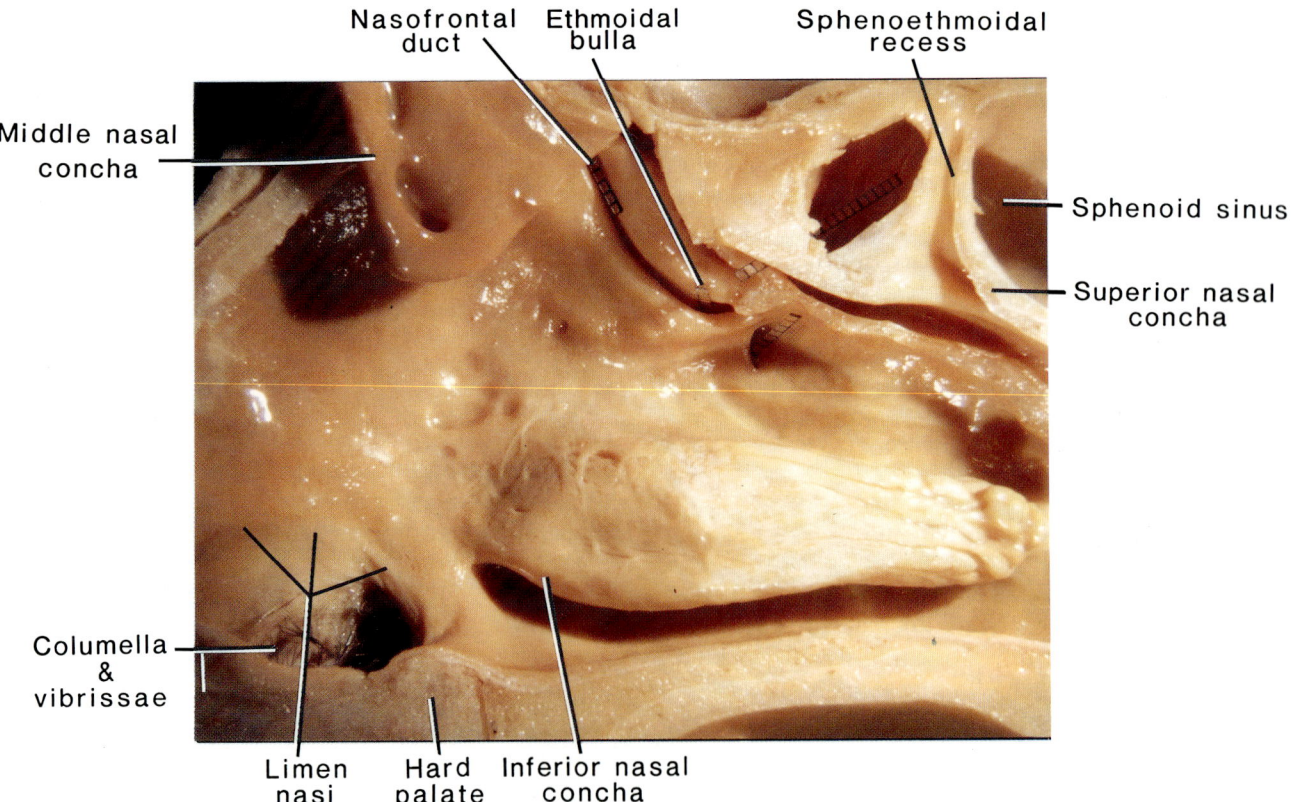

FIG. 2. Lateral wall of the nose after resection of the middle nasal concha.

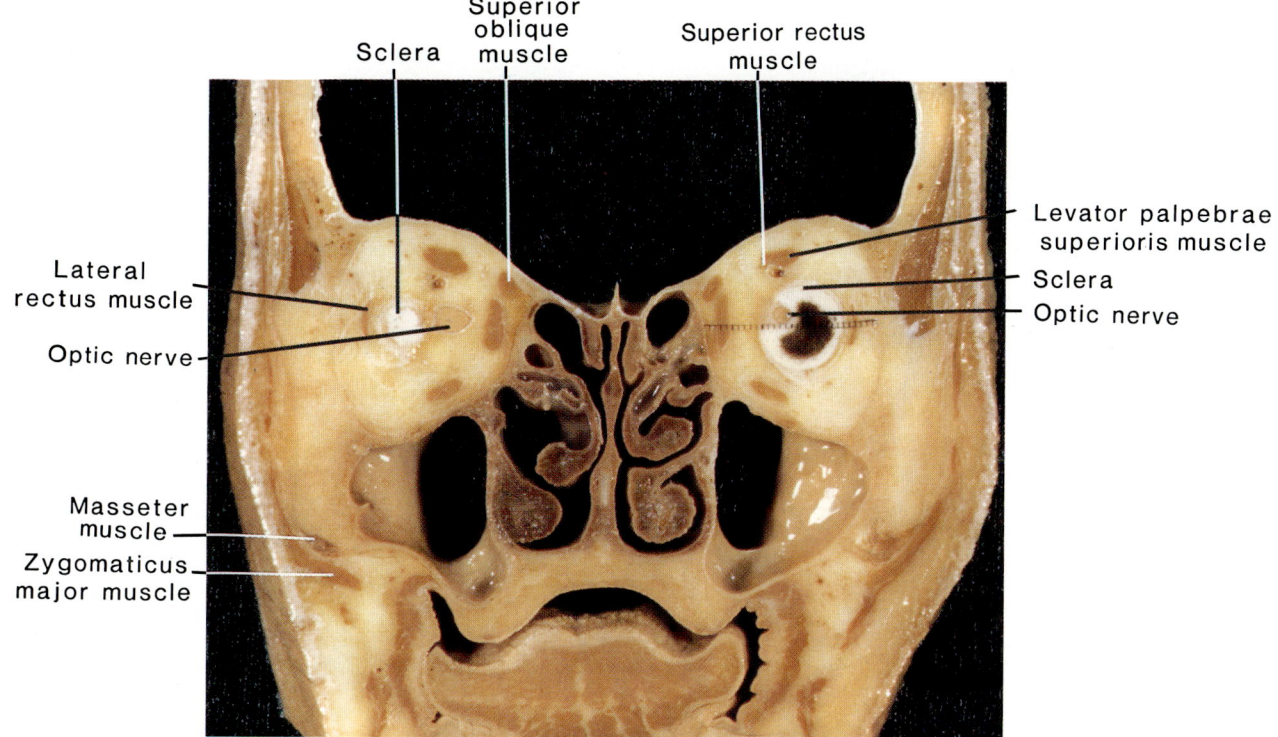

FIG. 3. Coronal section of the head, frontal view.

MAXILLARY SINUS

The relative size of the *maxillary sinus* is quite small in infancy and becomes progressively larger with increasing age (Fig. 3). In the specimens studied (13) the maxillary sinus was 2.5 mm wide in one 39-mm fetus. In neonates it is 5.3 mm high, 10 mm long, and 3.5 mm broad (20). At this age it does not reach the infraorbital canal laterally. In a 4-year-old boy the maxillary sinus was seen to be 7 mm wide, 17 mm long, and 12 mm high. The infraorbital canal and sulcus lay immediately lateral to its lateral wall. In adults the anterior segment of the maxillary sinus was 26.2 mm (range 16.4–37.9 mm) broad on the right, and 26.9 mm (range 16.1–39.8 mm) on the left side. Its medial side was 38.4 mm (range 30.1–49.2 mm) long on the right side, and 39.1 mm (range 31.1–45.8 mm) on the left. The cavity was 40.0 mm (range 29.3–56.2 mm) high on the right side and 40.8 mm (range 31.3–56.9 mm) on the left side (13).

HALLER'S CELLS

Haller's cells (Fig. 4) may lie lateral to the *ethmoidal infundibulum* (an area superolateral to the middle turbinate, which communicates with the frontal recess, maxillary sinus, and ethmoid sinus) and open into the middle nasal meatus. Stupka (24) thought that Haller's cells arose from a cell protruding from the ethmoidal bulla between the layers of the orbital floor, bulging the roof of the maxillary sinus. They project below the floor of the orbit over a variable distance. These Haller's cells can restrict access to the maxillary sinus or the anterior ethmoidal cells during endonasal procedures (15). Schlungbaum (21) described a bipartite antral cavity: the smaller anterior chamber opened into the middle nasal meatus and the posterior chamber into the superior nasal meatus. The latter could of course be regarded as a posterior ethmoidal cell projecting downward. A second type of secondary maxillary sinus is classified as a Haller's cell if it is due to a posterior ethmoidal cell projecting far forward in an inferior direction under the floor of the orbit. The transmaxillary route for opening and clearance of the ethmoidal cells is easier in such cases (9). If Haller's cells are particularly well developed, they border the orbit on one side, and the medial part of the superior wall of the maxillary sinus on the other (25). The maxillary sinus then does not meet the ethmoidal labyrinth or the orbit (maxilloethmoidal angle) in the frontal plane at an acute angle but appears to be flattened

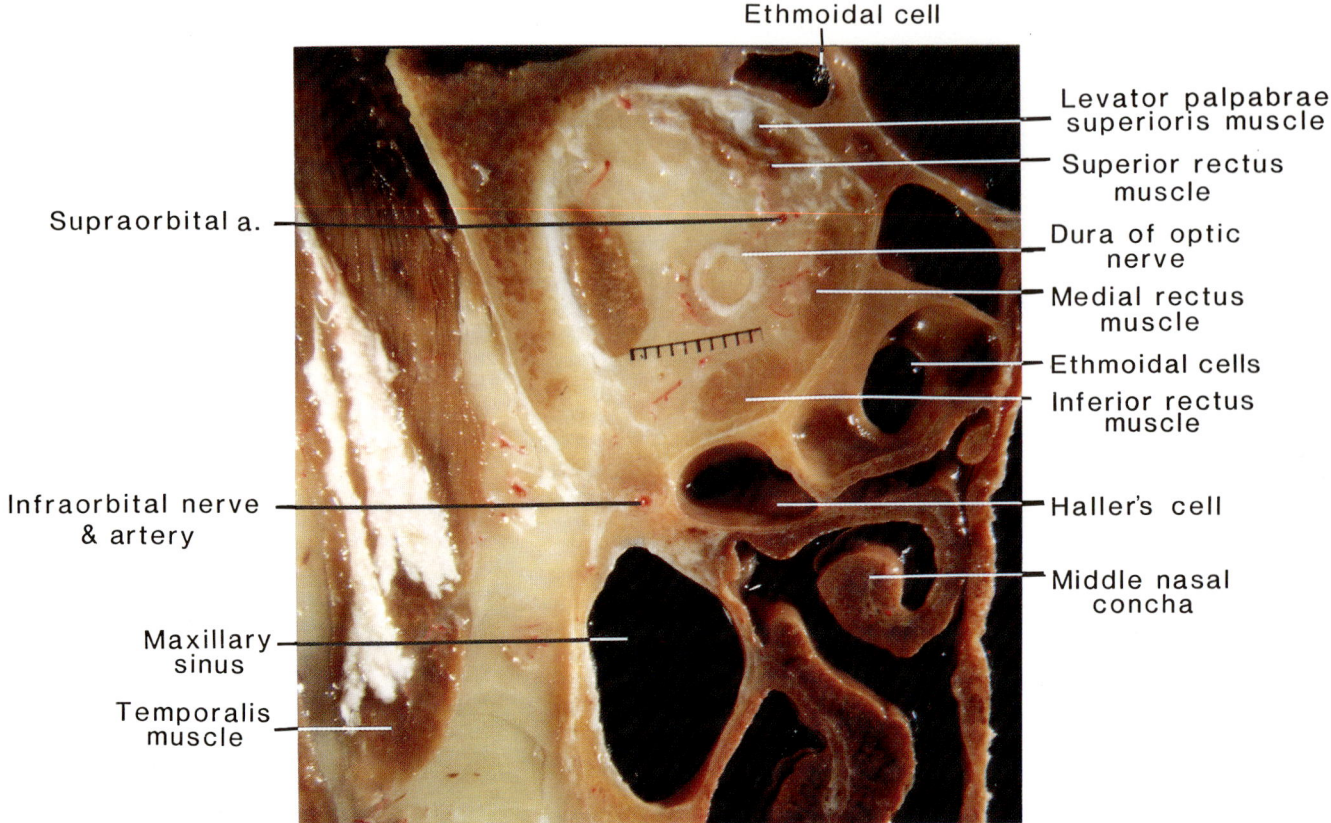

FIG. 4. Coronal section through the orbit and paranasal sinuses.

out in this area by the Haller's cells. The medial wall of the maxillary sinus may be displaced laterally if the nasal cavity and the ethmoidal labyrinth are well developed. There is then a danger of injury to the orbit during transmaxillary ethmoidectomy.

FRONTAL SINUS

The *frontal sinus* reaches a height of 24.3 mm (range 5–66 mm) within the frontal bone (16). The lateral wall of the frontal sinus lies 29.0 mm (range 17–49 mm) from the midline in adults (12). The longitudinal extent of the frontal sinus between the anterior and posterior end (in the orbital roof) was 20.5 mm (range 10–46.5 mm). Flesch (4) described one frontal sinus that extended posteriorly as far as the optic canal, the roof of the orbit being completely duplicated. Witt (26) found a duplicated orbital roof in almost 40% of his skulls (23% on both sides and 16% on one side). Division of the frontal sinuses into three or more chambers has been described by several authors. Boege (1) found two frontal sinuses on one side in 1.5% of his material. Jovanovic (7) reported an incidence of 21% but did not give an accurate definition. This extra sinus lay in the medial third or quarter of the orbital roof, being more common on the left side than the right. We found this cell in 17% of our material. In 23% of cases the frontal sinus had an inferior indentation that reached the nasal bone.

Frontonasal Duct

The length of the *frontonasal duct* (measured in 66 specimens) was 6.2 mm (range 3.2–14.9 mm). Based on our definition, a frontonasal duct was present in 77% of cases and an ostium of the frontal sinus in 23% (for details see ref. 11).

Opening of the Frontonasal Duct

The frontonasal duct opens into the semilunar hiatus in 67% of cases. The opening of the frontonasal duct lay outside the semilunar hiatus in 33% of cases, being anterior to the semilunar hiatus in 24%, anterior and lateral to it in 2%, in the region of an agger cell in 4%, and superior to the anterior end of the middle nasal concha, but still within the middle meatus, in 4%. In 23% of cases it was found that a *frontal ostium* met our criteria. Probing showed that the ostium led to the anterior part of the

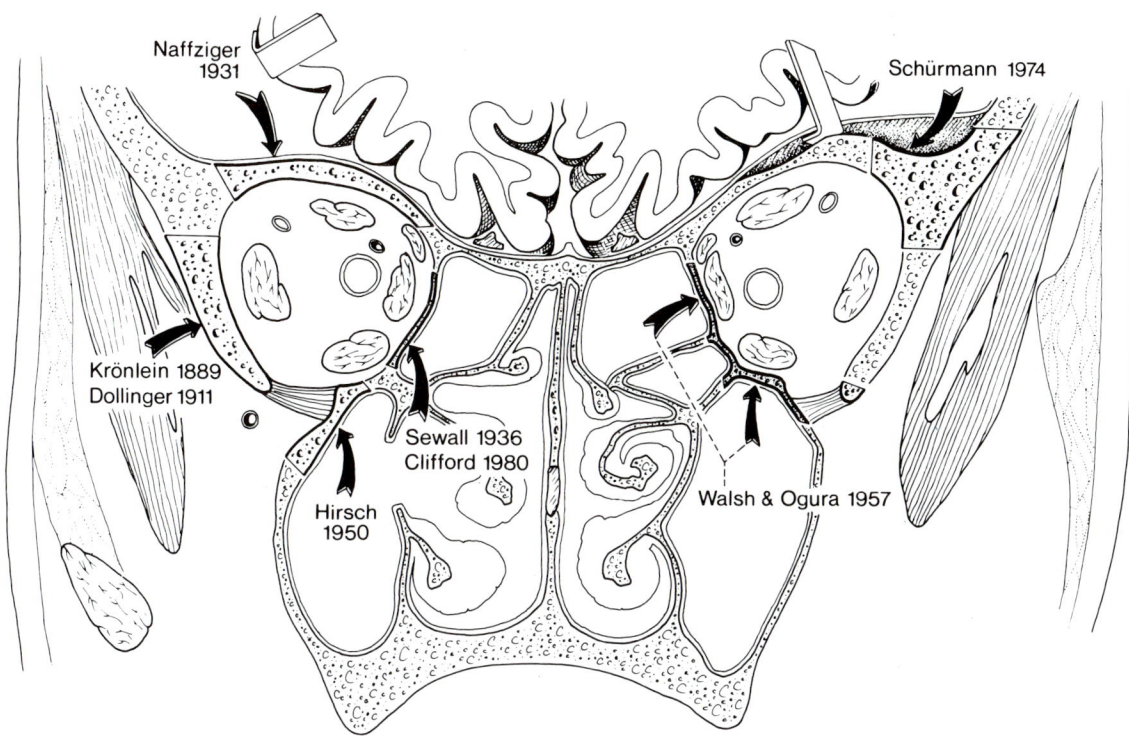

FIG. 5. Various described approaches to the orbit and surrounding structures.

semilunar hiatus in 47% of cases; in 40% the opening lay in front of the semilunar hiatus, in 7% lateral to it, and in 7% the ostium opened into an anterior ethmoidal cell.

Ethmoidal Canals and Their Contents

The *ethmoidal canals* (Fig. 5) carry vessels and nerves between the *orbit* and the *anterior cranial fossa* and the *nasal cavity*. The position of the ethmoidal canals in relation to the cribriform plate is important in diagnosis, in intranasal surgery, and in closure of CSF fistulae. The course of the *anterior ethmoidal canal* was determined in 54 subjects. This canal runs medially and anteriorly through the ethmoidal labyrinth, lying between 2 mm (1.1 mm) below and 4 mm above the cribriform plate. In 93% of cases, 6.9-mm (range 1.8–13.5 mm) long dehiscences of the walls of the anterior ethmoidal canal were found. Vessels and nerves pass through these dehiscences to the ethmoidal cells.

Tertiary ethmoidal canals (between the anterior and posterior canals) were present in 33% of the material, lying 1 mm (range 1.1–3.3 mm) above the cribriform plate. In 39% of cases there were dehiscences 2 mm (range 0.75–3.8 mm) long in the walls of the tertiary ethmoidal canals.

A *posterior ethmoidal canal* was seen in all specimens. The greatest part of the course lay 1.5 mm (range 0–3.1 mm) above the cribriform plate, running in an anteromedial direction. Dehiscences measuring 3.6 mm (range 1.1–7.7 mm) long were found in these canals in 59% of cases.

In our material the orbital opening of the posterior ethmoidal canal was not less than 1 mm from the orbital aperture of the optic canal, not only medially but also from above and laterally.

SPHENOID SINUS

The *sphenoid sinus* (Figs. 6–8) of elderly subjects was 13.5 mm (range 5–20.5 mm) wide in its superior segment, 16.9 mm (range 8.5–24 mm) in the center, and 18.7 mm (range 6.5–26.5 mm) in its lower segment. The sphenoid was 19.4 mm (range 6.5–32 mm) long in its upper part, 24.8 mm (range 9–36 mm) long in the center, and 18.5 mm (range 7–31 mm) long in the lower part. The vertical height between the floor and roof measured 16.4–20.4 mm, and the greatest width was between 15.3 and 17.1 mm in men. The dimensions in women were somewhat less.

Septum of the Sphenoid Sinus

The septum of the sphenoid sinus often deviates from the midline. It may be oblique or transverse, as described

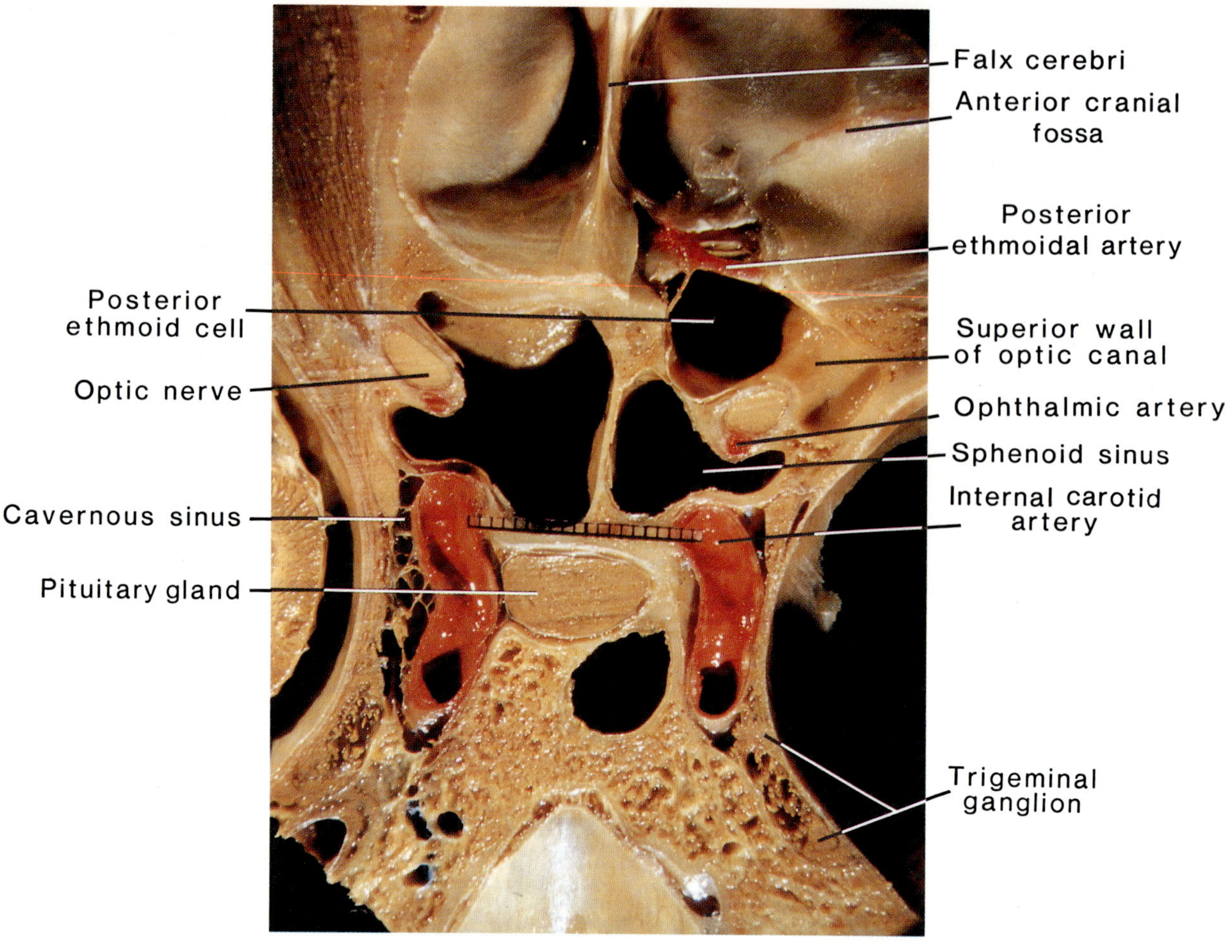

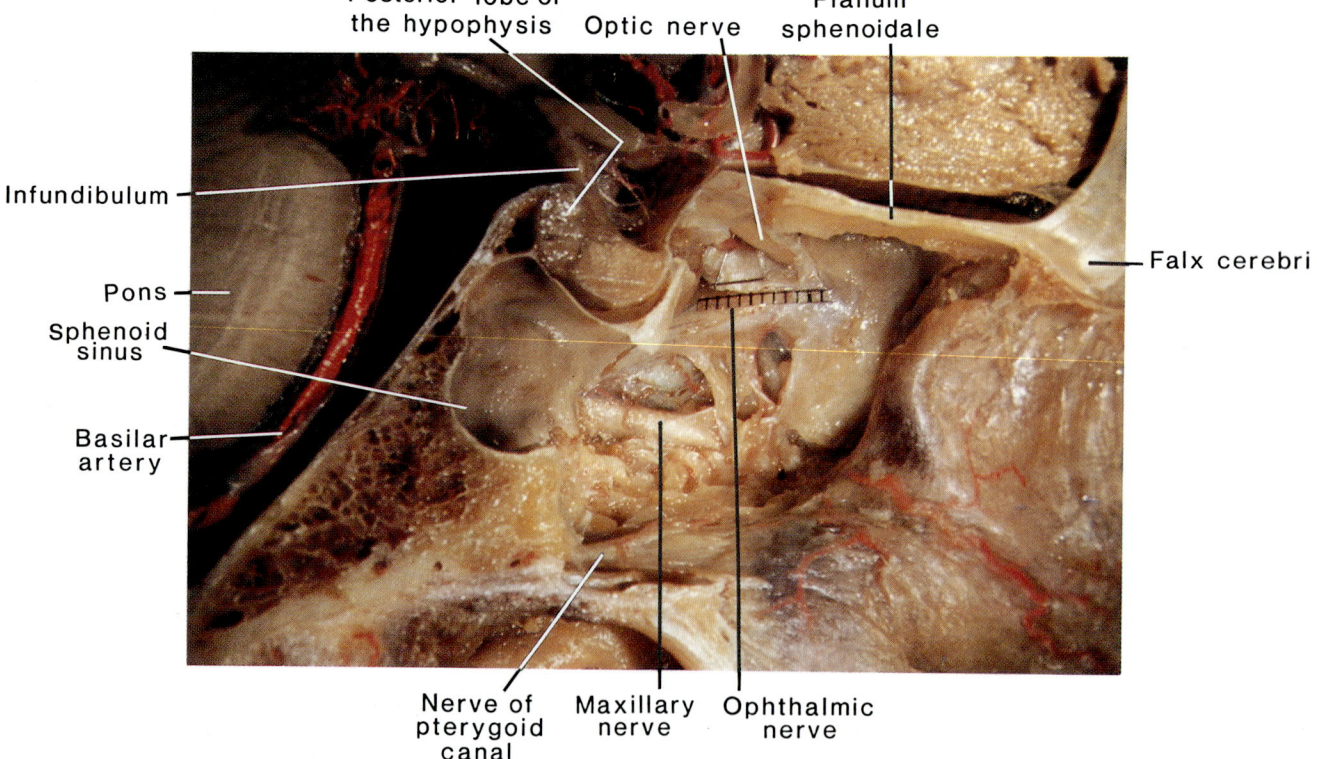

FIG. 6. Section showing the carotid canal completely surrounded by air cells.

FIG. 7. Large sphenoid sinus. The anterior and lateral walls have been dissected. The cavernous carotid artery has been removed.

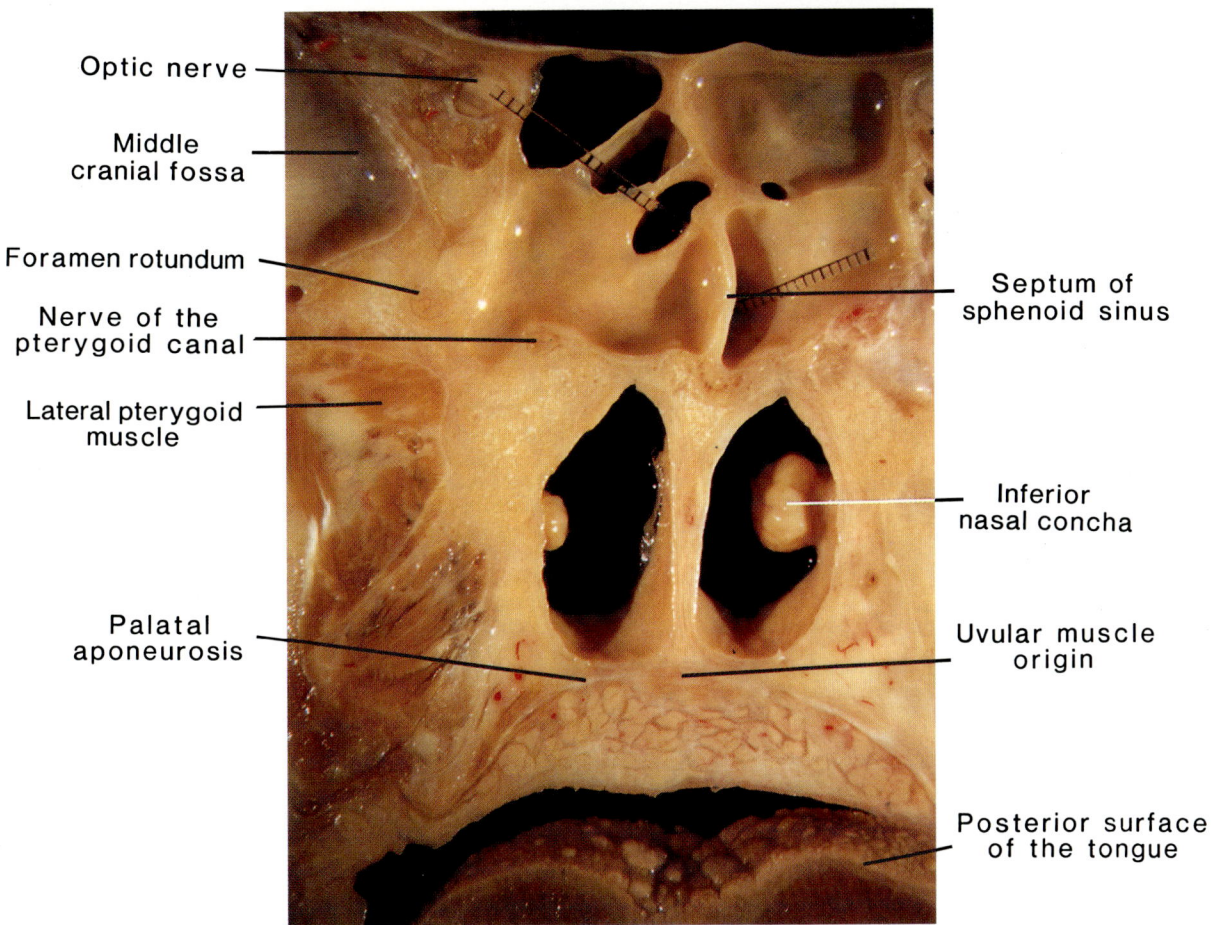

FIG. 8. Apertures of the sphenoid sinus.

many years ago by Morgagni (1682–1771), and is vertical in only 25% of cases (6). Accessory septa, arising from synchondroses of the sphenoid, are often found within the sinus. The septum of the sphenoid sinus lies in the midline in 27% of cases. In 43% of cases only the anterior part lies in the midline, whereas in the rest the septum is S-shaped, C-shaped, or has other shapes. Accessory septa are found in 76% of cases, of which 48% are unilateral and 28% bilateral (3).

Recesses of the Sphenoidal Sinus

The posterior septal recess is termed the sphenovomerine bulla. If the sphenoidal sinus grows inferolaterally, the rostrum of the sphenoid bone is completely pneumatized and projects downward between the alae of the vomer into the nasal septum.

Ethmoidal Recess

The sphenoidal sinus rarely extends into the posterior part of the ethmoid bone. More commonly, it extends into its posteroinferior angle, the orbit, the maxilla, and rarely into the supraorbital region.

Superior and Inferior Lateral Recess

A diverticulum of the sphenoidal sinus can encompass the optic canal laterally and above as far as the lesser sphenoid wing. The sphenoidal sinus can also extend laterally, below the optic canal (10).

Palatine Recess

The orbital process of the palatine bone may be pneumatized not only from the maxillary sinus but also from the sphenoidal sinus. Occasionally, the posterior ethmoidal cells also extended into the orbital process of the palatine bone. According to Cope (2) the recess of the sphenoidal sinus (termed by him the anterior recess) abuts on cells of the orbital process of the palatine bone but never communicates with them. In his material, an anterior recess was found in 5%, contacting the posterosuperior wall of the maxillary sinus in 2–3% of cases.

Inferolateral Recess

The lower part of the sphenoidal sinus can extend laterally into the orbital face of the greater wing of the sphenoid and pneumatize the posterolateral segment of the orbital wall. Rarely, the sphenoid sinus reaches the foramen rotundum and ovale. Peele described a sphenoid sinus extending as far as the mandibular nerve, the trigeminal ganglion, the apex of the petrous bone, and into the greater wing of the sphenoid bone.

Pterygoid Recess

A sphenoid sinus that has developed inferiorly and laterally often extends into the pterygoid process. The sinus can then reach the eustachian tube (14,22).

REFERENCES

1. Boege K. Zur Anatomie der Stirnhöhlen (Sinus frontalis). Dissertation, Königsberg. *Jber Fortschr Anat Entwicklungesch* 1903; 8(III):22.
2. Cope VZ. The internal structure of the sphenoid sinus. *J Anat (Lond)* 1917;51:127–136.
3. Elwany S, Yacout YM, Talaat M, El-Nahass M, Gunied A. Surgical anatomy of the sphenoid sinus. *J Laryngol* 1983;97:227–241.
4. Flesch M. Varietäten-Beobachtungen aus dem Präpariersaale zu Würzburg in den Wintersemestern 1875/76 und 1876/77. *Verh Phys Med Ges (Würzb)* 1879;13:1–38.
5. Grünwald L. Deskriptive und topographische Anatomie der Nase und ihrer Nebenhöhlen. In: Denker A, Kahler O. *Die Krankheiten der Luftwege und der Mundhöhle.* Berlin: Springer, 1925;S.1–95.
6. Hammer G, Radberg C. Sphenoidal sinus. An anatomical and roentgenological study with reference to transsphenoid hypophysectomy. *Acta Radiol. (Stockh)* 1961;56:401–422.
7. Jovanovic S. Supernumerary frontal sinuses on the roof of the orbit. Their clinical significance. *Acta Anat (Basel)* 1961; 45:133–142.
8. Killian G. Zur Anatomie der Nase menschlicher Embryonen. *Arch Laryngol Rhin (Berl)* 1895/96;3:17–47.
9. Krmpotić-Nemanić J, Draf W, Helms J. *Chirurgische Anatomie des Kopf-Hals-Bereiches.* Berlin: Springer, 1985.
10. Lang J. Optic nerve, topographic anatomy. In: Samii M, Jannetta PJ, eds. *The cranial nerves.* New York: Springer, 1981;76–84.
11. Lang J. *Clinical anatomy of the nose, nasal cavity and paranasal sinuses.* New York: Thieme Medical Publishers, 1989.
12. Lang J, Haas R. Neue Befunde zur Bodenregion der Fossa cranialis anterior. *Verh Anat Ges (Jena)* 1979;73:77–86.
12a. Lang J, Haas A. Über die Sagittalausdehnung des Sinus frontalis, dessen Wanddicke, Abstände zur Lamina cribrosa, die Tiefe der sogenannten Olfactorius-Rinne und die Canales ethmoidales. *Gegenbaurs morphol Jahrb* 1988;134:459–469.
13. Lang J, Papke J. Über die klinische Anatomie des Paries inferior orbitae und dessen Nachbarstrukturen. *Gegenbaurs Morphol Jahrb* 1984;130:1–47.
14. Mayer X. Beschreibung eines Sinus pterygoideus und jugalis beim Menschen. *Schmidts Jahrb Ges Med* 1841;31:12–21.
15. Messerklinger W. Schwierigkeiten bei der Kieferhöhlenspülung. *J Laryngol Rhinol Otol* 1980;59:22–29.
16. Milosslawski M. Die Sinus frontales. Dissertation, Moscow. 1903.
17. Myerson MC. Natural orifice of the maxillary sinus. *Arch Otolaryngol* 1932;15.
18. *Nomina Anatomica,* 6th ed. Edinburgh: Churchill Livingstone, 1989.
19. Peter K. Atlas der Entwicklung der Nase und des Gaumens beim Menschen mit Einschluß der Entwicklungsstörungen. *Fischer (Jena)* 1913.
20. Peter K. Die Nase des Kindes. In: *Handbuch der Anatomie des Kindes,* vol II. Munich: Bergmann, 1938.
21. Schlungbaum. Über die Bildung mehrerer Nebenräume der Nasenhöhle im Oberkiefer und ihre Deutung, mit Berücksichtigung der Beziehungen der Zähne zu ihnen. *Vierteljahrhundertschr Zanheilkunde* 1921;43.
22. Sluder G. The relations of the sphenoid sinus to the eustachian tube and their possible clinical importance. *Trans Am Laryngol Assoc* 1916[x]:281–287.
23. Soemmering STh. *Abbildungen der menschlichen Organe des Geruches.* Frankfurt: Varrentrapp & Wenner, 1809.
24. Stupka W. *Die Missbildungen und Anomalien der Nase und des Nasenrachenraumes.* Wien: Springer, 1938.
25. Terrahe K, Mündnich K. Gefahren und Komplikationen bei der transmaxillären Siebbein-Keilbeinhöhlenausräumung. *Arch Klin Exp Ohr-, Nas- Kehlkopfheilkunde* 1973;205:284–285.
26. Witt E. *Ausbreitung der Stirnhöhlen und Siebbeinzellen über die Orbita.* Medical Dissertation, Rostock, 1908.
27. Zuckerkandl E. *Normale und pathologische Anatomie der Nasenhöhle und ihrer pneumatischen Anhänge,* vol 2, part I. Wien: Braumüller, 1893.

CHAPTER 11

Anatomy of the Posterior Cranial Fossa

Johannes Lang

ROOF OF THE POSTERIOR CRANIAL FOSSA

Tentorium Cerebelli and Venous Sinuses

Bridging veins from the lateral, inferior and medial surfaces of the cerebrum frequently run into the upper surface of the tentorium cerebelli and continue as *superior tentorial sinuses* and drain either into the transverse or the sigmoid sinus.

Bridging Veins

On the superior surface of the tentorium there are approximately three (range 1-8) bridging veins with an average length of 11 mm (2). Bridging veins are also present on the inferior surface of the tentorium (Fig. 1). The posterior superior cerebellar vein drains into the medial inferior tentorial sinus. Occasionally, two inferior tentorial sinuses are present. In the substance of the tentorium (mainly collagen fibers) run the tentorial arteries and Arnold's nerve.

Clivus

The average length of the clivus (between the dorsum sellae and basion) is 45 mm (range 37-52 mm) in adults (Fig. 2). Part of the clivus formed by the sphenoid bone has a rough surface, while the part formed by the occipital bone is smooth and presents the depression of the clivus.

The dorsum sellae is occasionally pneumatized by air cells extending from the sphenoid sinus and may have defects in advanced age.

The thickest part of the floor of the posterior cranial fossa (except the petrous) is situated in the vicinity of the jugular tubercle. The length of the hypoglossal canal is about 4 mm and it is about 9.7 mm (range 6-15 mm) away from the occipital condyle.

BLOOD SUPPLY OF THE BONE AND DURA OF THE POSTERIOR CRANIAL FOSSA

The anterior and superior parts of the clivus belong to the vascular territory of the branches of the carotico cavernous truncs. The posterior and inferior parts of the clivus and anterolateral borders of the foramen magnum are supplied by twigs from the ascending pharyngeal artery entering the posterior cranial fossa through the jugular and hypoglossal canal. Contribution to the supply of this area is also made by the anterior meningeal branch of the vertebral artery. The dorsal part of the squamous occipital bone and the posterior margins of the foramen magnum are supplied by the posterior meningeal branch of the vertebral artery. The lateral part of the floor of the posterior cranial fossa is usually supplied by a twig from the occipital artery, which enters through the mastoidal emissary foramen. Small posterior emissary arteries and veins are frequently found in the vicinity of internal and external occipital protuberances. The tentorium cerebelli is supplied by the medial and lateral tentorial arteries, which arise from the branches of the carotico cavernous truncs or from the internal carotid artery itself. The petrosquamous branch of the middle meningeal artery contributes to the blood supply of the posterior cranial fossa together with vessels arising directly from the parietal branch of the middle meningeal artery. Branches of the ascending pharyngeal artery supply paramedian areas of the posterior cranial fossa.

NERVE SUPPLY OF THE DURA MATER OF THE POSTERIOR CRANIAL FOSSA

According to Kimmel (16) the floor of the posterior cranial fossa is supplied by twigs from the sympathetic

---

J. Lang: Institute of Anatomy, University of Würzburg, W-8700, Würzburg, Germany.

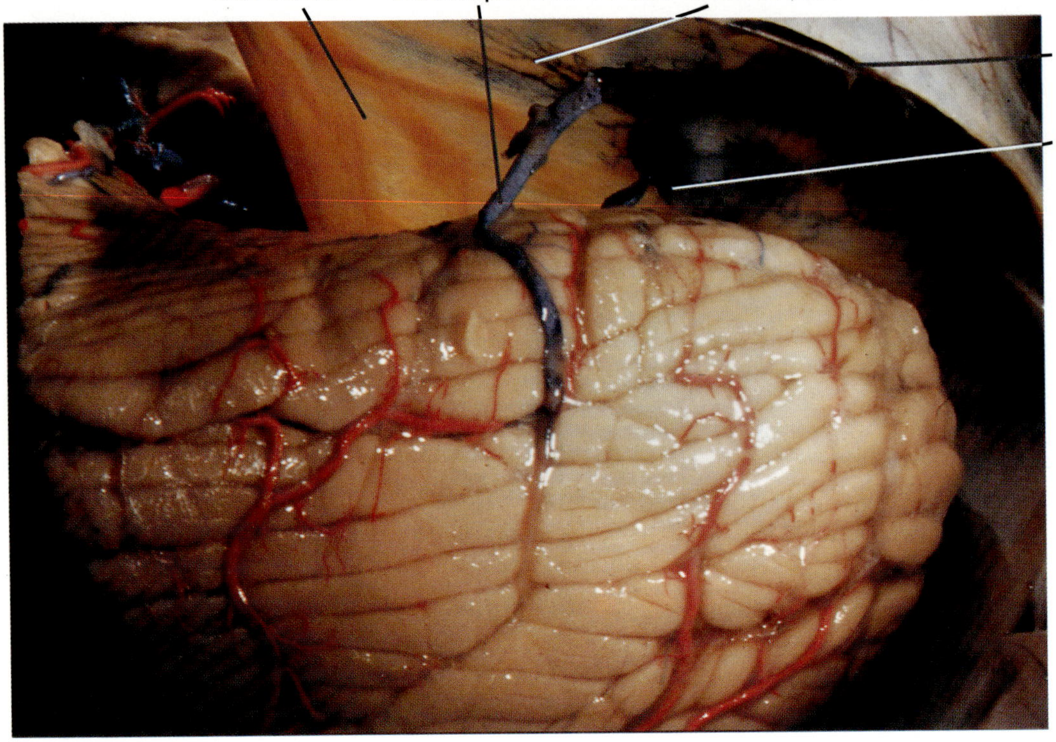

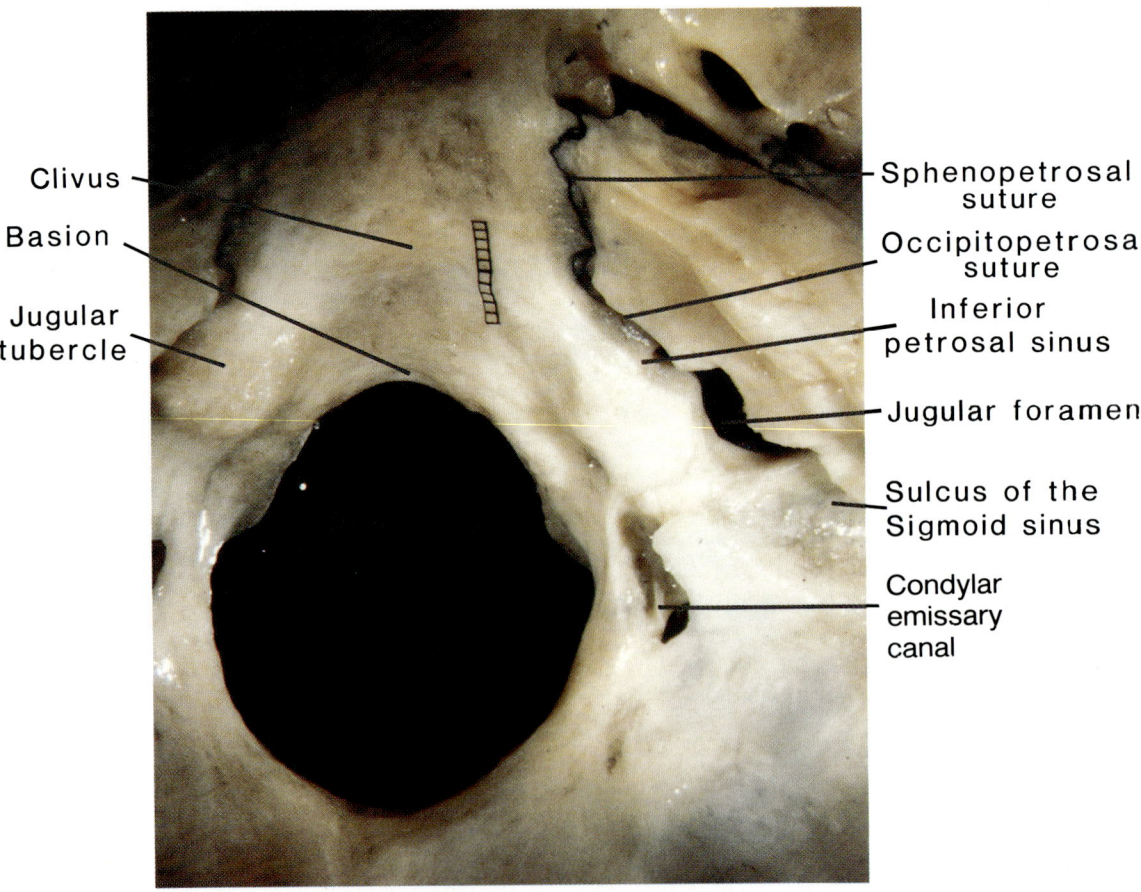

FIG. 1. Picture showing the bridging vein, cerebellar hemispheric vein, and its confluence into the lateral tentorial sinus.

FIG. 2. The petroclival and foramen magnum region from a superior view.

trunk and from the upper three cervical nerves. These nerves run into the posterior cranial fossa through the foramen magnum, the hypoglossal canal, and the jugular foramen. The nerves running through the foramen magnum arise from the upper three cervical nerves and from their ascending branches. These nerves supply the territory as far as the posterior clinoid process.

There are three to four dural branches that run through the jugular foramen together with the vagus nerve. Most of these twigs leave the vagus in the jugular foramen and run along the wall of the superior bulb of the jugular vein into the skull. Within the posterior cranial fossa these nerve fibers run backward in the wall of the sigmoid sinus to end near the transverse sinus. Meningeal branches entering through the hypoglossal canal accompany the twigs of the ascending pharyngeal artery and form a well developed nerve plexus within the hypoglossal canal, which also ramifies in the neighboring venous plexus. One of these fine nerves then runs anteriorly, while the others run dorsally within the external layer of the dura mater under the lateral border of the foramen magnum in the vicinity of the dural veins. Then they depart from the blood vessels. The anterior branch proceeds to the region of the inferior petrosal sinus and the posterior surface of the petrous temporal bone. The posterior branches innervate the margins of the foramen magnum and the medial part of the floor of the posterior cranial fossa (think of reflexes and opisthotonus).

GREAT CEREBRAL VEIN AND SINUSES

Great Cerebral Vein

The great cerebral vein (Fig. 3) is approximately 10 mm (range 5–15 mm) long and 3–5 mm in diameter. It curves around the posterior surface of the splenium of the corpus callosum and usually runs at a right angle into the transition zone between the inferior sagittal sinus and the straight sinus. The vein passes within a subarachnoid space (the cistern of the great cerebral vein) traversed by numerous dense bundles of connective tissue. These bundles hold the vein and its tributaries in position. The vein is formed by the union of the two internal cerebral veins. In approximately 60% the vein terminates at a right angle in the transition zone between the inferior sagittal sinus and the straight sinus; in 30% the junction is at an acute angle against the bloodstream, and in 10% it is at an obtuse angle. Occasionally, both internal cerebral veins drain separately into the sinus.

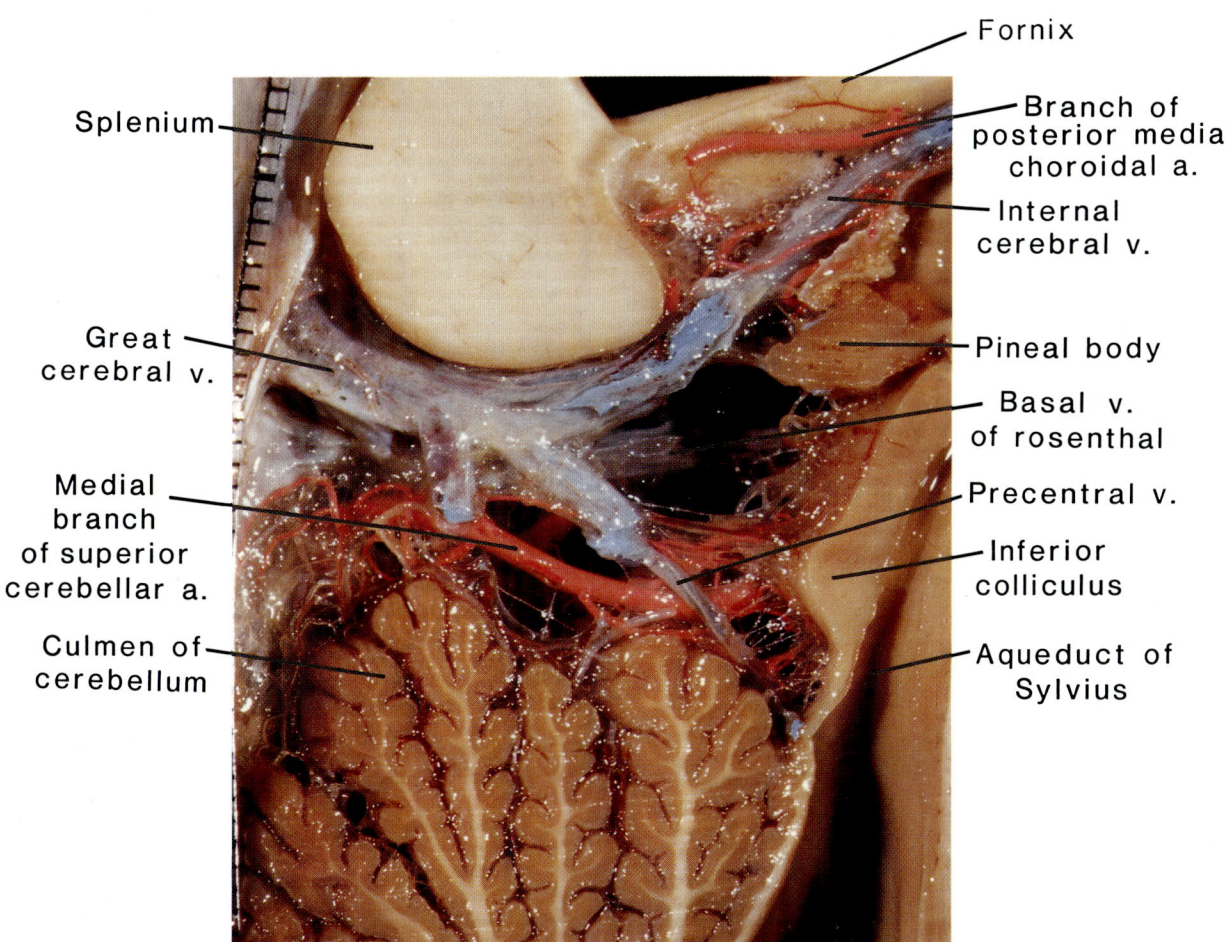

FIG. 3. Great cerebral vein (of Galen) and its tributaries.

Straight Sinus

The straight sinus has an average length of 50 mm (range 40–69 mm) and a width of about 4 mm (range 2–5 mm) (37). It forms an average angle of 51.5° (range 40°–71°) with the Frankfurt horizontal plane. In cross section it is almost triangular with the base below and the apex above. In the initial part of the straight sinus there is a lacuna or dilatation that measures 2–30 mm in height and 3–45 mm longitudinally. It is believed that this is an embryological remnant of the original drainage channel to the superior sagittal sinus. The tentorial sinuses drain into the straight sinus from both sides and superior cerebellar veins drain into it from below.

The terminal part of the straight sinus merges into the right and left transverse sinuses usually in the form of a bifurcation of variable diameter. In other cases it may drain exclusively to the left or to the right side. Alternatively, there may be a plexiform terminal segment of the straight sinus or it may drain into the occipital sinus.

Transverse Sinus

The right transverse sinus is usually larger in caliber than the left. In the vicinity of the attachment of the tentorium cerebelli the transverse sinus runs forward and laterally in its groove to the upper bend of the sigmoid sinus. The posterior part of the sinus runs on the inner surface of the squamous occipital bone and then in the vicinity of the mastoid angle of the parietal bone, continuing rostrally to the temporal bone. The greatest diameter of the right transverse sinus averages 7.9 mm and the left measures 7.7 mm (1). In addition to the tentorial sinuses, meningeal veins from the middle cranial fossa, the inferior superficial cerebral vein, and veins from the cerebellum drain into the transverse sinus.

According to Lack (18) the junction of the transverse sinus and the sigmoid sinus is situated an average of 5.97 mm above the Frankfurt horizontal plane. According to Howieson and Norrell (12) the confluence of sinuses is situated approximately midway between the lambda and the posterior lip of the foramen magnum. They point out that the posterior part of the transverse sinus runs approximately horizontally, the middle third then proceeding forward in a curve convex upward.

Sigmoid Sinus

The mean value of the angle made anteriorly between the line of the transverse part of the groove for the sigmoid sinus and the median sagittal plane in adults was about 96° on the right and 97.4° on the left. The range was from 80°–114°. In most age groups the mean value for the right side exceeded that for the left, perhaps because of the greater backward inclination of the petrous part of the right temporal bone. Nevertheless, the difference between the right and left sides was not statistically significant. The mean thickness of the skull behind the upper bend of the sinus (least distance between the inner and outer surfaces) was 2.7–16.2 mm in adults (30). Occasionally, the bone was paper thin. This point for the retrosigmoidal approach is 45 mm behind the suprameatal spine and 7 mm below the Frankfurt horizontal plane in 92%.

Petrosquamous Sinus

Zuckerkandl (46) observed bony grooves running lateral to the trigeminal impression from the foramen spinosum to the upper margin of the petrous temporal bone. He believed that they connected the superior petrosal sinus with the main trunk of the middle meningeal vein. Short petrosquamous sinuses connect the companion vein of the posterior division of the middle meningeal artery with the superior petrosal sinus and run along the tegmen tympani.

Squamopetrosal Sinus

Occasionally, there is a small sinus that runs in the angle between the petrous part and the squamous part of the temporal bone and plunges into the transverse sinus from the front. Rostrally, there is a communication through the squamous part of the temporal bone with the deep temporal veins, in the neighborhood of the zygomatic process of the temporal bone. The squamopetrosal sinus was first described by Sir Charles Bell (quoted from Knott) and was named the anterior petrosal sinus. Knott (17) demonstrated this sinus on both sides in 7 out of 44 bodies and on one side (more frequently left than right) in 19 of them.

Accessory Sinus

The accessory sinus is a sinus that runs backward from the sphenoidal fissure over the superior border of the petrous temporal bone and drains into the superior petrosal sinus and then into the transverse sinus. In its anterior part it anastomoses with the veins from the orbit. The term paracavernous sinus is used to denote a sinus that follows this course, and also the blood channel on the floor of the middle cranial fossa, which Hyrtl (13) termed the ophthalmopetrosal sinus. The superior petrosal sinus is of variable caliber and drains into the anterior upper part of the transverse sinus or into the upper curve of the sigmoid sinus.

Inferior Petrosal Sinus

In its superior longitudinal segment the inferior petrosal sinus is between 7 and 10 mm in diameter and communicates with the basilar plexus through numerous channels. In its inferior part (transverse limb) it has an average diameter of 2.85 mm (range 0.5–5 mm). More commonly (48%), the inferior petrosal sinus enters the jugular foramen between nerve IX and nerve X. In 30% of cases it runs into the jugular foramen in front of the IXth cranial nerve and in 6% between the Xth and XIth cranial nerves. Sometimes there are more than one outflow or the sinus drains into the internal jugular vein after it exits from the skull. The transverse limb of the sinus forms an average angle of 28° with the transverse plane. In approximately 46% of cases there is a medial intrapetrosal vein that arises in the formation area of the internal carotid venous plexus, runs downward through the region of the apex of the petrous temporal bone, and terminates in the inferior petrosal sinus at a point situated an average of 11 mm medial to its terminal segment. In 50% of specimens there was a lateral intrapetrosal vein that ran from the internal carotid venous plexus (region of the genu) through the petrous temporal bone to the termination of the inferior petrosal sinus. According to Denecke (6) glomus tumors spread along the veins of the petrous temporal bone.

EMISSARY VEINS

Mastoid Emissary Foramen

The internal opening of the mastoid emissary foramen is most commonly situated in the descending limb of the sigmoid sulcus at its upper curve. The canal then runs to the base of the mastoid process, in a line that is sometimes straight and sometimes convoluted. It opens at the outer wall of the skull at the level of the external acoustic meatus. In one-third of cases it was seen that the opening was in the vicinity of the suture. At the external opening the mastoid emissary vein running in the canal anastomoses with the occipital vein or the posterior auricular vein or with both. In the specimens analyzed, the canal was absent on the right in 4.5%, on the left in 11.5%, and on both sides in 20%. The average length of the mastoid canal was 11.6 mm (range 5–19.8 mm) on the right side and 11.9 mm (range 5.0–22.2 mm) on the left. Its intracranial opening had an average diameter of 3.4 mm (range 0.5–6.0 mm) on the right side and 3.2 mm (range 0.5–6.2 mm) on the left. The emissary vein was not uncommonly divided near the extracranial opening, with the result that there were two orifices on the exterior of the skull, and there may occasionally be three. The external opening of the mastoid foramen measured an average of 3.2 mm (range 0.5–10.0 mm) on the left. The mastoid foramen carries the mastoid emissary vein, and in addition the meningeal branch of the occipital artery usually passes through it into the skull.

Condylar Emissary Vein and Jugular Foramen

In 36% the condylar emissary vein was missing on the right side and in 32% on the left. In 38.46% it communicated with the jugular vein lateral to the intrajugular process of the petrous temporal bone (Fig. 4); in 25% the communication was situated exactly at the margo terminalis sigmoidea; in 7.69% the vein joined the terminal segment of the sigmoid sinus lateral to the margo terminalis sigmoidea; in 3.84% it joined the hypoglossal venous plexus in its canal medial to the jugular foramen; and in a further 3.84% (low confluence) it joined the internal jugular vein below the actual jugular foramen. If the roof of the emissary canal is rarefied, the vein may even run on the floor of the posterior cranial fossa.

Venous Plexus of the Hypoglossal Canal

In 34% the hypoglossal venous plexus communicated with the inferior petrosal sinus and in the same percentage with the marginal plexus of the foramen magnum and the basilar plexus. In 13.46% it communicates with the terminal segment of the sigmoid sinus and in 11.53% with the bulb of the jugular vein. In 5.76% of specimens there was an extracranial communication with the vertebral vein via a prevertebral vein.

Jugular Foramen: Passage of Nerves and Vessels

Contrary to what is stated in most textbooks, nerves IX, X, and XI do not traverse the medial and anterior part of the jugular foramen. Instead, they run through a connective tissue septum set obliquely at a variable angle in this major vascular portal of the posterior cranial fossa. Furthermore, a posterior meningeal artery regularly runs from the ascending pharyngeal artery through the jugular foramen to the floor of the posterior cranial fossa. As a rule, small twigs of this posterior meningeal branch can be seen through the thin endothelium of the jugular foramen and the sigmoid sinus (and other sinuses).

In the specimens studied (10), there was only one instance in which the meningeal branch of the ascending pharyngeal artery was not found (approximately 2%). In 50% there was one meningeal artery, in 37% there were two meningeal branches, and in 10.5% three meningeal branches from the ascending pharyngeal artery were seen running into the jugular foramen. Right–left differences in numbers and diameters of these vessels are common.

Termination of the Inferior Petrosal Sinus

In 23.07% the inferior petrosal sinus runs into the middle plane of the jugular foramen, and in 32.69% into

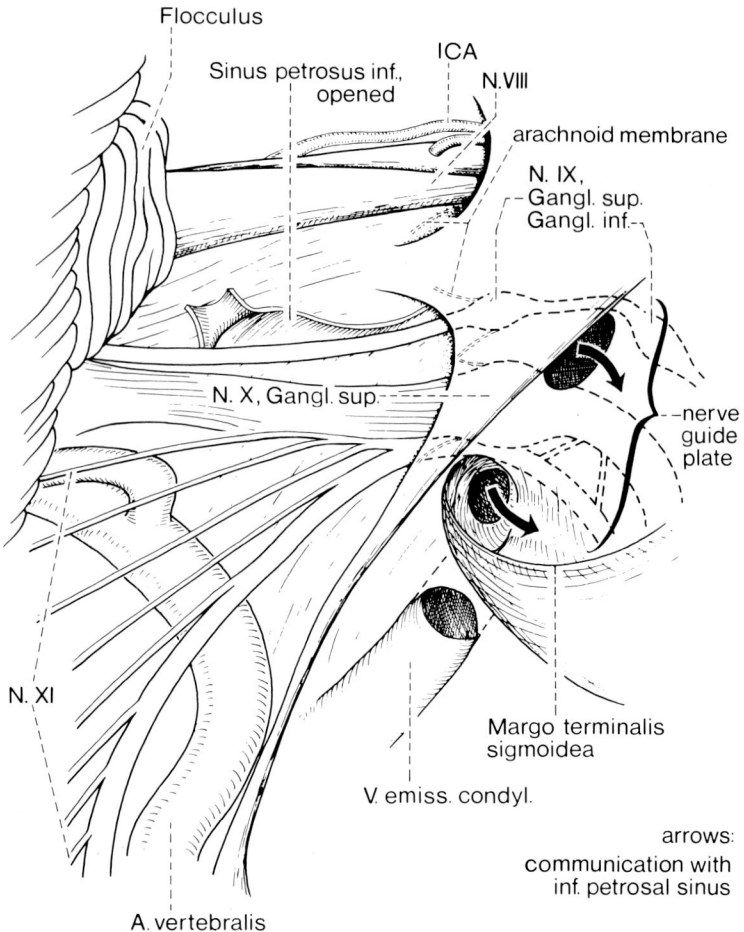

FIG. 4. The jugular foramen region.

the lower zone of the foramen. In 21.15% the inferior petrosal sinus terminates extracranially in the internal jugular vein, and in 17.3% in the jugular bulb. In approximately 7% there was no demonstrable connection between the inferior petrosal sinus and the jugular foramen or jugular bulb (low confluence into the internal jugular vein); in 24%, arrangements of this kind were present in addition to the main outflow.

The margo terminalis sigmoidea marks the transition between the sigmoid sinus and the jugular bulb. On the right side, this transition forms an average angle of 76° (range 51°–110°) with the median sagittal plane, the corresponding angle on the left side being 72° (range 40°–100°).

In the specimens studied, the dome of the jugular bulb was situated at an average of 8.8 mm (range 5–14 mm) above the margo terminalis sigmoidea on the right side, and 8.2 mm (range 5–13 mm) on the left. The jugular bulb had an average diameter of 11.5 mm (range 5–18 mm). According to Gabrielsen and Bookstein (8) the average diameter of the internal jugular vein below the bulb was 9.5 mm (range 6–16 mm) on the right side and 8.0 mm (range 5–13 mm) on the left. The highest point of the jugular fossa in the specimens studied was situated laterally from the median plane 33.4 mm (range 27–40 mm) to the right and 32.1 mm (range 26–38 mm) to the left.

PONS

In the specimens studied the average length of the pons (Fig. 5) was 28.6 mm (range 22.0–33.0 mm) (38). Situated in the median sagittal plane is the basal sulcus of the pons, which does not correspond to the course of the basilar artery. The lateral border of the pons formed by the entry zone of the sensory roots of the trigeminal nerve was situated at an average of 14.8 mm (range 12–20 mm) from the most rostral point of the pons. The transverse grooves on the surface of the pons and the basal sulcus of the pons are produced by the bundles of pontocerebellar fibers.

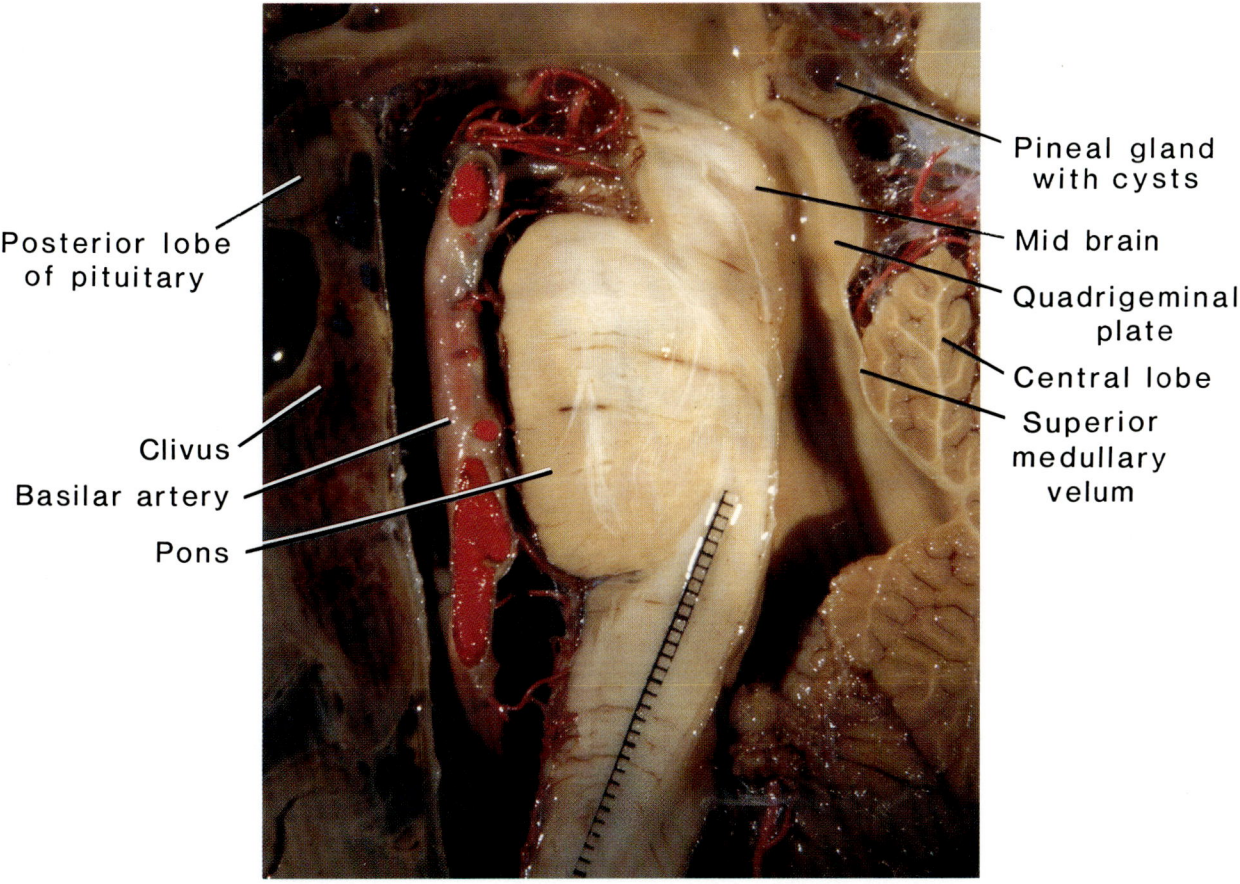

FIG. 5. Median sagittal section through the aqueduct of Sylvius and fourth ventricle.

RETRO-OLIVARY AREA AND CRANIAL NERVES

Pyramid

The superior border of the ventral surface of the medulla is formed by the inferior border of the pons, while its inferior border is marked by the decussation of the pyramids or by the uppermost ventral root fibers. At the lower border of the pons the median ventral fissure of the medulla oblongata deepens to form the foramen cecum. The pyramids project on either side of the fissure and carry corticospinal tracts. In the specimens studied the average width of the pyramids was 5.48 mm (range 4.0–7.0 mm).

Inferior Olive

The inferior olive is situated lateral to the pyramid, its upper border being an average of 0.96 mm (range 0.5–2.5 mm) below the caudal margin of the pons. The average length of the olive was 14.0 mm (range 9.5–16.0 mm) and its average breadth 5.61 mm (range 4.5–7.0 mm).

Parolivary Area

Lateral to the olive, the retro-olivary sulcus forms the medial boundary of the parolivary (retro-olivary) fossa, a smooth area averaging 3 mm in width (Fig. 6).

Exit Zones of the Lower Cranial Nerves

Abducent Nerve

The abducent nerve (Fig. 7) frequently emerges in the form of two bundles, an average of 3.93 mm (range 2.0–6.5 mm) from the median plane (39).

Facial Nerve

The VIIth cranial nerve leaves the brain in the cranial part of the parolivary fossa, at the border between the pons and the middle cerebellar peduncle. The exit zone is at an average of 11.81 mm (range 9.5–14.5 mm) from the median plane. It quite frequently traverses the transverse fibers of the middle cerebellar peduncle. Its maxi-

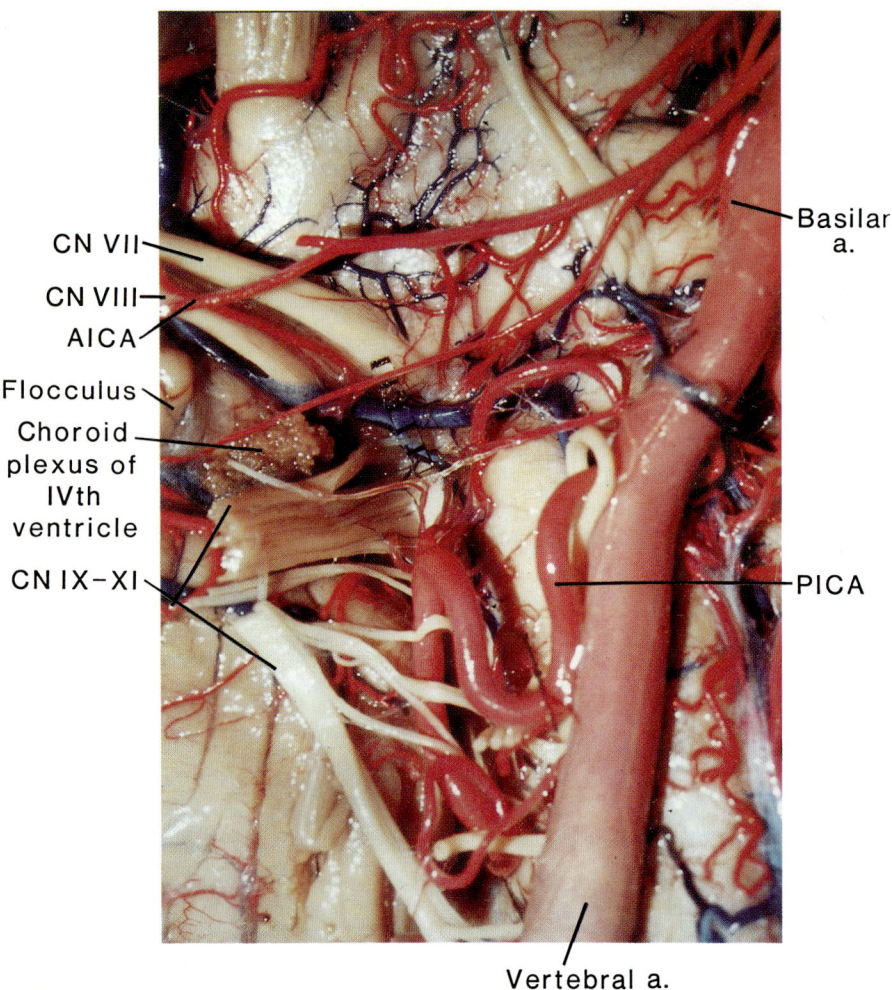

FIG. 6. Retro-olivary area.

mum diameter averaged 1.77 mm (range 1.0–2.0 mm), the average measurement being 1.82 mm on the right side and 1.72 mm on the left.

Vestibulocochlear Nerve

The vestibulocochlear nerve is usually oval (94%), averaging 3.05 mm (range 2.0–5.0 mm) in width and 1.3 mm (range 1.0–2.5 mm) in thickness. Its entry zone is situated at an average of 15.04 mm (range 13.0–17.5 mm) from the median plane, somewhat caudally and 1.36 mm (range 0.5–2.0 mm) lateral to the facial nerve. Within the internal auditory meatus, the cochlear root (35,000–50,000 fibers) runs anteromedially, the superior vestibular root laterally and superiorly, and the inferior vestibular part laterally and inferiorly. The fiber bundle undergoes rotation in the posterior fossa, so that upon entering the brain the cochlear part is positioned laterally with the inferior vestibular part medial to it and the superior vestibular part still farther medially. The vestibular part contains about 18,346 (range 4200–24,000) fibers, of which approximately 200 are efferent. The length of its central part is 8–12 mm. The transition zone is situated near the internal acoustic pore.

Nervus Intermedius

The nervus intermedius emerges from the brain between the facial nerve and the VIIIth nerve, closer to and often united with the latter. Its central segment is very short.

Exit Zone of Nerves IX, X, and XI (Cranial Roots)

The IXth and Xth cranial nerves (Fig. 7) and the central part of the XIth nerve emerge from the brain at the lateral border retro-olivary area (parolivary fossa), caudal to the pontomedullary sulcus. The IXth cranial nerve emerges an average of 3.19 mm (range 1.5–5.0

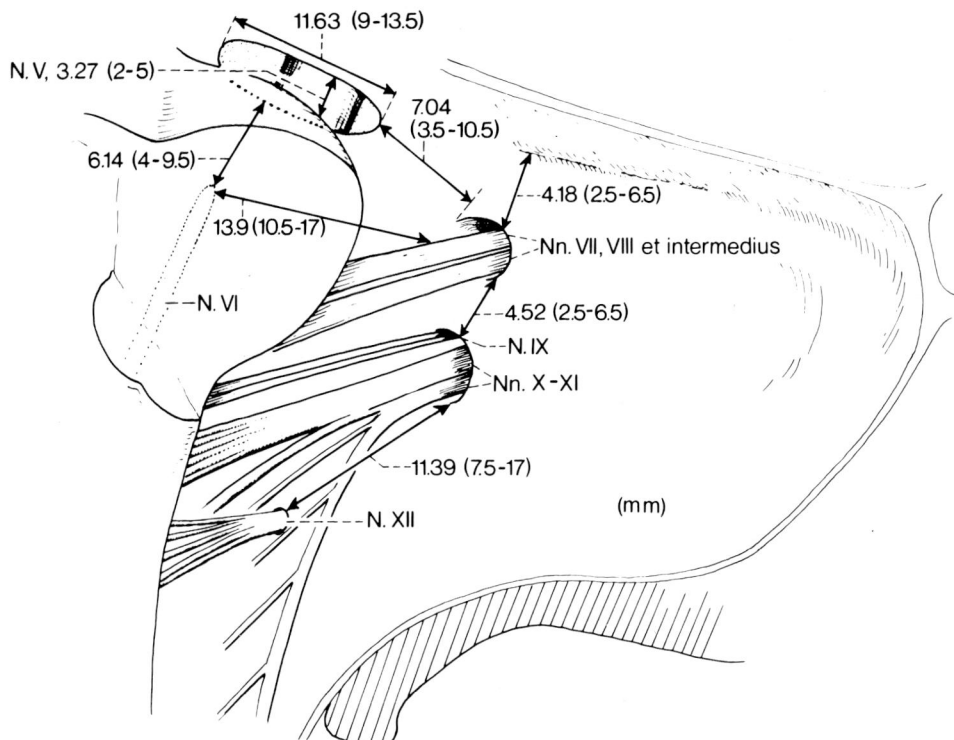

FIG. 7. Portals for lower cranial nerves.

mm) lateral to the lateral border of the olive and 1.79 mm (range 1.0–3.0 mm) caudal to the pontomedullary sulcus. It has numerous fine root fibers that usually unite to form two delicate bundles. Of these fine root fibers, the medial ones are possibly motor, the lateral ones sensory (21,44,45). The vagus nerve consists of 4–15 fine root fibers and emerges from the lateral part of the retroolivary area in the same line as the 6–16 cranial roots of the XIth nerve. Its exit zone has an average length of 4.07 mm (range 2.5–6.0 mm). Rostrally, it is situated 2.70 mm (range 1.5–4.0 mm) and caudally 3.62 mm (range 2.0–4.0 mm) from the lateral border of the olive.

Hypoglossal Nerve

As a rule, the XIIth cranial nerve has 7–26 root fibers that emerge from the groove between the pyramid and olive, which forms a continuation of the ventrolateral sulcus of the spinal cord. Each of these rootlets consists of 2–4 fine fiber bundles, which may emerge from the lateral part of the pyramid or the medial part of the olive. The beginning of the exit zone is situated 3.6 mm (range 1–5 mm) below the pontomedullary sulcus on the right side, the corresponding measurement on the left side being 3.8 mm (range 2.4–6.0 mm). The length of the exit zone on the right side was 12.5 mm (range 8–20 mm) and on the left side was 12.7 mm (range 9–16 mm). After a course of variable length the bundles unite into 4–6 trunklets, which run laterally and dorsally over the surface of the olive to the dural portal or portals of the XIIth nerve. In 65% there are two, sometimes three, root bundles.

Intracisternal Course of the Lower Cranial Nerves

Abducent Nerve

In the material examined by Stopford (40) the intracisternal course of the abducent nerve (Fig. 6) averaged 15 mm from the brain to its exit portal in the dura. In 16% of specimens the anterior inferior cerebellar artery ran dorsal to the abducent nerve, not basal to it, and in 5% it ran between two fiber bundles, the nerve being duplicated (19). In one case the artery divided and reunited, forming a ring through which the abducent nerve ran.

Trigeminal Nerve

The average length of the pars compacta of the trigeminal nerve (course within the posterior cranial fossa) was found to be 12.3 mm (range 9–17 mm) at the sensory and 14.1 mm (range 9–20 mm) at the motor roots (27). It forms an angle of 10°–35° with the median plane and an angle of 60°–65° with the clivus.

Topography of the Trigeminal Nerve: Trigeminal Portal

The dural exit portal (Figs. 7 and 8) of the trigeminal nerve from the posterior cranial fossa to the middle cranial fossa and into the cavum trigeminale is oval in shape, its long axis being transverse. It is situated under the furthest anterior and medial surface of the tentorium cerebelli. The average width of the exit portal in adults was seen to be 11.63 mm (range 9–15 mm) and its average height was 3.27 mm (range 2–5 mm) (5). The distance from the medial lip of the internal acoustic meatus averaged 7.04 mm (range 3.5–10.5 mm). In the vicinity of the upper anterior wall of the trigeminal portal, the superior petrosal sinus runs laterally and dorsally from the cavernous sinus. Occasionally, this channel is divided into two parts, and one vein passes beneath the pars triangularis of the trigeminal nerve. Apart from the neighboring petrosal vein, the course of the superior cerebellar artery in the vicinity of the trigeminal nerve is of clinical importance. In 30.7% of 215 cases of trigeminal neuralgia, Dandy (4) found that the artery was situated between the trigeminal nerve and the brain stem or along the lateral surface of the latter. According to Hardy and Rhoton (9) there are contact zones between the superior cerebellar artery and the nerve in approximately one-half of all cases. In six instances this contact zone was situated at the pontine entry zone of nerve V. They also noted contact of this area with the anterior inferior cerebellar artery in 8% of specimens. In one instance both the superior cerebellar artery and the anterior inferior cerebellar artery were in contact with the Vth cranial nerve. The segment of the superior cerebellar artery between its origin and the contact zone with the nerve has an average length of 28.0 mm (range 15.0–32 mm) (9). When the superior cerebellar artery does not come in contact with the nerve its average distance from the nerve is 3.2 mm (range 0.5–8.0 mm).

Situation of the Contact Zone

In most cases it is the superior and medial surface of the trigeminal nerve that comes into contact with the superior cerebellar artery (Fig. 8). Not uncommonly, a few fascicles of the nerve are displaced by the artery. This point is situated an average of 3.7 mm anterior to the entry zone of the nerve into the pons; it may occasionally be as far as 12 mm from the pons, and frequently immediately at its entry. The posterior inferior cerebellar artery and the basilar artery, or even occasionally a primi-

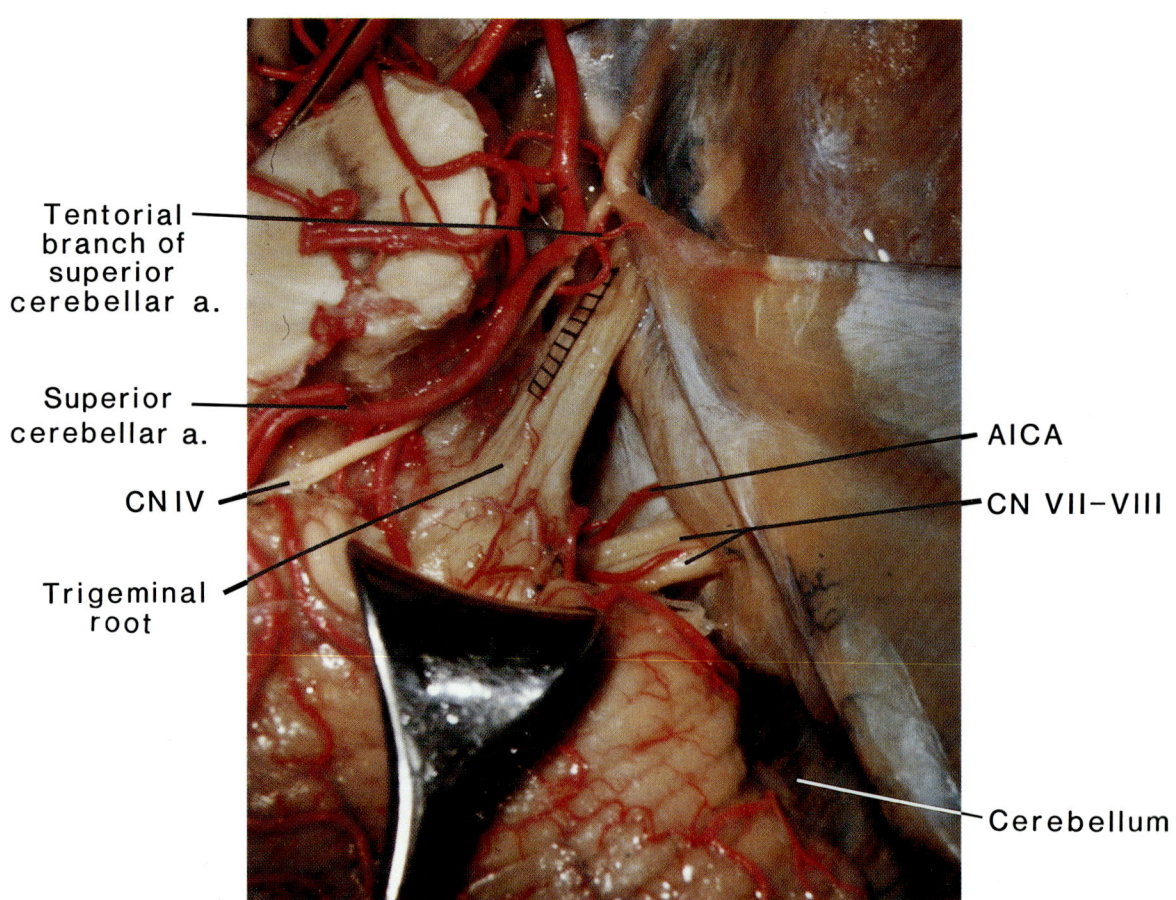

FIG. 8. Trigeminal nerves and the neighboring structures.

tive trigeminal artery, may come in contact with the root fibers of the Vth cranial nerve.

According to Jannetta (15) there is evidence of root compression by the superior cerebellar artery in most cases of trigeminal neuralgia. This chiefly affects the second and third divisions of the trigeminal nerve and, less commonly, the first and second divisions.

Facial Nerve

The average length of the intracisternal course of the facial nerve from the brain stem to the internal acoustic meatus was seen to be 15.80 mm (range 9–26 mm). The VIIth cranial nerve usually runs medial to the VIIIth and is not visible to the surgeon during the lateral approach to the posterior cranial fossa.

Vestibulocochlear Nerve

The intracisternal course of the vestibulocochlear nerve from the brain stem to the internal acoustic meatus was found to be 14.9 mm (range 9–22 mm) in length.

Nervus Intermedius

Rhoton et al. (35) found that in 20% of cases it was impossible to identify the nervus intermedius during its intracisternal course, because its separation from the vestibular part of the vestibulocochlear nerve frequently does not occur until the internal acoustic meatus is reached.

Glossopharyngeal, Vagus, and Accessory Nerves

The glossopharyngeal and vagus nerves run for an average of 15.6 mm (range 10–22 mm) within the posterior basal cisterns in their course laterally and anteriorly to their dural portals. The courses of the cranial roots of nerve XI within the common subarachnoid space are extremely variable. The spinal roots from segments C3 to C6 (C3–C7) run upward. In the specimens studied it was seen that the cranial roots have an average course of 20.71 mm (range 10–34 mm) in length (28).

Hypoglossal Nerve

After emerging from the brain the root fibers coalesce to form usually 13.6 (range 7–26) bundles, which run laterally round the olive in a gentle curve and usually rearrange themselves into two bundles within the subarachnoid space. Nine to 14 mm lateral to the median plane they enter the posterior basal cistern and run to the dural portal or portals of nerve XII. The intracisternal length of the upper root bundle is 13.3 mm (range 7–24 mm) and the length of the lowest is 11 mm (range 5.5–18 mm).

NERVES IX, X, XI, AND XII, POSTERIOR INFERIOR CEREBELLAR ARTERY, AND VERTEBRAL ARTERY

When the vertebral artery is atheromatous and thickened, it may project into the region between the inferior olive medially and flocculus laterally and may displace nerves IX, X, XI, and XII backward, pressing them against the medulla or against their dural portal. Sunderland (42) also draws attention to the variability of the course of the loop of the posterior inferior cerebellar artery between the nerve roots. In the specimens studied it was seen that the root fibers of the hypoglossal nerve were comparatively frequently stretched and damaged by the vertebral artery or the inferior cerebellar artery. In most cases the fiber bundles of the hypoglossal nerve run superior to the vertebral artery and, in rare cases, anterior or through a hole of this vessel.

Posterior Fossa, Arteries

The subarachnoid length of the vertebral artery was measured to be $25.4\bar{x}$ mm (3). In older people especially, there were sharply curved vertebral arteries, which occasionally displaced and stretched the hypoglossal nerve fibers. The first intracisternal part of the vessel in older people often shows degenerative wall changes. In very rare cases, duplicated vertebral arteries (22), persistent primitive hypoglossal arteries, or fenestrations through which some or all fibers of the cranial nerve XII were running were encountered (20). Fenestration of the vertebral artery is rarely associated with any clinical effects (11).

The first larger branch of the vertebral artery in 81.5–90% of specimens examined is the posterior inferior cerebellar artery (PICA). The posterior inferior cerebellar artery was absent on one side in 6–8.5% of cases (24,26) and in 3.6% it was missing on both sides of specimens (3). In 0.9% of cases this vessel is duplicated. It was seen that the origin zone of the posterior inferior cerebellar artery is situated in 50% of specimens in the lower third of the vertebral artery, in 27.6% in the middle part, and in 15.3% in the upper part of the vertebral artery near the junction with the opposite vessel. In 7.1% it was seen that the origin of this vessel was on the basilar artery. In approximately 4% the artery had its origin extradurally (23). Takahashi (43) demonstrated an origin of this artery at the axoatlantal part of the vertebral artery. After its origin from the vertebral artery, the loop of this vessel was seen to extend cranially in 52% and in 15.5% the loop reached the lower border of the VIIth and VIIIth nerves. In 26.7% the loop reached the level of the IXth nerve and in 37.8% the level of the Xth nerve. The loop was in relation to the fibers of the glossopharyngeal nerve in 8.9% and below the roots of the XIIth nerve in 11.1% (3). In 48% the posterior inferior cerebellar artery runs at first caudally after its origin, but in only 10% it forms a loop. In the remainder (38%) it runs dorsally at the lateral side of the medulla and nerves into the lateral medullary segment. In most cases, the vessel runs between the fibers of the accessory nerve from the anterior to the posterior medullary course. In about 25% it runs between the IXth and Xth nerves. It should be pointed out that, especially in older people who have curved vertebral arteries, the origin zone of the PICA can be found far laterally or medially placed. The loops of the PICA were found to be more marked in these people. In some cases we saw stretched and distorted nerve fibers of the XIIth and other caudal cranial nerves due to the loop. Jannetta (14) pointed out that lesions created by this artery can involve the Vth, VIIth, VIIIth, IXth, and Xth cranial nerves (especially their central segments) and cause trigeminal neuralgia, hemifacial spasm, tinnitus, vertigo, glossopharyngeal neuralgia, and high blood pressure. It should be noted that in some preparations the loop of the posterior inferior cerebellar artery reaches caudally down to the posterior arch of the atlas (22).

Smaller branches of the vertebral arteries are the anterior spinal artery, which has an outer diameter of 0.5 mm and an origin zone of 5.8 mm proximal to the union of the two vertebral arteries (3). In about 13% of specimens no union of the anterior spinal arteries was seen and in about 10% the vessel on one side was absent. It should be noted that the anterior spinal arteries have branches directed in the cranial direction in 55% of specimens. In 38% an accessory spinal artery exists, arising also from the vertebral artery with branches upward to the pyramids and to the pontomedullary sulcus. The posterior spinal artery origin was found in 43% on the PICA, in 20% on the vertebral artery, and in 36% the vessel was absent and replaced by branches of the vertebral, the PICA, or radicular C_1 arteries. The diameter of this vessel was found to be 0.38 mm. It supplies especially the nuclei gracilis and cuneatus and neighboring structures.

Basilar Artery

In 54–80% of specimens from older people, the basilar artery runs in a straight line. In 9–30%, it is concave to the right, and in 6.4–10%, it is concave to the left. Von Mitterwallner (33) found S-shaped arrangements in 1.4%, while Muller (34) saw this in 6%. It may be assumed that the tortuosity of the basilar artery increases with advancing age. The vessel was most frequently between 29 and 31 mm in length; extremes were 23 and 41 mm (24,25). The diameter of the vessel is between 1.8 and 3.8 mm (36). The inner diameter of this vessel in our material was measured to be 3.2 mm (range 1.73–4.86 mm) (29).

Anterior Inferior Cerebellar Artery (AICA)

The AICA (Fig. 9) arises from the lower third of the basilar artery in 52%, from the middle third in 46%, and from the upper third in 2% of the specimens studied. According to Lang and Kollmannsberger (24) the distance between its origin and the point of union of the two vertebral arteries varies between 4 and 25 mm (25). In the specimens studied the vessel was duplicated in 11.1% (inferior middle cerebellar artery). After its origin from the basilar artery it forms an angle of approximately 45° with the basilar artery (opened downward) in 50% of cases. Four arrangements of the main branches of the AICA are described.

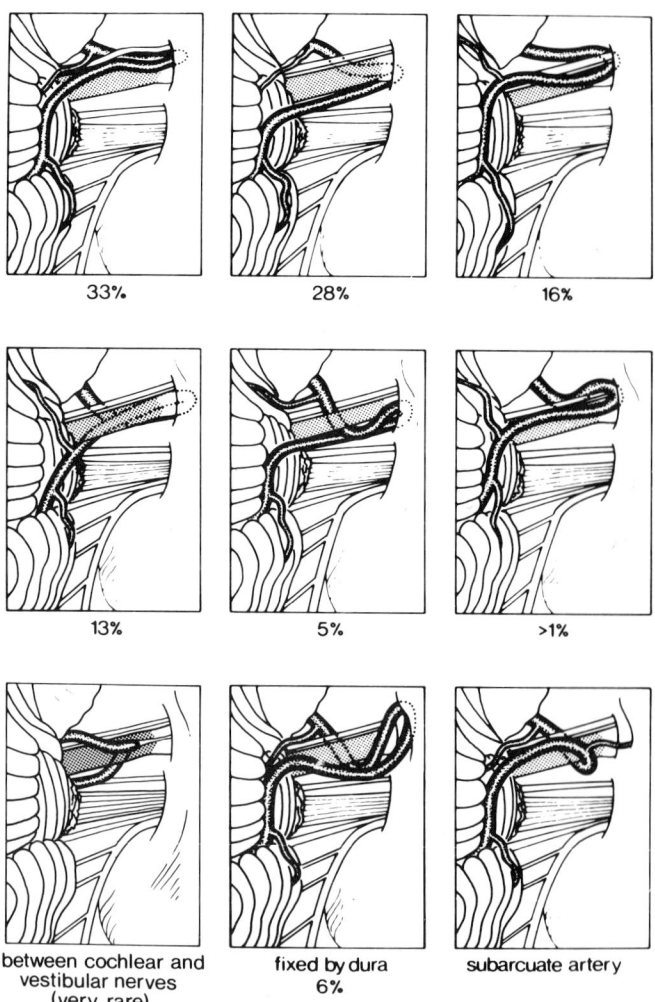

FIG. 9. Anterior inferior cerebellar artery and its variations on or in meatus. (64% Sunderland 1945, 67% Mazzoni 1969—relations to nn. VII, intermedius, and VIII; no relation to meatus—11% Sunderland, 33% Mazzoni).

Type I

The AICA runs ventrally to the abducent nerve in 79%, dorsally in 16%, and through the duplicated abducent nerve in 5% of the specimens studied. In type I (54% of the total of 101 arteries studied), the vessel runs almost as far as the cerebellopontine angle, giving off a thin twig to the latter, and then runs to the flocculus, forming one or two loops in the direction of the internal acoustic meatus. One or two fine labyrinthine arteries arise from the crest of the loop and the subarcuate artery. The main vessel then breaks up into three branches: one runs into the fissure between the superior semilunar lobule and the lobulus simplex, another into the horizontal fissure, and the third into the dorsolateral fissure of the cerebellum.

Type II

In 14% the artery runs between the pons and medulla to the cerebellopontine angle, courses over the flocculus, and then ramifies on the underside of the cerebellum. Occasionally, it gives off a narrow branch to the dorsolateral fissure in its course. This pattern is most commonly seen in cases where the PICA is thin, and its supply territory is to a greater extent taken from the AICA. Combinations of types I and II are frequent.

Type III

Type III is a combination of types I and II (26%). In these cases the AICA supplies the middle part of the cerebellum and part of its inferior surface.

Type IV

The course of the artery in type IV (6%) is the same as that in type II, but the artery gives off twigs to both fissures and to the upper side of the cerebellum. In these cases the PICA is always poorly developed in comparison to the AICA.

There exist large anastomoses between the AICA and the PICA, and sometimes between the PICA and posterior meningeal arteries (25). Occasionally, loops of the AICA and PICA are seen near the exit and entry zones of the facial and VIIIth nerves. Sometimes the vessel loops dorsally between the VIIth and VIIIth nerves near the brain stem. In these cases the AICA (or the PICA) may cause hemifacial spasm because of the central vulnerable segment of the VIIth nerve. The loop of the AICA was found in the meatus in 67% of specimens examined by Mazzoni (31,32) and in about 40% examined by Sunderland (41). The loop was found at the internal acoustic pore in 39% of specimens examined by Sunderland (41). It was not related to the internal acoustic pore or meatus in 11% (41) and in 33% of specimens (31,32). In the specimens studied by our group similar relations were seen. In about 20% of specimens the artery bifurcates proximal to or at the pore into two branches. It was noted that if the cerebellum is removed during examination from the posterior surface of the petrous part, the loop can be displaced and cause different results.

The returning limb of the AICA can course between the VIIth and VIIIth nerve (31) in 35%, below nerves VII and VIII in 18%, above nerves VII and VIII in 1%, anterior to the nerves in 8%, and between nerves VII and VIII and on the posterior wall of the meatus in 5%. For further details please see Fig. 9. It should be noted that the artery can be fixed in the area of the internal acoustic pore at the labyrinthine arteries and the subarcuate artery, sometimes embedded in dura mater, and can also pierce the petrous bone for a short looped way.

Mazzoni (31) also studied the origin, supplying areas, and relations of the subarcuate artery (for details see ref. 35). A primitive trigeminal artery is found in 0.1–0.2% of cases. In one case it was seen that the persistent trigeminal artery traversed first in the posterior fossa, piercing the dura medial after the trigeminal pore. The vessel looped in Meckel's cave and, after leaving the cave lateral to the Vth nerve, it joined the basilar artery and supplied a large part of the cerebellum (23). In this rare case, attempted thermocoagulation for trigeminal neuralgia could have resulted in arterial puncture and hemorrhage.

Superior Cerebellar Artery

In the specimens studied it was seen that when the artery arose as a single trunk, the inner diameter was 1.33 mm (range 0.77–2.26 mm). It divided into two main branches in 94% and into three main branches in 6%. In 50% the division was situated in relation to the peripeduncular cistern, and in the remainder distal to it (Fig. 8). Arising at the division, there is a lateral branch (marginal branch), which usually breaks up into two branches and runs on to the upper surface of the cerebellum. Less commonly, the artery may continue as a single trunk until it reaches the cerebellar surface (38%), or there may be secondary branches (11%). In 86% a twig runs in immediate relationship to the lateral border of the hemisphere. In 50% the vessel runs on the superior surface, in 6% on the inferior surface, and in 12% it alternates between both surfaces of the cerebellum.

The medial branch runs on the superior surface of the cerebellum, more commonly in the form of two twigs (45%); in 38% there are three twigs, in 12% it is a single trunk, and in 5% there are four twigs. In 1.5% no such twig on either side was identified. The distance across the median plane to the opposite branch ranges between minus 2 mm (opposite side) and plus 7 mm (same side). In 13% of the specimens studies the origin of the artery was in the form of their branches (28).

CEREBELLAR ARTERIES, WHOLLY OR PARTIALLY REPLACED BY OTHER CEREBELLAR ARTERIES

In only 60.5% of specimens the lower surface of the cerebellum was supplied by the posterior inferior cerebellar artery alone; in 16% the anterior inferior cerebellar artery, and in 3% the superior cerebellar artery participated.

The anterior inferior cerbellar artery varies inversely in size with the posterior inferior cerebellar artery. When the anterior inferior cerebellar artery has a large supply territory, the posterior inferior cerebellar artery is usually small.

In 67% of specimens the upper surface of the cerebellum is supplied by the superior cerebellar artery alone. In 26% this surface is supplied also by the anterior inferior cerebellar artery, and in 2.5% by both superior cerebellar and anterior inferior cerebellar arteries. As a rule, the cerebellar arteries anastomose freely with one another through small twigs. A large anastomotic circle at the base of the brain under the designation of circulus arteriosus cerebelli was described by Lang and Muller (25).

TOPOGRAPHY OF THE CEREBELLOPONTINE ANGLE AND THE INTERNAL ACOUSTIC MEATUS

The cerebellopontine angle is bordered anteriorly by the dura mater, which covers the posterior surface of the petrous bone, posteriorly by the anterior surface of the inferior part of the pons and middle cerebellar peduncle, inferiorly by biventral lobule, and inferomedially by the medullary olives. In this angular area, the exit zones of the VIIth and VIIIth cranial nerves are located more cranially and those for cranial nerves IX, X, and XI more caudally. Two important structures in this area are the flocculus and lateral aperture of the fourth ventricle.

Tumors of the VIIIth cranial nerve arise in most cases in the peripheral segment of the vestibular part or from the Obersteiner–Redlich (junctional) zone. The latter is located in the posterior fossa, near the internal acoustic meatus (IAC), or inside the internal acoustic meatus. To remove most acoustic neurinomas, the posterior lip of the IAC must be drilled away. Figure 10 shows the results of measuring a temporal bone cut transversely through the axis of the internal auditory canal. We found air cells in the posterior wall of the IAC in 17% of specimens, and behind the sigmoid sinus in 42%. Figure 11 also shows the relationships of the medial wall of the vestibule to the internal auditory meatus, dimensions of the lateral semi-

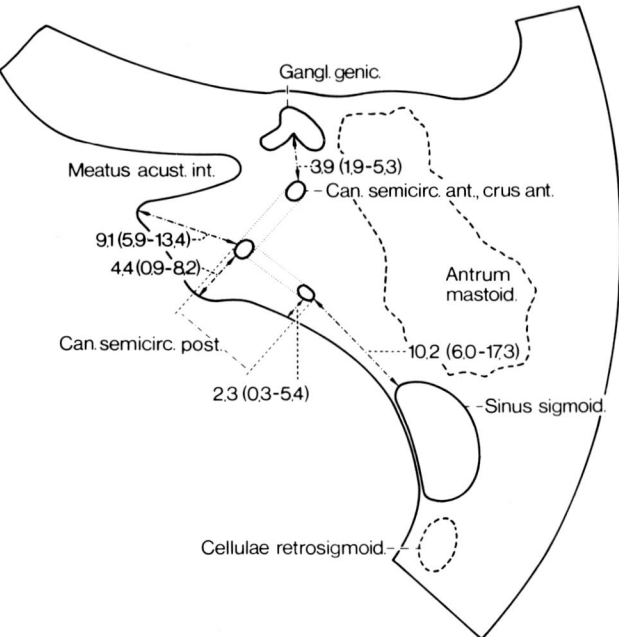

FIG. 10. Transverse section of the petrous bone through the region of the roof of the internal auditory meatus.

circular canal, distance between the cochlea and the facial nerve canal, the vestibule, and the facial nerve canal.

In Fig. 10 the double-headed arrows at the top show the relationships of the posterior semicircular canal to the posterior lip of the IAM. Also shown are distances between the anterior crus of the anterior semicircular canal and geniculate ganglion, between the lateral crus of the posterior surface of the petrous bone, and between the lateral crus and the sigmoid sinus.

By studying the coronal sections along the axis of the internal auditory canal, it was found that the meatus is

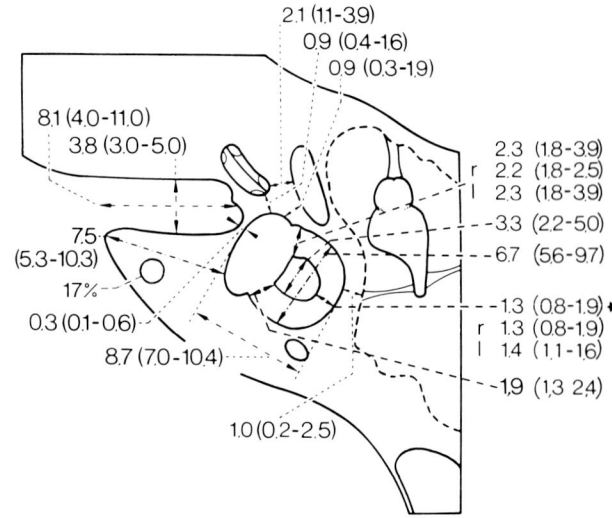

FIG. 11. Relationship of the internal auditory meatus to the surrounding structures of the petrous bone.

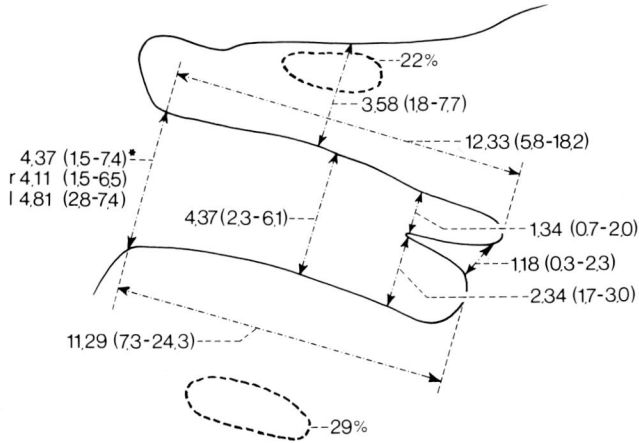

FIG. 12. Measurements (in mm) of the internal auditory meatus.

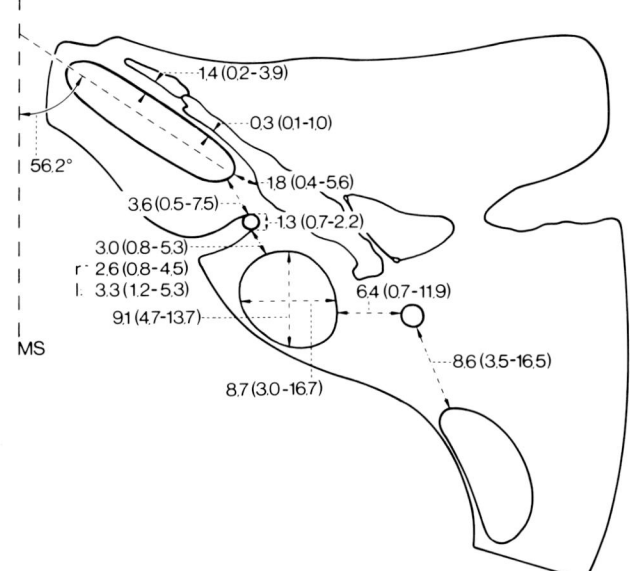

FIG. 13. Transverse section through the temporal bone at the level of the horizontal portion of the internal auditory canal.

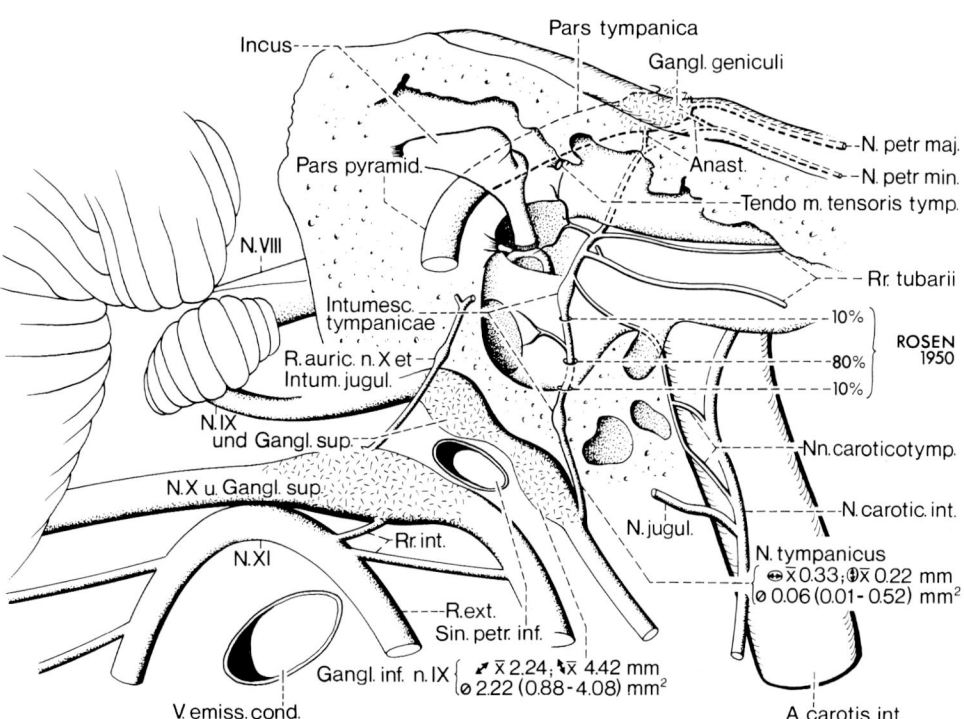

FIG. 14. Cranial nerves VII to XI in relation to the petrous bone.

4.37 mm (range 1.5–7.4 mm) high. The length of the canal, including the distance behind the transverse crest, was found to be 12.33 mm (range 5.8–18.2 mm) on the superior side and 11.29 mm (range 7.3–24.3 mm) on the inferior side. Figure 12 also shows measurements of the upper and lower fundus, with suprameatal and inframeatal air cells. The axis of the internal auditory canal turned laterally about 15° (5°–35°) away from the transverse plane.

Figures 13 and 14 show the relationships of the canals and nerves in the petrous bone. As is well described, aneurysms may arise in the intrapetrous part of the internal carotid artery.

After parts of the temporal and occipital bones have been removed, the course of the cranial nerves IX to XI in the area of the jugular foramen and below the skull base may be seen. The internal jugular vein in this preparation was removed, as was the external carotid artery at its origin. The diameters of the nerves and the lengths of the inferior ganglion of the Xth cranial nerve and the superior ganglion of the sympathetic trunk were measured, as were various distances between these structures. In most cases, glomus tumors are found in the tympanic cavity, but they may also be found in the area of the jugular fossa or elsewhere in the petrous bone. They are supplied by many vessels, the principal one of which is the ascending pharyngeal artery and its twigs.

REFERENCES

1. Arnold G, Lang J. Masse des Schadels, Korrelation von Leitungsbahnen und Beispiele ihrer praktischen Bedeutung. *Acta Anat* 1969;73:98–108.
2. Bertl Ch. *Praktisch-anatomische Befunde zu den Bruckenvenen und zu den Sinus tentorii.* Medical Dissertation, Wurzburg, 1981.
3. Brunner FX. *Uber die Arterien des Hirnstammes, Vorkommen, Zahl, Durchmesser und Variationen.* Medical Dissertation, Wurzburg, 1978.
4. Dandy WE. Concerning the cause of trigeminal neuralgia. *Am J Surg* 1934;24:447–458.
5. Dausacker J. *Praktisch anatomische Befunde an der mittleren und hinteren Schadelgrube.* Medical Dissertation, Wurzburg, 1974.
6. Denecke HJ. Zur Chirurgie ausgedehnter Glomustumoren im Bereich des Foramen jugulare. *Arch Klin Exp Ohr- Nas- Kehlkheilkd* 1966;187:656.
7. Fischer G. *Neue Befunde zu den Rami diencephalici und den Mittelhirnvenen.* Medical Dissertation, Wurzburg, 1987.
8. Gabrielsen TO, Bookstein JJ. Jugular venography by catheter approach from the arm. *Radiology* 1968;91:378–379.
9. Hardy DG, Rhoton AL Jr. Microsurgical relationship of the superior cerebellar artery and the trigeminal nerve. *J Neurosurg* 1978;49:669–678.
10. Heilek E. *Urprsungs- und Verlaufsvariationen der Arteria pharyngea ascendens.* Medical Dissertation, Wurzburg, 1977.
11. Helling M. *Hat die Fensterung der Arteria vertebralis eine klinische Bedeutung?* Medical Dissertation, Wurzburg, 1977.
12. Howieson J, Norrell H. Angiographic findings in congenital infantile hydrocephalus. *Acta Radiol Diagn (Stockh)* 1969;9:322–326.
13. Hyrtl J. Der Sinus ophthalmo-petrosus. *Wien Med Wochenschr* 1862;19:291–292.
14. Jannetta PJ. Arterial compression of the trigeminal nerve at the pons on patients with trigeminal neuralgia. *J Neurosurg* 1967;26:159–162.
15. Jannetta PJ. Observations on the etiology of trigeminal neuralgia, hemifacial spasm, acoustic nerve dysfunction, and glossopharyngeal neuralgia. Definitive microsurgical treatment and results in 117 patients. *Neurochirurgia (Stutta)* 1977;20:145–154.
16. Kimmel DL. Innervation of spinal dura mater and dura mater of the posterior cranial fossa. *Neurology* 1961;11:800–809.
17. Knott JF. On the cerebral sinuses and their variations. *J Anat Physiol* 1881;16:27–42.
18. Lack H. The endocranial equivalents of the Frankfurt plane and the exocranial position of the internal auditory meatus. *J Anat* 1930/31;65:96–107.
19. Lang J. Eintritt und Verlauf der Hirnnerven (III, IV, VI) "im" Sinus cavernosus. *Z Anat Entwicklungesch* 1974;145:87–99.
20. Lang J. In: Lanz von T, Wachsmuth W, eds. *Praktische Anatomie: ein Lehr- und Hilfsbuch der anatomischen Grundlagen arztlichen Handelns.* Fortgef und hrsg con J Lang, W Wachsmuth. Teil 1 Kopf. Teil B Gehirn- und Augenschadel, von Lang J, in Zsarb. mit K-A Busche, W Buschmann, D Linnert. Berlin: Springer, 1979.
21. Lang J. Uber Bau, Lange und Gefassbeziehungen der "zentralen" und "peripheren" Strecken der intrazisternalen Hirnnerven. *Zentralbl Neurochir* 1982;43:217–258.
22. Lang J. Clinical anatomy of the head. In: Wilson RR, Winstanley DP, trans. *Neurocranium–orbit–craniocervical regions.* Berlin: Springer, 1983.
23. Lang J. Uber einen bisher nicht beschriebenen Verlauf und Verzweigungstyp einer persistierenden A. primitiva trigemini. *Anat Arz* 1985;158:33–38.
24. Lang J, Kollmannsberger A. Beitrag zur Anatomie der Kleinhirnarterien. *Gegenbaurs Morphol Jahrb* 1961;102:170–179.
25. Lang J, Muller J. Uber bisher unbekannte topographische Beziehungen von Kleinhirnarterien. *Verh Anat Ges* 1975;69:823–828.
26. Lang J, Muller J. Weitere Befunde uber Kleinhirnarterien. *Verh Anat Ges* 1977;71:713–717.
27. Lang J, Reiter U. Uber die intrazisternale Lange des N. trigeminus. *Neurochirurgia (Stuttg)* 1984;27:159–161.
28. Lang J, Reiter U. Uber die intrazisternale Lange der Hirnnerven VII–XII. *Neurochirugia (Stuttg)* 1985;28:153–157.
29. Lang J, Schaffrath H, Fischer G. Weiters Befunde zu den Rami diencephalici. *Neurochirurgia (Stuttg)* 1987;30:103–107.
30. Lang J Jr, Samii A. Retrosigmoidal approach to the posterior cranial fossa. An anatomical study. *Acta Neurochir (Wien)* 1991;111:147–153.
31. Mazzoni A. Internal auditory canal arterial relations at the porus acusticus. *Ann Otol Rhinol Laryngol* 1969;78:797–814.
32. Mazzoni A. The subarcuate artery in man. *Laryngoscope* 1970;80:69–79.
33. Mitterwallner F von. Variationsstatistische Untersuchungen an den Hirngefassen. *Acta Anat* 1955;24:51–88.
34. Muller J. *Uber Lage und Ursprungszonen der Kleinhirnarterien und deren Quellgefasse.* Medical Dissertation, Wurzburg, 1975.
35. Rhoton AL, Kobayashi S, Hollinshead HW. Nervus intermedius. *J Neurosurg* 1968;29:609–618.
36. Ring A, Waddington M. Intraluminal diameters of the intracranial arteries. *Vasc Surg* 1967;1/3:137–151.
37. Saxena RC, Beg MAQ, Das AC. The straight sinus. *J Neurosurg* 1974;41:724–727.
38. Schubert M. *Praktisch-anatomische Befunde in der Fossa cranii posterior.* Medical Dissertation, Wurzburg, 1980.
39. Seith CH. *Uber Lage und Grosse bestimmter Hirnstrukturen und der unteren Hirnnerven.* Medical Dissertation, Wurzburg, 1980.
40. Stopford JSB. The arteries of the pons and medulla oblongata. *J Anat Physiol* 1916;50:131–164.
41. Sunderland S. Arterial relations of the internal auditory meatus. *Brain* 1945;68:23–27.
42. Sunderland S. Neurovascular relations and anomalies at the base of the brain. *J Neurol Neurosurg Psychiatry* 1948;11:243–257.
43. Takahashi M. *Atlas of vertebral angiography.* Berlin: Urban & Schwarzenberg/Tokyo: Igaku Shoin Ltd, 1974.
44. Tarlov IM. Structure of the nerve root. I. Nature of the junction between the central and peripheral nervous system. *Arch Neurol Psychiatry* 1937;37:555–583.
45. Tarlov IM. Structure of the nerve root. II. Differentiation of sensory from motor roots; observations on identification of function in roots of mixed cranial nerves. *Arch Neurol Psychiatry* 1937;37:1338–1355.
46. Zuckerkandl E. Beitrage zur Anatomie des Schlafenbeins. *Mschr Ohreinheilkd* 1873;7:101–108.

CHAPTER 12

Anterior and Anterolateral Craniofacial Resection

Ivo P. Janecka and Laligam N. Sekhar

Anterior and anterolateral craniofacial surgery encompasses structures of the midline and paramedian skull base (Fig. 1). The cribriform plate and corresponding ethmoid labyrinth superiorly, anterior wall of the sphenoid sinus posteriorly, frontal sinus anteriorly, and nasopharynx inferiorly are included in the surgical perimeter of the *anterior* craniofacial resection.

Anterolateral craniofacial resection includes the orbitomaxillary and infratemporal fossa region, as well as the floor of the middle cranial fossa (Fig. 2). The shape of this three-dimensional resection resembles a pyramidal form with its apex pointing toward the region of the cavernous sinus and lateral sphenoid sinus wall.

Anterior and anterolateral craniofacial resections have certain surgical limits beyond which their benefit rapidly diminishes. It is thus essential that the right approach is selected for specific tumor perimeters and biology.

PLANNING

Conceptually, anterior and anterolateral craniofacial resections are designed to encompass tumors along the anterior and the middle cranial fossae. The segmental nature of the craniofacial skeleton lends itself to schematic compartmentalization of neoplasms involving this region. The interorbital compartment, limited by medial walls of the orbits, the cribriform plate, and the dura, encompasses the usual specimen removed during anterior craniofacial resection. Any lateral extension of the perimeter of excision would then constitute anterolateral craniofacial resection.

The goals of anterior craniofacial resection include treatment of primarily ethmoid neoplasms. The anterolateral resection is usually applied to orbital and extensive maxillary sinus neoplasia. In addition, extensive transcranial middle fossa tumors (e.g., meningiomas) can be removed through the anterolateral craniofacial approach.

Preoperative determination that the tumor extent is confined to the interorbital space permits selection of an anterior craniofacial approach. In such cases, the soft tissue of the orbital cones is not involved by tumor, and in most instances, the lamina papyracea of the medial orbital wall is intact as well. This bony wall serves as a lateral surgical margin. For the anterolateral craniofacial resection where the orbital content is often included in the specimen, the lateral perimeter of the resection extends to the infratemporal fossa.

SURGICAL STEPS

The *anterior craniofacial resection* is performed through bicoronal scalp and paranasal facial incisions (Fig. 3). Following facial bone exposure, the medial walls of both orbits are explored, identifying and cauterizing the anterior and posterior ethmoidal vessels. This establishes the lateral perimeter of the resection. Horizontal osteotomies can be performed at this point using a reciprocating saw blade through the medial wall of each orbit at the junction with the orbital floor. Also, posteriorly with an angled oscillating saw blade, a vertical cut can be

---

I. P. Janecka: Center for Cranial Base Surgery, University of Pittsburgh School of Medicine, Presbyterian University Hospital, and Department of Otolaryngology, Eye and Ear Institute, Pittsburgh, Pennsylvania 15213.

L. N. Sekhar: Department of Neurosurgery, Center for Cranial Base Surgery, University of Pittsburgh School of Medicine, Presbyterian University Hospital, Pittsburgh, Pennsylvania 15213.

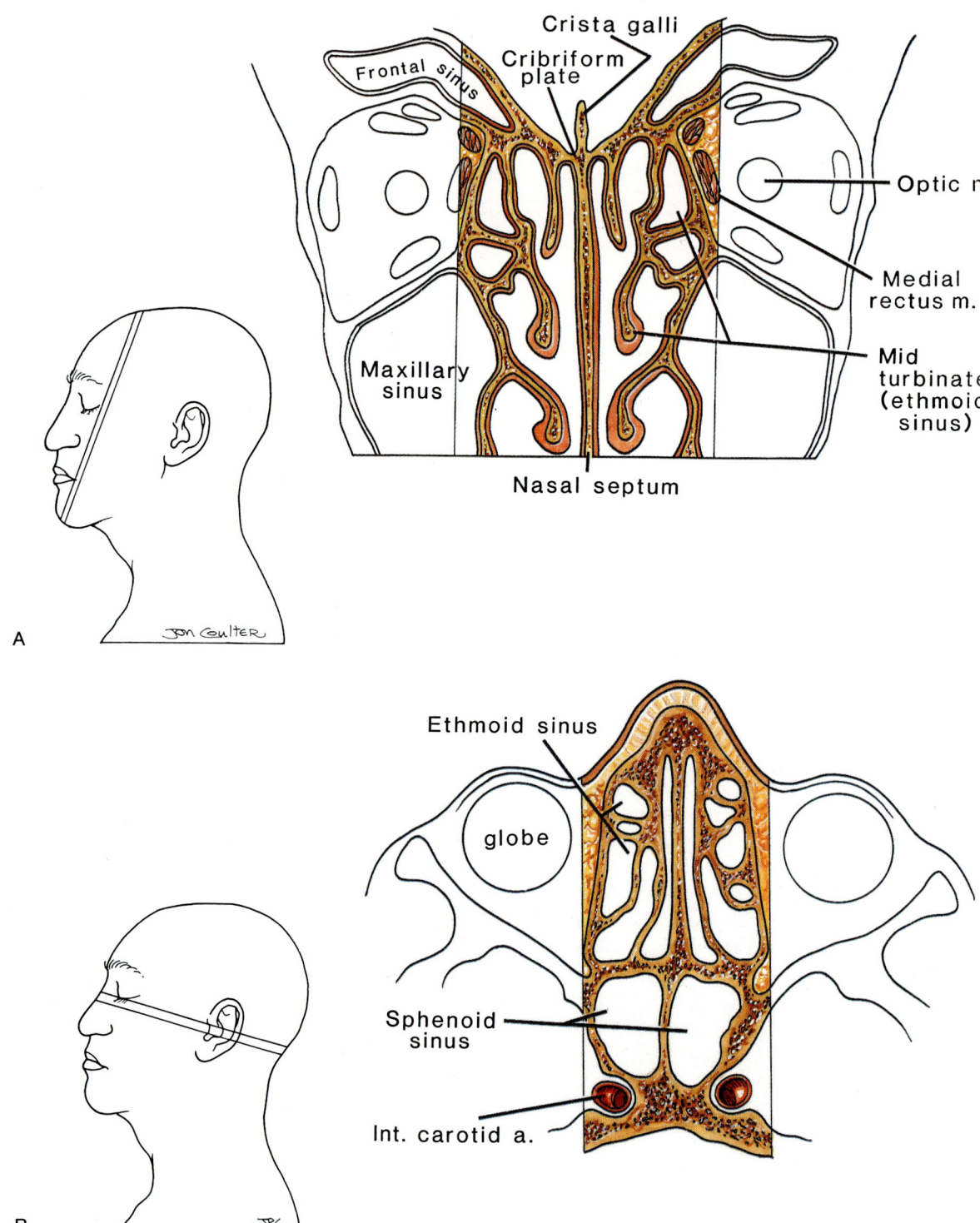

FIG. 1. A: Coronal CT scan view depicting midline anatomic structures of the anterior cranial base. **B:** Axial view.

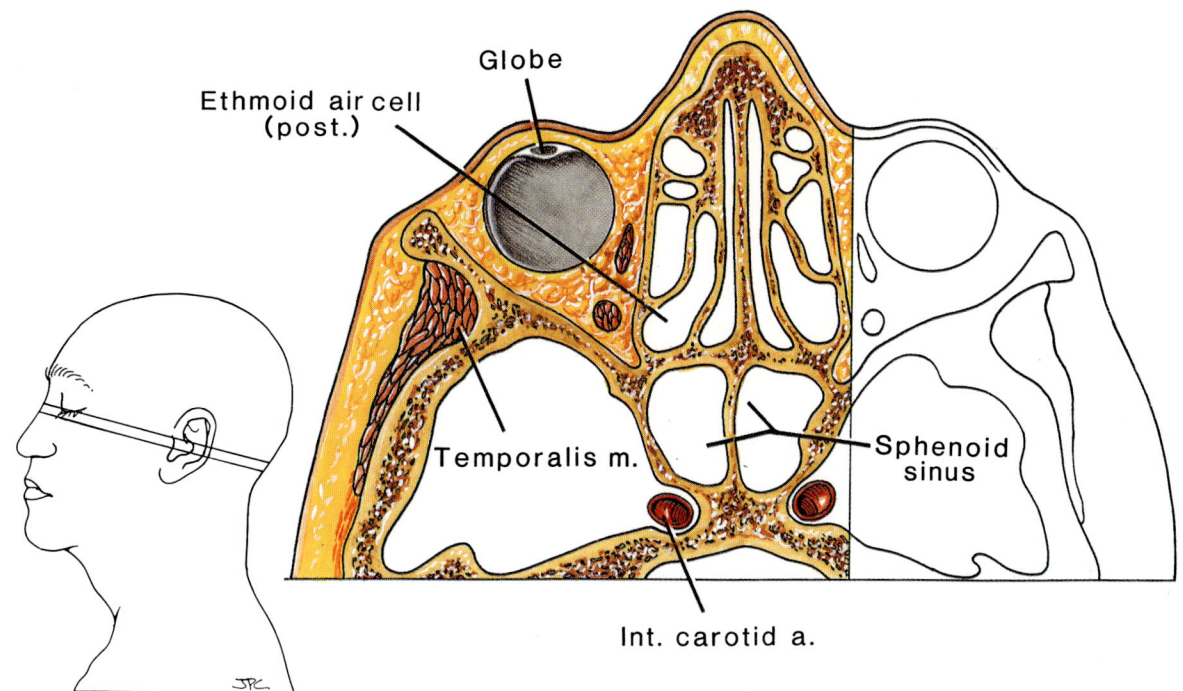
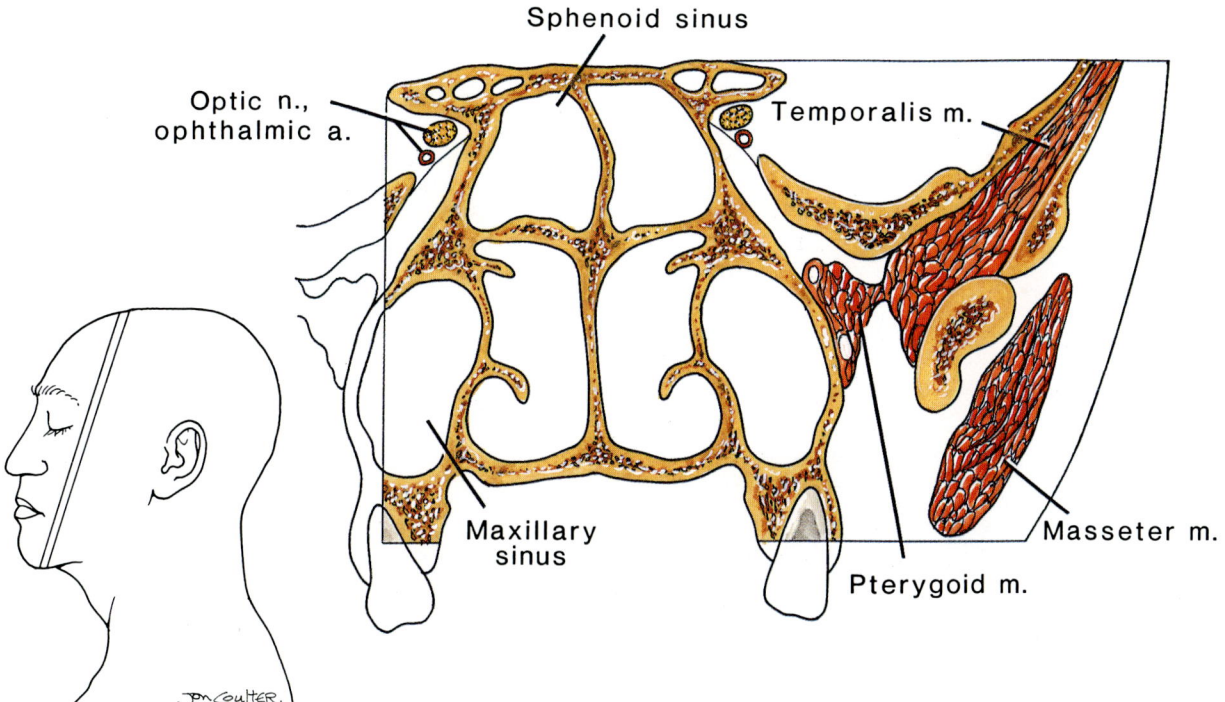

FIG. 2. A: Axial CT scan image demonstrating midline and paramedian anatomic structures of the anterolateral skull base. **B:** Coronal view.

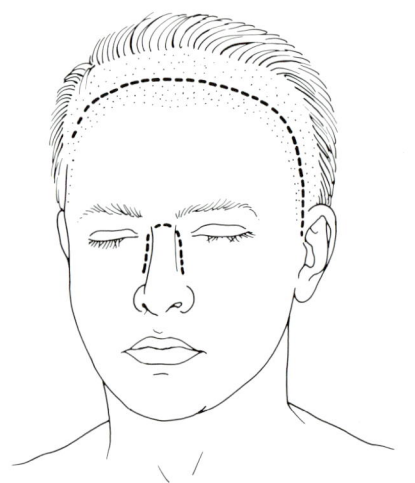

FIG. 3. Skin incisions used for anterior craniofacial resection.

performed at the level of the posterior ethmoidal foramen. Anteriorly, similar vertical cuts can be made from the level of the lacrimal fossa to the level of the nasion. At this point, a bifrontal craniotomy is performed, reflecting the basal dura along the cribriform plate to the planum sphenoidale. Depending on the extent of the tumor, both optic nerves can be decompressed at this point and an entry through the planum sphenoidale into the sphenoid sinus identifies the most posterior extent of the resection (Fig. 4). The central anterior portion of the frontal bone, from the nasion to the inferior extent of the bifrontal craniotomy, can be incorporated into the specimen (Fig. 5A) or removed separately. This permits a very inferior (basal) approach to the anterior cranial fossa without significant brain retraction. The vomer is transected in the nasopharynx and, with a curved osteotome,

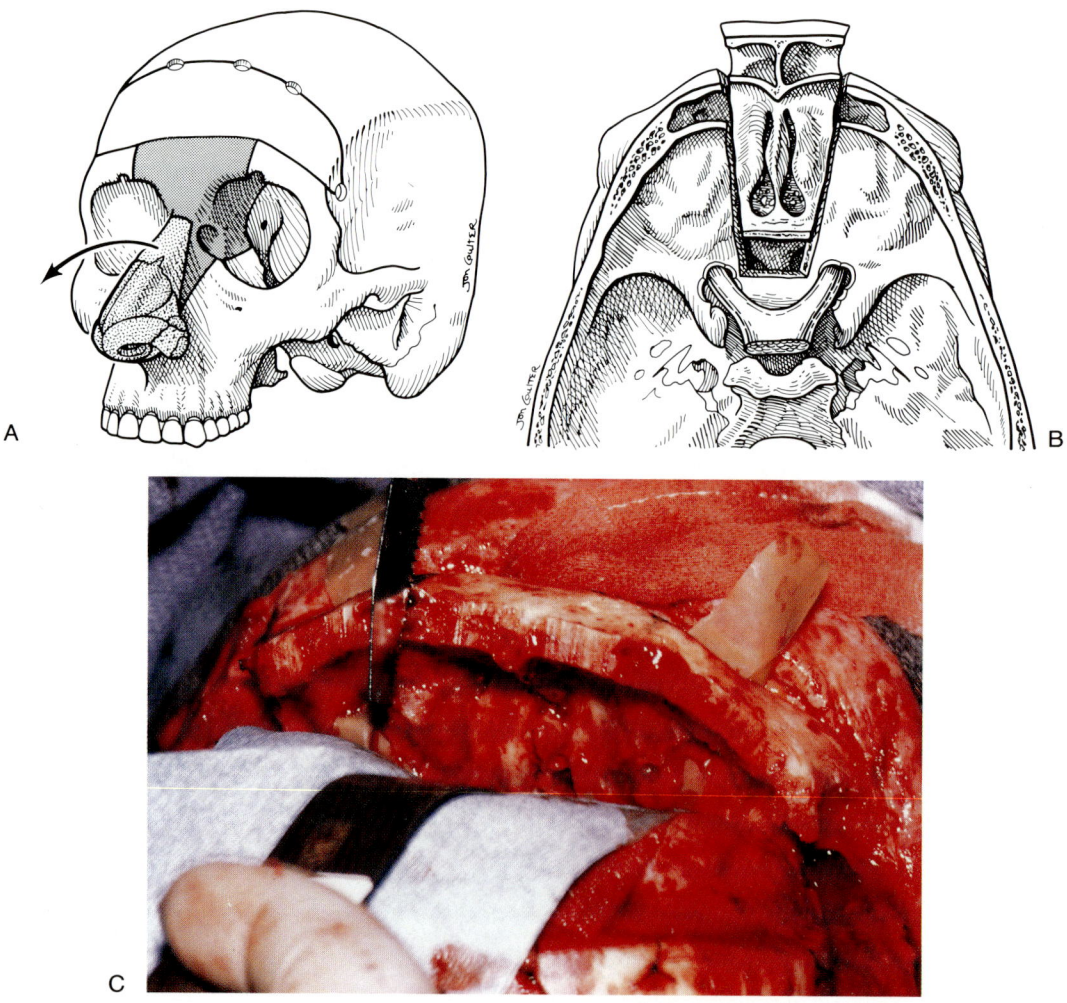

FIG. 4. A: Schematic outline of orbital and frontonasal osteotomies as well as bifrontal craniotomy. **B:** Removal of the central compartment of the anterior cranial base; both optic nerves are seen decompressed. **C:** Clinical photograph of exposed anterior cranial fossa with initiation of left vertical osteotomy.

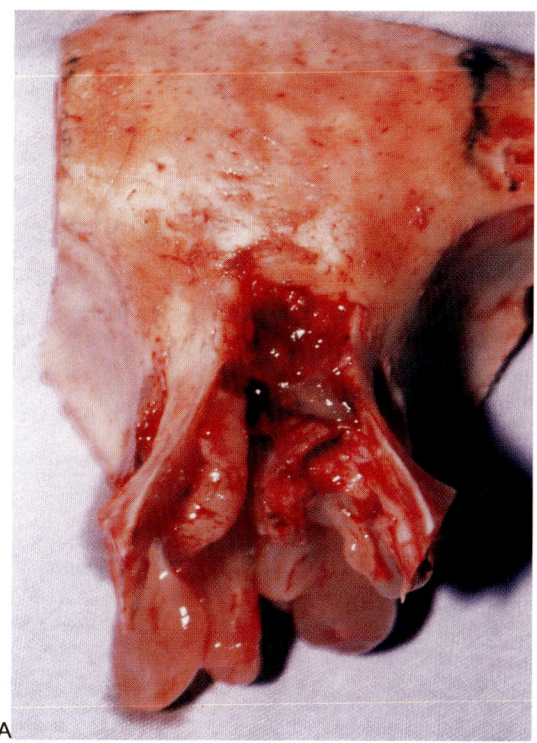
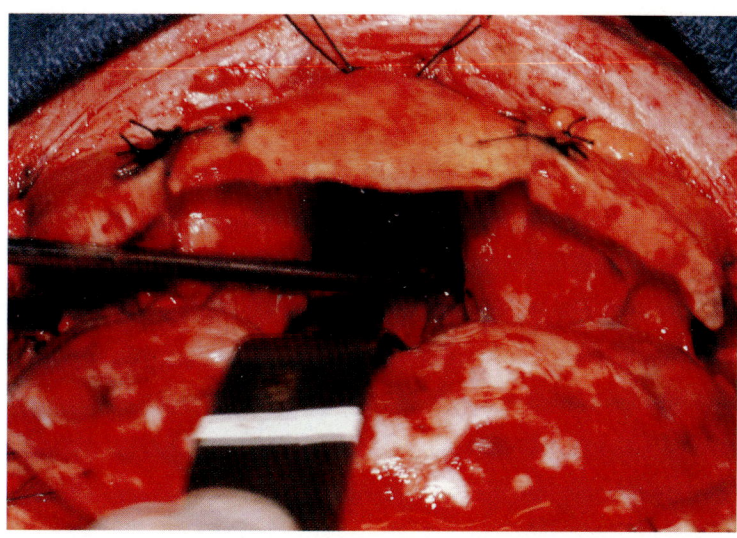

FIG. 5. A: Surgical specimen following anterior craniofacial resection. **B:** Defect in the anterior cranial fossa.

posterior cuts are completed from the sphenoid sinus to the nasopharynx.

Following anterior craniofacial resection, the defect (Fig. 5B) has, as its posterior margins, the remaining portion of the sphenoid sinus and optic nerves posteriorly and the periorbita laterally. Inferiorly, the defect is open to the nasopharynx.

Reconstruction is begun with repair of the frontal dura. This may be done with the use of a pericranial *graft*, usually obtained from the region of the skull posterior to the line of the bicoronal scalp incision.

The bicoronal scalp *flap* serves as a donor site for harvesting of a pericranial flap (Fig. 6A). This flap is raised in a rectangular fashion with its base at the supraorbital region and receives its blood supply from the supraorbital and supratrochlear vessels. The dissection is done at the level of the galea (Fig. 6B). It is essential that this thin flap not be permitted to desiccate during surgery. Insertion of the flap intracranially is done through roofs of the orbits and sutured to the basal dura (Fig. 6C). This provides a carpetlike resurfacing of the anterior cranial fossa. The frontal lobes are subsequently permitted to expand and assure contact between the basal dura and the flap. If the bony defect in the floor of the anterior cranial fossa is judged large enough to potentially permit brain herniation, a split cranial bone graft can be placed between the pericranial flap and the dura to provide basal support. Anteriorly, the central portion of the frontal bone above the level of the nasion is then reconstructed with a bone graft or if this bone was uninvolved with tumor, it is then replaced as a free graft. The exposed intranasal and orbital soft tissues are not grafted and are permitted to undergo secondary healing.

The *anterolateral craniofacial resection* is also done through a bicoronal or modified bicoronal scalp incision. The facial incisions are usually paranasal with possible lip split and eyelid incisions. If the orbital content is to be included in the specimen, incisions are then made near the eyelid margins (Fig. 7). The extent of facial osteotomies (Fig. 8) depends on the size of the tumor. In general, they are made within the orbit along the medial and lateral wall as well as across the zygoma. The craniotomy may extend from the bifrontal to the ipsilateral temporal region or be limited to a frontotemporal area. The dural elevation may extend to the region of the optic nerve and cavernous sinus, where, depending on the extent of the tumor, the posterior incision is made. Resection of the cavernous sinus requires disposition of the internal carotid artery either by prior elective balloon embolization or intraoperative clipping in selected patients. In most cases, however, the most posterior extent of the anterolateral craniofacial resection is the superior orbital fissure and the optic nerve (Fig. 9).

Following dural repair, the preserved craniofacial skeleton is replaced and affixed with multiple miniplates (Fig. 10). For soft tissue repair, the temporalis muscle (Fig. 11) and pericranial flap are very useful or a free microvascular flap can be used (Fig. 12). The intraoral portion of the exposed temporalis muscle may be skin grafted. If a hard palate is also resected, a prefabricated prosthesis provides excellent support in the postoperative period. The orbital defect, following orbital exenter-

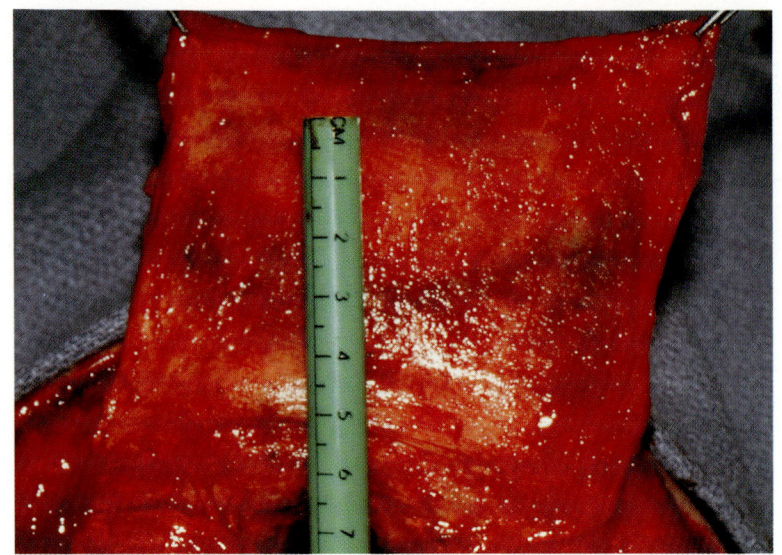
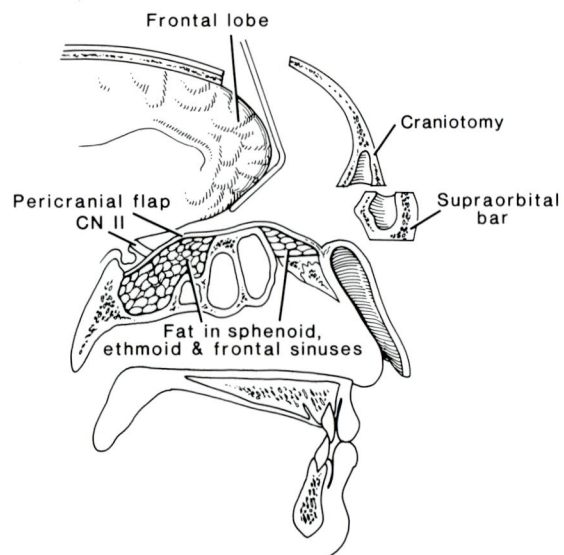
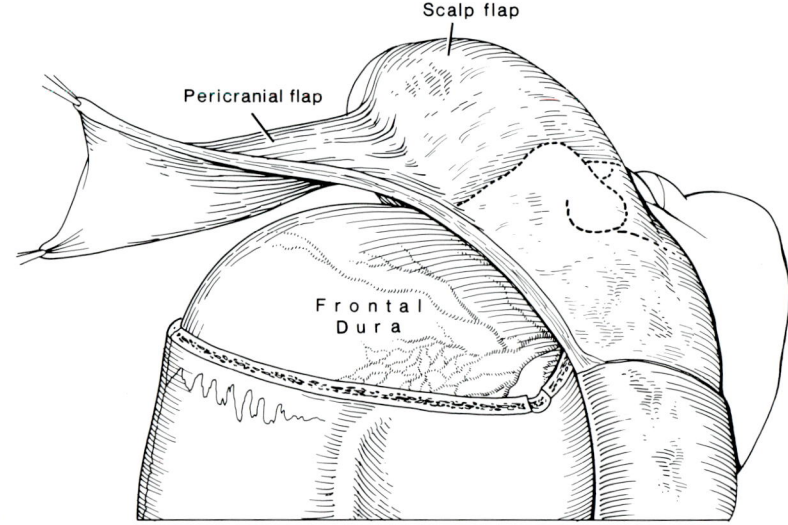

FIG. 6. A: Pericranial flap. **B:** Pericranial flap raised from scalp flap. **C:** Inset of pericranial flap at the level of orbital roofs under replaced supraorbital bone.

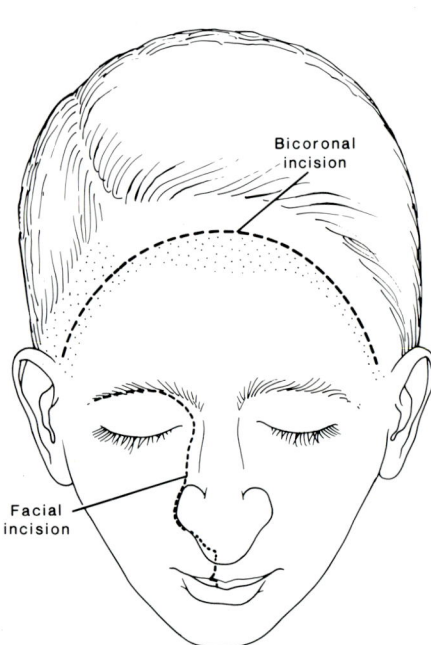

FIG. 7. Available incisions for anterolateral craniofacial resection.

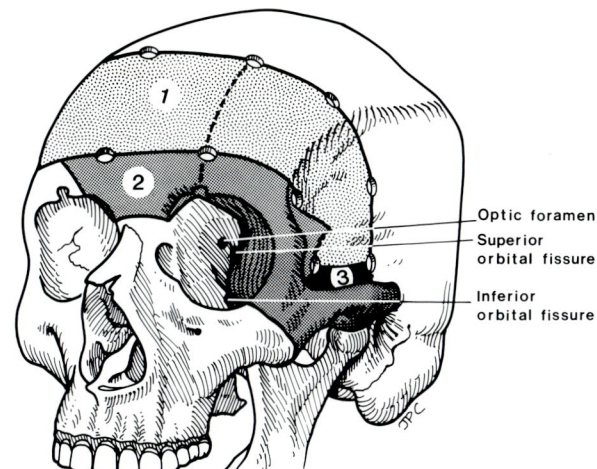

FIG. 8. Craniofacial osteotomies used for exposure in anterolateral craniofacial resection.

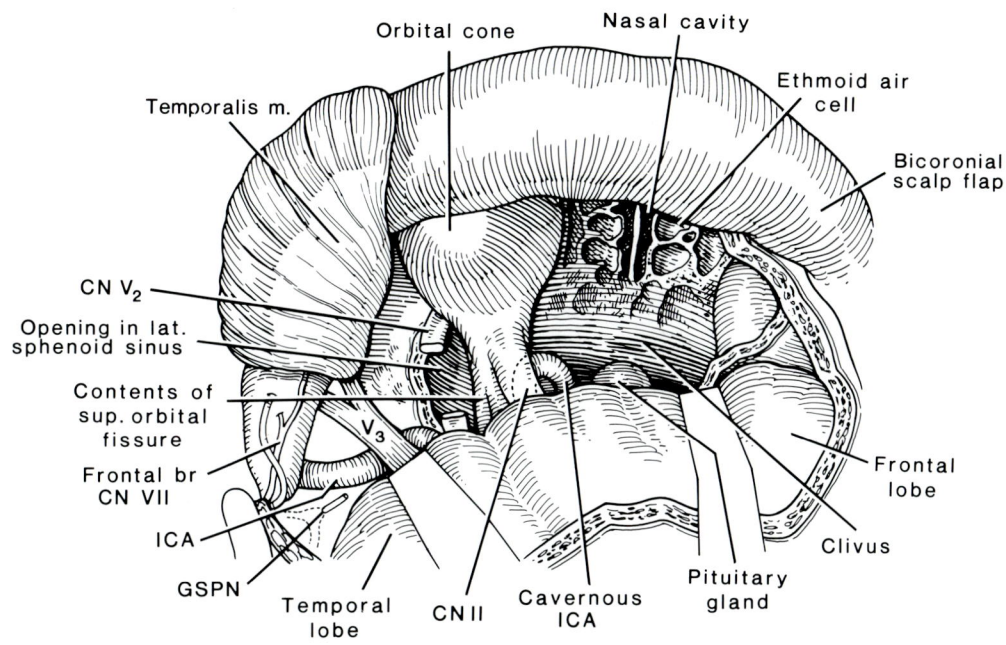

FIG. 9. Potential exposure of anterolateral skull base.

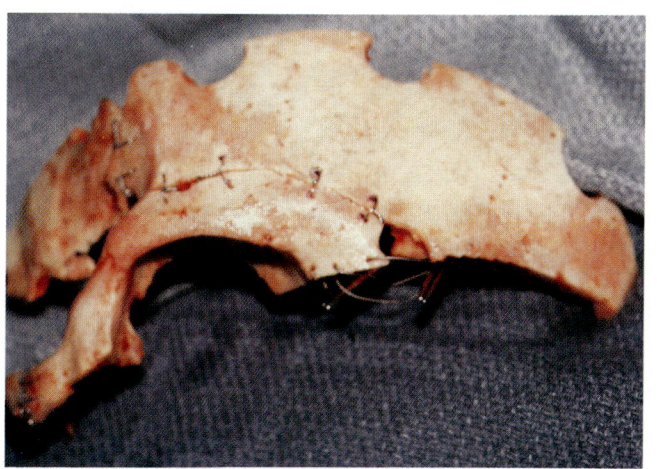
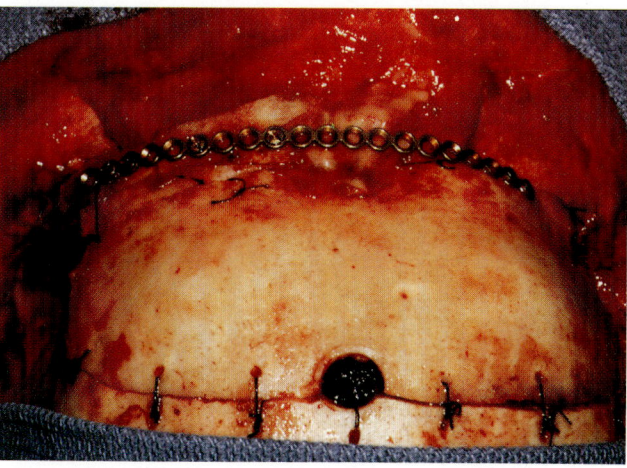

FIG. 10. A: Craniofacial bones removed during exposure. **B:** Miniplate fixation of replaced craniofacial skeleton.

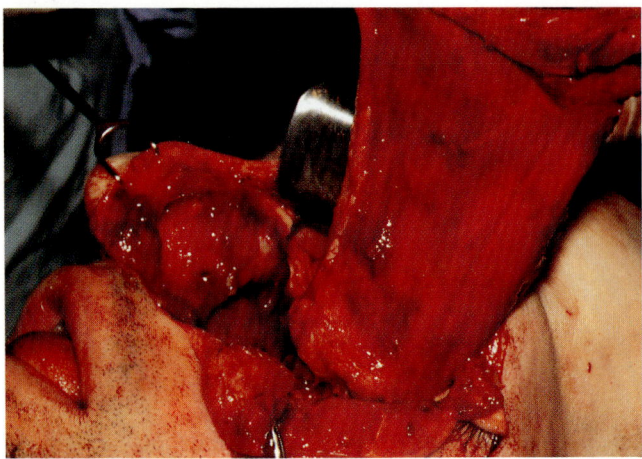

FIG. 11. Rotation of temporalis muscle for reconstruction.

ation, can be lined with the remaining eyelid skin. In cases where the globe is preserved, the orbital support has to be reestablished to prevent ocular dystopia. Again, bone grafts and miniplates are useful. The nasolacrimal duct may be stented or a permanent dacryocystorhinostomy is performed. If the temporalis muscle is used for soft tissue repair of the surgical defect, the subsequent depression of the temporal fossa may be lessened by a free abdominal fat graft.

Specific Concerns

Facial *scars* placed in the paranasal and periorbital region usually heal quite well. Selection of the optimal direction for the incisions prevents scar contracture, which may become visible as an epicanthal fold or hypertrophic scar. The bicoronal scalp incision should be placed approximately 10 cm from the level of the supraorbital rims in order to maintain adequate length of the eventual pericranial flap. The direction of the incision through the scalp should respect the position of the hair follicles to minimize the frequent hair loss along scalp scars.

Facial *osteotomies* can be done with standard maxillofacial instrumentation except for the posterior vertical orbital osteotomy, which is best done with a small angulated oscillating saw. This osteotomy may also be done from above, following bifrontal craniotomy, with an osteotome.

The creation of the bifrontal craniotomy must include consideration of the frontal sinus. The extent of the sinus can be anticipated from the preoperative scans. If a large sinus is present, an osteoplastic flap may be developed first, following outlining of the sinus perimeter on the frontal bone utilizing a template from a six-foot Caldwell x-ray. Removal of the anterior sinus wall then permits direct access to the posterior wall. With a high-speed drill, separation of the posterior table and the dura is performed. In smaller sinuses, the craniotome may cut directly across the sinus in the supraorbital area. The final disposition of the frontal sinus usually requires obliteration of the nasofrontal duct and cranialization of the sinus. In smaller sinuses, it may also be possible to obliterate them, following mucosal removal, with free abdominal fat.

In addition to intracranial confinement of *CSF,* a good seal of the anterior cranial fossa, with a pericranial flap, is also essential in order to prevent pneumocephalus in the postoperative period.

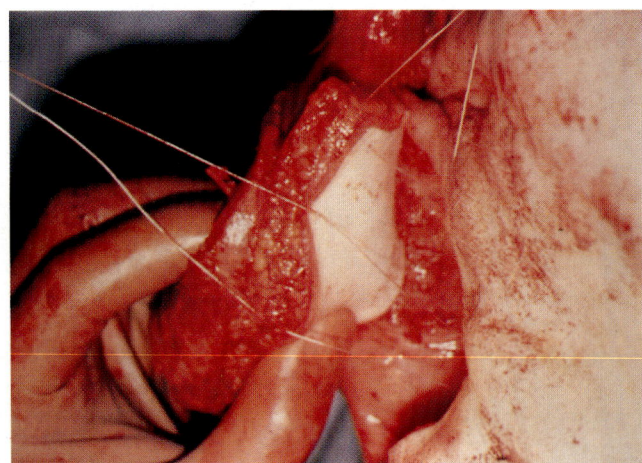
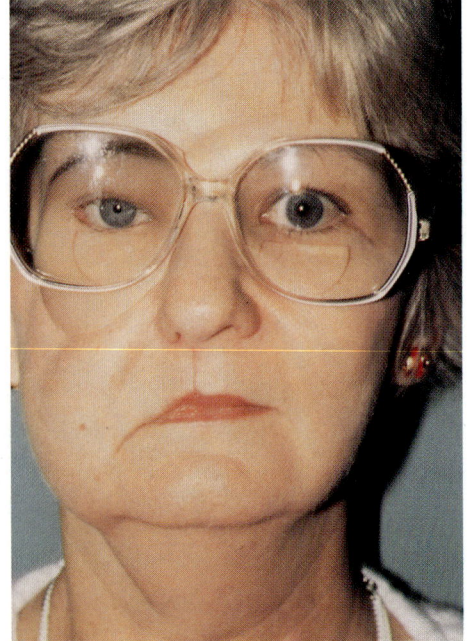

FIG. 12. A: Inset of a microvascular myocutaneous flap into craniofacial defect. **B:** Postoperative appearance with right orbital prosthesis.

In the anterolateral craniofacial resections, the reestablishment of the lateral orbital and zygomatic contour with replaced skeleton requires excellent stabilization in three planes. Any movement of this segment of the craniofacial skeleton will very likely result in incomplete healing and subsequent need to remove this segment of bone. The craniotomy is replaced and stabilized.

Preoperative Care

Attention to scalp hygiene with Phisohex shampoo as well as intranasal care is important (especially in patients who had radiation to the nasopharyngeal region). Shaving of hair is optional. However, long hair attached to a scalp flap presents a technical problem during surgery, and for that reason may have to be shaved preoperatively. Patients with previous surgical procedures in the craniofacial region need assessment of the scalp vascularity. The extent of the previous incisions determines our options for any new flaps. Also, determination of temporalis muscle innervation and its approximate bulk helps to estimate its usefulness for reconstruction. Antibiotics are started in all cases within an hour prior to surgery. In most cases we have used a single agent (third generation cephalosporin).

Postoperative Care

Patients are placed on anticonvulsant medication, and a spinal drain is used for a period of 3–4 days. On the average, 50 cc of spinal fluid are removed every shift. Soft tissue drains are removed when drainage significantly diminishes (down to 10–20 cc/24 hr). Once the external drains are removed, the antibiotics are stopped. Most of our patients undergo CT scanning within the first 24 hr postoperatively. This is done in order to establish an immediate postsurgical baseline in terms of the amount of intracranial air, blood, and CSF collections. Any subsequent change in the patient's mental status is evaluated by CT scanning and compared to the original 24-hr scan. Any oral packing used to stabilize a skin graft over the temporalis muscle is removed within 7 days.

Follow-up

Following the patient's discharge, continued attention to nasal hygiene on a weekly basis is important to facilitate uncomplicated secondary healing of interorbital, nasal, and oral surfaces. This is best accomplished with direct nasal irrigation utilizing modified waterpik and mechanical cleansing. Once a mucosal surface is reestablished intranasally, only maintenance hygiene is needed. At approximately 3 months following surgery, CT or MRI scans are obtained to serve as a baseline for oncological follow-up. These studies are then repeated at gradually lengthening intervals.

COMPLICATIONS

Maximum intraoperative visualization significantly lessens the potential for intraoperative complications. Clear visualization of optic nerves and limited frontal lobe and ocular retraction are aided with wide surgical exposure. Intraoperative monitoring of cranial nerve VI as well as visual evoked responses have so far not been standard for every anterolateral craniofacial resection. Postoperatively, a CSF leak and the presence of intracranial air or blood can be encountered. In extensive anterolateral craniofacial resections, a limited amount of pneumocephalus is present for the first 24–48 hr. However, any progression in the volume of air should be an indication for consideration of surgical reexploration. A certain amount of CSF leak may be encountered in the first few days postoperatively but that often undergoes spontaneous seal. However, any significant, gravity-dependent leak should be actively investigated and treated. Supine position and functioning spinal drain represent the first line of defense. Persistence of the leak requires surgical reexploration. Occasionally, a degree of upper airway obstruction may force air intracranially. This may be overcome with nasopharyngeal airway stenting. If the eye is preserved following anterolateral craniofacial resection, a tarsorrhaphy provides the best protection for the globe.

CONCLUSION

Anterior and anterolateral resections are done primarily as oncological procedures. The esthetic and functional importance of the craniofacial region intensifies the demands for surgical safety, limitation of surgical morbidity, and critical esthetic reconstruction. The pericranial and temporalis muscle flaps assist greatly in soft tissue reconstruction and separation of extracranium and intracranium. The elective use of craniofacial osteotomies and split cranial bone grafts with miniplate fixation assures stability of the craniofacial skeleton and thus reestablishment of important esthetic facial contours.

SUGGESTED READING

1. Sekhar LN, Janecka IP, Jones NF. Subtemporal–infratemporal and basal subfrontal approach to extensive cranial base tumors. *Acta Neurochir* (*Wien*) 1988;92:83–92.
2. Janecka IP, Sekhar LN. Surgical management of cranial base tumors: a report on 91 patients. *Oncology* 1989;3:69–74.
3. Janecka IP, Sekhar LN. Cranial base tumors. In: Myers EN, Suen J, eds. *Cancer of the head and neck,* 2nd ed. New York: Churchill Livingstone, 1989;337–382.
4. Janecka IP. Cancer of the orbit. In: Myers EN, Suen J, eds. *Cancer of the head and neck,* 2nd ed. New York: Churchill Livingstone, 1989;711–734.

5. Janecka IP, Sekhar LN, Jones NF, Shestak KC. Treatment of cancer of the skull base. Head and neck cancer. Proceedings of the Second International Conference. In: Fee WE, Goepfert H, Johns ME, Strong EW, Ward P, eds. *Head and neck cancer,* vol II. New York: BC Decker, 1990;382–384.
6. Snyderman CH, Sekhar LN, Sen CN, Janecka IP. Malignant skull base tumors. In: Rosenblum ML, ed. *Neurosurgery clinics of north america.* Philadelphia: Saunders, 1990;243–259.
7. Sekhar LN, Janecka IP. Intracranial extension of cranial base tumors and combined resection: the neurosurgical perspective. In: Jackson CG, ed. *Surgery of skull base tumors.* New York: Churchill Livingstone, 1991;211–250.
8. Al-Mefty O. The supra-orbital pterional approach to skull base lesions. *Neurosurgery* 1987;21:474–477.
9. Derome PJ, Akerman M, Anquez L, et al. Les tumeurs spenoethmoidales. *Neurochirurgie [Suppl]* 1972;18:1–164.
10. Hakuba A, Liu SS, Nishimura S. The orbitozygomatic infratemporal approach: a new surgical technique. *Surg Neurol* 1986;26:271–276.
11. Jackson IT, Marsh WR, Hide TAH. Treatment of tumors involving the anterior cranial fossa. *Head Neck Surg* 1984;6:901–913.
12. Ketcham AS, Hoye RC, Van Buren JM, et al. Complications of intracranial facial resection for tumors of the paranasal sinuses. *Am J Surg* 1966;112:581–596.
13. Persing JA, Jane JA, Levine PA, Cantrell RW. The versatile frontal sinus approach to the floor of the anterior cranial fossa. *J Neurosurg* 1990;72:513–516.
14. Schramm VL Jr, Myers EN, Maroon JC. Anterior skull base surgery for benign and malignant disease. *Laryngoscope* 1979;89:1077–1091.
15. Sekhar LN, Janecka IP, Jones NF. Subtemporal–infratemporal and basal subfrontal approach to extensive cranial base tumors. *Acta Neurochir (Wien)* 1988;92:83–92.
16. Sundaresan N, Shah JP. Craniofacial resection for anterior skull base tumors. *Head Neck Surg* 1988;10:219–224.
17. Van Buren JM, Ommaya AK, Ketcham AS. Ten years' experience with radical combined craniofacial resection of malignant tumors of the paranasal sinuses. *J Neurosurg* 1968;28:341–350.

CHAPTER 13

Anterior, Anterolateral, and Lateral Approaches to Extradural Petroclival Tumors

Laligam N. Sekhar, Chandranath Sen, Carl H. Snyderman, and Ivo P. Janecka

Extradural, clival, and petroclival neoplasms may be benign (e.g., meningioma, epidermoid cyst, and cholesterol granuloma), of a low-grade malignancy (e.g., chordoma, chondrosarcoma), or of a high-grade malignancy (e.g., squamous cell carcinoma, osteogenic sarcoma). In this chapter, five surgical approaches that we normally use in the operative resection of these lesions are described. These include: the subtemporal, transcavernous, and transpetrous apex approach; the subtemporal and preauricular infratemporal approach; the extended frontal approach; the combination of the subtemporal, infratemporal and extended frontal approaches; and the extreme lateral, transcondyle, and transjugular approach. Although the transethmoidal, transmaxillary, transnasal, transsphenoidal, total petrosectomy, and transoral approaches are used by us for some lesions in this area, they are not discussed here since they are detailed extensively in other chapters (1–3,7–9,13–15,25).

APPROACH SELECTION FOR EXTRADURAL CLIVAL TUMORS

The clivus may be divided conveniently into three anatomical regions (Figs. 1 and 2). The upper clivus is the area above the petrous apices and above the crossing points of the trigeminal and the abducens nerves from the posterior to the middle cranial fossa. It includes the dorsum sellae and the posterior clinoid processes. It is bounded *laterally* by the intracavernous carotid arteries and the cavernous sinuses with contained structures, the structures in the tentorial notch area, and the temporal lobes; *posteriorly* by the basilar artery and its branches and the midbrain; and *anteriorly* by the sella turcica and the sphenoid sinus. The *midclivus* extends from the sixth cranial nerve down to the exit foramina (pars nervosa of the jugular foramen) of the ninth, tenth, and eleventh cranial nerves. The midclivus is related *posteriorly* to the basilar artery and branches, the vertebrobasilar junction, and the pons; *laterally,* by the inferior petrosal sinuses, the petrous apices, and the seventh and eighth cranial nerves; and *anteriorly,* by the nasopharynx and retropharyngeal tissues. The *lower clivus* is the area below the ninth, tenth, and eleventh cranial nerves and includes the occipital condyles, the foramen magnum, and the hypoglossal canals. *Posteriorly,* the lower clivus is related to the vertebral arteries, the pontomedullary junction, the medulla, and the spinomedullary junction; *laterally* to the hypoglossal nerves, the sigmoid sinus, and the jugular bulb; and *anteriorly,* to the nasopharynx and retropharyngeal tissues. This type of division of the clivus into upper, middle, and lower areas is helpful to the surgeon to plan the surgical approaches based on the anatomical location of the tumor.

For lesions of the upper clivus, the subtemporal, transcavernous, and transpetrous apex approach is used. For lesions of the midclivus, the surgical approach used will depend on the tumor location with respect to the midline. When one-half of the clivus and the petrous apex region are involved, the subtemporal and infratemporal approach is optimal. When the entire midclivus, petrous apex, and the sphenoid area are involved, we use either the subtemporal and infratemporal approach with the division of V_3, or the subtemporal and infratemporal approach in combination with the basal frontal ap-

---

L. N. Sekhar: Department of Neurosurgery, Presbyterian University Hospital, Pittsburgh, Pennsylvania 15213.

C. Sen: Department of Neurosurgery, Mt. Sinai Medical Center, New York, New York 10029.

C. H. Snyderman: Department of Otolaryngology, Eye and Ear Institute, Pittsburgh, Pennsylvania 15213.

I. P. Janecka: Center for Cranial Base Surgery, Presbyterian University Hospital, and Department of Otolaryngology, Eye and Ear Institute, Pittsburgh, Pennsylvania 15213.

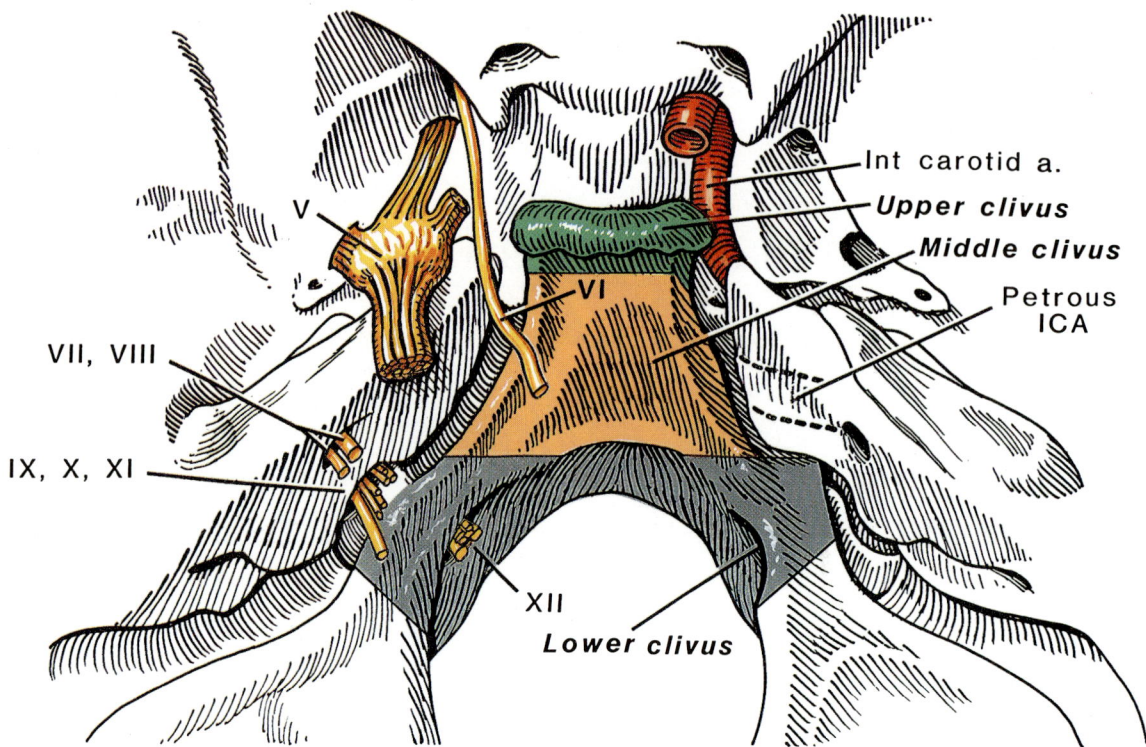

FIG. 1. The anatomical divisions of the clivus into upper, mid, and lower regions.

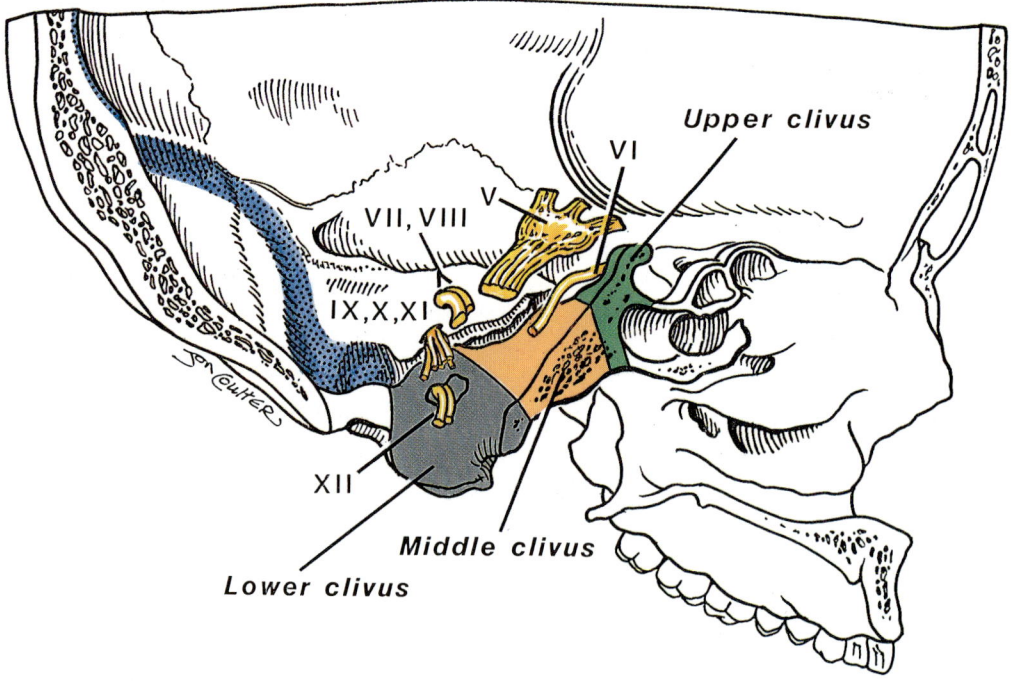

FIG. 2. Adjacent cranial base structures of clivus are shown.

TABLE 1. *Approach selection for extradural clival neoplasms*

Region	Subregion	Approach(es)[a]
Upper clivus	Transpetrous apex	Subtemporal, transcavernous
Midclivus	Petrous apex + adjacent half of clivus	Subtemporal–infratemporal approach
	Petrous apex + entire midclivus, sphenoid sinus	Subtemporal–infratemporal approach with V₃ division, or subtemporal–infratemporal + basal frontal approach
Lower clivus	+ Jugular foramen, condyle	Extreme lateral, transjugular, and transcondyle approach with/without subtemporal–infratemporal approach
Upper, middle, and lower clivus	Midline only	Basal frontal approach

[a] *Alternative approaches* (discussed in other chapters): transethmoidal approach, transnasal–transseptal approach, transmaxillary approach, facial translocation approach, transoral approach.

proach. When the neoplasm is confined to the midline only and involves the upper, middle, and lower clivus, it can be removed entirely through a basal frontal approach, which also allows removal of some of the petrous apices. When the lesion involves the lower clivus, jugular foramen, and the condyle area, the extreme lateral, transjugular, and transcondyle approach is optimal (Table 1).

SUBTEMPORAL, TRANSCAVERNOUS, AND TRANSPETROUS APEX APPROACH

This is an intradural approach suitable for lesions of the upper clivus, which arise from the upper clival bone and the petrous apex area on one side, with extension into the ipsilateral cavernous sinus. It is a modification of the transpetrous apex approach of Kawase et al. (11). The side selected for the approach will be the side on which the petrous apex or the cavernous sinus is involved by tumor. If there is no such involvement, the right side is selected. The critical anatomical structures that lie in the area include the temporal lobe, the brain stem, the basilar artery and its branches, the intracavernous and intrapetrous internal carotid artery, cranial nerves III, IV, V, and VI, the sphenoid sinus, and the pituitary gland. Another operative approach available to reach these tumors is the transseptal, transsphenoidal approach, but with this approach, the exposure is deep and narrow with little room to maneuver in case of trouble. The basal frontal approach can also be used for lesions of this area but the reach of this approach is limited superiorly by the pituitary gland and laterally by the petrous apices.

The patient is placed in the supine position with a roll under the shoulder to minimize neck stretch, and a spinal drain may be used if a considerable mass is not present in the tentorial notch. Neurophysiological monitoring of cranial nerves III, VI, and VII is employed. The patient's head is turned 60° away from the surgeon, slightly extended, and held in three-point pin fixation. A curvilinear incision is made starting in the temporal region curving inferiorly above the pinna of the ear and extending to the preauricular area. The skin flap is dissected along with the superficial layer of the temporal fascia. Below the level of the zygoma, dissection is performed in layers to preserve the superficial temporal artery and to get to the masseteric fascia. The periosteum is elevated from the zygomatic arch posteriorly to the external ear canal and anteriorly to the zygomaticomaxillary suture. The temporalis muscle is elevated from the temporal fossa. The deep layer of temporal fascia is detached anteriorly from the orbital rims and inferiorly from the zygomatic arch. A temporal craniotomy is performed, with its posterior extent just above the mastoid process (Fig. 3). The capsule of the temporomandibular

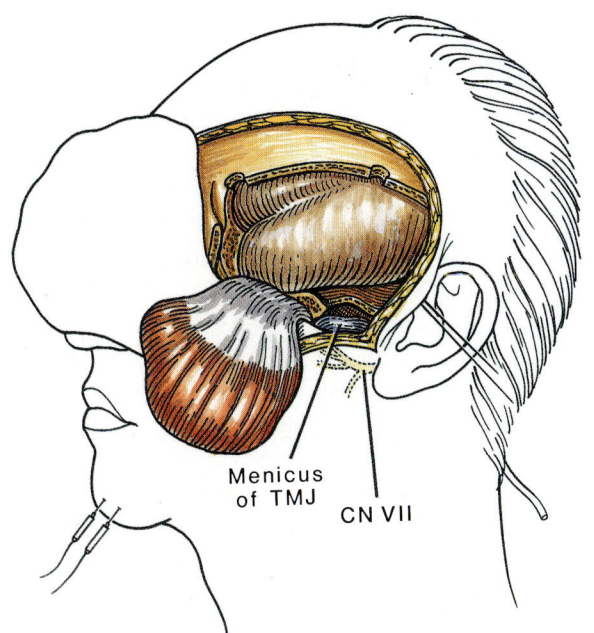

FIG. 3. The temporal craniotomy and zygomatic osteotomy for a subtemporal, transcavernous, and transpetrous apex approach are shown.

joint (TMJ) is opened and the meniscus is dissected from the condylar fossa and depressed. Extradural middle cranial fossa dissection is then performed from a lateral to medial, and from a posterior to an anterior direction to identify the following landmarks: the tegmen tympani, arcuate eminence, lesser superficial petrosal nerve (LSPN), greater superficial petrosal nerve (GSPN), middle meningeal artery, mandibular nerve (V_3), and the horizontal segment of the petrous internal carotid artery (if it is uncovered by bone). The GSPN may be distinguished from the LSPN by the fact that the LSPN nerve joins the middle meningeal artery at the foramen spinosum, and by electrical stimulation of the GSPN as far posteriorly as possible with the observation of resulting contraction of facial musculature on EMG. A zygomatic osteotomy is then performed including the condylar fossa posteriorly, and anteriorly just lateral to the orbit (Fig. 3). Posteriorly, the surgeon stays just lateral to the medial extent of the condylar fossa to avoid entry into the eustachian tube and into the petrous carotid canals. Care must also be exercised not to enter the middle ear cavity, which lies posterior to the TMJ.

The dura is opened and the temporal lobe is gently retracted after splitting the sylvian fissure widely, working with the aid of the surgical microscope (Fig. 4). The arachnoid membrane of the perimesencephalic cistern is opened, taking care not to injure the posterior cerebral or the superior cerebellar artery, which lie immediately under the arachnoid in this area. The fourth cranial nerve is identified and the tentorium is divided just posterior to the entrance of the fourth cranial nerve. The division of the tentorium is extended posterolaterally just posterior to the superior petrosal sinus. The trigeminal root is identified. The lateral wall of the cavernous sinus is peeled away from a posterior to an anterior direction, over the trigeminal ganglion and cranial nerves IV and V_1. If patent, some of the cavernous sinus is packed between cranial nerves IV and V, and the superior petrosal sinus will have to be packed with Surgicel anteriorly and posteriorly as it will be divided during this process. The dura is also opened all the way forward along the lower border of the trigeminal root, trigeminal ganglion, and V_3, and the lateral wall of Meckel's cave is opened completely. It may be essential to dissect the fourth cranial nerve in the lateral wall of the cavernous sinus and move it superiorly to allow the surgeon to work between cranial nerves IV and V in Parkinson's triangle. The surgeon may also work in the cavernous sinus between cranial nerves III and IV and between rootlets of cranial nerve V in Meckel's cave. The tumor in the prepeduncular area is usually extradural and the clival dura will have to be opened to allow adequate tumor resection. Occasionally, tumor may also be in the subdural space, intimately intertwined with the branches of the basilar ar-

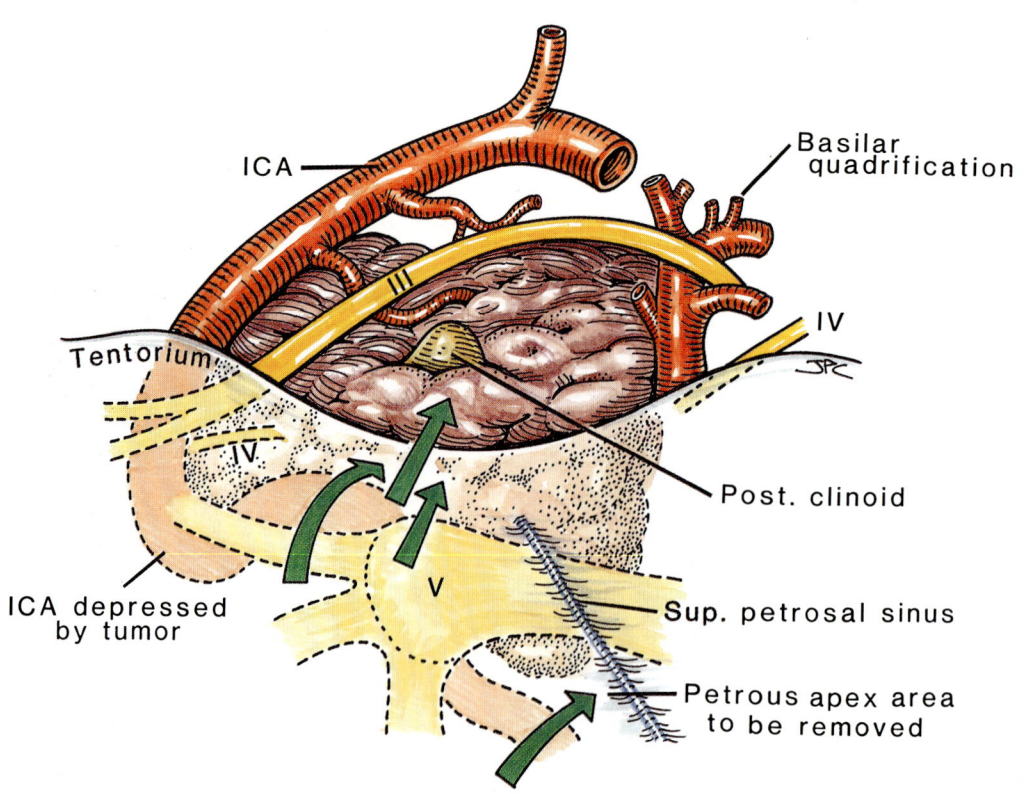

FIG. 4. The important anatomical structures encountered during the subtemporal, transcavernous, and transpetrous apex approach are shown. Also seen is the tumor. The arrows show the different approaches to the tumor.

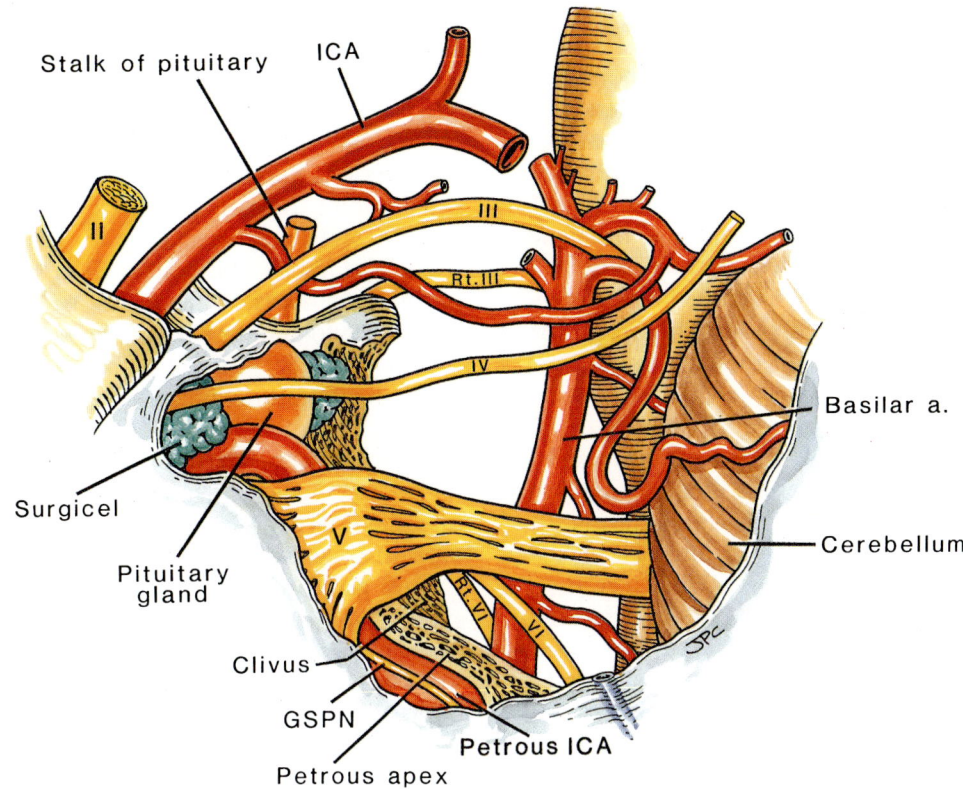

FIG. 5. The tumor has been removed. The tentorium has been divided and the cavernous sinus opened to remove the tumor. The petrous apex and the clival origin of the tumor have been drilled away.

tery, and these will have to be dissected with great care. The petrous apex bone is removed with a high-speed drill, lateral to the trigeminal root and the ganglion, *working intradurally*. The lateral border of the removal of the petrous apex is the horizontal segment of the petrous internal carotid artery. It is easier to do this intradurally rather than extradurally since the surgeon is not limited by the temporal dura. The sixth cranial nerve will be identified just medial to the trigeminal root and can be followed into the cavernous sinus at this time and care has to be taken not to damage it. The surgeon has to remove all the bone of the dorsum sellae, both posterior clinoids and the floor of the sella turcica, and any of the involved sphenoid and petrous apex bone (Fig. 5).

Reconstruction

Autologous fat obtained from the thigh or the abdomen is packed through the holes in the dura. A fascia lata graft is then laid over the openings in the dura and anchored with a few sutures circumferentially. Autologous fibrin glue may be employed to close the openings further. If the sphenoid sinus is opened by this operation, it is better to widen the opening to remove the mucosa, and pack it with autologous fat, before the fascial repair.

A wider opening in the sphenoid sinus may necessitate the application of a pericranial flap by a subfrontal approach (10,24).

If there is any question of tumor remnant in the petroclival bone or in the sphenoid bone, an anterior approach, either transnasal–transseptal or a basal frontal, is needed in a separate operation to complete the tumor resection.

SUBTEMPORAL AND INFRATEMPORAL APPROACH

The subtemporal and preauricular infratemporal approach was first described in 1987 (17–19). It was developed as a modification of the middle fossa extradural approach and the infratemporal approach (5,6). More recently, the approach has been successfully combined with a basal frontal approach and the extreme lateral transcondylar, transjugular approach to treat cranial base lesions (16,20,21). The application of this approach to intradural lesions has also been described (23). Approximately 150 operations have been performed in our institution using the subtemporal–infratemporal approach. Many variations of this approach are currently being described in the literature for smaller lesions, which usually involve a zygomatic osteotomy, and less clival bone resection (12,26).

This approach is particularly suited for lesions that involve the petrous apex and midclival area, reaching just beyond the midline, with minimal to moderate invasion of the sphenoid sinus. When V_3 is divided, this approach can be extended to lesions of the lower clivus, sphenoid, the opposite petrous apex, and the ipsilateral lower cavernous sinus. It is also useful for tumors involving the infratemporal and pterygopalatine fossae, for lesions of the nasopharynx extending into this area, such as juvenile angiofibromas, and for the excision of some intradural midclival lesions.

A spinal drain is used if the procedure is purely extradural. However, if the drain does not work adequately, an intradural opening of the cisterns will be necessary to relax the brain further. The patient is placed during the operation in the supine position, with the head turned 45°–60° to the opposite side, extended, and placed either in pins or a horseshoe head rest. If it is anticipated that the patient's head position will need to be changed during the operation, the endotracheal tube should be attached to the teeth of the lower jaw by means of fine stainless steel wire passed interdentally.

The skin incision can be bicoronal with extension into the preauricular area or it can be curvilinear in the temporal region with a preauricular parotidectomy type of extension (Fig. 6). Above the superior temporal line, the incision is extended through the pericranium to the bone. Below the superior temporal line, the pericranium blends with the superficial layer of the temporal fascia. Dissection is performed between the superficial and deep layers of temporal fascia, the deep layer being the shiny layer. Fatty tissues are often found on either side of the deep layer of temporal fascia and are not reliable landmarks. The lateral orbital rim and the zygomatic arch are denuded of periosteum anteriorly to the zygomaticomaxillary suture and posteriorly to the external ear canal. Below the zygomatic arch, the incision and dissection are kept very close to the ear to about the level of the earlobe. Dissection is performed in line with the incision in a layer by layer fashion, carefully preserving the superficial temporal artery and getting quickly down to the masseteric fascia and the capsule of the temporomandibular joint. Anteriorly, the facial tissues are dissected away, keeping the dissection plane just superficial to the masseteric fascia. This will avoid injury to the branches of the facial nerve, which travel in the substance of the parotid gland and then in the superficial fascia and fatty tissues of the face (Fig. 7).

If a parotidectomy type of incision is used and further mobilization of the mandible is anticipated, the extratemporal facial nerve should be located. The landmarks for finding the facial nerve are the tympanomastoid suture, the external ear canal cartilage ("the pointer"), and the digastric muscle. The facial nerve is followed into the parotid gland, where it branches into two major divisions. The distal branches, especially the upper ones, may be traced forward (Fig. 8).

The deep layer of the temporal fascia is divided along the orbital rim and the upper border of the zygomatic arch, and the entire temporalis muscle is elevated from the temporal fossa, taking care not to enter the external ear canal posteroinferiorly. The masseteric fascia and muscle are also detached from the zygomatic arch. A temporal craniotomy is performed. The posterior extent of the craniotomy will depend on how much clival tumor is present and usually is just above the mastoid process. It is preferable to do the craniotomy first before performing the zygomatic osteotomy. Following the reverse sequence resulted in the craniotome slipping into the orbit on one occasion, since the orbital tissues were not being protected by the curving lateral bony wall of the orbit.

An extradural middle cranial fossa dissection is performed as detailed previously. A zygomatic osteotomy is

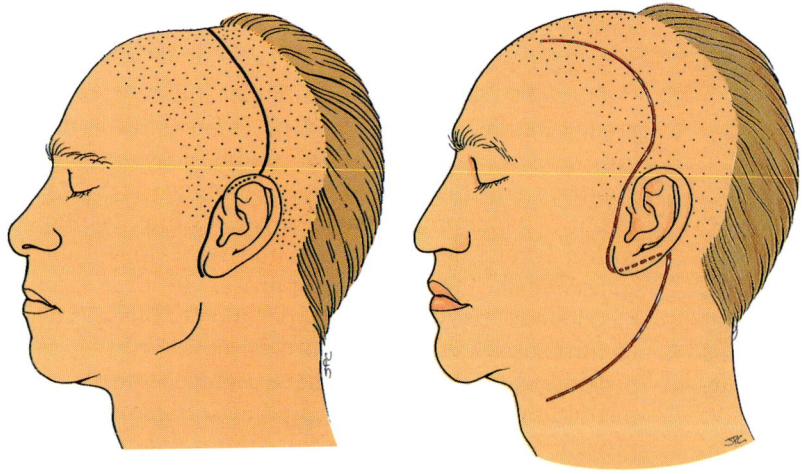

FIG. 6. The two types of skin incision for the subtemporal–infratemporal approach are shown. **A:** The bicoronal incision with extension into the preauricular area is preferred. **B:** However, if neck dissection is desired for tumor removal, or for cervical ICA control, a preauricular and cervical extension may be employed as shown.

A,B

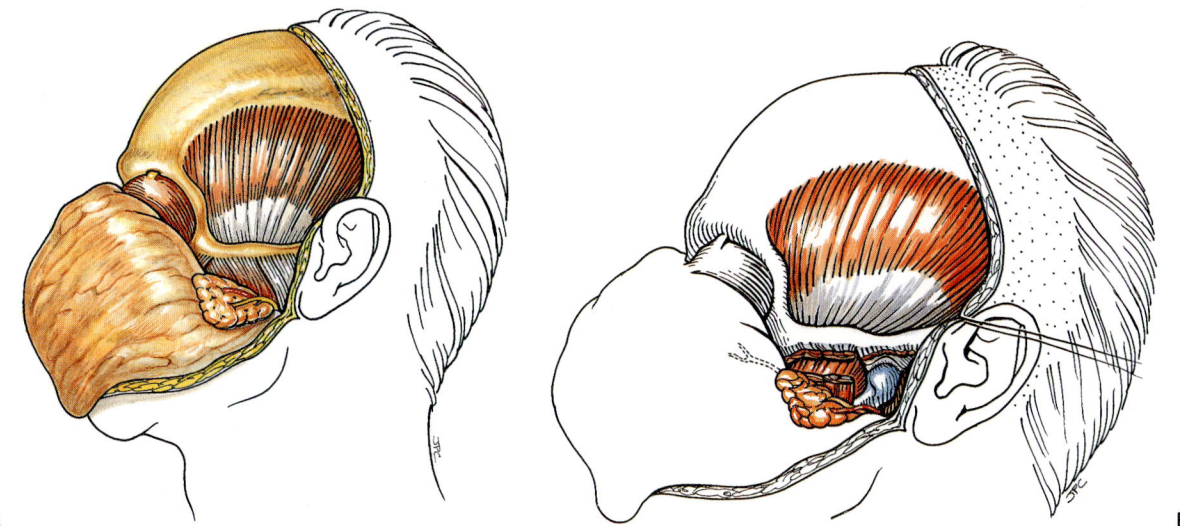

FIG. 7. Subtemporal and infratemporal approach, bicoronal incision. **A:** The exposure after the reflection of the scalp, and the facial tissues is seen here. **B:** The division of the masseter muscle from the zygomatic arch, and the opening of the temporomandibular joint.

then performed either including or excluding the condylar fossa. If more posterior room is needed or if the condyle is to be resected, it is better to include the condylar fossa. This provides a better exposure and also will be better if prosthetic replacement of the TMJ is elected at a later time (Fig. 9). The temporomandibular joint capsule is opened and the meniscus is dissected from the mandibular fossa and depressed.

In order to resect the condyle of the mandible, the attachments of the pterygoid muscles are divided. The soft tissues are dissected and the condyle is divided at the neck, with the help of a reciprocating saw or Midas Rex instrumentation, and removed. The remaining soft tissues of the condylar fossa are excised, taking care not to injure the external ear canal posteriorly. The styloid process is a good landmark in the infratemporal fossa and

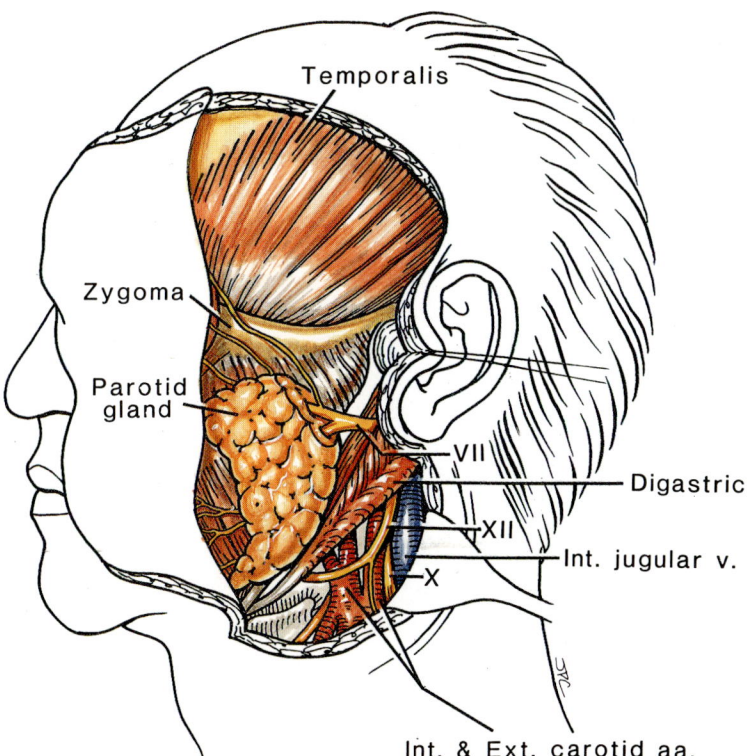

FIG. 8. Subtemporal and infratemporal approach. Exposure after a temporal, and preauricular–cervical incision. The facial nerve and its upper branches have been dissected and mobilized from the underlying masseteric fascia. The upper cervical vessels and the cranial nerves have been exposed.

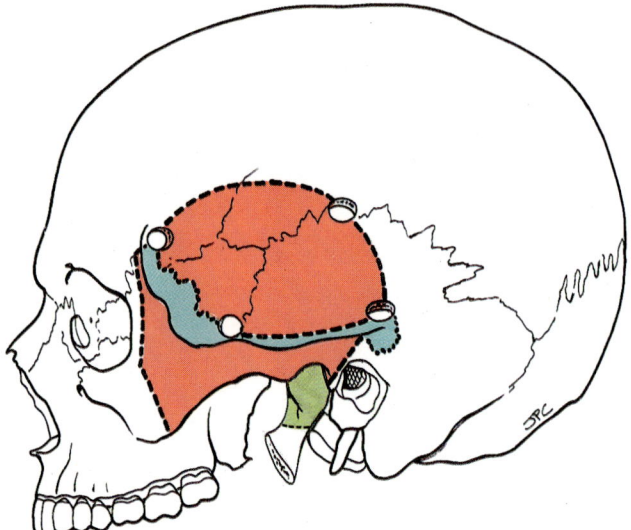

FIG. 9. A temporal craniotomy and zygomatic osteotomy are shown. If only a limited exposure of the petroclival area is required, or if the mandibular condyle is not being resected, the posterior osteotomy cut is made in front of the condylar fossa.

the surgeon should not go to a deeper plane at this point. The zygomatic osteotomy can also be performed after the condyle resection.

The next step is to identify and expose the petrous and the upper cervical internal carotid artery. It is best to start in an area where the artery is not involved by tumor. In order to find the horizontal segment of the petrous ICA, the GSPN is located again and divided. The middle meningeal artery is coagulated and divided. The remaining bone of the greater wing of the sphenoid is removed in order to completely unroof V_2 and V_3. The horizontal segment of the petrous ICA often lies partially exposed without any bony covering just posteromedial to V_3 and the middle meningeal artery, and inferior to the GSPN (Fig. 10). If it is not exposed, bone will have to be removed with the aid of high-speed drills and rongeurs to expose the artery in this area. In order to expose the genu of the petrous ICA, bone will have to be removed at the junction between the middle cranial fossa floor and the mandibular fossa. The surgeon will come across the tensor tympani muscle and eustachian tube (at the junction of the bony and cartilaginous portions) and the petrous ICA lies just medial to these structures (Fig. 11). Care must be taken not to injure the cochlea or the geniculate ganglion of the facial nerve, which lie immediately posterosuperior to the genu of the petrous ICA. The GSPN is a good landmark for these structures. The distance between the genu of the petrous ICA and the cochlea is variable and can be well appreciated on the preoperative bone-window CT scans. In order to identify the vertical segment of the petrous ICA, the tympanic bone lying medial to the temporomandibular joint is removed progressively with a high-speed drill, the last stage

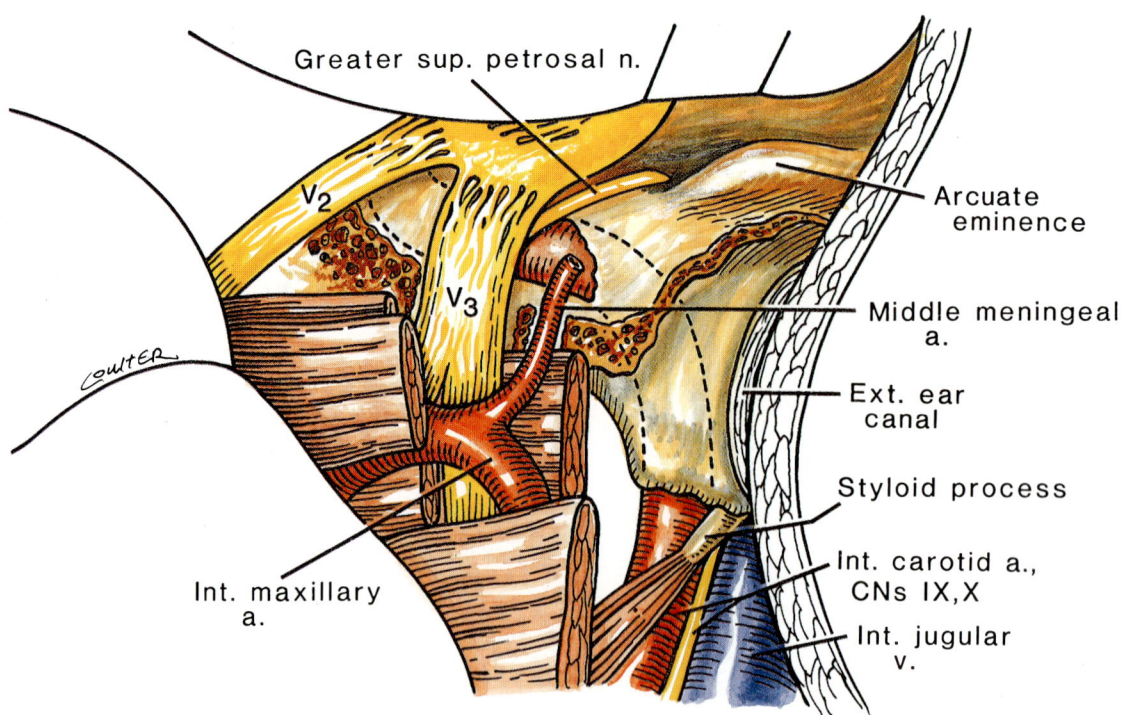

FIG. 10. The mandibular condyle has been resected. Extradural middle fossa dissection has been performed and a subtemporal resection of the greater wing of the sphenoid bone has been performed to unroof the maxillary nerve (V_2), the mandibular nerve (V_3), the middle meningeal artery, greater superficial petrosal nerve, and the arcuate eminence.

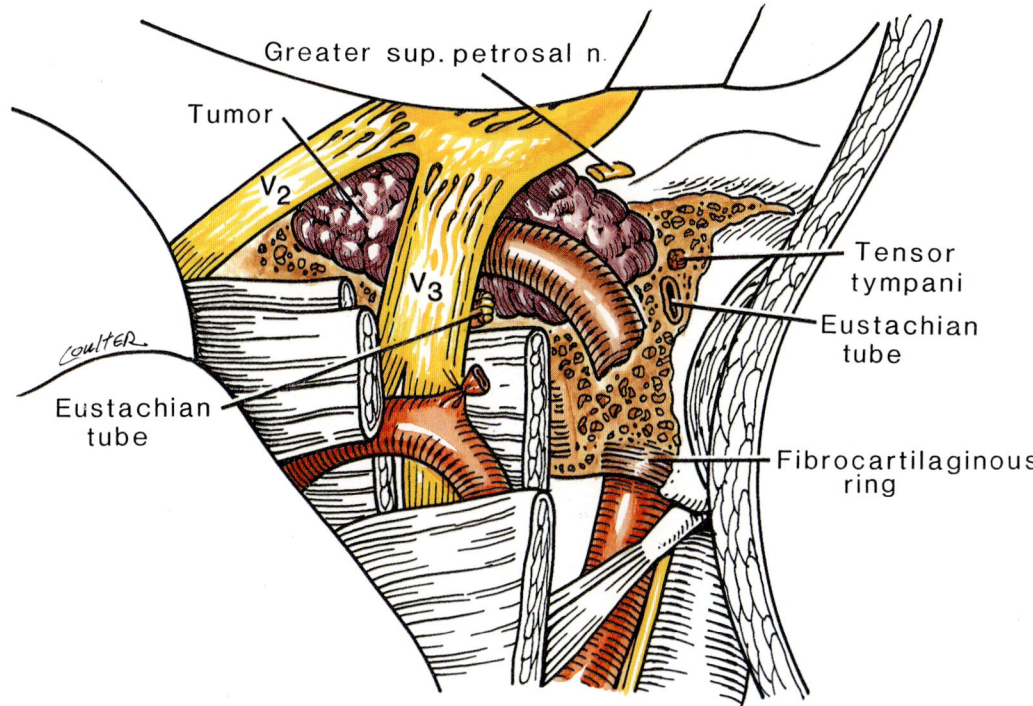

FIG. 11. In this drawing, the genu of the petrous ICA has been exposed, the tensor tympani and the eustachian tube have been divided, and the fibrocartilaginous ring at the entrance of the petrous ICA into the carotid canal is partly exposed. Some tumor is seen medial to the petrous ICA. The eustachian tube has been sutured shut.

of bone removal being completed with fine curettes and rongeurs. To find the upper cervical segment of the ICA, the lower border of the tympanic bone and the styloid process are identified by palpation. The styloid process is resected at its base and its inferior attachments to the stylohyoid and stylomandibular muscles and the stylomandibular ligament are divided. Dissection is performed through the soft tissues in this region to identify the upper cervical ICA.

Once the petrous ICA is identified in one area, the entire petrous ICA is progressively exposed and unroofed (Figs. 12–15). The petrous ICA has a covering of a venous plexus and then the periosteum of the carotid canal. The sympathetic nerve lies in the plane of the venous plexus. At the entrance to the carotid canal, there is a dense fibrocartilaginous ring to which the periosteal layer is firmly attached. The fibrocartilaginous ring will have to be opened and excised at least over half of the circumference and the attachment of the periosteal layer to it will have to be divided. The upper cervical ICA also has to be completely mobilized free of soft tissues around it. Superiorly, the bone medial to V_3 and lateral to the petrous ICA must be removed so that the artery can be mobilized to the point where it enters the cavernous sinus. Anterior to the vertical segment and the genu of the petrous ICA there are dense fibrocartilaginous tissues that have to be excised. The cartilaginous

eustachian tube is divided just medial to V_3. At this time, the lumen of the eustachian tube is cauterized, packed with either muscle or fat, and closed with two sutures of 4-0 Neurolon. The petrous ICA can now be mobilized forward and either gently retracted or sutured to the pterygoid muscles in a new position. However, the surgeon may have to work alternately in front or behind the petrous ICA (Fig. 16).

Immediately posterior to the vertical segment of the petrous ICA and the upper cervical ICA lie the jugular bulb and cranial nerves IX, X, and XI. The petrous apex bone medial to the petrous ICA is progressively drilled away, taking care not to damage the cochlea, the facial nerve, or the semicircular canals. In the normal situation, the change from the petrous to the clival bone is indicated by a sudden change in the denseness of the bone, the clival bone being cancellous. The midclival and petrous apex dura can be completely exposed. The surgeon can enter the inferior aspect of the cavernous sinus following the petrous ICA. Anteriorly, the surgeon can work between V_2 and V_3 going through the base of the pterygoid process, which allows entry into the sphenoid sinus laterally. Superior to V_2 and between V_2 and V_1 the removal of the sphenoid bone will also allow entry into the sphenoid sinus. The surgeon can also follow V_1 and V_2 posteriorly into the region of the cavernous sinus. Medial to the vertical segment of the petrous ICA, pro-

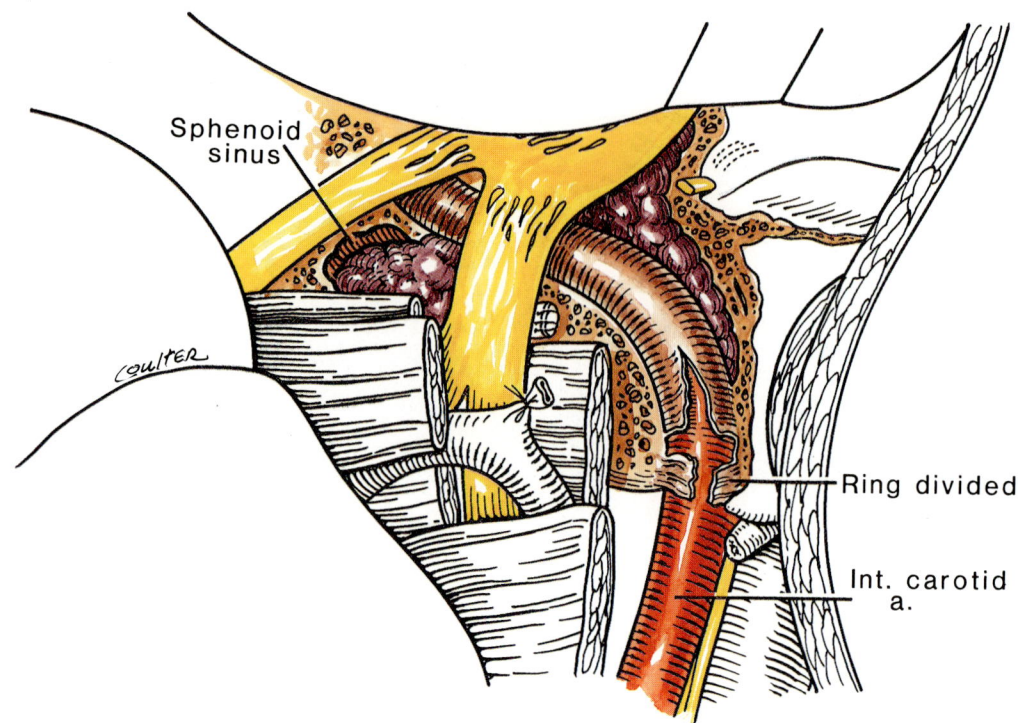

FIG. 12. The entire petrous ICA and the upper cervical ICA have been dissected from the fibrocartilaginous ring. The base of the pterygoid process has been removed between V_2 and V_3 to enter the sphenoid sinus.

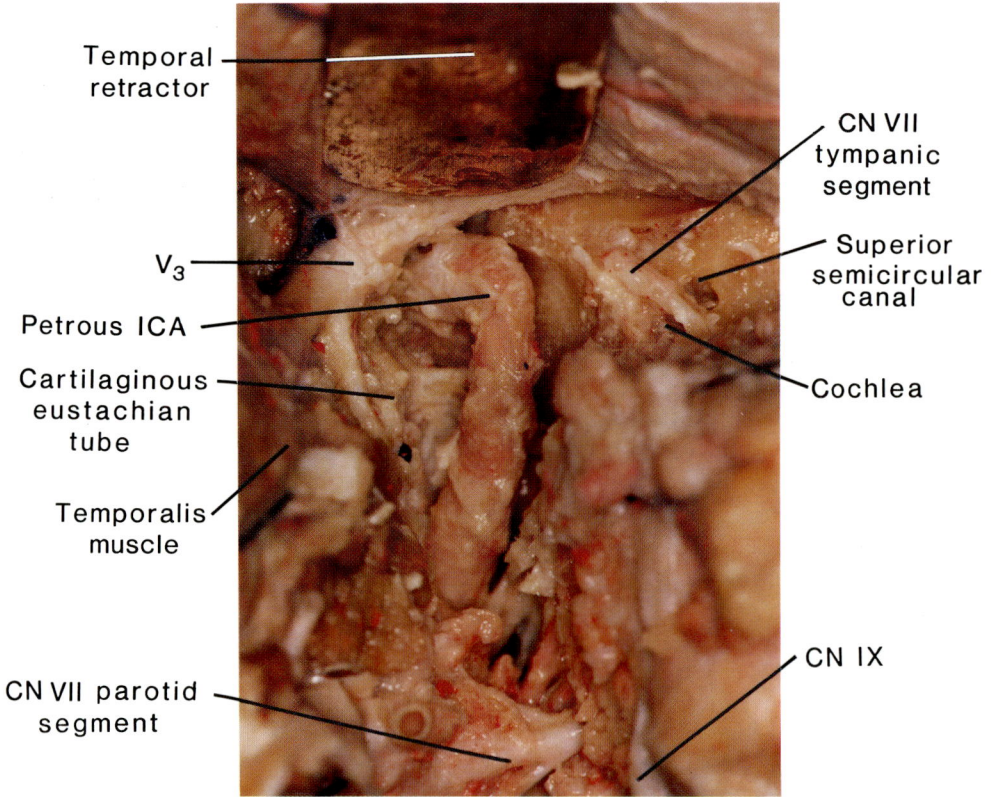

FIG. 13. Cadaver dissection showing the exposure of the entire petrous ICA. The facial nerve and cochlea have been opened to show their relationship.

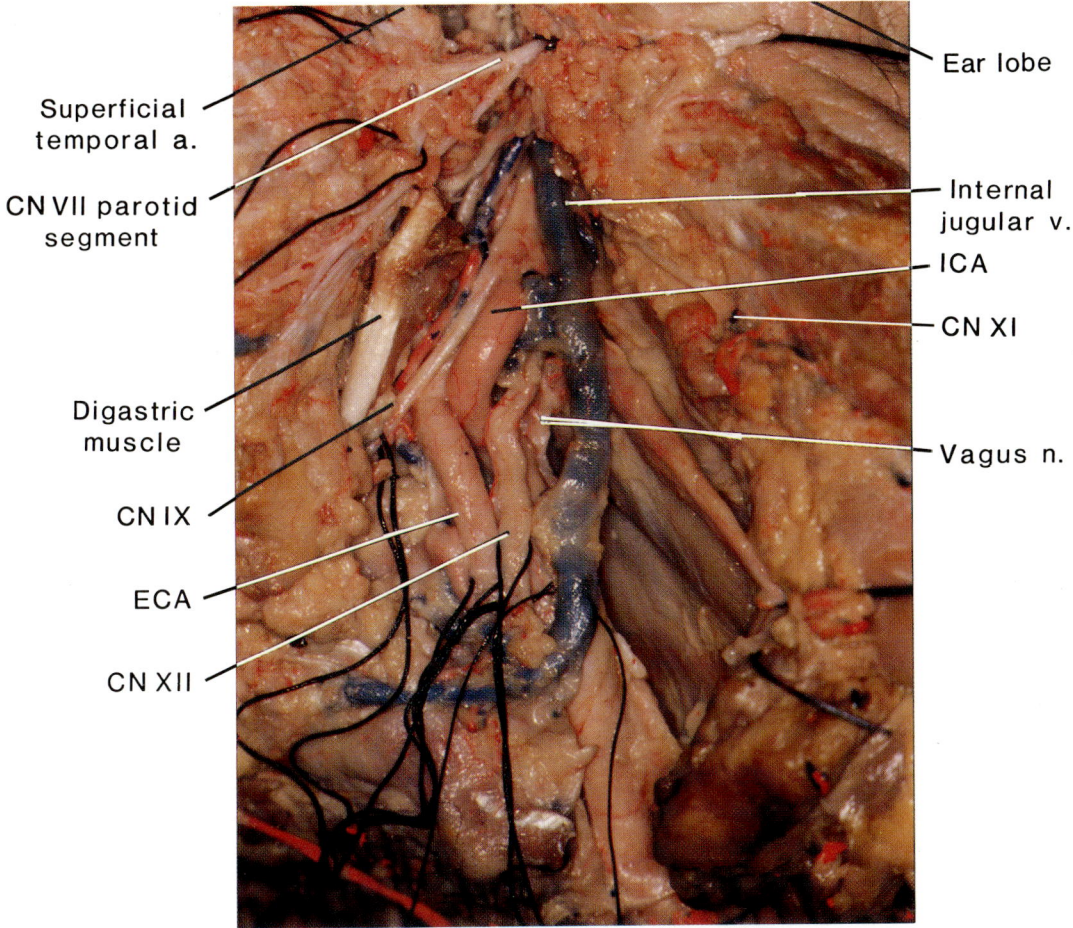

FIG. 14. This photograph shows the anatomy of the neurovascular structures in the upper cervical area.

gressive removal of the bone will allow the unroofing of the hypoglossal nerve in its canal extradurally and also the removal of the anterior two-thirds of the occipital condyle. If tumor extends into the jugular bulb and there is good communication between the two transverse sinuses across the torcula, the surgeon can enter the jugular bulb posterior to the vertical segment of the petrous ICA and remove tumor, packing off any venous bleeding by means of rolls of Surgicel.

Division of V_3

In order to further extend the exposure by the subtemporal–infratemporal approach, V_3 has to be divided at its exit through the foramen ovale. The temporal lobe can now be further retracted and the petrous ICA can be further mobilized into the cavernous sinus. It can be retracted upward with the temporal lobe, as needed. The surgeon can work anterior, posterior, or inferior to the petrous ICA, reaching across the clivus, all the way to the opposite petrous ICA canal. However, there is no definite landmark for identifying the opposite petrous ICA and great caution has to be taken to avoid its injury. Tumor extension within the sphenoid sinus can also be removed more easily after the division of V_3 (Figs. 17 and 18).

Reconstruction

At the conclusion of the tumor resection, any holes in the dura are closed primarily or patched with fascia lata grafts. The ends of V_3 are anastomosed by means of epineural sutures. If there is not an extensive opening into the nasopharynx, and if the temporalis muscle has a normal bulk and vascularity, reconstruction can be performed by the use of a temporalis muscle flap and autologous fat. The temporalis muscle is split into two halves and packed into the cavity of the tumor both anterior and posterior to V_3. Autologous fat is used to fill any remaining dead space. The posterior opening of the divided eustachian tube into the middle ear must be closed either by means of the temporalis muscle or the fat. The

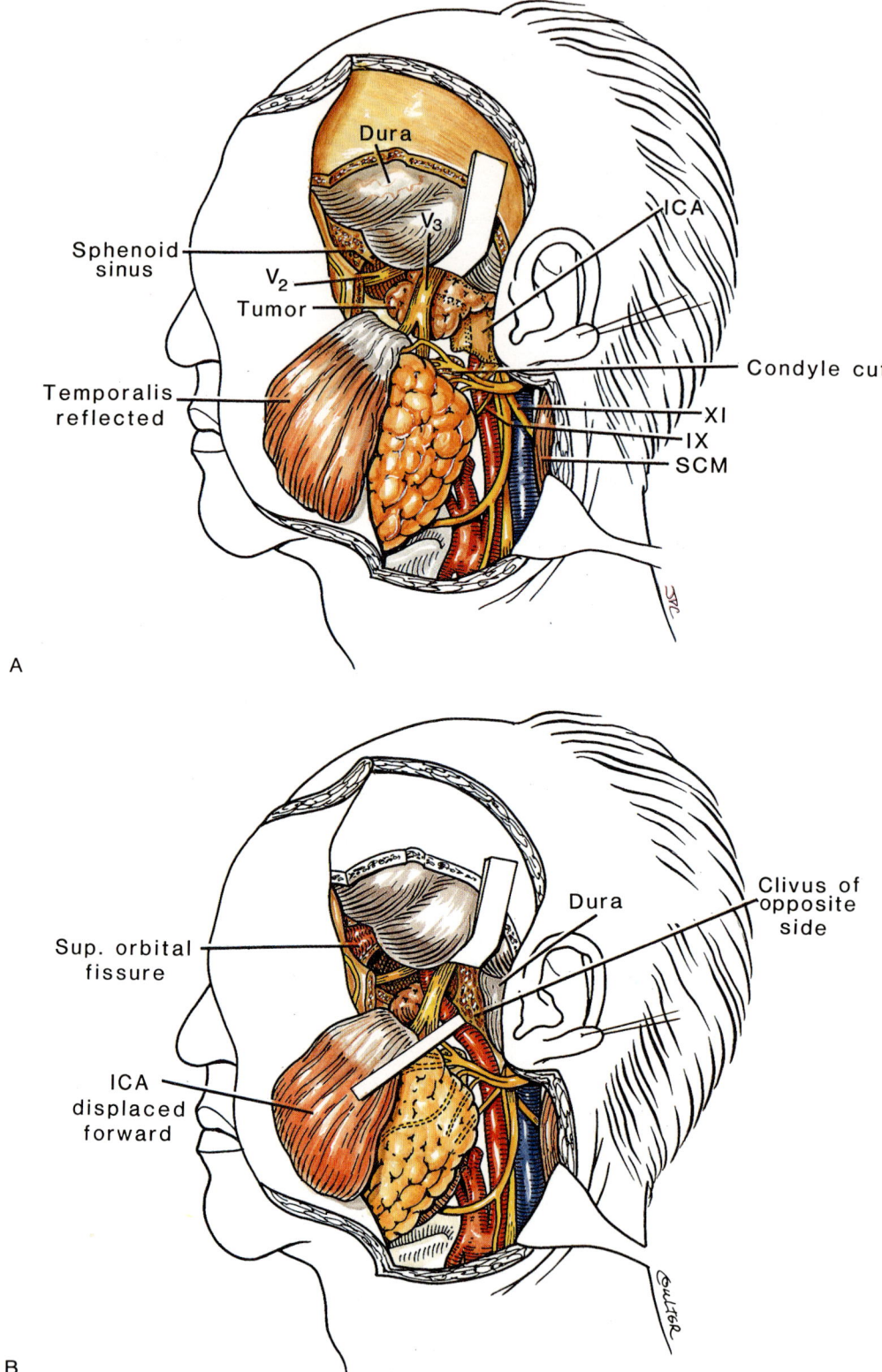

FIG. 15. A: The exposure obtained where a subtemporal–infratemporal approach is combined with an upper cervical dissection. Since the upper portion of the petrous ICA is involved by tumor, dissection will be started in the vertical petrous segment or the upper cervical ICA. **B:** The petrous ICA has been mobilized forward with petroclival dura exposed.

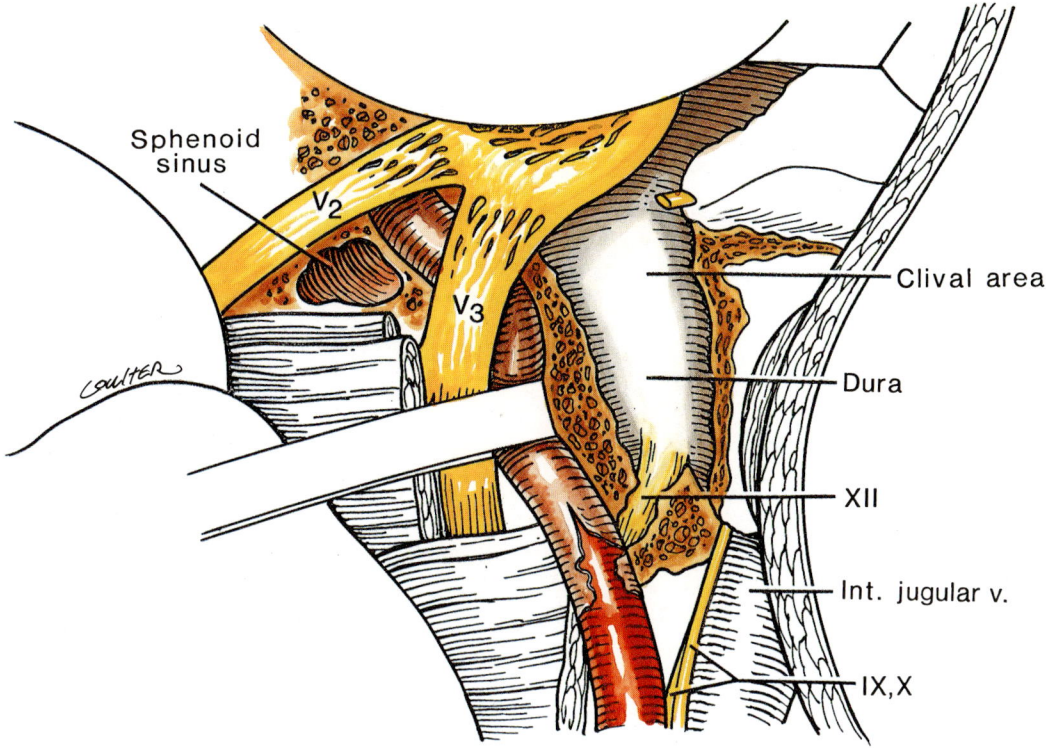

FIG. 16. The petrous and upper cervical ICA has been mobilized forward and the tumor has been removed. The petroclival dura is exposed. Note the hypoglossal nerve in its extradural canal.

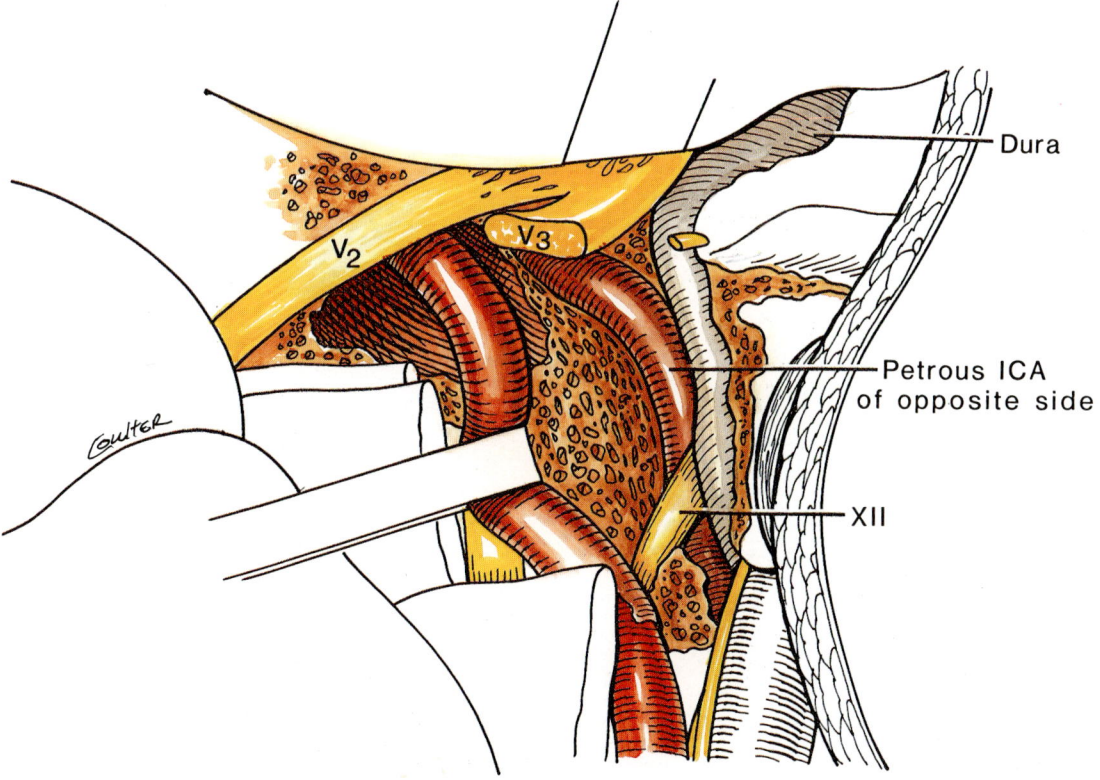

FIG. 17. V₃ has been divided and retracted upward. The ipsilateral petrous ICA has been completely mobilized. Most of the midclival and lower clival bone has been removed, and the contralateral petrous ICA is exposed. Caution has to be exercised here since there are no good landmarks to indicate the contralateral petrous ICA with this approach, as one removes the bone progressively.

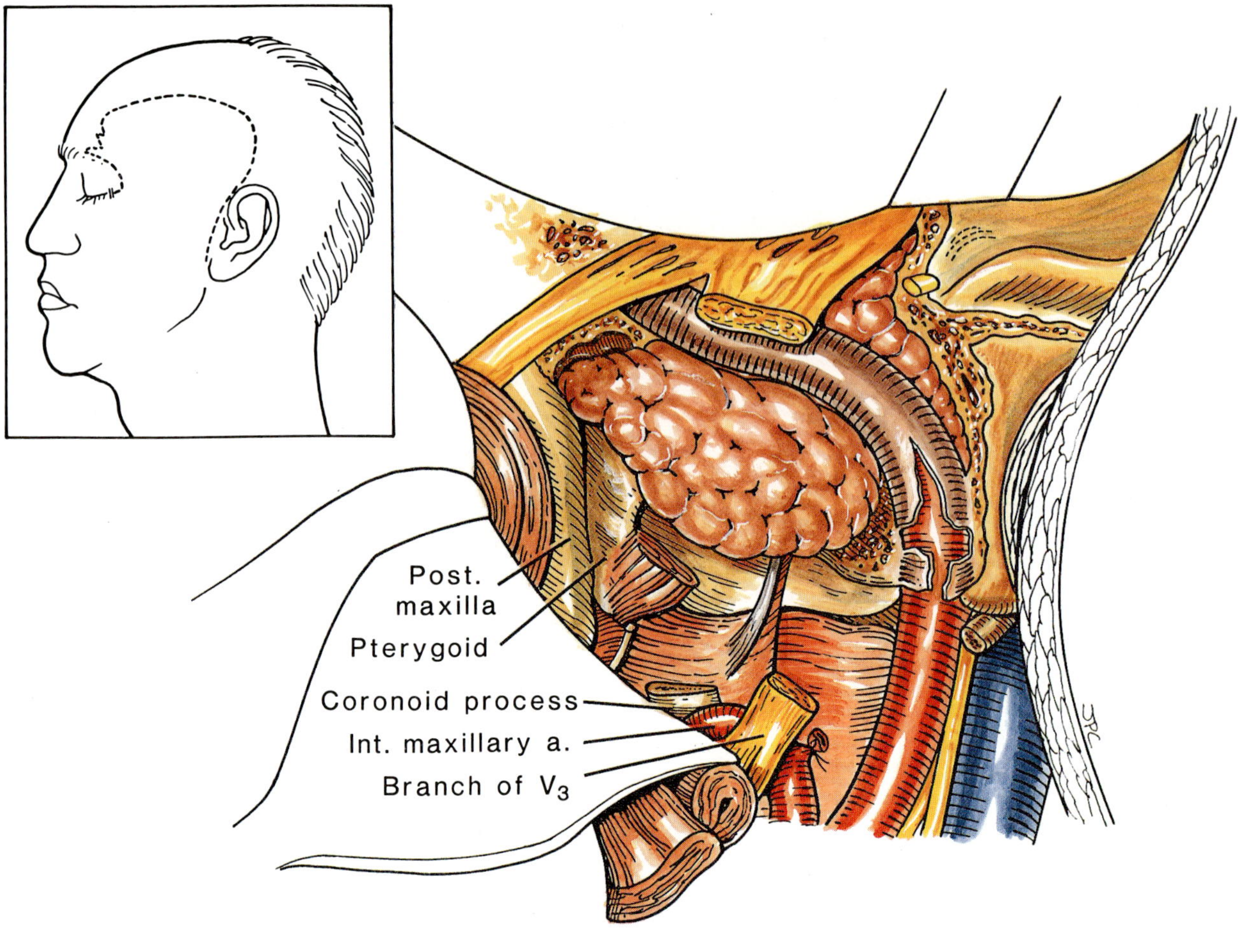

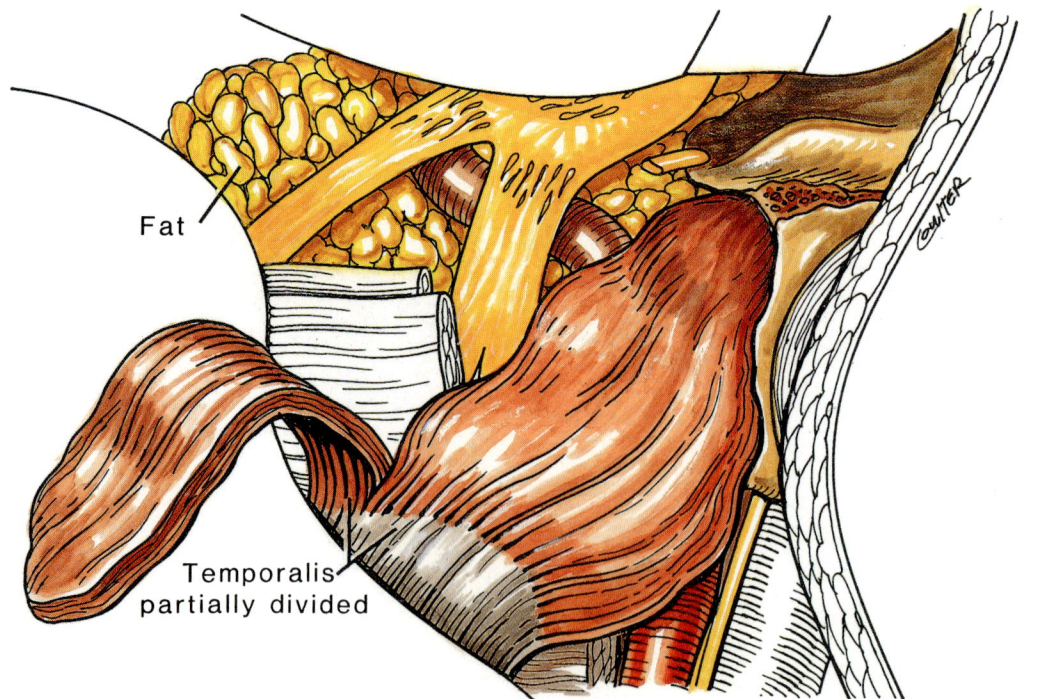

FIG. 18. This figure shows an anterior extension of the subtemporal and infratemporal approach. The approach allows a further exposure of the pterygoid fossa, and an approach through the maxillary sinus is also possible.

FIG. 19. Reconstruction has been accomplished with autologous fat and a temporalis muscle flap.

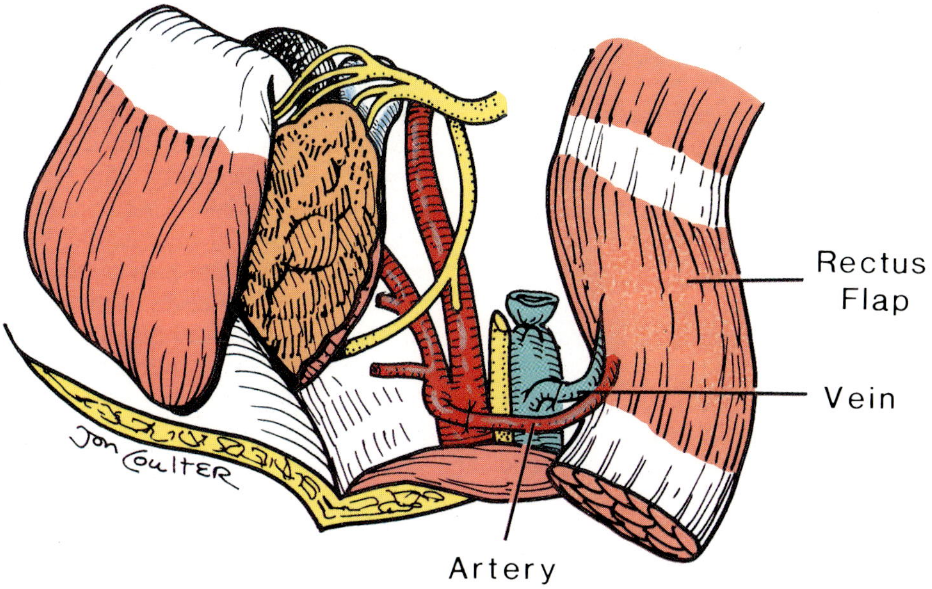

FIG. 20. A rectus abdominis microvascular flap has been connected by microanastomosis to the cervical vessels for the purpose of reconstruction.

petrous ICA must be covered, preferably by vascularized tissues (Fig. 19).

If the temporalis muscle is atrophic or avascular at the end of the operation, if there is a large dead space, or especially if the nasopharynx is open, reconstruction using a vascularized free flap may be necessary (10). The subtemporal–infratemporal approach allows the reconstruction using a rectus abdominis or latissimus dorsi free flap transferred by microvascular anastomosis to the area (Fig. 20). If the patient has a short neck, a pectoralis myocutaneous flap denuded of epithelium can be used for the reconstruction.

Disadvantages

The disadvantages of a full-fledged subtemporal and infratemporal approach include the loss of one eustachian tube and the temporomandibular joint. There is also a possibility of injury to the petrous ICA and to cranial nerves VI–XII. The potential for CSF leakage through the sphenoid sinus or the eustachian tube exists if the dura is opened, but this complication is more easily managed than when it occurs following an anterior approach.

EXTENDED FRONTAL APPROACH

The extended frontal approach (or the basal frontal approach) is a modification of the transbasal approach of Derome, with the addition of a orbito-fronto-ethmoidal osteotomy (4,8,16,20). The osteotomies minimize brain retraction (Fig. 21).

Midline tumors involving the clivus and the sphenoid sinus extending from the base of the dorsum sellae to the foramen magnum, with some involvement of the petrous apices, can be removed by this approach. The major sequel to this approach is the complete loss of olfaction and the resultant loss of some taste sensation. This approach is limited laterally by the optic nerves, the cavernous and petrous and internal carotid arteries, and the

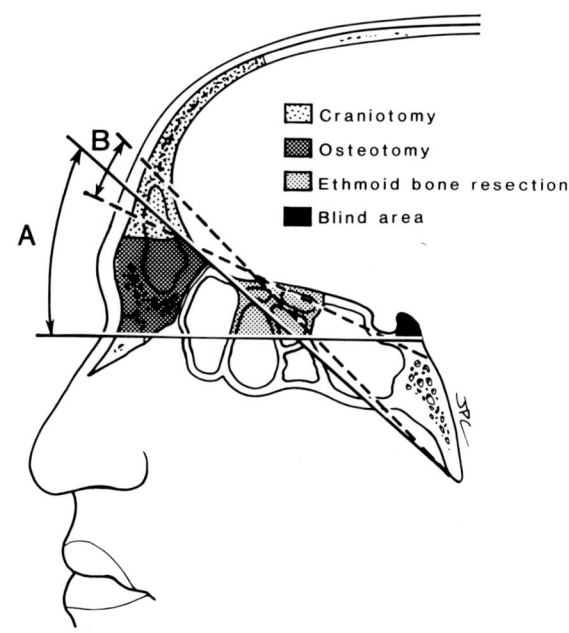

FIG. 21. Extended frontal approach. This figure illustrates how the orbito-fronto-ethmoidal osteotomy allows the surgeon to reach lower in the clivus while minimizing brain retraction.

hypoglossal nerves. The lowest possible reach of this approach is down to C1, although it becomes restricted at and below the foramen magnum.

A major advantage of this approach is that the upper aerodigestive tract is not violated significantly, and the air sinuses can be occluded at the end of the operation by a pericranial or a galeofrontalis flap and autologous fat. The sphenoid and ethmoid sinuses are opened but these structures are not normally colonized by virulent bacterial organisms unless they have previously been communicated by means of an ethmoidectomy or a maxillectomy to the oronasal cavities.

To perform this operative approach, the patient is placed in the supine position, with the head resting on a horseshoe rest or in pins. The two pins of the Mayfield clamp should be turned to the vertical position and placed just behind the ear. A bicoronal skin incision is made starting just in front of the ear, extending vertically up to the opposite side. The incisions can be curved forward slightly near the zygomatic arches if necessary, but care must be taken not to interrupt the superficial temporal arteries or the frontal branches of the facial nerves. The incision is taken down to the bone and the pericranium is divided along the line of the skin incision. However, if a longer pericranial flap is desired, the pericranium can be dissected from the skin flap posteriorly and divided approximately 3–4 cm behind the line of the skin incision. The superficial temporal fascia is dissected from the deep layer and reflected forward along with the skin flap and dissection is performed to expose the superior orbital rims bilaterally, and in the midline down to the frontonasal suture. The supraorbital nerves and vessels can usually be dissected from the supraorbital notch; however, if in a foramen, they may have to be liberated by notching the foramen, either with an osteotome and mallet, or by the use of a reciprocating saw. The periorbita is dissected from the superior walls of the orbit at least 3 cm posterior to the supraorbital ridges. The periorbita is also dissected from the lateral wall of the orbit and the upper medial walls of the orbit down to the level of the lacrimal sacs bilaterally.

A unilateral frontal craniotomy is then carried out, extending 6 cm up from the nasion and just to the edge of the superior sagittal sinus at the midline. This craniotomy often results in dural tears in older individuals with hyperostosis frontalis interna. The superior sagittal sinus is then separated under direct vision from the midfrontal bone and an additional frontal craniotomy is then carried out on the contralateral side, extending to the junction of the middle third and lateral third of the superior rim of the orbit. This technique of making the craniotomy in two pieces avoids injuries to the superior sagittal sinus. Both craniotomies must be cut as low as possible and will include the upper portions of the frontal sinuses. The frontal sinus mucosa is exenterated at this time or later.

Cerebrospinal fluid is removed either via a previously inserted spinal drain or by opening the chiasmatic cisterns to relax the brain. The subfrontal dura is then separated from the roofs of the orbit bilaterally on either side of the cribriform plates, back to the limits of the anterior cranial fossa posteriorly, and medially to include the planum sphenoidale. This is preferably done with the help of the surgical microscope. The dura is also separated from the crista galli in the midline, which is resected. The dural sleeves of the olfactory nerves passing through the cribriform plates are then divided as low as possible bilaterally. A dural and arachnoidal opening in this area is impossible to avoid, at least in places, and the dural openings should be closed watertight.

Orbito-fronto-ethmoidal Osteotomy

Self-retaining retractors are used for subfrontal retraction, taking care to keep the retraction to a minimum and to remove the retractors whenever they are not necessary during the procedure. The orbital osteotomy (Figs. 22 and 23) cuts are then made. It is easiest to start from the keyhole burr hole area on the ipsilateral frontal side. The orbit can easily be opened in this region and a coronal cut through the roof of the orbit on the ipsilateral side is made at least 2½ cm back from the supraorbital rim. This cut is then extended across the posterior aspect of cribriform plates of the ethmoid to the contralateral side as shown in the figure. A specially designed reciprocating saw blade or the Midas Rex angled attachment is useful in making these cuts. The cuts are preferably made from above down, protecting the subfrontal dura with self-

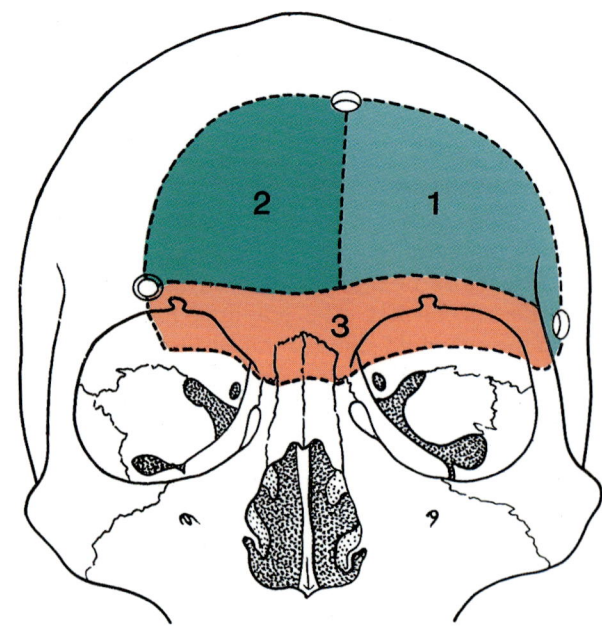

FIG. 22. Steps in the osseous exposure for the extended frontal approach. Steps 1 and 2 are craniotomies, and step 3 is the orbito-fronto-ethmoidal osteotomy.

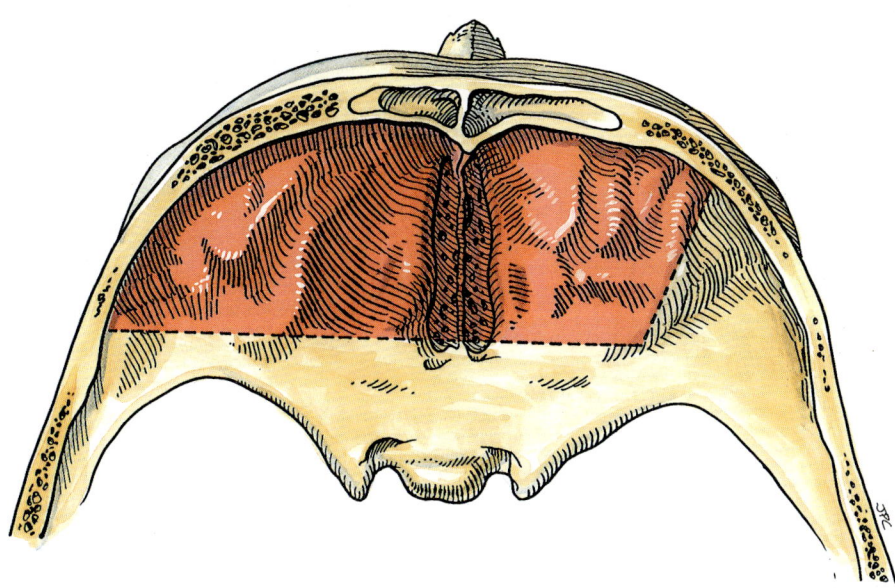

FIG. 23. Superior view illustrating the orbito-fronto-ethmoidal osteotomy. The coronal and sagittal cuts are shown.

retaining retractors and the periorbita with manual retraction. The coronal cut is then extended forward sagittally on the contralateral side to meet limits of the frontal craniotomy. Horizontal cuts are now made starting at or just below the frontonasal suture and extending posteriorly approximately 3 cm to meet the coronal cuts made from above. The horizontal cuts will extend approximately to the anterior ethmoidal foramen. Some bleeding is to be expected at this point because of the laceration of the mucosa of the upper nasal–ethmoidal area by the osteotomies. The orbito-fronto-ethmoidal osteotomy piece may have to be freed up with an osteotome and a mallet and removed.

Entry into the Sphenoid Sinus

Hemostasis is achieved by bipolar coagulation of the bleeding mucosa and the ethmoidal air cells are packed with rolls of Surgicel. Gentle subfrontal retraction is used for the remainder of the work, and generally a single retractor at or near the midline is adequate. The remainder of the planum sphenoidale is removed with the aid of rongeurs and a drill. The optic nerves are unroofed bilaterally or unilaterally (depending on the location of the tumor) on their superior, lateral, and medial aspects. However, no attempt is made to resect the anterior clinoid processes completely, since it is difficult from an extradural approach and unnecessary for this operation. More of the medial orbital wall can be removed just inferior to the optic nerves. The sphenoid septum and the mucosa are resected (Fig. 24).

Tumor Resection

The middle and posterior ethmoidal cells are resected, and as more of these cells are resected, the lower down the clivus the surgeon can reach, and more room becomes available to work (Fig. 21). The superior wall of the body of the sphenoid bone is now removed and the sellar dura is unroofed completely. The lateral walls of the body of the sphenoid bone are also removed in a progressive fashion from an anterior to a posterior direction. The anterior bend of the intracavernous carotid artery will usually be identified just inferior and posterior to the optic nerves. The cavernous sinuses have a thin dural covering on the medial aspect, which may be preserved if not involved by tumor, but when this dura is resected to remove tumor within or if its torn during bone removal, the cavernous sinus has to be packed with Surgicel as needed. The resection of the lateral wall of the sphenoid body is extended posteriorly until one can see the posterior vertical segment of the intracavernous carotid artery extending up from the petrous apex region. Posteriorly, the sphenoclival bone is removed progressively from above downward with the aid of a high-speed drill and rongeurs. The tumor in this region can be resected easily; however, the bone has to be removed at least 1 cm beyond tumor margins since the tumor often infiltrates through the bone beyond what is apparent microscopically. Bony resection margins should also conform to the tumor margins seen on MRI scans.

The clival dura is quite thick and is often easily separated from tumor. However, tumors may infiltrate the dura or may attenuate the dura considerably, especially in older individuals, and in such cases, the dura may have to be resected along with the tumor. Considerable venous bleeding may be encountered from the basilar venous plexus, which is controlled by packing with Surgicel. When the clival dura is resected, care has to be taken not to injure branches of the basilar artery or the brain stem. The petrous apices can be removed partially on either side. It is best to follow the posterior vertical

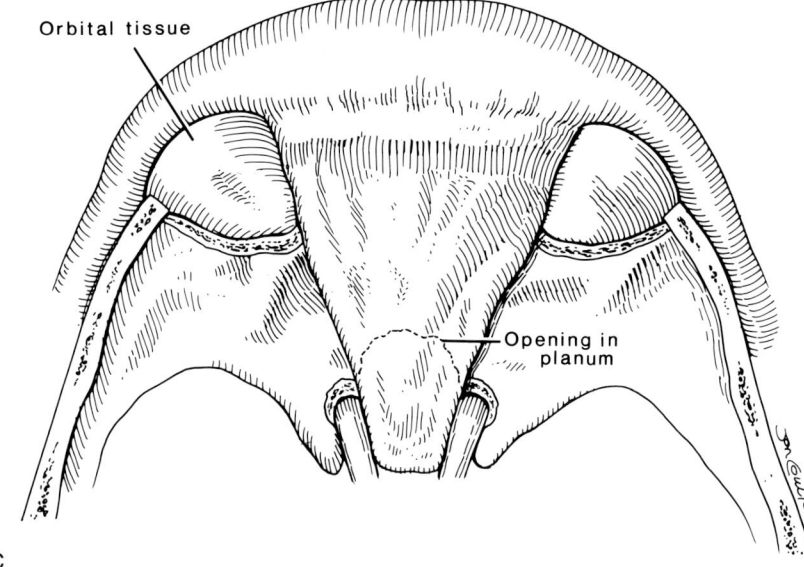

FIG. 24. A: The view obtained anteriorly after a fronto-orbital-ethmoidal osteotomy; optic nerve decompression (on the left) and sphenoidotomy are shown. **B, C:** The reconstruction after an extended frontal approach with a pericranial flap and autologous fat is shown.

segment of the cavernous carotid artery back all the way to the second bend of the petrous ICA into the cavernous sinus. However, it is not possible to expose the horizontal segment of the petrous ICA from this approach. If extensive involvement of the petrous apex is present, then the basal subfrontal approach has to be combined with a subtemporal–infratemporal approach to ensure complete tumor resection. In this region, the sixth cranial nerve can also be seen extradurally as it travels from the posterior fossa to enter Dorello's canal in the cavernous sinus. Great caution has to be exercised not to damage this segment of the nerve.

Inferiorly, the tumor resection can be extended down to the margins of the foramen magnum. Inferiorly and laterally, the resection can be extended to the hypoglossal foramina, but there is no definite way to identify the hypoglossal nerves from this approach. Injury to cranial nerve XII may be avoided by limiting the resection to bony structures only. The medial aspect of the occipital condyle can also be removed with this approach. Better exposure of cranial nerve XII and the occipital condyle generally requires the addition of the extreme lateral transcondylar approach.

The anterior wall of the body of the sphenoid bone can also be removed with this approach if there is concern about involvement by tumor, but care must be taken not to penetrate the nasopharyngeal mucosa or retropharyngeal tissues in doing this.

At the end of the tumor resection, the Surgicel packing must be removed sequentially to inspect and ensure the absence of any residual tumor. After this, some of the packing will have to be replaced to stop the venous bleeding but the amount of packing is kept to the minimum needed.

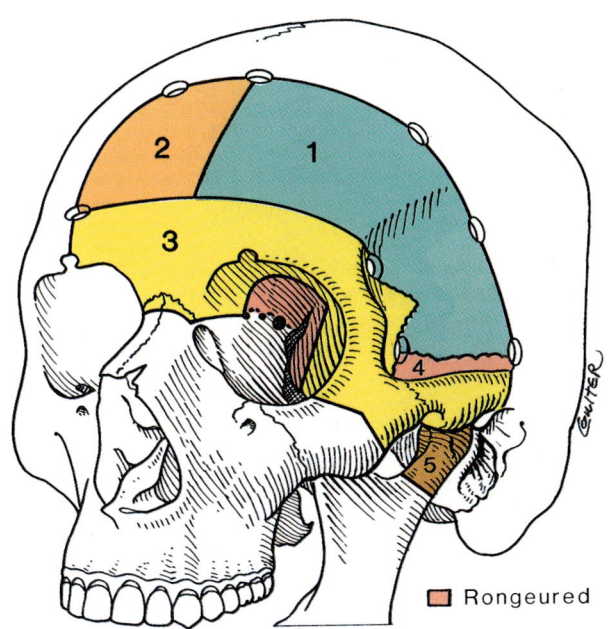

FIG. 25. Combined anterior and lateral approach. Craniotomy and orbital-zygomatic osteotomy are shown.

Reconstruction

Any holes in the clival dura are patched with fascia lata, which is anchored with a few sutures, generally not in a watertight fashion. The dural opening in the olfactory area should also be sutured or patched. A pericranial or a galeopericranial flap based on the supraorbital and supratrochlear vessels is then developed. The flap is brought into the cavity of the tumor inferior to the orbital osteotomy piece if a more posterior reach is needed, or superior to the orbital osteotomy piece if a limited posterior reach is adequate. Autologous fat extracted from the thigh or abdomen is packed into the sphenoidal area to lie within a pocket of the pericranial flap so that the flap lines the anterior, inferior, and posterior walls of the defect. If the flap is not long enough to enable this, the fat should be packed posterior to the flap to enable the flap to lie posteriorly, close to the clival dura. The surgeon must ensure that the fat does not compress the optic nerves. If the flap was brought inferior to the orbital rims, the surgeon usually has to excise a thin sliver of bone inferiorly to prevent compression of the flap and loss of vascularity when the bone is reapproximated.

The orbito-fronto-ethmoidal osteotomy piece is now anchored on either side to orbital rims by means of 2-0 Neurlon sutures. If the pericranial or galeopericranial flap was brought superior to the osteotomy piece, sutures can also be placed to anchor the osteotomy to the nasal bones. Dural tack up sutures are placed and tied. The craniotomy pieces are replaced. Closure of the scalp is then carried out with gravity drainage for about 2 days. The spinal drain is removed at the end of the operation.

Disadvantages

The main disadvantage of the basal subfrontal approach is the bilateral olfactory denervation, which can be initially troublesome to some patients, due to the associated change in taste. There is also a potential for injury to the frontal lobes and cranial nerves II and VI.

COMBINED ANTERIOR AND LATERAL APPROACH

The combination of the subtemporal–infratemporal and the extended frontal approach allows the resection of some very extensive clival tumors (16,20) (Fig. 25). The surgeon is afforded exposure both in the lateral and anterior aspects of the sphenoclival area, as shown in Figs. 26 and 27, and the division of V_3 is not needed. Both the subtemporal–infratemporal and basal frontal approaches need not be as extensive as discussed earlier but are modified to suite the tumor. At the end of the tumor resection, reconstruction can be performed with the help of a pericranial or galeopericranial flap, temporalis muscle, and fat (Fig. 28). Some patient examples are provided.

EXTREME LATERAL, TRANSCONDYLE, AND TRANSJUGULAR APPROACH

This approach, which has been used in our institution since 1985, has recently been published (21). The details of this approach are provided in the chapter by Sen and Sekhar. The extreme lateral, transcondyle, and transjugular approach is particularly suited for lesions that involve the lower clivus and extend into the occipital condyles and the jugular bulb on one side. Obviously, even if there is extension of the tumor into the jugular bulb, a good demonstration of crossover patency of venous drainage across the torcular Herophili is essential in order to occlude one sigmoid sinus. It is not usually possible to resect the jugular bulbs bilaterally. This approach is often used to complement the lower reach of the subtemporal–infratemporal approach, or of the basal frontal approach, and when residual tumor remains in the occipital condyle, in the jugular bulb area, or in the lower clivus region.

To perform the operation, the patient is placed in the lateral position with the lower arm hanging off the edge of the table and supported by means of padding on the horizontal bars of the Mayfield table attachment and an arm board (Sugita position). This position allows the patient to be operated for many hours without any risk of pressure sores or stretch injuries. An L-shaped incision is usually employed, but a C-shaped curvilinear incision can also be used. If a preauricular incision has previously been used, care must be taken to preserve the vascularity

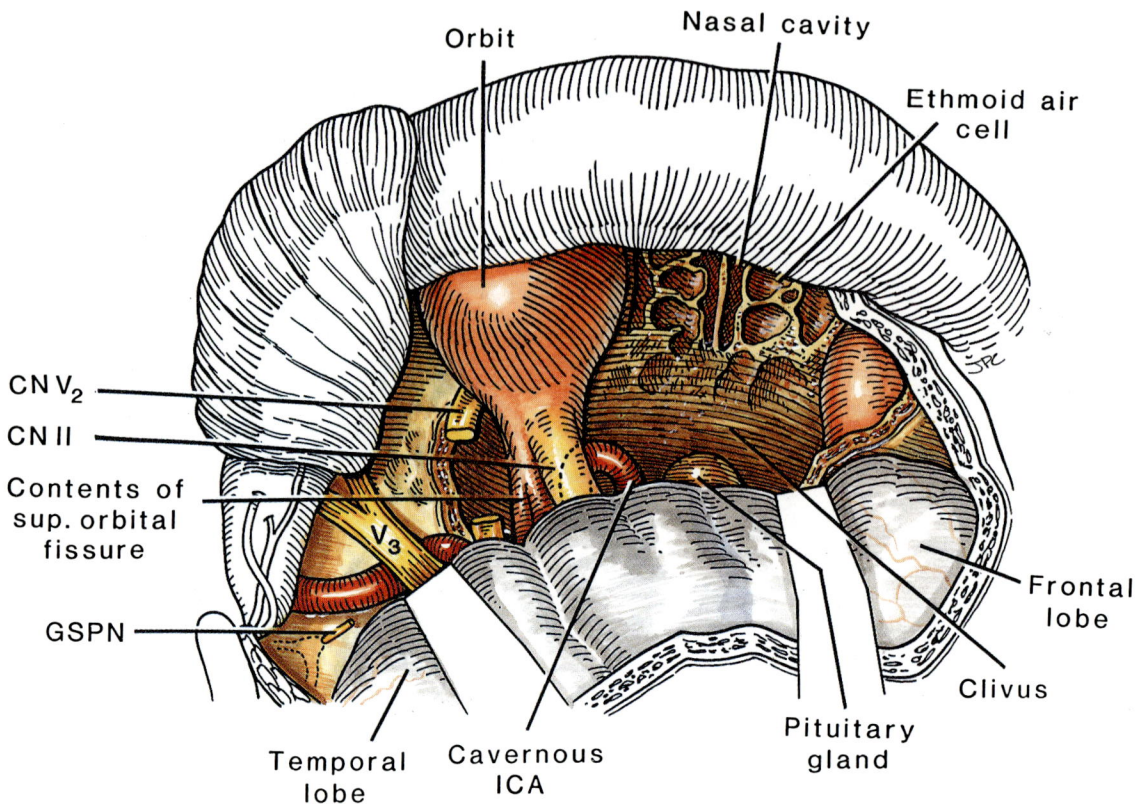

FIG. 26. Combined anterior and lateral approach. The exposure from the anterior aspect is shown.

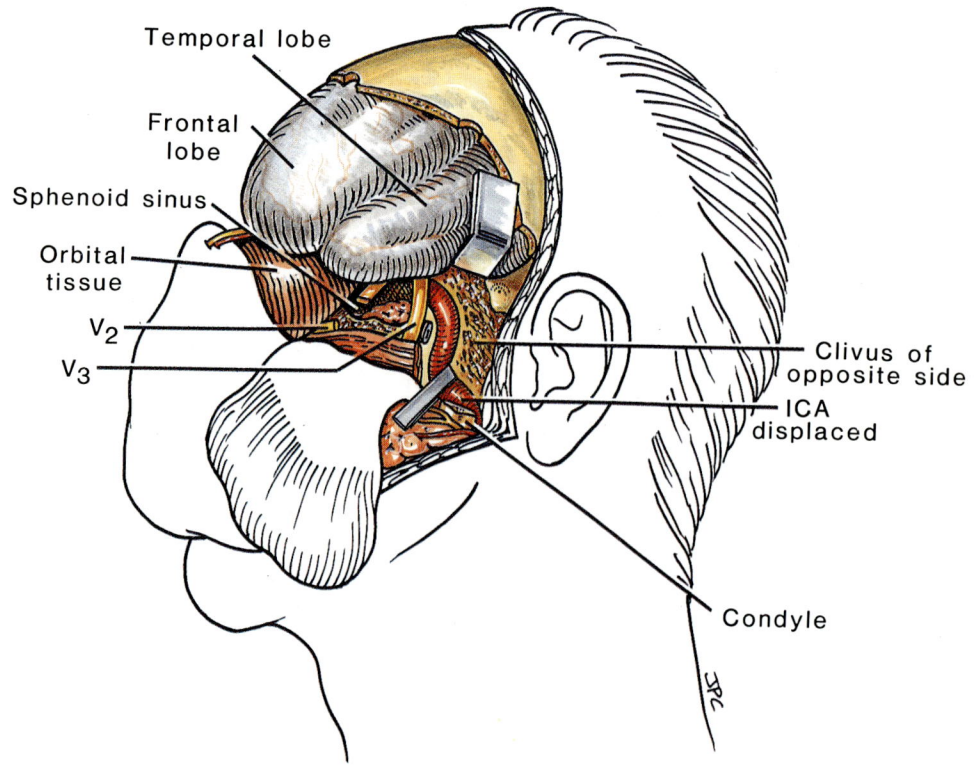

FIG. 27. Combined anterior and lateral approach. The exposure from the lateral aspect is shown.

of the pinna of the ear by leaving an adequate island of skin and subcutaneous tissues to keep the pinna vascularized. With a C-shaped incision, the greater occipital nerve may have to be divided. The lesser occipital nerve will always have to be divided with either incision. The greater auricular nerve can generally be preserved with both incisions. Any divided nerves are tagged and reanastomosed at the end of the operation.

The sternomastoid muscle is detached and reflected inferiorly and posteriorly from the mastoid process. The C1 and C2 transverse processes are identified by inspection and palpation. Just anterior to this area, the jugular vein and cranial nerve XI can be identified. The identity of cranial nerve XI should be confirmed by electrical stimulation. The semispinalis capitis and splenius capitis muscles are elevated from the suboccipital bone and reflected posteroinferiorly. The oblique muscles are detached from the C1 transverse process and the muscle layers are reflected medially. The extradural segment of the vertebral artery can be found in this area, from the foramen transversarium of C1 to the suboccipital membrane, and carefully dissected. If necessary, the artery can also be dissected from the C2 foramen to the C1 foramen. The C1 foramen is unroofed posteriorly and laterally. There is a venous plexus that surrounds the vertebral artery, which also warns the surgeon of the location of the artery here. The vertebral artery is dissected from the groove on the superior surface of C1, mobilized completely from C2 to the dura, and displaced inferomedially. A C1 laminectomy is performed from the transverse process to the midline, either with the aid of a reciprocating saw or with rongeurs, carefully protecting the vertebral artery (Fig. 29).

A small laterally placed occipital craniotomy is carried out to the foramen magnum. A low mastoidectomy is performed, extending anteriorly to the level of the fallopian canal of the facial nerve, and posteriorly to unroof the sigmoid sinus and the jugular bulb. At this point, the posterior two-thirds of the occipital condyle is resected in a piecemeal fashion with the aid of a high-speed drill. If necessary, the posterior half or two-thirds of the articular process of C1 can also be resected. The sigmoid sinus is divided well above the location of the tumor and the outside wall is sutured to the inner wall with 4-0 Neurolon sutures. The jugular bulb is now opened and tumor is removed from within. The internal jugular vein can either be ligated or packed with Surgicel. Cranial nerves XII, IX, and X are unroofed extradurally, working through the jugular bulb. However, if there is a doubt about their locations, the dura can be opened to identify the nerves intradurally and then follow them out extradurally (Fig. 30). The dura of the jugular bulb area may be infiltrated by tumor or markedly adherent to it and may need to be resected with tumor. The vertebral artery may be followed from its extradural course into the intradural segment and dissected from the tumor if necessary. The medial wall of the jugular bulb is resected, and the surgeon can work between the extradural sleeve of cranial nerves IX, X, XI, and XII, as well as inferior to the sleeve of cranial nerve XII, to resect the lower clival bone and tumor. The remaining occipital condyle can be resected completely (Fig. 31).

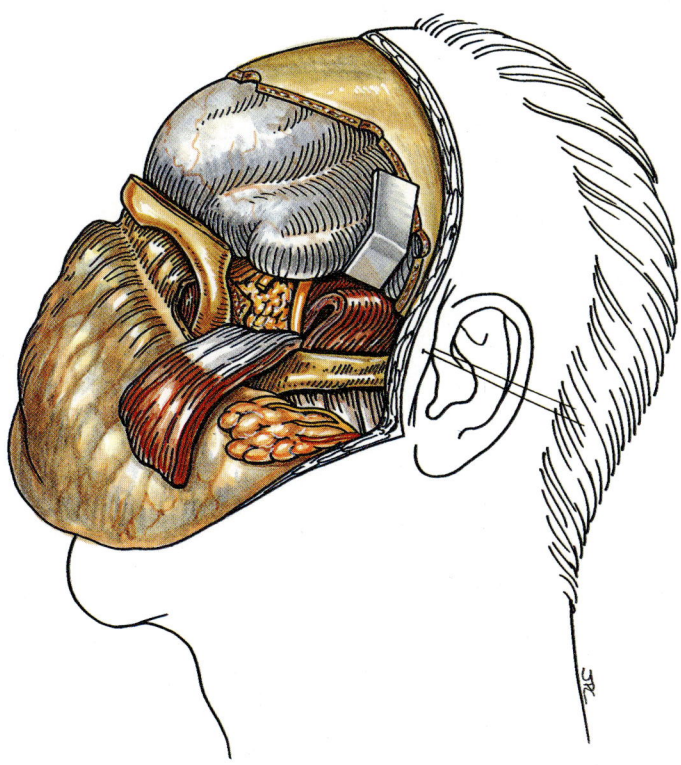

FIG. 28. Combined anterior and lateral approach. The reconstruction with a galeopericranial flap and temporalis muscle is shown.

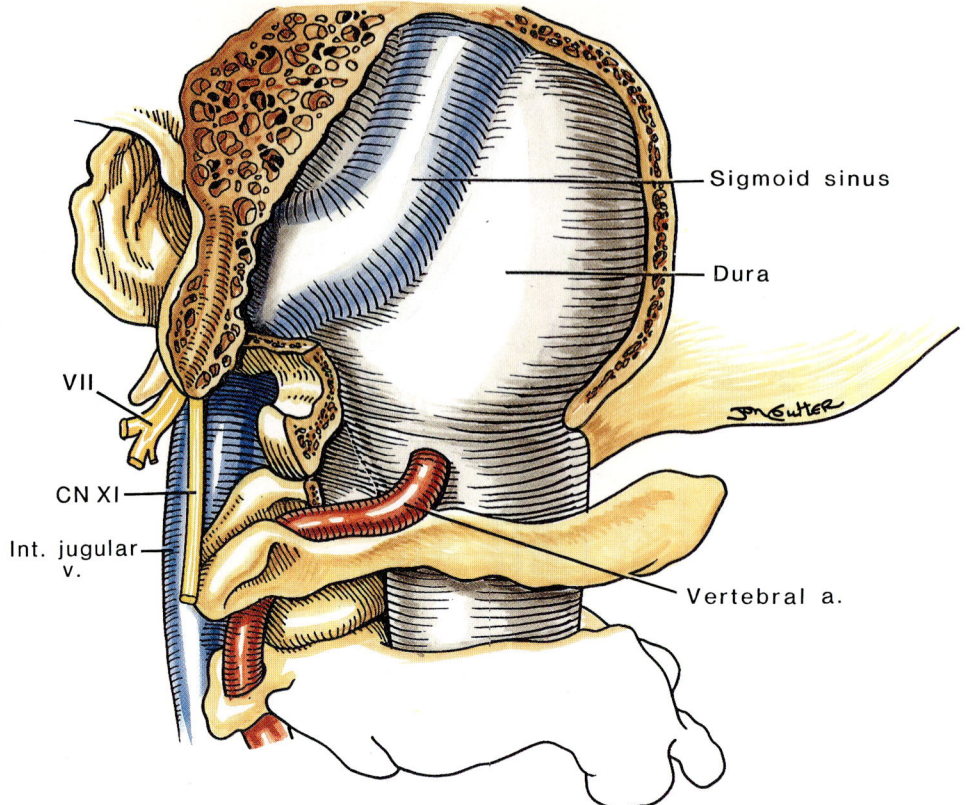

FIG. 29. Extreme lateral approach. The extradural vertebral artery has been exposed. A retrosigmoid craniotomy has been performed and a mastoidectomy has unroofed the sigmoid sinus and the jugular bulb partially. The occipital condyle and the articular process of C1 have been partially removed.

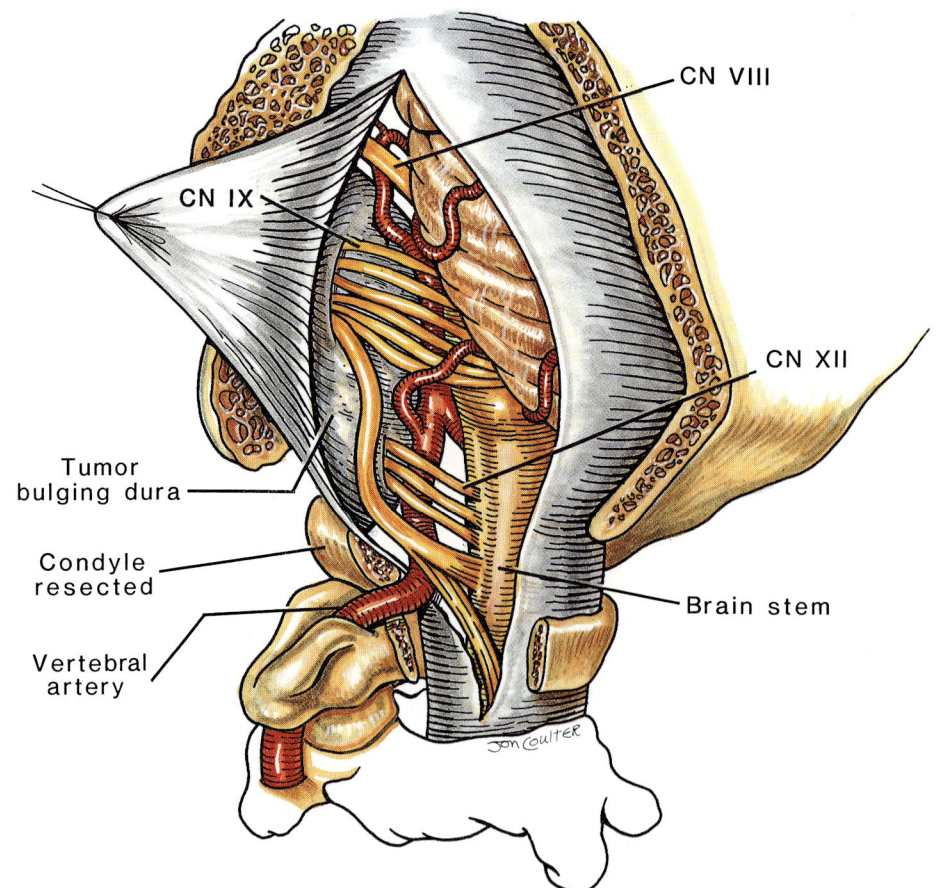

FIG. 30. Extreme lateral approach. The dura has been opened to help in the identification of cranial nerves IX–XII extradurally, to look for intradural tumor, and to allow the safe resection of dura when involved by the tumor.

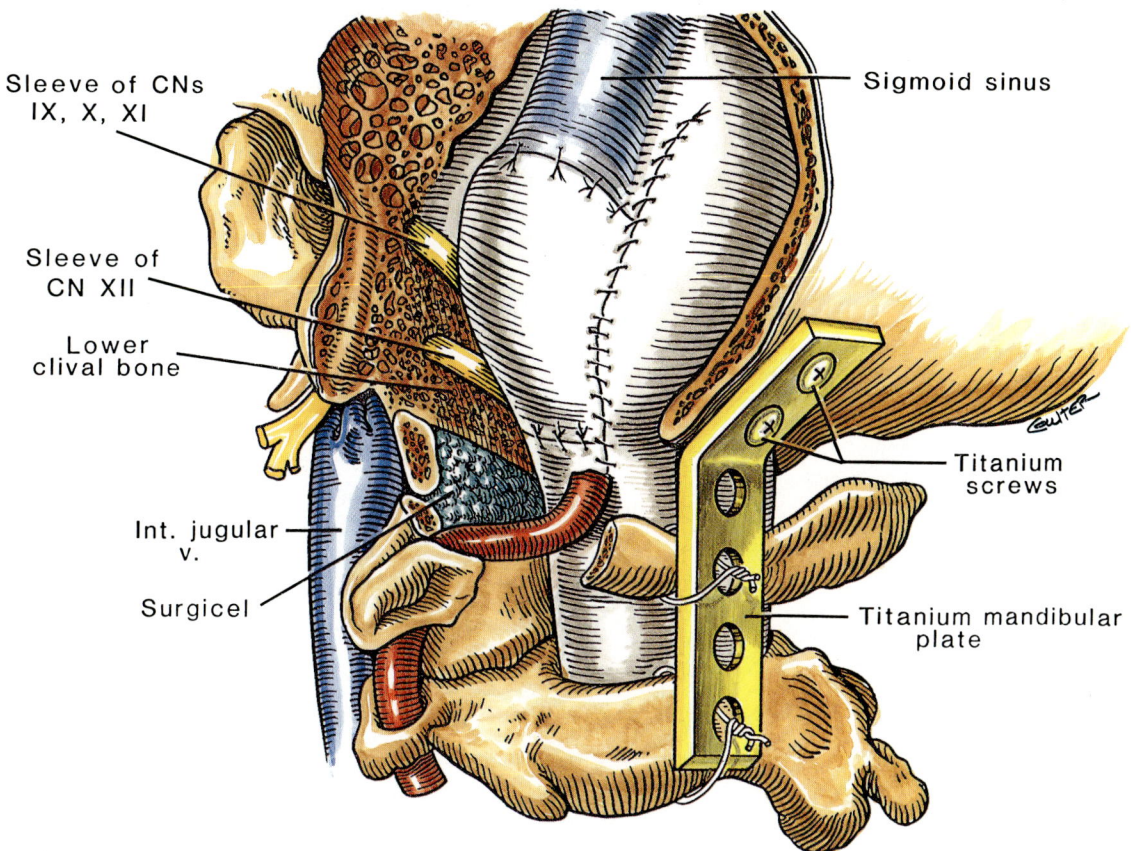

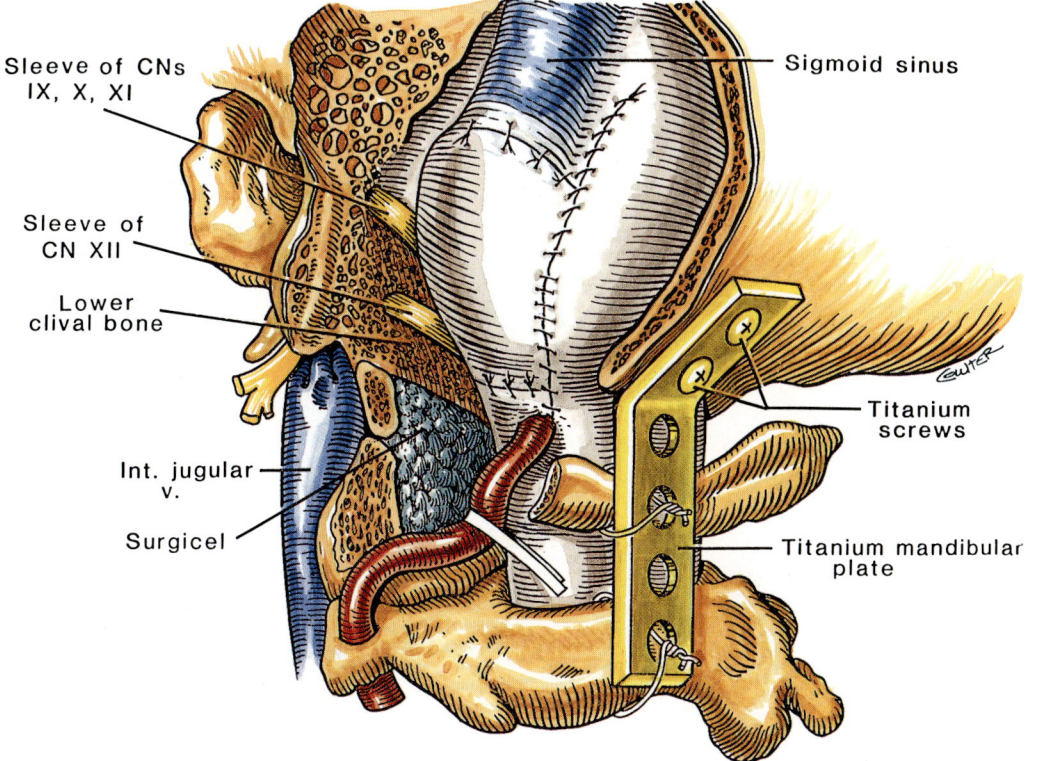

FIG. 31. A: The conclusion of the operation, extreme lateral approach. The sigmoid sinus and the internal jugular vein have been ligated. Tumor has been resected, including the occipital condyle and the extradural sleeves of cranial nerves IX, X, XI, and XII. A titanium plate fixation from the occiput to C1 and C2 arches has been performed. Bone grafts will subsequently be applied to obtain a bony fusion. **B:** The vertebral artery has been mobilized completely from C2 to the dura.

Reconstruction

Any dural defect is reconstructed with the aid of a fascia lata graft with circumferential sutures and a fat graft is used to occlude the dead space. If the entire occipital condyle has been resected, a titanium plate is fixed from the occiput to C1 and C2 laminae and bone grafts are laid to allow a bony fusion to occur.

The upper limit of bony resection with this approach is the labyrinth and the internal auditory canal (Fig. 32). When this approach is combined in the same operation or in a separate operation with a subtemporal–infratemporal approach, it is possible to leave the facial nerve, the labyrinth, and the middle ear entirely intact and remove all the midclival and lower clival tumor and the tumor involving the petrous apices. The combination of the

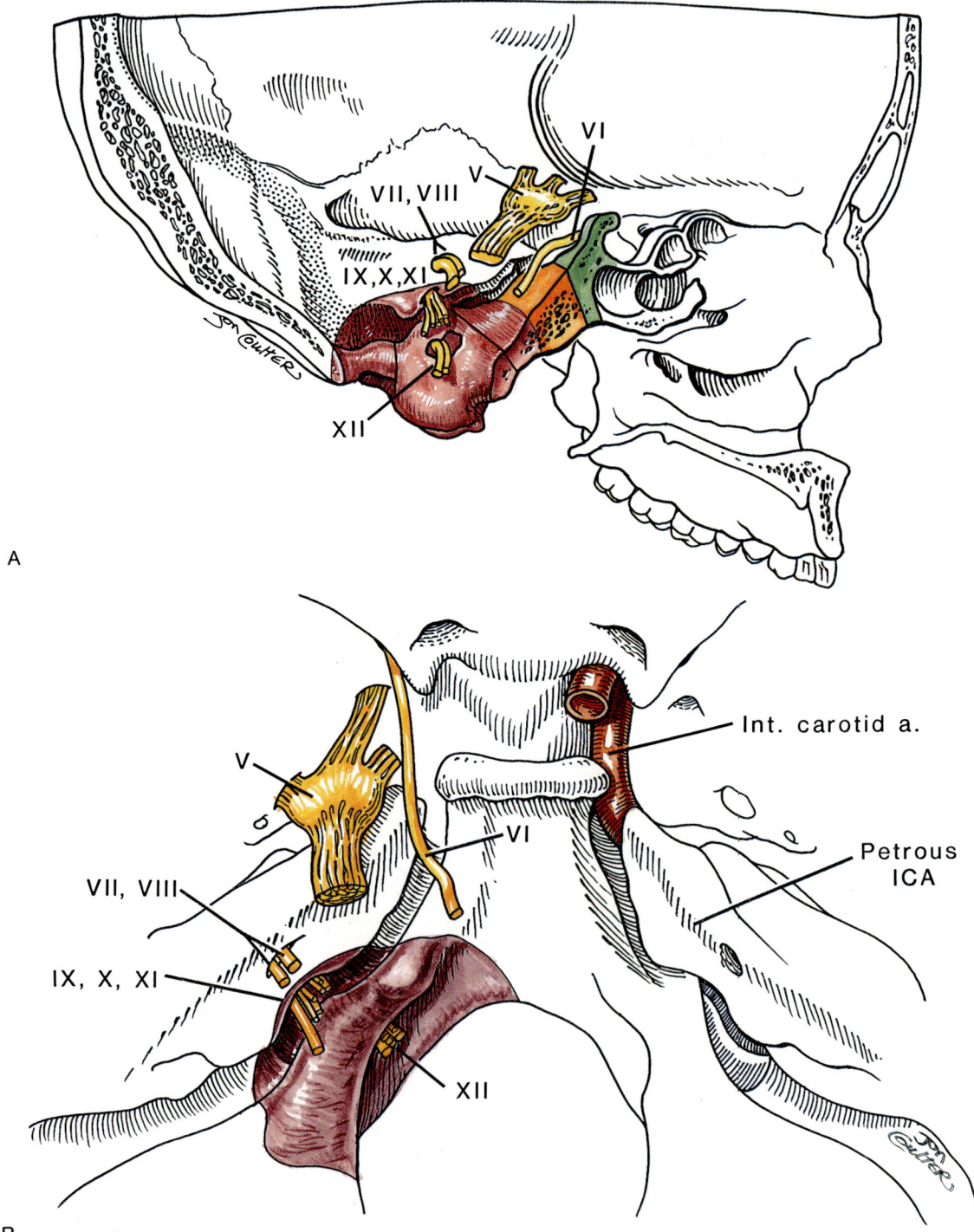

FIG. 32. The area from which tumor can be removed by an extreme lateral transcondyle and transjugular approach is shown in the lateral (**A**) and dorsal (**B**) views.

two approaches also allows further tumor resection across the midline and, if necessary, the resection of the clival dura across to the opposite side.

Disadvantages

The drawback of the extreme lateral approach as described here is the destruction of the occipital condyle and the jugular bulb. Without occlusion of the jugular bulb, this approach is still useful, but less clival bone resection is possible.

Illustrative Cases

In figures 33 through 68, eight con examples are shown to illustrate the various surgical operations described above.

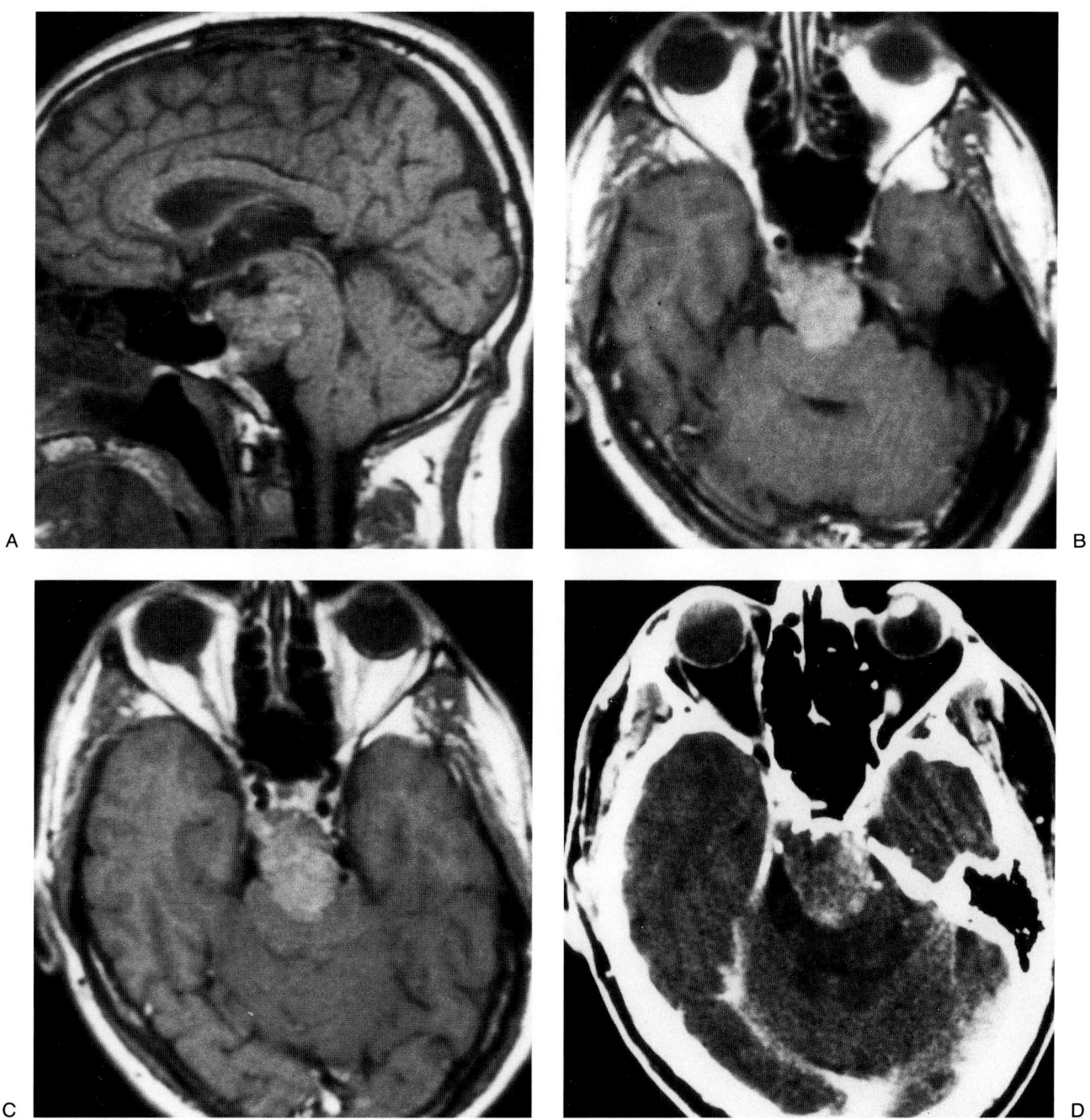

FIG. 33. R.V.–This 42-year-old patient presented with headaches and a right cranial nerve VI palsy. Preoperative MRI scans (**A–C**) and axial CT scan (**D**) reveal a tumor involving predominantly the upper clivus with some extension into the cavernous sinus on the right.

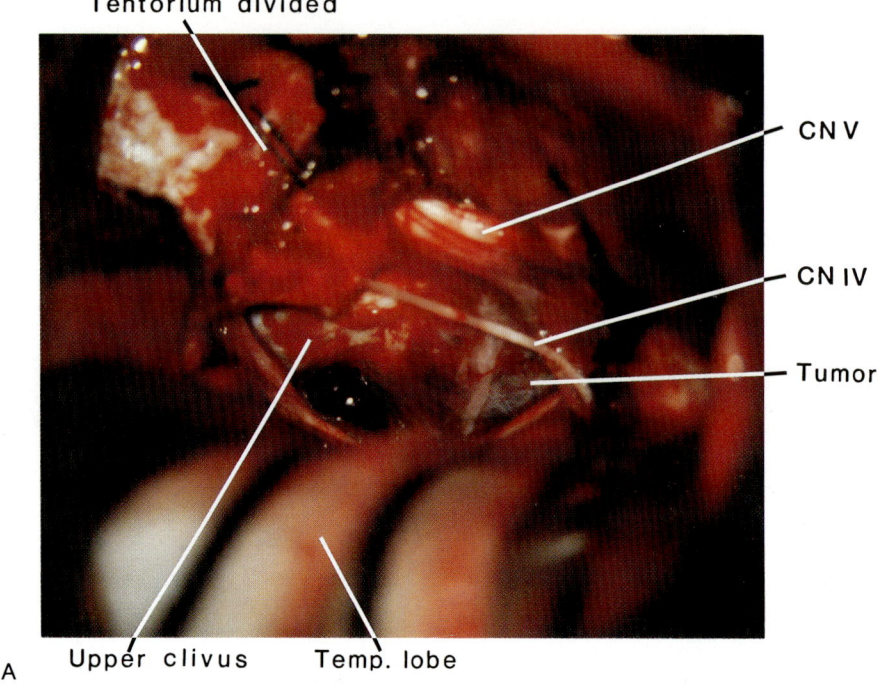

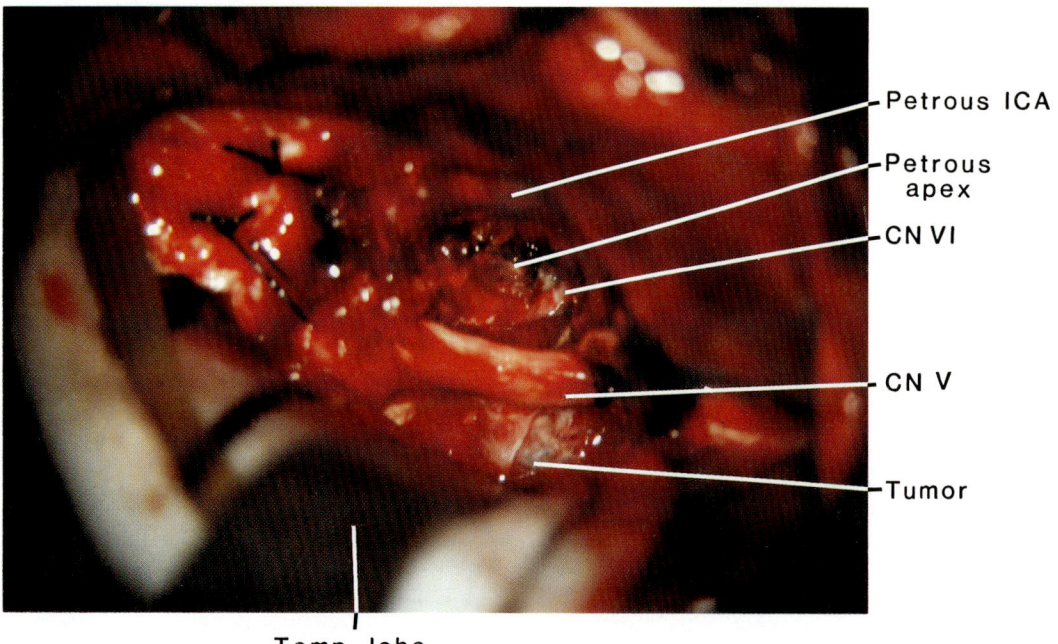

FIG. 34. R.V.–The patient underwent tumor resection in two stages. The first operation was by a right subtemporal, transzygomatic, transpetrous apex and transcavernous approach. **A:** The operation photograph shows the initial intradural tumor exposure after the division of the tentorium. The tumor had penetrated the clival dura, with evidence of prior subarachnoid hemorrhage. **B:** The petrous apex removal, the horizontal petrous ICA, and the early visualization of the ipsilateral cranial nerve VI.

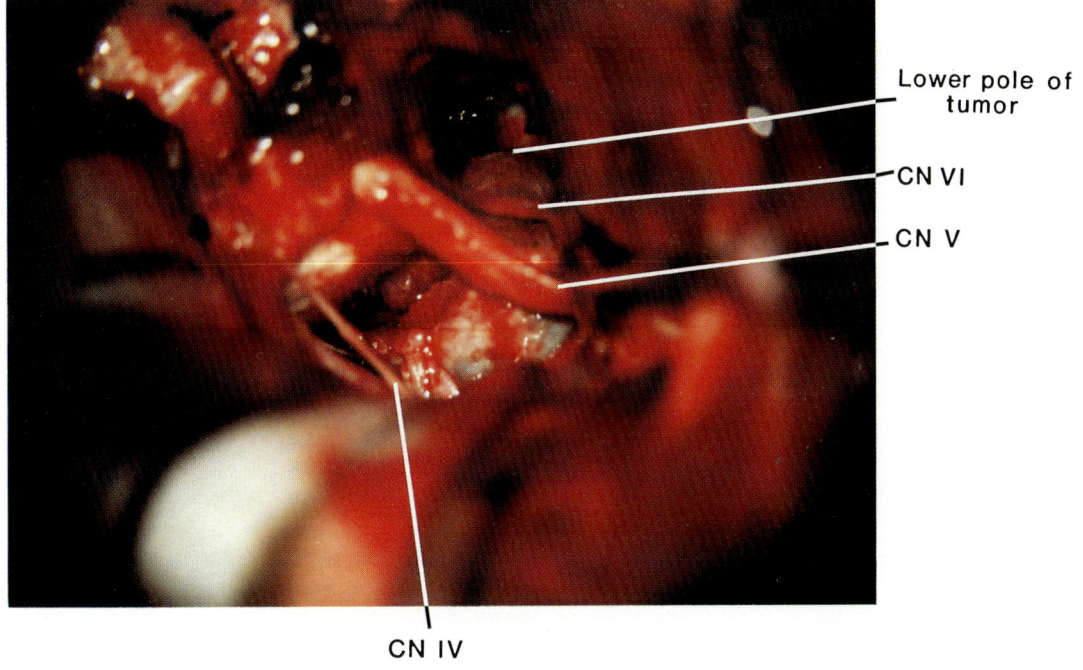

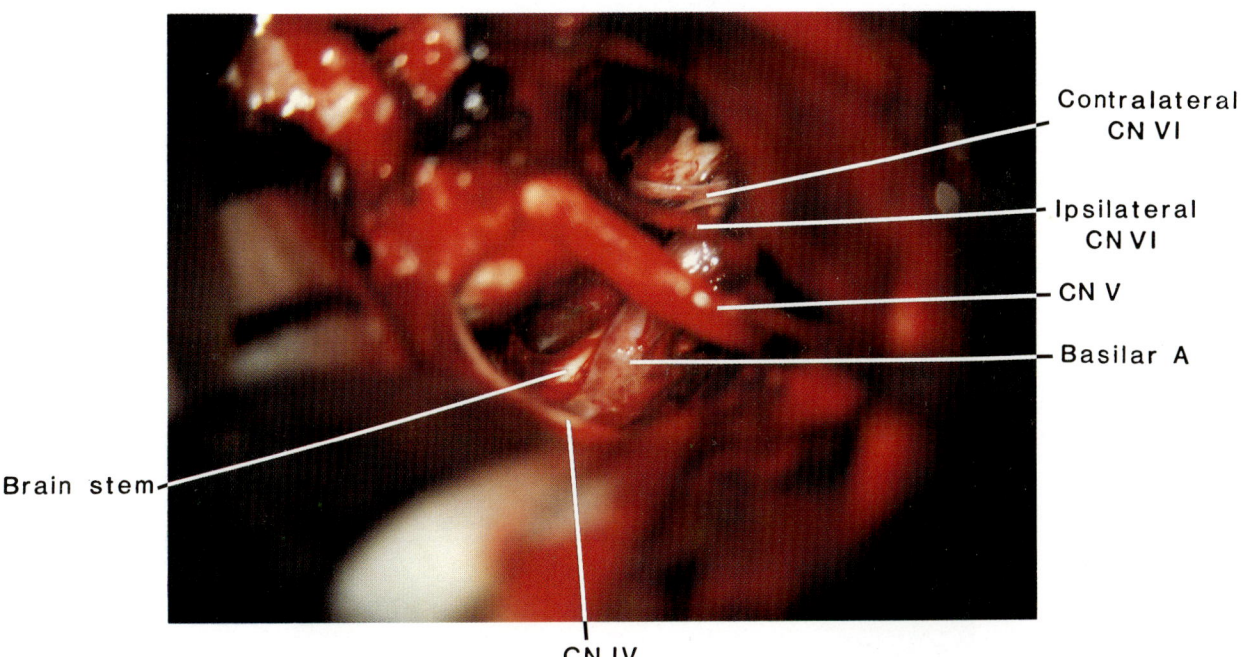

FIG. 34. *Continued.* **C:** Removal of the petrous apex has been completed, and the lower pole of the tumor is seen. **D, E:** The appearance at the conclusion of dual tumor resection by this approach. Some of the basilar artery branches had to be carefully dissected from tumor. Both the ipsilateral and contralateral cranial nerve VI are seen. Tumor removal from the cavernous sinus area is not shown in these photographs.

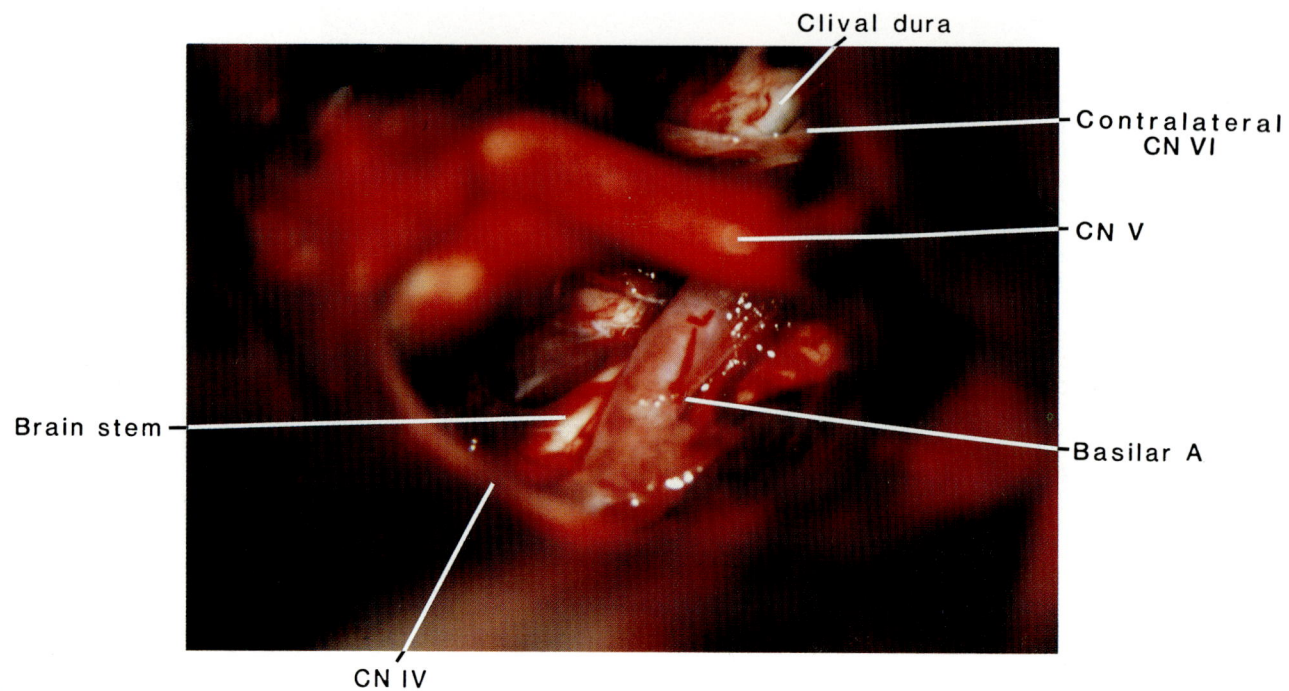

FIG. 34. *Continued.*

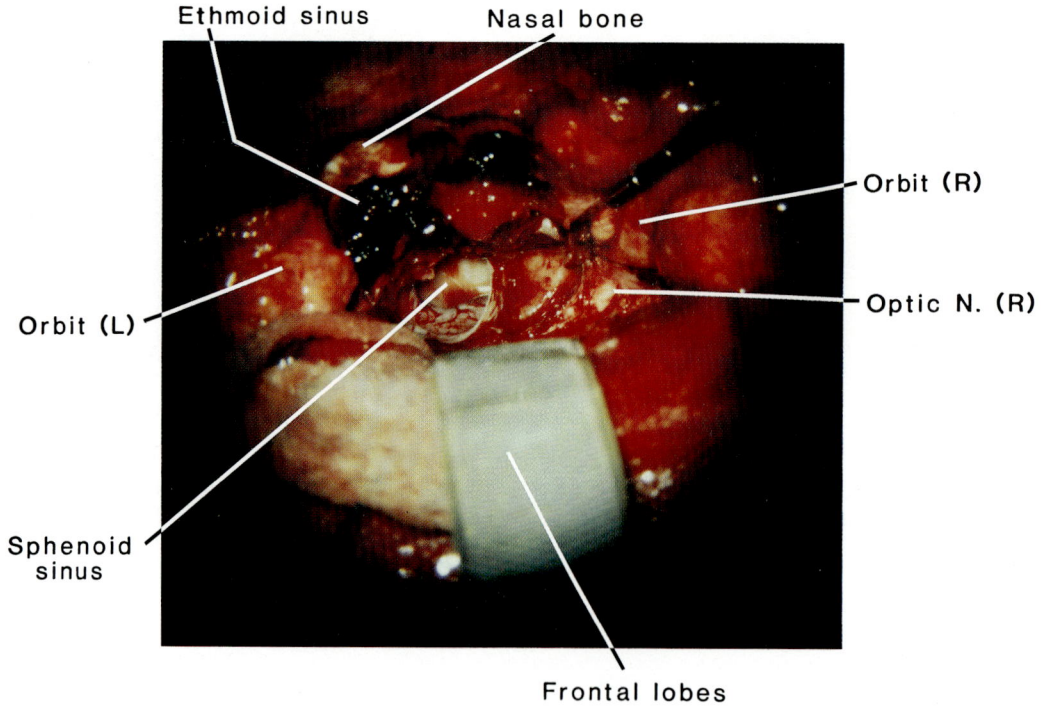

FIG. 35. R.V.–In order to remove the remaining root of the tumor in the clival bone, a basal frontal approach was employed, 6 weeks later. **A:** Entry into the sphenoid sinus, the ethmoid sinuses, the right optic nerve and orbit, and the left orbit.

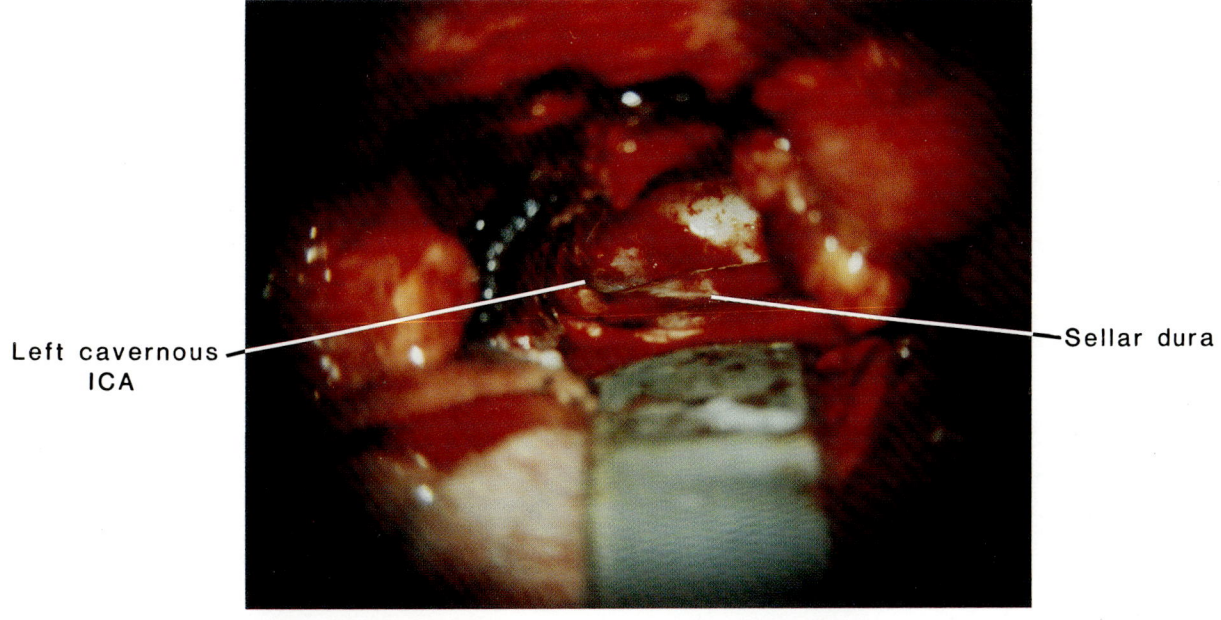

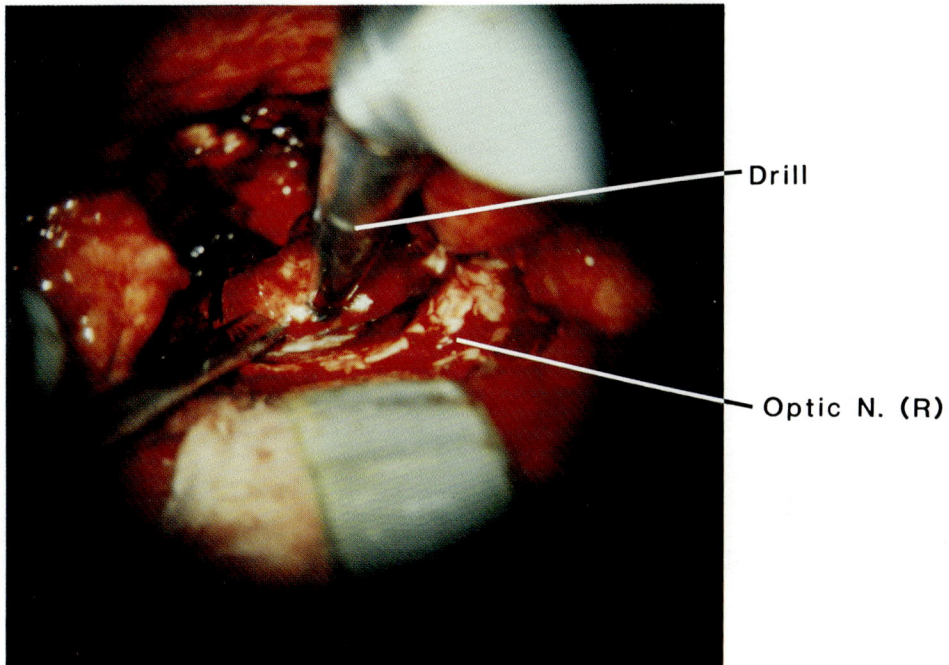

FIG. 35. *Continued.* **B:** The unroofing of the sellar dura and the left cavernous sinus. **C:** The sphenoclival bone is being drilled away.

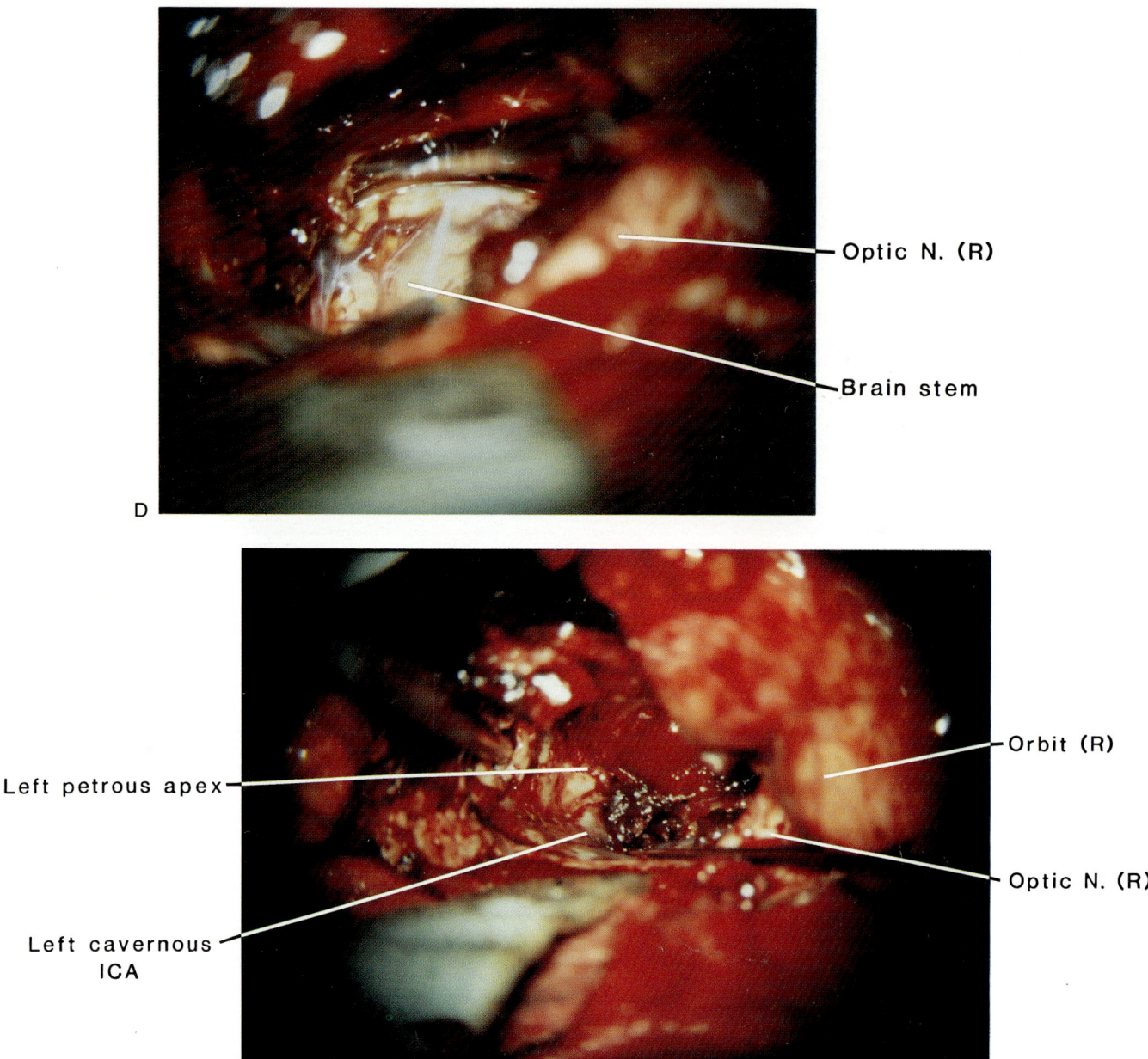

FIG. 35. *Continued.* **D:** Since the clival dura has been resected, the anterior surface of the brain stem is well seen. **E:** At the conclusion of tumor resection, the left cavernous ICA has been completely unroofed, and the left petrous apex is visible.

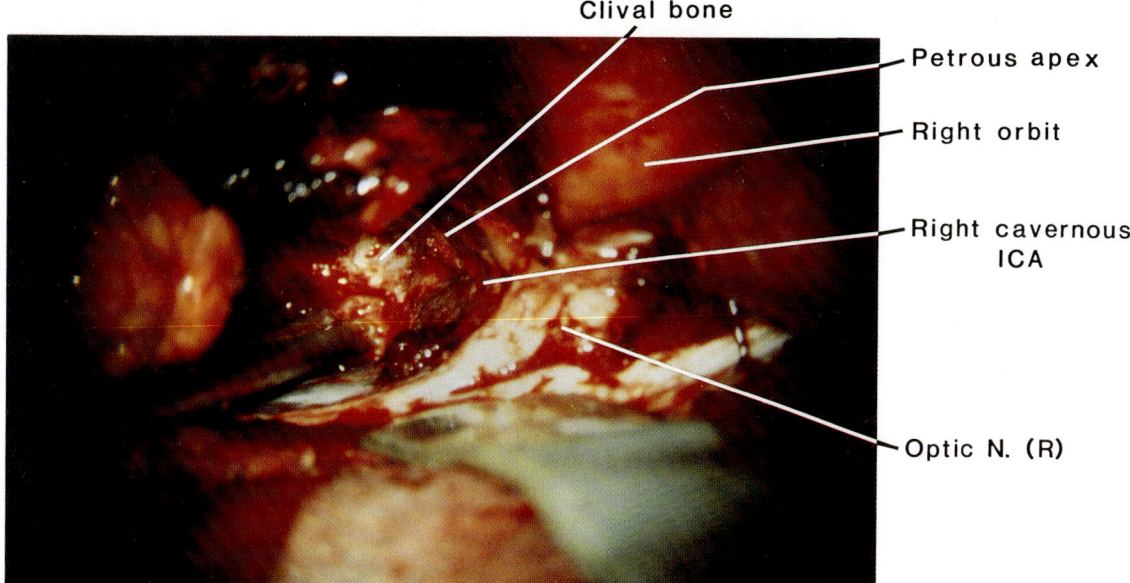

FIG. 35. *Continued.* **F:** The right cavernous ICA, the petrous apex, and the clival bone are visible. Reconstruction was accomplished with a fascia lata graft for the dural defect, a galeopericranial flap, and autologous fat.

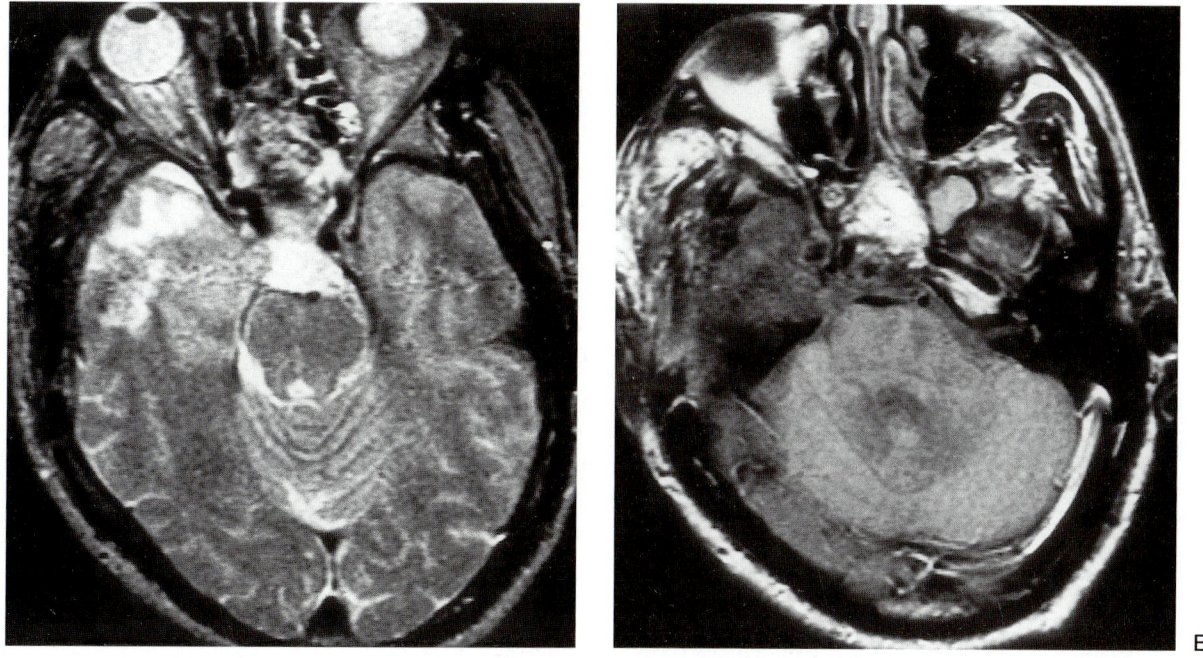

FIG. 36. Postoperative T2-weighted axial (**A**) and enhanced axial (**B, C**) MRI scans and nonenhanced CT scan (**D**) of the patient shows an apparently total tumor resection and the fat packing of the sphenoid sinus.

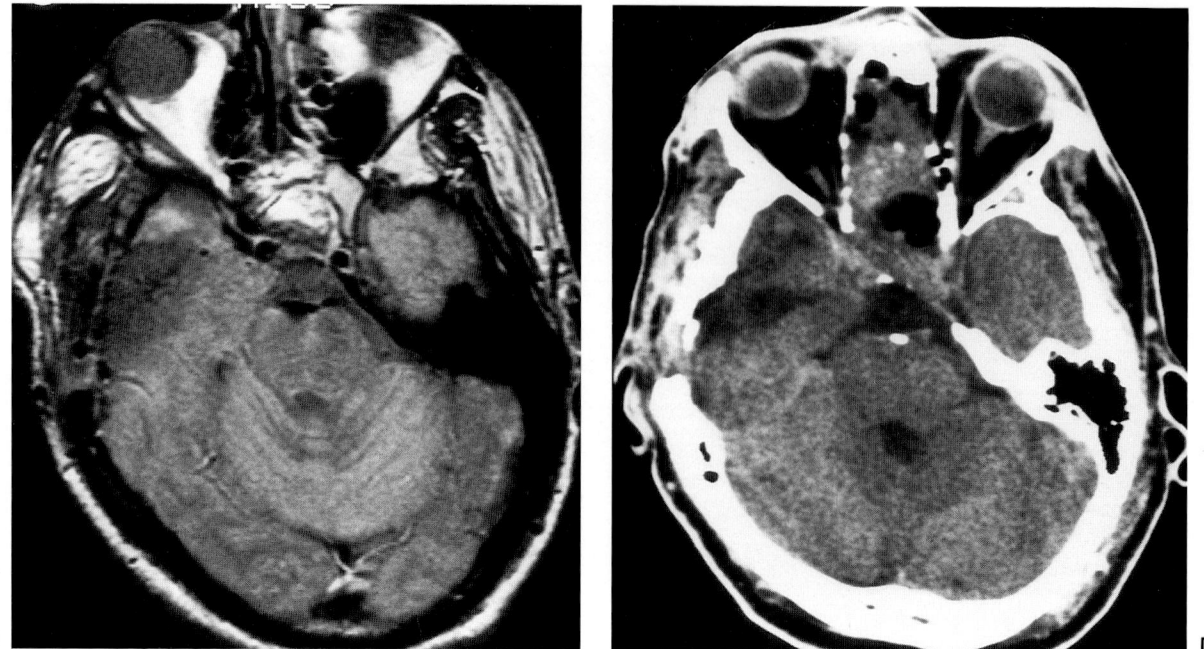

FIG. 36. *Continued.*

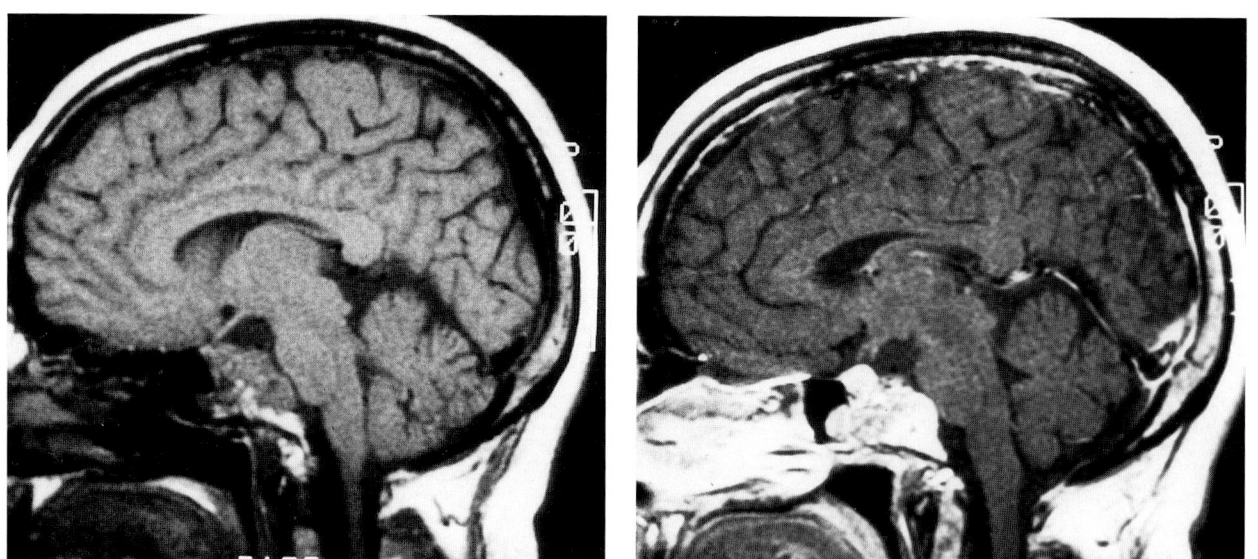

FIG. 37. M.C.–This 43-year-old patient presented with a complete ophthalmoplegia for the past 2 months and a prior history of transnasal–transsphenoidal resection of a chordoma, followed by external beam radiation therapy. Preoperative nonenhanced (**A**), enhanced (**B**), and sagittal MRI scans and enhanced coronal MRI images (**C, D**) reveal a recurrent clival chordoma of the upper clivus and midclivus and the right cavernous sinus.

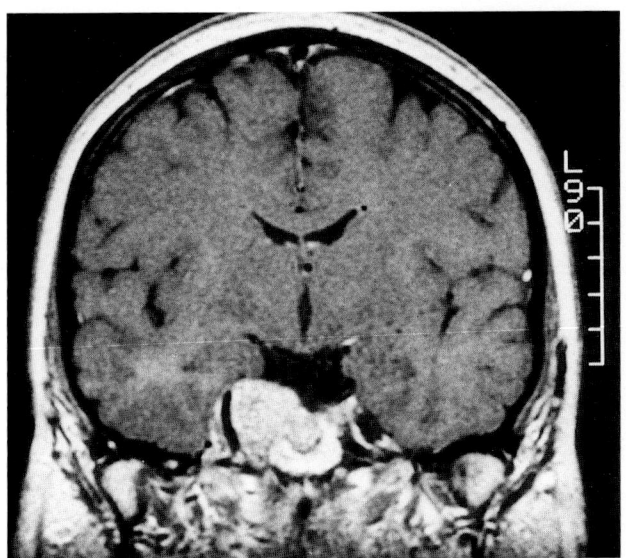
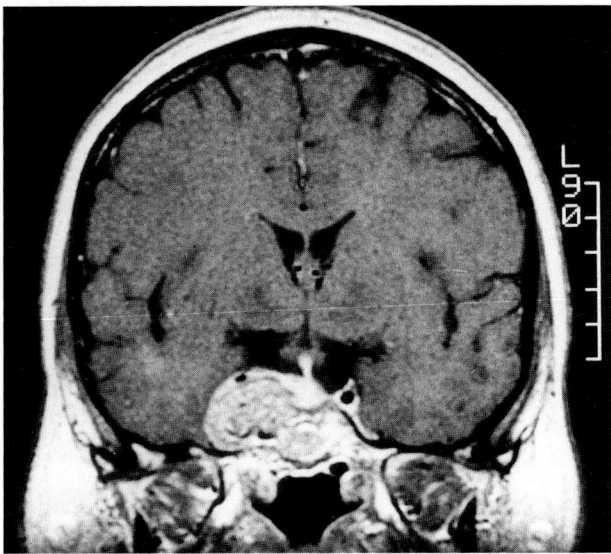

FIG. 37. *Continued.*

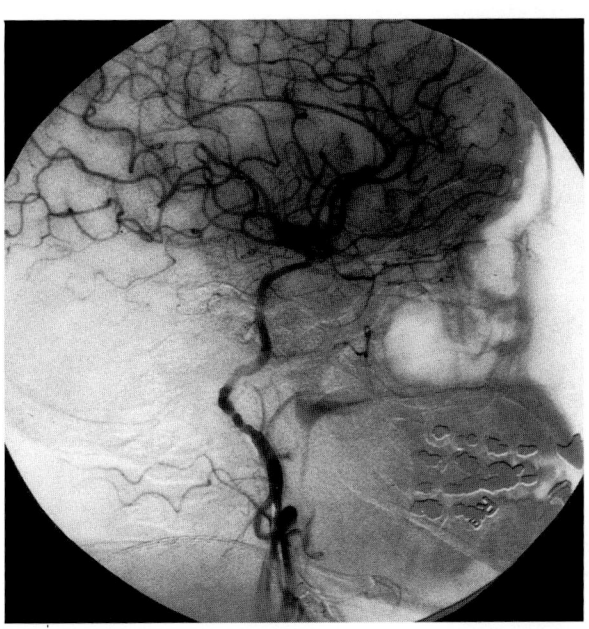

FIG. 38. M.C.–The preoperative angiogram reveals the posterior and upward displacement and narrowing of the intracavernous ICA. The patient failed the BTO-ICA clinically but operative resection was still elected.

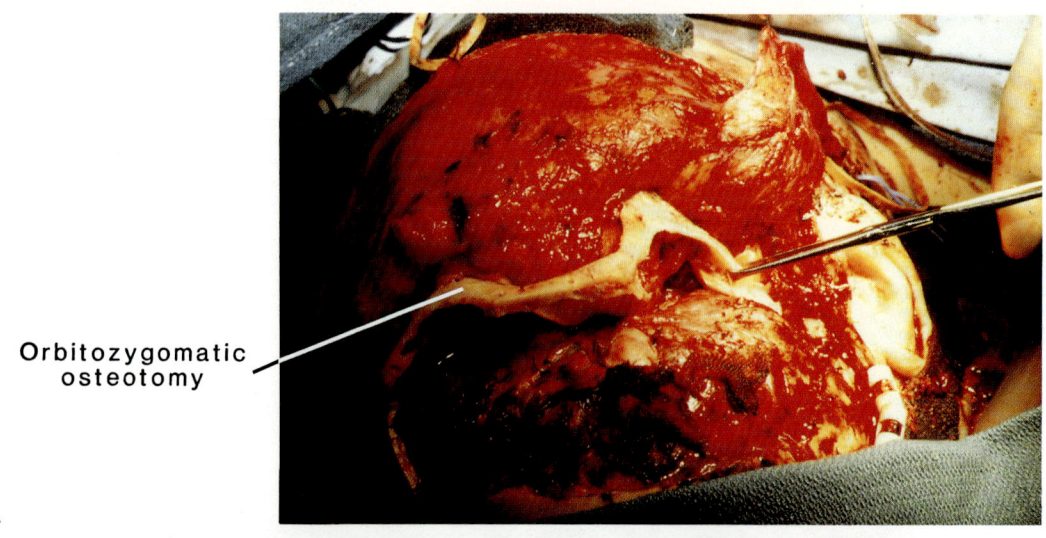

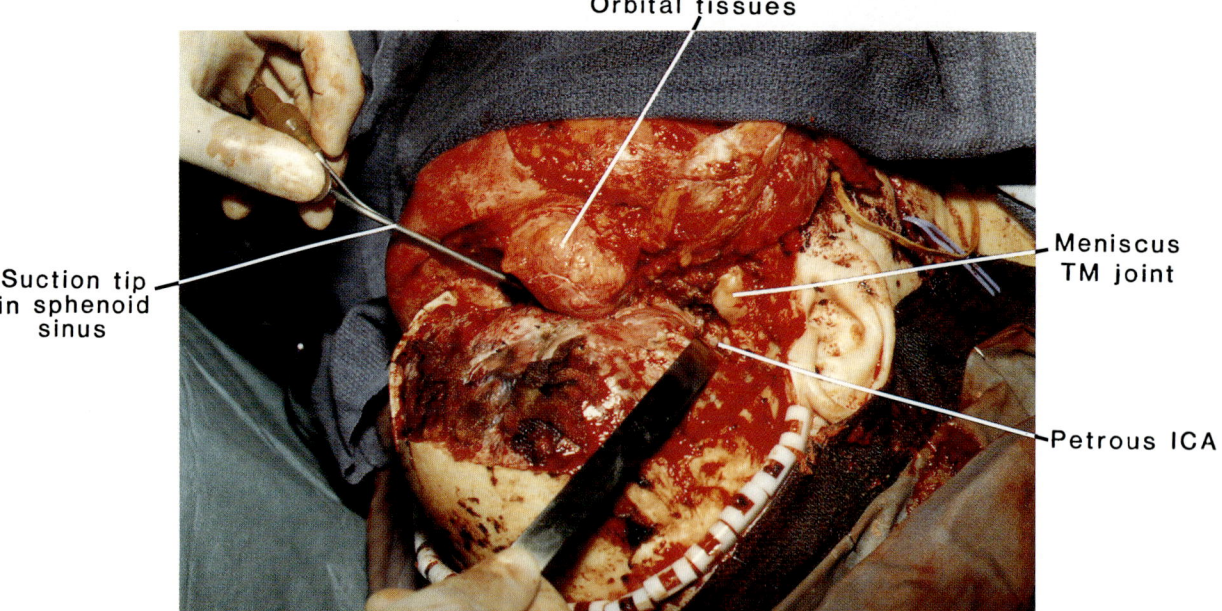

FIG. 39. This patient was operated by a basal frontal, subtemporal–infratemporal, and transcavernous approach to remove tumor. **A:** A frontotemporal craniotomy has been performed, and a zygomatic osteotomy and an orbital osteotomy extending across the midline have been performed. **B:** The orbitozygomatic osteotomy piece. **C:** This photograph, taken at the conclusion of the operation, shows the combined anterior and lateral exposure, the completely decompressed orbit, the horizontal petrous ICA, and the meniscus of the temporomandibular joint. The mandibular condyle did not need to be resected in this patient.

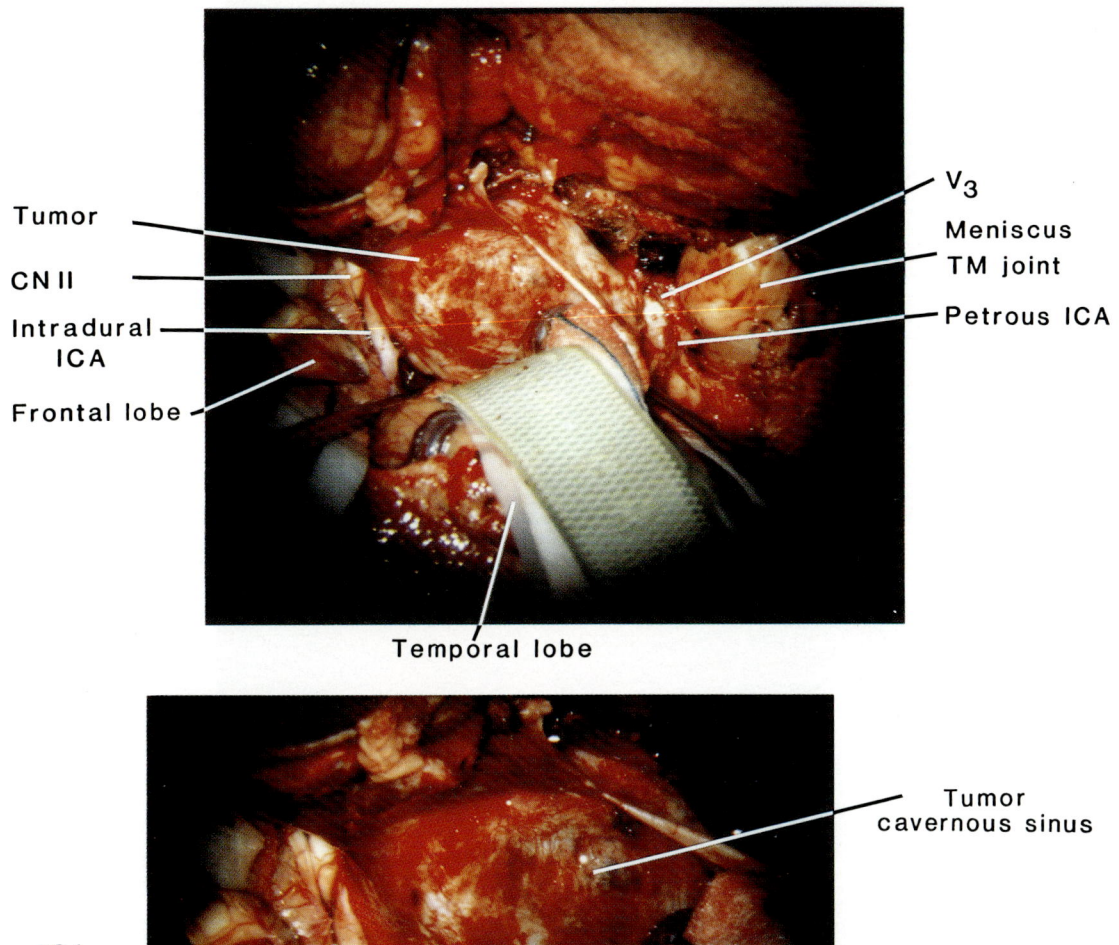

FIG. 39. *Continued.* **D:** This photograph, taken after the dura was opened, shows the tumor bulging the cavernous sinus laterally, the intradural optic nerve and ICA, frontal and temporal lobes, and, extradurally, V_2, V_3, petrous ICA (horizontal segment), and the meniscus of the TM joint. **E:** At higher magnification, this photograph shows the intradural optic nerve, ICA, cranial nerve III, and the CS bulging with tumor. The tumor was removed laterally working between V_1 and V_2 and the intracavernous ICA are seen.

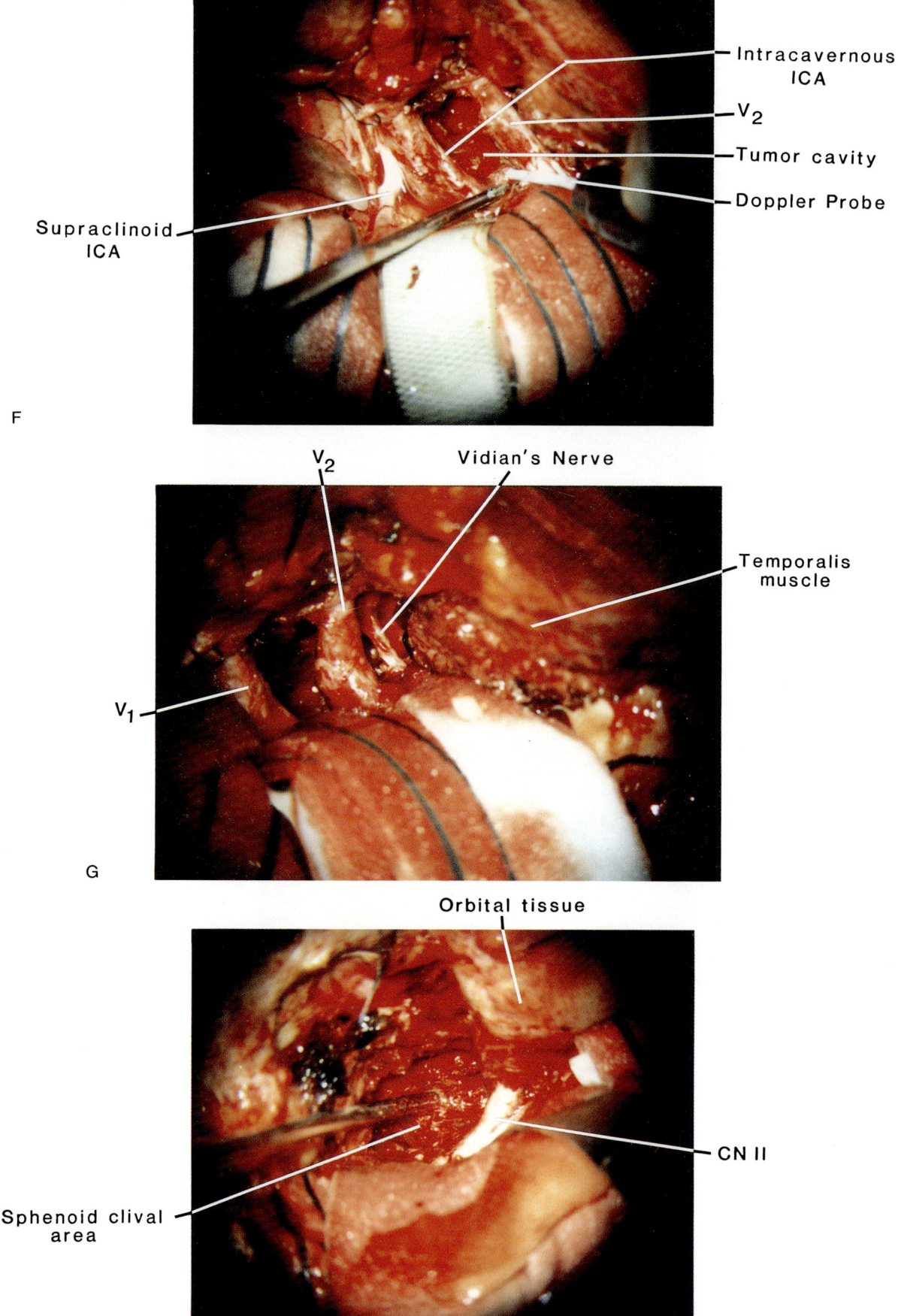

FIG. 39. *Continued.* **F:** Patency of the ICA is being verified by an intraoperative Doppler. **G:** One can see V_1, V_2, and Vidian's nerve, which has been unroofed by tumor resection in the sphenoid bone. **H:** The entry into the sphenoid sinus to remove tumor is shown. Note the right optic nerve (extradural) and the suction tip on the clivus.

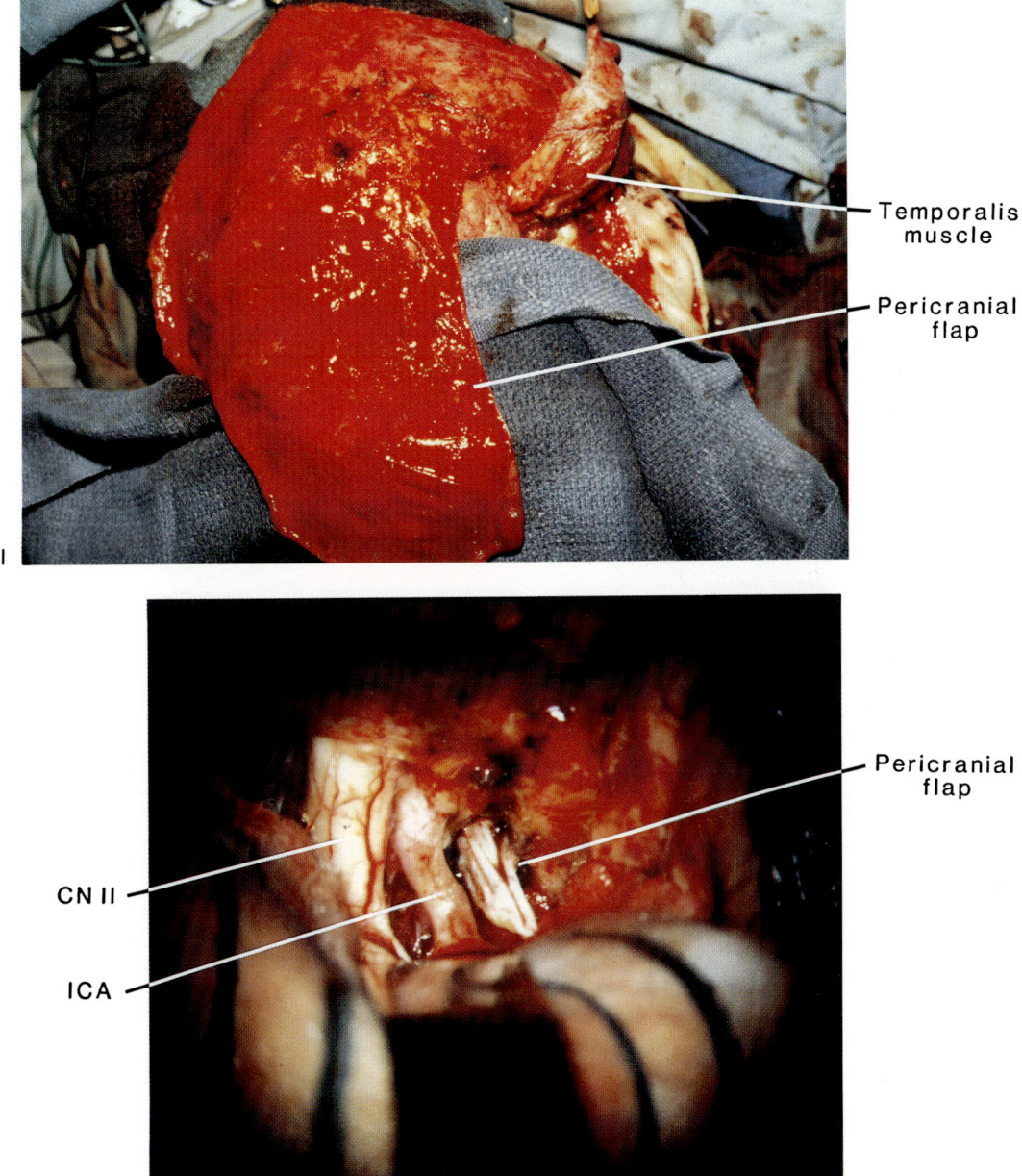

FIG. 39. *Continued.* **I:** The very vascular pericranial flap and the temporalis muscle used for reconstruction. A fascia lata patch and autologous fat were also used for reconstruction. **J:** Postoperatively, some enhancement was noted along the posterosuperior aspect of the cavernous sinus, and the patient was reexplored to remove a possible tumor residue with CS entry through the superior wall. The enhancing lesion was found to be the pericranial flap. The patient developed CSF leakage through this superior opening into the CS and due to hydrocephalus, which was controlled by packing some fat through this opening and with a ventriculoperitoneal shunt.

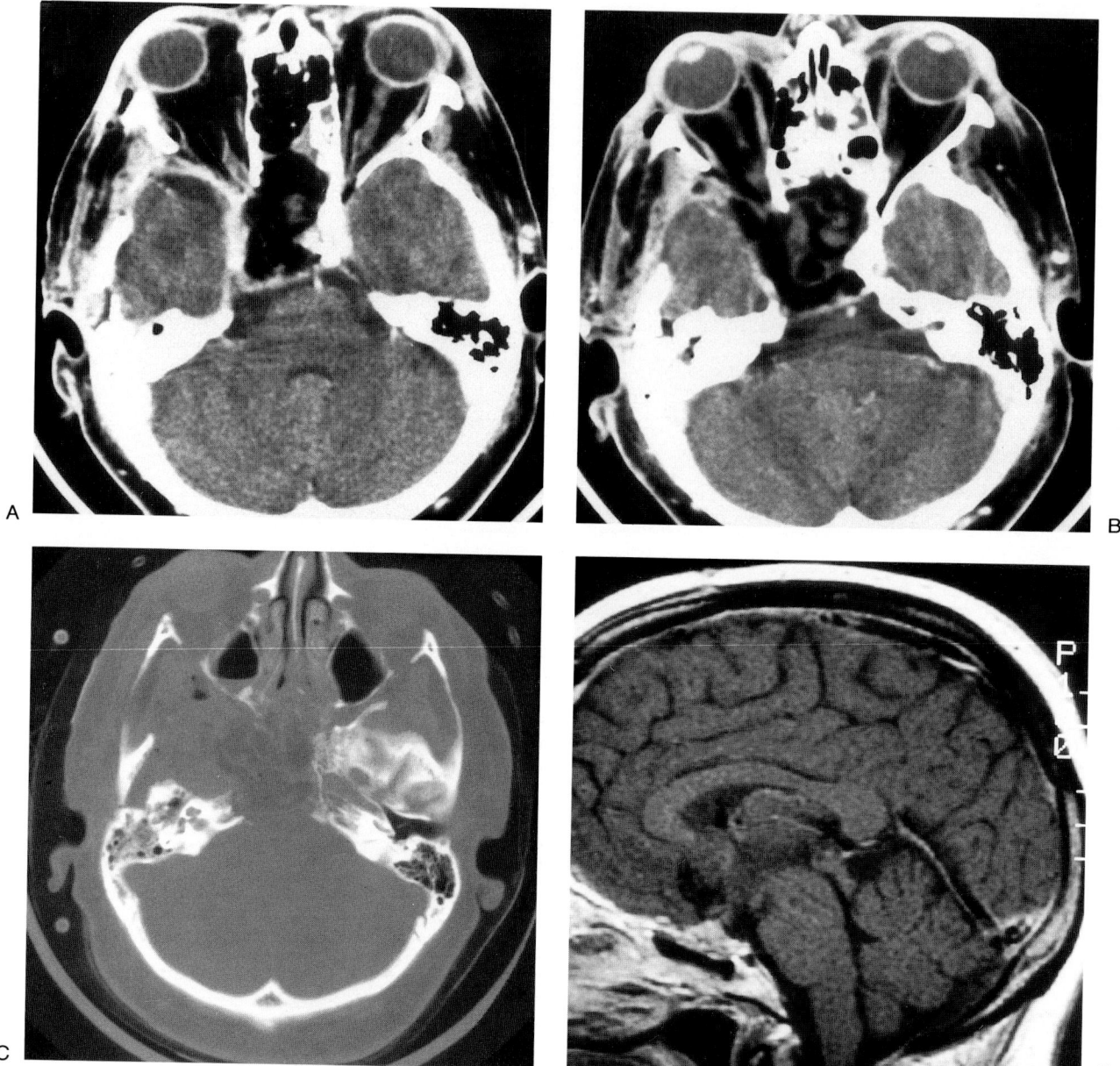

FIG. 40. Postoperative CT scans in soft tissue (**A, B**) and bone window (**C**) and a postoperative enhanced sagittal MRI scan (**D**) reveal the extent of bone resection and the fat used for reconstruction. At 6 months follow-up, the patient had made a near complete recovery of eye movements and had returned to full-time employment.

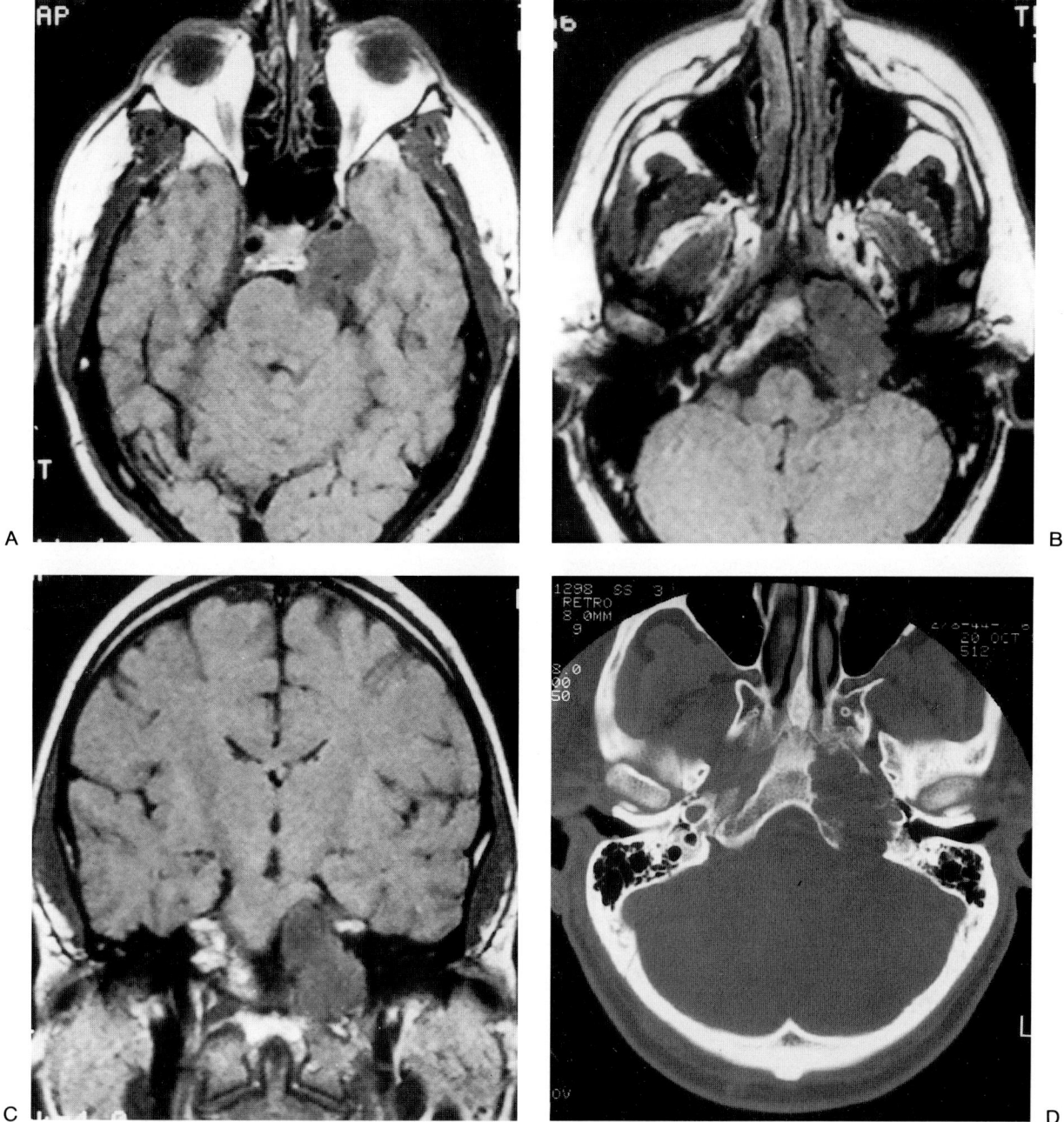

FIG. 41. D.Z.–This 33-year-old man presented with sixth cranial nerve paralysis. Preoperative axial (**A, B**) and coronal (**C**) MRI scans and bone window CT scan (**D**) reveal a tumor involving the petrous apex, the basal cavernous sinus, the midclivus and lower clivus, and the left jugular bulb area. The lesion was removed completely by a subtemporal and infratemporal intradural approach.

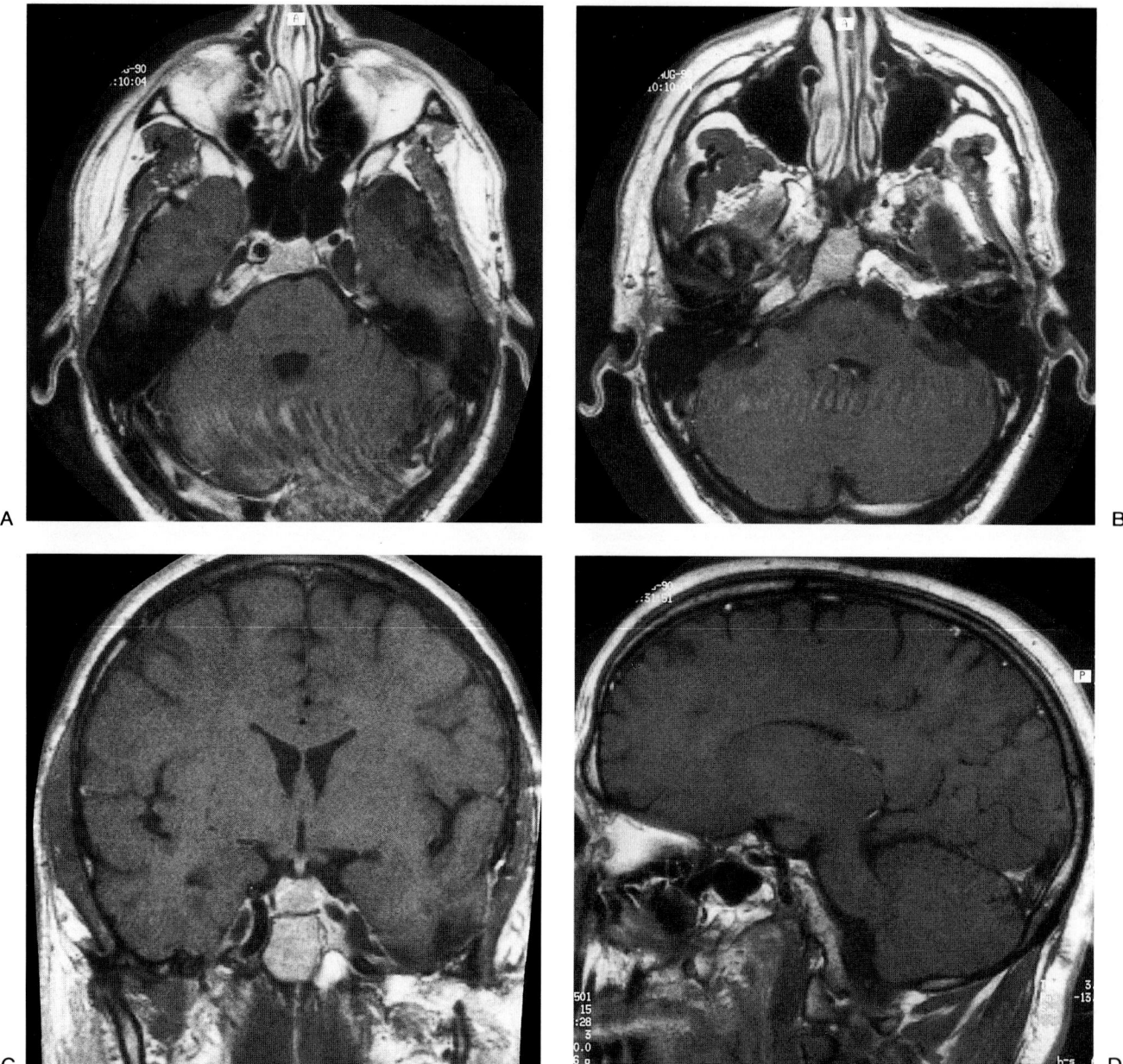

FIG. 42. D.Z.–A postoperative MRI scan showing scar tissue in the tumor bed and the fat that was packed in the tumor bed for reconstruction (**A–D**).

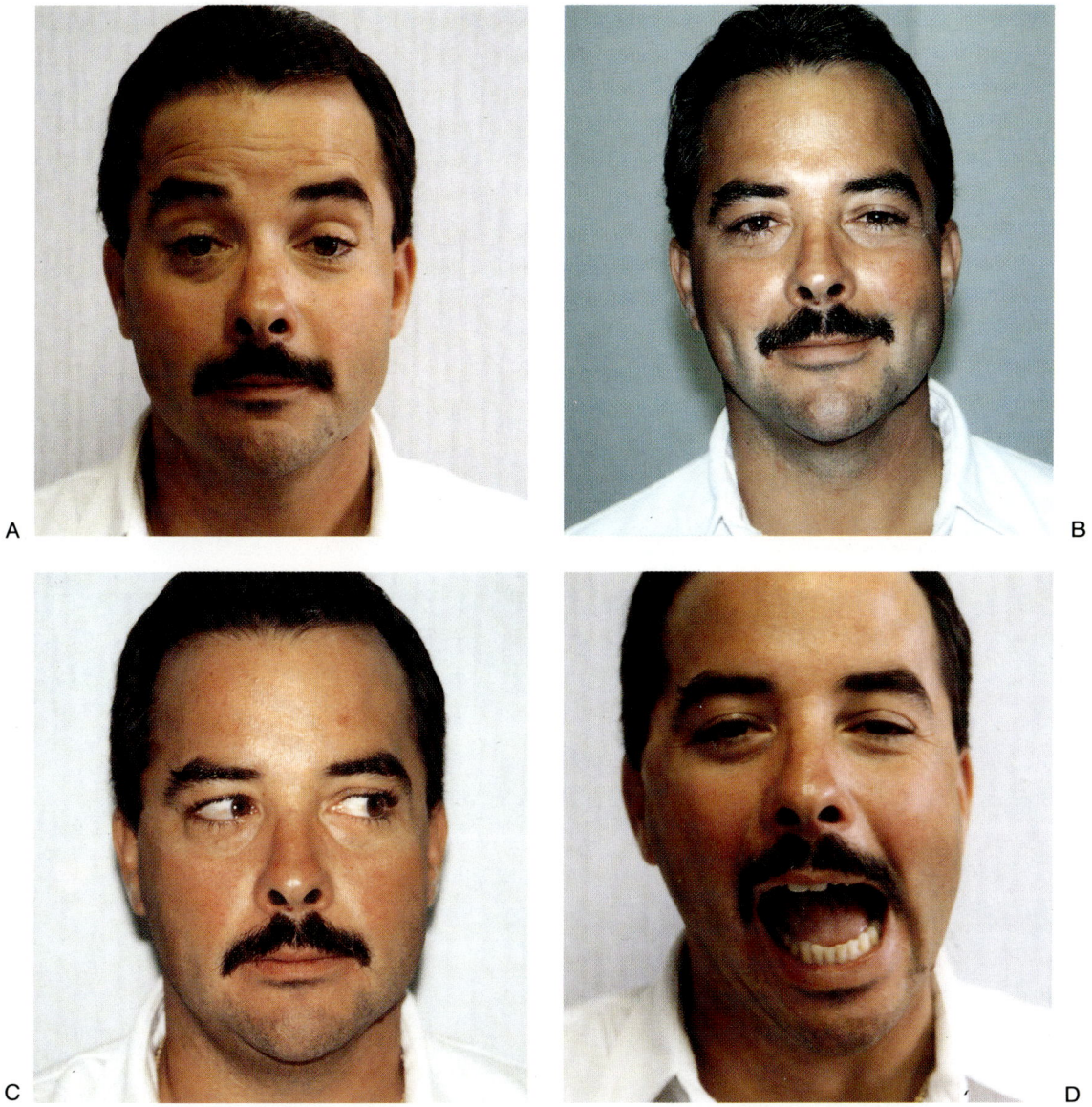

FIG. 43. D.Z.–Postoperatively, the patient is seen to have normal facial movements (**A, B**), complete recovery of abducens function (**C**), and jaw deviation caused by the condyle resection (**D**). (Reproduced with patient's permission.)

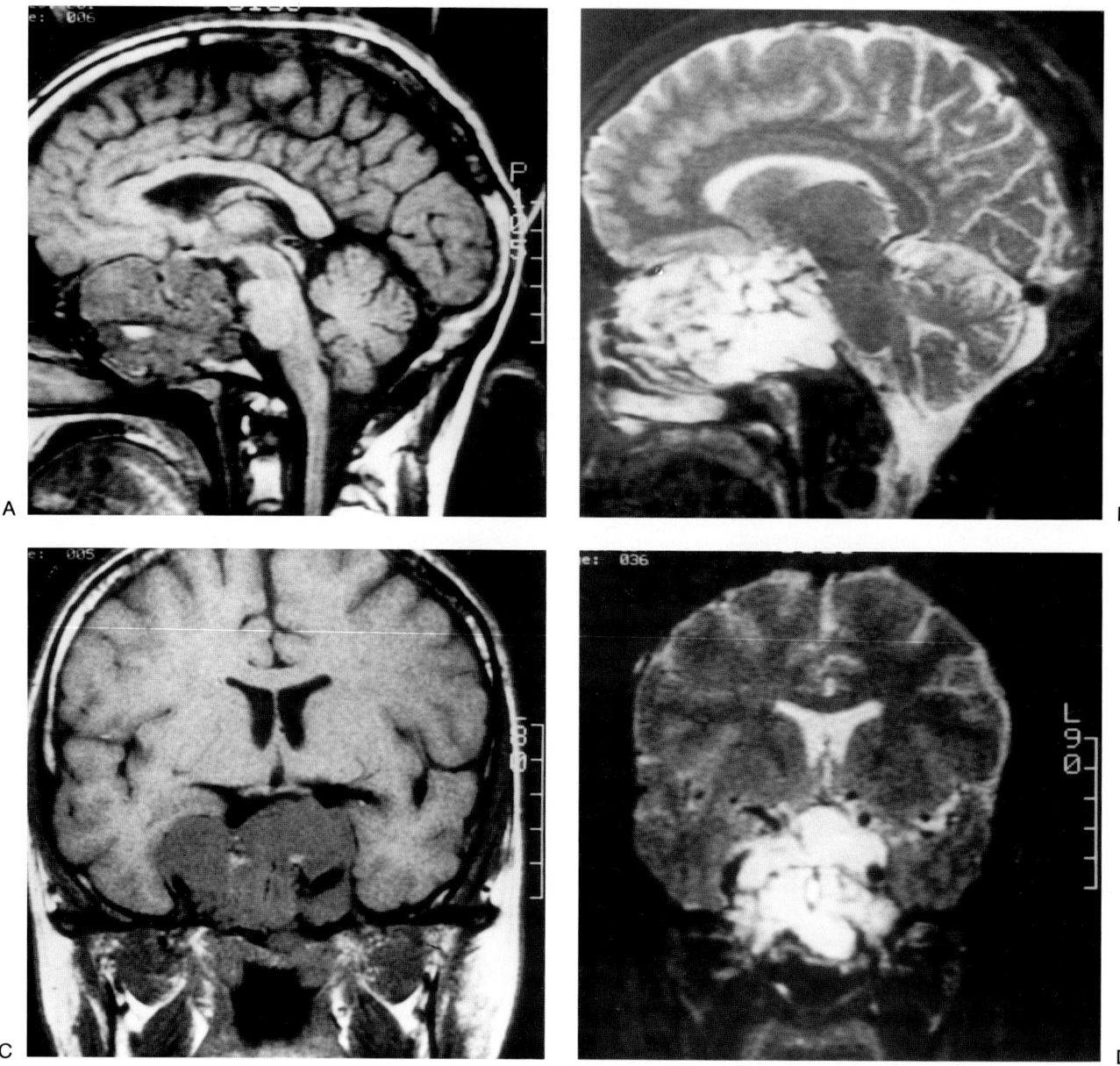

FIG. 44. T.E.–This 25-year-old man was discovered after a minor head injury to have a very large tumor of the clivus, ethmoid and sphenoid sinus, both cavernous sinuses, and the suprasellar area. A transoral biopsy revealed this to be a low grade chondrosarcoma. His right eye was amblyopic from birth, and this had presumably masked the patient's sixth cranial nerve paresis. Preoperative MRI scans in T1- and T2-weighted images reveal this large tumor (**A–D**).

FIG. 46. T.E.–Postoperative photographs reveal excellent recovery of eye movements. (Reproduced with patient's permission.)

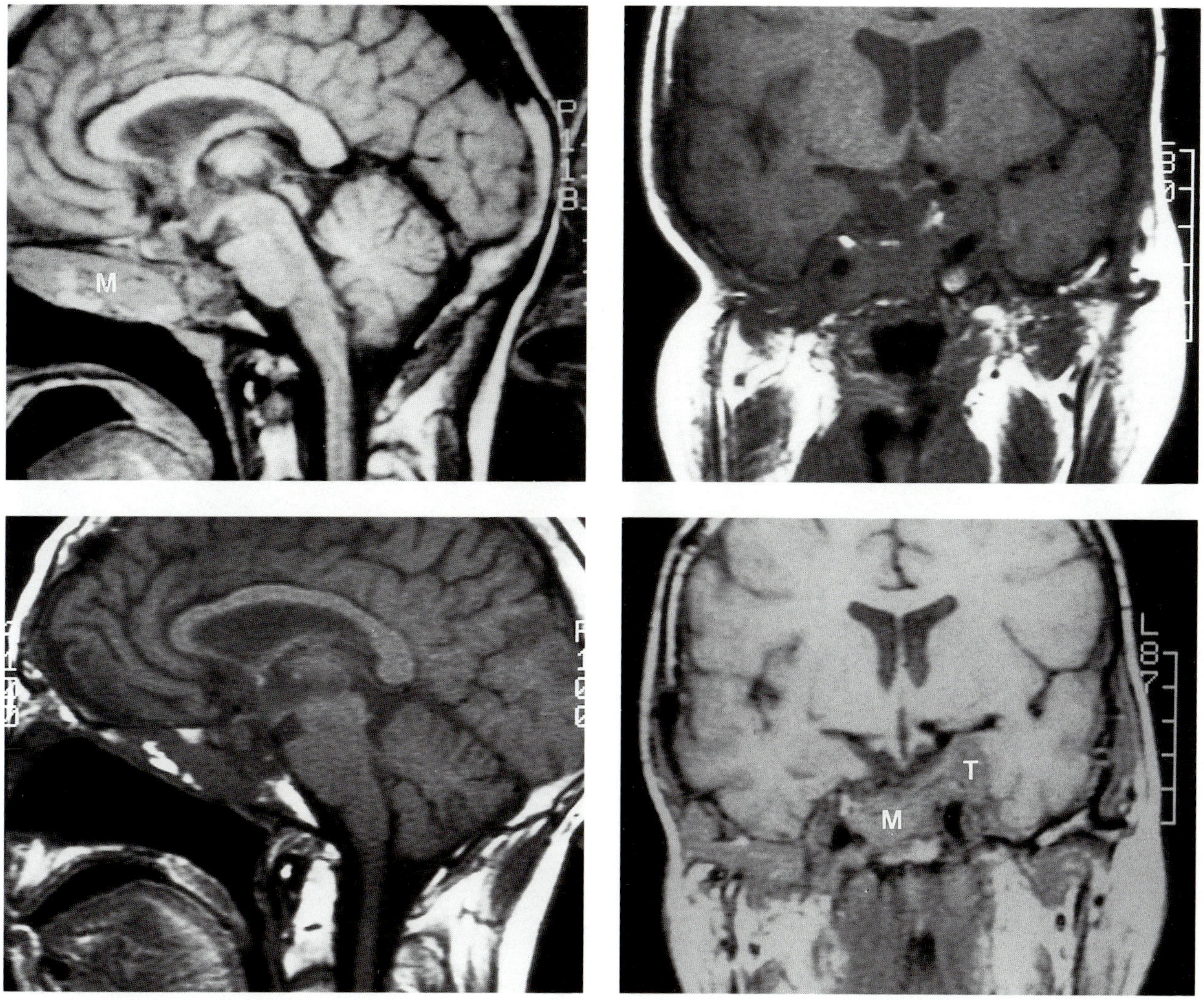

FIG. 45. T.E.–The patient's tumor was removed in two stages. During the first operation, a subtemporal–infratemporal lateral approach and a transethmoidal anterior approach were combined. All but the tumor in the left cavernous sinus and the suprasellar area could be removed by this operation. A rectus abdominis muscle flap was used for the reconstruction of the tumor bed (M, muscle flap). The patient required reexploration for a CSF leak from the subfrontal area. The tumor remnant was removed by an intradural frontotemporal approach, but a small residue remained in the CS (T, tumor residue) **(A–D)**. The patient's postoperative recovery was excellent. Adjuvant radiation therapy was given, and no tumor recurrence was seen after 5 years.

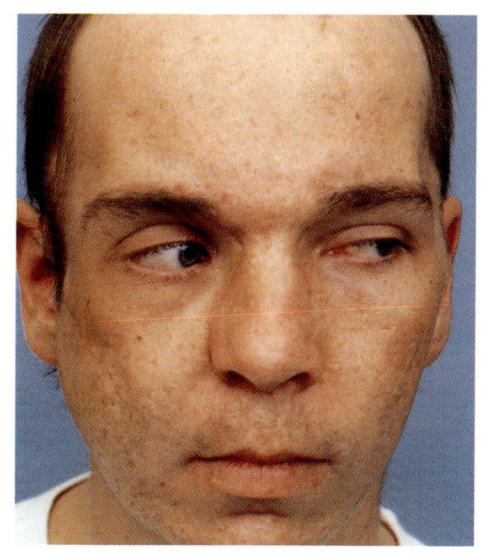
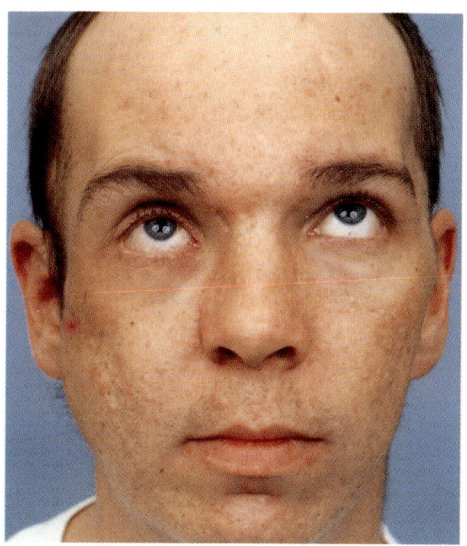

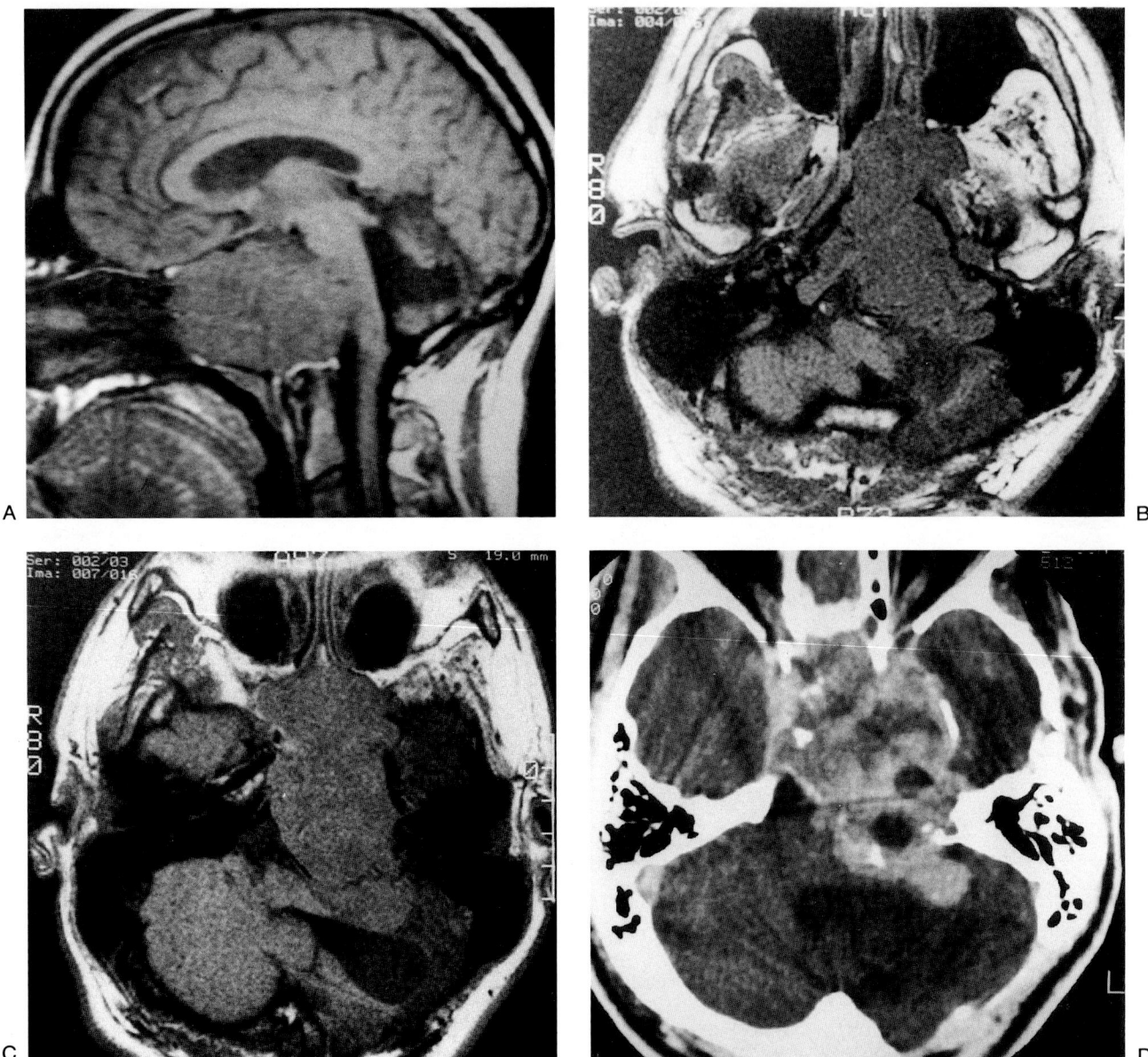

FIG. 47. K.P.–This 30-year-old patient had previously undergone two operations by a retrosigmoid approach with the partial resection of the giant neurilemoma. He presented with progressive growth of the tumor. Preoperative deficits included a partial facial paralysis (House Grade III function) and a complete hearing loss on the left side. Preoperative sagittal (**A**) and axial (**B, C, D**) scans reveal the extensive tumor.

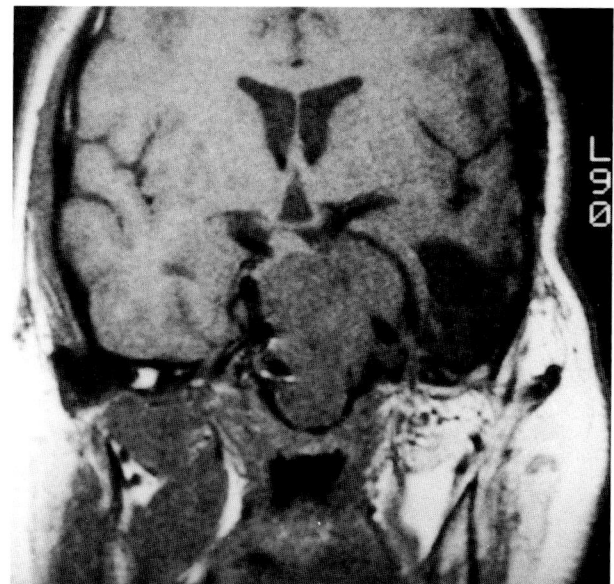 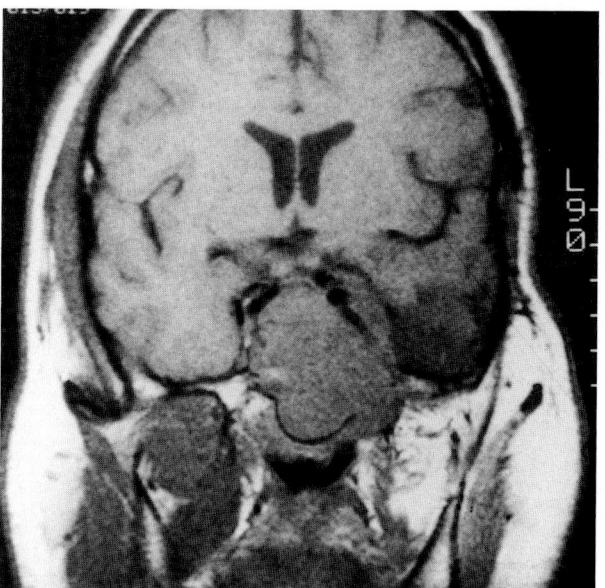

FIG. 48. A, B: K.P.–The coronal MRI scans show the extensive involvement of the right cavernous sinus. He was operated initially by a combined subtemporal–infratemporal approach and a basal frontal approach. Tumor remained in the cerebellopontine angle and petrous bone. At operation, the facial nerve was found to be tumor invaded. A total petrosectomy was therefore performed and the remaining tumor resected. Cranial nerve VII was reconstructed with a greater auricular nerve interposition graft. The patient eventually recovered House Grade III facial function.

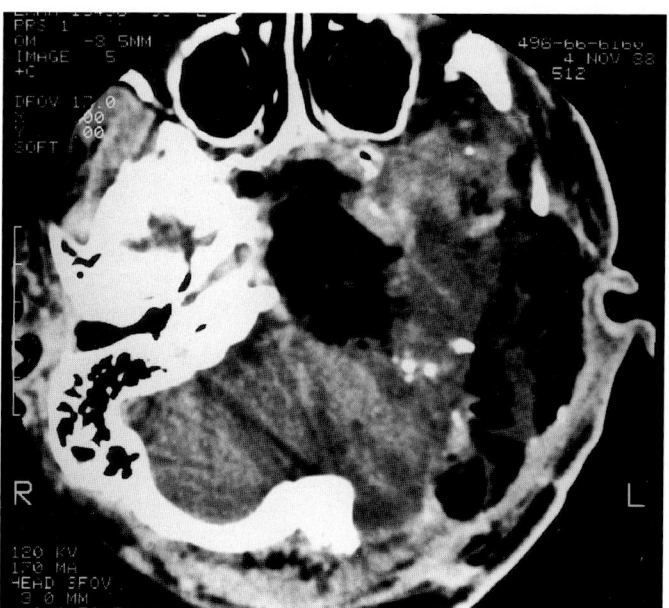 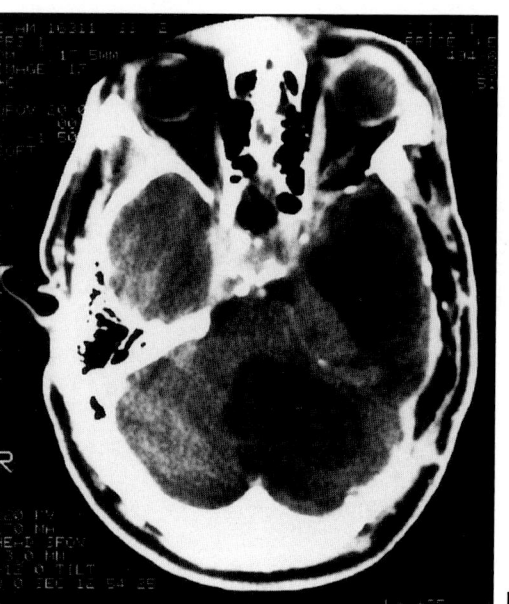

FIG. 49. A, B: K.P.–Postoperative CT scans show no tumor recurrence and a complete excision.

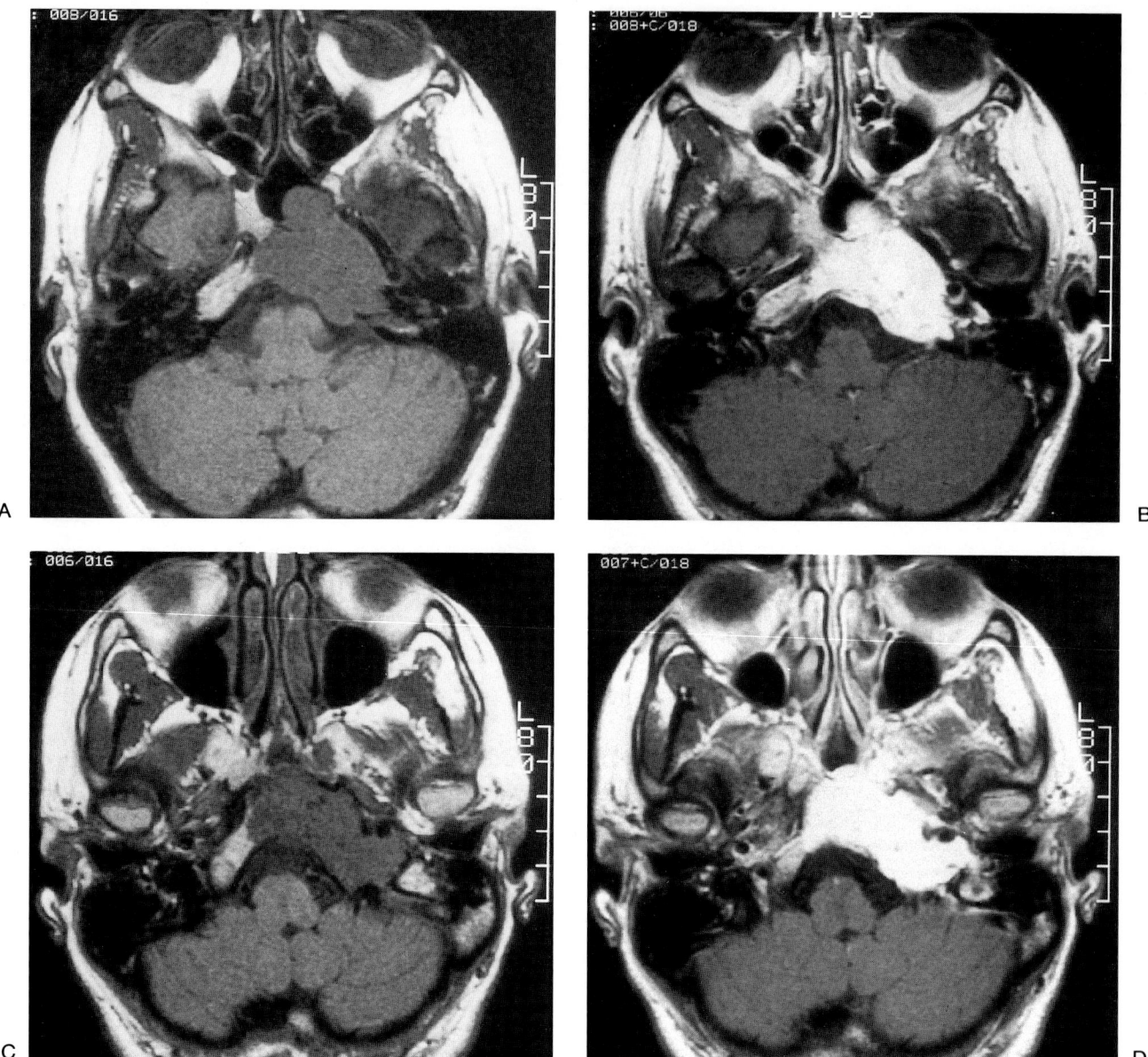

FIG. 50. B.W.–This 40-year-old patient presented with a sixth cranial nerve paresis and a previous history of removal of a chordoma by an intradural–subtemporal approach. Preoperative nonenhanced and enhanced MRI images reveal a large neoplasm involving the petroclival area (**A–D**).

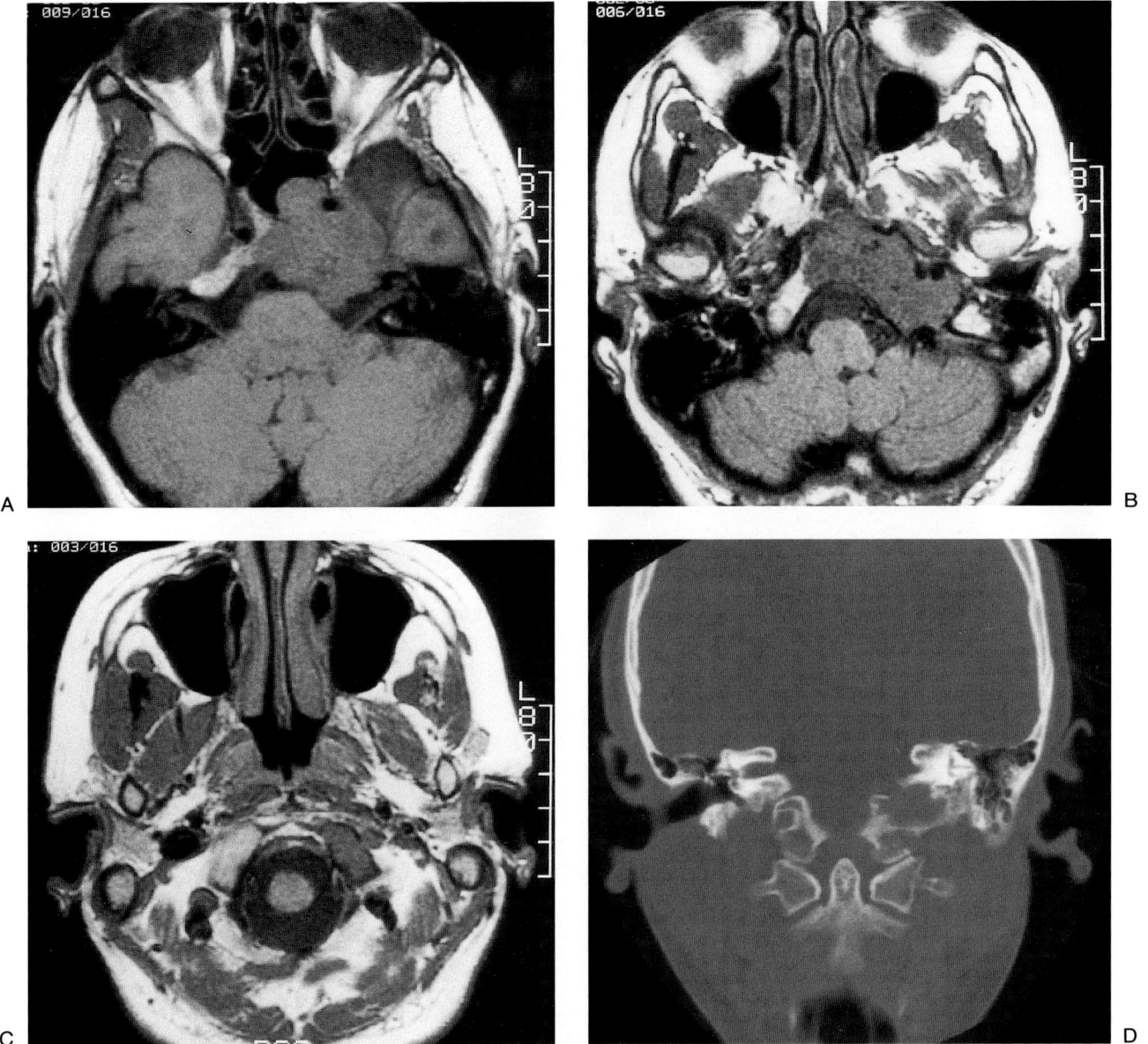

FIG. 51. B.W.–Further preoperative nonenhanced MRI scans (**A–C**) and the preoperative coronal CT image (**D**) show the involvement of the petroclival bone and the left occipital condyle.

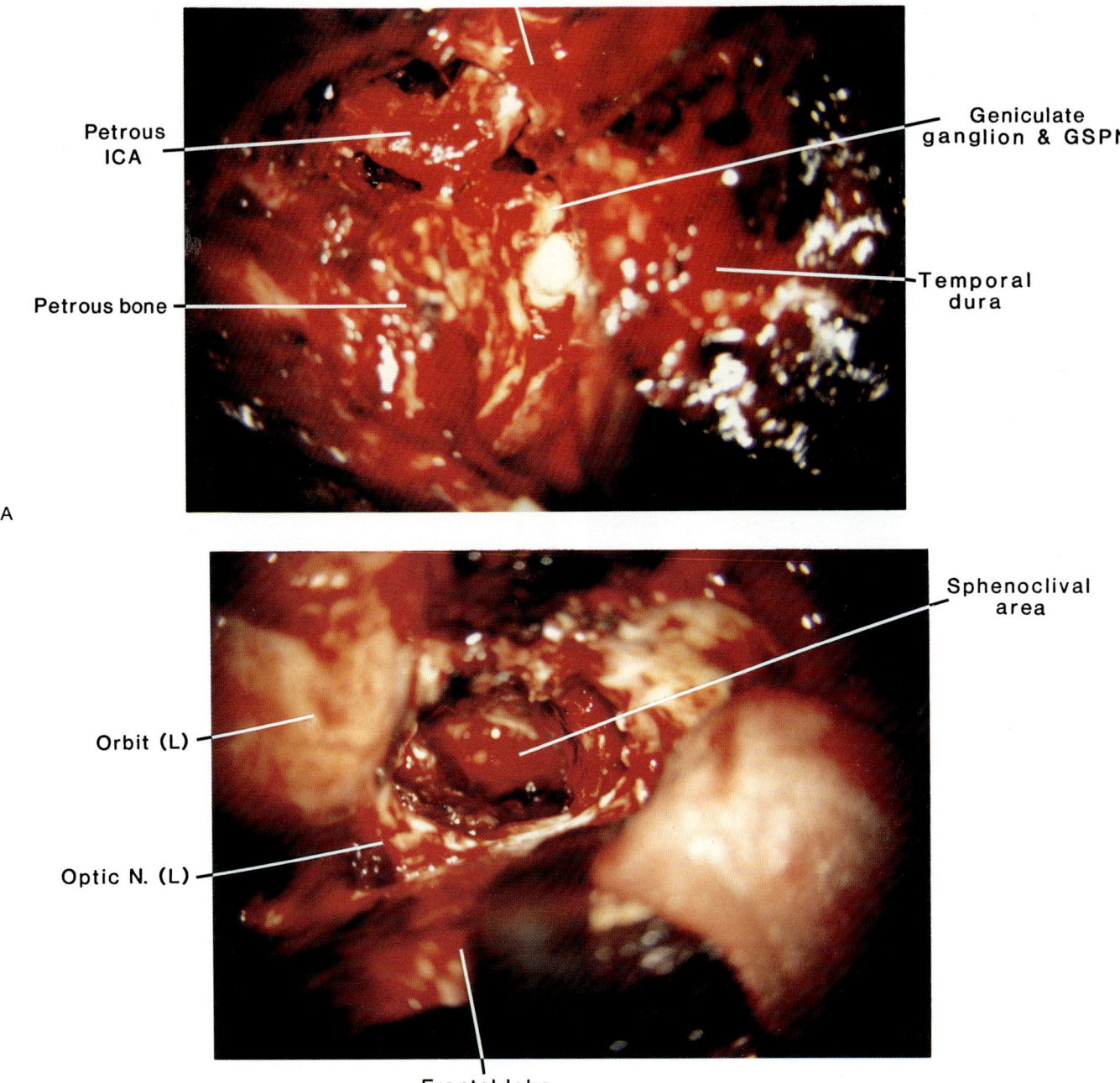

FIG. 52. During the initial operation, a subtemporal–infratemporal approach was combined with a basal frontal approach to remove the majority of the tumor. **A:** The subtemporal–infratemporal exposure of the lesion. **B:** The basal frontal exposure of the lesion.

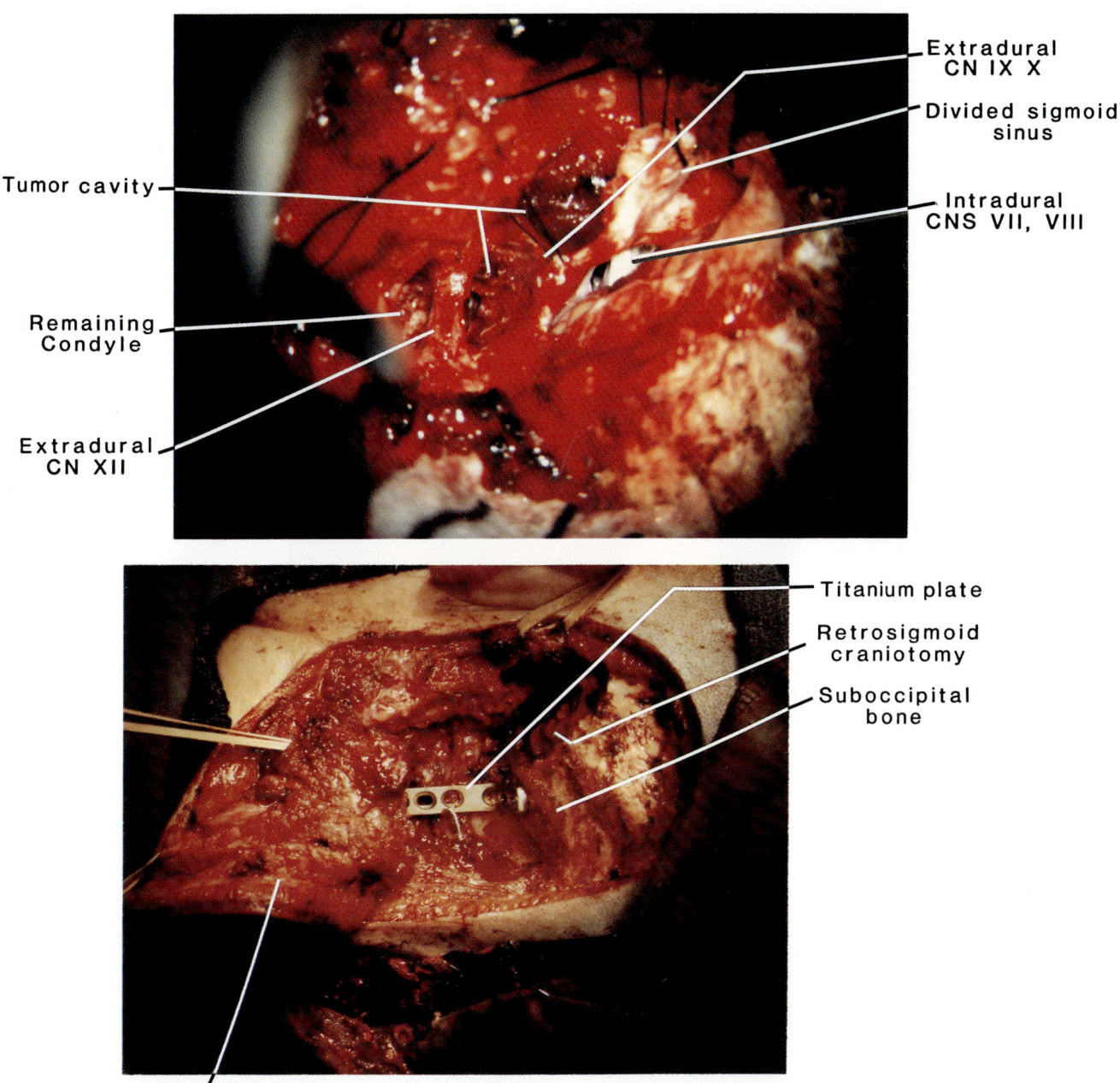

FIG. 53. During the next stage of the operation, a tumor remnant in the jugular foramen, occipital condyle, and lower clival area was removed by an extreme lateral, transcondylar, transjugular approach. At the same time, an occiput to C1–C2 fusion was performed with a titanium plate and bone graft because of complete excision of one condyle. **A:** The exposure after tumor resection. The dura has been partially opened to aid the identification of cranial nerves. **B:** The titanium plate fixation.

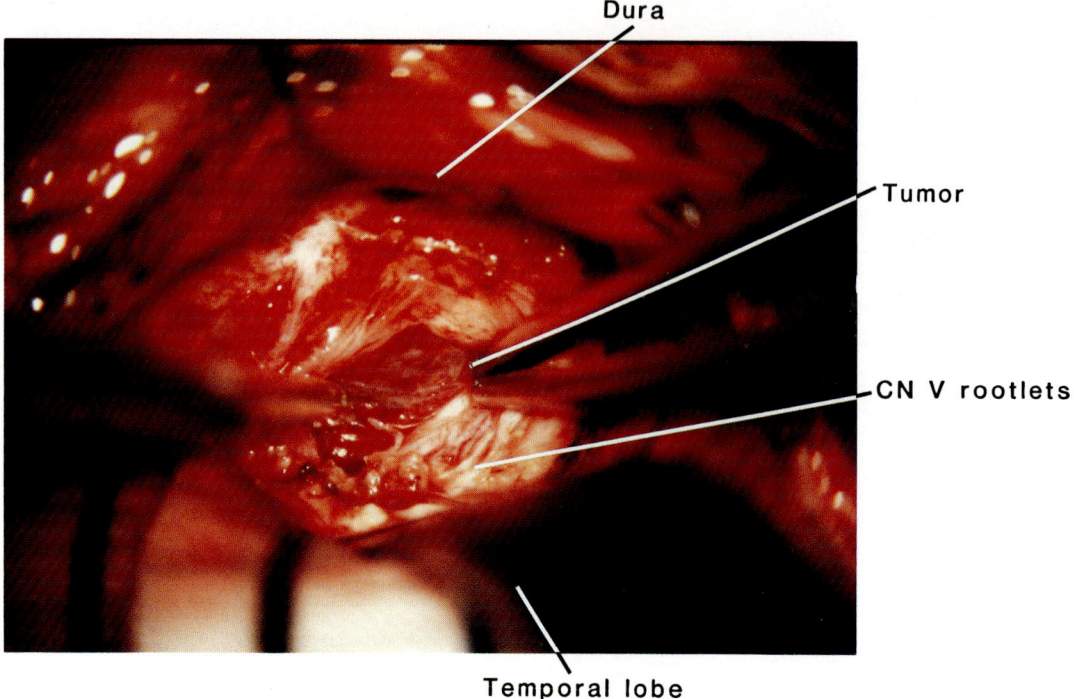

FIG. 54. A small tumor remnant was found in the posterior aspect of the cavernous sinus. This was removed by a very big operation by a subtemporal approach through Meckel's cave. The fibers of the trigeminal root were split to approach the tumor in this area. Photograph shows the rootlets of cranial nerve V_1 and the tumor medially.

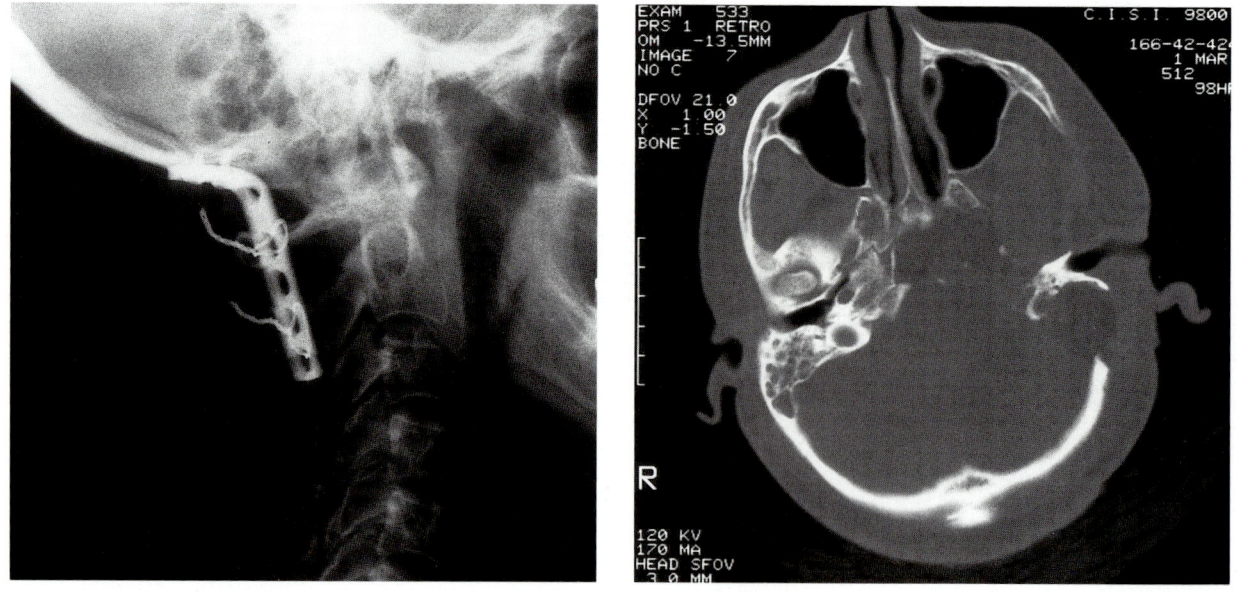

FIG. 55. Postoperative cervical spine radiograph (**A**) shows the fusion and the bone-window CT scan shows the bone resection (**B**).

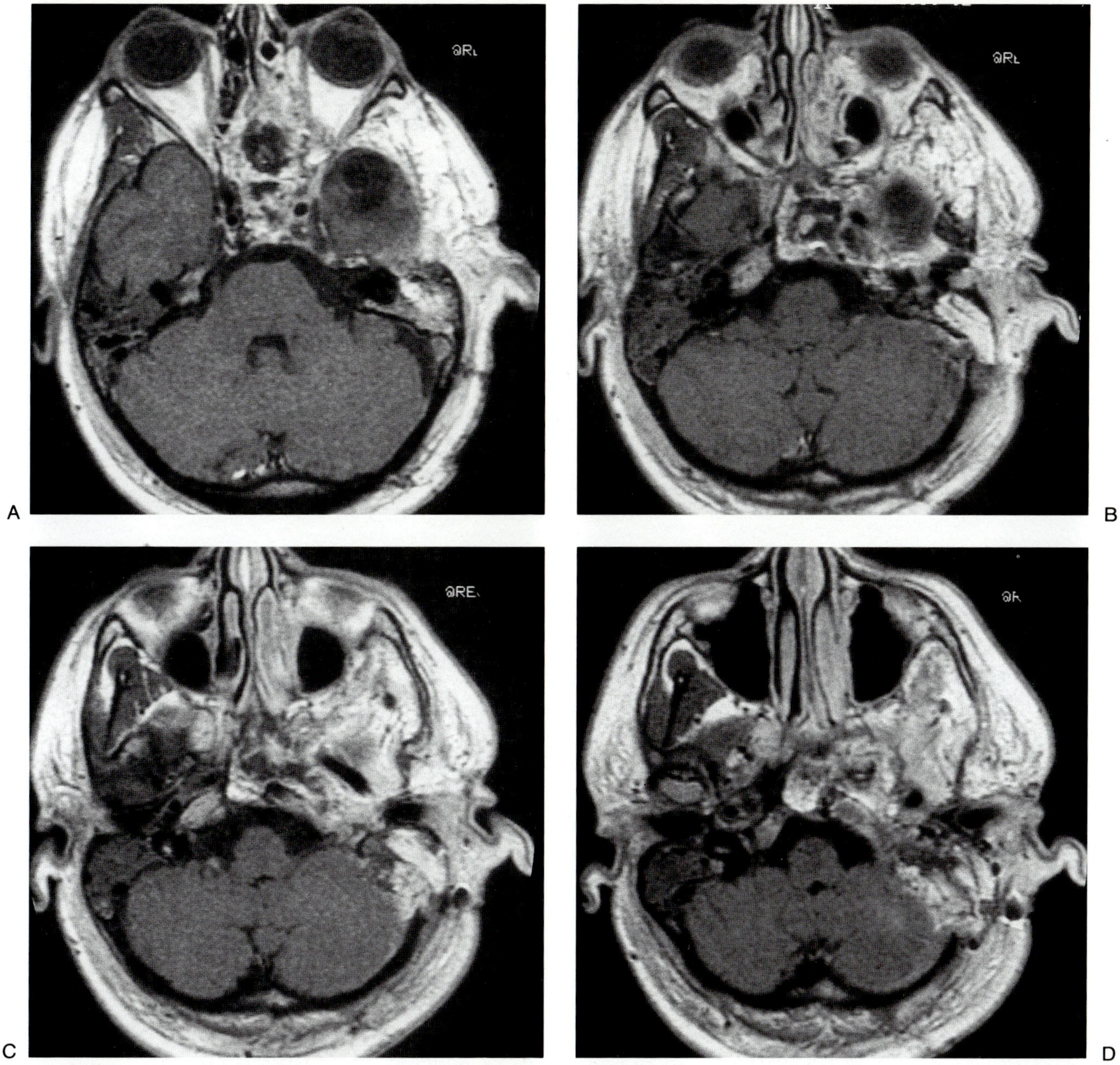

FIG. 56. A–D: Postoperative enhanced MRI scan shows complete tumor excision and enhancement of the vascularized flaps.

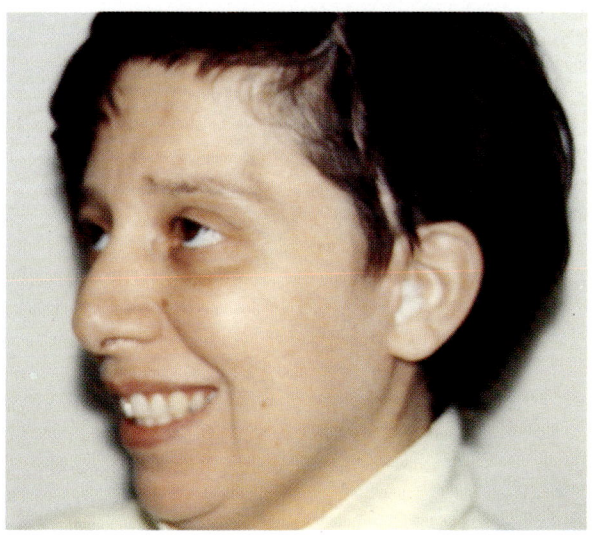

FIG. 57. Postoperative patient photograph. (Reproduced with patient's permission.)

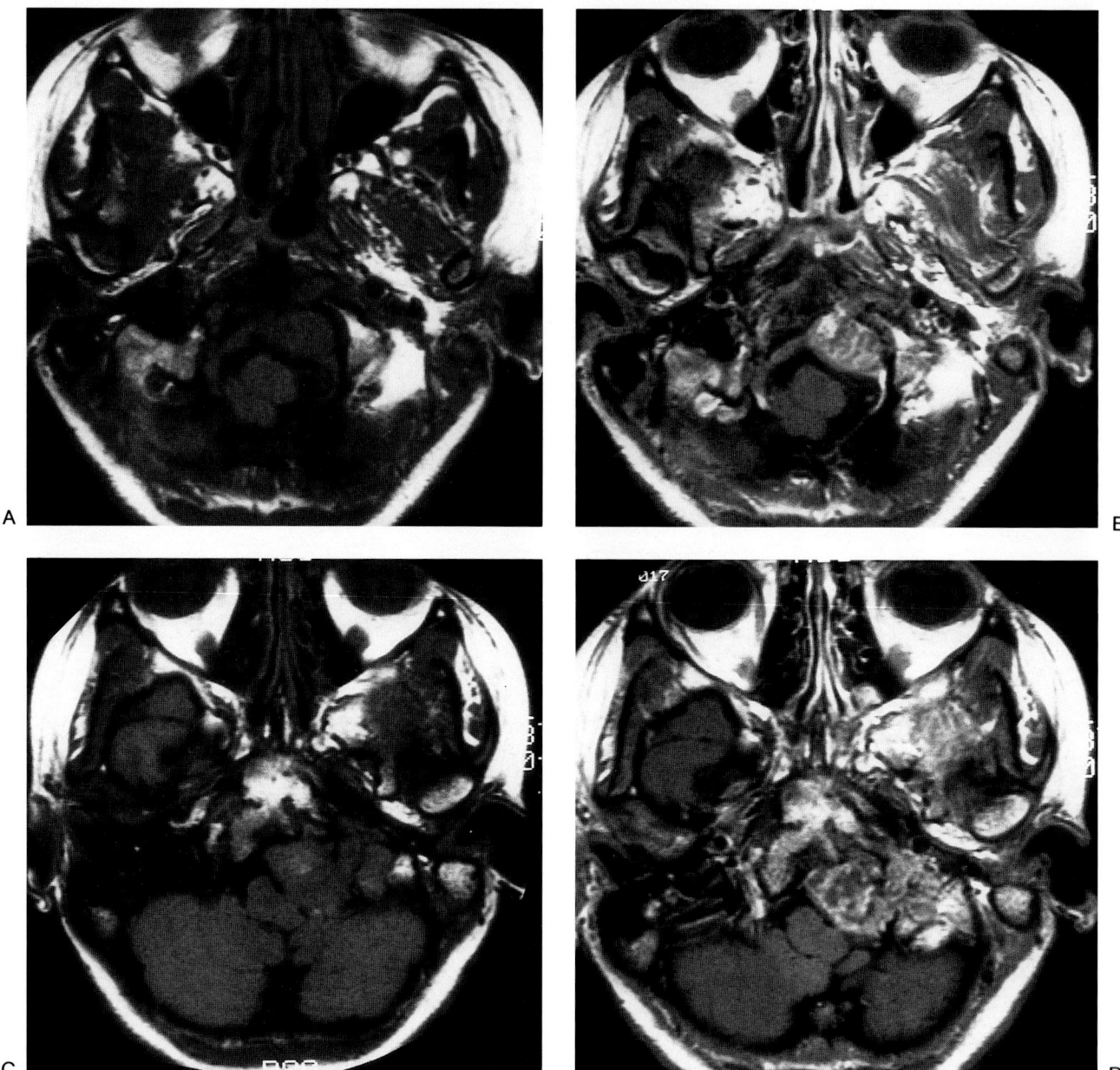

FIG. 58. A–D: A.G.-L.–This 19-year-old girl had undergone the transoral excision of a clivus chordoma 2 years previously. She presented with a recurrent tumor involving the lower clivus, jugular foramen posterior fossa, and the ipsilateral occipital condyle area. Tumor extent and brain stem compression are revealed in the nonenhanced preoperative MRI scans.

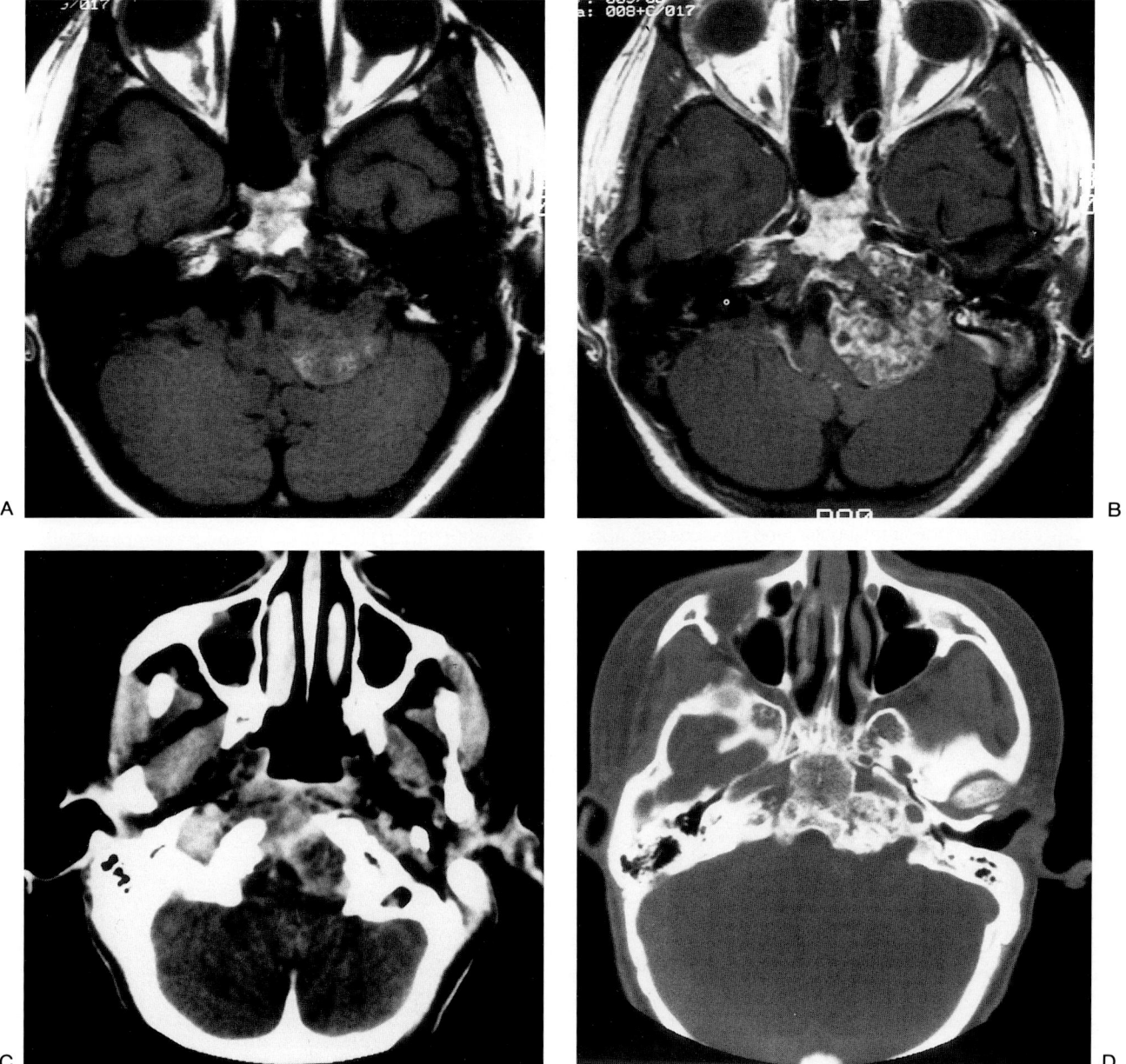

FIG. 59. A.G.-L.–Enhanced preoperative MRI scans (**A, B**) and CT scans (**C, D**) reveal the tumor extent and the brain stem compression.

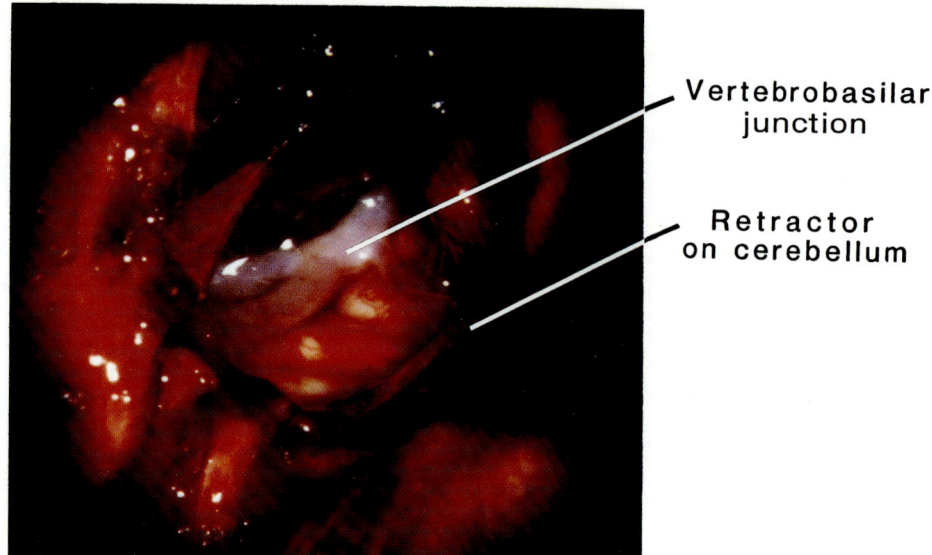

FIG. 60. Intraoperative photograph shows the vertebrobasilar junction after tumor resection by an extreme lateral, transjugular, and transcondyle approach. The dura had to be resected to ensure complete tumor removal.

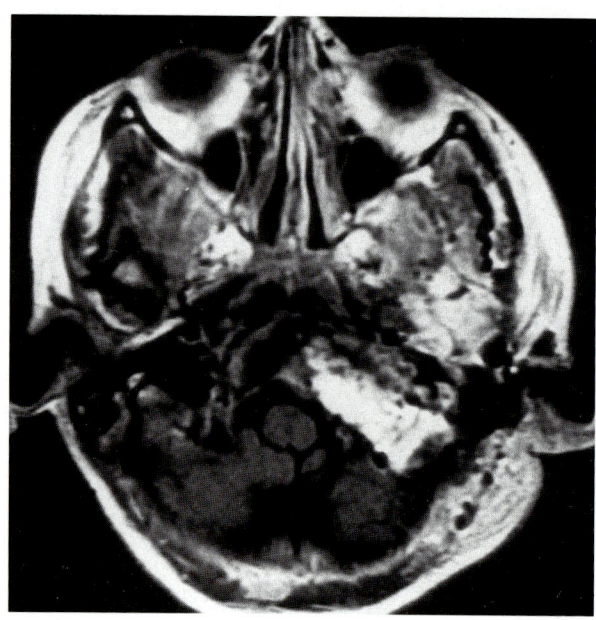

FIG. 61. Fascial lata was used for repair. Postoperative MRI scan shows the extent of tumor resection with this approach, and the fat used for reconstruction.

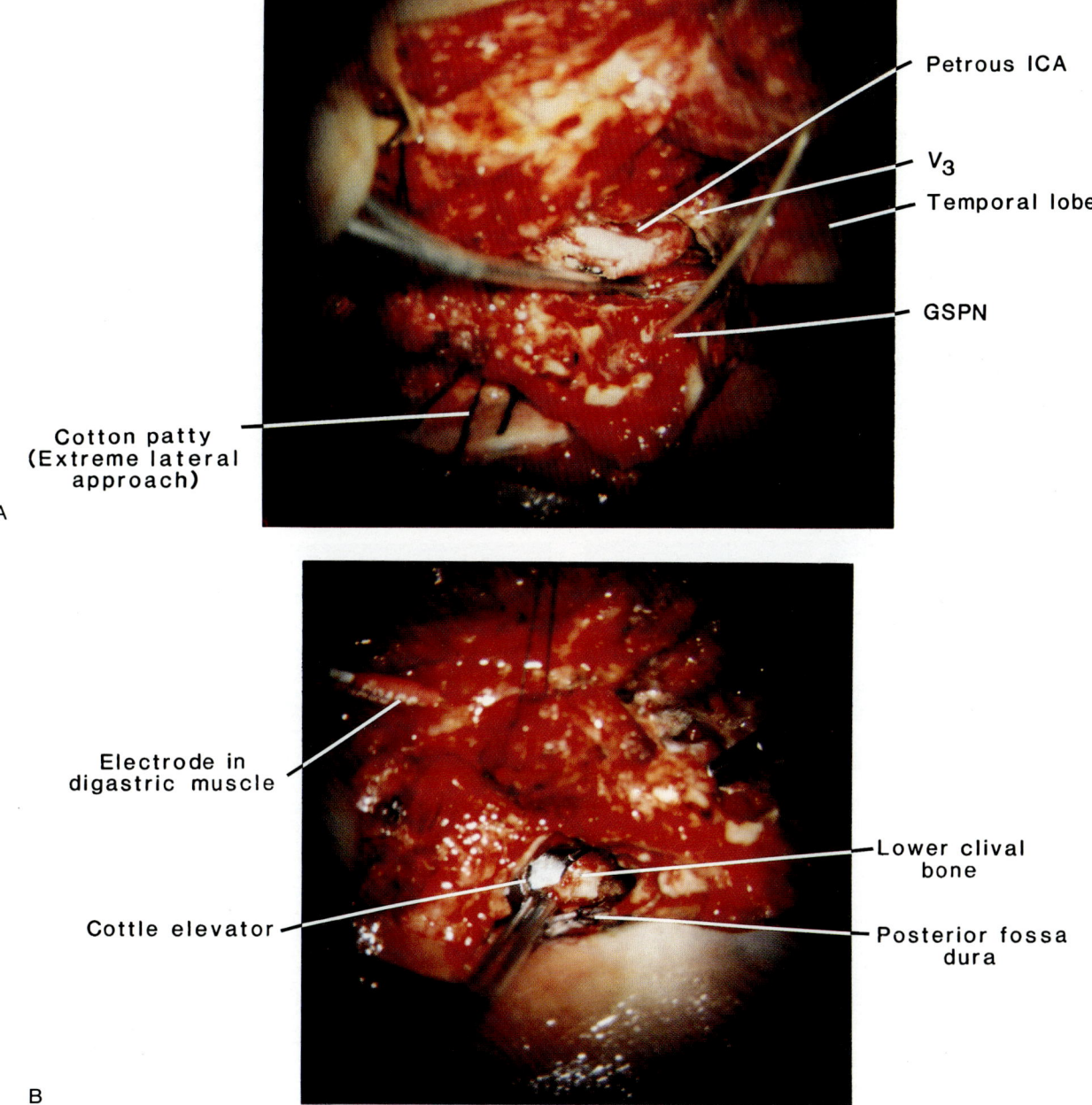

FIG. 62. During the second stage of tumor resection, a subtemporal–infratemporal approach was used to resect the remaining tumor. **A:** A monopolar electrode stimulating the greater superficial petrosal nerve (GSPN). Also seen are the petrous ICA, V_3, and the suction tip indicating the clivus. The intratemporal facial nerve has not been mobilized. The cottonoid has been inserted by the extreme lateral approach. **B:** A cottle elevator passed from the subtemporal–infratemporal approach medial to the petrous bone. The repaired dura and the electrode for monitoring electromyography from the digastric muscle are shown. The patient sustained a paresis of cranial nerves VII, IX, and X postoperatively but with quick recovery.

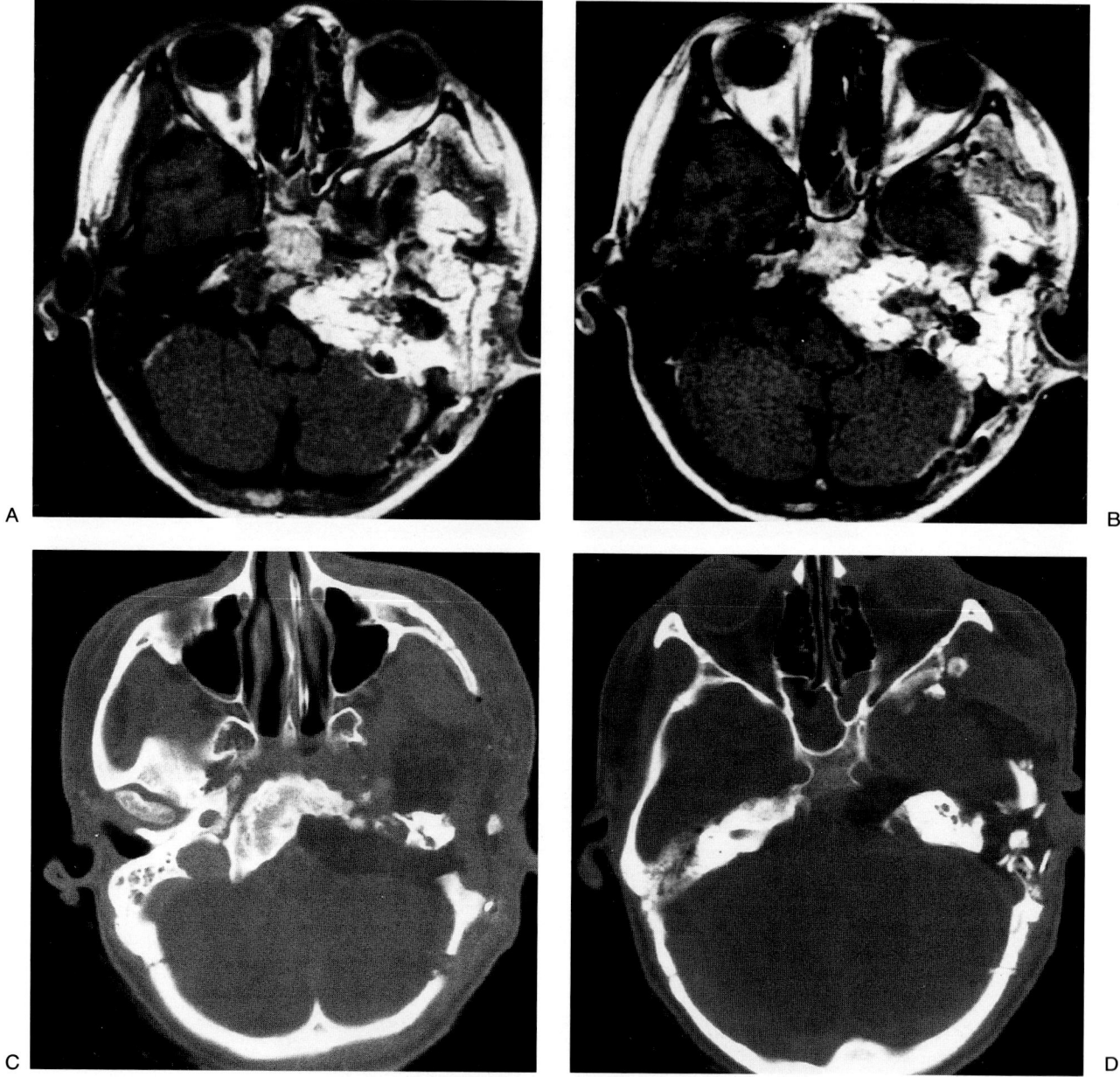

FIG. 63. A, B: Postoperative MRI scans document the tumor resection and the autologous fat used for reconstruction. **C, D:** The extent of bone resection with the sparing of the cochlea and labyrinth.

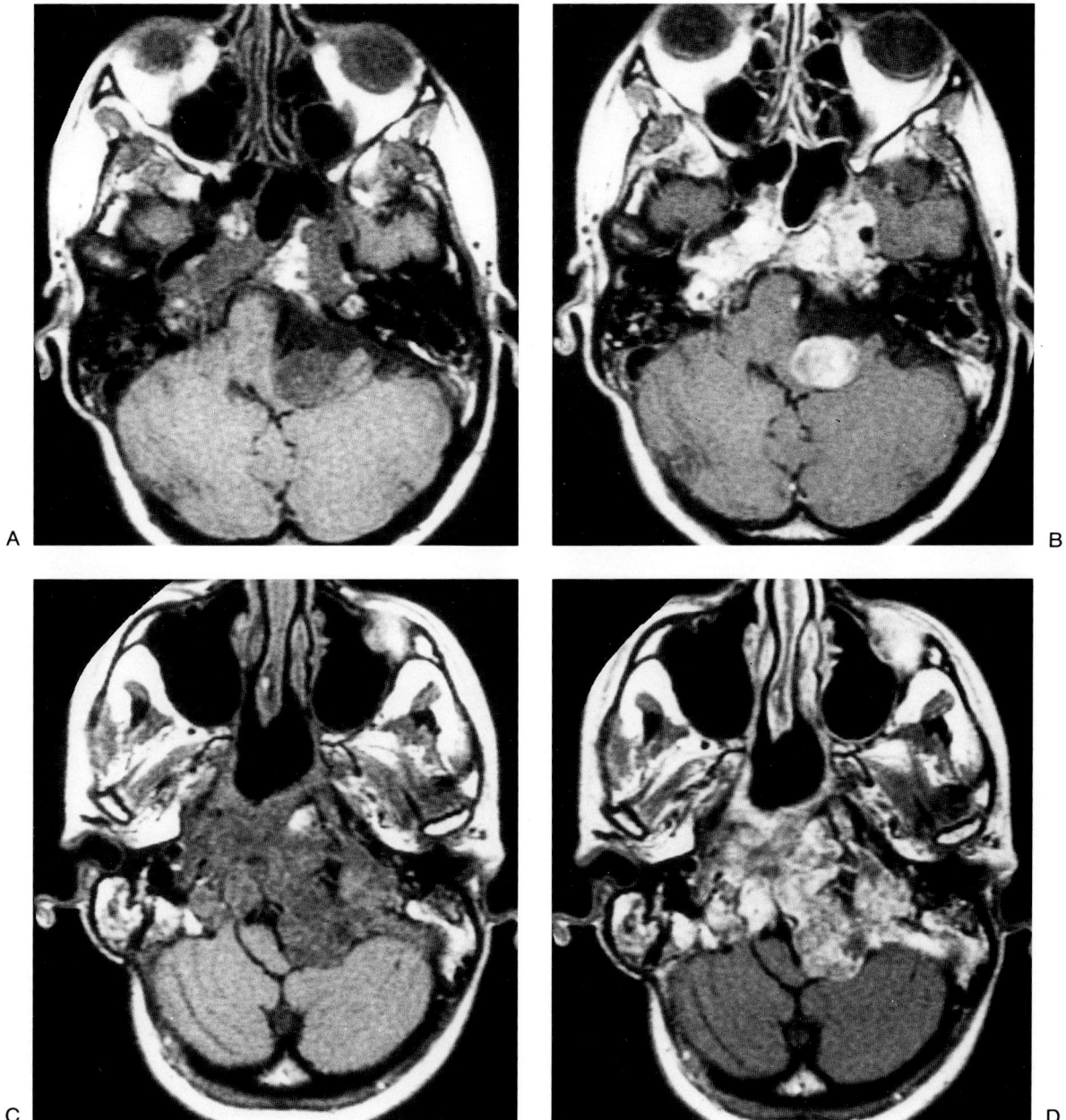

FIG. 64. A–D: K.K.–This 19-year-old woman had previously undergone two transoral approaches and one retrosigmoid approach to surgically resect this clivus chordoma, along with radiation therapy. She presented with significant deficits of cranial nerves IX, X, and XII. Preoperative nonenhanced and enhanced axial MRI scans show the tumor.

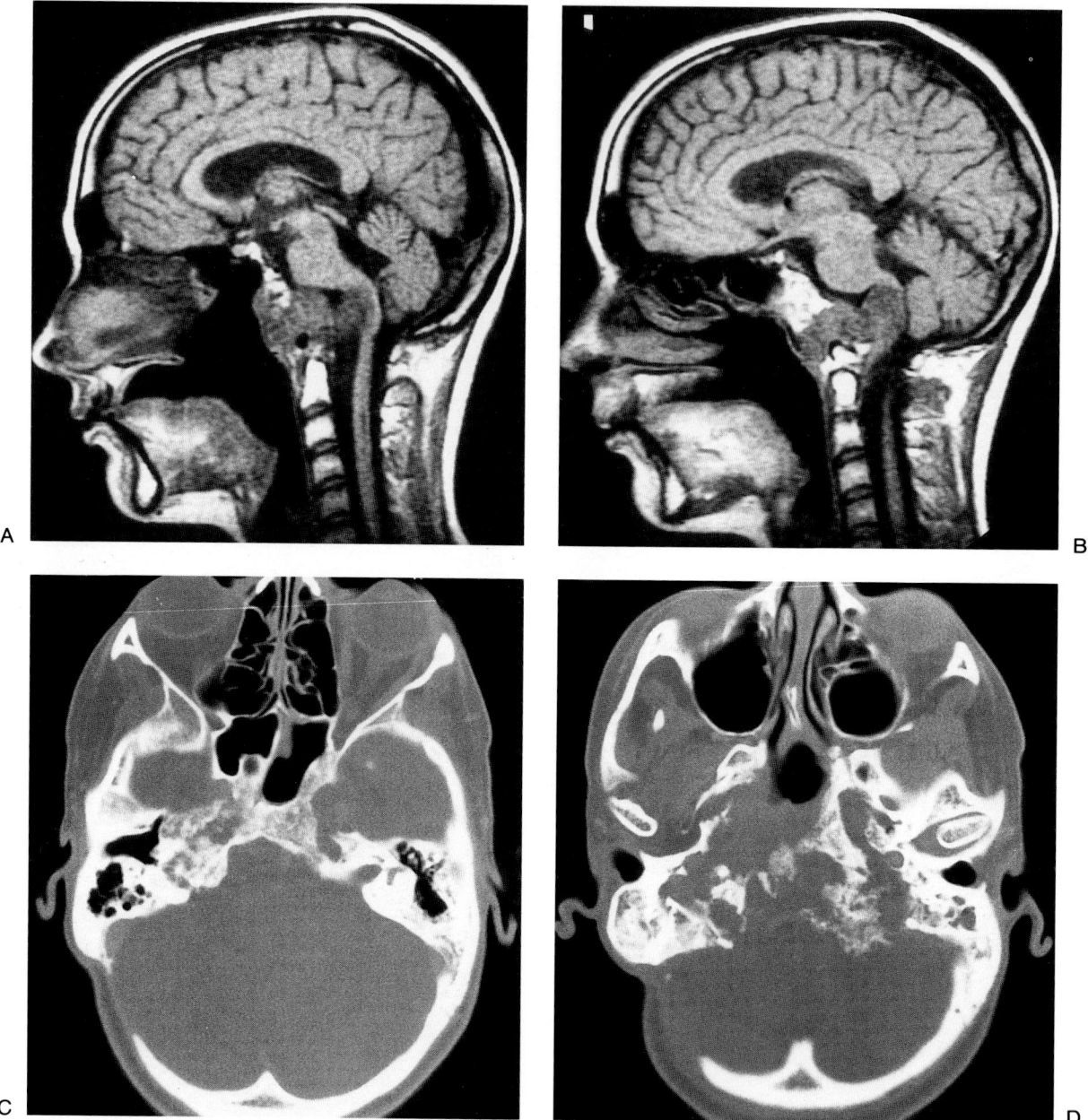

FIG. 65. K.K.–Sagittal MRI scans (**A, B**) and bone-window CT scans (**C, D**) show the tumor.

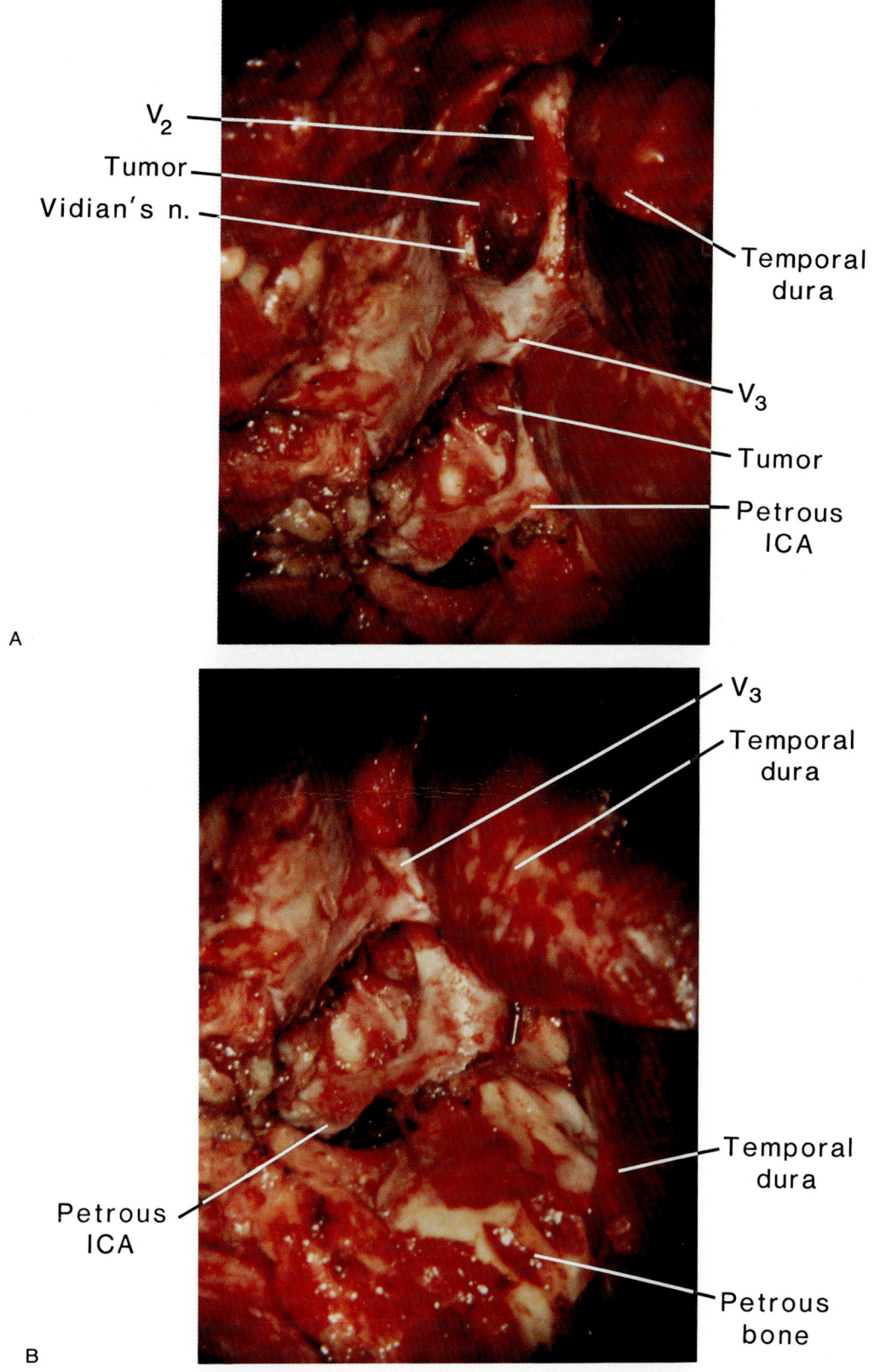

FIG. 66. The patient initially underwent an extreme lateral, transjugular, and transcondyle approach, and subsequently a subtemporal–infratemporal approach with division and reconstruction of V_3. A postauricular incision was made but the pinna was divided and resutured, resulting in the preservation of the conductive hearing mechanism. This series of photographs show the exposure by the subtemporal–infratemporal approach. **A:** The petrous ICA, V_3, tumor in the sphenoid sinus, and the vidian nerve are seen. **B:** A more magnified view of the petrous ICA and V_3 is seen.

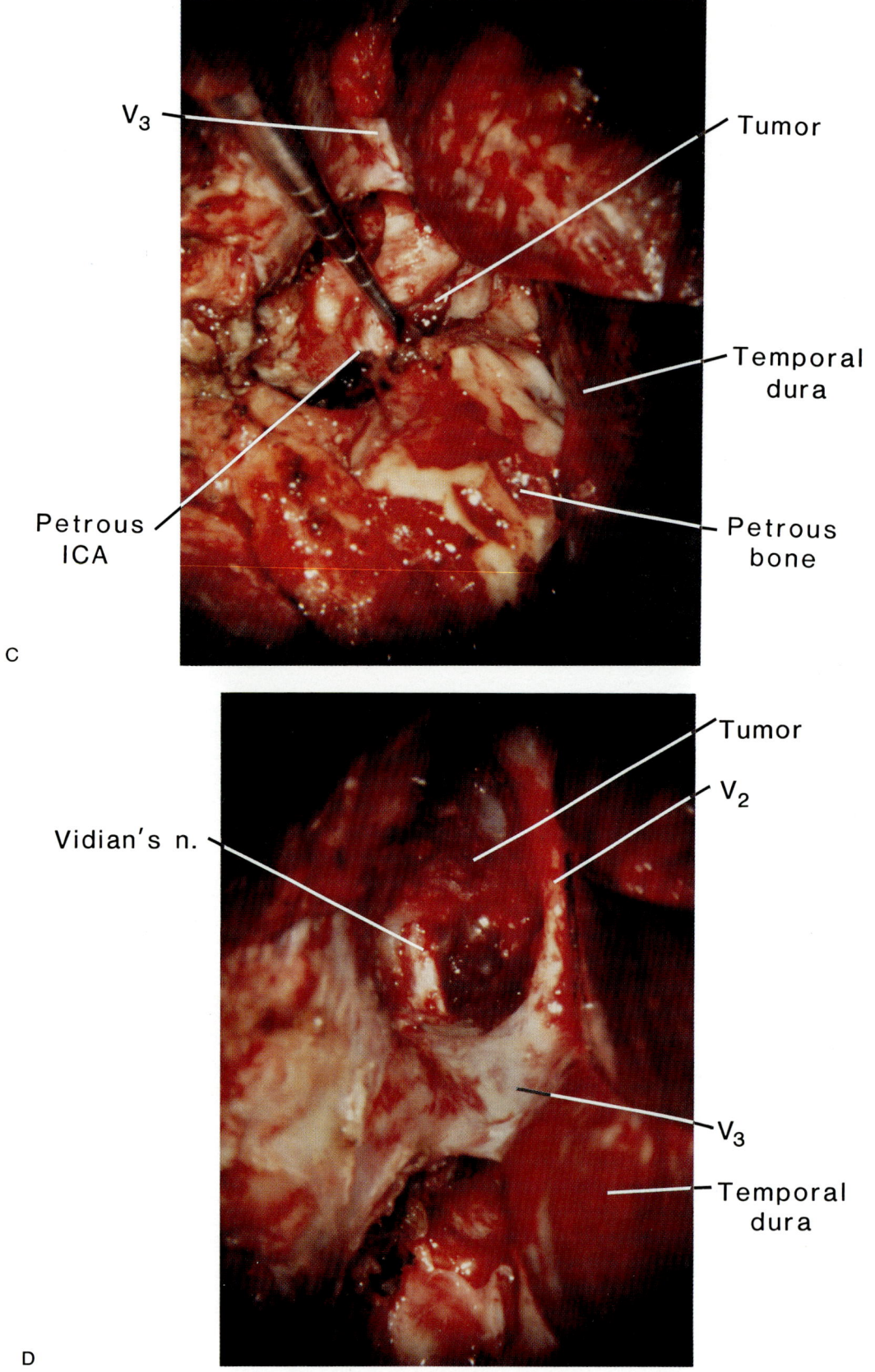

FIG. 66. *Continued.* **C:** The petrous ICA is being displaced, to show the tumor medial to it. **D:** Detail of the vidian nerve and tumor in the sphenoid sinus area.

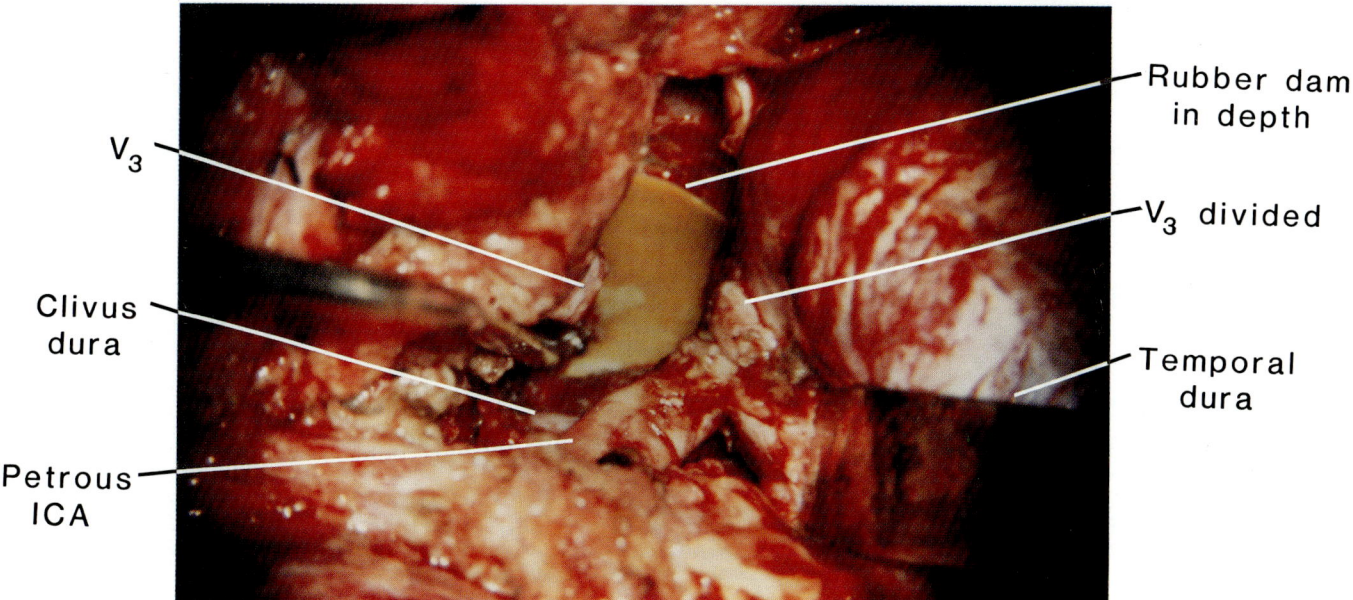

FIG. 66. *Continued.* **E:** V_3 has been divided, and the petrous ICA has been mobilized completely up to the cavernous sinus. This allows removal of tumor in the sphenoid sinus and the contralateral petrous apex. V_3 is resutured at the end by epineural sutures. The surgical defect was reconstructed with temporalis muscle and autologous fat.

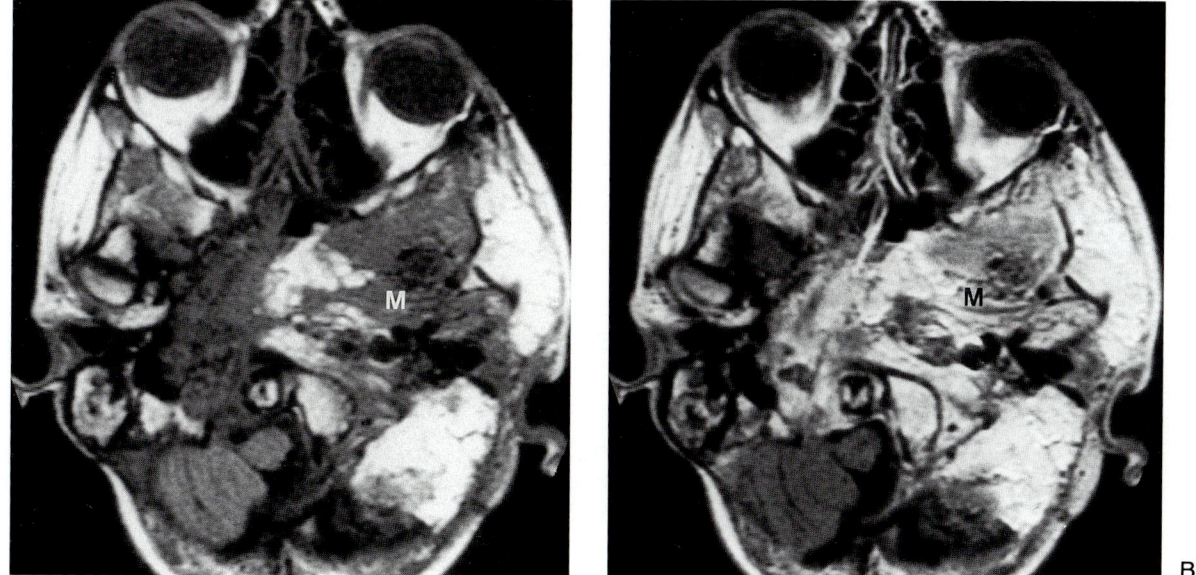

FIG. 67. The patient suffered a postoperative meningitis due to transient hydrocephalus and cerebrospinal fluid leakage. This resolved with antibiotics and spinal fluid drainage. The nonenhanced and enhanced postoperative MRI scans (**A–D**) show the absence of tumor in the midline–clival area, left petrous bone, and the left jugular foramen region. The muscle flap (M) is enhancing. There appears to be tumor residue in the left side of the clivus and petrous apex region, but biopsy of this region revealed only radiation-induced bone changes.

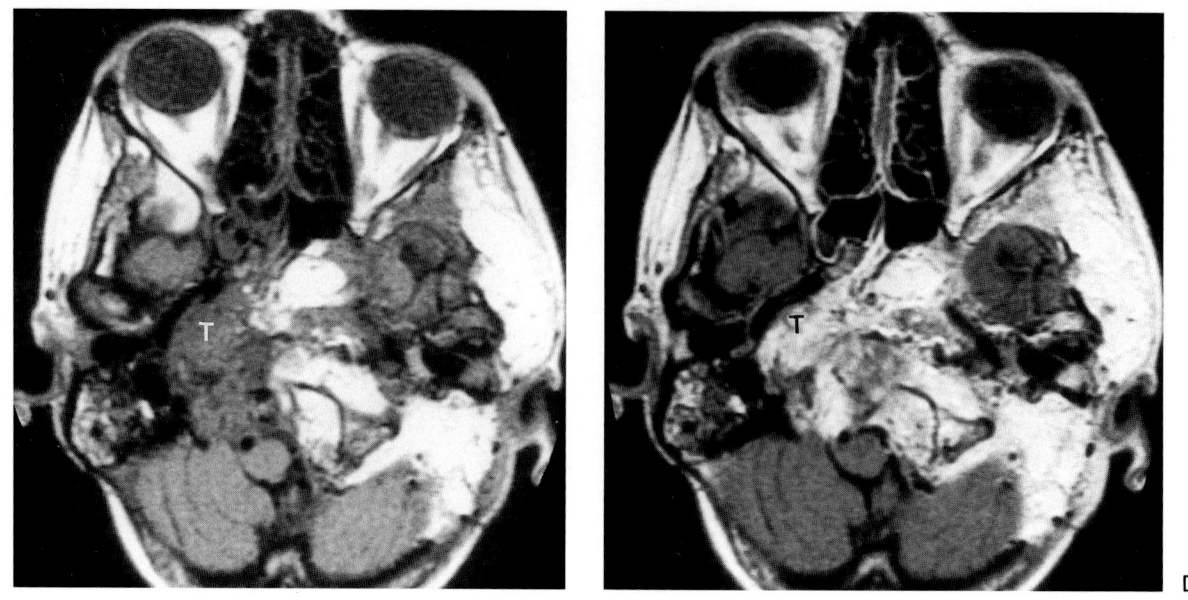

FIG. 67. Continued.

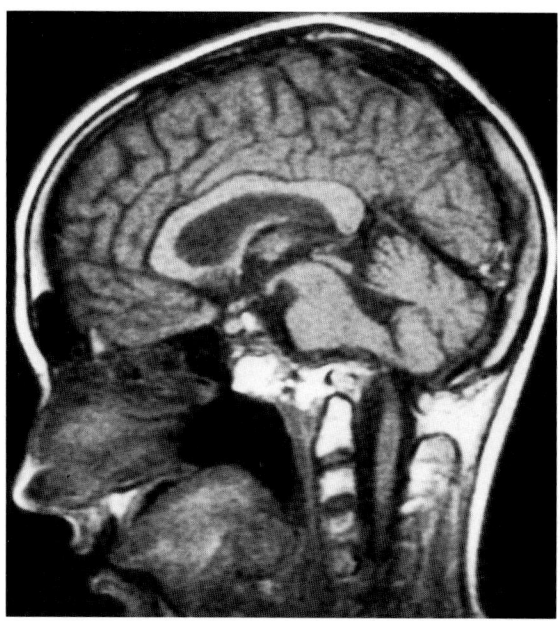

FIG. 68. A sagittal postoperative MRI showing fat in the area of previous tumor. This will subsequently undergo further shrinkage.

TABLE 2. *Extradural petroclival neoplasms operated 1983–1990: tumor resection and disease status*

Tumor type	Total	NED	AWD	DOD	DOC
Benign lesions					
Cholesterol granuloma	3	3	—	—	—
Epidermoid cyst	1	1	—	—	—
Chondroblastoma	1	1	—	—	—
Neurilemoma IX, X	4	4	—	—	—
Meningioma	4	2	—	1	1
Glomus jugulare	4	4	—	—	—
Teratoma, benign	1	1	—	—	—
Carniopharyngioma	2	1	—	1	—
	20	17	—	2	1
Low grade malignancies					
Chordoma	18	9	8	1	—
Chondrosarcoma	11	5	6	—	—
Cardiac myxoma (metastatic)	1	1	—	—	—
Pituitary adenoma (invasive)	5	4	1	—	—
Adenoid cystic carcinoma	5	2	2	1	—
	40	21	17	2	—
High grade malignancies					
Squamous cell carcinoma	4	—	—	4	—
Adenocarcinoma	1	—	—	1	—
Basal cell carcinoma	1	1	—	—	—
Osteogenic sarcoma	2	1	1	—	—
	8	2	1	5	1

EXPERIENCE WITH EXTRADURAL PETROCLIVAL NEOPLASMS

The authors' experience with surgical resection of extradural petroclival neoplasms during the years 1983–1990 is summarized in Table 2. In addition to approaches described here, transtemporal approaches requiring the mobilization of cranial nerve VII were also used in some patients. In four patients, CN VII was resected because of prior tumor invasion, or intraoperative injury, and reconstructed with an interposition graft. The tumors are considered under three categories: benign, low grade malignant, and high grade malignant (Table 2). *Benign lesions* were quite varied in their histology. Included in this group were meningiomas and glomus jugulare tumors with major extradural petroclival involvement. *Low grade malignancies* were predominantly chordomas and chondrosarcomas, but also included are some invasive pituitary adenomas, and adenoid cystic carcinomas (22). *High grade malignancies* were varied, including squamous cell cancer, adenocarcinoma, basal cell carcinoma, and osteogenic sarcoma.

Many of these tumors were very extensive and had been previously operated. In some patients, staged operations were essential to achieve complete tumor resection. With increasing experience, our ability to achieve apparently complete tumor resection (based on postoperative CT or MRI studies) has improved steadily, and the morbidity has declined. The follow-up ranges from a few months to 7 years, with a median of 3.5 years. As can be seen from Table 3, when total resection was achieved, local recurrence was very uncommon, occurring only in two highly malignant lesions (Table 3). However, when overall patient status was considered, patients with highly malignant lesions fared poorly, due to the development of metastatic disease (Table 2). It therefore appears that, in future, success in the treatment of highly malignant lesions involving the clivus will depend on the availability of improved methods of adjuvant therapy.

Complications

The complications encountered during operative management of extensive petroclival tumors and their

TABLE 3. *Petroclival neoplasms operated 1983–1990: extent of resection versus local recurrence*

Neoplasm	Resection	Local recurrence
Benign		
Total excision	17	0
Partial excision + radiation	3	2
Low grade malignancy		
Total excision	20	2
Partial excision + radiation	20	8
High grade malignancy		
Total excision	7	2
Partial excision + radiation or chemotherapy	1	0

TABLE 4. Extradural petroclival neoplasms, 1983–1990: operative complications

Death (infection, bilateral ICA rupture)	1	
Cerebral infarct		
Delayed ICA occlusion, moderate recovery	1	
Basilar perforator occlusion, no recovery	1	
Basilar perforator injury, thalamic hemorrhage	1	
Temporary hemiparesis, internuclear ophthalmoplegia (recovered)	1	
Pneumocephalus 2° to postoperative spinal fluid drainage	2	
Subdural hematoma, chronic (related to above)	2	
Cerebrospinal fluid leakage (all reoperated)		
Eustachian tube	2	
Wound	2	
Ethmoid sinus	1	
Sphenoid sinus	5	
Hydrocephalus, needing shunt	3	
Infection		
Wound (excluding above case)	1	
Meningitis (CSF leak associated)	2	
Pharyngotympanic fistula (reoperation)	1	
Cranial nerve palsies	Temporary	Permanent
CN III	5	—
CN IV	5	—
CN V	2	—
CN VI	10	—
CN VII	12	—
CN IX, X	6	4
CN XII	3	1

causes are discussed below (Tables 4 and 5). Retraction-induced brain swelling or hematoma is a potential complication that was not observed in our series.

One early patient with extensive squamous cell carcinoma and bilateral ICA encasement was operated, with the idea of debulking the tumor considerably before treatment with radiation therapy (Fig. 68). The ipsilateral upper cervical ICA was intraoperatively injured and repaired. The patient did well initially postoperatively but sustained a massive hemorrhage from the ICA a week later since the temporalis muscle flap used for reconstruction was avascular and failed to exclude the ICA from the nasopharynx. The patient was initially salvaged with ICA repair and a rectus abdominis free muscle flap. A few days later, the contralateral ICA ruptured and was occluded, and the patient recovered. But she eventually succumbed to uncontrolled sepsis. In retrospect, this patient's tumor was unsuitable for operation. However, this and two other instances of carotid or vertebral artery rupture (in patients without petroclival tumors) reinforce our caution against the use of operative approaches through the upper aerodigestive passage (e.g., transoral or transmaxillary approach), which may leave arteries exposed at the end of the operation to the virulent bacterial flora that inhabit these areas. When such approaches expose the arteries, the vessel should be protected with a vascularized flap.

Three patients suffered cerebral infarction. A 2-year-old child had the delayed occlusion of the ICA opposite to the side of the operation, presumably caused by excessive head turning during the operation, kinking of the ICA by the styloid process, and perioperative hypercoagulability. In two other cases, brain stem perforator injuries occurred in patients who had large previously operated tumors with extensive involvement of the basilar artery from tumor and/or scar tissue. In one of these patients with a very heavily calcified tumor, this injury occurred even though we did not actually remove tumor near the basilar artery, presumably due to rocking the remaining tumor against the arteries. Although the patient recovered well from this initially, this was followed by an unfortunate cascade of complications including severe hypertension and thalamic hemorrhage, sepsis, and hypotension (Fig. 69). He remains severely disabled.

CSF leaks occurred in patients in whom the tumor was both intradural and extradural, or wherein the dura was excised along with the tumor. They were successfully repaired.

Cranial nerve palsies were, for the most part, temporary. Facial nerve palsy was usually associated with mobilization of the nerve in its intratemporal segment or its resection and graft reconstruction. When cranial nerve VII was not mobilized from the temporal bone, temporary cranial nerve VII palsy was followed by an early

TABLE 5. Outcome of operative complications

Died	1
Mild disability, died of disease	1
Severe disability, living	2

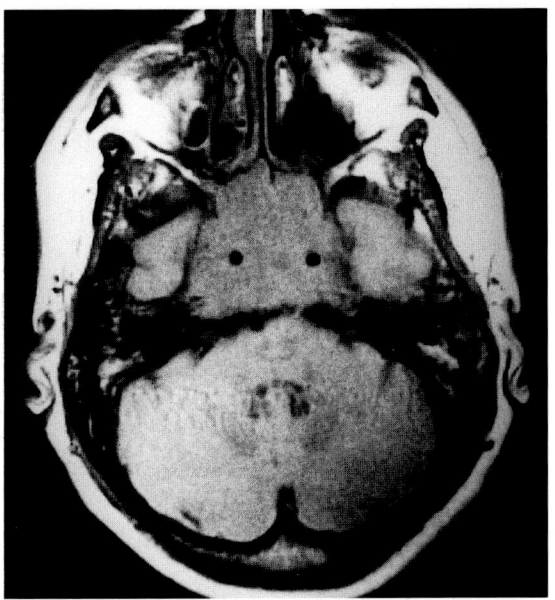 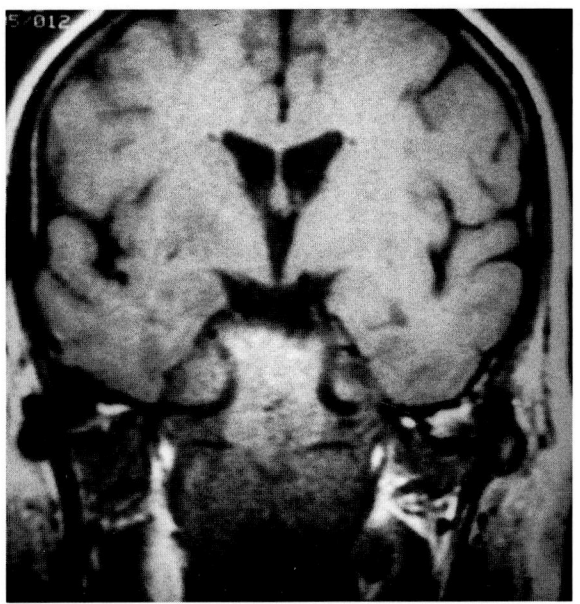

FIG. 69. A, B: Patient with an extensive squamous cell carcinoma encasing both petrous internal carotid arteries and with extension into both cavernous sinuses. This patient suffered bilateral ICA rupture and died eventually because of infection.

recovery to a House Grade I or II function. When cranial nerve VII was displaced from the temporal bone or grafted, the recovery was usually to a House Grade III. Deficits of cranial nerves IX and X were due to tumor invasion.

Except for the case reported above, infections were generally easily treatable, including two cases of meningitis following CSF leakage through the wound. One patient who had an extensive chordoma involving the clival, sphenoidal, and cavernous sinus areas was referred to us after a transoral biopsy. The tumor was initially removed by a combined anterior and lateral approach, reconstruction being performed with a galeopericranial flap and autologous fat. The fat necrosed and she developed a pharyngotympanic fistula about 2 months postoperatively (Fig. 70). She was reoperated by an extreme

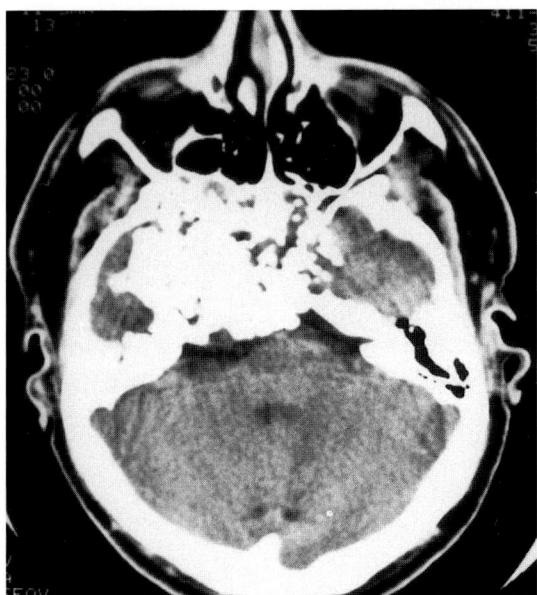 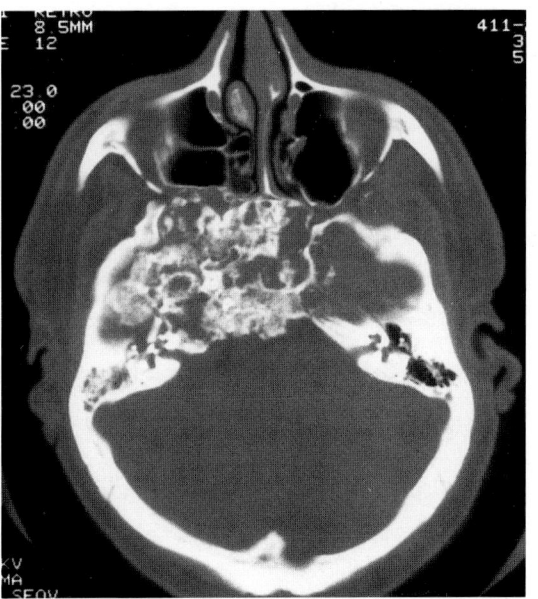

FIG. 70. Patient with a very extensive, recurrent, petroclival chondrosarcoma who suffered a brain stem infarction postoperatively and is significantly disabled as a result (A, B). The pictures show nonenhanced CT scans in soft tissue and bone windows (C, D).

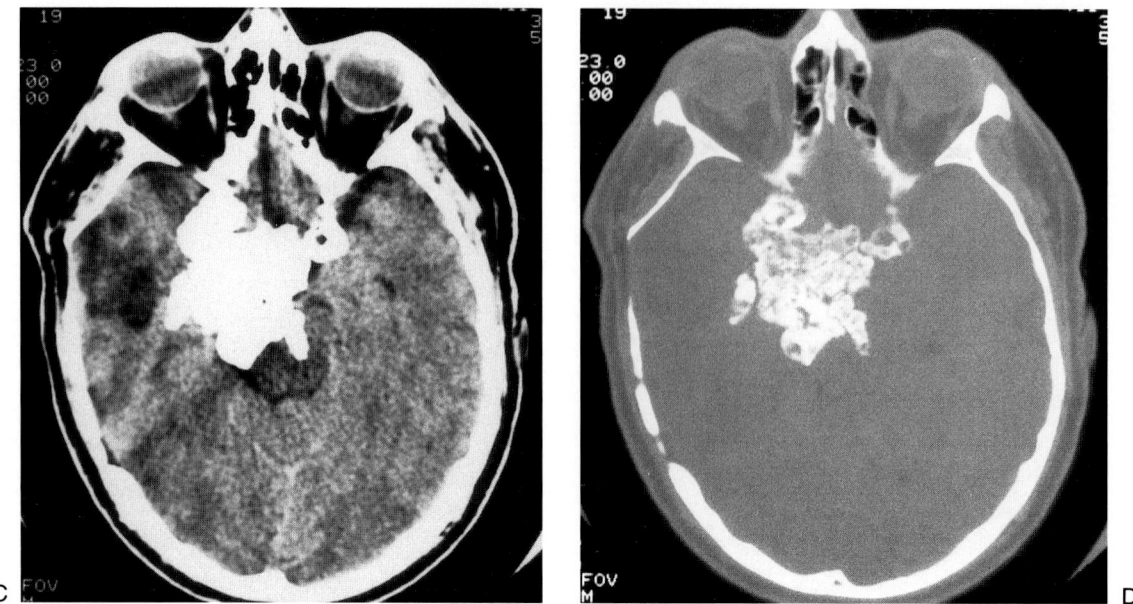

FIG. 70. *Continued.*

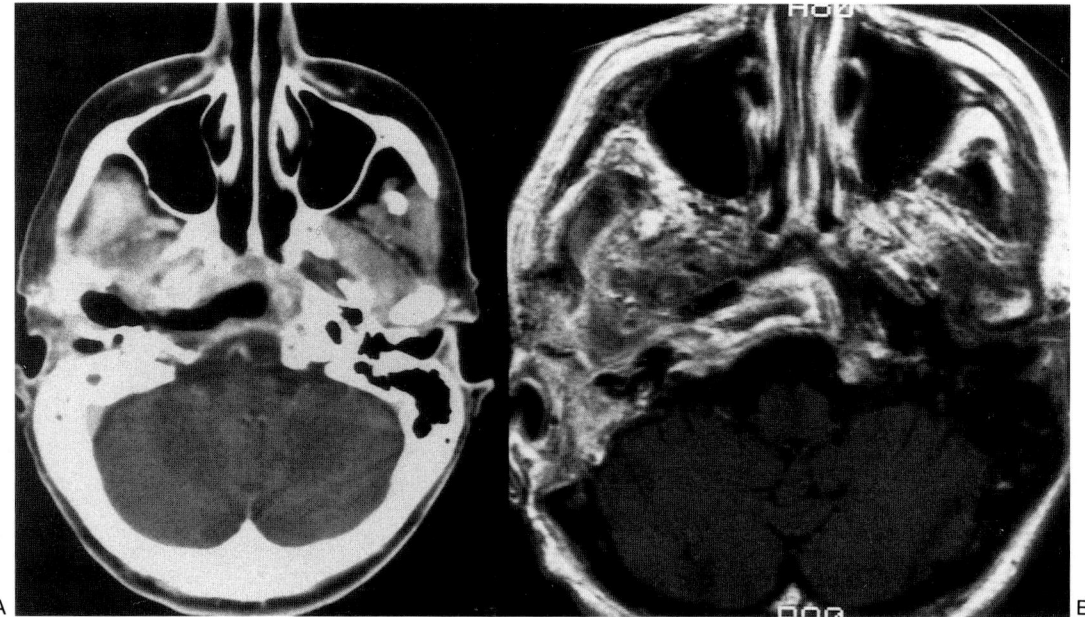

FIG. 71. A patient with an extensive petroclival chordoma developed a pharyngo-spheno-tympanic fistula after a combined anterior and lateral approach seen in the CT scan (**A**). This was successfully repaired with the aid of a temporalis muscle flap (**B**), seen in a T1-weighted MRI scan.

lateral, transcondyle, and transjugular approach combined with the previous exposure. The fistula was debrided and closed successfully with a temporalis muscle flap. The previous transoral approach probably contributed to the development of the pharyngotympanic fistula (Fig. 71).

We observed an increased complication rate in patients who had previously been operated (especially through anterior approaches), patients with giant sized tumors, and patients with intradural and extradural tumors.

CONCLUSION

While anterior approaches, such as the transoral and transmaxillary, have an important role in the management of extradural petroclival neoplasms, the majority of these lesions can be managed optimally by the approaches described in this chapter. The choice of the approach to an individual tumor will depend equally on the experience of the individual surgeon and personal preferences.

REFERENCES

1. Archer DJ, Young S, Uttley D. Basilar aneurysms: a new transclival approach via maxillotomy. *J Neurosurg* 1987;67:54.
2. Cocke EW, Robertson JH, Robertson JT, et al. The extended maxillotomy and subtotal maxillectomy for excision of skull base tumors. *Arch Otolaryngol Head Neck Surg* 1990;116:92–104.
3. Crockard HA, Bradford R. Transoral transclival removal of a schwannoma anterior to the craniocervical junction. *J Neurosurg* 1985;62:293.
4. Derome PJ, Visot A, Monteil JP, Maestro JL. Management of cranial chordomas. In: Sekhar LN, Schramm VL Jr, eds. *Tumors of the cranial base: diagnosis and treatment.* Mount Kisco, NY: Futura, 1987;607–622.
5. Fisch U, Kumar A. Infratemporal surgery of the skull base. In: Rand RW, ed. *Microneurosurgery,* 3rd ed. St. Louis: Mosby, 1985;398–420.
6. House WF. Middle cranial fossa approach to the petrous pyramid. Report of 50 cases. *Arch Otolaryngol* 1963;78:460–469.
7. House WF, Hitselberger WE. The transcochlear approach to the skull base. *Arch Otolaryngol* 1976;102:334.
8. Jackson IT, Hide TH. A systematic approach to tumours of the base of the skull. *J Maxillofac Surg* 1982;10:92–98.
9. Janecka IP, Sen CN, Sekhar LN, Nuss D, Arriaga M. Facial translocation. A new approach to the cranial base. *Otolaryngol Head Neck Surg* 1990;100:413–419.
10. Jones NF, Schramm VL, Sekhar LN. Reconstruction of the cranial base following tumour resection. *Br J Plast Surg* 1987;40:155–162.
11. Kawase T, Toya S, Shiobara R, et al. Transpetrosal approach for aneurysms of the lower basilar artery. *J Neurosurg* 1985;63:857–861.
12. Lesoin F, Authricque A, Villette L, et al. Anteroexternal approach to the internal carotid artery at the base of the skull and intrapetrously. In: *Proceedings of the International Symposium on Cavernous Sinus.* Ljubljana, Yugoslavia: University Medical Centre, 1986;265–274.
13. Miller E, Crockard HA. Transoral transclival removal of anteriorly placed meningiomas at the foramen magnum. *Neurosurgery* 1987;20:966.
14. Mullan S, Naunton R, Hekmat-panah J, Vailati G. The use of an anterior approach to ventrally placed tumors in the foramen magnum and vertebral column. *J Neurosurg* 1966;24:536.
15. Sano K, Kinko M, Saito I. Vertebro-basilar aneurysms, with special reference to the transpharyngeal approach to the basilar artery aneurysms. *Brain Nerve (Tokyo)* 1966;18:1197.
16. Sekhar LN, Janecka IP, Jones NF. Subtemporal–infratemporal and basal subfrontal approach to extensive cranial base tumors. *Acta Neurochir (Wien)* 1988;92:83.
17. Sekhar LN, Schramm VL Jr, Jones NF. Operative management of large neoplasms of the lateral and posterior cranial base. In: Sekhar LN, Schramm VL Jr, eds. *Tumors of the cranial base: diagnosis and treatment.* Mount Kisko, NY: Futura, 1987;655–682.
18. Sekhar LN, Schramm VL Jr, Jones NF. Subtemporal–preauricular infratemporal fossa approach to large lateral and posterior cranial base neoplasms. *J Neurosurg* 1987;67:488.
19. Sekhar LN, Schramm VL Jr, Jones NF, et al. Operative exposure and management of the petrous and upper cervical internal carotid artery. *Neurosurgery* 1986;19:967.
20. Sekhar LN, Sen CN. Anterior and lateral basal approaches to the clivus. *Contemp Neurosurg* 1989;11:1–8.
21. Sen CN, Sekhar LN. An extreme lateral approach to intradural lesions of the cervical spine and foramen magnum. *Neurosurgery* 1990;27:197–204.
22. Sen CN, Sekhar LN, Schramm VL Jr, et al. Chordoma and chondrosarcoma of the cranial base: an 8-year experience. *Neurosurgery* 1989;25:931–941.
23. Sen CN, Sekhar LN. The subtemporal and preauricular infratemporal approach to intradural structures ventral to the brain stem. *J Neurosurg* 1990;73:345–354.
24. Snyderman CH, Janecka IP, Sekhar LN, et al. Anterior cranial base reconstruction: role of galeal and pericranial flaps. *Laryngoscope* 1990;100:49.
25. Stevenson GC, Stoney RJ, Perkins RK, et al. A transcervical transclival approach to the ventral surface of the brain stem for removal of a clivus chordoma. *J Neurosurg* 1966;24:544.
26. Suzuki T, Tokuno H, Hakuba A. The orbito-zygomatic infratemporal approach (a new surgical technique). In: *Proceedings of the International Symposium on Cavernous Sinus.* Ljubljana, Yugoslavia: University Medical Centre, 1986;390–398.

CHAPTER 14

Transoral Approach to Intra/Extradural Tumors

H. Alan Crockard

The transoral approach to intradural and extradural lesions is but one of the routes with which the skull base surgeon should be acquainted so that the optimal surgical approach may be chosen for individual pathology. In general terms, lesions anteriorly placed to the neuraxis are best approached anteriorly and, while this is easily accepted in the lower cervical spine and now increasingly in the thoracic and lumbar spinal regions, there has been, understandably, a degree of reluctance to apply the rule to tumors of the clivus, the craniocervical junction, and the upper two cervical vertebrae. With improved radiological definition of the lesion and recent advances in instrumentation and exposure, it is my contention that the rule can be applied uniformly even to the craniocervical junction. In this chapter the approach is recommended for lesions of the lower third of the clivus, the craniocervical junction, and the anterior segments of the first two cervical vertebrae, either as the sole operative procedure or in combination with posterior surgery for further tumor removal or posterior surgery to provide stabilization of the craniocervical junction following extraction of the anteriorly placed lesion.

SPECIFIC DIAGNOSTIC CONSIDERATIONS

With currently available scanning techniques, it is possible to be fairly certain of the exact pathology of the lesion and to define accurately its relationship to major blood vessels, the neuraxis, and the craniocervical articulations. With the recent availability of sophisticated three-dimensional image analysis, it is possible for the surgeon to "rotate" the pathology in any direction and thus evaluate the possibilities of various surgical approaches to the lesion without ever inserting the surgical knife (Fig. 1). Soft tissue abnormalities are probably best visualized using magnetic resonance imaging (MRI) (Fig. 2). The bony abnormalities, however, are still very much better defined on computed tomography (CT); computed myelotomography (CMT) is still, in our experience, a most valuable tool in assessing the effects of flexion and extension on the craniocervical junction and neuraxis (Fig. 3). Conventional polytomography has only a limited place in our practice and is most useful in identifying the midline in the more bizarre congenital anomalies associated with odontoid translocation. Vertebral angiography is important, particularly if the tumour is suspected of being vascular, and secondly, if there is a degree of rotation of the atlas on C1 which may rotate a vertebral artery into the surgical field of view.

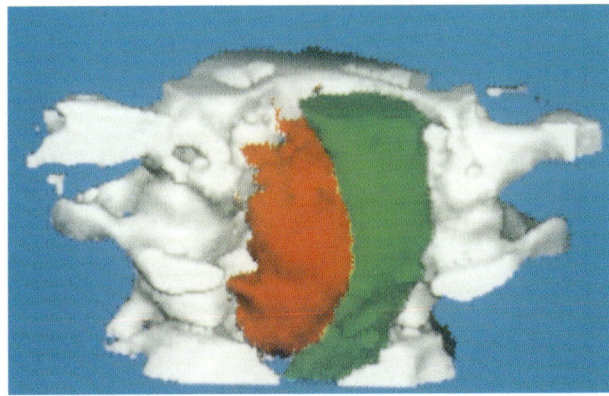

FIG. 1. A craniocervical meningioma showing lateral computed myelotomogram of the lesion. Three-dimensional reconstructions show the tumor (*red*) compressing the spinal cord (*green*).

H. A. Crockard: Department of Surgical Neurology, The National Hospital for Neurology and Neurosurgery, London W9 1TL, England.

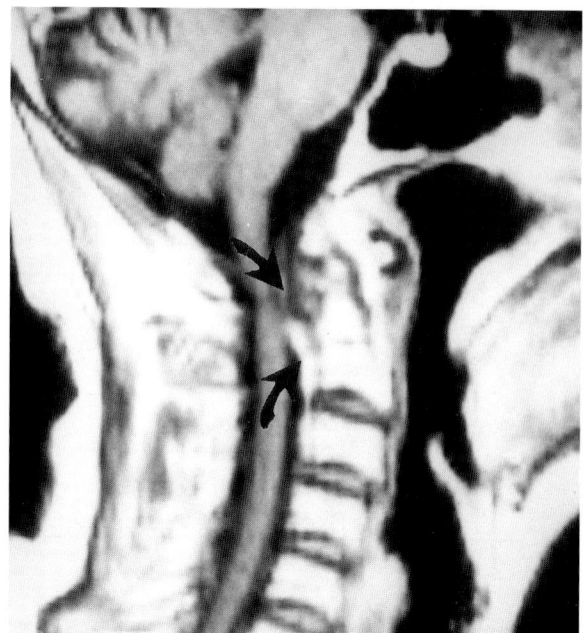

FIG. 2. Magnetic resonance image of an extradural compressive mass involving C2 in a 67-year-old woman. The posterior longitudinal ligament is intact, and there is no instability. The lesion (*arrows*) was a metastasis from an unidentified gastrointestinal primary.

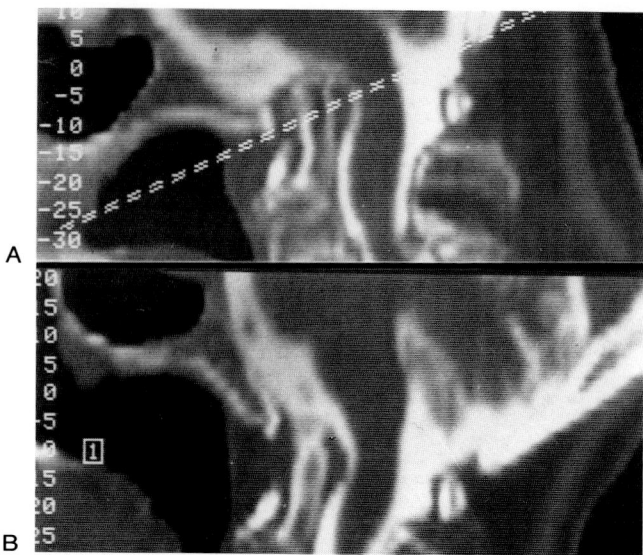

FIG. 3. Dynamic computed myelotomography provides essential information in deciding on anterior surgery and whether or not the area is stable in rheumatoid arthritis. Note the brain stem distortion with flexion due to the translocation of the odontoid peg: (**A**) flexion and (**B**) extension.

Needle biopsy has not been very useful and this Unit's practice is to expose the lesion, obtain a frozen section on the open pathology, and then decide the extent of the individual procedure based on that knowledge.

PATIENT SELECTION

The transoral approach is chosen for lesions confined to the midline of the lower third of the clivus, the craniocervical junction, and the upper two cervical vertebrae. It is ideal for *extradural lesions* confined to these surgical boundaries; but for those extending beyond the limits, a transoral procedure might be considered as part of a staged approach to a radical excision of the lesion. For malignant extradural lesions, more amenable to radiotherapy, a transoral approach would still be the most direct method for decompression and tissue diagnosis. Only in those lesions in which craniocervical junction instability is a major problem, associated with a malignant tumor, would one consider a posterior approach both to obtain the tissue and to provide stabilization for the short lifespan allotted to that patient. The decision to use the approach for entirely *intradural lesions* such as schwannomas (Fig. 4), epidermoids, and meningiomas must be based on the exact location of the lesion, the probable tissue diagnosis, and the experience of the surgical team involved. Lower and middle third basilar ar-

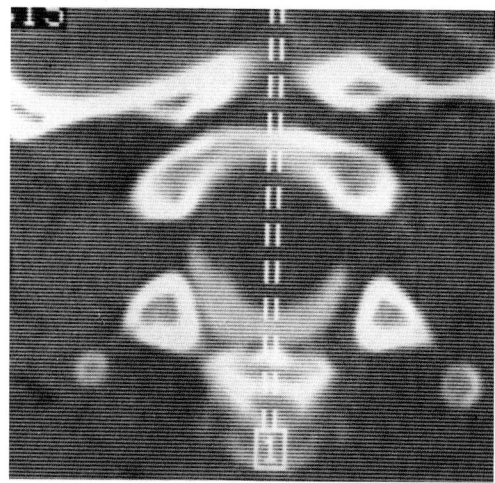
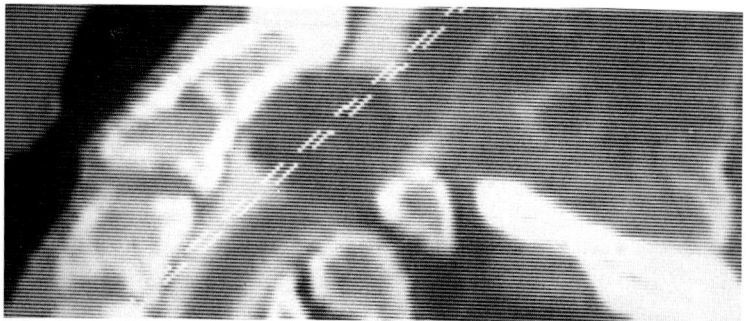

FIG. 4. Intradural schwannoma at the craniocervical junction demonstrated by computed myelotomography: (**A**) transverse and (**B**) sagittal.

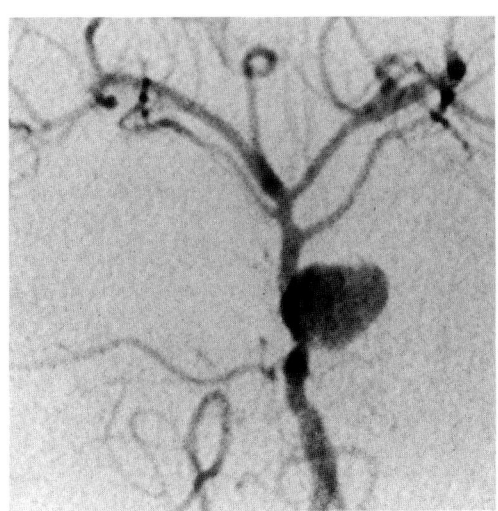

FIG. 5. A giant, partially clotted midbasilar aneurysm buried within the brain stem, which was clipped successfully transorally using an Orbiting aneurysm clip applier.

tery *aneurysms* are particularly amenable to a transoral approach but a specialized aneurysm clip applicator is required (Fig. 5).

The *general physical state* of the patient is most important and, in particular, the respiratory function with particular attention to the vital capacity. If the respiratory function is reduced as a result of brain stem compression, then there is every chance that the patient's condition will improve following surgery provided there has been no undue intraoperative medullary compression. If, however, the patient's general physical state is such that the vital capacity is less than 1 liter, the patient may never be weaned off the ventilator.

Evaluation of the mouth is important. If the jaws do not open more than 25 mm, anesthetic and surgical inaccessibility may preclude the procedure. However, I have used the midline mandibular split in such cases, which allows the lateral retraction of the individual mandible components and permits the tongue to be retracted downward into the hypopharynx. The state of the teeth, the presence of gum disease, and the bacteriological swabs of the nose and throat are all part of the routine evaluation of patients for this procedure.

OPERATIVE TECHNIQUE

Anesthesia

Routine *tracheostomy* on all patients is not required; in some, a tracheostomy may be more dangerous and difficult to perform than the techniques about to be described. However, in any situation where it is believed that there will be a long period of postoperative airway problems, or if there will be an extensive intradural procedure where gastric or pulmonary soiling would be a disaster, then it is our practice to proceed directly to tracheostomy. For lesions of the upper cervical vertebrae and below the foramen magnum, a *nasotracheal tube* may be passed and retracted out of the surgical field with the transoral retraction system. It is more comfortable for the patient in the postoperative period compared to an orotracheal tube.

For any lesion in which there is craniocervical junction instability, a *fiberoptic laryngoscopy* is recommended.

A *nasogastric tube* is inserted to empty the stomach before and after surgery.

Patient Position

The patient is placed in the *lateral position* on the operative table with the head held in the Mayfield head holder, the head slightly elevated compared to the feet and with a degree of cervical extension, provided this does not compromise the craniocervical junction (Fig. 6). The advantage of the lateral position is that the blood, drilled fragments, and washings will flow from the operative site to the dependent tonsillar fauces and thus allow continuous visibility in a way that is not possible with the supine patient. While the surgeon has to "relearn" the anatomy of the region rotated through 90°, it is rewarded in terms of the superior visibility. It also allows the surgeon to sit during the procedure with the support of the elbows, should this be necessary. The lateral tilt facility on the operating table may allow the operative site to be horizontal at the end of the procedure when the dural repair with thrombin fibrin glue is being effected, yet to have it in the lateral position for the actual surgery when it is at its greater advantage.

Prior to surgery, bacteriological swabs should be taken and the sensitivity of any organisms known. The mouth is cleaned with a weak aqueous cetavalon solution. With the induction of anesthesia, antibiotics (cephalosporin

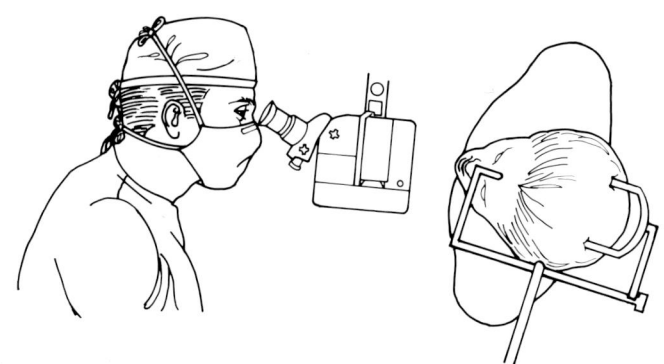

FIG. 6. The lateral operative position affords good exposure with gravity drainage of blood and washings from the operative site. The surgeon is seated. **A:** Seated surgeon. **B:** Position on table.

and metronidazole) are given and continued for 2 days. To prevent postoperative swelling of the tongue and lips, a hydrocortisone cream is applied prior to the insertion of the retractor and at 6-hr intervals for 2 days following the operation. Scrupulous postoperative mouth care is also essential every 4 hr. The nasogastric and nasotracheal tubes prevent physical soiling and reduce the incidence of wound infections.

Exposure

A tongue retractor of suitable proportions is inserted and care is taken to ensure that the lip or tongue is not caught between itself and the teeth (Fig. 7). The retractor is gently opened to expose the soft palate. If the upper jaw is edentulous with a great deal of gum recession, then the retractor should be angled "outward" by packing gauze swabs or a towel underneath the bottom of the tongue retractor blade; this will also improve the exposure of C2 and C3 (Fig. 8).

For lesions below the foramen magnum, the soft palate need not be split; the soft palatal retractors attached to the retraction system will allow access and preserve the integrity of the structure. The curved soft palatal retractor is hooked round the nondependent side of the soft palate (with the patient on their side). The blade is held in position with a 7-in. artery forcep and the locking nut tightened into position (Fig. 7). If a nasotracheal tube has been used, this plus the nasogastric tube are retracted into the dependent tonsillar fauces with the right angled palatal retractor. The *tubercle* on the anterior surface of C1 is the *surgical key* to the area (Fig. 9); if there is any doubt about the surface landmarks, an intraoperative radiograph should be performed. Lignocaine and 1:200,000 adrenaline is injected at the tubercle on C1 to dissect off the pharyngeal tissues from the deeper structures and to provide some hemostasis.

In the author's practice, a midline incision is used, and the pharyngeal retractor is then inserted, converting the vertical incision into a hexagonal exposure (Fig. 10). The two pharyngeal retractor blades, the tongue blade, and the soft palatal blades act as a "ring of steel" around the area in which the surgery is being carried out, preventing damage from inadvertent instrument slippage during the dissection. It is most important to keep the pharyngeal tissues untraumatized; this contributes to good postoperative healing.

A midline raphe exists between the longus coli muscles as they insert into the tubercle of C1; the anterior longitudinal ligament also arises from this point. The arch of C1 and the odontoid peg are exposed by "cutting" diathermy of the muscles and ligaments in the area.

The bone in the area is removed using the angled high-speed airdrill with a 3- or 4-mm cutting burr down through the cancellous bone; when the cortical bone appears, a diamond burr is used. The arch of C1 is removed

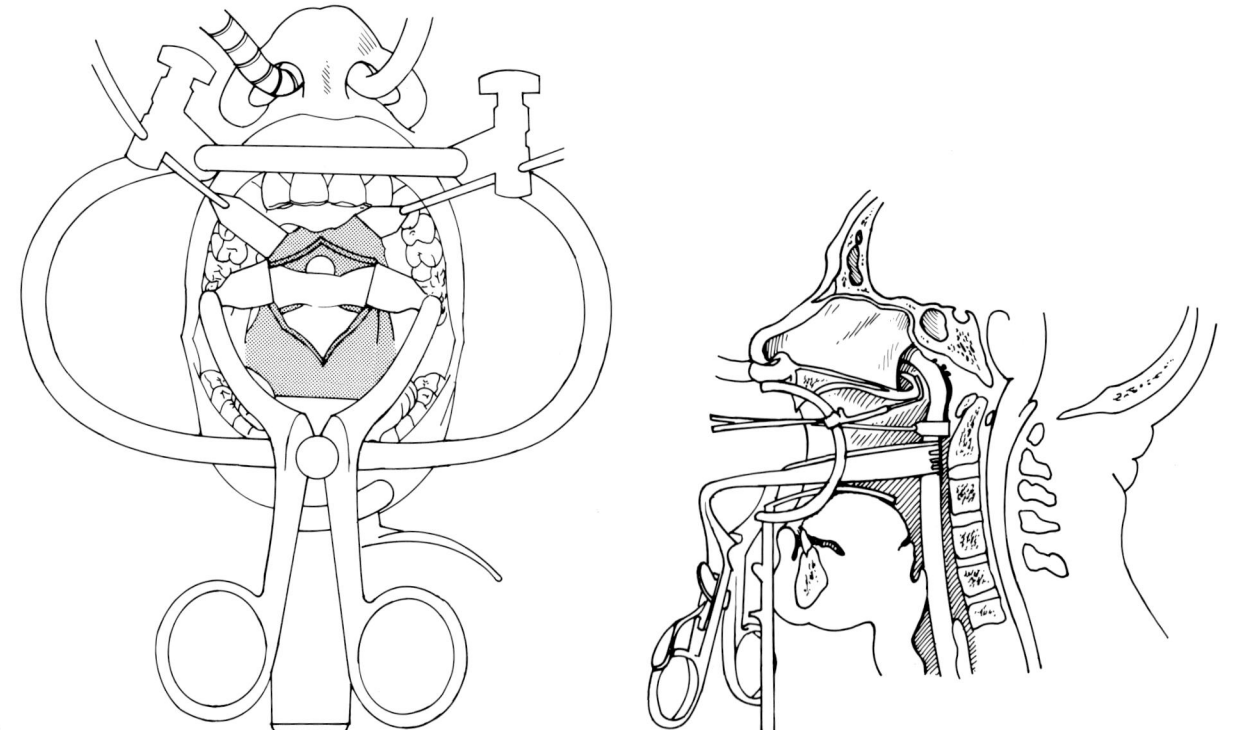

FIG. 7. The soft palate may be retracted without division for lesions below the clivus. The nasogastric tube may also be retracted with the same instrumentation: **(A)** transoral view and **(B)** lateral view.

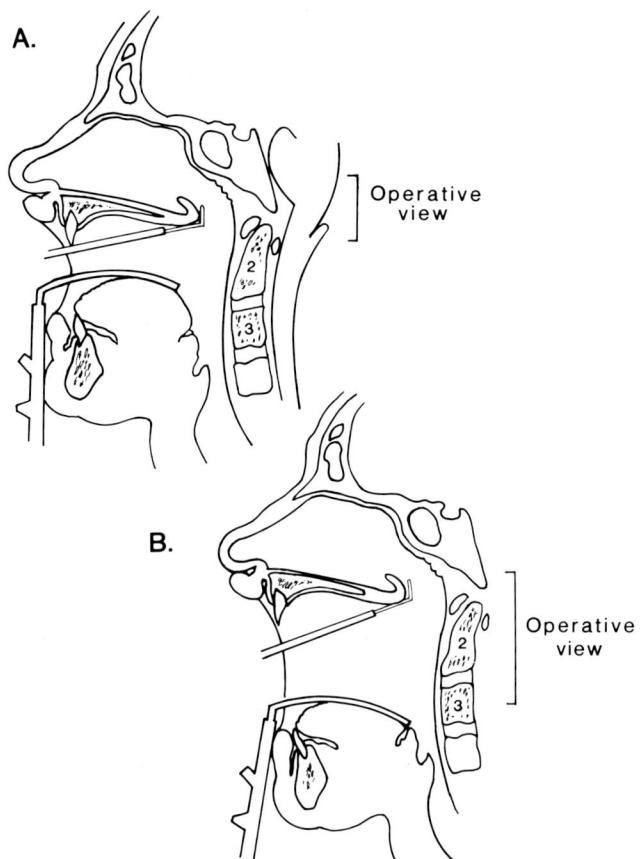

FIG. 8. A: A lateral view of the craniocervical junction with tongue retractor in position. **B:** The caudal end of the exposure may be increased by holding the retractor handle away from the body, which in turn exposes the lower pharynx.

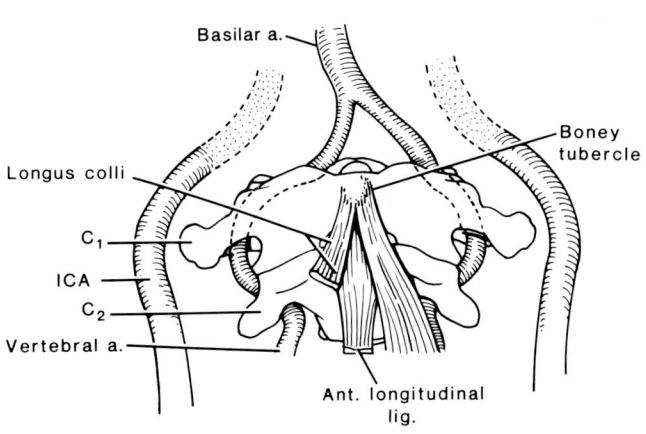

FIG. 9. The key to surgery at the craniocervical junction is the tubercle on C1 to which is attached the anterior longitudinal ligament and longus coli muscles.

and the odontoid peg is exposed. This is "hollowed-out" and thinned until transparent. At this stage the odontoid peg is divided using the angled dissector and the 1-mm and 2-mm foot plate Kerrison "upcuts" to allow the distal tip of the odontoid peg to be "delivered" into the wound by intradural pressure. The odontoid peg grasping forceps (Fig. 11) are used to hold the distal fragment and pull it "out and down," identifying the alar and apical ligaments, which are then divided. The odontoid peg forceps are also used to hold the unstable peg while the drilling is carried out. The transverse ligament and the posterior longitudinal ligament may be divided to ex-

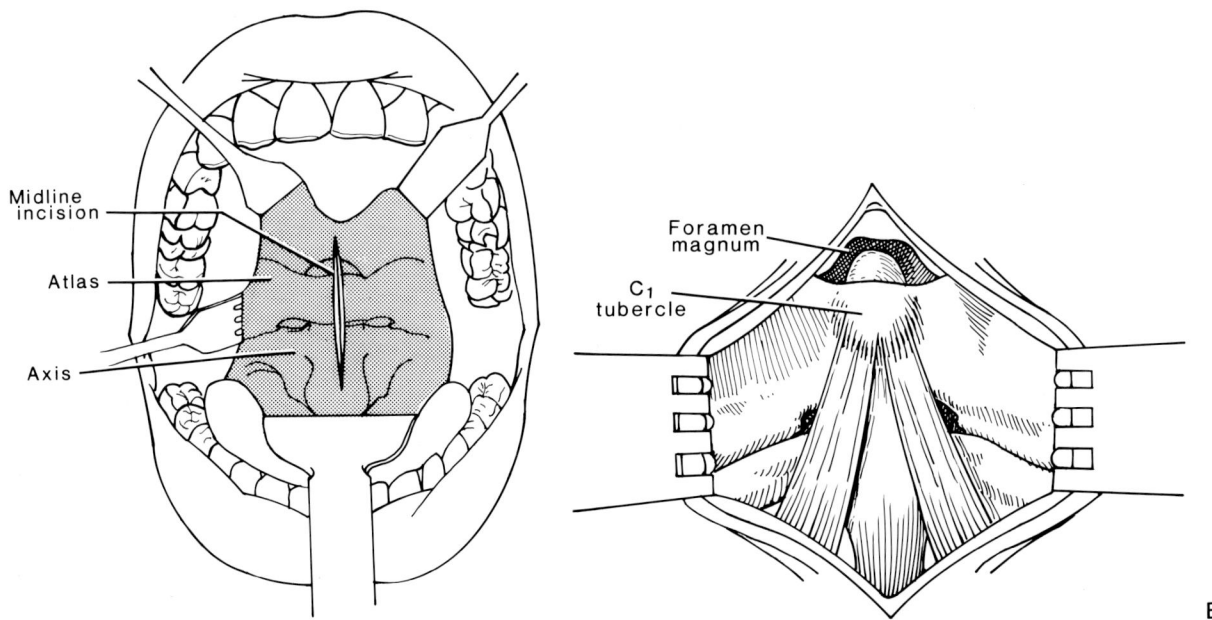

FIG. 10. A: The soft palate has been elevated to expose the posterior pharynx and a midline vertical incision. The positions of C1 and C2 are outlined. **B:** The vertical incision is converted into a hexagon to expose the C1 tubercle with muscle and ligament attachment.

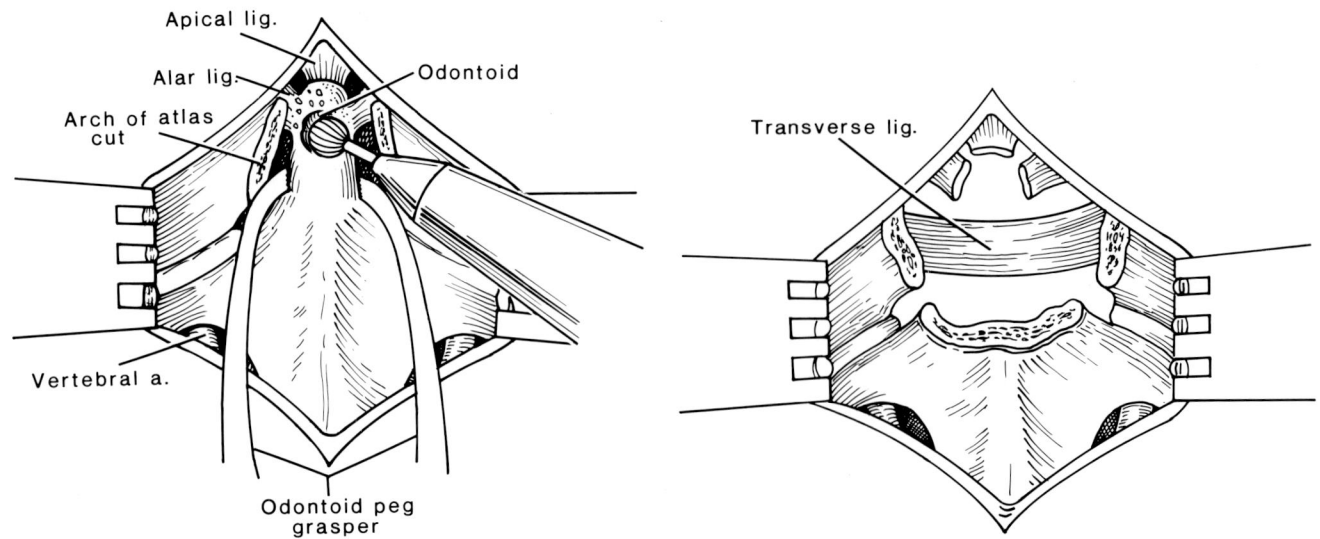

FIG. 11. A: Removal of odontoid peg. The arch of C1 is divided and the peg held firmly with special forceps if there is any instability. **B:** The ligaments are subsequently divided and further bone may be removed.

pose dura. If the exposure extends down to the C2–C3 interspace, the disc space should be removed and the endplate of the upper surface of C3 removed. Angled bayonetted curettes (Carlin), the angled dissector (Crockard), and various sizes of straight and curved suction tubes are used to remove, piecemeal, *extradural tumor* in the area. The currently available ultrasonic aspirators have not been useful in the area due to the dimensions of the handpiece, but the laser is helpful in excision and hemostasis.

Lesions Above the Foramen Magnum

The transoral approach to this area requires division of the hard and soft palate and the line of the incision chosen is shown in Fig. 12 with preservation of the

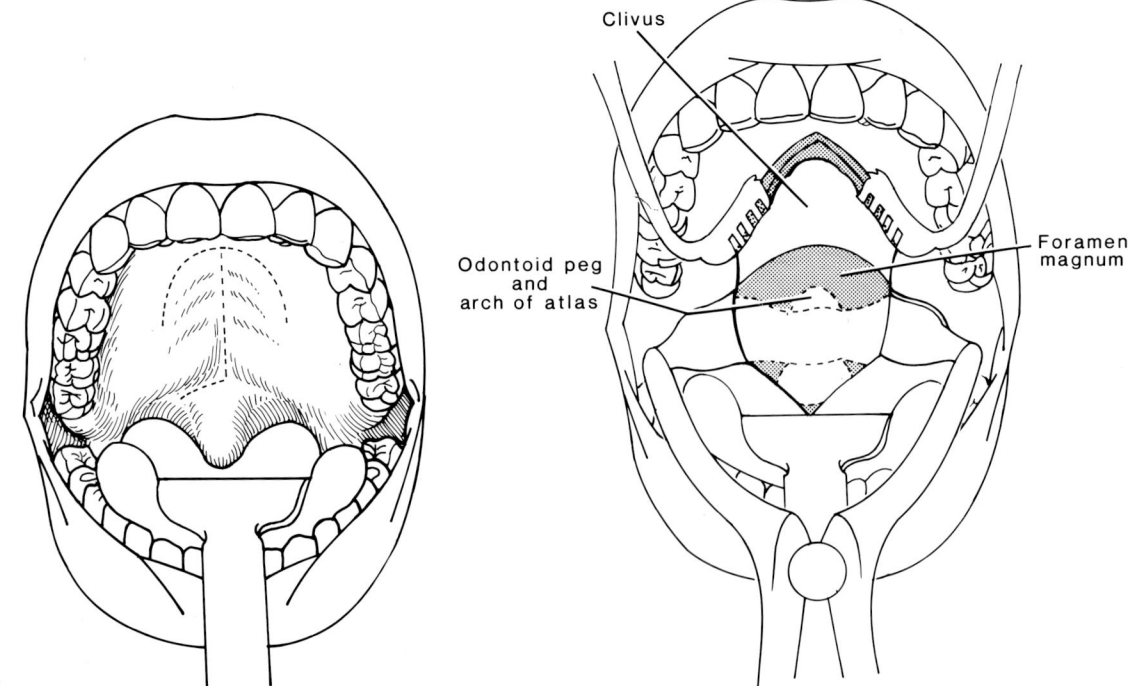

FIG. 12. The transpalatal approach is used for lesions above the foramen magnum. **A:** The soft and hard palate incision. **B:** The lower third of clivus C1 and C2 are exposed using the specially designed instruments.

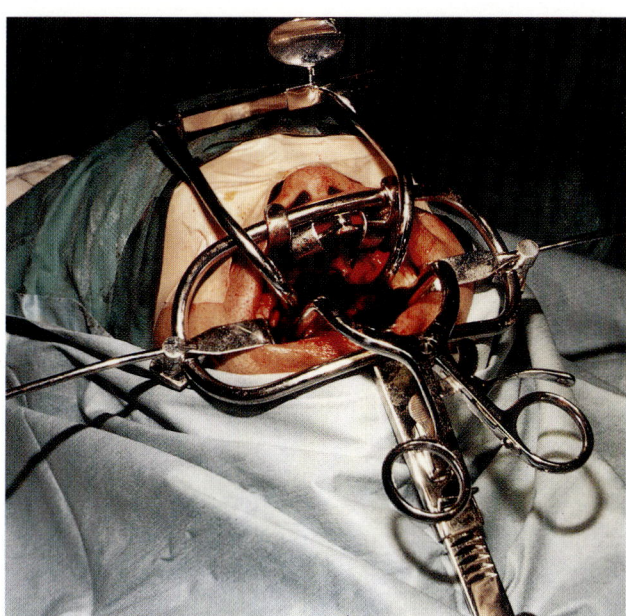

FIG. 13. The hard palate retractor, pharyngeal retractor, and mouth gag are designed to "lie low" on the patient's face.

uvula. A fine "side cutting" drill or a reciprocating saw is used to incise the palate in the midline and to the sides behind the superior alveolar margins. The vomer is removed and the two sides of the hard palate "infractured" into the nasal cavity. The turbinates and vomer are removed and the hard palate retractor is inserted to produce maximum exposure. The instrument is designed to lie on the contours of the face, out of the surgeon's way (Fig. 13). The nasal mucosa is divided and with readjustments of the palatal retractor will expose the clivus. The incision may be extended into the pharynx and the pharyngeal retractor used in the lower portion of the wound below the foramen magnum. The bone is generally thinned until it is transparent before the final removal, as previously described. Dural bleeding from intercommunications between the cavernous sinuses and the marginal sinus at the level of the foramen magnum may be quite troublesome. Bipolar coagulation, gentle pressure with a Surgicel pack, and the laser may control it.

The lateral limits of the surgery are 11–14 mm from each side of the midline at the foramen magnum, where the jugular foramen and the vertebral arteries are at risk and, higher up along the clivus, the carotid artery and cavernous sinus.

INTRADURAL SURGERY

Prior to surgery, a lumbar drain is inserted for planned intradural procedures to drain blood products postoperatively and to reduce CSF pressure, thus improving the chances of a watertight closure. Once the appropriate amount of bone has been removed and the dura exposed, it is divided in the usual way with a sharp hook and knife. Retraction stitches are often difficult to insert but may hold the edges apart to expose the intradural lesion.

Removal of a schwannoma in the area begins in the conventional way with debulking the tumor, separating the capsule from surrounding tissue, identifying the position of the vertebral arteries, identifying early on the feeding vessels into the tumor, and, finally, separating the capsule from the brain stem to remove the lesion.

WOUND CLOSURE

Dural Closure

Closure of the dura is very important if meningitis is to be avoided. Surgicel is used and then thrombin fibrin glue, either obtained commercially or prepared from the patient's own blood products, is applied over the Surgicel. Fascia and fat, obtained either from the abdomen or the lateral aspect of the thigh, are then placed in layers and further thrombin fibrin glue is used between layers. The pharynx is closed with interrupted vicryl sutures above this. Below the foramen magnum it is possible to identify two distinct layers, the deeper being the superior constrictor and the pharyngobasilar fascia. Tight closure of this layer will prevent wound breakdown. Interrupted

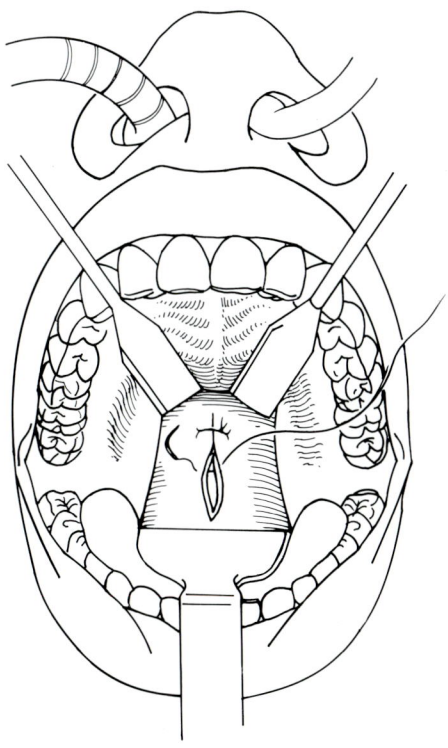

FIG. 14. Closure of the pharyngeal mucosa is in two layers of interrupted absorbable sutures.

mucosal stitches in the nasopharynx and oropharynx are used. A 9-in. Rogers Heany (Codman and Shurtleff) aortic aneurysm needle holder is useful and the transoral bayonetted toothed forceps have also a needle grasping facility. The needle is bent from its curve into a "J" to allow its passage in the narrow confines (Fig. 14).

Closure of the Hard and Soft Palate

The palatal osteomucosal flaps are reflected "downward" into their original position using the Howarth dissector passed through the nostrils. The mucosa of the hard palate is sutured with interrupted vicryl stitches. The soft palate is reconstituted in two layers with vicryl.

TECHNICAL PROBLEMS

Bleeding

Epidural bleeding and bleeding from the venous sinuses can be very troublesome during transoral surgery. The rapid widespread exposure of the area is one way to take the pressure off the veins and coagulate them with diathermy or laser. Bone bleeding may be controlled with bone wax and the diamond burr. Inadvertent straying into the vertebral artery may be a major problem but the bleeding may be controlled in the vertebral foramen with Surgicel and bone wax packing. Intradural bleeding is extremely difficult to control and is to be avoided at all costs.

Bone Grafting

Transoral bone grafting is possible and there is good evidence of sound bony fusion. However, suspended struts from clivus to the base of C2 will only work provided there is firm immobilization, either by screwing or by a Halo Body immobilizer. Bone grafting has been used in association with posterior occipitocervical fixation inserted under the same anesthetic; in this situation, there has been good bony fusion. The iliac crest has been chosen; fibular and tibial struts anteriorly seem unnecessary and may not fuse so easily.

POSTOPERATIVE MANAGEMENT

Details of the postoperative management are given elsewhere but the most important aspects are set out below.

The *airway* is paramount in all the postoperative management problems. The tube is not removed if there is any problem with respiration or tracheal secretions. In the uncomplicated case, the nasotracheal tube is removed at 24–48 hr after a lateral cervical x-ray has confirmed the lack of posterior pharyngeal swelling. If there is a great deal of pharyngeal swelling, the airway is kept in position. If there is to be a second operation within a few days, the airway is again left in position. If the patient is hypoventilating or hypothermic, a period of elective ventilation may be required.

Swelling of the tissues is controlled with hydrocortisone cream, applied locally.

A *lumbar drain* is required for all those who have had a CSF leak or in whom the dura has been deliberately opened. The drain is kept in position for about 5 days and, if there has been an extensive intradural procedure, it is converted into a lumboperitoneal shunt after this period.

Chest physiotherapy and *mobilization* are most important. The patient is usually put in the sitting-up position within 48 hr and moved out of bed as soon as possible.

Cephalosporin and *metronidazole* are given for a period of 3 days.

Antiemetics and metoclopramide are administered every 6-hr for 48 hr. *Analgesia* is provided with a pump infusion of morphine 1–2 mg/hr with a careful check on respiratory rate.

COMPLICATIONS

The important complications are those associated with the airway and respiratory function. Great attention is placed on the care of the airway and mouth with diversion of tracheal secretions and stomach contents. If this is carefully attended to, there have been few problems with the wound. Careful suturing of the palate will prevent palatal breakdown. CSF leakage will require a lumbar drain. Postoperative bleeding is usually a reactive hemorrhage and the wound will require debridement and evacuation.

ILLUSTRATIVE CASES

C1/C2 Chordoma

A 38-year-old psychiatrist presented with a 4-year history of neck and occipital pain, a 4-month history of weakness in his right hand, and a recent history of stiffness in his legs. He had complained of 6 weeks of dysphagia and, while gargling, had noticed a large soft tissue mass in the back of his own pharynx.

The CT scan showed a large multilobulated mass around the lateral mass and the base of C2. There was a large soft tissue mass and intradural compression due to the lesion (Fig. 15).

A MRI showed the soft tissue extent of the lesion (Fig. 16). Angiography revealed that the vertebral artery ran through the tumor on the right side. It was decided to do

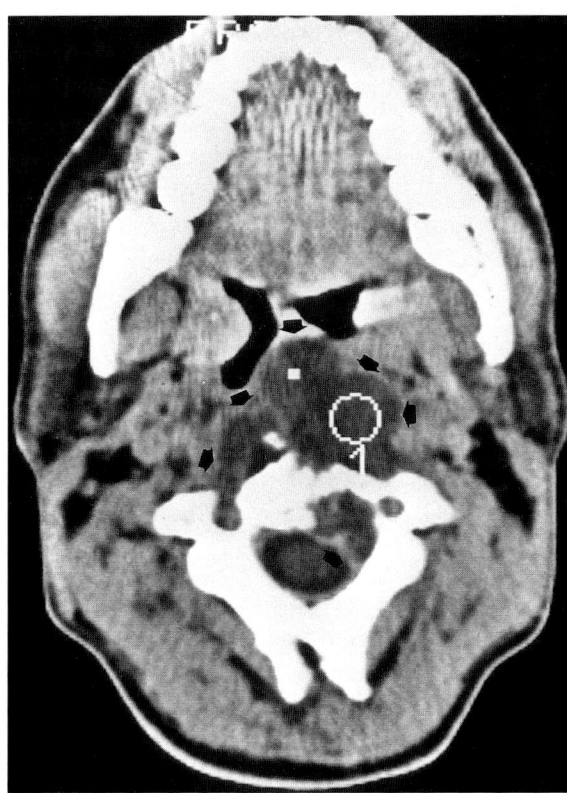

FIG. 15. Computed tomography scan of chordoma at C2 with marked soft tissue extension, bony erosion, and cord compression. *Arrows* indicate the extent of the lesion retropharyngeally.

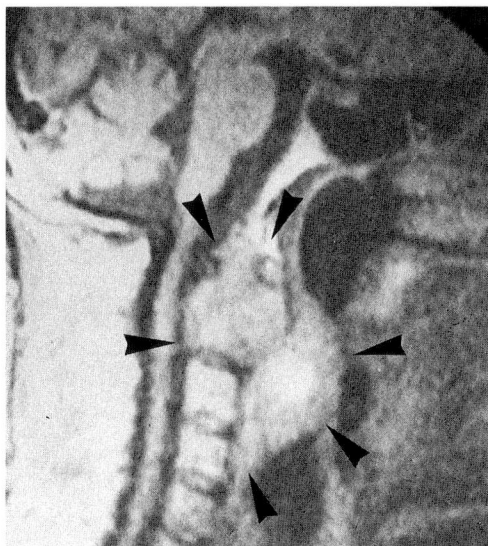

FIG. 16. Magnetic resonance image of the same lesion shown in Fig. 15, in a sagittal reconstruction. *Arrows* indicate the extent of the lesion extradurally and retropharyngeally.

a radical resection and stabilization. A transoral approach was used with a midline incision of the pharynx from the anterior tubercle on to the upper border of C3. All the soft tissue mass was removed. The base of C2 and the tumor extending around the vertebral artery on the right side were removed. The arch of C1 was carefully preserved and the tip of the odontoid peg left untouched. All the tumor that was visible anteriorly was removed and the wound closed.

Posteriorly, under the same anesthetic, the mass coming around the lateral mass of C2 on the right side was dissected off the vertebral artery. The lateral aspect of the lamina was also removed but the spinous process and the left sided lamina were left intact. An occipitocervical Hartshill Ransford loop was inserted. Bone was obtained from the iliac crest and used as a bone graft. The wound was closed in layers.

A nasogastric tube and tracheostomy were left in position for a few days. He was out of bed in 2 days. The wounds healed well and he was discharged from hospital 9 days after the operative procedure.

Neurenteric Cyst

A 35-year-old man presented with a 4-year history of occipital pain and a more recent rapid history of stiffness in his legs. He was transferred to The National Hospitals for Nervous Diseases as an emergency, quadriplegic, and breathing on one lung, having deteriorated rapidly over 48 hr. The MRI scan showed a large cystic mass in-between the vertebral arteries and distorting the craniocervical junction (Fig. 17). A preoperative diagnosis of a cystic schwannoma was made and for that reason it was decided to approach the lesion transorally. A transoral procedure with a split of the hard and soft palate was carried out. The lower third of the clivus, the arch of C1, the odontoid peg, and the base of C2 were drilled out. As described, the dura was exposed and a long midline dural

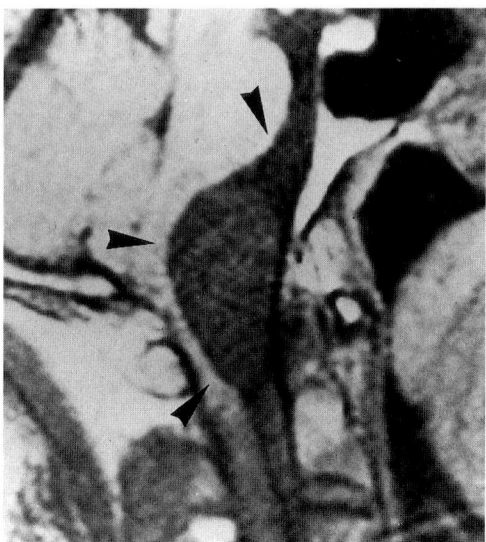

FIG. 17. An intradural neurenteric cyst at the craniocervical junction. *Arrows* indicate the extent of brain stem distortion by the lesion.

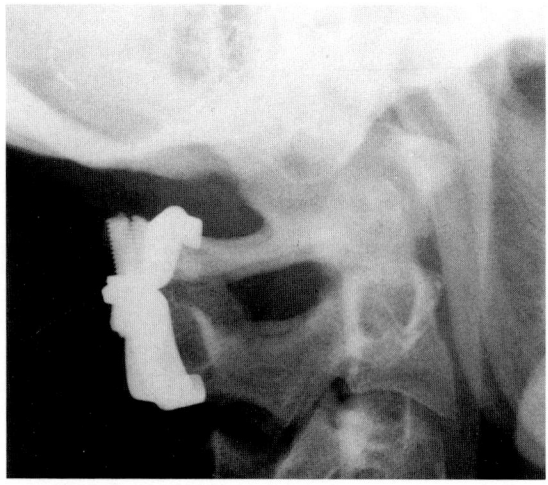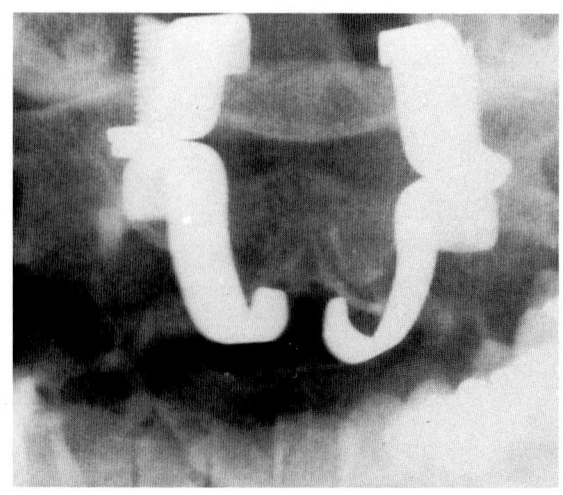

FIG. 18. Posterior stabilization by Halifax interlaminar clamp: **(A)** lateral and **(B)** anteroposterior.

incision was made to extend above and below the lesion. The cystic lesion was identified in-between the vertebral arteries. The cystic fluid and capsule were removed. There was little or no solid component and pathological examination revealed it to be a neurenteric cyst. A lumbar drain was inserted. The wound was closed as described for dural closure. The lumbar drain was converted into a lumboperitoneal shunt at 5 days. He was out of bed and walking prior to his lumboperitoneal shunt but about 8 days after the procedure he felt a great deal of occipital pain and flexion and extension radiographs revealed considerable movement at the craniocervical junction consequent on the bony removal. A C1/C2 Halifax clamp fixation with bone in the area was used, regaining his stability (Fig. 18). He was discharged from hospital with no signs of increased tone and normal neurological function 10 days after the posterior stabilization.

CONCLUSION

The technique has obviously evolved over the last 5 years and that which we recommend now has changed greatly from our original experience. With over 250 transoral cases, for a variety of pathology, it is my belief that the transoral route is a safe, reliable, and effective method for dealing with anteriorly placed pathology at the craniocervical junction, whether intradural or extradural. If appropriate care is taken, the risk of meningitis is very low.

The key to the area is imaging of the highest quality, good retraction, and instruments appropriately designed to perform the surgery. A team approach is required, and unless there is intensive care and anesthesia of the highest quality, horrendous complications will occur.

ACKNOWLEDGMENTS

The author is most grateful to Dr. I. Calder, Consultant Anesthetist at The National Hospitals for Nervous Diseases, and Dr. J. Stevens and Dr. B. Kendall, Consultant Neuroradiologists at The National Hospitals for Nervous Diseases for all their help.

The manuscript was prepared by Michelle Green.

FURTHER READING

Ashraf J, Crockard HA. Transoral fusion for high cervical fractures. *J Bone Joint Surg* [*Br*] 1990;1.
Calder I. Anaesthesia for transoral surgery and craniocervical surgery. In: Jewkes D, ed. *Balliere's clinical anaesthesiology.* London: Saunders, 1987;441–457.
Crockard HA, Calder I, Ransford AO. One stage transoral decompression and posterior fixation in rheumatoid atlanto-axial subluxation: a technical note. *J Bone Joint Surg* [*Br*] 1990;72B:682–685.
Crockard HA, Koksel T, Watkin N. Transoral transclival clipping of anterior inferior cerebellar artery aneurysm using new rotating applier. Technical note. *J Neurosurg* 1991;75:483–485.
Miller E, Crockard HA. Transoral transclival removal of anteriorly placed meningiomas at the foramen magnum. *Neurosurgery* 1987;20:966–968.
Crockard HA, Sen CN. The transoral approach for the management of intradural lesions of the craniovertebral junction: a review of 7 cases. *Neurosurg* 1991;28(1):88–98.

CHAPTER 15

The Transmaxillary Approach to the Clivus

H. Alan Crockard

As the clivus is relatively inaccessible, a wide variety of surgical approaches have been developed; many put cranial nerves and major vessels at risk. The advantage of the transmaxillary approach to the area is that no major vessel or cranial nerve is put at risk by this anteroinferior approach. It requires teamwork from several disciplines to allow entry and for a good cosmetic reconstruction. Its chief advantage is that it is particularly suitable for lesions of the upper and middle third of the clivus, for removing lesions that extend beyond the lateral boundaries of the clivus, and if there are congenital deformities around the oral cavity for an approach to the deformed skull base in profound basilar invagination. The approach is not useful for lesions at the craniocervical junction itself as the hard palate, while tilting downward anteriorly, tilts upward posteriorly, obscuring the lower third of the clivus. In this chapter, the techniques of the transmaxillary approach are described followed by the extended maxillectomy.

SPECIFIC DIAGNOSTIC CRITERIA

Magnetic resonance imaging (MRI) and *computed tomography* (CT) are absolutely essential for visualizing this area. The recent development of *three-dimensional reconstruction* interrogation packages provides an unparalleled view of lesions in this complicated area (Fig. 1). Four-vessel *angiography* is also required to outline the position and distortion, if any, of the carotid and vertebral arteries.

PATIENT SELECTION

The route is particularly suitable for *extradural lesions* extending into the sphenoid and of the upper and middle part of the clivus (Fig. 2). It is also very useful for lesions that, though primarily extradural, extend intradurally, and the approach is very suitable for aneurysms of the midbasilar region. It is also suitable for removal of metastases in the extradural region in this area. It is not suitable for large clival meningiomas. It would rarely be suitable for an extensive intradural approach to this very selected area, as the lateral boundaries are limited by third, fourth, fifth, and sixth cranial nerves and the venous intercommunications between the cavernous sinuses.

OPERATIVE TECHNIQUE

Anesthesia

The nasotracheal route is not suitable in this situation for the anesthetic tube. Instead, an orotracheal tube may

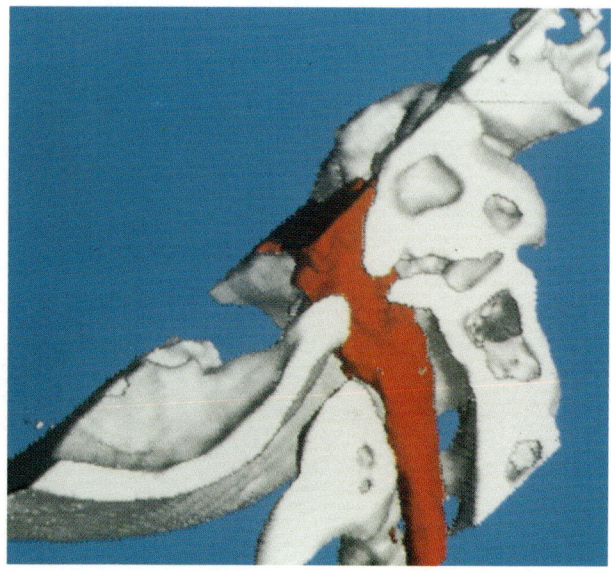

FIG. 1. Three-dimensional reconstructions of congenital basilar invagination with marked neuraxial compression.

H. A. Crockard: Department of Surgical Neurology, The National Hospital for Neurology and Neurosurgery, London WC1N3BG, England

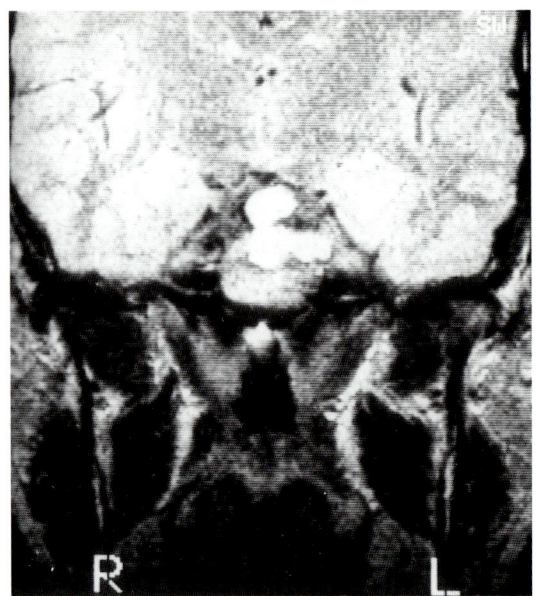

FIG. 2. A chordoma extending into the pituitary fossa and laterally into the cavernous sinus and middle third of the clivus.

Patient Position

As with the other transoral procedures, a three-quarter supine position is preferred. This is achieved by placing the patient in the lateral position on the operating table with the head held in the Mayfield head holder (see Crockard, Transoral Approach to Intra/Extradural Tumors). Head extension is produced and, with the lateral tile facility, the patient can be put almost horizontal, should that be required during the period of dural repair. This allows the blood and washings from the wound to drain to the dependent parts of the exposure out of the direct surgical field.

Exposure

Preoperatively, the bacteriological flora of the nose and throat should be obtained and the appropriate antibiotics, usually cephalosporin and metronidazole, are commenced with the induction of anesthesia, and continued for 48 hr only. The whole area is cleaned with a weak aqueous cetavalon solution.

An *incision* is made along the upper alveolar margin, extending right round to the molars on both sides, and the mucosa is stripped off the bone (Fig. 3). The maxillary buttress on both sides is identified and the floor of the nasal cavity is also identified. The dissection must go back to behind the last molar to expose the bone in the region. The position of the saw cut is then marked out. A pantorthogram of the dentition is advisable to identify the position and height of the dental roots and the incision planned to avoid these. The incision may go into the maxillary sinus on both sides. Care is taken to avoid the maxillary branch of the trigeminal on the maxilla. Having marked out the incision, the titanium (arthrodax) plates are placed in position over the maxillary buttress

be inserted. The disadvantage of this is that the downward palatal retraction may clamp the orotracheal tube between the teeth and compromise the airway lumen. It has been our practice to perform an *elective tracheostomy* on most of the patients requiring maxillectomy for their approach. The tracheostomy stays in position for about 2 or 3 days. Craniocervical stability is not usually a problem with these patients and thus a conventional anesthetic approach, initially, is acceptable. Instead of a nasogastric tube, a *pharyngogastric tube* is inserted. The tube is passed into the stomach in the usual way and a stab incision is made in the lateral fauces to one side and through this the tube is pulled.

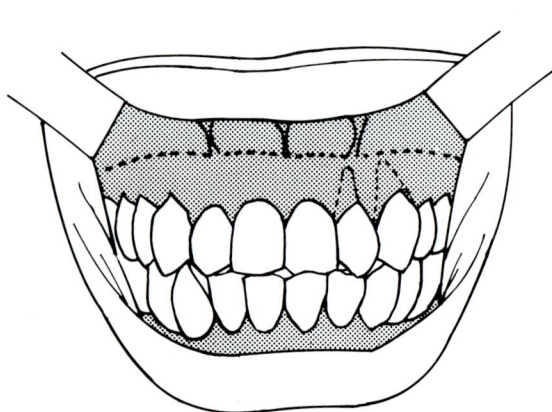
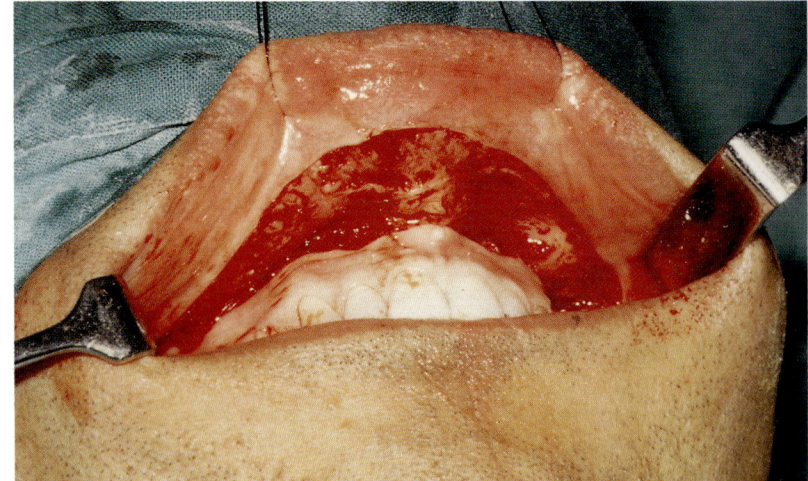

FIG. 3. The transmaxillary approach: superior alveolar mucosal incision, **(A)** drawing and **(B)** operative photograph.

on both sides and the small titanium screws placed in such a manner as to avoid the future saw cut (Fig. 4). The reason for inserting the plates at this stage is so that there is perfect dental occlusion following the procedure; if there is less than perfect occlusion when the jaw is reconstituted, it will significantly affect dental occlusion.

After positioning the plates, they are then removed and the oscillating saw is used to make the incision to disarticulate the hard palate (Fig. 5). Care is taken to preserve the palatine nerve and arteries on both sides as this provides the blood and nerve supply to the disarticulated palate. The hard palate is then "down-fractured" into the oral cavity (Fig. 6). The mucosa on the nasal surface is gently dissected off, and the vomer is removed. The nasal surface is reflected upward and laterally and as much as possible is preserved. The turbinates may be removed to improve the exposure. The septum is removed or reflected to one side. The transoral retractor, with its transmaxillary plate adaption (Fig. 7A), is then inserted into the wound. The transmaxillary plate is inserted and allowed to grip firmly onto the exposed undersurfaces of the maxillary sinus on both sides (Fig. 7B). The small tongue blade is applied to the upper surface on the now depressed hard palate and this is then gently opened to expose the area (Fig. 7C). The large tongue retractor is not suitable for this retraction maneuver. During the operation, the retractor is released from time to time to ensure return of circulation to the palate and prevent any serious postoperative complications with the palatal wound and its healing. The undersurface of the sphenoid sinus and the upper portion of the clivus are then identified. The mucosa is retracted gently to each side. A midline incision is made in the clival mucosa and the pharyngeal retractors, long or short, are inserted to retract the soft tissue laterally and expose the midline structures of the sphenoid and upper and middle part of the clivus (Fig. 8). Usually, if there is a prominent sphenoid sinus, the floor of the sphenoid is removed and

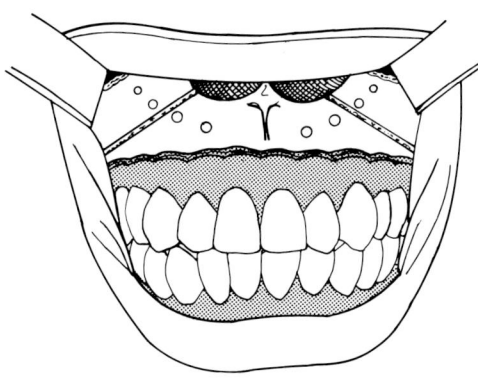

FIG. 5. The plates are removed and the saw cut made.

the posterior wall of the sinus identifies the upper margin of the undersurface of the clivus (Fig. 9).

Using the high-speed airdrill with a 3-mm cutting burr on the angled handpiece, the bone of the clivus is drilled away. In the upper and middle clivus region, the bone is extremely thick; it may be 14–18 mm thick and will require considerable dissection. There are often intercommunication veins in the lateral portion of the clivus, going into the cavernous sinuses; these may have to be packed with bone wax from time to time. The clivus is about 20 mm wide and 20–30 mm thick (Fig. 10). The drilling is continued until the cortical bone is noted on the deep surface. No attempt is made to remove any of the bone until it is all thinned out. The final thinning of the cortical bone on the inner surface of the clivus is effected using the diamond burr (3-mm diameter). The thinned bone is then gently removed with the transoral dissector and 1- and 2-mm Kerrison "upcuts." Sometimes there is a great deal of bleeding at this stage from intercommunications between the cavernous sinuses. There are also an unpredictable and variable number of venous channels in the dura in this area between the

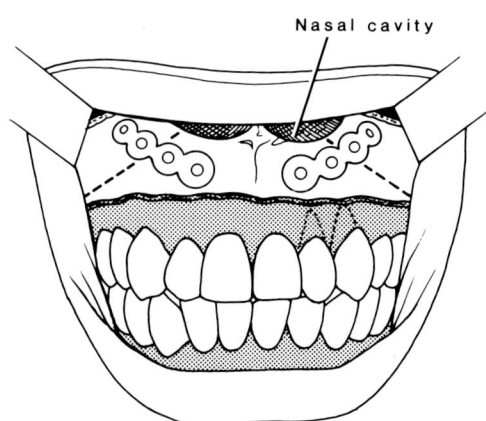

FIG. 4. The position of the fixation plates on the maxillary buttresses is determined before the saw cut to provide perfect dental occlusion.

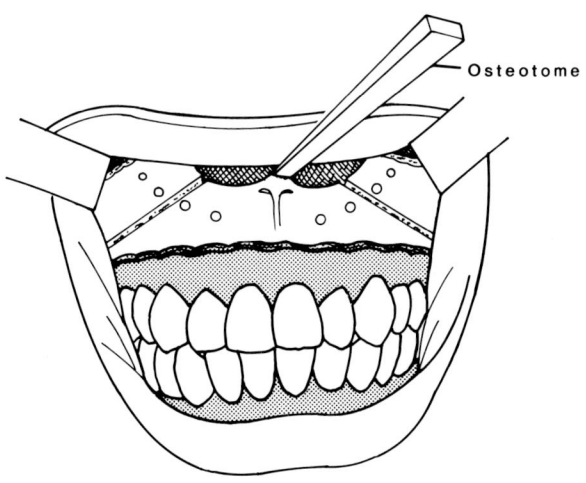

FIG. 6. The hard palate is "down-fractured" into the oral cavity.

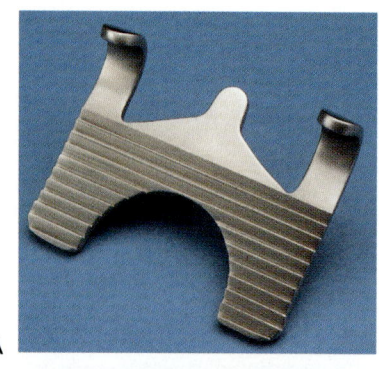
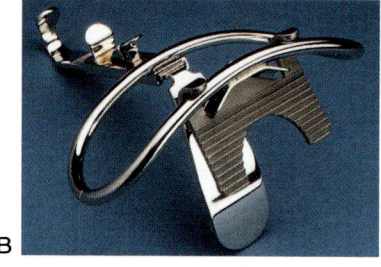
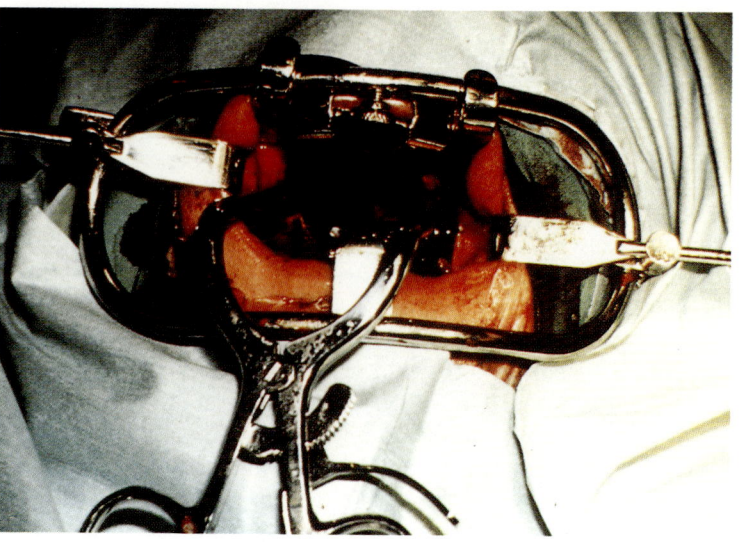

FIG. 7. The addition of a specially designed plate (**A**) to the transoral retractor (**B**) allows it to be fixed in position. The small tongue plate is applied to the upper surface of the hard palate to retract it downward (**C**). The "palatal" retractors may also be used to retract the corners of the mouth. (Transoral instruments by Codman and Shurtleff.)

venous sinuses and communication with the marginal sinus and petrosal sinuses. If the dissection is entirely extradural, great care is taken not to damage these, as the bleeding may obscure vision. The position of the carotid canals should be very carefully identified in the patient's radiographs. The rostral ends of the canals are 20 mm apart while the caudal positions are at least 50 mm apart. Thus it is the portion of the carotid entering the cavernous sinus that is most at risk.

For extradural tumors, the area is well exposed now

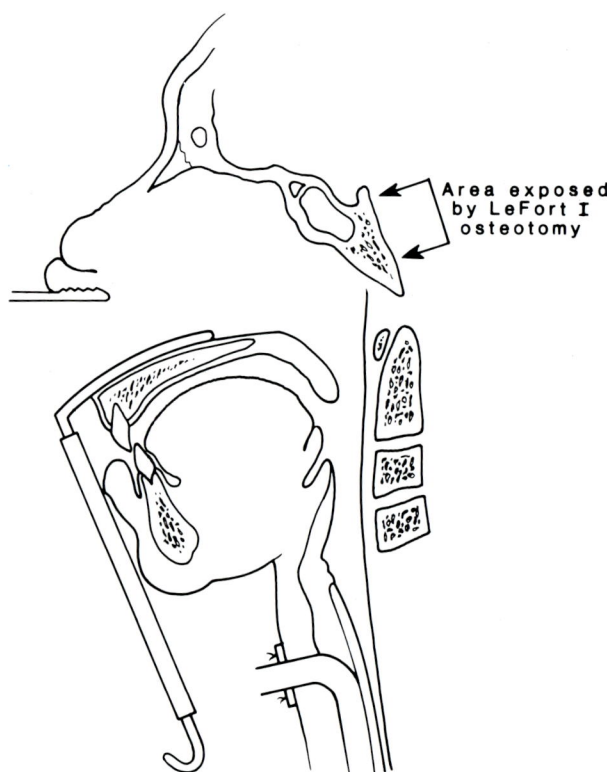

FIG. 8. The upper and middle third of the clivus are well exposed in this procedure.

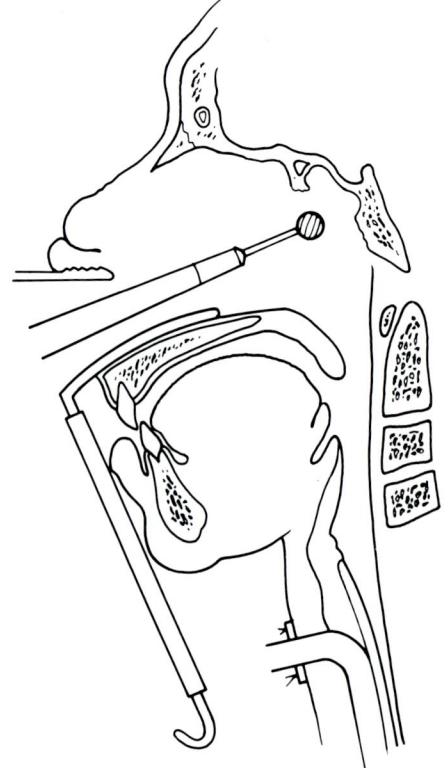

FIG. 9. The angled high-speed airdrill is used to remove the sphenoid and clivus.

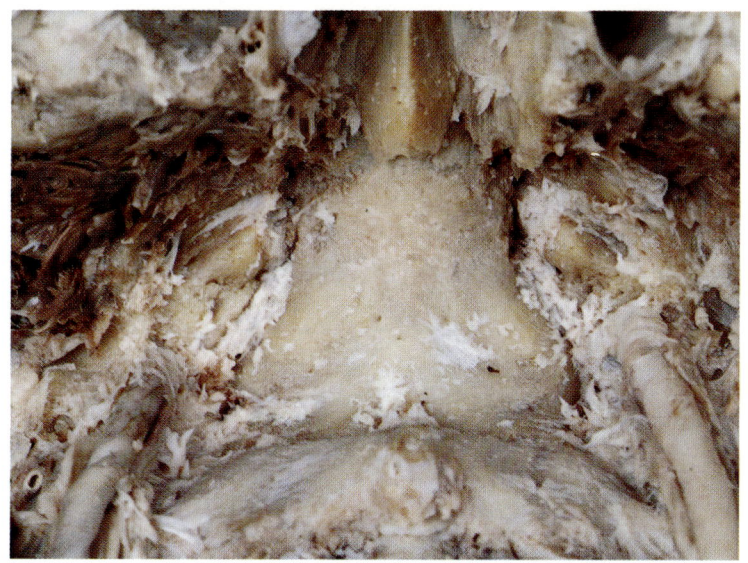

FIG. 10. A cadaveric preparation to show the clivus. Inferiorly is the arch of C1 with its prominent tubercle. Laterally are the carotid arteries entering the carotid canals. The vomer appears superiorly.

and, with angled curettes, angled Orbiting (Codman and Shurtleff) instrumentation, and angled dissectors, the tumor can be removed with suction. The laser may also be used, but the current ultrasonic aspirators are too bulky to be useful in the confines of this exposure. The dissection may be carried out laterally, provided one is aware of the position of the carotid. It is usual that the cranial nerves are pushed laterally by an extradural mass in this region.

For intradural tumors the dura is opened in the usual way. Often there is bleeding from the venous sinuses and this may be stopped with coagulation on the cut edges rather than coagulation on the intact venous sinus in the dura.

Closure

Closure of the wound in this area, if it is an intradural, is as described in Crockard (Transoral Approach to Intra/Extradural Tumors). Fascia, fat, thrombin fibrin "glue" (Tisseel/Immuno, Austria, or manufactured from the patient's own blood), and Surgicel are used in layers as described in Crockard (Transoral Approach) and this effects a good closure. No sutures are inserted in this area, partly because of inaccessibility and partly because of the tearing effect of the needle in the thin dura in this region. The mucosal flaps are approximated over with vicryl sutures. A nasal pack is used to hold the graft and the mucosal flaps in position, when the retractors are removed. The mucosa of the maxillary sinuses and any debris therein are removed. The hard palate is approximated back to its position and the titanium plates are reinserted to hold the upper jaw in its exact anatomical position. The oral mucosa is then closed with interrupted vicryl sutures.

TECHNICAL PROBLEMS

Bleeding

There are several areas from which bleeding may cause a problem. The first of these is from the exposed cut bone surfaces and also the mucosa during the maxillectomy. The septal artery is sometimes a troublesome bleeding point.

Drilling of the bone may reveal some intercommunications between the cavernous sinuses. They can usually be stopped by using the diamond drill and with Surgicel and bone wax. Bleeding from the venous sinuses or the intercommunications between them is a major problem from time to time. It may be controlled with Surgicel and a pattie but it produces an irritating loss of visibility.

Intradural bleeding from an artery is extremely difficult to control and everything should be done to prevent that problem.

Access to Tumor

Occasionally, the tumor may penetrate the pons (Fig. 11). In this example, the instruments were just not long enough to cope with the distances involved. Although the transoral equipment is designed to work at great depth, some of the tumor may be inaccessible. An important point is illustrated here; namely, surgical flexibility to choose and use more than one approach in the attempt to eradicate such pathology.

The Basilar Artery

The tumor may be found wrapped around the basilar artery. Great care should be taken in case the perforating

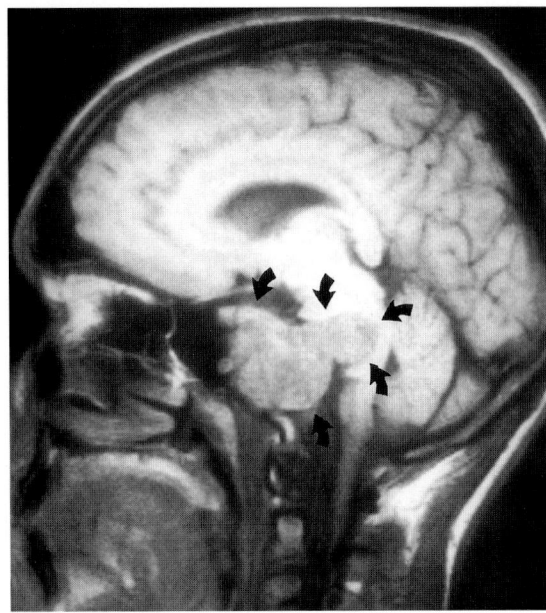

FIG. 11. A chordoma that has extended deep into the pons may be too "deep" even for this exposure.

vessels are damaged with dire consequences. Usually, however, the vessel is pushed to one side and, with careful attention to the angiogram and scans, its position is accurately determined before surgery.

Accurate Replacement of the Upper Jaw

This is critical as far as the patient is concerned and the technique that has been described has been developed to reduce the risks of malocclusion.

POSTOPERATIVE MANAGEMENT

1. *General mouth and nasal care.* As with all the other transoral procedures, great care is taken with the nose and mouth. There will probably be packs in the nose. These should be kept in for 5 days. Mouth care every 4 hr is given and careful attention is paid to the wound. No food is given orally for 5 days and gastric contents and tracheal secretions are diverted by the relevant tubes. When there are bowel sounds, food may be passed with the pharyngogastric tube.

2. *The airway.* Usually, a tracheostomy has been inserted and this will be kept in place for 2 days.

3. *The pharyngogastric tube.* The tube that was inserted preoperatively is kept in position for at least 5 days for feeding and also for ensuring that there is no vomiting or gastric regurgitation into the wound.

4. *Antibiotics.* Cephalosporin and metronidazole are prescribed for 2 days.

5. *Antiemetics.* Metoclopramide is administered every 6 hr for 2 days. An H2 antagonist is administered to reduce gastric acidity.

6. *Analgesia.* An infusion pump is used to deliver a slow continuous morphine dose. Unlike the patients who are unstable at the craniocervical junction, pain is not a major postoperative problem.

7. *Nasal packs.* These are kept in position for 5 days and then removed.

8. *The lumbar drain.* If the dura has been breached, the drain is kept for 5 days. If there has been a major dural tear, then the lumbar drain is converted into a lumboperitoneal shunt to keep the CSF pressure low until the wound is healed.

COMPLICATIONS

The complications of this type of operation have already been covered in the technical problems section. These are basically bleeding, CSF leaks, and malposition of the upper jaw. Infection within the meninges is always a major complication and should be guarded against very carefully. The intraoral incisions do not seem to suffer from infection in a major way following this procedure.

THE EXTENDED MAXILLECTOMY

As mentioned, the transoral approach is ideal to expose the craniocervical junction, but it is limited in its upward and lateral extension and the alveolar margins limit the retraction of the hard palatal flaps. The maxillectomy has the advantage of good vision at the upper end of the wound but cannot expose adequately the craniocervical junction. For extensive congenital anomalies producing basilar invagination (Fig. 12), or for extensive tumors in the area, we have devised a technique —the *extended maxillectomy*—which combines the Le

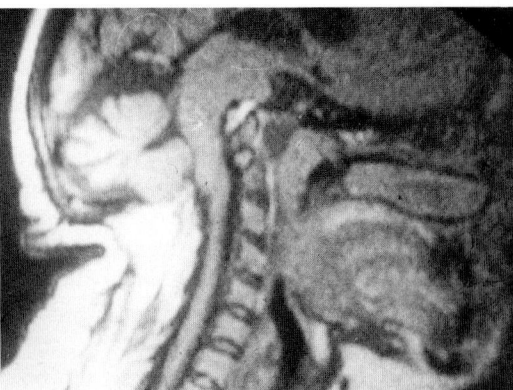

FIG. 12. Extensive congenital basilar invagination causing marked neuraxial compression. The extended maxillectomy will allow adequate exposure.

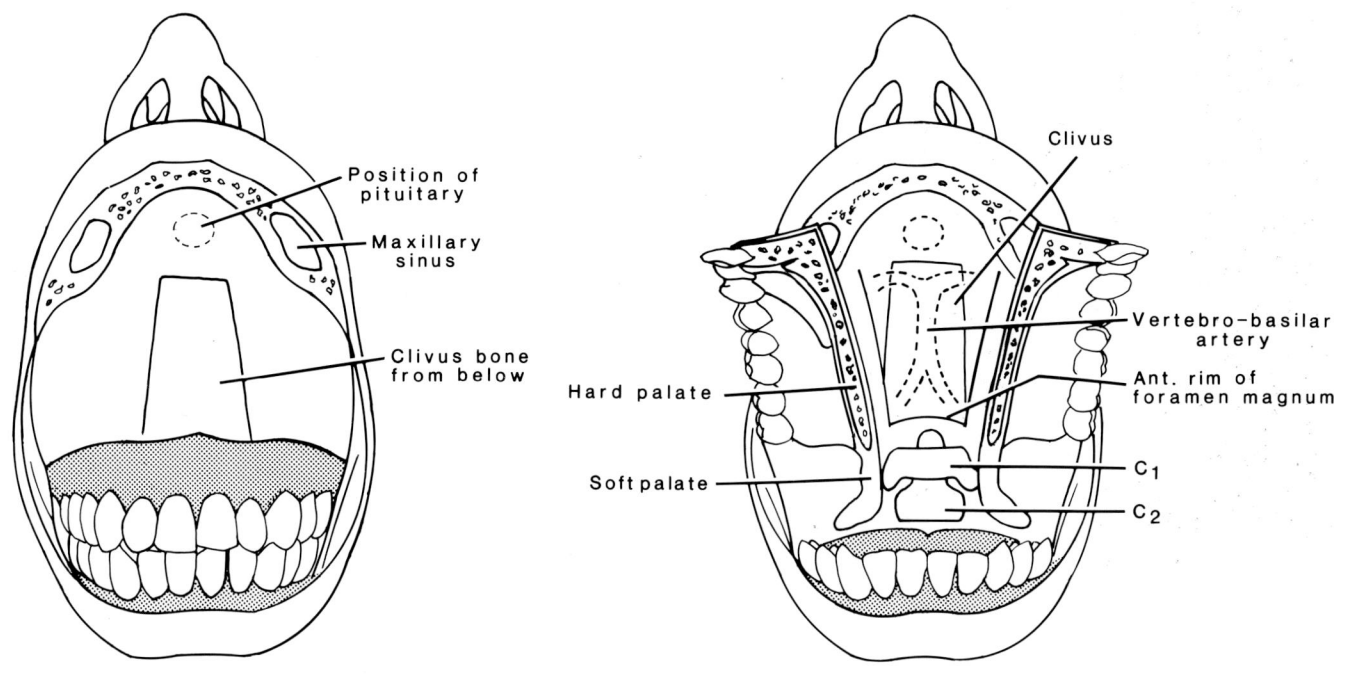

FIG. 13. The relative exposures of the Le Fort maxillectomy (**A**) and the extended maxillectomy (**B**) are shown.

Fort osteotomy with a midline incision of the hard and soft palate and this allows a "swinging" laterally of the two flaps of the hard palate based on their own palatine artery and nerves (Fig. 13). The advantage is extensive exposure; the disadvantage is the length of the procedure and the intricacy with which the wound must be closed to effect good occlusion and proper functioning of the hard and soft palate again.

OPERATIVE TECHNIQUE FOR EXTENDED MAXILLECTOMY

The same mucosal incision is made on the superior alveolus and the bone is exposed to allow a cut on the superior alveolus above the dental roots. As already described, the titanium plates are placed in position and fixed in position prior to the saw cut to allow perfect occlusion postoperatively. A midline incision is made in the hard and soft palate down to the uvula and then to one side of the uvula, as described in Crockard (Transoral Approach). Depending on the shape of the hard palate, a titanium plate may be applied to the nasal or oral surface of the hard palate and fixed in position, and then a midline saw cut along the hard palate and between the upper incisors is made to allow the flaps to swing laterally.

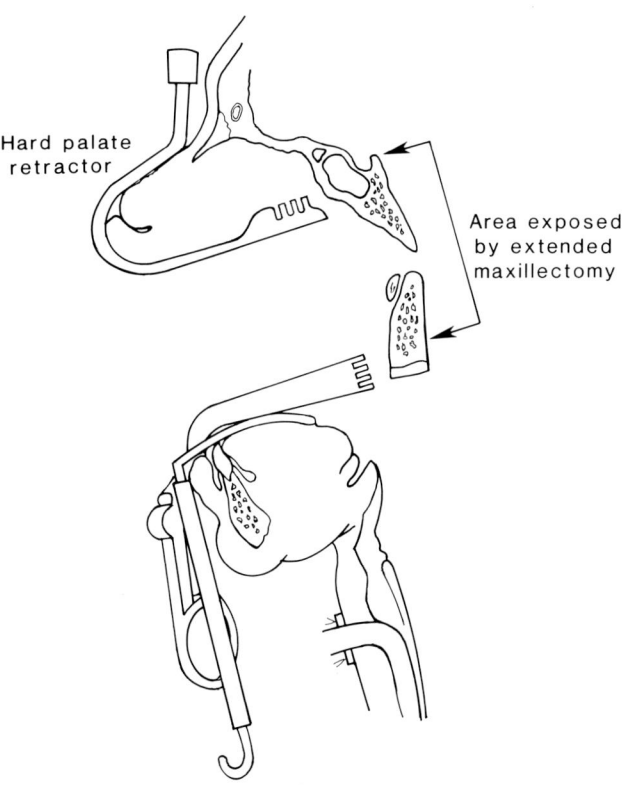

FIG. 14. A lateral diagram to show the extensive midline exposure produced by the extended maxillectomy.

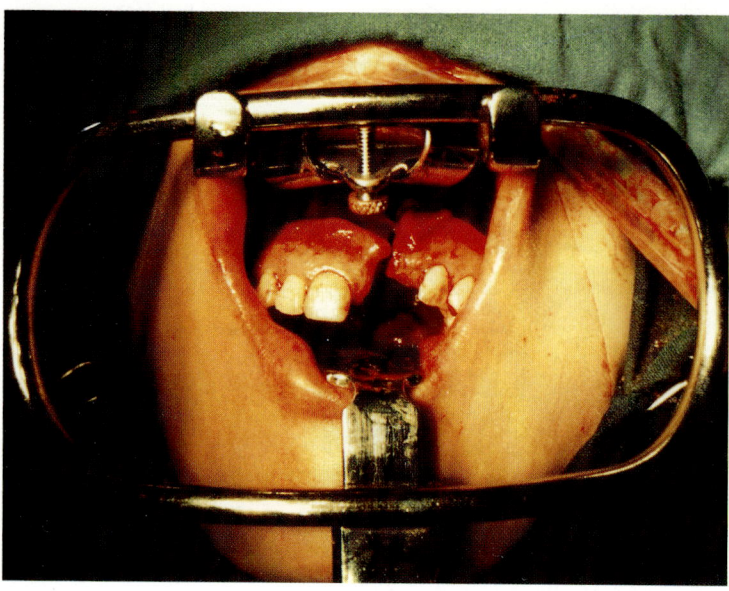

FIG. 15. An operative illustration after maxillectomy and midline palatal division and prior to the retraction of the segments.

The transoral retractor (Fig. 7A, B) with the transmaxillary plate adaption is inserted in position to allow for retraction (Fig. 14). The pharyngeal retractor is used to hold the palatal flaps laterally and after the division of the nasopharyngeal and oropharyngeal mucosa, the pharyngeal retractors are readjusted to keep this out of the way and expose the bone in the area of surgical interest. The transpalatal retractor may be useful in retracting the palatal flaps and the combination of pharyngeal and hard palatal retractors can be used to erect the best exposure depending on the individual shape of the base of the skull and the oral cavity. The corners of the mouth are retracted by using the soft palatal retractor applied to the transoral retractor frame (Fig. 15).

Surgery proceeds as previously described in this chapter and in Crockard (Transoral Approach). The closure of the extended maxillectomy is an extension of the material already described in this chapter.

ILLUSTRATIVE CASES

Myeloma of the Clivus

A 48-year-old man presented with progressive cranial nerve palsies and a MRI scan showed a complete resorption of the bone of the clivus and replacement by tumor. A preoperative diagnosis of either chordoma or metastasis was made (Fig. 16). A maxillectomy was performed as

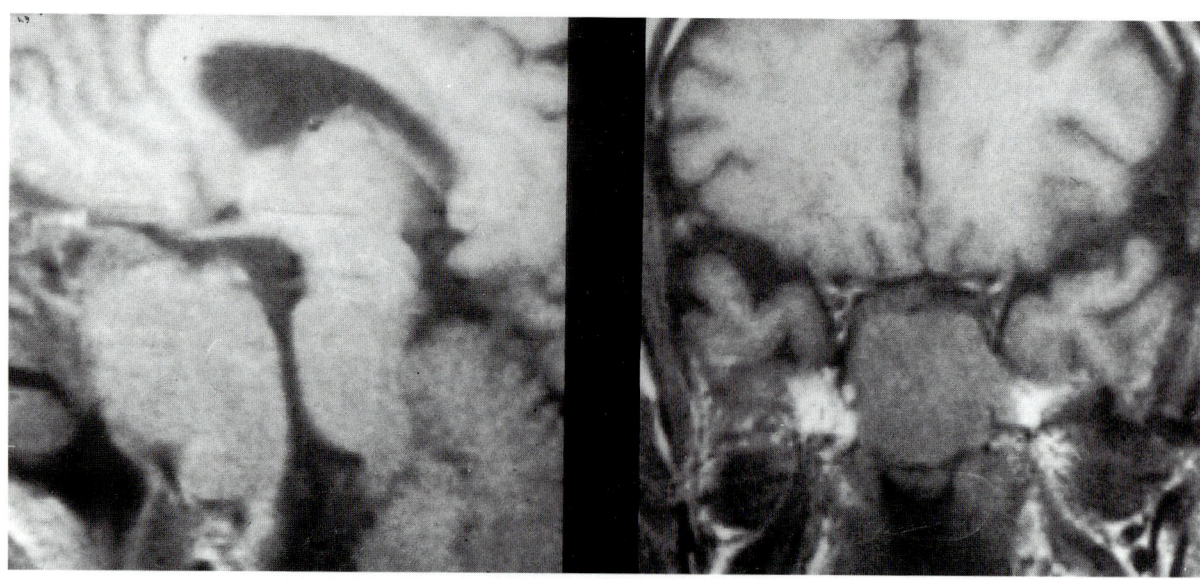

FIG. 16. An isolated plasmacytoma of the clivus.

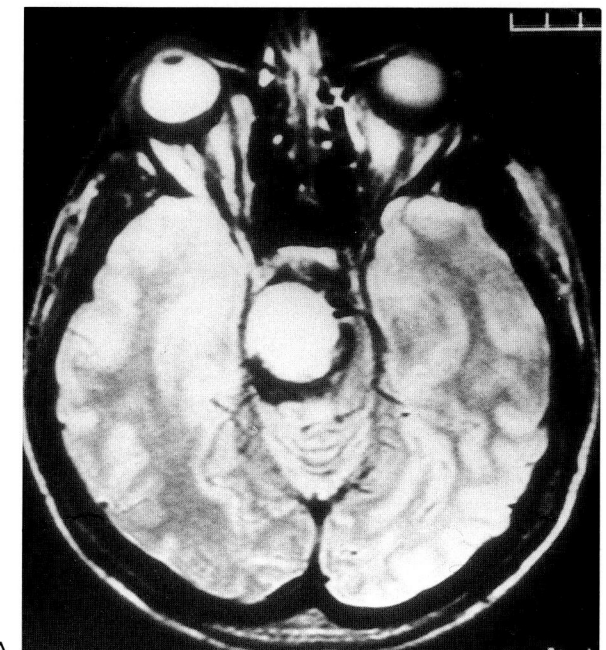 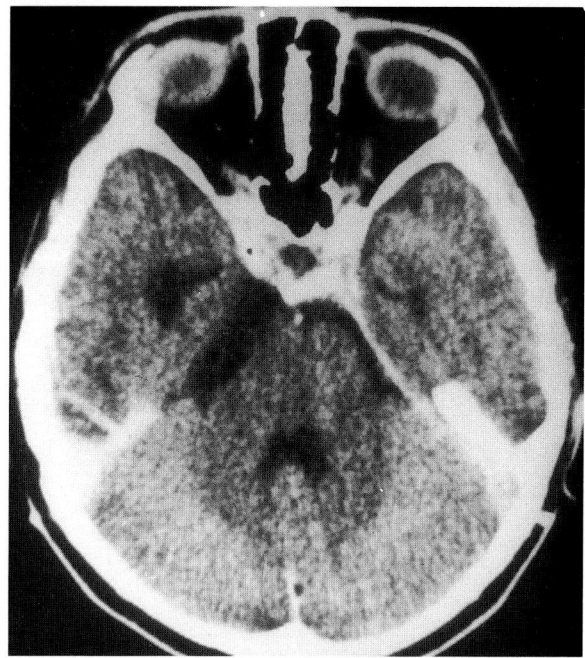

FIG. 17. Preoperative (**A**) and postoperative (**B**) scans of a chordoma extending into the cavernous sinus and intradurally successfully excised using the techniques described.

described in the first part of this chapter. The bony shell of the clivus was still intact in places, but this was easily removed with the dissector and curettes and deep to this was extremely soft and vascular tumor, which was removed with the angled and straight suction tubes. The patient was discharged from hospital 8 days after the transmaxillary approach to the lesion. The cranial nerve palsy resolved within 2 weeks. Histology revealed a plasmacytoma and further investigation has excluded any other site of plasmacytoma deposit. He has had local radiotherapy, and 2 years later there is no evidence as yet of any further development of his myeloma.

Intradural and Extradural Chordoma

A 42-year-old man presented with progressive sixth nerve, fifth nerve, and fourth nerve palsies. Magnetic resonance images revealed a mass at the junction of the petrous apex and the clivus. CT scan density and MRI suggested that the lesion was a chordoma (Fig. 17). Angiography excluded a giant aneurysm.

A tracheostomy and lumbar drain were inserted prior to surgery, and the transmaxillary approach was used. The outer surface of the clivus was intact, but in the sphenoid sinus there was one area where the bone was so thin that tumor could be seen. The intact bone was removed with the high-speed airdrill and the characteristic features of the chordoma noted. The tumor itself was soft and removed with angled curettes, angled dissector, congeurs, and suction. The tumor had breached the dura and was extending through just medial to the left cavernous sinus. There were large intercommunications between the cavernous sinuses in this area and the petrosal sinus. With the widening of the dura opening to effect the total excision, there was a great deal of bleeding. This was controlled with bipolar coagulation with tamponading with Surgicel packs. Eventually, visibility was restored, and the whole of the chordoma as seen in the operative field was removed. After hemostasis, the dura was repaired. Nasal packs were placed in position and the wounds closed in the usual way. In this case, it was decided not to convert the lumbar drain into a lumboperitoneal shunt and the drain was removed at 5 days without subsequent CSF leakage. He was discharged from hospital on the 10th postoperative day. Postoperative CT scan showed no obvious residual tumor.

CONCLUSION

The transmaxillary approach is a useful and necessary adjunct to midline surgery of the clivus. The extended maxillectomy provides wide exposure for extensive tumor or bony abnormalities in the area. Both procedures are commended.

Clearly, a great deal of teamwork is required and intensive care of the highest level. A great deal of new surgical anatomy is required, but, having learnt it, the technique will be found to be a most useful adjunct for skull base surgery.

ACKNOWLEDGMENTS

The author is grateful to Mr. D. James, FRCS, Consultant Maxillofacial Surgeon, University College Hospital, London, and Dr. I. Calder, Consultant Anesthestist, The National Hospitals for Nervous Diseases, London. Without their unstinting help, none of this work would be possible.

The author is also indebted to Michelle Green for the preparation of this manuscript.

FURTHER READING

Archer DJ, Young S, Uttley D. Basilar aneurysms: a new transclival approach via maxillotomy. *J Neurosurg* 1987;67:54–58.

Ashraf J, Crockard HA. Transoral fusion for high cervical fractures. *J Bone Joint Surg [Br]* 1990;1.

Crockard HA. Anterior approaches to lesions of the upper cervical spine. *Clin Neurosurg* 1988;34:389–416.

Crockard HA, Calder I, Ransford AO. One stage transoral decompression and posterior fixation in rheumatoid atlanto-axial subluxation: a technical note. *J Bone Joint Surg [Br]* 1990;72B:682–685.

Crockard HA, Sen CN. The transoral approach for the management of intradural lesions of the craniovertebral junction: a review of 7 cases. *Neurosurgery* 1991;28:88–98.

James D, Crockard HA. Surgical access to the base of skull and upper cervical spine by exterior maxillotomy. *Neurosurg* 1991;29(3):411–416.

Harkey HL, Crockard HA, Stevens JM, Smith R, Ransford AO. The operative management of basilar impression in osteogenesis imperfecta. *Neurosurg* 1990;27(5):782–786.

CHAPTER 16

Facial Translocation Approach to Nasopharynx, Clivus, and Infratemporal Fossa

Ivo P. Janecka, Chandranath Sen, Laligam N. Sekhar, and Daniel W. Nuss

Nasopharynx, clivus, and infratemporal fossa represent important segments of the cranial base. Anatomically, these complex areas comprise the structural as well as functional junction of the splanchnocranium and neurocranium, as it can be well delineated on coronal and axial CT scans (Fig. 1). Satisfactory surgical access to these areas has always been difficult to achieve. This was primarily due to the presence of complex but oncologically uninvolved craniofacial anatomy, which represented a barrier between the surgeon and the pathology.

The large number of surgical approaches to these areas described in the literature attests to the difficulties of surgical access. For example, the transbasal, transsphenoidal–transoral, and subtemporal–preauricular approaches do reach individual parts of this region of the cranial base, but none provides a simultaneous access to all three areas within a single wide surgical field (1–5).

The facial translocation approach permits a direct access to this area (6,7). It provides a surgical field extending from the contralateral eustachian tube to the ipsilateral cervical ICA encompassing nasopharynx, clivus, and sphenoid sinus as well as the cavernous sinus. Also, anterior and middle cranial fossae and orbital fissures are reachable. It may also be extended further in a horizontal as well as vertical plane. Conceptually, this procedure satisfies the need for temporary displacement of normal craniofacial anatomy along esthetic and functional planes in a systematic disassembly of soft tissue and the skeleton. The obtained surgical field is wide enough in three dimensions to permit advanced oncological surgery as well as systematic reconstruction of the defect with autogenous tissue; especially the dural repair along the floor of the middle cranial fossa.

PLANNING

The selection of a specific approach to the cranial base is primarily determined by the location of the tumor and its shortest distance to the skin surface. Alternate routes are designed to bypass critical structures (e.g., eye) not planned for inclusion in the oncological resection or structures essential to the patient's homeostasis (the temporal lobe or ICA where there is a significant dependence of cerebral circulation on this vessel).

The facial translocation approach to nasopharynx, clivus, and infratemporal fossa can especially be used in treating the following lesions at these sites:

1. Extensive angiofibromas extending through the skull base to the middle cranial fossa and cavernous sinus.
2. Nasopharyngeal carcinomas originating primarily on the lateral wall of the nasopharynx.
3. Chordomas of the clivus and the surrounding structures, especially those with extension across the midline and to the craniovertebral junction.
4. Sarcomas of the sphenoid rostrum.
5. Transcranial lesions (e.g., meningiomas, nerve sheath tumors, congenital tumors) extending to the infratemporal fossa and nasopharynx.
6. Extensive parotid salivary gland neoplasms with intra-

I. P. Janecka: Center for Cranial Base Surgery, University of Pittsburgh School of Medicine, Presbyterian University Hospital, and Department of Otolaryngology, Eye and Ear Institute, Pittsburgh, Pennsylvania 15213.

C. Sen: Department of Neurosurgery, Mt. Sinai Medical Center, New York, New York 10029.

L. N. Sekhar: Department of Neurosurgery, Center for Cranial Base Surgery, University of Pittsburgh School of Medicine, Presbyterian University Hospital, Pittsburgh, Pennsylvania 15213.

D. W. Nuss: Department of Otolaryngology, Louisiana State University School of Medicine, New Orleans, Louisiana 70112.

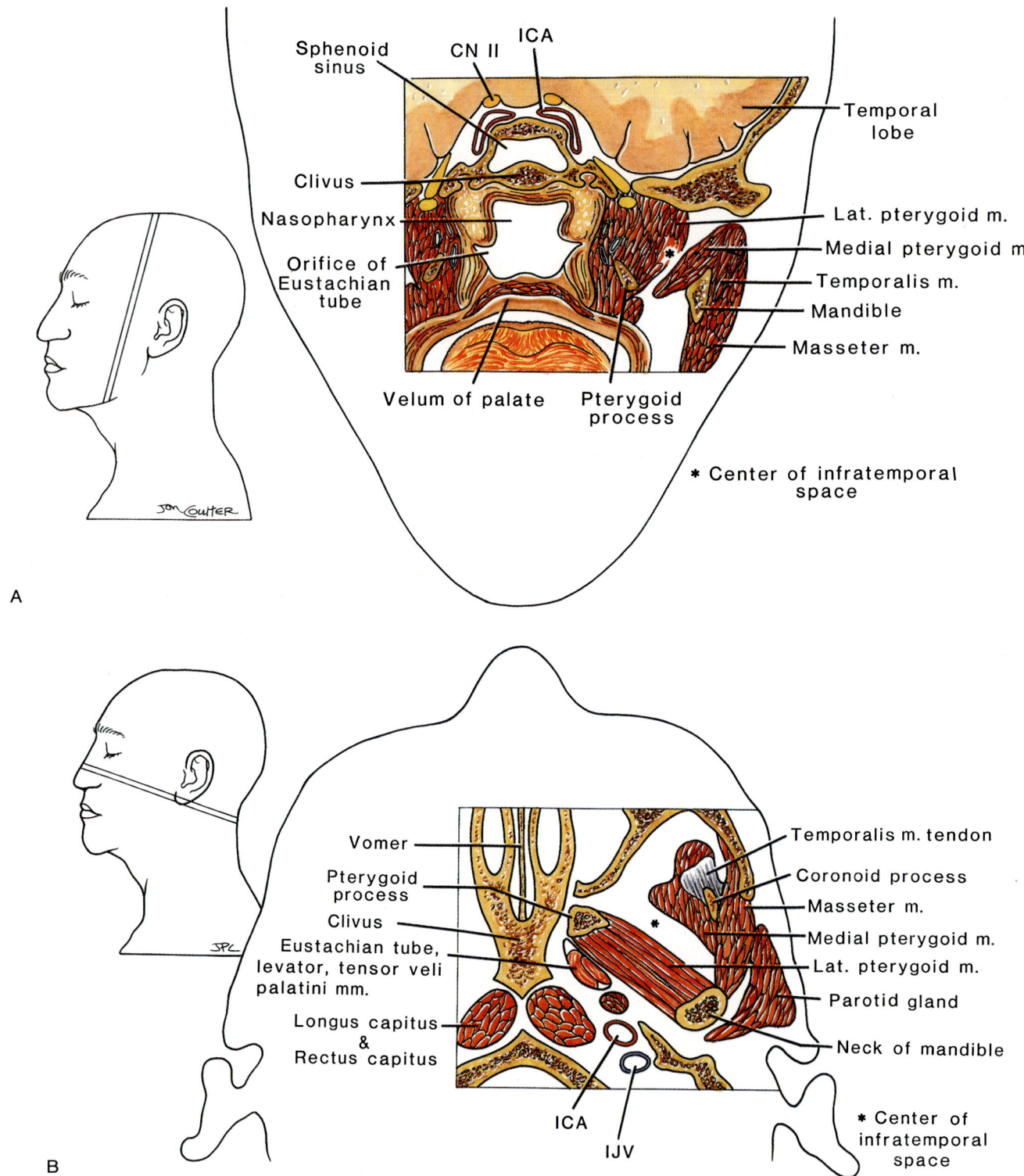

FIG. 1. Outline of the anatomy of the nasopharynx, clivus, and infratemporal fossa schematically illustrated on coronal and axial CT sections.

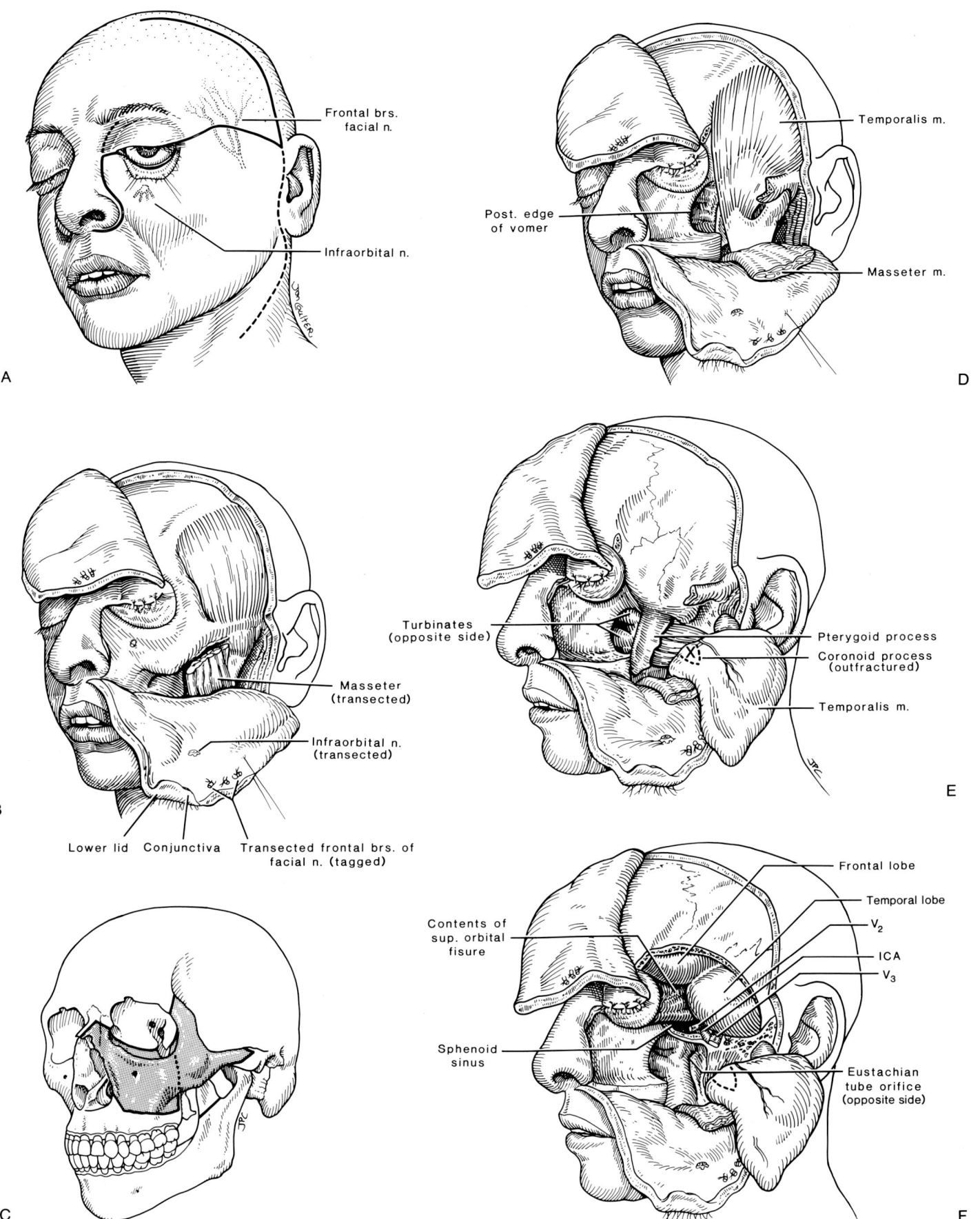

FIG. 2. Surgical steps depicted in drawings of facial translocation procedure.

cranial, infratemporal fossa as well as lateral pharyngeal extent.

SURGICAL STEPS

1. Facial incisions (paranasal, conjunctival, temporal) join the hemicoronal and preauricular with optional neck extension. Both medial and lateral canthi are divided. Postauricular as well as midline extensions are feasible as well (Fig. 2A).
2. The forehead branches of the facial nerve are isolated under magnification with the use of a nerve stimulator and under EMG control (4–6 branches are usually identified above the level of the zygomatic arch). Nerve branches are tagged with 7-0 nylon and sectioned. The infraorbital nerve is also isolated, tagged, and transected; the nasolacrimal duct is sectioned as well.
3. The craniofacial skeleton is exposed and freed from the temporalis and masseter muscles (Fig. 2B).
4. The soft tissue cheek flap is reflected inferiorly (including lower lid) to the level of the palate (dissection is done under the masseteric fascia in order to protect the main branches of the facial nerve) (Fig. 2B).
5. Elective osteotomies are performed permitting temporary removal of the craniofacial skeleton (Fig. 2C).
6. The posterior wall of the maxillary sinus (Fig. 2D) and the pterygoids (Fig. 2E) are removed (with the help of two horizontal osteotomies of the pterygoid plates at the level of the hard palate and the skull).
7. A subperiosteal osteotomy of the coronoid process permits further inferior rotation of the temporalis muscle to the palatal plane. Final exposure is achieved (Fig. 2E, F).
8. Additional optional steps, dictated by tumor extent, may include:
    a. Isolation of the main trunk of the facial nerve.
    b. Isolation of upper cervical and petrous ICA.
    c. Isolation of V_{2-3}.
    d. Opening of the sphenoid sinus.
    e. Dissection of the medial wall of the orbit to the level of the posterior ethmoid foramen.
    f. Further temporary removal of maxillofacial skeleton (ipsilateral or contralateral).
    g. Frontotemporal craniotomy.
    h. Intradural dissection.

SPECIFIC CONCERNS

Vascularity

The soft tissue flap (facial skin with lower eyelid) is well vascularized with preserved facial, superficial temporal, and labial arteries. Even with upper lip division, the vascularity of this flap should be adequate. Preexisting preauricular or postauricular scars may compromise external ear blood supply following the new procedure in this region. This is best avoided by incorporating the scars in the new flap design and preserving the preauricular segment of superficial temporal artery. Sometimes previous neurological procedures (e.g., frontotemporal craniotomy) leave a vertical midforehead scar. Reelevation of the frontotemporal scalp with a new horizontal inferior temporal incision potentially further diminishes blood supply to the original flap. Preservation of the supraorbital/supratrochlear vascular system as well as the contralateral superficial temporal artery should be sufficient for adequate scalp perfusion following facial translocation. Microvascular anastomosis of the superficial temporal artery is also feasible (Fig. 3).

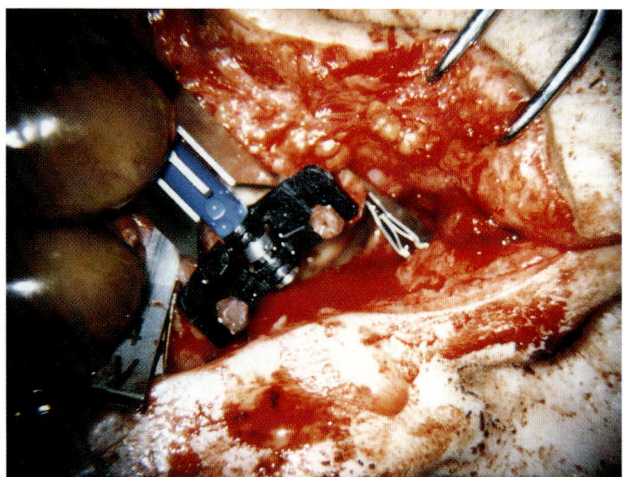 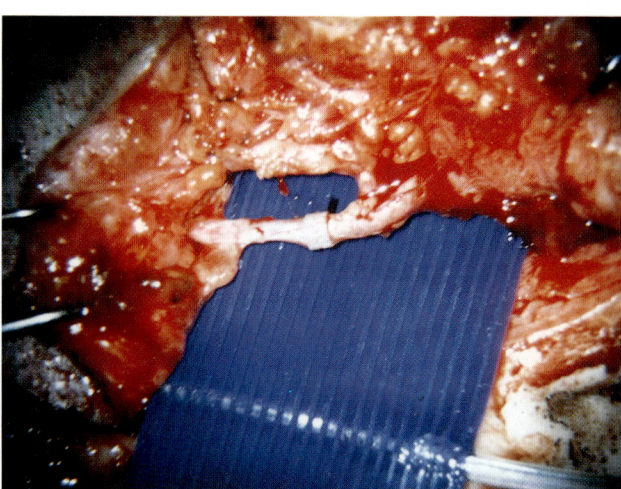

FIG. 3. A: 3M (St. Paul, MN) microvascular anastomotic device ready for vessel approximation. **B:** Reconnected superficial temporal artery with 2.0-mm rings.

Facial Nerve

The ophthalmic branch of the facial nerve is considered its most important branch. The facial translocation procedure preserves this nerve as well as its attachments to the orbicularis muscle. The inclusion of the entire lower lid in the translocation soft tissue flap protects this neuromuscular unit. Flap elevation at the level of the maxillary periosteum and under the level of the masseteric fascia protects the other main branches of the facial nerve as well as the main trunk.

The elective transection of the numerous branches of the facial nerve above the zygomatic arch is done under magnification. Individual nerves are placed in 6-mm-long soft silicon tubing, tagged with 7-0 nylon at each end, and transected in the middle. At the completion of the entire procedure, slight telescoping of one end of the silicon tubing into the other permits nerve stabilization and longitudinal alignment. Additional 7-0 nylon, across the invaginated segments of the tubing, is sufficient for nerve approximation (Fig. 4). Recovery of forehead function begins at 6–9 months (Fig. 5).

Facial Incisions/Scars

The paranasal incision is a variation on the well-accepted rhinotomy incision. By placing it about halfway between the nasal bridge and the lateral nose, the eventual scar seems to be even less visible (Fig. 6). This may be due to the uniformity of the skin composition within the midportion of the lateral nasal skin (it is a part of the same "esthetic unit" of the nose) as opposed to the site of the "standard" lateral rhinotomy incision, which is at the junction of the nasal and cheek skin (here the dermis representation in the skin is different between those two sites).

Medial and lateral canthal incisions fall into a category of canthotomies that have also been previously used and are considered esthetically acceptable, as is the con-

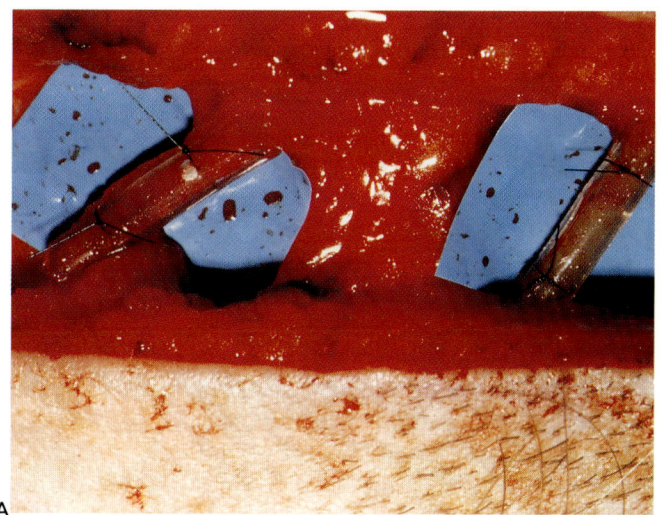

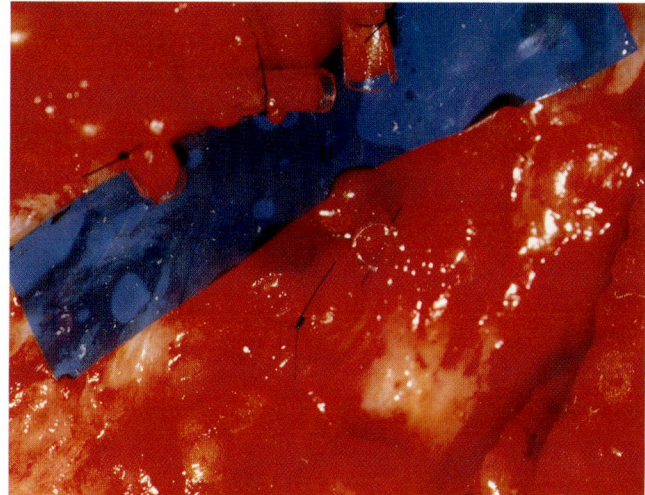

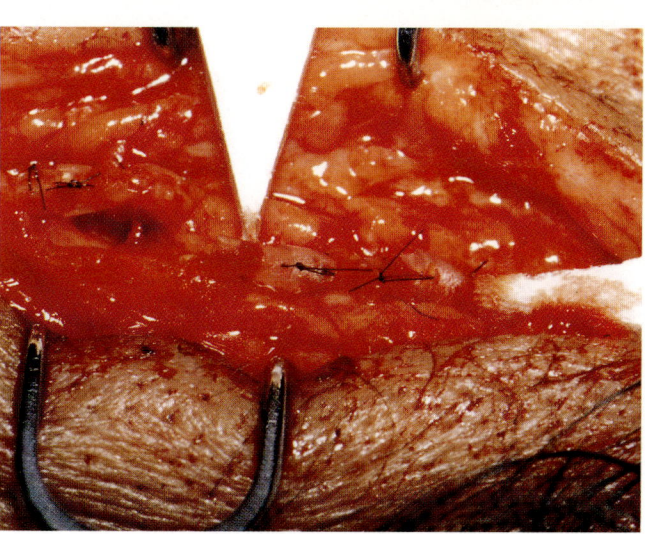

FIG. 4. A: Isolated facial nerve branches above the zygomatic arch ensheathed in silicone tubings. **B:** Transected tubings with nerve. **C:** Reapproximation of nerve/tubing units.

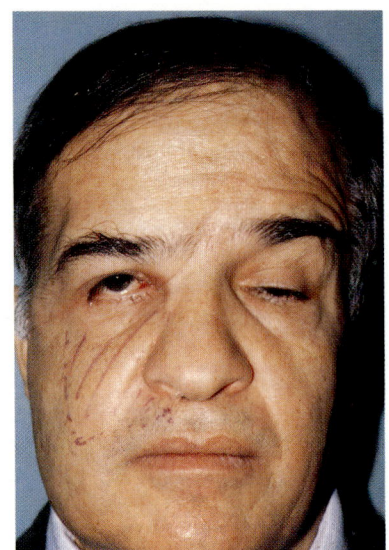
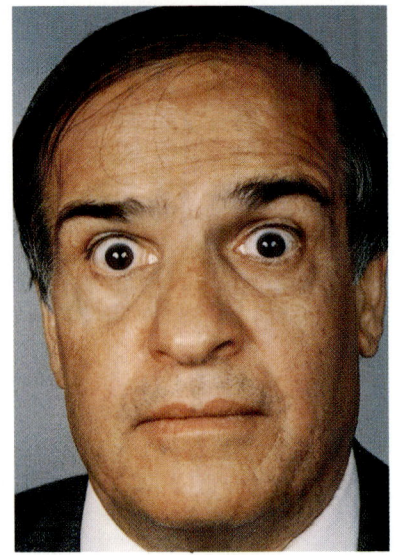

FIG. 5. A: Absence of forehead function shortly following surgery. **B:** Forehead function 9 months later.

junctival incision in the inferior fornix. Reestablishment of the canthal balance (especially the medial) can be made easier by marking the attachment of the medial canthal ligament to the nasolacrimal bony crest at the time of canthal detachment. At the completion of the entire procedure, temporary tarsorrhaphy (with mattress sutures) is performed to assist in proper vertical orientation of the lid soft tissue during the early healing phase. The sutures are removed in 7–10 days. By then, the entire orbicularis oculi muscle functions and is able to support the low lid position (Fig. 7).

Nasolacrimal Duct

The reestablishment of the continuity of this drainage system is done by direct stenting with the use of soft silicon tubing (e.g., Crawford nasolacrimal stent, which is commercially available and already comes with attached metal probes) (Jedmed, 1430 Hanley Industrial Court, St. Louis, MO 63144). The tubing is passed through both canaliculi into the nose where it is tied (Fig. 8). It is left in place for 6–8 weeks. The majority of the patients have adequate lacrimal drainage following removal of this stent.

Infraorbital Nerve

Full elevation of the cheek flap (as in the standard procedure for maxillectomy) requires transection of this nerve. If not involved by tumor, elective transection and tagging with 6-0 nylon permits neurorrhaphy at the completion of the procedure. The preservation of this nerve proximal segment, during the approach phase of the translocation procedure, is done by enlarging the infraorbital foramen (with a small currette); the nerve can then be brought into the orbit and protected during the subsequent osteotomies of the orbital floor.

At the completion of the entire procedure, the proximal nerve segment is tagged with a long 6-0 nylon suture, which is brought through the enlarged infraorbital fora-

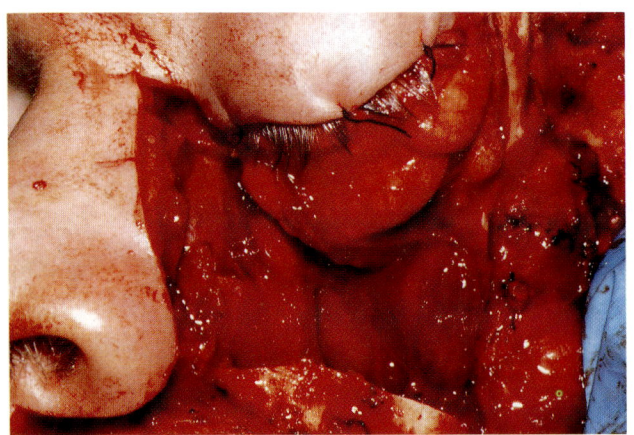
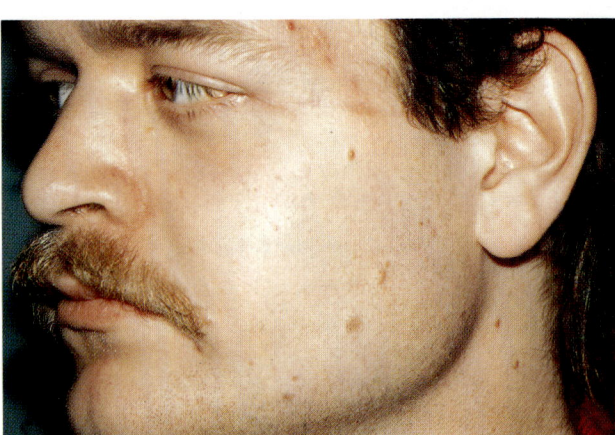

FIG. 6. A: Exposure achieved with facial incisions. **B:** Healed face.

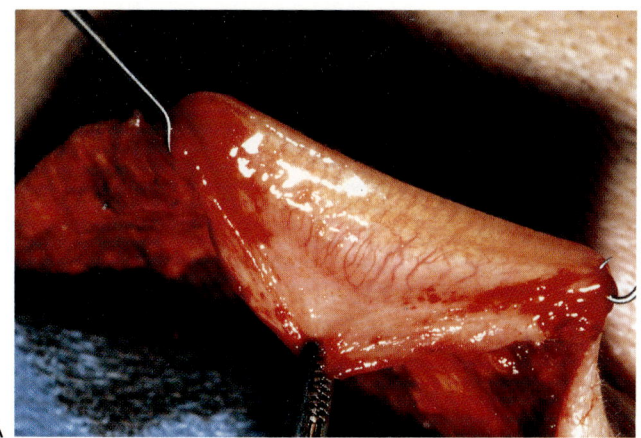
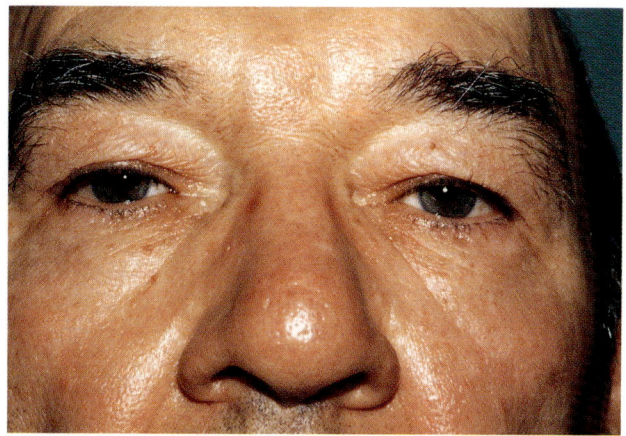

FIG. 7. **A:** Surgical view of displaced left lower lid with conjunctiva. **B:** Patient's appearance following reconstruction (left face).

men of the replaced maxilla. It is sutured to the most distal part of the nerve in the cheek flap. Recovery of cheek sensation is expected within 6–9 months (Fig. 9).

Craniofacial Skeleton

The osteotomies of the skeleton are performed in a "key–keyhole" pattern so as to minimize potential movement following replacement. The Le Fort I osteotomy is done horizontally in endentulous patients but should respect the prominent canine root where present. The intraorbital cuts originate from the inferior orbital fissure. They extend laterally to include the lateral orbital wall (this is done with a reciprocating saw). The orbital floor cut is done with an oscillating saw using a modified right angle blade, which permits access into a narrow space (between the bone and the orbital content) for precise bony cuts. Medially, the osteotomies end up at the posterior lacrimal crest. At the completion of the surgery, most of the lacrimal bone is removed to facilitate nasolacrimal drainage. The fixation of replaced craniofacial skeleton following oncological surgery is done with a mini or micro-plating system following removal of remnants of maxillary sinus mucosa (Fig. 10).

Nasal Mucosa

The mucosa of the lateral nasal wall (including inferior turbinate) is elevated before making the osteotomy along the medial maxillary wall. This mucosal flap can be based anterosuperiorly and is used for reconstruction of the lateral nasal wall. It is subsequently attached to the transferred temporalis muscle.

Along the vomer and clivus, the soft tissue can also be elevated in a lateromedial direction. It serves as a valuable attachment for the distal portion of the transferred temporalis muscle. Early reestablishment of the mucosal coverage in the postoperative period is thus enhanced.

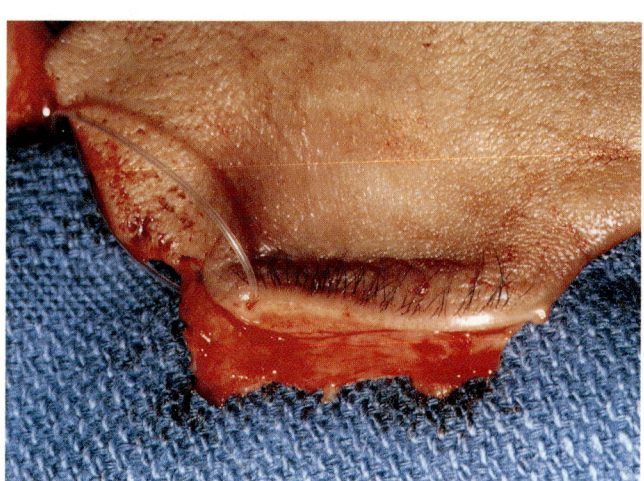

FIG. 8. Stenting of the lacrimal canaliculi.

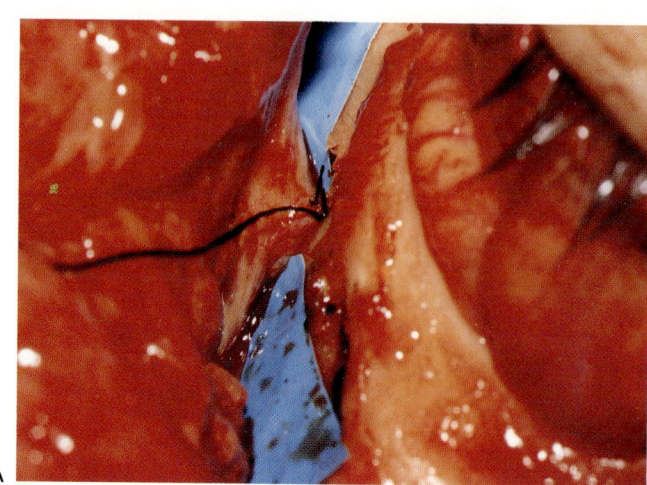
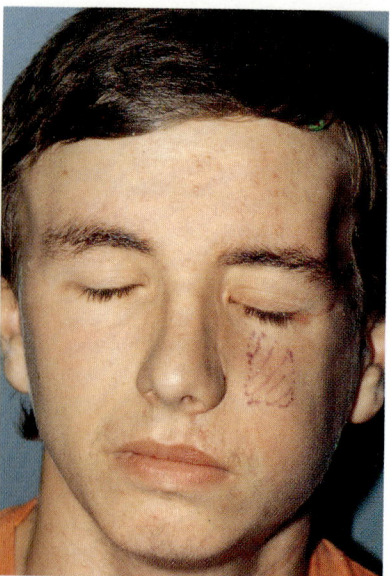

FIG. 9. A: Neurorrhaphy of the left infraorbital nerve. **B:** Remaining zone of decreased sensation on patient's cheek 5 months later.

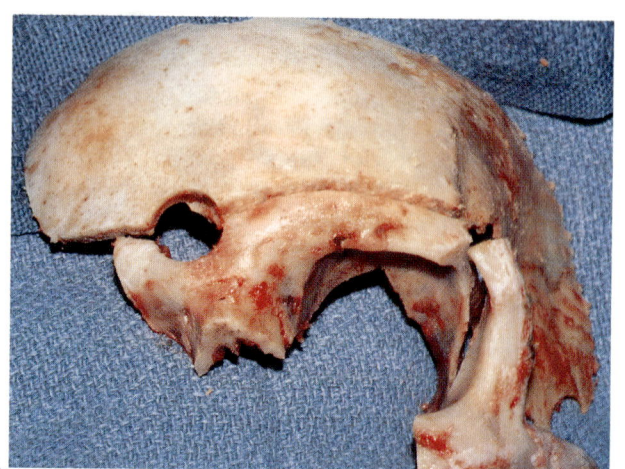
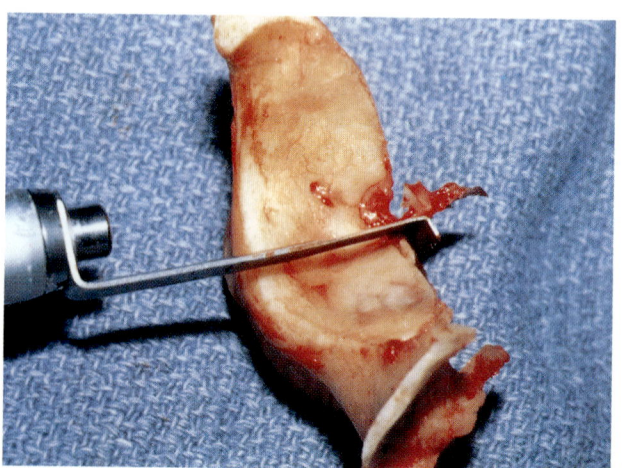
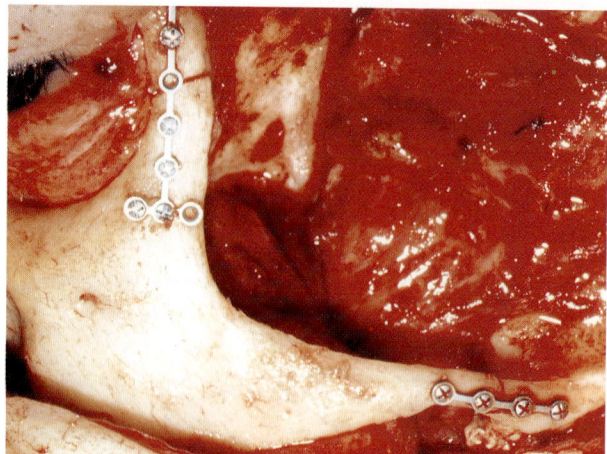

FIG. 10. A: Temporarily removed craniofacial skeleton. **B:** Modified right angle blade used for cutting the orbital floor. **C:** Replaced left facial skeleton with miniplate fixation.

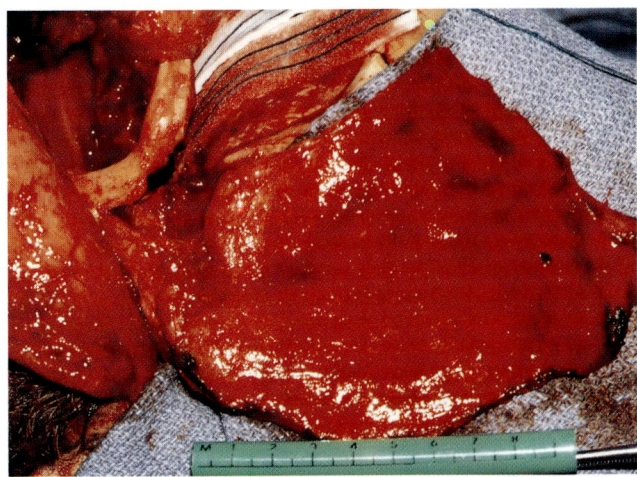 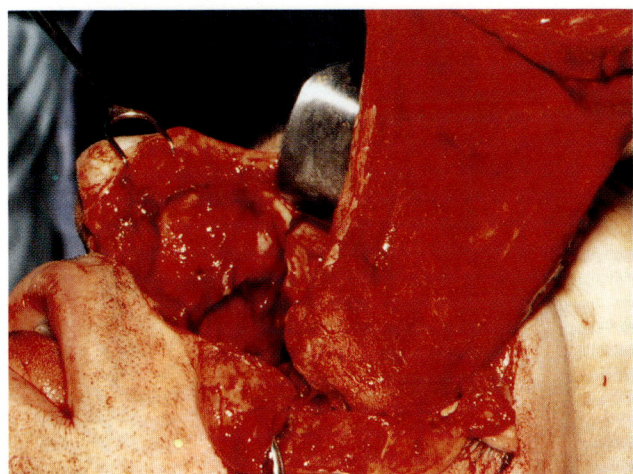

FIG. 11. **A:** Raised left temporalis muscle. **B:** Rotation of temporalis muscle into the surgical defect.

Temporalis Muscle

The protection of the temporalis muscle blood supply is an important aspect in the facial translocation sequence. This muscle is very valuable in the reconstructive phase (Fig. 11). It provides strong autogenous as well as vascularized protection of the temporal dura and can obliterate the sphenoid sinus and the "dead space" created by tumor and maxillary sinus removal. The elevation of the muscle and its temporary displacement from the center of the surgical field are enhanced by subperiosteal osteotomy of the coronoid process. This permits right angle rotation of its insertion. This maneuver exposes the lateral pterygoids and assists in early identification of the internal maxillary artery. This is very helpful in surgery for vascularized tumors, especially angiofibromas, and potentially diminishes the need for preoperative tumor embolization.

Occasionally, the tumor resection requires transection of the proximal course of the internal maxillary artery. If, however, the distal communications (e.g., palatine vessels) are intact, it may still be possible to transfer this muscle on its now reversed distal blood supply.

PREOPERATIVE CARE

Hospital Unit

1. External skin/scalp is washed with Phisohex and the hair is shampooed the night before.
2. Any suspected draining site is cultured.
3. Oral/nasopharyngeal rinsing with a bacitracin/neomycin solution mouth wash three times may be of benefit in patients with previous radiotherapy to these sites.

Operating Room

1. Neuroanesthesia setup.
2. Broad spectrum antibiotics are administered. (Cefuroxime 750 mg every 8 hr is currently used and is started approximately 1 hr before surgical incision.)
3. Patient is placed in a supine position on the operating table with head resting on a Mayfield headrest.
4. Endotracheal tube is wired to the opposite dentition or affixed with a circummandibular wire.
5. Neurophysiological monitoring leads (for somatosensory potentials) are placed on the scalp (outside the planned sterile area).
6. Both lower extremities are placed in automatic compression stockings.

TABLE 1. *Indications for facial translocation in the first 20 patients*

Tumors		Follow-up (14 months)	Remarks
Angiofibromas	4	4/4 NED	1/4 CT suggestive of possible recurrence
CSF leaks	3	3/3 NED	
Carcinomas	7	1/7 DOD	
Sarcomas	5	1/5 DOD	
Chordoma	1	1/1 NED	Reop for recurrence; postop RT
Total	20		

TABLE 2. *Complications encountered among our patients*

Complications		Treatment	Remarks
Infection	2/20	Surgery and antibiotics	One bone graft One tumor recurrence
Nasolacrimal duct obstruction	2/20	Surgery	

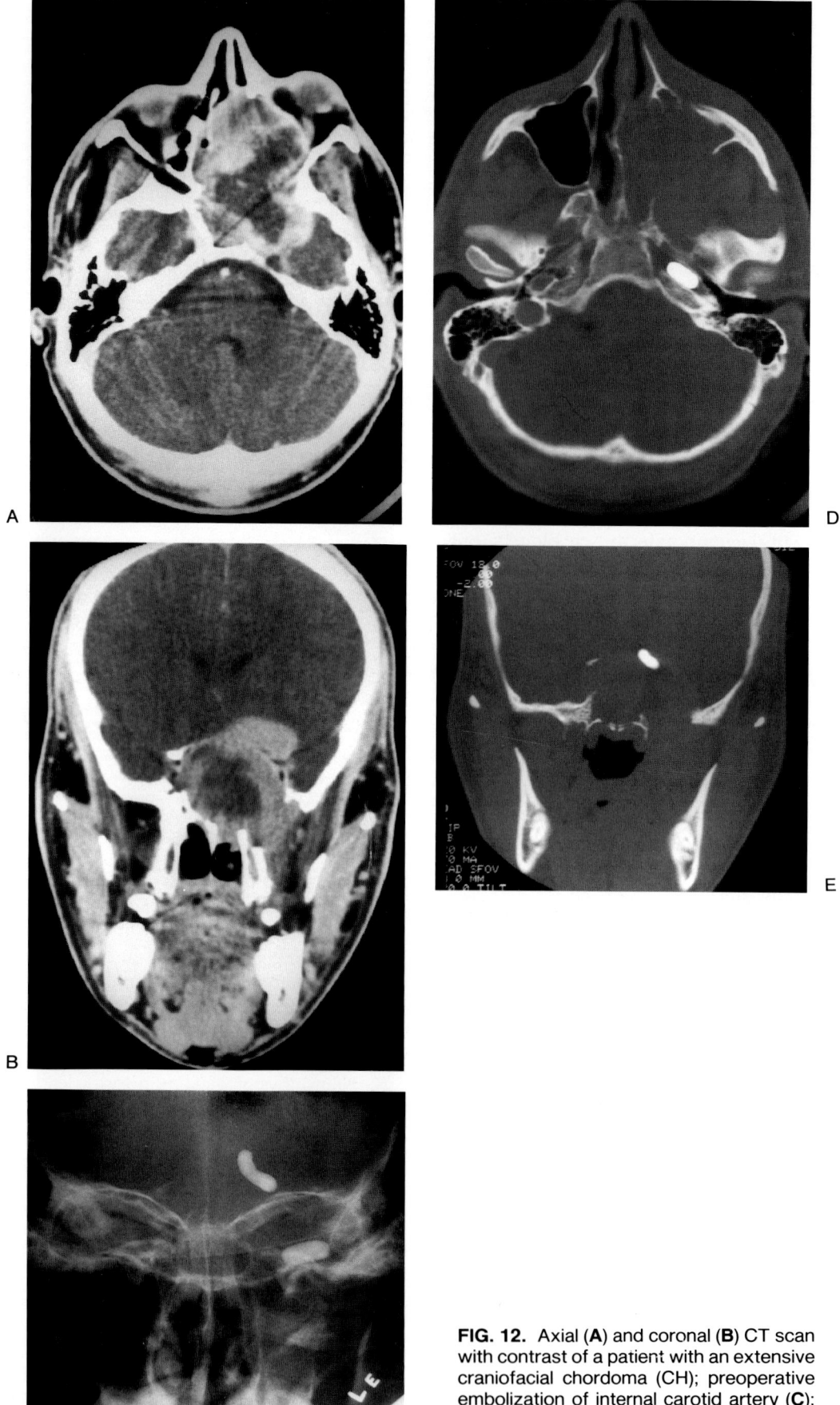

FIG. 12. Axial (**A**) and coronal (**B**) CT scan with contrast of a patient with an extensive craniofacial chordoma (CH); preoperative embolization of internal carotid artery (**C**); in the petrous (**D**) and supraclinoid (**E**) segment.

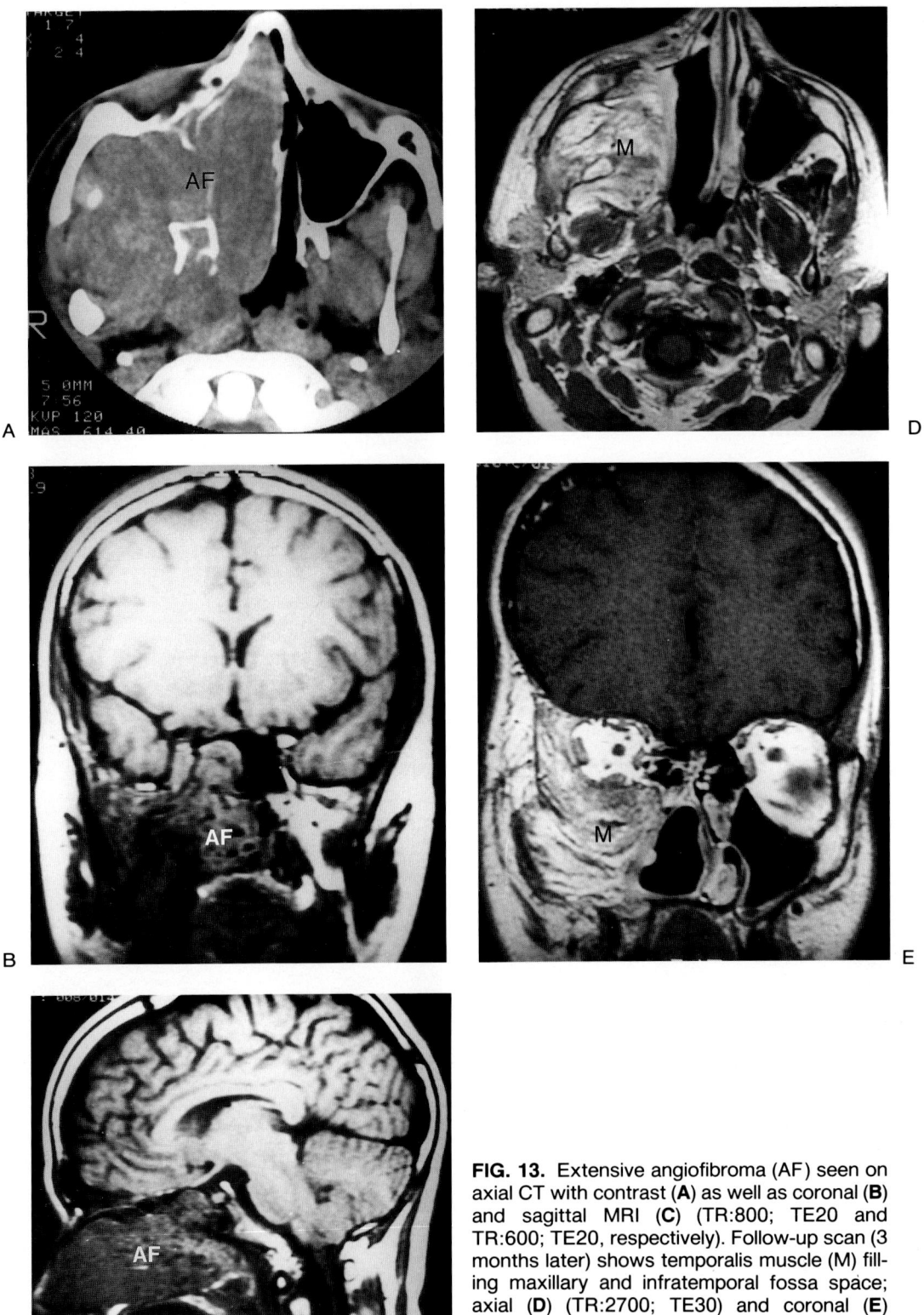

FIG. 13. Extensive angiofibroma (AF) seen on axial CT with contrast (A) as well as coronal (B) and sagittal MRI (C) (TR:800; TE20 and TR:600; TE20, respectively). Follow-up scan (3 months later) shows temporalis muscle (M) filling maxillary and infratemporal fossa space; axial (D) (TR:2700; TE30) and coronal (E) (TR:800, TE20) MRI with contrast.

7. Betadine/alcohol prep of head/neck area is done as well as other sites (e.g., abdomen for a possible microvascular rectus abdominis flap or a free-fat graft; or thigh is prepped for possible saphenous vein graft harvesting or obtaining a fascia lata graft; calf may be prepped if a sural nerve graft is needed).
8. Draping of all needed sites is done as well as placement of the facial nerve monitoring electrodes in designated sterile areas.
9. Facial incisions are marked and tissue is injected with $\frac{1}{4}$% xylocaine with 1:400,000 epinephrine, except for the region of facial nerve branches planned to be monitored.

POSTOPERATIVE CARE

There are some general concerns in the postoperative period that are universal to all cranial base procedures: airway hemostasis, CSF containment, and CNS and cranial nerve functionality, as well as systemic homeostasis. CT scan is obtained on the first or second day to assess intracranial extent of air and blood. If significant manipulation of petrous carotid artery was performed intraoperatively, a postoperative angiogram determines the intraluminal flow status as well as potential aneurysm formation.

The facial translocation procedure does not require any specific postoperative measures. The temporary tarsorrhaphy sutures are removed in about 10 days or when the lower lid portion of the orbicularis oculi muscle begins to demonstrate function. The nasal stent is removed then as well. The nasolacrimal stent is kept in for at least 6 weeks. At 3 months postoperatively, a baseline CT is obtained, which is used as a reference for future CTs. If the eustachian tube has been resected, a PE tube is inserted.

COMPLICATIONS

Possible complications associated with the facial translocation procedure are similar to other cranial base procedures (e.g., CSF leak, meningitis, hematomas). Specific consideration must be given to the internal carotid artery and the cavernous sinus. Adequate access to these vascular structures minimizes potential injury and assists in control. Cavernous sinus bleeding can be controlled with oxidized cellulose (e.g., Oxycel; Becton Dickinson Acute Care, One Becton Drive, Franklin Lakes, NJ 07417) and Surgicel (Johnson & Johnson Hospital Services, P.O. Box 4000, New Brunswick, NJ 08903).

Late complications may include some degree of enophthalmos. This may result from incomplete orbital reconstruction and/or atrophy of periorbital fat. Full nasolacrimal duct obstruction may need modified dacryocystorhinostomy. The appearance of temporal fossa depends on the degree of free-fat graft survival. Some graft is expected to survive, minimizing the concavity of this temporalis muscle donor site.

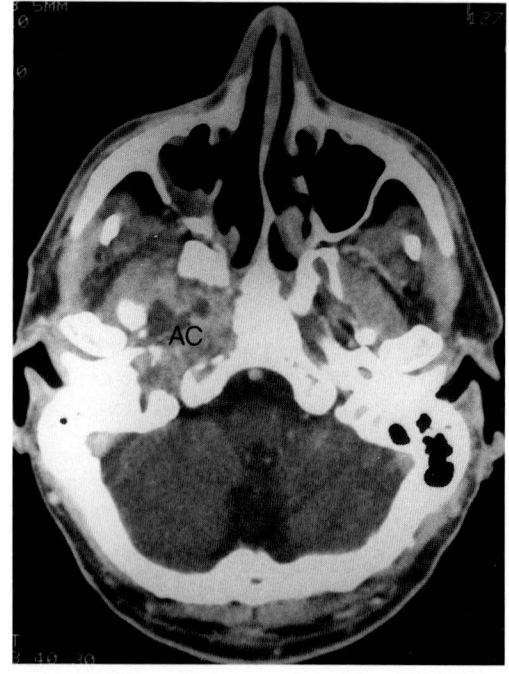 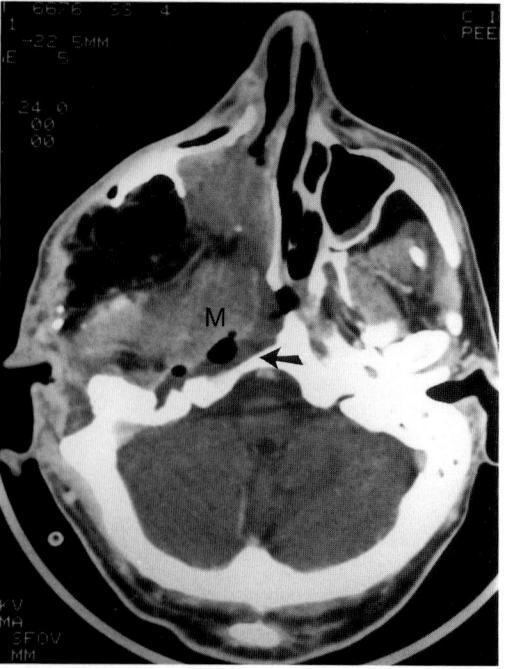

FIG. 14. Axial CT with contrast demonstrating a recurrent adenoid cystic (AC) carcinoma (**A**) at the skull base; a similar CT cut (**B**) 1 month postoperatively with removal of a portion of the clivus (*arrow*); microvascular rectus abdominis muscle (M) transfer was used for repair of the surgical defect.

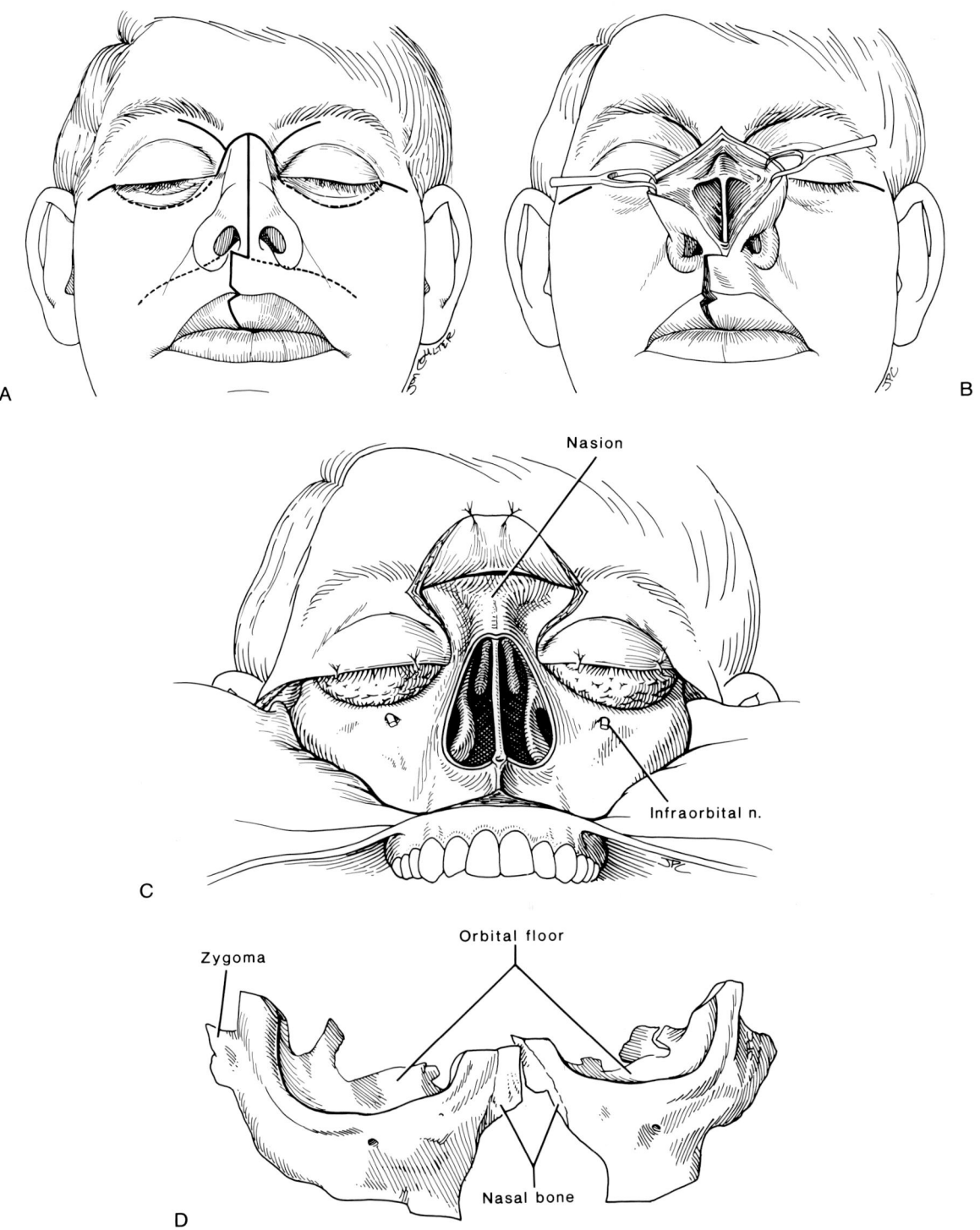

FIG. 15. A: Outline of incisions for midfacial split approach to central and paracentral cranial base. **B:** Nasal split. **C:** Outline of exposed maxillofacial skeleton following midfacial splitting of soft tissues. **D:** Extent of temporarily removed maxillofacial skeleton. **E:** Exposure of key structures in central cranial base. **F:** Transfer of right temporalis muscle into cranial base defect of central skull base following midfacial split technique.

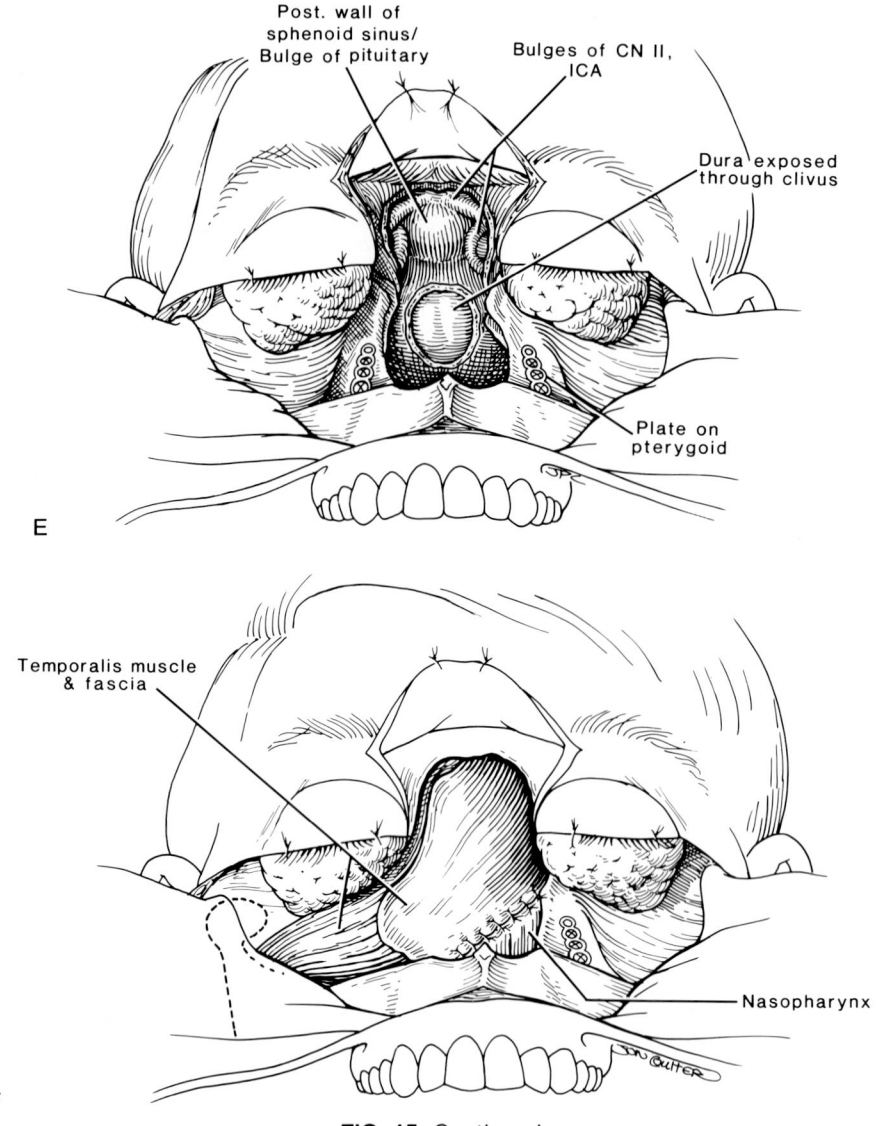

FIG. 15. *Continued.*

FOLLOW-UP

Primary healing following the facial translocation approach is expected. An exception may be severely radiated and previously operated-on patients. In most patients oncological evaluation is performed by CT/MRI scanning done at 6-month intervals during the first 1–2 years. The frequency of scans is determined by the tumor histology as well as clinical suspicion. Areas of concern may be biopsied directly or with CT guidance. Prosthetic rehabilitation may include external eye prosthesis following exenteration or dental appliance if hard palate had to be resected as well. The frontalis muscle is expected to begin functioning at 8–9 months.

DISCUSSION

There is no perfect approach to the cranial base. The facial translocation approach to lesions in the nasopharynx, clivus, and the infratemporal fossa offers significant technical as well as oncological advantages. The wide exposure, simplified control of essential structures, and functional and esthetic reconstruction are the hallmarks of the procedure.

We have reviewed the first 20 patients who underwent a facial translocation procedure (Tables 1 and 2). Most were done for oncological reasons (Figs. 12–14). All patients healed per primum. The frontal branches of the facial nerve showed signs of recovery at 8–9 months and continued to improve. The new nasolacrimal passage had to be reexplored in two patients.

An expansion of the facial translocation includes the midfacial split approach to the central and paracentral cranial base (Fig. 15).

CONCLUSION

The facial translocation approach and its potential for further multidirectional expansion permit extension of oncological surgery at the anterolateral cranial base.

REFERENCES

1. Derome PJ. The transbasal approach to tumors invading the base of the skull. In: Schmidek MH, Sweet WH, eds. *Operative neurosurgical techniques,* 2nd ed, vol. 1. Orlando: Grune and Stratton, 1988;619–633.
2. Hardy J. Transsphenoidal hypophysectomy. *J Neurosurg* 1971;34:582–594.
3. Fisch U. Infratemporal fossa approach to tumors of the temporal bone and base of the skull. *J Laryngol Otol* 1978;92:949–967.
4. Sekhar LN, Janecka IP, Jones NF. Subtemporal–infratemporal and basal subfrontal approach to extensive cranial base tumors. *Acta Neurochir* 1988;92:83–92.
5. Crockard HA, Bradford R. Transoral transclival removal of a schwannoma anterior to the craniocervical junction. *J Neurosurg* 1985;62:293–295.
6. Janecka IP, Sen CN, Sekhar LN, Arriaga MA. Facial translocation: a new approach to the cranial base. *Otolaryngol Head Neck Surg* 1990;103:413–419.
7. Arriaga MA, Janecka IP. Surgical exposure of the nasopharynx: anatomic basis for a transfacial approach. *Surg Forum* 1989;40:547–549.

CHAPTER 17

The Transmandibular–Transcervical Approach to the Skull Base

Yosef P. Krespi and Gady Har-El

The middle compartment of the skull base, especially the extracranial surface of the middle cranial fossa between the carotid arteries, has always been a difficult region to approach surgically (Fig. 1). This compartment has been exposed either through the sinonasal region (sublabial–transseptal, transethmoidal, lateral rhinotomy) with a very limited exposure, through the mouth (transoral, transoral–transpalatal, medial labiomandibuloglossotomy) with a better exposure to midline structures but limited exposure lateral to the sphenoid sinus, or through the neck (trancervical retropharyrngeal). The introduction of the transmandibular–transcervical approach (without glossotomy) gave the skull base surgeons a technique that provides excellent exposure of the middle compartment of the skull base from the foramen magnum and clivus to the sphenoid sinus and sella turcica together with lateral exposure of the infratemporal fossa, inferior surface of the petrous bone, and the parapharyngeal space with its major neurovascular structures.

The combined transmandibular–transcervical approach has been used for management of neoplastic lesions such as chordomas, pituitary tumors, glomus vagale, high vascular schwannoma, choroid plexus tumor, and benign as well as malignant tumors of the nasopharynx. Tumors that originated in the parapharyngeal space and extended medially with displacement of the oropharyngeal/nasopharyngeal walls (e.g., parotid deep lobe tumors or neurogenic tumors) have also been managed via this approach. Nonneoplastic lesions were also treated with the same technique. Examples are invagination of the odontoid process, teratogenic cyst of the brain stem, internal carotid aneurism, and foreign bodies (bullets). The need for decompression, reduction, and realignment of the occipito-atlanto-axial complex is another indication.

SURGICAL TECHNIQUE

Under general anesthesia (unless intubation is contraindicated by unstable cervical spine or large pharyngeal tumor), with the patient in a supine position and the

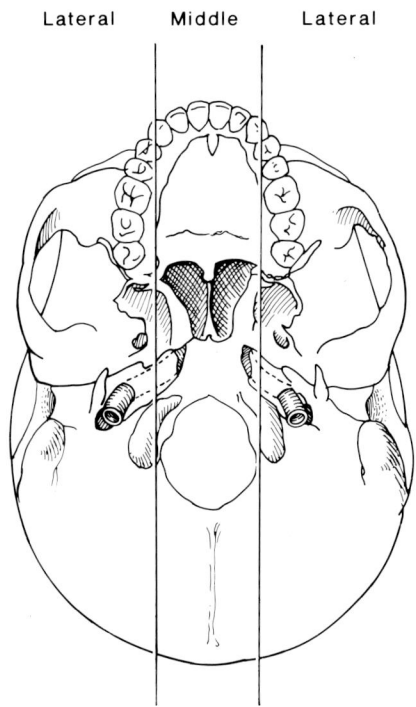

FIG. 1. The compartments of the extracranial surface of the skull base.

Y. P. Krespi: Department of Otolaryngology, Head and Neck Surgery, St. Lukes/Roosevelt Hospital Center, New York, New York 10019.

G. Har-El: Department of Otolaryngology, SUNY-Health Sciences Center at Brooklyn, and the Long Island College Hospital, Brooklyn, New York 11201.

neck slightly extended, a tracheotomy is performed. After the airway is secured, a curvilinear incision is made, extending from the mastoid tip to the submental region (Fig. 2). The incision should pass 4–5 cm below the mandible. The platysma muscle is divided and limited subplatysmal flaps are developed superiorly and inferiorly. The inferior border of the submandibular gland is identified and the dissection is carried below and deep to the gland. Low skin incision and avoiding unnecessary dissection between the platysma and the gland will prevent injury to the marginal mandibular nerve. The digastric tendon is now identified. This structure, together with the stylohyoid muscle, is released from the hyoid attachment and reflected superiorly with the submandibular gland. Care is taken to avoid injury to the hypoglossal nerve, which lies deep to the digastric tendon after it leaves the carotid sheath.

The sternocleidomastoid muscle is retracted posterolaterally and the major neurovascular structures of the neck are now exposed. These are identified and followed toward the skull base as they pass deep to the posterior belly of the digastric muscle. There is no need at this time to complete the dissection deep and around the carotid sheath all the way up to the skull base. This will be easier to do later through the transmandibular part of the surgery.

The common and internal carotid arteries and the tenth, eleventh, and twelfth cranial nerves are identified and preserved. The internal jugular vein is preserved unless contraindicated by the disease. The external carotid artery is followed toward the mandible. This artery may be ligated at this time distal to the superior thyroid artery in order to diminish blood loss. Vascular loops may be passed around the common and internal carotid arteries. These are tagged and kept loose.

The skin incision is extended superiorly toward the lower lip (Fig. 2). A midline lip-splitting incision is made and the anterior mandible is exposed between the mental foramina. The mandibular periosteum is incised in the midline and elevated laterally and an oscillating power saw is used to mark a stair-step anterior mandibulotomy between the medial incisors (Fig. 3). In patients with poor dentition, one medial incisor is extracted and the cut is marked through the tooth socket. Four holes for wire closure are drilled, one on each side of both steps, before the mandibulotomy. The mandible is then divided with the oscillating saw or the Gigli's wire saw. Care should be taken not to damage the apexes of the medial incisors. Beveling the mandibulotomy cuts will allow the stabilization of the reapproximated segments in all directions. The tongue is grasped with a towel-clip and retracted contralaterally. An incision is made in the floor of the mouth, starting in the midline between the orifices of Wharton's ducts and extending posteriorly toward the anterior tonsillar pillar (Fig. 4). The lingual nerve should be identified and preserved, except for its postganglionic fibers to the submandibular and sublingual glands, which are transected. Wharton's duct is also

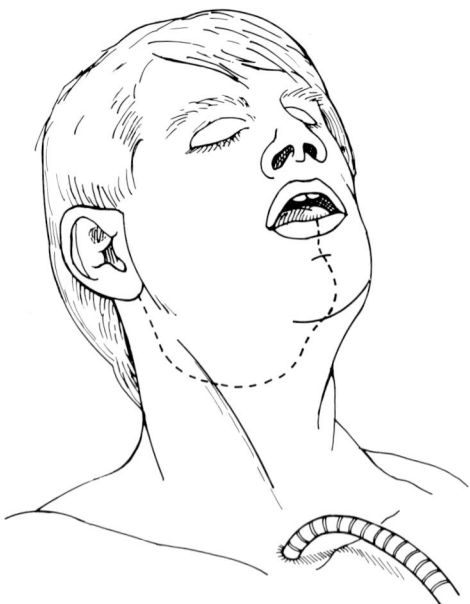

FIG. 2. Skin incision. The mental and lip-splitting part of the incision are performed only after the cervical part of the operation is completed.

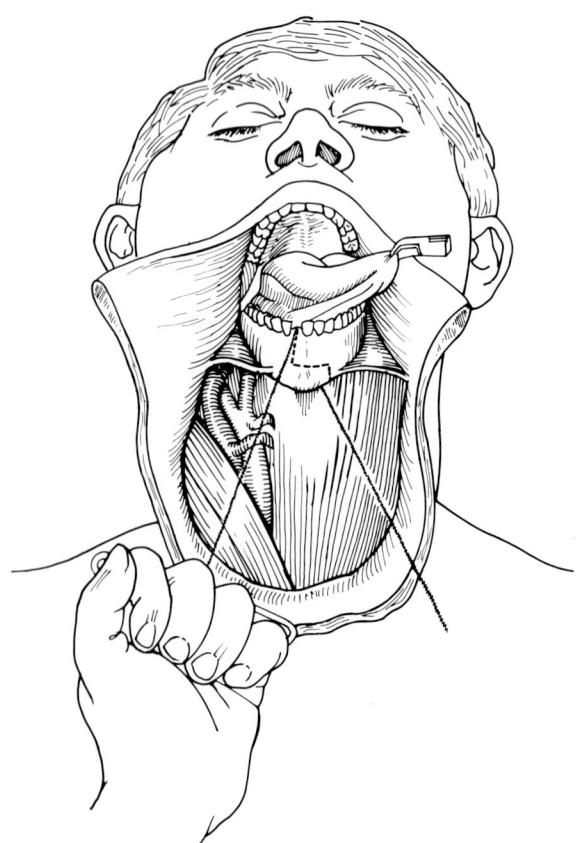

FIG. 3. Stair-step median mandibulotomy.

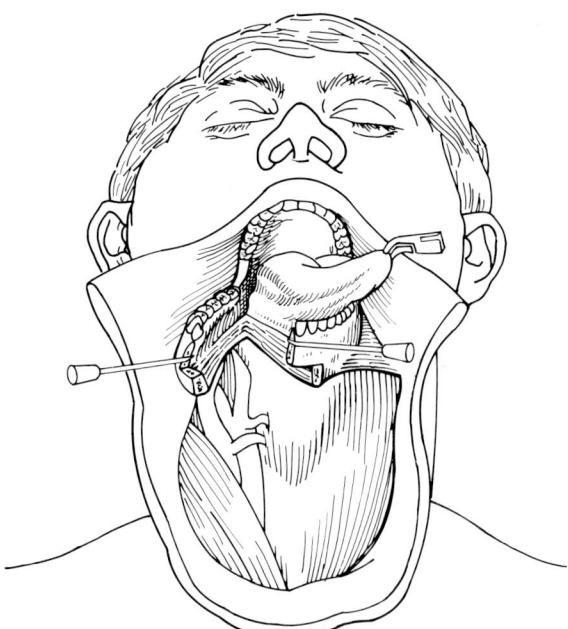

FIG. 4. The incision in the floor of the mouth. After the muscles are divided, the oral and cervical surgical fields are connected.

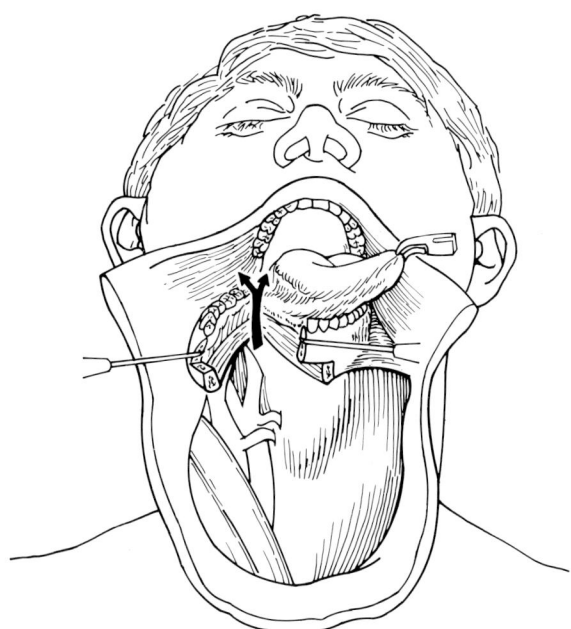

FIG. 5. The basic part of the operation is completed. Dissection may be continued toward the middle and/or the lateral compartment.

divided. With the hemimandible retracted laterally and the tongue and opposite hemimandible retracted contralaterally, the incision is carried deeper in the floor of the mouth. The supporting musculature (mylohyoid, anterior belly of the digastricus) with its nerve supply is divided, thus connecting the neck and oral incisions, creating one surgical space, and allowing the hemimandible to swing even further laterally. This is still limited by the external carotid artery. The division of this artery distal to its lingual branch allows maximal lateral retraction of the hemimandible together with the contents of the submandibular triangle.

The parapharyngeal space is now exposed. The styloid musculoligamentous complex is identified running in an antero-infero-medial direction and divided. If the styloid process is elongated, it is fractured. This allows the complete dissection all around the major neurovascular structures toward the carotid canal and jugular foramen in the skull base. The basic part of the operation is now completed. Depending on the exact location of the lesion and the procedure to be performed, the surgeon may continue in dissection and exposure of the middle compartment of the cranial base and/or the lateral compartment, which includes the infratemporal and parapharyngeal spaces (Fig. 5).

If the lesion or the area to be exposed is within the lateral compartment between the mastoid process, glenoid fossa, and sternocleidomastoid laterally and the constrictor muscles medially, then the major dissection has been completed and the surgeon should be able by now to follow the lesion. If the area to be exposed is more medial (i.e., medial to the major vessels) and the pharynx itself makes the access difficult, then the oral incision is continued into the soft tissues lateral and behind the oropharyngeal mucosa and blunt dissection is then carried out between the oropharynx and nasopharynx and the spine. The nasopharynx is detached from the prevertebral fascia and the longus colli muscles and retracted to the contralateral side without violating the circumferential mucosal integrity. This maneuver may be limited by the eustachian tube and the tensor and levator veli palatini, which should therefore be divided.

If the medial compartment, the clivus, the sphenoid sinus, the posterior nasal mucosa, or the pterygopalatine space need to be explored, or if the entire two-thirds of the cranial base of the middle fossa (i.e., the middle compartment and one lateral compartment) needs exposure, then a few more surgical steps are required.

The oral mucosal incision is continued through the palatoglossus muscle and medial to the retromolar trigone onto the soft and hard palate, passing 8–10 mm medial to the gingival margin (Fig. 6). This incision may be extended, if necessary, toward the anterior midline. A hemipalatal (soft palate and the mucoperiosteum of the hard palate) flap can be elevated, exposing the hard palate and posterior maxilla. This requires the sacrifice of the ipsilateral greater palatine vessels. With the hemipalatal flap retracted contralaterally and with the use of the osteotome and rongeur, limited posterior palatectomy and posterior maxillectomy may be performed

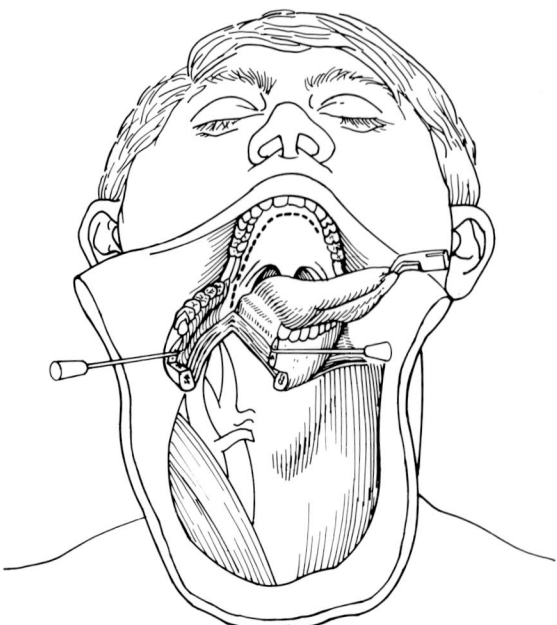

FIG. 6. Hemipalatal flap is outlined.

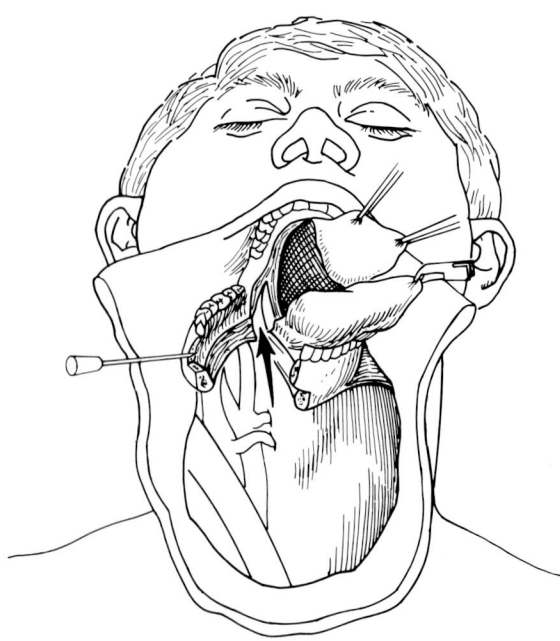

FIG. 8. Retropharyngeal dissection. This is followed by detachment of the nasopharynx from the skull base.

(Fig. 7). This maneuver is combined with the dissection through the soft tissues lateral and behind the oropharynx, followed by blunt dissection and detachment of the middle and superior constrictors from the spine (Fig. 8). Contralateral retraction of the nasopharynx will bring the cartilaginous eustachian tube and the veli palatini muscles into view. These are divided under direct vision by placing blunt scissors medial to the internal carotid artery. The nasopharynx is then detached from the skull base (Fig. 9). If needed, the posterior choanae are exposed by removing more palatal bone and excising the posterior nasal mucosa (Fig. 10). The lingual nerve is followed superiorly. This helps to identify the medial pterygoid muscle, on which the nerve lies, and the foramen ovale, through which the mandibular division of the trigeminal nerve (which is joined by the lingual

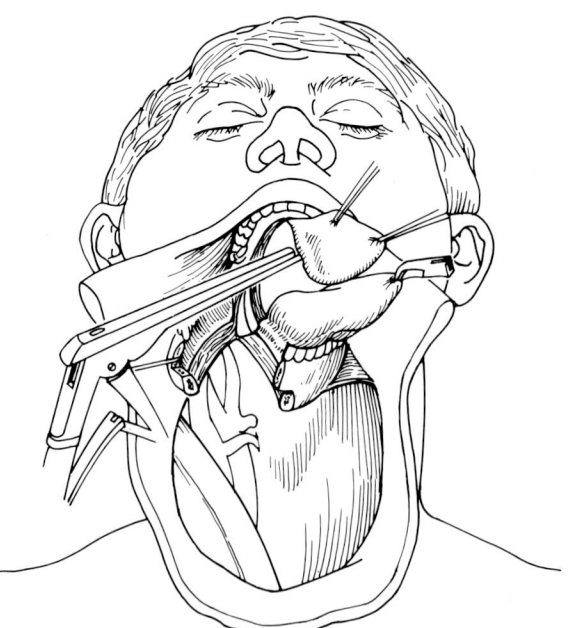

FIG. 7. With the hemipalatal flap retracted contralaterally, posterior palatectomy and posterior maxillectomy are performed in order to expose the posterior choanal, nasopharynx, and pterygoid plates.

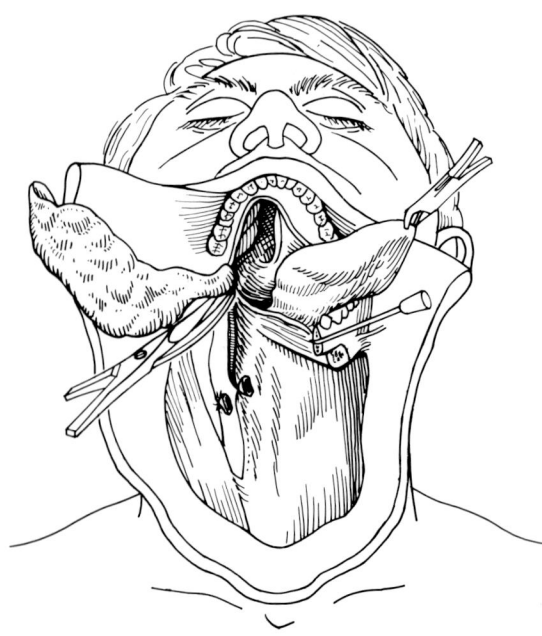

FIG. 9. Division of the cartilaginous portion of the eustachian tube and the palatine muscles.

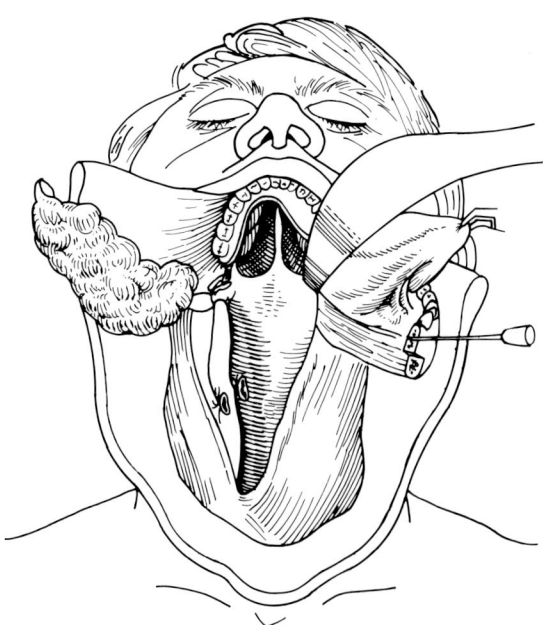

FIG. 10. Retraction of the oropharynx and nasopharynx provides wide exposure to the middle compartment and the cervical spine, with full neurovascular control.

nerve) passes into the cranium. By removing the pterygoid plates the pterygopalatine space is exposed, and by dividing the pterygoid muscles the infratemporal fossa is reached. At this stage the entire medial and lateral compartments become one surgical space.

Resection of the osseous cranial base may be performed at this stage with the use of osteotomes, rongeurs, or drill. It is possible to drill the carotid canal with preservation of the internal carotid artery. In cases where the entire thickness of the bone needs to be removed, a combined approach is recommended, with the neurosurgical team controlling the bone resection from within the cranium.

Closure is begun with the reattachment of the oropharynx and nasopharynx to the prevertebral fascia. If there is a significant pharyngeal defect due to tumor resection, then a myocutaneous flap (usually pectoralis major or rhombotrapezius) is rotated for reconstruction. A nasogastric tube is placed and a cricopharyngeal myotomy is routinely performed to prevent long-term swallowing difficulties. The hemipalate flap is reattached to the maxillary gingiva. A palatal splint may be used to hold the flap in place and to avoid its separation from the palatine bone. A figure-of-eight closure, using #25 wire, is recommended for reapproximation of the mandibular segments. It is better to close the floor of the mouth after the mandible is wired together. This closure is supported by the approximation of the mylohyoid muscle. A soft suction catheter is placed vertically with its tip at the skull base and its exit through a stab wound in the lower neck. The neck incision is then closed with meticulous approximation of the vermillion border and three-layer closure of the lip.

The need for carotid coverage with muscle flap or dermal graft is determined by the nature of the lesion and by the existence or the possibility of infection. It is routinely performed when radical neck dissection was included in the procedure and when radiation therapy has been or would be given.

COMPLICATIONS

The most common significant complication is conductive hearing loss due to negative middle ear pressure and serous otitis media. It is usually ipsilateral but may be bilateral. It is managed by the insertion of tympanostomy tubes. Depending on the exact location of the lesion, the extent of skull base dissection and resection, and the duration of pharyngeal and tongue retraction during the procedure, dysphagia and recurrent aspirations are possible complications. Very few cases will require prolonged tracheostomy and/or temporary gastrostomy tube. Intensive swallowing exercises and early maxillary prosthetic rehabilitation should be started as soon as possible.

Mild to moderate hematoma and wound infection are possible complications as in any other major head and neck surgery, but major vessel hemorrhage has not been observed. The possibility of intracranial infection due to direct extension from the mouth does exist, but in reality it is very rare. Antibiotic coverage is begun preoperatively and is continued for 3–5 days postoperatively. Orocervical fistula, mandibular malunion, parapharyngeal or retropharyngeal abscess, and vagal, accessory, or hypoglossal nerve deficits are other possible complications.

CHAPTER 18

Transtemporal and Infratemporal Approach for Benign Tumors of the Jugular Foramen and Temporal Bone

Barry E. Hirsch, Laligam N. Sekhar, and Donald B. Kamerer

Benign tumors that involve the jugular foramen and temporal bone considered in this chapter are paragangliomas, neurilemomas of the lower cranial nerves, and meningiomas. The following considerations are important in planning the operation.

1. Age of the patient; general medical condition.
2. Preoperative neurological deficits.
3. Goal of the operation: total resection versus partial removal.
4. Patency of the sigmoid sinus and collateral flow.
5. Involvement of the petrous ICA.
6. Areas involved by the tumor:
   Temporal bone
     Jugular foramen
     Middle ear
     Inner ear
     Carotid canal
     Facial nerve canal
   Posterior fossa
   Clivus
   Occipital condyle, C1 area
   Vertebral artery
   Infratemporal fossa
   Cavernous sinus
   Transverse sinus, sigmoid sinus, and the internal jugular vein

7. Vascularity of the tumor and source of blood supply (external or internal carotid artery).

PREOPERATIVE EVALUATION

The patient must be carefully examined for neurological deficits, especially with regard to hearing, facial function, and the lower cranial nerves. If the patient has no neurological deficits preoperatively, there should be definite evidence of tumor growth in order for an operation to be recommended to the patient. Patients with preexisting lower cranial nerve palsies usually have already adapted considerably and are thus able to better tolerate the effects of lower cranial nerve dysfunction postoperatively. Although attempts are made to preserve hearing during the operation, total unilateral hearing loss is a possibility, and the patient should be prepared for this. A temporary facial paralysis with eventual recovery to a House grade II–III function is common following procedures in this area. Patients should be informed and psychologically counseled for this as well.

A bone windowed CT scan with 1.5-mm sections through the temporal bone is essential to adequately evaluate the bone changes. MR imaging reveals the presence of a tumor more thoroughly and also provides information about encasement of the internal carotid and vertebral arteries, and patency of the internal jugular vein and sigmoid sinus.

Cervical and cerebral angiography is very essential. This provides information about the blood supply to the tumor, which may be derived from the external and internal carotid circulation, extracranial branches of the vertebral artery, and intracranial branches of the verte-

---

B. E. Hirsch and D. B. Kamerer: Department of Otolaryngology, University of Pittsburgh School of Medicine, Eye and Ear Institute, Pittsburgh, Pennsylvania 15213.
L. N. Sekhar: Department of Neurosurgery, Center for Cranial Base Surgery, University of Pittsburgh School of Medicine, Presbyterian University Hospital, Pittsburgh, Pennsylvania 15213.

brobasilar circulation. When the petrous ICA is significantly involved by the tumor, a balloon occlusion test of the ICA should be performed to evaluate the adequacy of the collateral circulation (see the chapter by Horton et al.). When the vertebral artery is involved, a balloon occlusion test is usually not performed since the risk of arterial dissection following test occlusion is higher. Instead, the relative size of the two vertebral arteries, their communication, and the size and connection of the posterior communicating arteries provide adequate information about the patient's tolerance to potential occlusion. The surgeon must be prepared to repair or reconstruct any artery that may be injured or resected. However, despite successful reconstruction, vascular occlusion may still be encountered.

In rare situations, the tumor may involve a sigmoid sinus which is solitary, dominant, or has poor connection with the other side. In such instances, it is better to wait until occlusion of the sinus occurs spontaneously because of tumor growth.

When feasible, all vascular tumors are embolized by an interventional neuroradiologist preoperatively. When the tumor is fed by branches of the external carotid artery alone, such embolization can be performed with minimal patient risk. However, when the feeding vessels originate from the internal carotid artery or from the vertebrobasilar arteries, the advantages of embolization must be carefully weighed against the potential neurological risks. Superselective embolization of the occipital and postauricular arteries may occlude the stylomastoid artery with subsequent facial paralysis. Some patients with paragangliomas can have severe hypertension due to the secretion of vasoactive substances. This should be evaluated preoperatively as it may cause serious problems intraoperatively. Paragangliomas may also involve multiple sites and can be bilateral. This may be found incidentally during angiography and would need to be considered when planning surgical therapy.

CHOICE OF SURGICAL APPROACH

The choice of surgical approach to the tumor depends on its anatomical location and the presence of vascular encasement (Fig. 1). When the tumor involves only the jugular bulb area, an upper cervical approach is com-

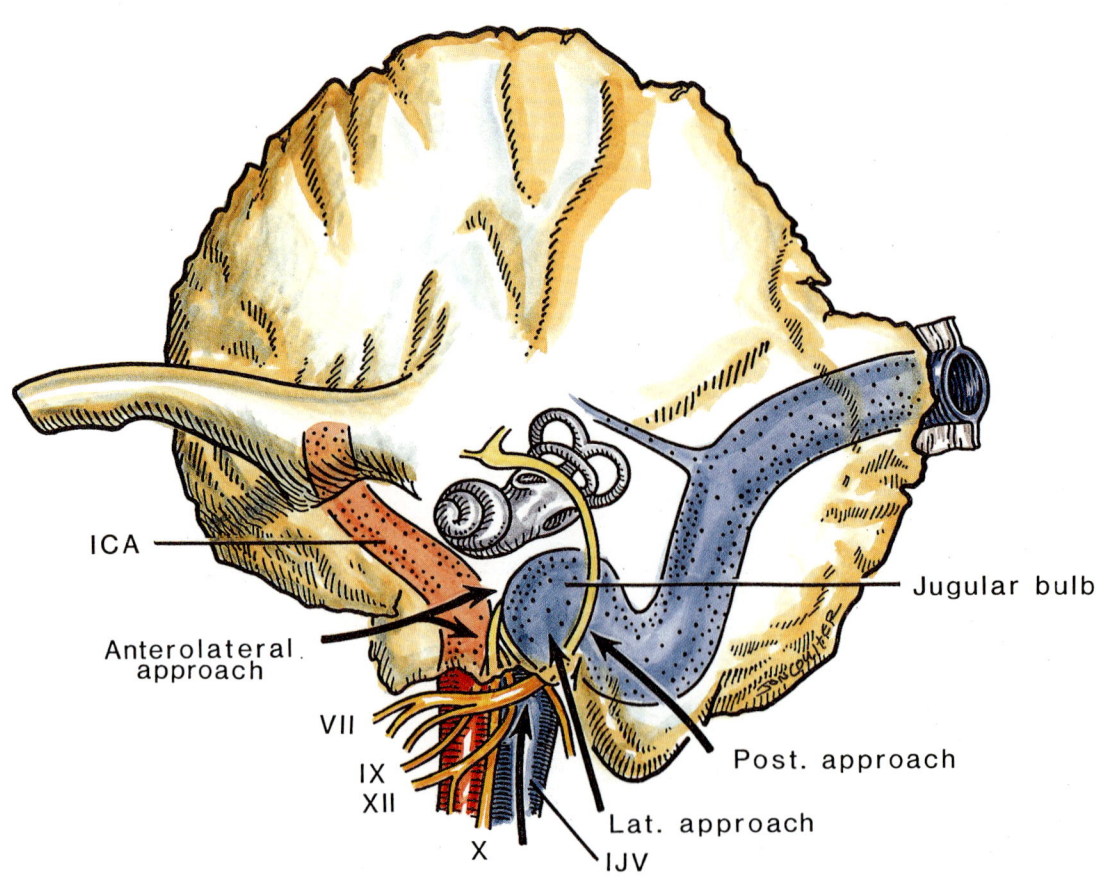

FIG. 1. This figure schematically illustrates the anatomy of the temporal bone and the important structures contained within. Depending on the surgeon's experience and need, several approaches to the jugular bulb area are possible, as shown by the *arrows*.

bined with a transmastoid approach, with or without the anterior translocation of the middle ear and mastoid segments of the facial nerve. When there is significant intradural invasion of the posterior fossa, a retrosigmoid craniotomy is performed and the posterior fossa dura is opened to perform tumor resection. When the clivus is involved in a limited fashion by tumor, a transmastoid approach with facial nerve translocation provides adequate exposure. When clival involvement is extensive, a subtemporal and infratemporal approach with dissection and displacement of the petrous ICA is necessary. When the petrous ICA is encased, complete exposure of the artery is performed. Usually by opening the periosteal sheath around the petrous ICA, the tumor can be completely dissected away from the artery. However, in some patients, resection and vein graft replacement of segments of the petrous ICA are necessary to achieve complete resection. When the cavernous sinus is involved by a benign tumor originating in the jugular foramen–temporal bone area, it may be necessary to remove this portion of the tumor at a second stage procedure.

ANESTHETIC CONSIDERATION

The anesthetic technique and choice of anesthetic agents for lateral skull base surgery must take into account certain factors. Requirements for the procedure include maintaining adequate cerebral blood flow, sedation, and analgesia with the avoidance of paralytic agents. Neurophysiologic monitoring during the procedure has significantly increased the safety to the patient and information available to the surgeon. Electromyographic monitoring of cranial nerve VII, and occasionally of cranial nerves X and XII, is critical to the transtemporal–infratemporal fossa approach. Therefore inhalation agents are predominantly used to provide safe and effective anesthesia. Details of the anesthetic technique are thoroughly reviewed in the chapter by Gonzalez. During most of the operation, the patient's head is fixed with head pins and a Mayfield head rest, and the head position is not changed during surgery. If head repositioning is necessary, the endotracheal tube is fixed to the mandibular teeth with fine stainless steel wire or, when edentulous, by circumferential mandibular wiring.

Patients with lesions involving the jugular foramen may incur injury to the lower cranial nerves. If not present preoperatively, involvement in the resection of the glossopharyngeal and vagus nerves compromises deglutition and laryngeal function. If resection of the lower cranial nerves is anticipated, a tracheotomy should be given serious consideration. Patients who have lower cranial nerve paralysis prior to surgery have often developed adequate compensation. In such patients, tracheotomy can be done subsequently if aspiration becomes a clinical problem.

PATIENT POSITION

After adequate general anesthesia has been commenced via an endotracheal tube or tracheotomy tube, head rotation away from the side of the lesion is necessary. Adequate rotation may not be achieved in a patient with a short neck in the supine position. A semilateral position with the ipsilateral shoulder depressed provides additional head rotation. The head is laterally extended toward the contralateral shoulder along with limited hyperextension. This position is then fixed with head pins secured to a Mayfield head rest. Anticipation of the potential surgical defect and the possible reconstruction allow adequate preparation of the donor areas at the start of the operation. The surgical field to be prepared may include the abdomen, if an abdominal fat graft or a rectus abdominal muscle free flap is needed. The ipsilateral thigh serves as a source for subcutaneous fat and fascia lata for grafting. The medial thigh gives access to the saphenous vein in the event that carotid resection and vein graft reconstruction are anticipated. The distal leg offers the sural nerve, should extensive facial nerve grafting be necessary. Elastic stockings and pneumatic compression stockings are routinely used.

OPERATIVE TECHNIQUE

Skin Incision

A large C-shaped incision is utilized (Fig. 2). The anterior extent of the incision is just superior to the pterion.

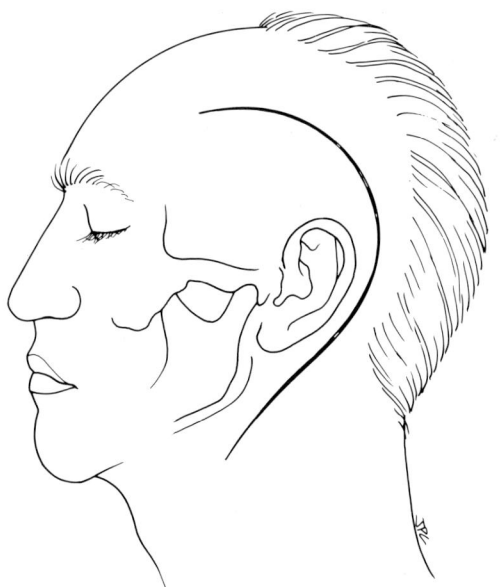

FIG. 2. Skin incision is C-shaped and placed 3–4 cm posterior to the postauricular sulcus. The superior limb extends just anterior to the frontotemporal hairline and inferiorly enters a neck crease approaching the greater cornu of the hyoid bone.

The anterior limit of the incision is usually at the hairline in women and in men with a normal hairline. This incision then extends superiorly and posteriorly in a curvilinear fashion to the postauricular area. Lesions limited to the middle and anterior aspect of the posterior fossa or the base of the temporal bone require 3–4 cm of skin between the incision and the postauricular crease. This affords adequate tissue for closure and blood supply to the pinna, which is included in the anteriorly based flap. For lesions that extend more into the posterior fossa, the incision should extend further posteriorly behind the ear. The incision then extends into the neck through an existing skin crease. The anterior inferior extent of the incision approaches the lateral aspect of the hyoid bone. Superiorly, the incision is deepened to the deep layer of the temporal fascia, and dissection is performed between the two layers of temporal fascia. In the postauricular area, dissection is performed superficial to the fibroperiosteal layer of the mastoid cortex. The dissection in this area extends anteriorly to the subcutaneous tissue of the posterior wall of the exterior auditory canal. Dissection of the cervical skin flap is performed deep to the platysma muscle. The greater auricular nerve is dissected for potential use as a nerve graft. Dissection continues anteriorly to the submandibular area. The inferior aspect of the incision is dissected off the lateral and anterior aspects of the sternocleidomastoid muscle.

The closure of the external auditory meatus is reinforced with the aid of a fibroperiosteal flap. This is performed by incising the fibroperiosteal tissue over the mastoid cortex with two parallel incisions, one above and below the limits of the external auditory canal. A vertical incision at its posterior limb creates an anteriorly based flap, which is used for the second layer of closure. The skin of the external auditory canal is then transected, going through the canal from posterior to anterior. The cartilaginous canal is dissected away from the skin of the lateral external canal. This cylinder of external canal skin is then everted and approximated with absorbable suture. Dissection is continued anteriorly, incising the periparotid fascia attached to the subcutaneous tissue of the anterior canal wall. The free edges of the fibroperiosteal flap are then secured to the subcutaneous tissue.

Soft Tissue Dissection

Large lesions extending into the petrous bone and encasing the ICA may require an infratemporal fossa approach. The superior dissection would then continue by developing the plane between the superficial and deep layers of the temporalis fascia. The dissection is continued by dissecting the periosteum off the zygomatic arch, and just superficial to the masseteric fascia. The parotid gland can be elevated off the masseteric fascia as well. In this fashion, the upper branches of the facial nerve (which course in the superficial fascia and fat of the face) are protected from injury. Retraction of the skin flap does put some traction on the upper facial nerve branches. Further dissection and management of the facial nerve are required with the transtemporal–infratemporal approach. The peripheral main trunk of the facial nerve is identified and dissected by elevating the fibrous fascia of the parotid gland away from the remaining cartilaginous and bony external auditory canal. Markers for the facial nerve include the digastric muscle, the cartilaginous "pointer" of the external canal, and, more medially, the styloid process. Identification of the tympanomastoid suture also leads the surgeon inferiorly to the stylomastoid foramen and the exit of the facial nerve from the temporal bone. With the nerve exposed at its main trunk, dissection is carried out toward the pes, or first bifurcation.

The sternocleidomastoid muscle is elevated off the mastoid tip and retracted posteriorly. The great vessels of the neck are then identified. Vessel loops are employed to separately tag the common carotid, internal carotid, and jugular vein. Identification and dissection of the vagus, spinal accessory, and hypoglossal nerves are performed. The structures are then dissected superiorly toward the skull base. The posterior belly of the digastric muscle is cut from the inferior aspect of the mastoid and retracted anteriorly to provide exposure of the vessels and central nerves up to the skull base.

Infratemporal Fossa Exposure

Extensive lesions invading the petrous apex require exposure of the petrous internal carotid artery. Infratemporal fossa dissection is necessary in order to isolate and manage the ICA. The text and figures that follow describe and illustrate the approach when this greater exposure is needed. Limited lesions isolated to the jugular bulb and posterior fossa are described later.

The exposure of the infratemporal fossa requires removal of the zygomatic arch. The temporalis muscle and fascia are elevated from the temporal fossa and freed up from its attachment to the medial surface of the zygomatic arch, which is now circumferentially isolated from soft tissue. Osteotomy cuts are made with a reciprocating saw to isolate and remove the zygomatic arch. Further subperiosteal dissection in the infratemporal fossa approaches the middle meningeal artery. Depending on the location of the tumor, inferior retraction or, when complete carotid exposure is needed, resection of the condyle of the mandible is often necessary. The lateral pterygoid muscle is elevated off the neck of the condyle with electrocoagulation. The condyle is then sectioned at the neck using the reciprocating saw and removed. Venous bleeding is often encountered in the pterygoid muscles, which is controlled with bipolar cautery and by packing with oxidized cellulose. Further dissection can then be continued toward the foramen or ovale and potentially the pterygoid maxillary fissure. If the tumor dissection requires isolation and mobilization of the carotid artery, a low frontotemporal craniotomy is performed. Burr holes are performed and a cranial bone flap is created after elevating the underlying dura between the burr holes. Further exposure is accomplished with the use of a rongeur, removing the inferior portion of the lateral sphenoid bone (Figs. 3 and 4). Extradural middle fossa dissection is then performed to identify and isolate the horizontal segment of the petrous ICA and subsequently to isolate the entire petrous ICA.

Transtemporal Dissection

A transcortical mastoidectomy is performed. Preservation of cochlear function is maintained by entering the middle ear through either a transtympanic or facial recess approach. The incudostapedial joint is separated and the structures lateral to the stapes are removed. The posterior canal wall is taken down to the level of the horizontal fallopian canal and facial ridge. The sigmoid sinus is skeletonized by removing bone anterior and posterior to the sinus and the posterior fossa dura is exposed. After the bone is removed from the sinus, ligation of the distal transverse or proximal sigmoid sinus will have to be performed prior to tumor removal from the jugular bulb area. The bone of the anterior middle ear is removed, communicating the middle ear with the glenoid fossa. Tumors located deep to the facial nerve may require transposition of the nerve. Facial nerve decompression with removal of the lateral fallopian canal allows dissection of the nerve from its bony compartment (Fig. 5). Leaving a fibrous tissue cuff around the facial nerve at the stylomastoid foramen facilitates this dissection and its fixation in an anteriorly transposed position. Further removal of the mastoid tip and styloid process will expose the ascending pharyngeal and occipital arteries, which may need to be ligated. The cranial nerves, jugular vein, and carotid artery are further dissected superiorly to the inferior aspect of the tumor. Identification

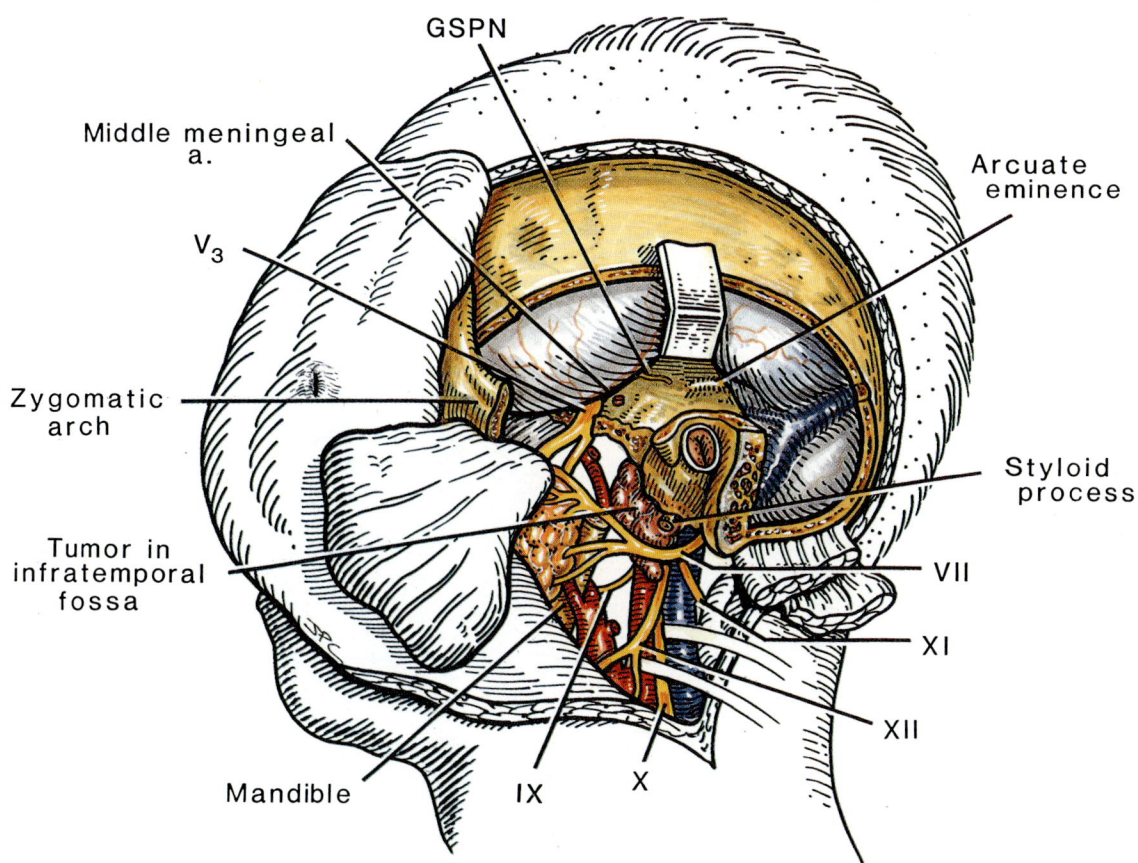

FIG. 3. Extensive tumors involving the petrous bone and ICA require greater exposure. The anteriorly based skin flap is retracted. The temporalis muscle flap is retracted inferiorly following removal of the zygomatic arch and glenoid fossa and the mandibular condyle. A frontotemporal craniotomy has been performed. Posterior and middle fossa dura and the infratemporal fossa are exposed. The sternocleidomastoid and splenius capitus muscles are reflected posteriorly. Neck dissection has isolated the carotid artery and jugular vein and cranial nerves X, XI, and XII.

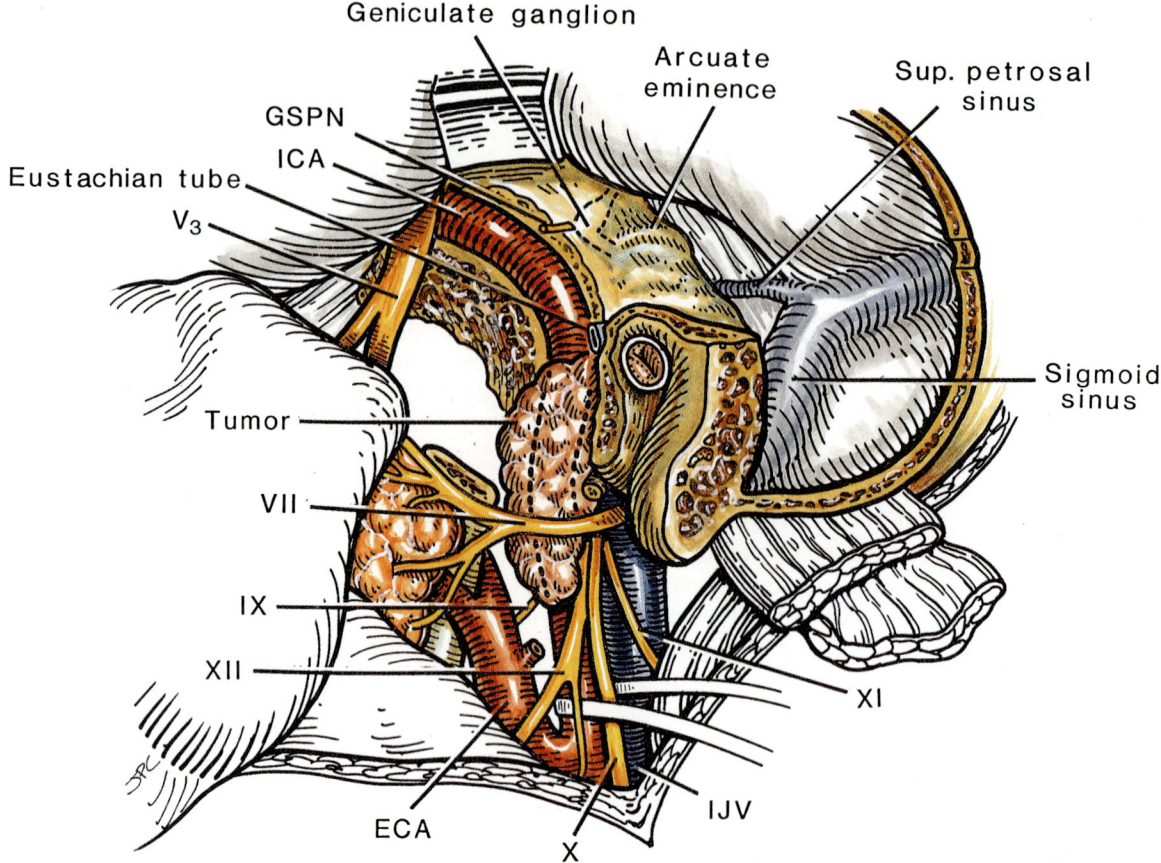

FIG. 4. Tumor exposure is facilitated by isolating the carotid artery through the petrous bone. V_3 is intact.

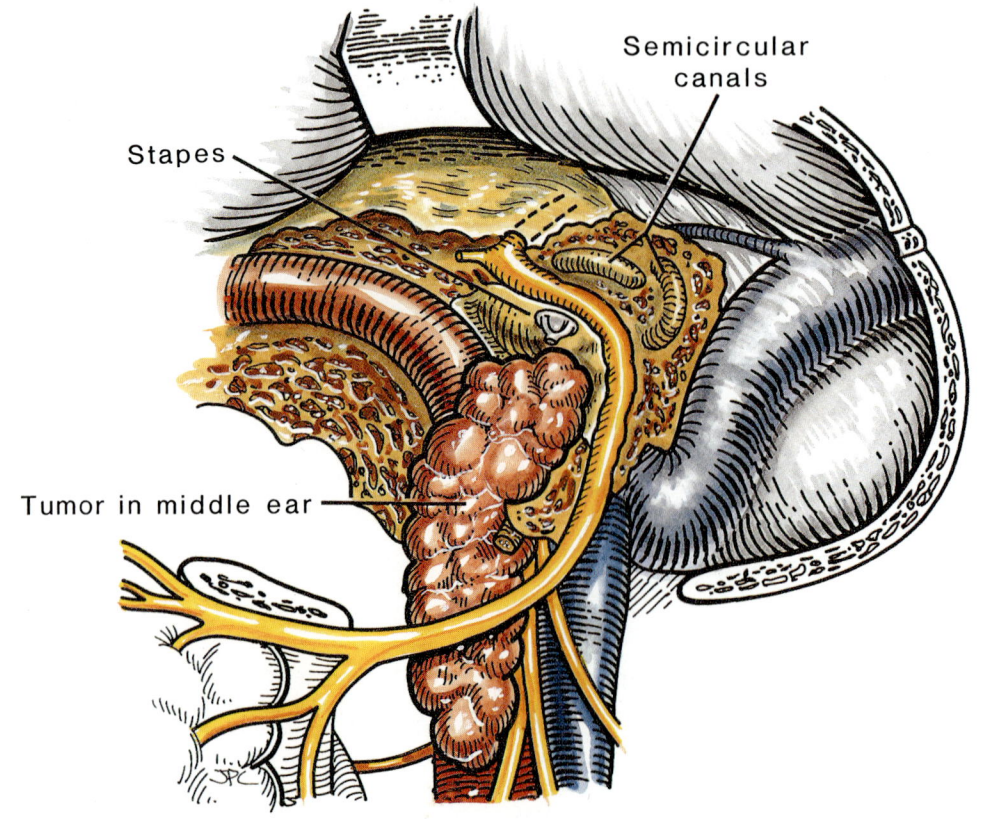

FIG. 5. Temporal bone dissection exposes lateral tumor surface. The fallopian canal is opened if facial nerve transposition is necessary.

of the vertebral artery may be necessary when the tumor lies close to the transverse process of the atlas.

Tumor Isolation

Tumor dissection is sequentially performed by isolating the limits of its extent. The ligation of the jugular vein in the neck is saved for the end so as to prevent tumor engorgement and excessive bleeding from the margins of the tumor to the center. If resection of the dura is necessary, the proximal sigmoid sinus is ligated entering into the posterior fossa. Bipolar cautery is the critical technique for hemostasis and tumor removal. Dissection is continued inferiorly toward the lateral portion of the foramen magnum. In the case of paragangliomas, tumor that has not extensively involved the posterior fossa may have as its medial limit the dural side of the sigmoid sinus and jugular bulb. Opening the sinus and dissecting from a posterior superior direction approaches the inferior petrosal vein. This must be plugged with oxidized cellulose to stop venous bleeding. The jugular vein is ligated and divided inferiorly and dissected upward from the lower cranial nerves and the ICA. Direct adherence of tumor onto the carotid may require dissection in a subadventitial plane. When the petrous ICA is encased by tumor, opening its periosteal sheath allows tumor removal in most patients. In some cases, small lacerations of the ICA may require resuture after temporary trapping. Rarely, vein graft reconstruction of the ICA may be needed, as described in the chapter by Linskey et al. Lesions that extend through the cochlea or internal auditory canal may enter into the cerebellopontine (CP) angle. Primary closure of the eustachian tube is performed so as to avoid CSF rhinorrhea.

Posterior Fossa Tumor Resection

When the tumor has a significant intradural extension into the posterior fossa, a retrosigmoid craniotomy or craniectomy is performed. The dura is opened medial to the sigmoid sinus, and the cerebellum retracted with self-retaining retractors, under the surgical microscope. The lateral cerebellomedullary cistern is drained, and the cranial nerves VI–XI are exposed by arachnoidal dissection.

Paragangliomas involving the posterior fossa are quite vascular and are sometimes supplied by branches of the posterior or anterior inferior cerebellar arteries. However, they are generally easily removed after bipolar coagulation of the feeding vessels and capsule. It is best to start the tumor removal and dissection of the lower cranial nerves after the entire extradural tumor has been isolated and devascularized. This allows the dissection of cranial nerves IX–XI and their preservation when the tumor is not invading these nerves (Fig. 6). The exception to this is in patients where the mass in the posterior fossa is considerable. If cranial nerves IX–XI are invaded by the tumor and injured by tumor dissection, reconstruction should be attempted with an interposition nerve graft or a direct nerve resuture.

For neurilemomas of cranial nerves IX–XI, the surgical strategy is similar to paragangliomas, but neurilemomas are generally less vascular. When the tumor is very large, it is usually impossible to tell the nerve of origin proximally, but it can often be identified distally. It is not possible to preserve the nerve of origin, but preservation of the remaining nerves should be attempted.

When meningiomas invade the jugular foramen, their growth pattern is similar to paragangliomas. In addition, these tumors also invade the temporal bone extensively. The removal of the intradural portion of the tumor is similar to other posterior fossa meningiomas. In addition, all the hyperostotic bone, dura, and extradural tumor must be removed.

Limited Lesions

Tumors located in the jugular bulb and posterior fossa require a more limited exposure. It is not necessary to perform a temporal craniotomy and an extradural middle fossa dissection or an infratemporal fossa dissection. The condyle of the mandible is undisturbed. Dissection is directed to the posterior fossa, sigmoid sinus, and middle ear through a transmastoid and retrosigmoid craniectomy approach. Bone is removed from the sigmoid sinus, posterior fossa dura, and the horizontal and vertical portions of the facial nerve (Fig. 7). The vertical portion of the carotid artery is isolated by working medial to the anterior wall of the external ear canal. Management of the facial nerve is dictated by the location and invasion of the tumor. If necessary, the facial nerve may need to be transposed anteriorly. Posterior fossa dura may have to be resected and repaired. Following complete tumor removal, the posterior and inferior exposure is similar to that of the previously described approach (Fig. 8).

Other Invaded Areas

The removal of tumors from the C1–occipital condyle area (extreme lateral, transcondylar, transjugular approach), from around the petrous ICA, and from the extradural petroclival area (subtemporal–infratemporal approach), and from the cavernous sinus (extradural and intradural approaches) has been extensively discussed in other chapters.

Reconstruction following tumor resection is dependent on the operative defect. If the facial nerve must be excised because of tumor invasion, primary repair is preferred when no tension on the anastomosis exists. Small defects are grafted with the great auricular nerve, but

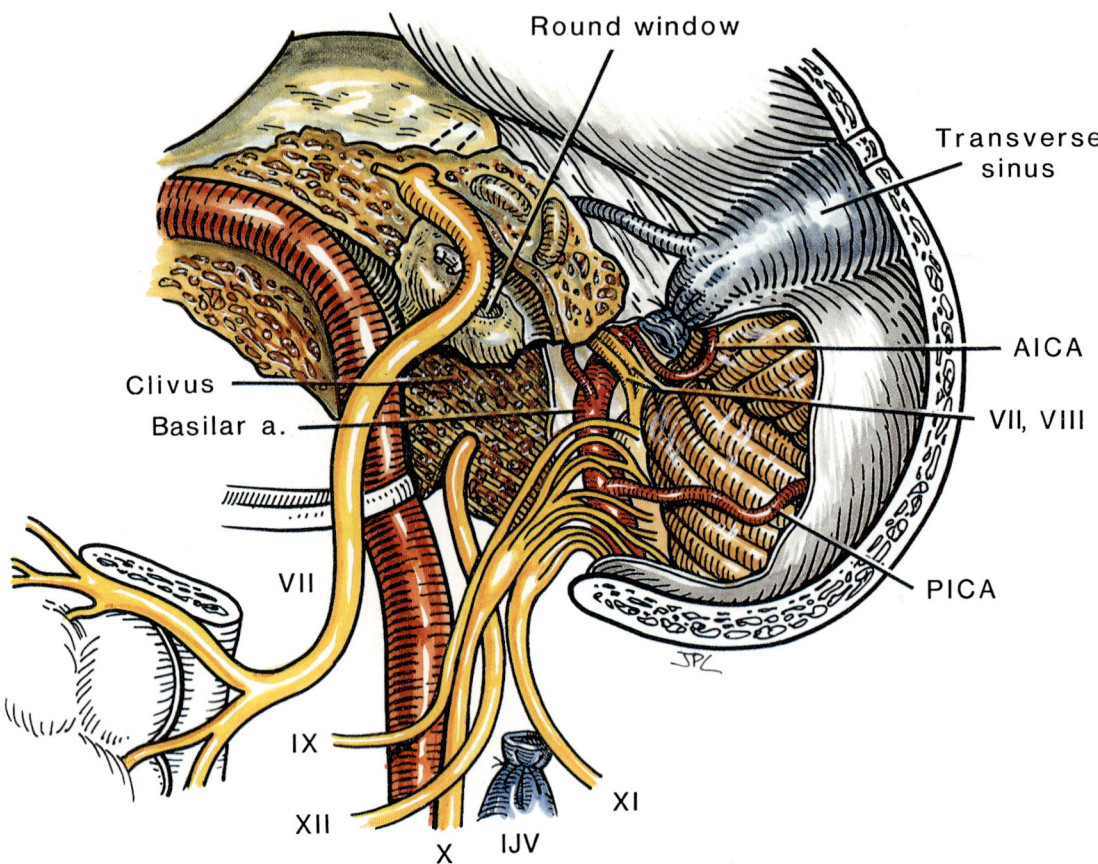

FIG. 6. Completed tumor excision. Facial nerve is anteriorly displaced from the fallopian canal. Petrous ICA is isolated at the anterior margin. Sigmoid sinus and internal jugular vein are ligated. The posterior fossa dura is open. Cranial nerves VII–XII have been preserved. Medial extent of exposure is the inferior lateral clivus.

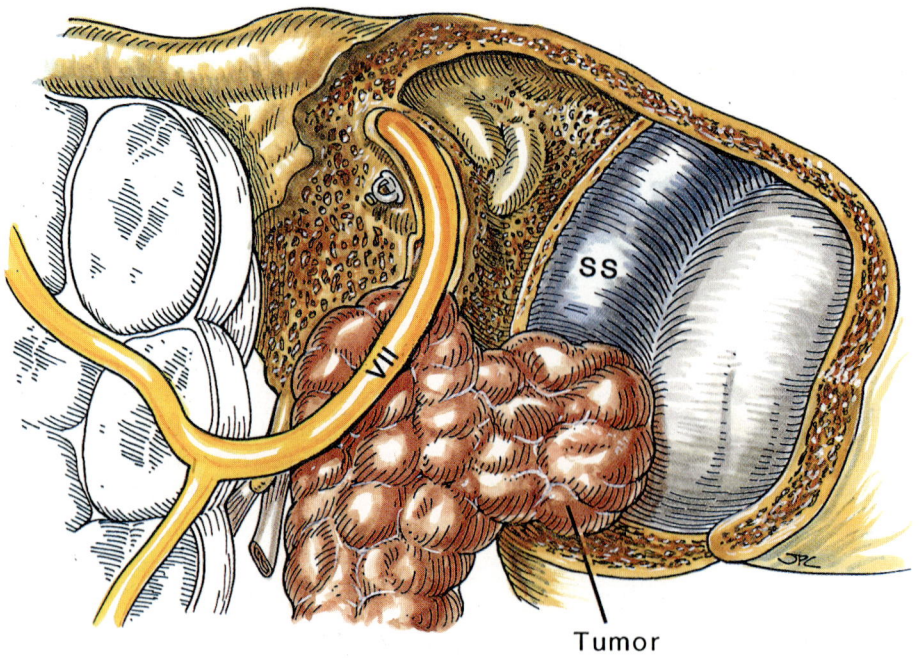

FIG. 7. Tumor involving the jugular bulb and upper cervical area. A mastoidectomy and retrosigmoid craniectomy have been performed. The sigmoid sinus (SS) has been skeletonized.

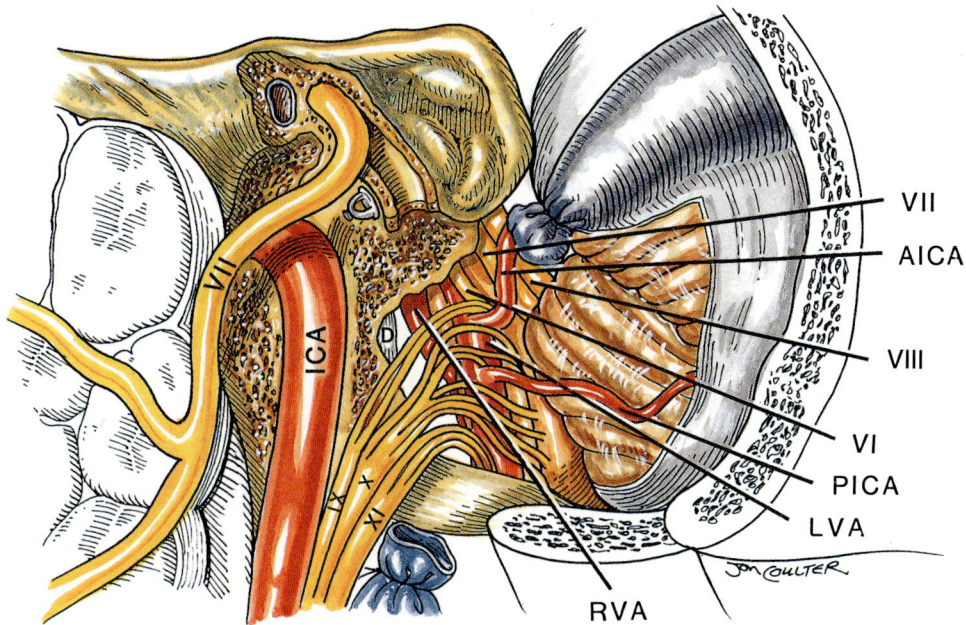

FIG. 8. The posterior fossa has been opened. Tumor has been removed after ligation of the sigmoid sinus and internal jugular vein. Cranial nerves VII–XI, the vertebral and basilar arteries, and the brain stem are exposed.

larger defects require a sural nerve graft. If such a large resection is necessary, the inner ear is often involved. Access to the proximal facial nerve in the cerebellopontine angle or the internal auditory canal may facilitate repair with a smaller cable graft. Obtaining a watertight closure is preferred; however, this is often difficult at the medial and inferior aspects of the posterior fossa. If dural resection was necessary, fascia lata, galea, or pericranium is employed for grafting. The craniotomy bone flap and the zygomatic arch are returned to their anatomic positions and secured with 2-0 braided nylon. Large surgical defects are filled with fat and temporalis muscle is rotated posteriorly and closed over the infratemporal, fossa, middle ear, and mastoid defect. The edges of the muscle are approximated to the sternocleidomastoid muscle, the semispinalis and splenius muscles, the parotid tissues, and the temporal dura. Hemovac or Jackson Pratt drains are tunneled through a stab incision in the posterior skin of the neck and occiput and connected to a bile bag, to drain by gravity. Suction drainage is avoided since the dura is not usually closed watertight.

Complications

Most of the complications that occur with the transtemporal-infratemporal fossa approach are identified in the immediate postoperative period. Cerebellar and brain stem injury or cerebral hemispheric ischemic injuries are major complications. These are fortunately rare with good neurosurgical techniques during the operation. Should they occur, management is in the usual fashion. Cranial nerve deficits following the resection are usually evident upon awakening. Potential compromise of cranial nerves V through XII exist given the location of the surgical resection. With larger lesions involving the trigeminal nerve, hypoesthesia of the cornea may not require opthalmologic supportive measures if the facial nerve is functioning normally. With paresis or paralysis due to compromise of the facial nerve, the prime concern is focused toward care of the potentially exposed cornea. Topical synthetic tears during the day and ointment at night are provided to the eye with inadequate corneal protection. Further comfort is provided by a clear plastic moisture chamber placed over the involved eye. Return of facial function following primary or cable grafting may take from 6 to 12 months depending on the proximal site of resection. For patients in whom a long period of recovery is anticipated, the use of an upper lid gold weight is an effective means for rehabilitation. In those patients with laxity of the lower lid and a tendency toward ectropion, a tarsorraphy or lower lid shortening procedure is most helpful.

Resection or injury of the lower cranial nerves poses significant compromise for pharyngeal and laryngeal function. Loss of the glossopharyngeal and vagal nerves renders the pharynx hypoesthetic with decreased tone, uncoordinated motor activity, and inability to protect the trachea from aspiration. In addition, vocal cord dysfunction is manifested by hoarseness and often the inability to produce an effective cough. This poses the problems of inability to resume an oral diet or handle one's secretions. Nutritional support in the short run is managed by nasal gastric feeding. If this situation may be prolonged, a gastrostomy or jejunostomy is performed. Vocal cord dysfunction, manifested by hoarseness, a weak cough, and inadequate tracheal protection, is rehabilitated with Gelfoam or a Teflon injection of the involved vocal fold. Compromise of the hypoglossal nerve adds an additional burden to the patient's handling of secretions and oral intake. The previously mentioned methods for rehabilitation are implemented much sooner if the hypoglossal nerve had to be sacrificed.

Cerebrospinal fluid (CSF) leak in the postoperative period adds to the patient's potential morbidity. The best means of handling such a problem is avoiding the occurrence through meticulous attention to surgical techniques. Despite efforts toward watertight closure, CSF leaks still occur. CSF leakage via the gravity drains is common. Drainage is continued until the fluid is relatively clear of blood or the drainage is minimal. This allows the wound to heal, preventing wound leakage. CSF leaks that occur through the wound or the eustachian tube at a later stage generally indicates hydrocephalus due to poor CSF absorption. This is managed by lumbar subarachnoid drainage. Goals for drainage are 50 cc per 8-hr shift. If after 5–7 days this should prove to be unsuccessful, then reexploration of the wound is warranted. A permanent ventriculoperitoneal shunt or a lumbar–peritoneal shunt is rarely needed.

The operative procedure described removes the amplifying mechanism of the tympanic membrane and ossicles and closes the external auditory canal. This obligates the patient to have a conductive hearing loss despite the presence of good cochlear function. Patients usually are accepting of this loss if normal auditory function exists on the contralateral side. Aural rehabilitation is possible with the use of a bone conducting hearing aid. Implantable subcutaneous hearing devices are available but at this time have not met universal acceptance.

Retraction of the mandible or the resection of the condyle may create crossbite deformity and malocclusion. Though a crossbite deformity initially is often present, return of occlusion may still occur in those patients with good dentition. This is aided by the use of nocturnal splints. Relining of dentures is effective in the edentulous patient. Serial adjustments of the denture are necessary in this situation.

Delayed postoperative complications include wound infection, hematoma, and rarely ischemia and breakdown of the suture line. The patient is managed using standard general and plastic surgery principles.

CASE 1

G.C., a 33-year-old male, presented with hoarseness for 1 year, right pulsatile tinnitus, conductive hearing loss, and right vocal cord paralysis. A erythematous mass was noted in the right middle ear. CT scan revealed a 3 × 3.5-cm destructive mass occupying the jugular bulb with extension into the middle ear (Fig. 9), posterior fossa, and petrous carotid canal (Fig. 10). Coronal images con-

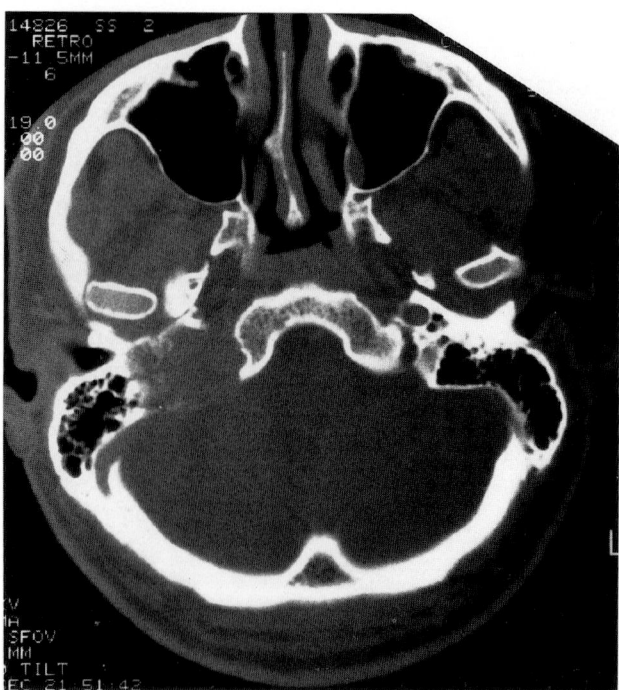

FIG. 9. G.C.—Preoperative CT scan. A 3.5-cm destructive lesion is seen in the jugular bulb area.

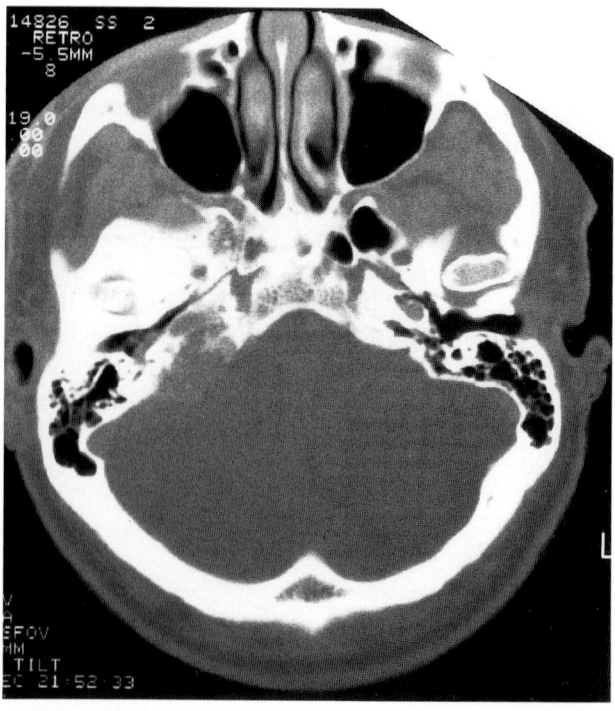

FIG. 10. G.C.—Lesion eroding into middle ear and the petrous carotid artery canal.

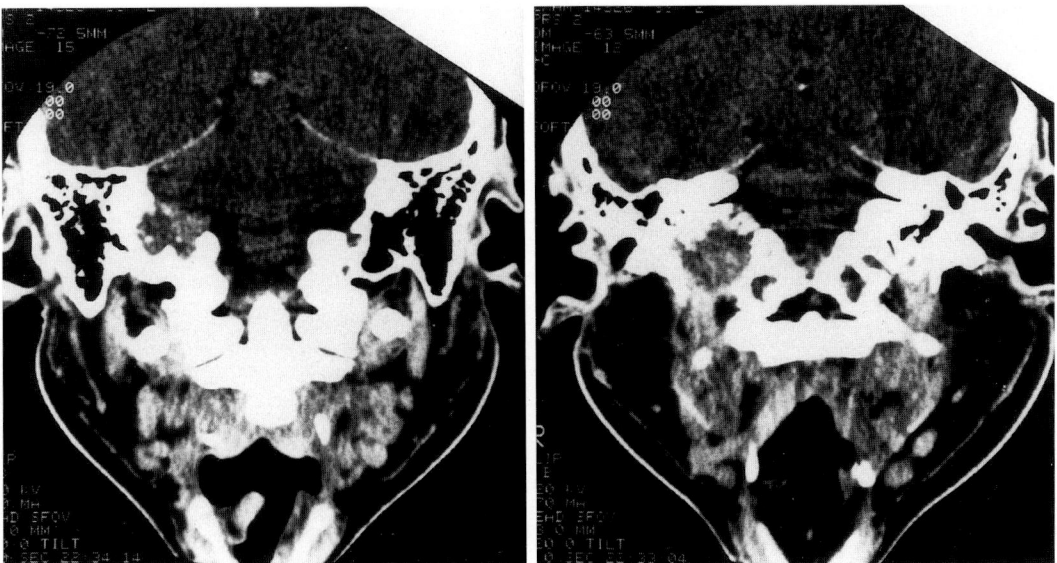

FIG. 11. G.C.—Coronal CT scan showing extension into the right posterior fossa and jugular bulb.

firmed the lesion to be centered in the jugular fossa with extension into the posterior fossa and proximal jugular vein (Fig. 11). Preoperative evaluation included cerebral angiography, balloon test occlusion, and embolization. Right carotid artery injection revealed extrinsic narrowing of its petrous portion (Fig. 12A). Injection of the right ascending pharyngeal artery localized the tumor blush to the temporal bone, which was then embolized (Fig. 12B). The patient clinically failed balloon occlusion of the carotid with symptoms of intermittent confusion during the inflation.

The procedure entailed a right retromastoid craniotomy, transtemporal–infratemporal fossa approach with transposition of the facial nerve. It was necessary to open the carotid sheath in the petrous segment in order to remove adherent tumor. The facial nerve sheath was infiltrated by the tumor. It was possible to dissect the tumor under magnification and remove it without injury to the nerve.

The wound was closed with abdominal fat and temporalis muscle flap. Postoperative scans shows the surgical bone defect (Fig. 13). This was obliterated with fat and the temporalis muscle (Fig. 14).

Teflon injection of the right vocal cord was necessary to minimize aspiration. Facial function remained normal, as did cranial nerves XI and XII (Fig. 15). A maxi-

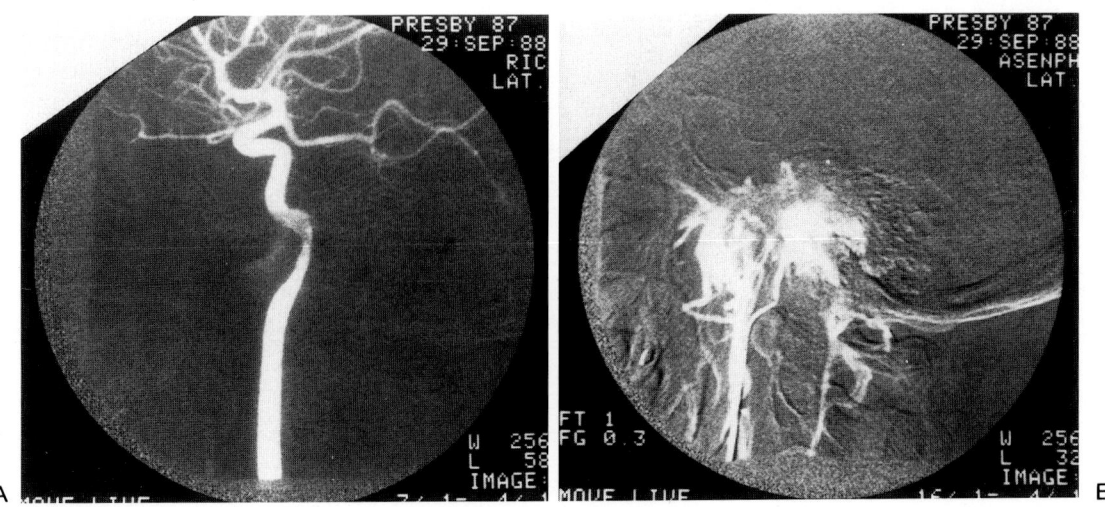

FIG. 12. G.C.—**A:** Right lateral carotid injection showing extrinsic compression and narrowing. **B:** Right lateral ascending pharyngeal artery injection showing tumor blush.

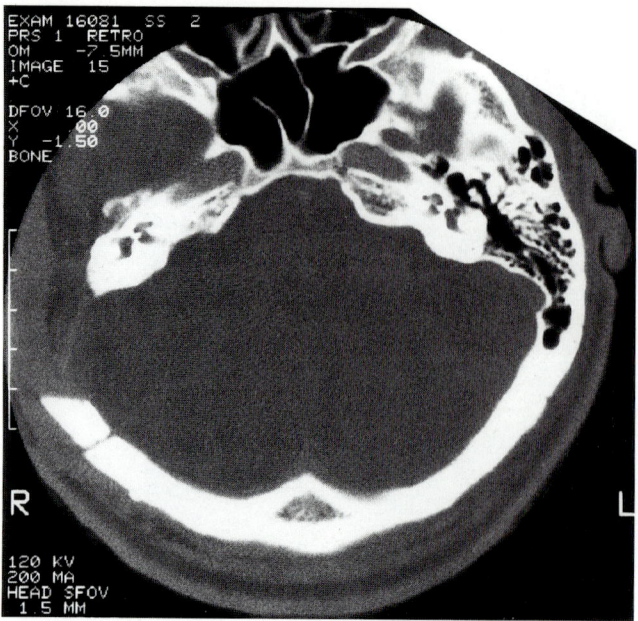

FIG. 13. G.C.—Postoperative CT scan of lateral temporal bone defect. No tumor noted.

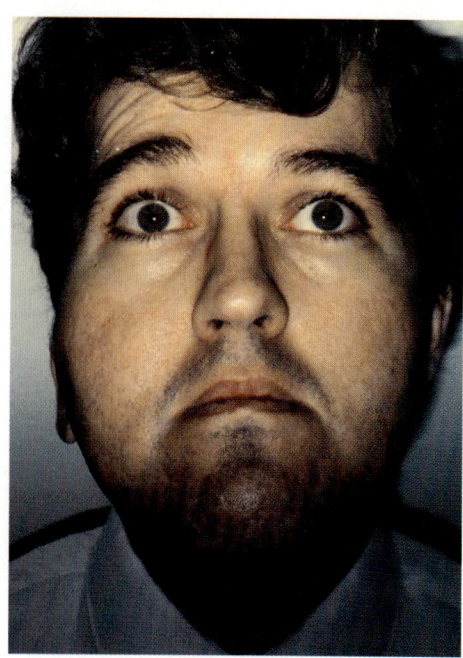

FIG. 15. G.C.—Postoperative, right glomus jugulare, with normal facial function (House grade I). Frontalis function is noted.

mum right conductive hearing loss occurred with normal cochlear reserve. He maintains a normal diet and resumed his previous profession as an engineer.

CASE 2

G.S., a 34-year-old draftsman, gave a 7-year history of right-sided hearing loss, progressive hoarseness, and tongue dysmotility. Examination revealed diminished right pharyngeal sensation with weak palatal elevation, atrophy, and fasciculations of the tongue. CT scan showed an extensive lesion of the jugular fossa. The inferior extent was at the level of C3 into the carotid space, with destructive extension into the occiput, clivus, and petrous temporal bone (Figs. 16 and 17).

The patient underwent a two-stage resection of a vagal neurilemoma separated by 6 weeks. The intracranial portion was initially removed via a suboccipital approach. The second procedure was a combined transtemporal and infratemporal approach with facial nerve transposition. The mandibular condyle was inferiorly displaced to provide access and exposure of the petrous ICA. Tumor extended superior and medial to the artery (Fig. 18). The lower limit of the lesion tapered into the vagus nerve in the upper neck (Fig. 19). The intracranial portion of the tumor was removed from the clivus by dissecting anterior and posterior to the ICA (Fig. 20). The postoperative CT scan shows the operative defect, which was reconstructed with a temporalis muscle flap (Fig. 21). The patient had return of facial function to a House grade III (Figs. 22 and 23).

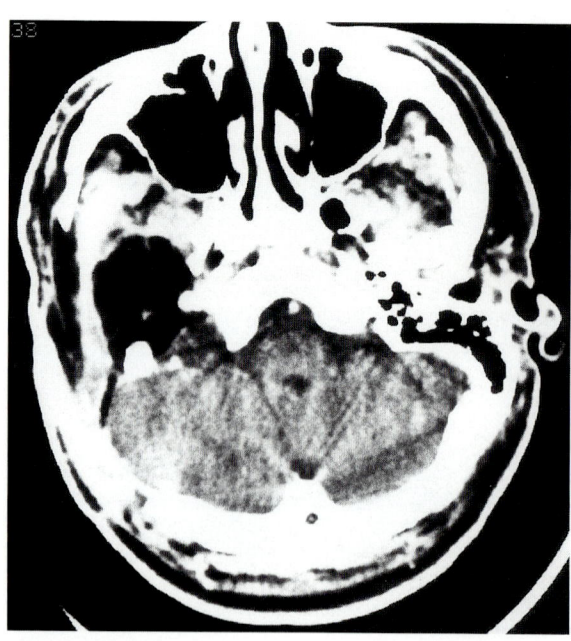

FIG. 14. G.C.—Postoperative CT scan showing reconstruction of the defect with fat and the temporalis muscle.

CASE 3

J.G., a 40-year-old female, was diagnosed with multiple sclerosis at age 30. Symptoms began with bilateral vision loss with subsequent improvement in the right eye but a residual left central scotoma remained. Eighteen

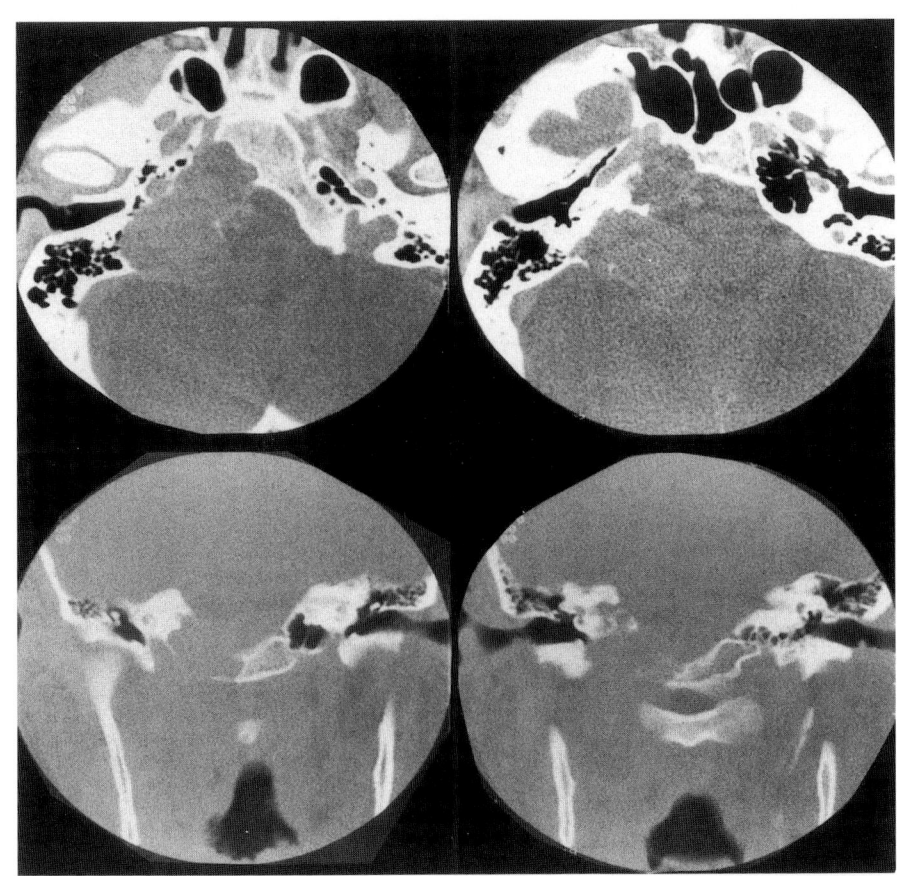

FIG. 16. G.S.—Bone algorithm CT scan showing a large destructive lesion of the petrous temporal bone, internal carotid artery, and clivus with extension into the neck.

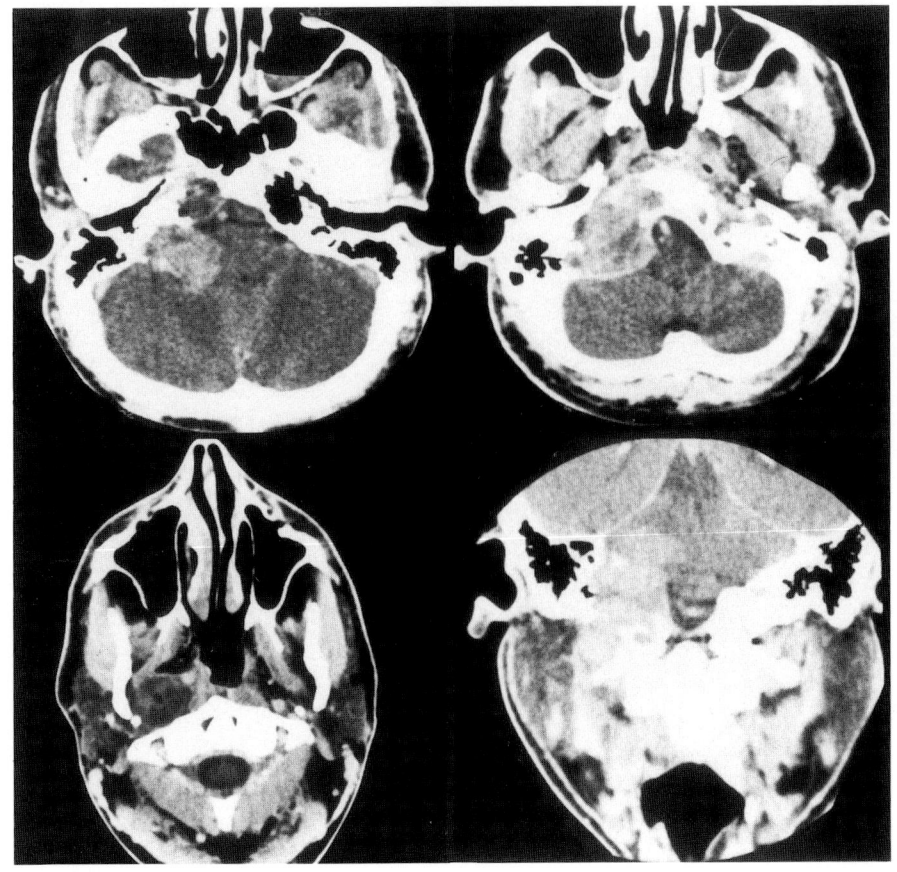

FIG. 17. G.S.—Enhanced CT scan showing intracranial portion and right parapharyngeal extension at C1.

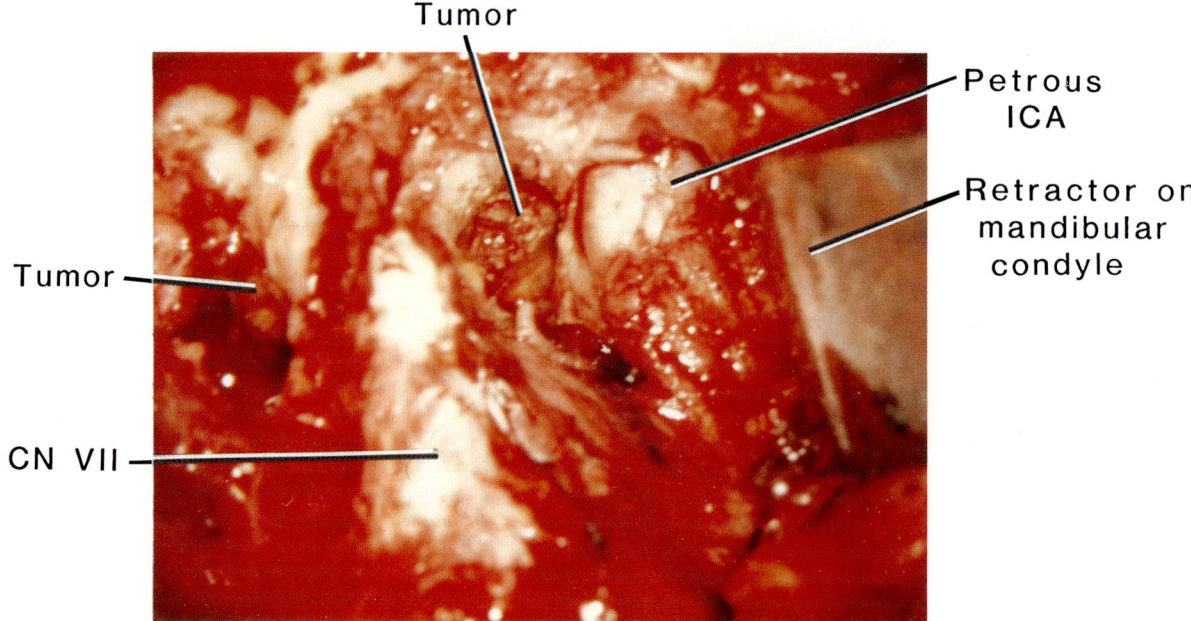

FIG. 18. G.S.—Operative exposure of the petrous internal carotid artery and facial nerve with tumor identified.

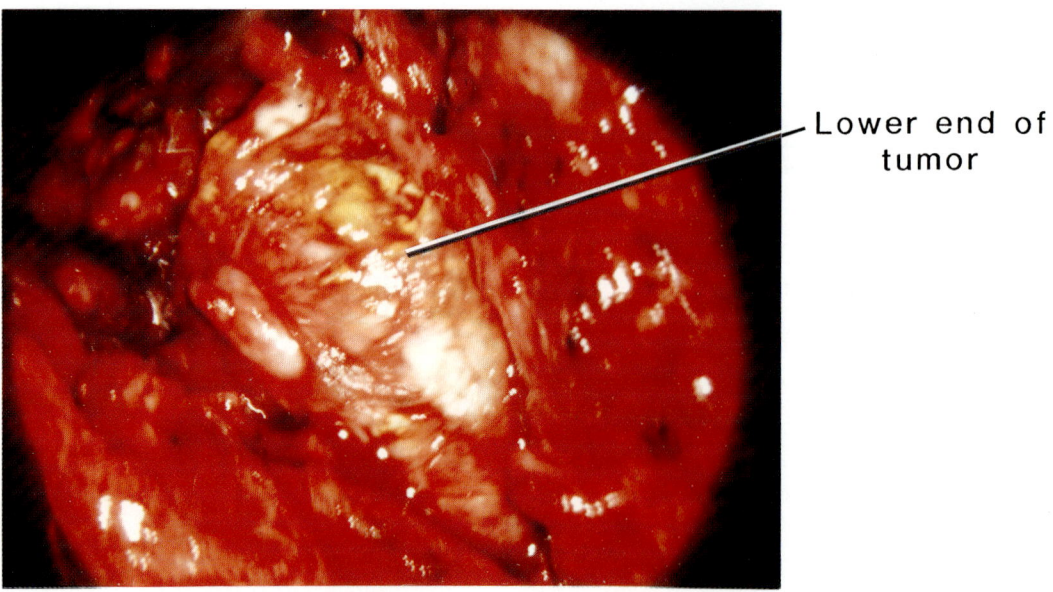

FIG. 19. G.S.—Lower limit of the vagal neurilemoma in the neck.

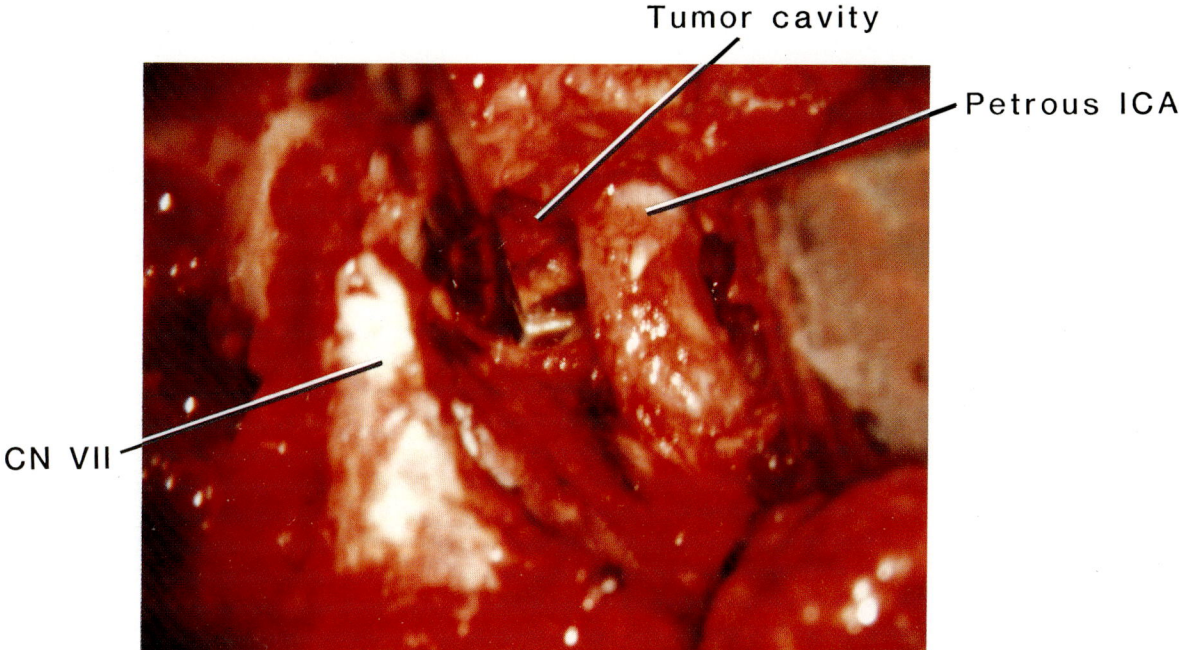

FIG. 20. G.S.—Total tumor resection from the clivus with isolation of the petrous ICA.

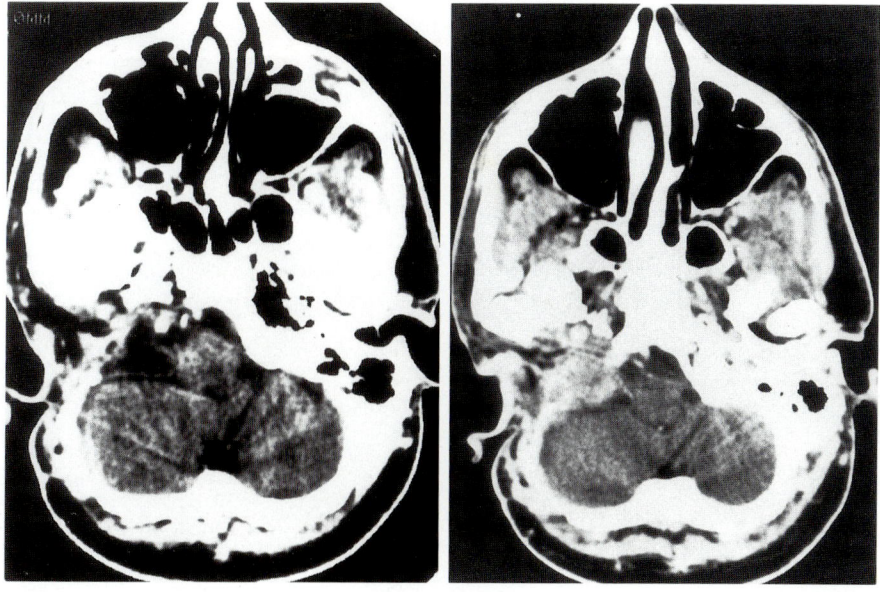

FIG. 21. G.S.—Postoperative CT scan following complete tumor removal and repair with a temporalis muscle flap.

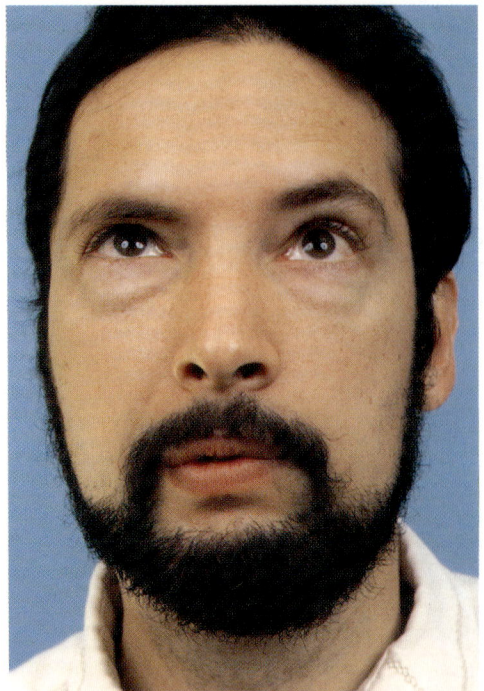

FIG. 22. G.S.—Postoperative, facial nerve transposition. Good facial tone with mild orbicularis oris weakness.

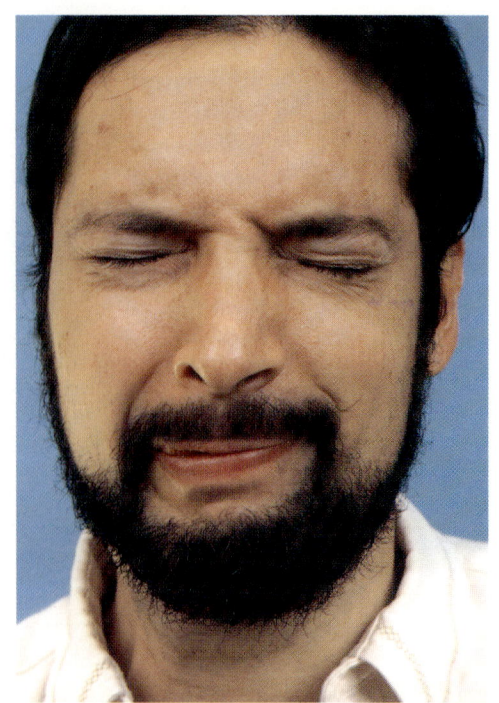

FIG. 23. G.S.—Mild synkinesis and facial weakness.

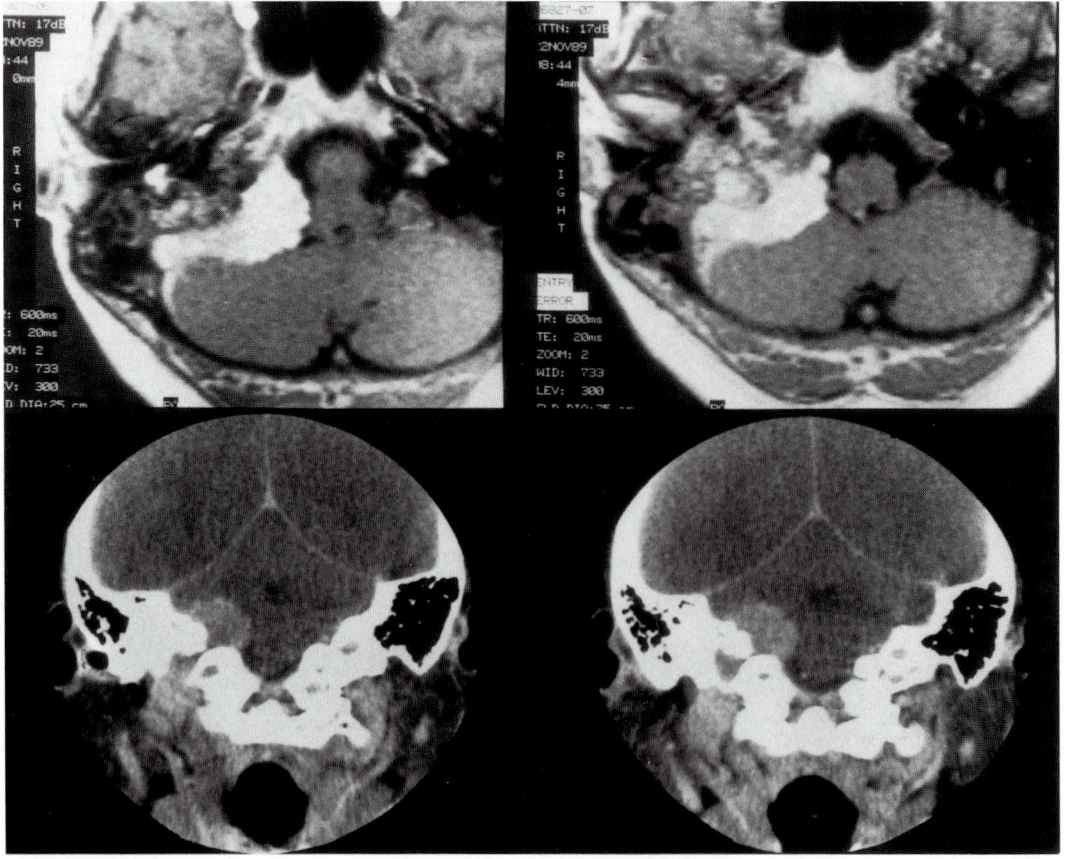

FIG. 24. J.G.—A 40-year-old female with posterior fossa, temporal bone, and high cervical meningioma.

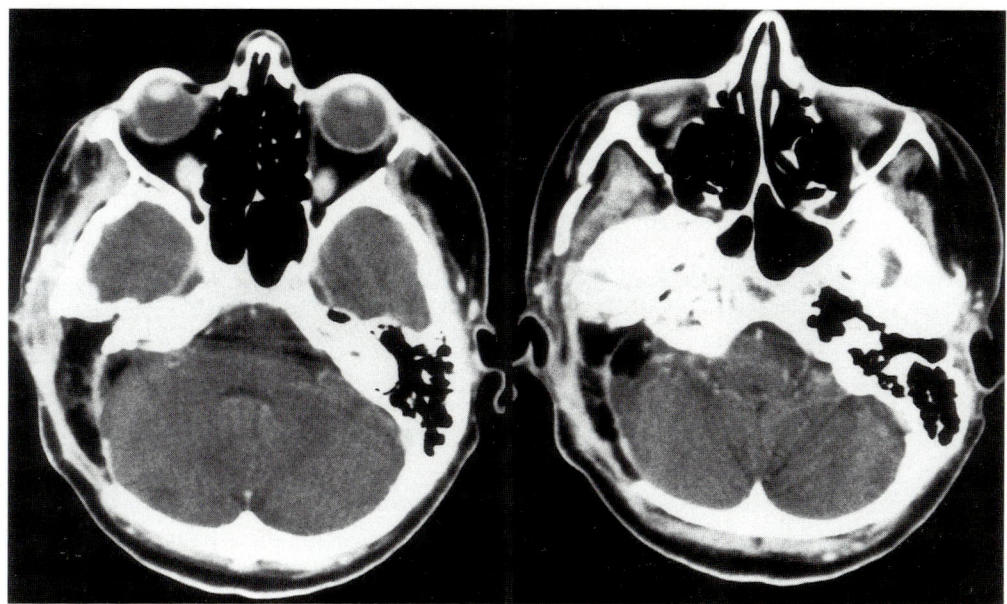

FIG. 25. J.G.—Postoperative CT scan following complete tumor resection. Fascia lata and abdominal fat were used for closure.

months prior to this evaluation she was involved in a motor vehicle accident and shortly thereafter experienced vertigo with nausea and vomiting, right pulsatile tinnitus, and hearing loss. She then developed symptoms of aspiration, dysphagia, and choking at night. Examination showed right facial hypoesthesia and a right mixed hearing loss. CT scan identified an enhancing lesion centered in the right petrous bone with extension into the middle ear, CP angle, and, inferiorly, into the jugular vein and carotid space (Fig. 24).

Arteriography and balloon test occlusion were obtained. A right common carotid study identified an enhancing lesion consistent with meningioma. The patient tolerated balloon occlusion of the right internal carotid artery. The operative procedure entailed a retrosigmoid craniectomy and a transtemporal–infratemporal approach with complete tumor resection. It was necessary to resect cranial nerves IX, X, and XI because of tumor invasion but cranial nerve XI was reconstructed with a graft. Tracheostomy was done at the start of the procedure. Abdominal fat and fascia lata were used for closure. Teflon injection of the right vocal cord and a gastrostomy were necessary. The patient resumed a full oral diet without the tracheotomy tube 4 months postoperatively. Spinal accessory nerve function recovered by regeneration. The CT scan shows the postoperative defect and reconstruction (Fig. 25). The patient maintained normal facial function (Fig. 26).

CASE 4

T.R., a 49-year-old male, had a previous partial resection of a large neurilemoma of the left temporal bone with extension into the clivus, CP angle, and petrous carotid. The patient had dysphagia and a left facial paralysis. Preoperatively, a CT scan identified extensive enhancing residual tumor (Figs. 27 and 28).

A postauricular transtemporal–infratemporal fossa approach achieved exposure for total tumor resection.

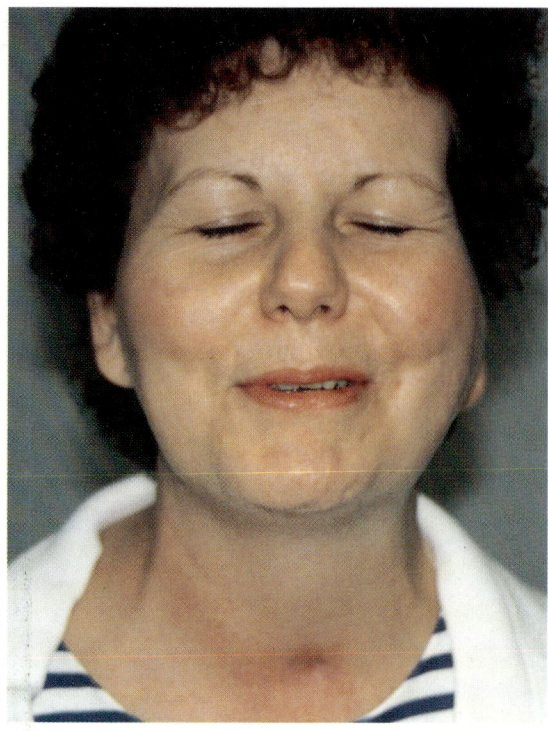

FIG. 26. J.G.—Tracheotomy tube is out. House grade I facial function.

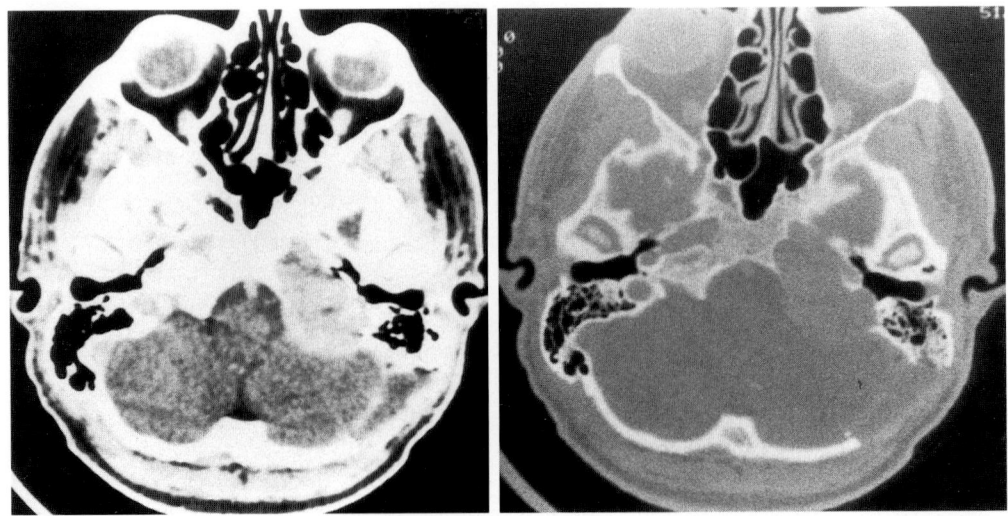

FIG. 27. T.R.—Axial CT scan identifying residual tumor in the posterior fossa petrous bone and clivus.

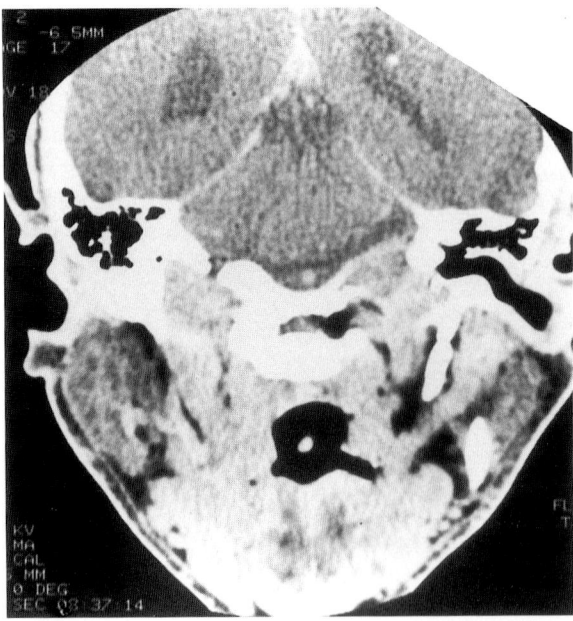

FIG. 28. T.R.—Coronal CT scan shows tumor filling the left jugular fossa.

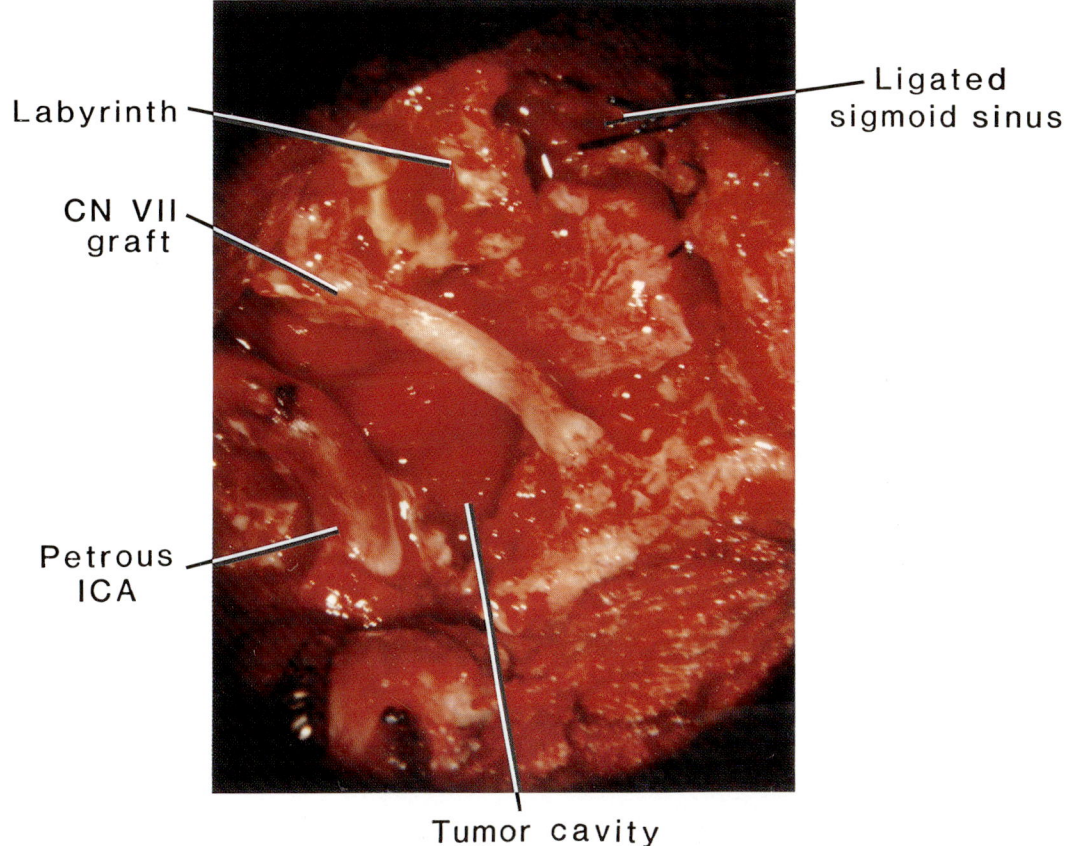

FIG. 29. T.R.—Left transtemporal resection of jugular fossa neurilemoma. Facial nerve repair with greater auricular nerve graft. Petrous internal carotid artery is freely dissected.

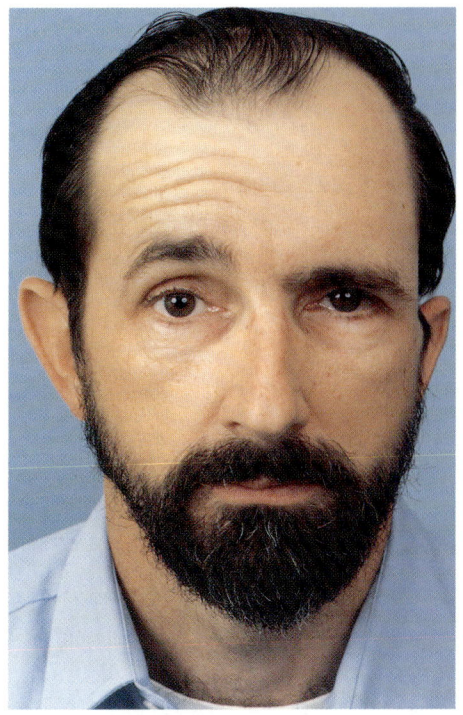

FIG. 30. T.R.—House grade III facial function following greater auricular nerve graft.

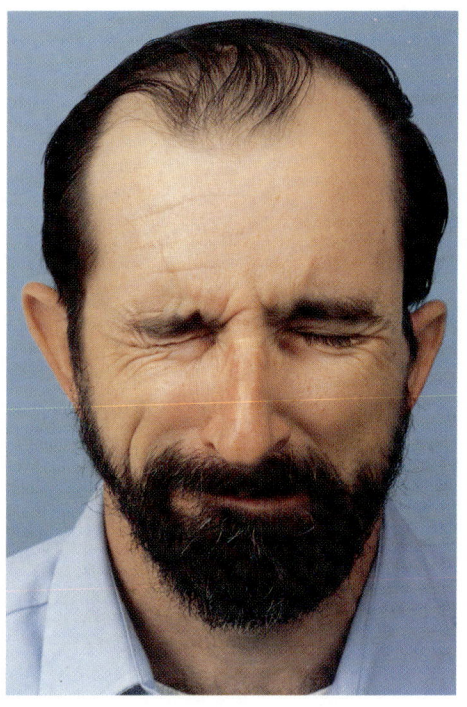

FIG. 31. T.R.—Same as Fig. 30.

The facial nerve was reconstructed with a greater auricular nerve graft (Fig. 29). Additional cranial nerve deficits included VIII, X, and XII. A tracheotomy placed at the time of the procedure was removed within 1 week. The patient had return of House grade III facial function (Figs. 30 and 31) and normal swallowing. He has returned to full-time employment as a registered nurse.

CASE 5

O.P., a 68-year-old female, had a right progressive hearing loss, dizziness, and ataxia. A 2.5 CP angle lesion was initially explored with the suspicion of acoustic neuroma. A smooth vascular mass thought to be an aneurysm was identified, the wound closed, and evaluated further. The CT scan identified a posterior fossa enhancing mass. Arteriography demonstrated a large right posterior fossa hypervascular lesion with inferior extension into the neck, displacing the carotid artery (Fig. 32). This was suggestive of a large glomus tumor.

An extended postauricular transtemporal–infratemporal approach with dissection of the petrous carotid artery was performed providing exposure for complete resection. Cranial nerves VII, XI, and XII were preserved, sacrificing IX and X because of paraganglioma tumor invasion. Tracheotomy and right Teflon vocal cord injection were necessary. The postoperative CT scan illustrated the surgical defect with no evidence of tumor (Fig. 33). The patient has a mild facial paresis, House grade II (Fig. 34).

CASE 6

G.F., a 40-year-old male, developed progressive right hearing loss. Sudden right facial paralysis prompted further evaluation, identifying a glomus jugulare tumor. The initial resection left residual tumor in the petrous apex and was complicated by right palatal and vocal cord paralysis and intermittent CSF otorrhea. Seven years later, evaluation for new pulsatile tinnitus revealed recurrent tumor. The patient was then referred to our service.

Imaging studies localized the lesion to the petrous

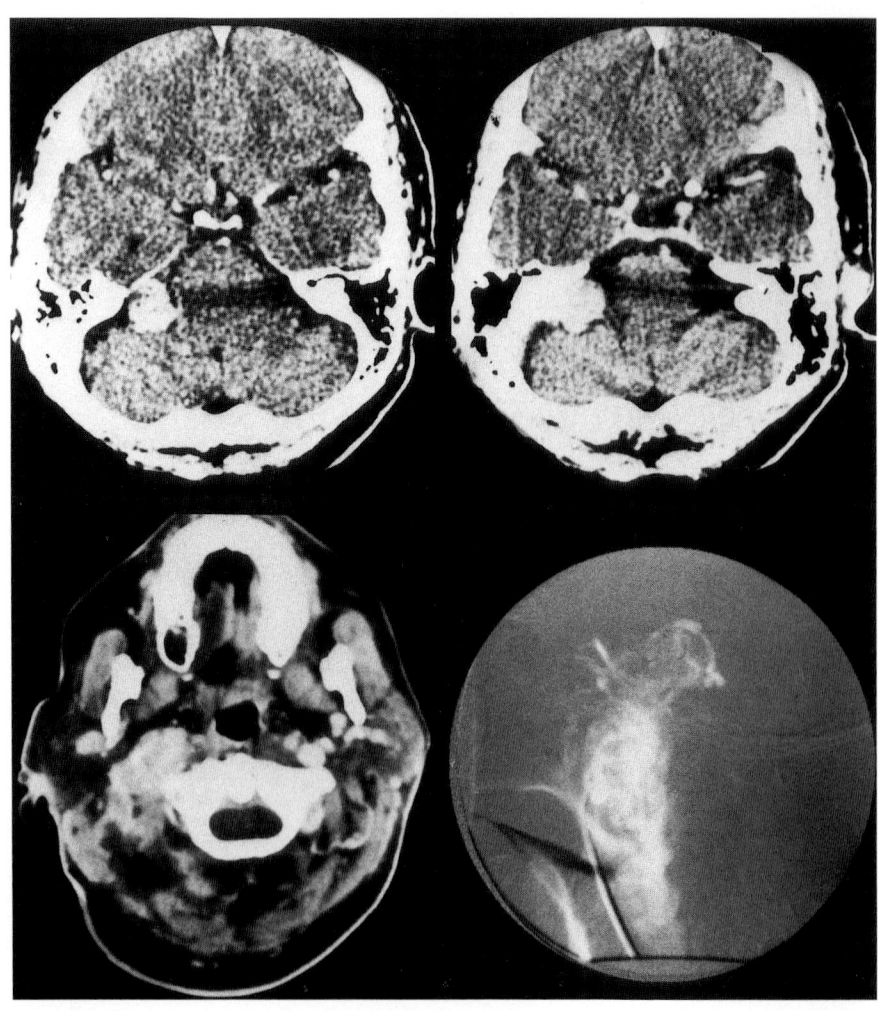

FIG. 32. O.P.—Right posterior fossa enhancing lesion with infratemporal extension. Hypervascularity is noted on arteriography.

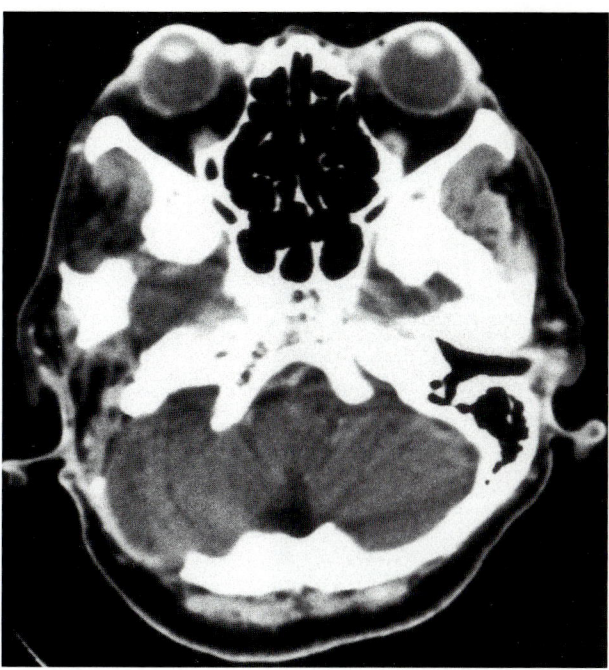

FIG. 33. O.P.—Postoperative CT scan following complete resection of glomus jugulare tumor.

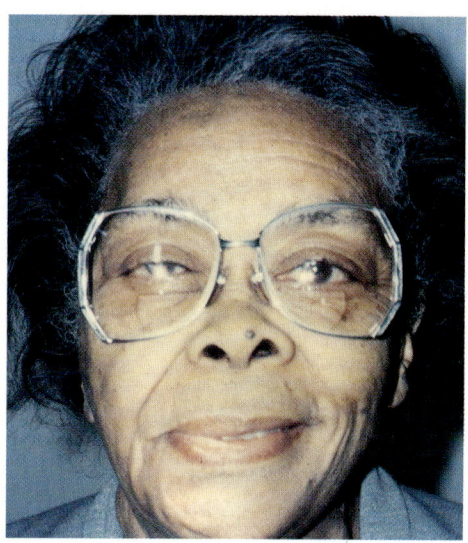

FIG. 34. O.P.—Mild facial paresis, House grade II, following resection of glomus jugulare.

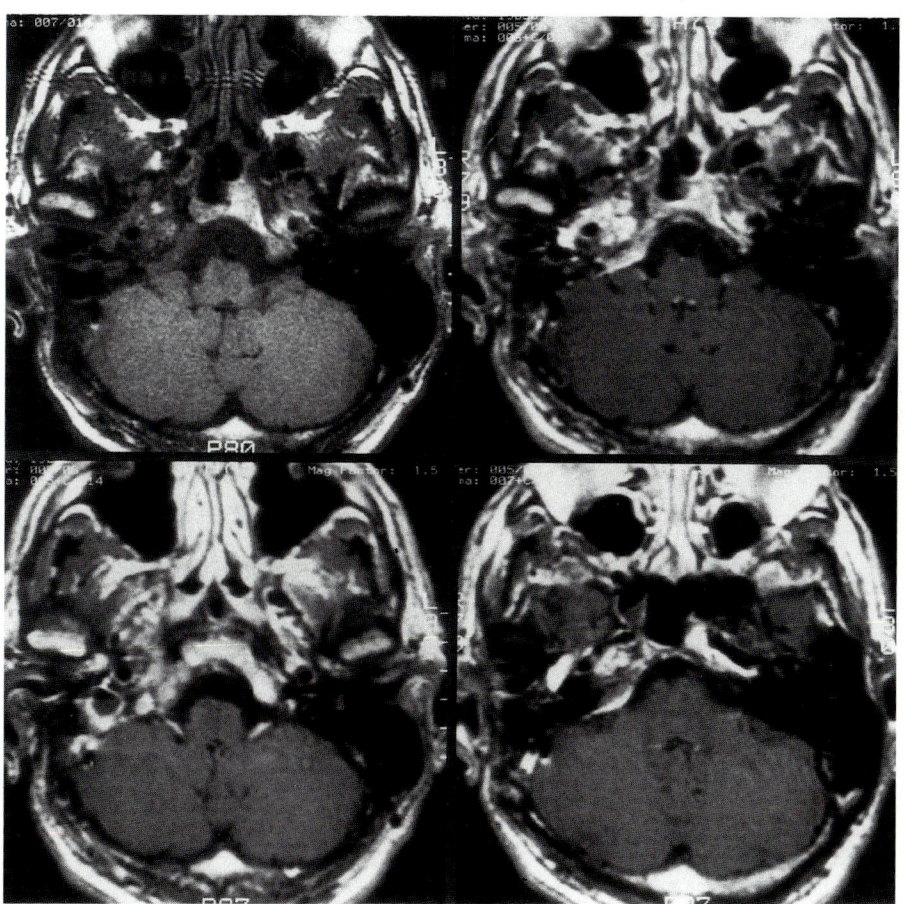

FIG. 35. G.F.—MRI showing glomus tumor in the right petrous bone, surrounding the carotid artery. Invasion into the clivus is seen.

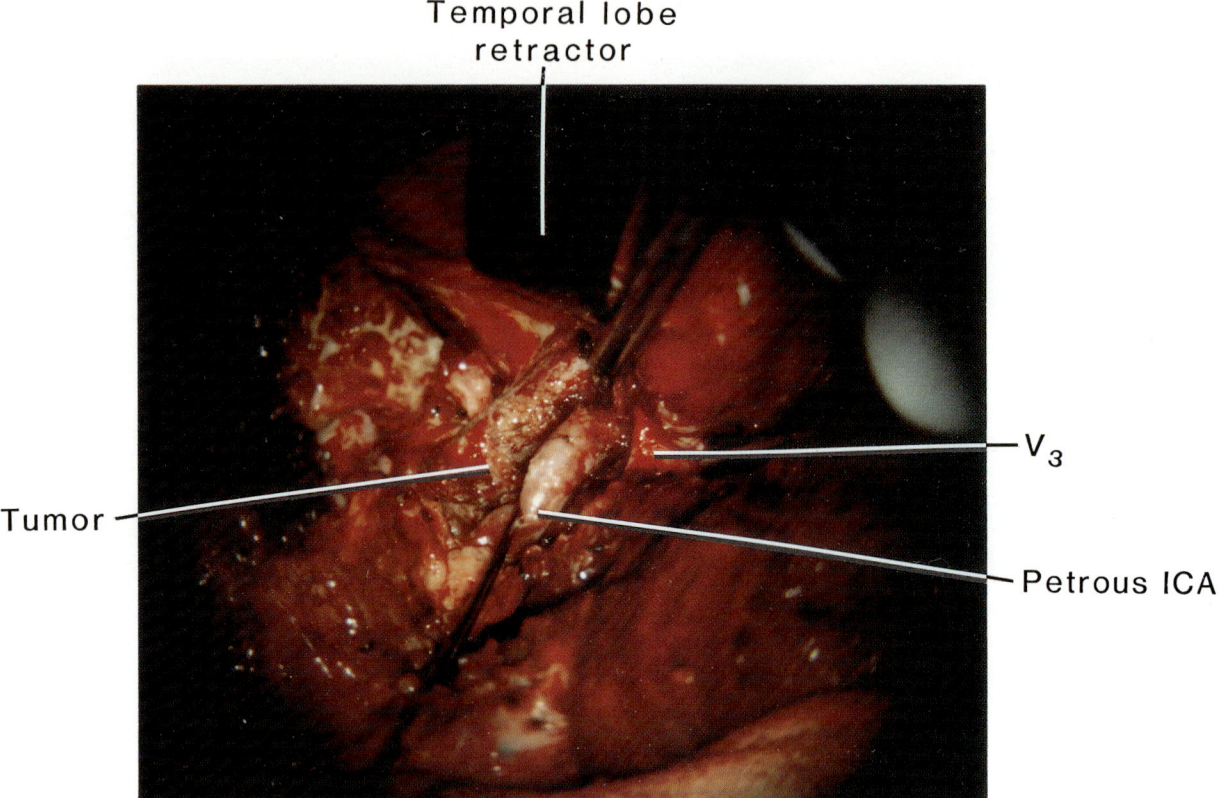

FIG. 36. G.F.—Transtemporal–infratemporal fossa exposure of petrous carotid being dissected away from tumor.

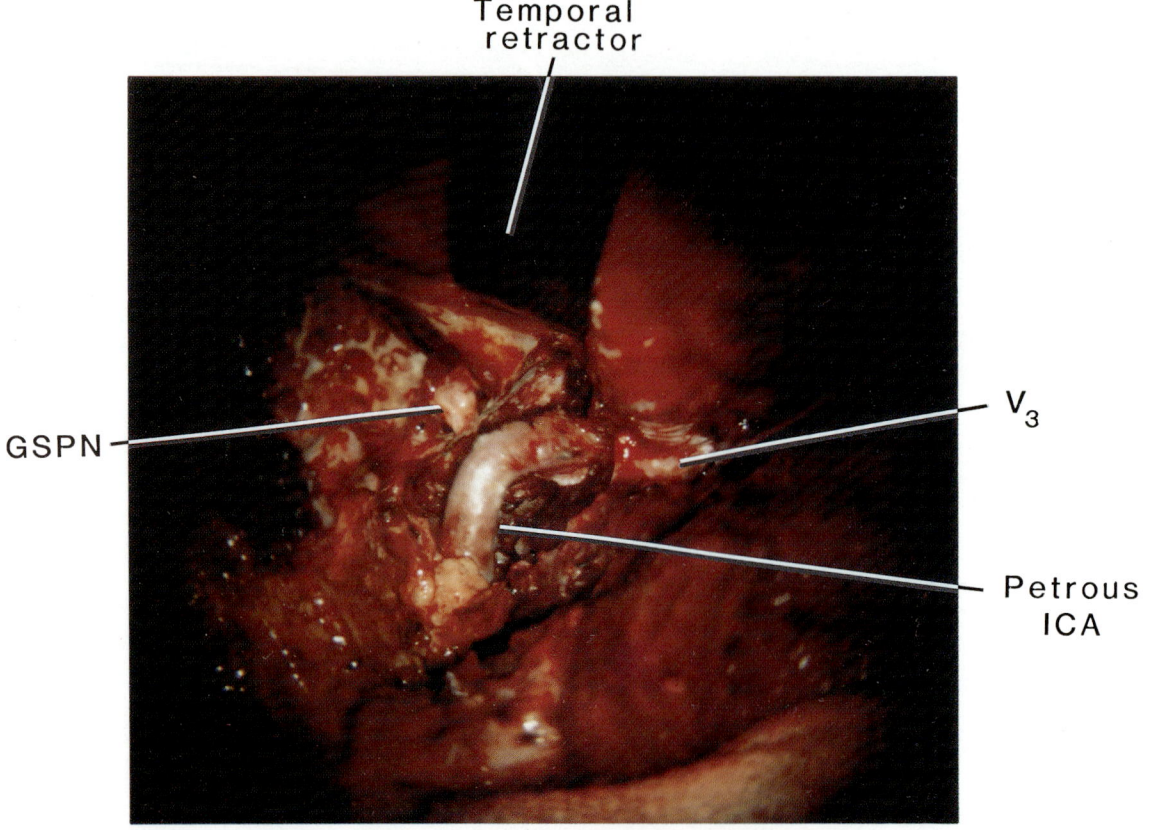

FIG. 37. G.F.—Superior limit of tumor has been removed by mobilizing the petrous ICA. Extradural middle fossa exposure identifies the greater superficial petrosal nerve (GSPN) and mandibular division of trigeminal nerve (V_3).

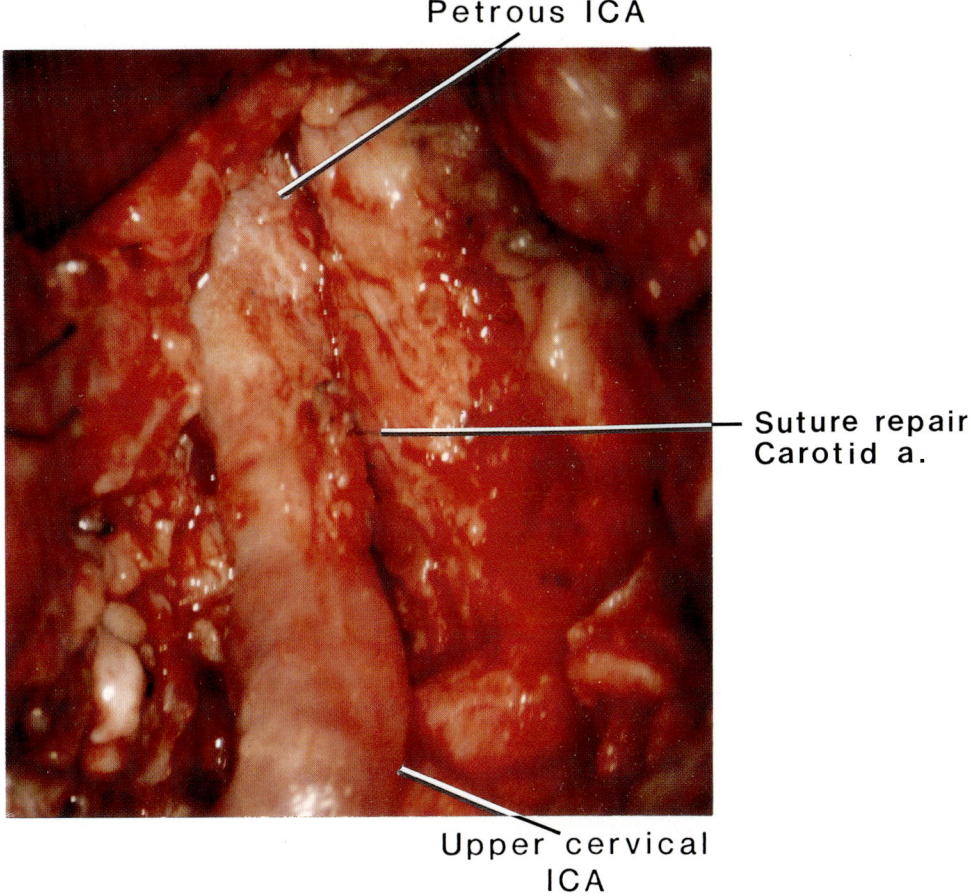

FIG. 38. G.F.—A pseudoaneurysm of the ICA was reexplored and repaired with suture.

apex encasing and narrowing the carotid artery, extending into the precavernous area (Fig. 35). Balloon test occlusion was well tolerated. The operation was done by a subtemporal and infratemporal approach to achieve complete tumor resection. By opening the periosteal sheath of the petrous ICA, tumor could be peeled away (Fig. 36). With anterior mobilization of the petrous ICA, the petrous apex and clival tumor could be removed (Fig. 37).

The patient sustained a small intimal dissection of the upper cervical ICA secondary to BTO, which became manifest as a pseudoaneurysm, and a delayed postoperative worsening of cranial nerve IX and X function. The wound was reexplored and the artery was repaired with trimming the intima and tacking it down with sutures (Fig. 38). The patient made a complete recovery with normal facial and lower cranial nerve function. No tumor recurrence has been evident upon follow-up.

CHAPTER 19

Surgical Excision of Petrous Apex Lesions

Ricardo Ramina, Joao Maniglia, and Carlos E. Barrionuevo

Petrous apex lesions are usually defined by the otologist and neurosurgeon in different ways. Otologists traditionally understand these lesions as those that produce bone erosion (e.g., congenital cholesteatomas, facial nerve neurinomas, and cholesterol granulomas). Neurosurgeons include other lesions related to the petrous apex, but not necessarily with bone erosion (e.g., petroclival meningiomas, trigeminal neurinomas, and chordomas). This led us to search for an anatomical definition of the petrous apex region and the lesions related to it. In 1986, a multidisciplinary group interested in the treatment of skull base lesions was founded in Curitiba. According to the "team-work concept" of this group, the skull base is formed by three components: an extracranial, an intracranial, and a transitional area (bone and foramina) between both.

Based on this definition, petrous apex lesions comprise those that, even if they do not produce bone erosion, maintain a close relationship to any of the three components of the skull base at the petrous apex. This region is like a pyramid having three surfaces: an anterior, a posterior, and an inferior. The anterior surface is limited by the foramen lacerum, sphenopetrous fissure, facial nerve hiatus, and the eminentia arcuata. The posterior surface is limited by the fissura petro-occipitalis (inferior petrosal sinus sulcus), superior lip of the jugular foramen, and the posterior border of the internal auditory canal. The inferior surface of the petrous apex is limited by the foramen lacerum, petro-occipitalis fissure, medial lip of the carotid canal, and the sphenopetrous fissure. These three surfaces point to the clivus region posteroanteriorly.

R. Ramina: Department of Neurosurgery, Curitiba Skull Base Foundation, Hospital das Nacoes, 80420 Curitiba, Brazil.
J. Maniglia: Department of Otorhinolaryngology, Hospital de Clinicas, University Federal of Paraná, 80420 Curitiba, Brazil.
C. E. Barrionuevo: Department of Otorhinolaryngology, Hospital de Clinicas, University Federal of Paraná, 80420 Curitiba, Brazil.

Lesions presented in this chapter are those arising in one of these three surfaces, inside the petrous apex bone, and those, even though they arise outside, having a portion that reaches this region, producing signs and symptoms. These are rare in children and are usually benign lesions, requiring surgical excision for definitive treatment. The combined surgical approach (neuro-otological) is the best option for total removal of the lesion, giving the patient the best chance for cranial nerve and vessel preservation or reconstruction. Five different surgical approaches are presented in this chapter.

DIAGNOSTIC CONSIDERATIONS

The most frequent symptoms presented by patients with petrous apex lesions are unilateral hearing loss, facial nerve paralysis, vestibular symptoms, trigeminal nerve manifestations, infection, and cerebellar symptoms. Ear infection may be the reason for initial consultation when the lesion reaches the external auditory canal. It is always preceded by hearing loss. Facial nerve paralysis preceding ear infection suggests the presence of a petrous apex lesion, such as a cholesteatoma. Vestibular symptoms may be absent due to long-standing nerve compression with simultaneous central compensation mechanisms.

At examination, several degrees of hearing loss may be observed. Frequently, the patient comes with severe sensory-neural hearing loss when the cochlea is affected. When the lesion is retrocochlear, hearing may be partially preserved. In acoustic neurinoma, the dissociation between hearing level and discrimination can occur in patients with acoustic neurinomas, but we have seen patients with good hearing and discrimination. Hearing is usually preserved in petroclival meningiomas, even though occasionally we can find abnormal evoked response audiometry. This method can objectively locate hearing loss within the auditory pathways. The analysis of waves I to V and the measurement of latencies can locate the lesion in the cochlea, auditory nerve, or central pathways.

Otoscopy may show tumor in the external auditory canal or middle ear. Eustachian tube blockage with serous otitis may be present due to tumor compression. Vestibular testing is important. The integrity of the vestibular response should be determined. Schirmer's test is performed to define the site of facial nerve lesion. If lacrimation is present, the lesion is lateral to the exit of the greater superficial petrosal nerve. Impedance testing shows the presence of stapedial muscle reflex or decay indicating disturbance of the sensory or motor portion of the reflex arc produced by a lesion of the cochlear or facial nerve, medial to the stapedial nerve.

Trigeminal nerve function may be impaired in cases of trigeminal neurinomas.

RADIOLOGICAL EXAMINATION

Conventional radiology and tomography may show erosion of the petrous apex and hyperostosis in meningiomas. Computerized tomography determines the location, extention, and in most cases the nature of the lesion. Cholesteatomas and cholesterol granulomas are usually hypodense, nonenhancing lesions. Meningiomas show enhancement by contrast and acoustic neurinomas show enlargement of the internal auditory canal. Magnetic resonance imaging (MRI) shows the location, extension, and possible nature of the tumor, giving additional information about the involvement of vessels. Angiography is performed to demonstrate the infiltration or compression of important arteries and occlusion of venous sinuses at the skull base. Balloon occlusion tests should be performed if there is need of surgical removal of vessels. A complete neuroradiological investigation is required to plan the surgical approach.

PATIENT SELECTION

Basically all patients with benign lesions of the petrous apex should be operated on. Contraindication to surgery should consider the relation risk/benefit of surgery to the patient. The natural history of the disease, the slow progression of symptoms, age, and the general condition of the patient are important factors. A partial tumor resection, reducing the compression to the brainstem and cranial nerves may be of value for high-risk patients.

We do not advocate surgery for histiocytosis, fibrous dysplasia, osteopetrosis, and malignant tumor. A biopsy establishes the diagnosis, and treatment follows with radiotherapy and/or chemotherapy.

SURGICAL APPROACHES

Surgical difficulties in the treatment of petrous apex lesions are related to the involvement of the internal carotid artery or basilar artery and their branches, brain retraction, Labbé's vein, tumor extension to the brain stem, and repair of extensive surgical defects for prevention of CSF fistula and infection.

The following factors should be considered in choosing the most appropriate approach: the nature and extent of the lesion, the presence of facial nerve paralysis, the status of hearing and vestibular function, and the presence of infection.

Five different approaches are used by our group: translabyrinthine with or without cavity obliteration, middle fossa, posterior fossa, combined (middle–posterior fossa with petrosectomy), and the occipito–transmastoid–cervical approach.

Approach 1: Translabyrinthine

With Marsupialization (Approach 1A)

Indication

This approach is used in the treatment of petrous apex cholesteatoma extending to the middle ear and external auditory canal with secondary infection and sensoryneural hearing loss (Figs. 1 and 2). This approach is performed by an otologist and is extradural.

Surgical Technique

The patient is operated on under general anesthesia and is placed in the supine position with contralateral head rotation. A retroauricular skin incision, 1 cm behind the posteroauricular sulcus is made. A radical mastoidectomy and a labyrinthectomy are performed. The lesion is removed as radically as possible. If infection is present, marsupialization of the cavity should be carried out. A wide meatoplasty is done using a retroauricular skin graft to facilitate postoperative care of the cavity. Incision of the dura mater is avoided because of risk of infection and CSF fistula.

With Cavity Obliteration (Approach 1B)

Indication

This technique is indicated in case of trauma (mostly gunshot wounds). These patients usually have hearing loss greater than 60 dB. For this reason, obliteration of the cavity may be performed. Surgical treatment that leaves an open cavity facilitates infection, which requires permanent care.

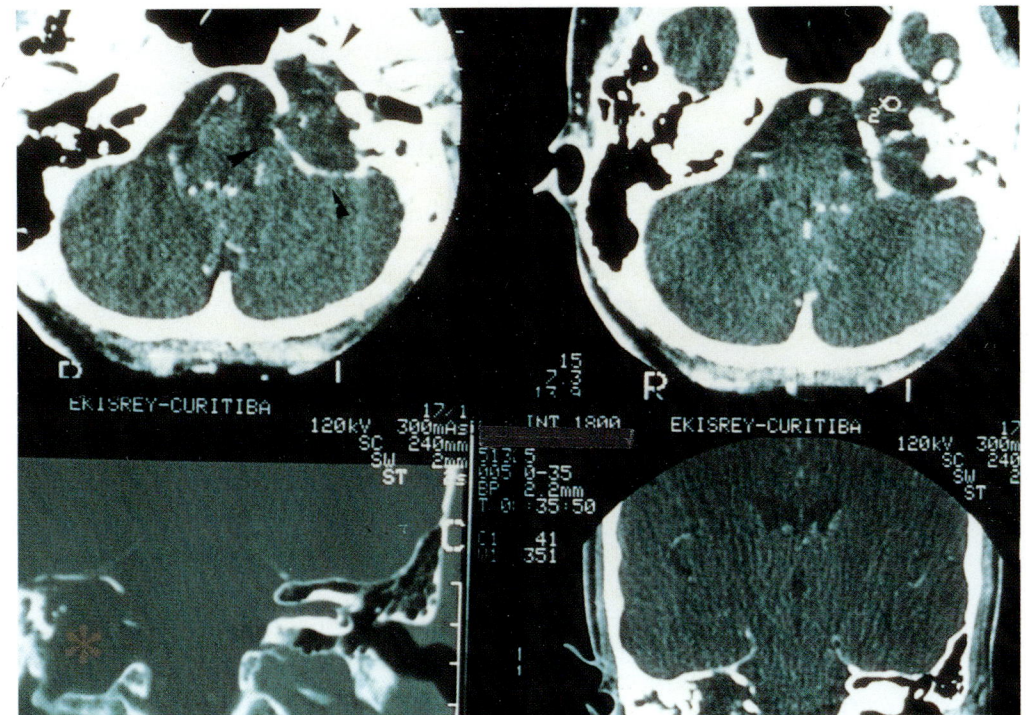

FIG. 1. Approach 1A. Preoperative CT scan showing petrous apex congenital cholesteatoma. **Top:** *Arrow* points to the dura mater limiting cholesteatoma to extradural space. **Bottom:** *Star* localizes petrous apex erosion.

Facial and acoustic neurinomas and vestibular nerve section may be performed by this approach (Fig. 3). The surgical cavity is obliterated to avoid chronic infection and CSF fistula. Cooperation between the otologist and neurosurgeons is mandatory in order to facilitate total removal, thus avoiding second stage procedures, and to reconstruct affected cranial nerves. We usually do not use the translabyrinthine approach to treat acoustic neurinomas.

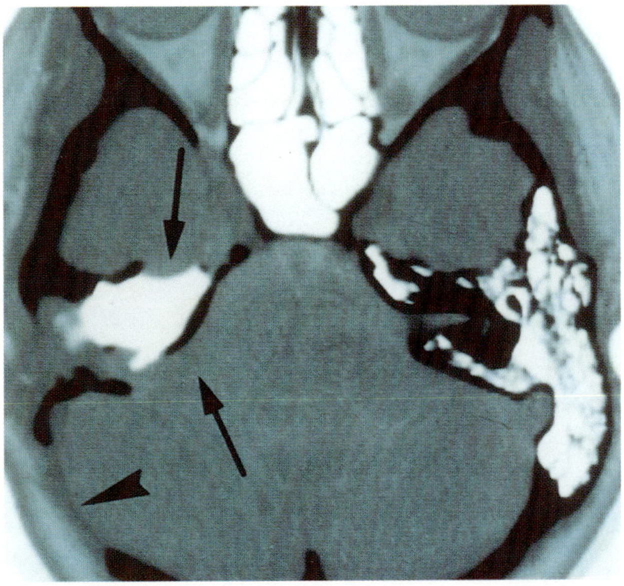

Surgical Technique

The patient is placed in the supine position with contralateral head rotation under general anesthesia. A postauricular skin incision is made 2 cm posterior to the sulcus. The mastoid cortex is exposed after periosteal incisions and a complete mastoidectomy is carried out. In cases of gunshot lesion, the mastoidectomy is extended (radical mastoidectomy) with removal of bullet fragments and bone sequestrum. Dura mater lacerations are repaired by suture or graft. Mastoid cavity is cranialized (tip removal). The cavity is obliterated using muscle–periosteal flaps.

In cases of facial nerve neurinomas when there is no useful hearing (usually destroyed by tumor extension to the inner ear), labyrinthectomy is completed as tumor is removed. After facial nerve reconstruction, the cavity is obliterated as above.

Facial Nerve Management

If facial nerve function is normal, the facial nerve may be translocated to a new position in the parotid region

FIG. 2. Approach 1A. Postoperative CT scan. *Arrows* point to the limit of translabyrinthine total petrosectomy. *Arrowhead* shows site of second stage posterior fossa craniectomy for an intracranial–extratemporal facial nerve anastomosis (Dott).

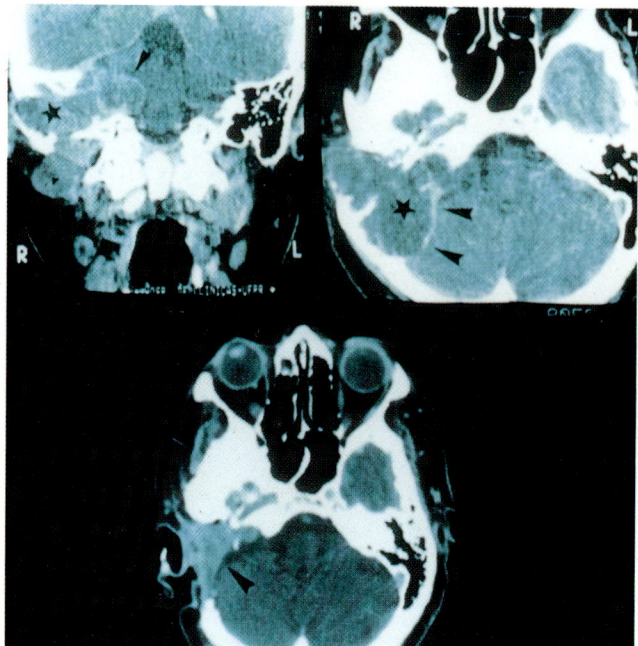

FIG. 3. Approach 1A. CT scan examination. **Top:** Preoperative. Facial nerve neurinoma with destruction of mastoid, middle ear, and petrous apex. *Arrow* shows tumor in posterior and middle cranial fossae. *Star* shows intratemporal tumor. **Bottom:** Postoperative. *Arrow* shows translabyrinthine petrosectomy obliterated by temporal periosteum flap and temporal muscle.

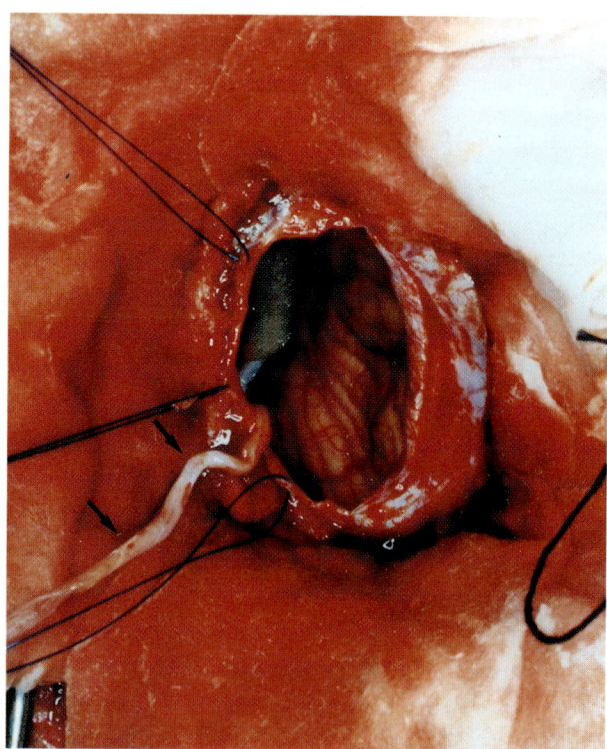

FIG. 4. Approach 1A. Posterior fossa craniotomy for facial nerve grafting at brainstem. Dura mater has been incised and cerebellum is seen through the incision. *Arrows* point to 14-cm sural nerve graft already anastomosed to proximal facial nerve stump. The distal portion will be sutured to distal facial nerve stump in the stylomastoid foramen region.

(rerouting) to facilitate the approach and, in the case of open cavity surgery, to permit better postoperative care. Two factors should be considered in cases of facial nerve reconstruction: the presence of infection and the proximal stump of the nerve. In the presence of infection, reconstruction of the seventh cranial nerve (intradural proximal stump) should be delayed and carried out in a second operation. If possible, a primary suture should be performed even in the presence of infection. Rerouting of the facial nerve may permit end-to-end anastomosis. In the presence of open infection, the use of nerve grafts should be avoided.

If the proximal nerve stump is intradural and there is no infection, we prefer to perform a facial-to-facial reconstruction. If an end-to-end suture is not possible, an intracranial-to-extratemporal anastomosis using nerve graft (sural nerve or great auricular nerve) is carried out. The proximal nerve stump is identified at the brain stem, and the graft is sutured with 10-0 nylon. The distal stump is usually identified at the stylomastoid foramen (Dott) (Figs. 4 and 5) or in the mastoid portion of the seventh cranial nerve (Samii–Draf). If a facial-to-facial reconstruction is not possible, a hypoglossal-to-facial anastomosis is carried out.

Approach 2: Middle Fossa

Indications

This approach is used to treat petroclival meningiomas, nonexteriorized congenital cholesteatomas, facial and trigeminal neurinomas, facial nerve lesions at or medial to the geniculate ganglion, CSF fistula, teratomas, and small acoustic neurinomas (with hearing preservation) (Figs. 6–9).

Through the middle fossa approach, the superior aspect of the petrous apex can be exposed widely intra-

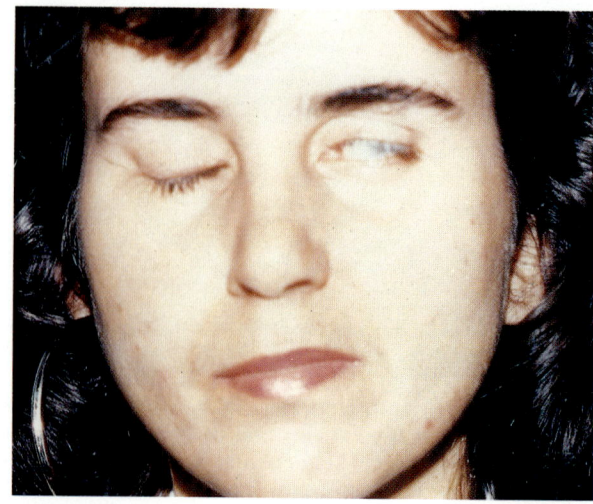

FIG. 5. Approach 1A. Postoperative result 9 months after intracranial–extratemporal facial nerve graft.

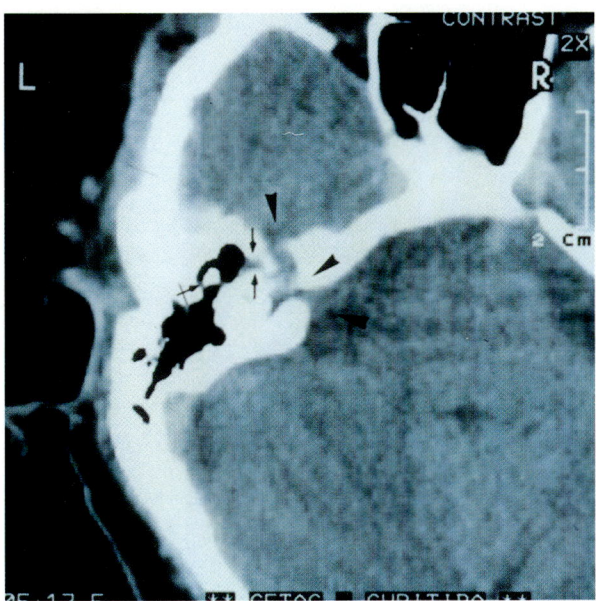

FIG. 6. Approach 2. CT scan examination of congenital cholesteatoma (petrous apex). *Arrows* point to the head of malleus (*crossed arrow*), fallopian canal (*small arrows*), cholesteatoma bone erosion, and internal auditory canal (*arrowheads*).

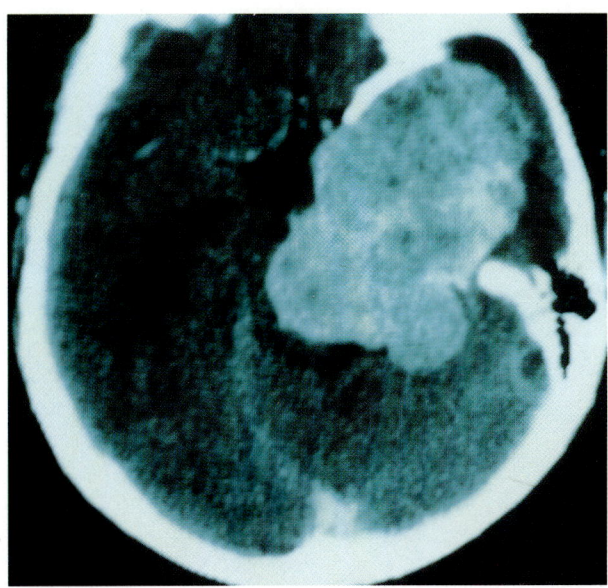

FIG. 8. Approach 2. CT scan of large trigeminal neurinoma in middle and posterior fossae, showing displacement of brain stem and the fourth ventricle.

durally and extradurally. The facial nerve can be reached in its meatal and intrapetrosal portions. The access can be extended to the infratemporal fossa to expose the petrosal portion of the internal carotid artery. The middle ear and mastoid can be entered by opening the tegmen. The posterior fossa is exposed by splitting the tentorium.

Surgical Technique

The patient is placed under general anesthesia, with dorsal decubitus and contralateral head rotation: the head is extended and held by a three-point skeletal device with the zygomatic arch at the highest point. A semicircular skin incision is made beginning at the tragus level and extending anteriorly to the frontal region behind the hairline. A temporalis fascia flap is developed by dissection from the zygomatic arch, remaining attached inferiorly to the skin flap. The zygomatic arch, the upper portion of the bony external auditory canal, and the temporal muscle are exposed. The temporal muscle is detached superiorly and the root of zygoma can be thinned out with a drill, or the zygomatic arch is temporarily removed for a more basal access when necessary (e.g., exposure of the infratemporal fossa or petrous carotid artery) to avoid excessive temporal lobe retraction. In selected cases, the glenoid fossa can be opened and rarely the mandibular condyle is resected for access to the infratemporal fossa. The excision of tumor can be completed by a transmaxillary approach (Fig. 10). Mannitol or lumbar CSF drainage can be used to reduce temporal lobe retraction.

A four burr-hole craniotomy is fashioned. The first hole is made in the parietotemporal region in the squamous suture, anterior to the transverse sinus, 6 cm above the external auditory canal. The second burr hole is placed in the parietotemporal region, posterior to the coronal suture. The third and fourth burr holes are made in the temporal area, above the zygomatic arch, one anterior and the other posterior at its root (Fig. 11). The temporal bone craniotomy is replaced at the end of the pro-

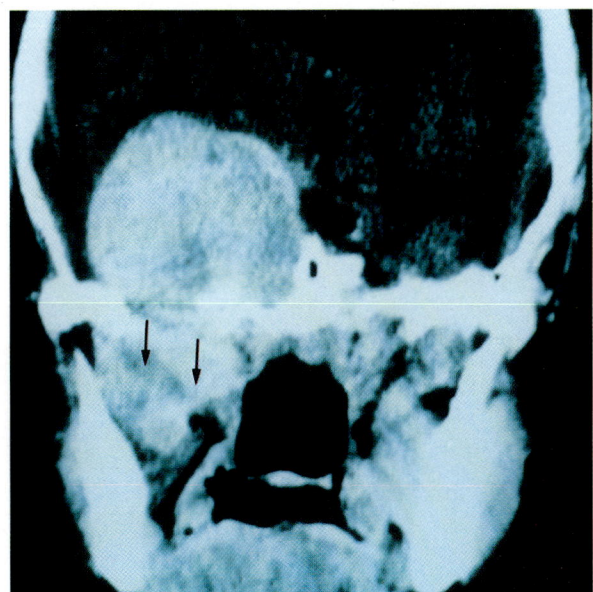

FIG. 7. Approach 2. Coronal CT scan showing a large trigeminal neurinoma in middle fossa. *Arrows* points out tumor extension to infratemporal fossa.

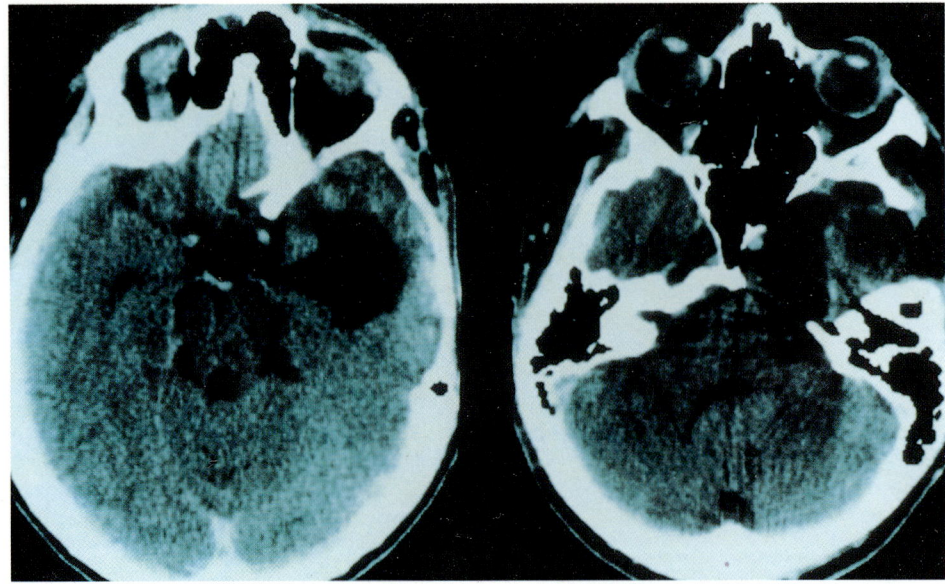

FIG. 9. Approach 2. CT scan showing total removal of trigeminal neurinoma.

cedure. Additional bone removal (craniectomy) is carried out at the temporal base, exposing the floor of the middle fossa.

The dura mater of the middle fossa is elevated from the bony floor, exposing the middle meningeal artery. This vessel is coagulated and sectioned and the foramen spinosum is obliterated with bone wax. Medial and perpendicular to this artery, the greater superficial petrosal nerve can be identified and is carefully separated from the dura mater and followed to its exit (hiatus facialis) in the superior aspect of the temporal bone. The facial nerve can be dehiscent in 5% of cases. With further posterior elevation of the dura mater, the arcuate eminence harboring the superior semicircular canal is exposed. The dura mater is elevated, medial and anterior to the foramen spinosum up to the entrance of the mandibular nerve in the foramen ovale. This extradural approach can be used to reach the internal auditory canal and the labyrinthine and tympanic portions of the facial nerve. The petrosal and horizontal portions of the internal carotid artery can be exposed by removal of bone with a diamond drill medial to the eustachian tube.

The dura mater is incised parallel to the sylvian fissure and two small cuts perpendicular to the cranial base are made. The temporal lobe is carefully retracted from ante-

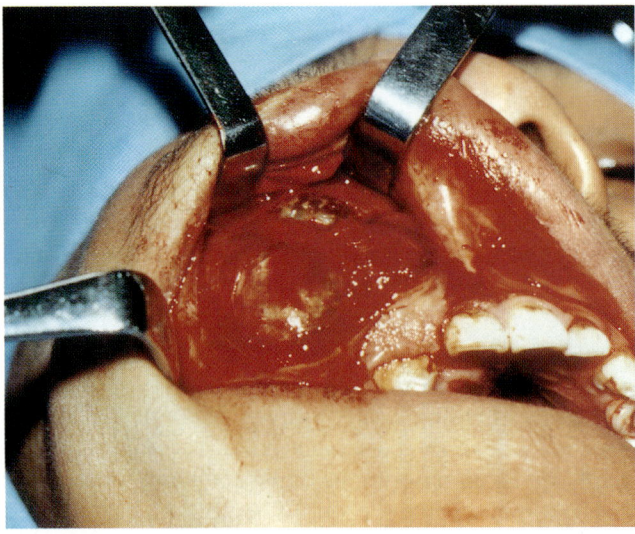

FIG. 10. Approach 2. Transmaxillary approach shows trigeminal neurinoma inside infratemporal fossa. This access is simultaneous with the middle fossa approach for radical tumor removal and cranial base reconstruction.

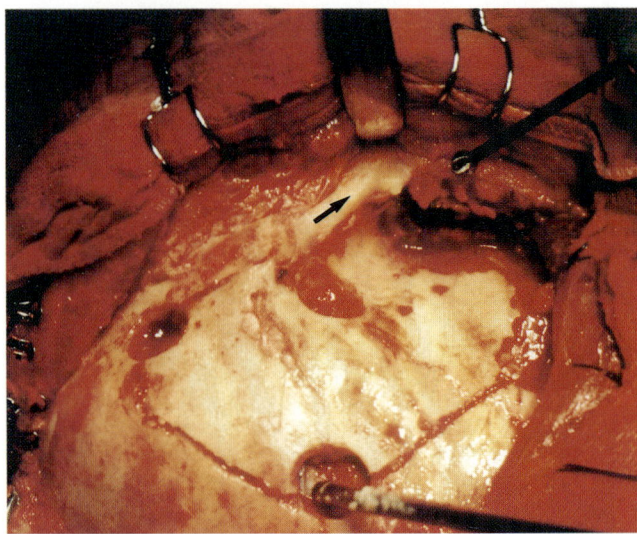

FIG. 11. Approach 2. Temporal craniotomy. *Arrows* show zygomatic arch temporarily sectioned for a more basal access.

rior to posterior, preserving Labbé's vein entering the lateral sinus a few millimeters behind the entrance of the superior petrosal sinus (Fig. 12). Tumor is exposed in the floor of the middle fossa. It is removed using microsurgical techniques, exposing the free border of tentorium. The fourth cranial nerve is identified at the margin of the tentorium and the third cranial nerve anterior and medial to the fourth, before it enters the cavernous sinus. The posterior communicating artery and its perforating branches, as well as the superior cerebellar artery, are identified. If necessary, the tentorial border is split posterior to the fourth nerve, exposing cranial nerves V, III, and VIII (Fig. 13). If a wider exposure is necessary, additional bone is removed with a drill from the petrous apex between the porus acousticus and the trigeminal nerve. The posterior fossa and clivus region are exposed in this way. Tumor removal is piecemeal using microsurgical techniques and ultrasonic aspiration. In large lesions, preservation of the trochlear nerve is very difficult. Branches of the basilar artery may be embedded in meningiomas and dissection should be very careful, using high magnification.

After tumor removal, the dura mater is closed in watertight fashion. Any open zygomatic and mastoid cells are closed with bone wax. The middle ear and mastoid cells, if open, are occluded with temporal muscle graft. The temporalis fascia flap is rotated into the cranial base. The craniotomy bone and zygomatic arch are secured in position and the skin is closed.

Approach 3: Posterior Fossa

Indications

This approach is used for petrous apex lesions located beneath the tentorium. The most common lesions are

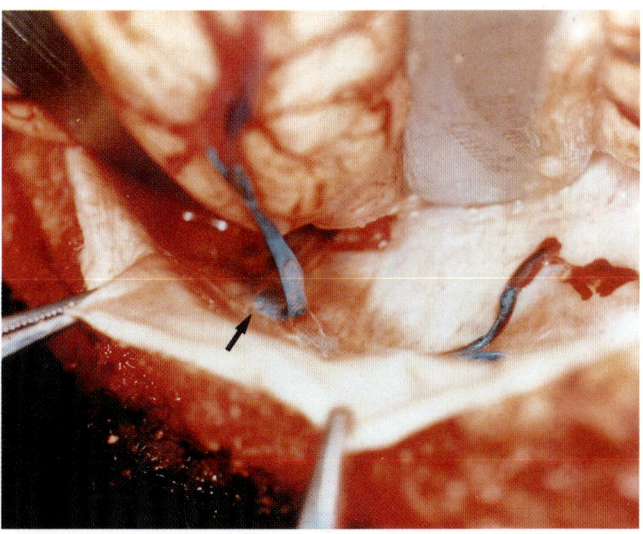

FIG. 12. Approach 2. Anatomical dissection. The temporal lobe is elevated showing middle fossa skull base and Labbés vein entering the superior petrosal sinus.

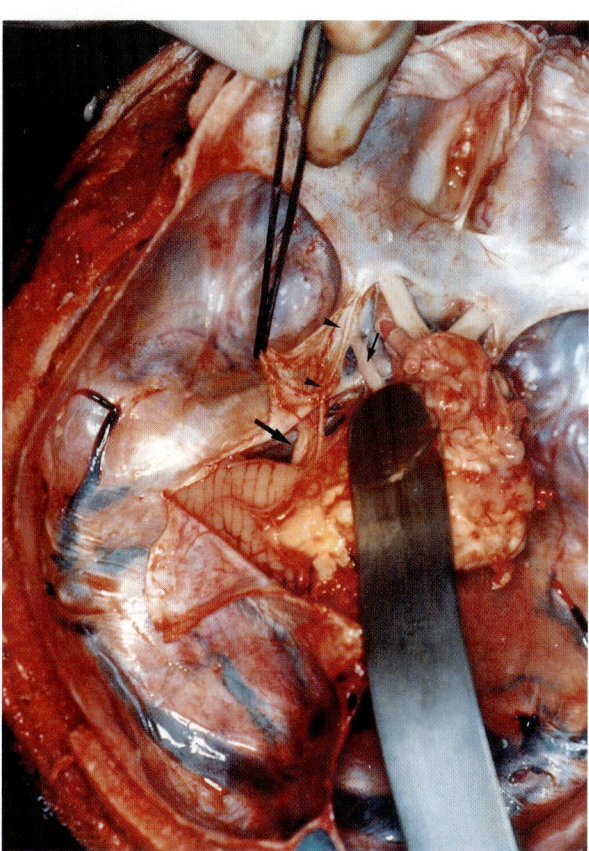

FIG. 13. Approach 2. Anatomical dissection. The tentorium was sectioned. Cranial nerves IV (*arrowhead*), III (*small arrow*), and V (*arrow*) are exposed. Forceps holds tentorium, showing posterior fossa contents.

meningiomas of the cerebellopontine angle, acoustic neurinomas, trigeminal neurinomas, epidermoid cysts, and teratomas (Figs. 14 and 15).

Surgical Techniques

The procedure is performed with the patient under general anesthesia. Two different positions may be used.

1. Semi-sitting position with a 30° contralateral head rotation. It has the advantage of gravitational drainage of blood and spinal fluid, making constant suctioning unnecessary. It has the disadvantage of possible arterial hypotension, air embolism, and discomfort to the surgeon in more prolonged operations. A central venous pressure catheter and Doppler monitoring for detection and treatment of embolization are routinely used. Ventilation with PEEP of 10–15 mm Hg can prevent air embolism.

2. Supine position with 60° degree contralateral head rotation with slight extension. This position is used for older patients or when a middle fossa approach is contemplated. This position is more comfortable for the surgeon and makes air embolism unlikely. The

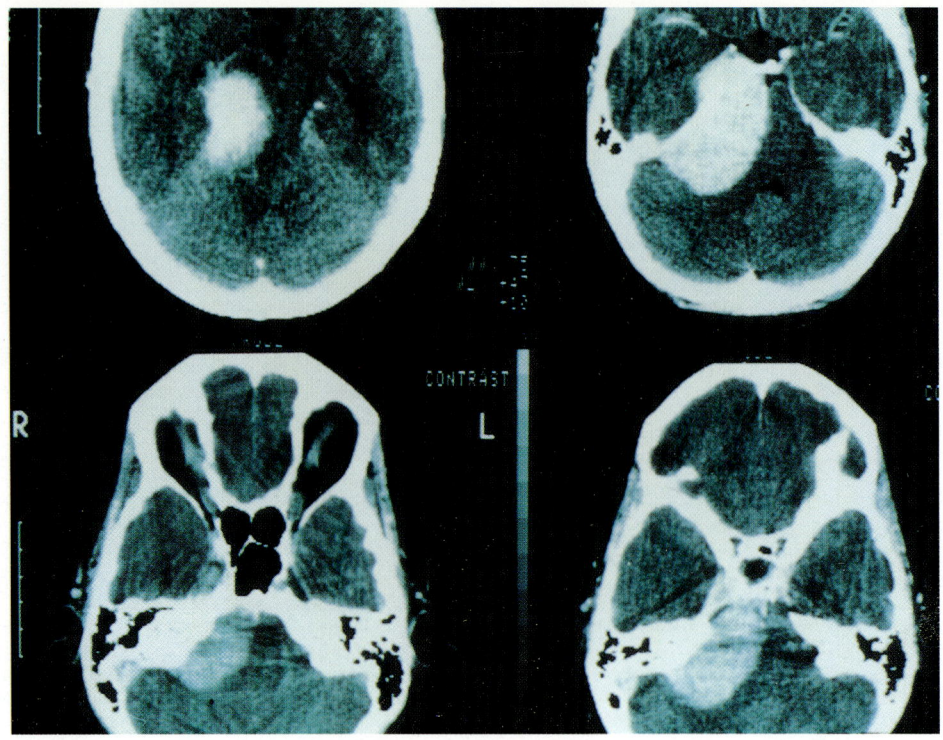

FIG. 14. Approach 3. CT scan of a petroclival meningioma. **Top:** Tumor in middle cranial fossa, tentorial border, and cavernous sinus. **Bottom:** Tumor extension to posterior fossa, displacing the brainstem.

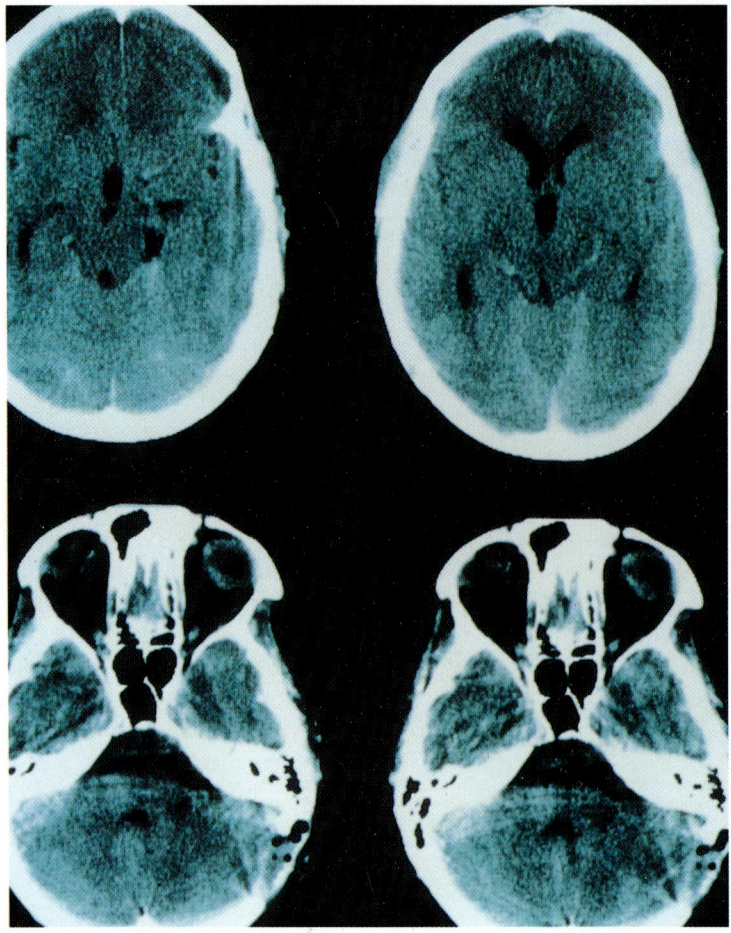

FIG. 15. Approach 3. Postoperative CT scan showing transmastoid, retrosigmoid posterior fossa craniotomy and radical removal of tumor.

disadvantage is the accumulation of blood and cerebrospinal fluid in the operative field, making cranial nerve dissection difficult.

A retroauricular skin incision 5 cm from the external auditory canal is performed.

The occipital artery and the mastoid emissary veins are located and coagulated. A Valsalva maneuver can facilitate location of the emissary veins.

A 4-cm diameter craniectomy is designed. Its superior limit is the lateral sinus and the anterior limit is the border of the sigmoid sinus (inside the mastoid cavity). Opened mastoid cells are occluded with bone wax to prevent spinal fluid fistula. The foramen magnum is opened only if there is a tumor extension within it. Dura mater is incised posteriorly to and parallel to the sigmoid and lateral sinuses. The sigmoid sinus is retracted anteriorly by two sutures placed in the anterior dural flap.

Cerebellar retraction is minimal and careful until the lower cranial nerves, the cerebellopontine angle, and the tentorium are identified.

The tumor is removed by intracapsular dissection to reduce its size and to expose cranial nerves V, VII, and VIII at the brain stem. The posterior wall of the internal auditory canal is drilled away for the removal of acoustic neurinomas (Fig. 16). The vestibular nerves are cut at the crista transversa level and Bill's Bar and facial nerve are identified. The nerve is dissected from the tumor capsule and preserved along with its vascular supply (Fig. 17).

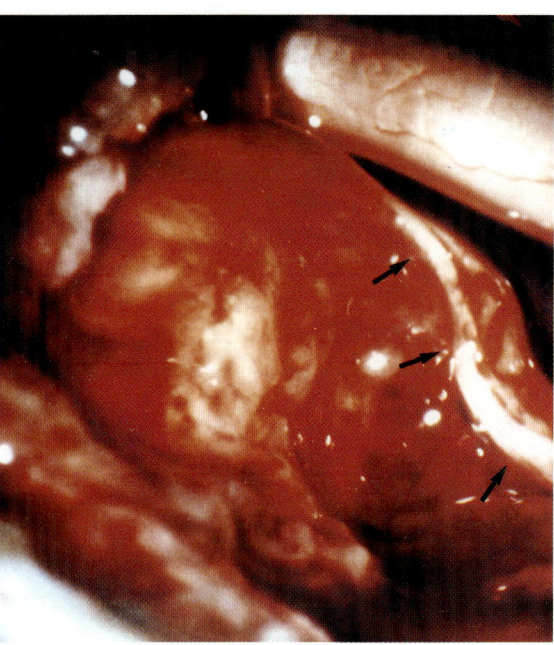

FIG. 17. Approach 3. Partial tumor resection. *Arrow* points to facial nerve dissected from superior tumor pole. Trigeminal nerve is above.

Trigeminal lesions can be repaired using a sural nerve graft.

The tentorium can be opened to combine the middle fossa approach for more extensive lesions.

Tumor removal can expose the prepontine region. Infiltrated dura mater and bone should be removed to avoid residual tumor. After careful hemostasis, the dura mater is closed watertight.

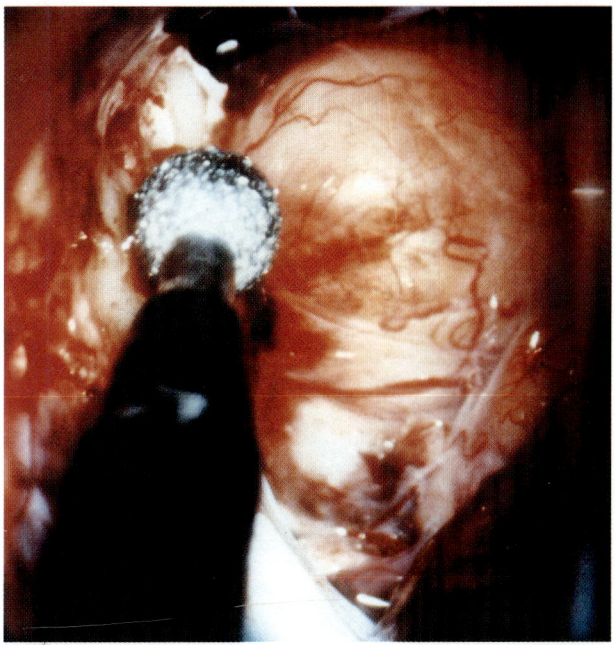

FIG. 16. Approach 3. Surgical picture of an acoustic neurinoma. Diamond burr in position to open the internal auditory canal.

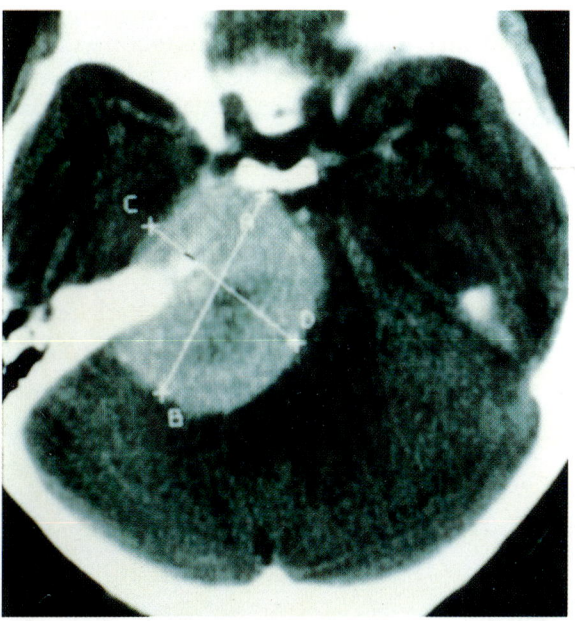

FIG. 18. Approach 4. CT scan of a large petroclival meningioma in middle and posterior fossae, reaching the clivus.

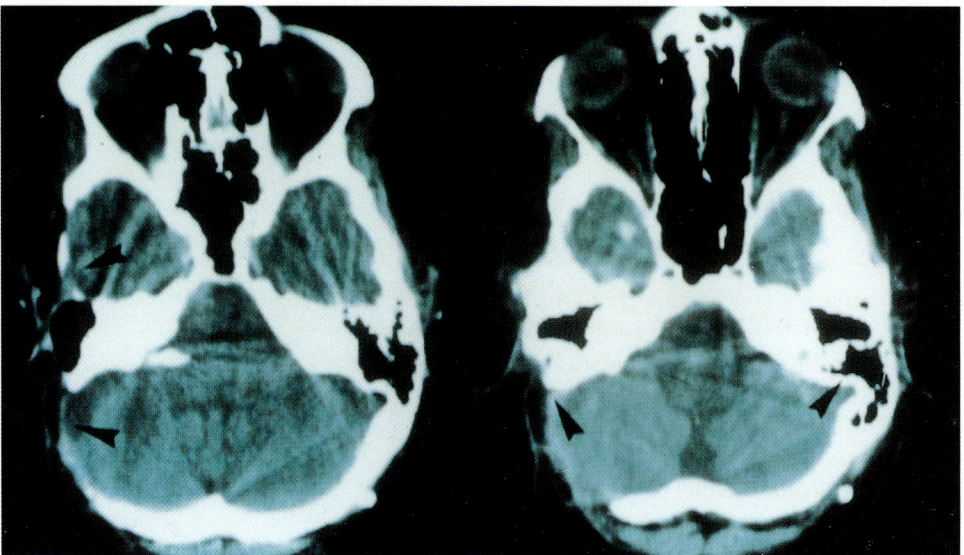

FIG. 19. Approach 4. Postoperative CT scan showing middle and posterior fossa craniotomy combined with a mastoidectomy. Total tumor removal is achieved.

Approach 4: Combined Middle–Posterior Fossa

Indication

Middle cranial fossa tumors with large posterior fossa extension or posterior fossa lesions with supratentorial extension may require a combination of approaches 2 and 3 for their safe removal in one stage, avoiding brain retraction.

The typical example is petroclival meningioma (Figs. 18 and 19).

Surgical Technique

The patient is in the dorsal supine position with contralateral head rotation under general anesthesia.

A basal access to the middle cranial fossa (approach 2) is performed, combined with a transmastoid retrosigmoid approach to the posterior fossa (approach 3) (Fig. 20).

If the lesion is large, the sigmoid sinus is sectioned after ligation and the tentorium is opened (Fig. 21). The temporal lobe is retracted anteriorly and the cerebellum is retracted posteriorly, with wide exposure of the petrous apex region (superior and posterior faces). Brain

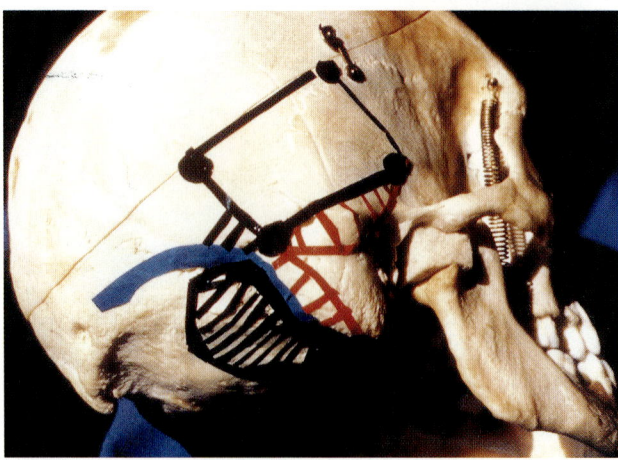

FIG. 20. Approach 4. Temporal craniotomy combined with posterior fossa craniectomy. In *red*, bone removal in the mastoid gives wider basal access.

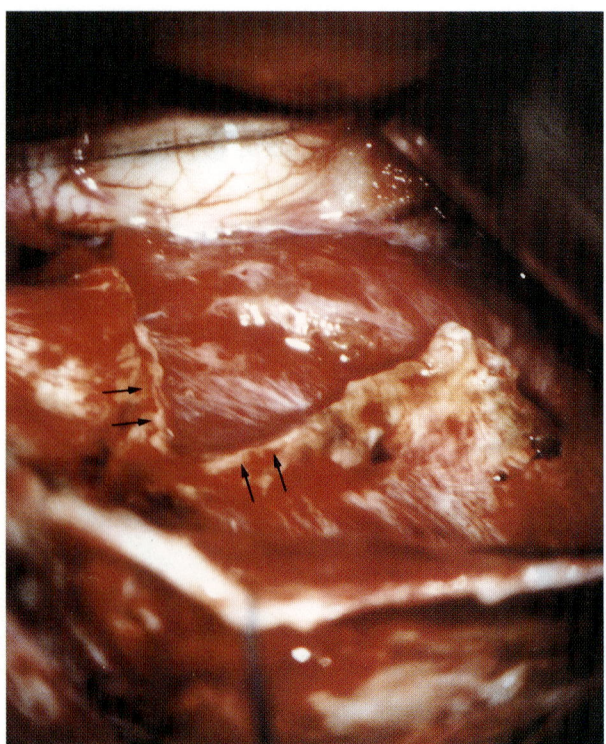

FIG. 21. Approach 4. Operative view of sectioned tentorium (*arrow*). Tumor is exposed at tentorial border.

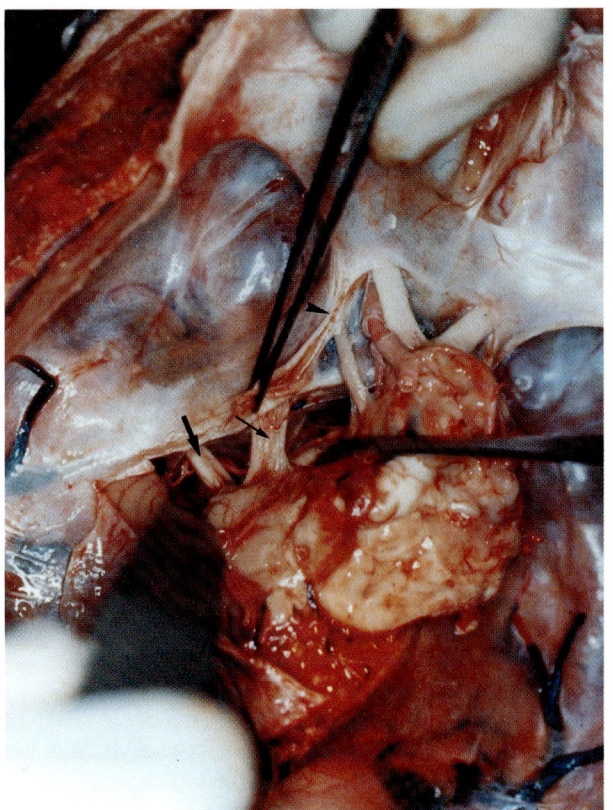

FIG. 22. Approach 4. Anatomical dissection. Tentorium is opened, exposing cranial nerves in posterior fossa and clivus. *Arrowhead* shows cranial nerve IV, *small arrow* shows cranial nerve V, and *arrow* shows cranial nerves VII and VIII.

cranial nerves V, VII, and VIII in the posterior fossa (Fig. 22). Tumors of this region (mostly meningiomas) are supplied by branches of the middle meningeal artery, the tentorial artery (Bernasconi–Cassinari), and branches from the meningohypophyseal trunk from the intracavernous internal carotid artery. We prefer to devascularize the tumor before its removal, trying to coagulate those vessels near the skull base and tentorium dura mater.

Tumor removal is initially intracapsular, reducing its size, and afterward the capsule is removed. Some tumors may produce an indentation in the brain stem with firm adhesions and shared vascular supply. Removal, even with microsurgical techniques and high magnification, may result in damage to the brain stem.

Cranial nerves VII and VIII are usually displaced and should be dissected from the tumor capsule and preserved.

Infiltrated dura mater should be removed and compromised bone can be drilled out. All pneumatized bone opened by surgery should be occluded by bone wax and temporal muscle graft.

Dura mater is closed watertight with nonabsorbable sutures.

Approach 5: Occipito–Transmastoid–Cervical

Indications

This approach is used for removal of tumors in the jugular foramen region with extension to the cervical and petrous apex region. Paragangliomas, neurinomas, and meningiomas are the most frequent lesions (Figs. 23 and 24).

retraction should be minimal and gentle with preservation of Labbé's vein to avoid temporal lobe edema. After identification of cranial nerves V, VII, and VIII, the petrous tip can be removed. Reference landmarks are cranial nerves III and IV in the free edge of tentorium and

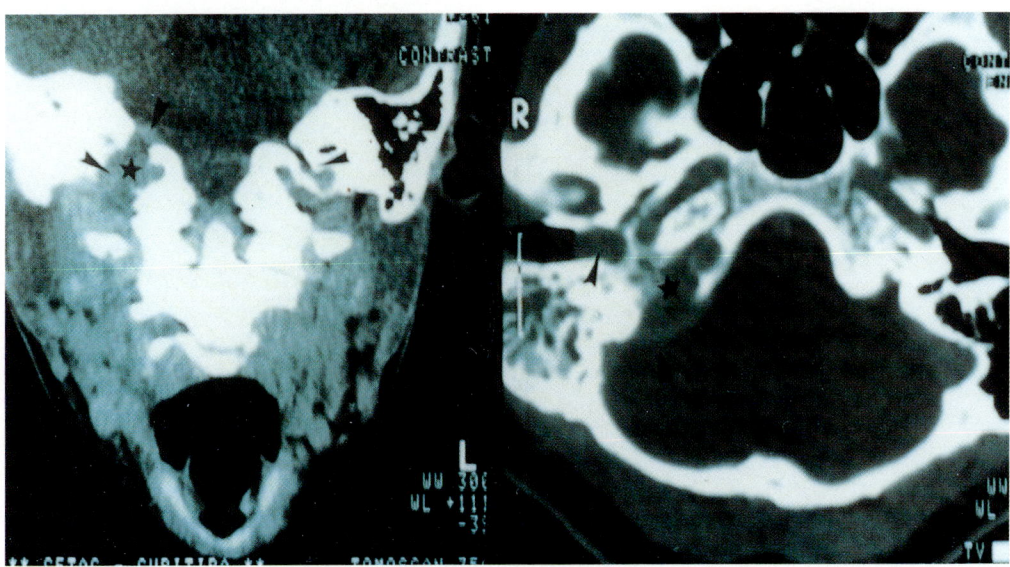

FIG. 23. Approach 5. Preoperative coronal CT scan shows tumor in jugular foramen (*star*). Axial CT scan view of tumor (*arrowheads*) in middle ear and posterior cranial fossa and in jugular foramen (*star*).

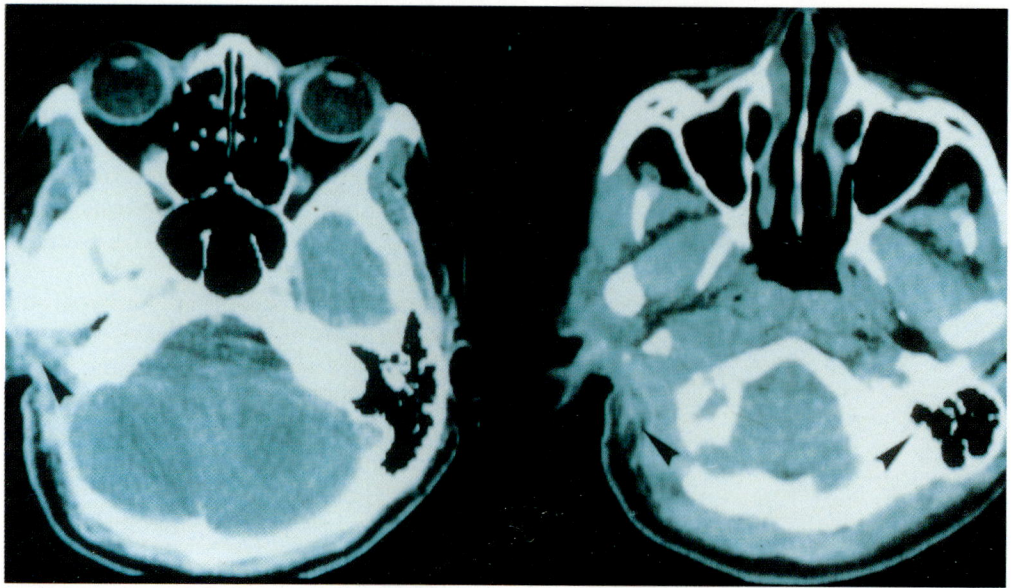

FIG. 24. Approach 5. Postoperative CT scan shows site of craniotomy and posterolateral access to jugular foramen (*arrowhead*).

Surgical Techniques

All patients are operated on under general anesthesia with endotracheal intubation. We had no need for tracheostomy in any of our patients. If intraoperative cranial nerve monitoring is planned, the use of muscle relaxants should be kept to a minimum. The patient is placed in the supine position, with the head turned away from the site of the lesion. The patient's hair is shaved in the retromastoid region.

The incision begins in the temporal region, circumscribes the outer ear, with a large scalp around the ear behind the mastoid tip (Fig. 25). It follows inferiorly the first cervical skin fold to the cricoid cartilage. We do not recommend the Y-shaped incision because it may produce ischemia of the inferior portion of the ear.

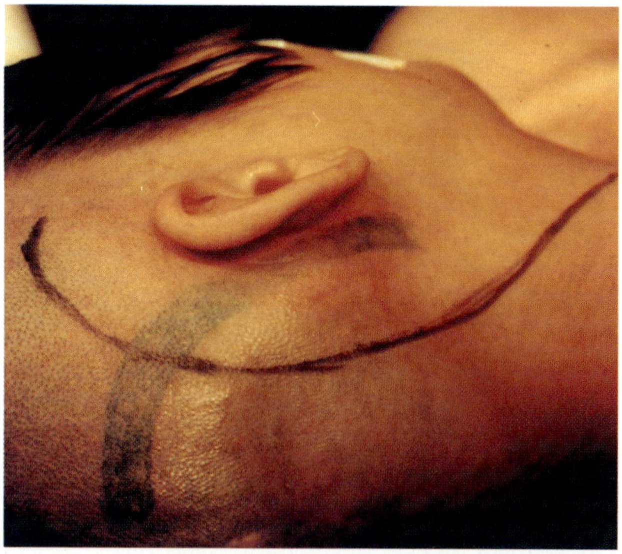

The flap is folded anteriorly. In the temporal region, a temporalis muscle flap is developed. It will be used at the end of the procedure to cover the opening of the dura mater. The next step is the identification of the greater auricular nerve. It should be dissected and, if necessary, used as graft for the reconstruction of the facial nerve (Fig. 26). The external auditory canal is severed at the

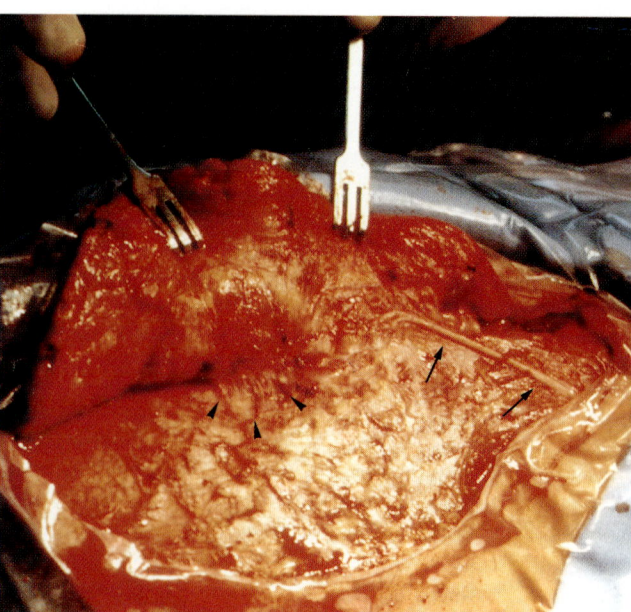

FIG. 26. Approach 5. Operative picture of anterior skin flap turned anteriorly. External auditory canal (*arrowheads*). Great auricular nerve crosses the sternocleidomastoid muscle (*arrow*).

FIG. 25. Approach 5. Skin incision for tumor in the jugular foramen region.

osteocartilaginous junction and closed with absorbable sutures. Usually, a small posterior auricular muscle flap is made to cover this suture line in order to avoid a postoperative CSF fistula. A neck dissection is the next step. The posterior edge of platysma is identified.

The anterior border of the sternocleidomastoid muscle and the posterior edge of the parotid gland are exposed and dissected. The sternocleidomastoid muscle is retracted posteriorly, exposing the upper cervical region. The internal jugular vein is identified and tagged with vessel loops. The common facial vein is ligated. Other small veins are coagulated with bipolar cautery. The common carotid artery is identified and followed to its bifurcation. Temporary ligation of the external carotid artery and its branches will reduce the vascular supply to the lesion. The branches of the external carotid artery are exposed and ligated. It is important in cases of glomus jugulare tumors to ligate the ascending pharyngeal and occipital arteries.

The next step is the identification of the cranial nerves in the cervical region. The hypoglossal nerve is exposed after identification of the digastric muscle. It courses below this muscle and crosses the external carotid artery. The hansa hypoglossi is exposed. The vagal nerve is dissected inferomedially to the common carotid artery. The accessory nerve is identified superolaterally below the sternocleidomastoid muscle (Fig. 27).

After exposing these structures, we identify the facial nerve in the stylomastoid foramen region. The key landmarks to identify this nerve are the digastric muscle, the "pointer," and the tympanomastoid suture line. The posterior border of the parotid gland is carefully retracted. The digastric muscle is followed upward to its insertion in the mastoid; the facial nerve courses medial to this muscle. The "pointer" is palpated and the stylomastoid suture is identified. The facial nerve is now dissected toward the stylomastoid foramen.

The mastoidectomy is carried out. The facial canal is identified. Contrary to other surgeons, we do not usually remove the facial nerve from its canal, if there is no sign of infiltration of the nerve. Enough space is provided for tumor removal, if a craniectomy and a canalplasty are performed. The sinus plate is identified. Very often the mastoid cells are infiltrated by tumor. The posterior fossa and the middle fossa dura mater are exposed. After removal of the ossicular chain, the internal carotid artery can be exposed medial to the eustachian tube and tympanic bone. Usually in cases of glomus jugulare tumors, bleeding from caroticotympanic vessels occurs and is controlled by packing the outer ear for a few minutes.

The next step is a retrosigmoid craniectomy. This craniectomy is about 4 cm in diameter, exposing the sigmoid sinus and the posterior fossa dura mater anteriorly to the sinus. Bone removal over the sigmoid sinus is carried out with a rongeur. Usually, the sinus wall is very thin, and bleeding can occur. The sites of sinus wall ruptures are occluded by light pressure of a gelfoam pack. The sigmoid sinus is ligated below the superior petrosal sinus. If necessary (depending on tumor extention), the foramen magnum is opened and the arch of C1 removed. The vertebral artery should be carefully dissected from the tumor in the C1/occipital condyle region. If this vessel is infiltrated by the lesion (determined by preoperative angiography) and the cross flow from the other vertebral artery is not good, a balloon occlusion test should be performed and a reconstruction of the vessel should be planned. In the majority of cases, however, the vessel can be dissected from the tumor.

This approach (mastoidectomy, craniectomy, and canalplasty) allows a very good exposure of the jugular foramen, petrous apex region, and internal carotid artery. The lateral wall of the jugular foramen is removed with a Kerrison punch. With this approach, the jugular foramen is more posterior, with the facial nerve in its canal and far from surgical manipulation.

The next step is the ligature of the internal jugular vein in the neck. In two-thirds of cases the internal jugular vein runs medial to cranial nerve XI. After its ligature, the accessory nerve is dissected from the vein wall, which is pulled back, leaving cranial nerve XI anterior to it. The outer wall of the sigmoid sinus is opened, exposing the tumor in this region. The jugular bulb with the tumor is now removed (Fig. 28). Total removal of this portion of the lesion is achieved. Bleeding from the inferior petrosal sinus usually occurs. The sinus is just inferior and anterior to the jugular bulb and is packed with a piece of gelfoam. The surgical microscope is used to ex-

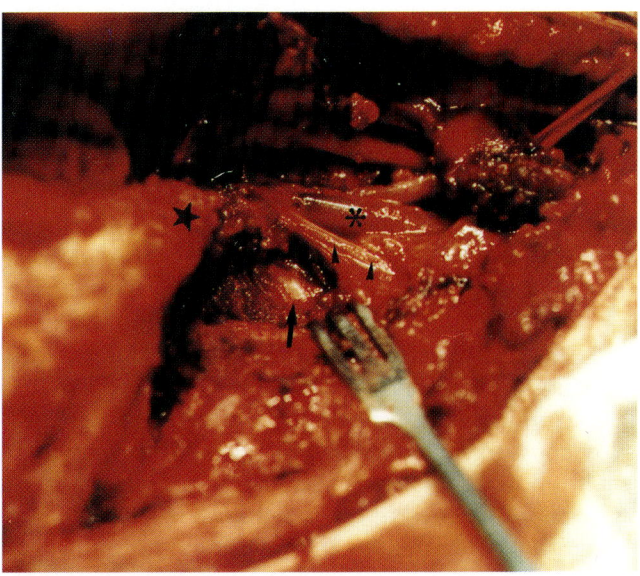

FIG. 27. Approach 5. Operative view of upper cervical dissection. Rake retracts splenius capitis muscle, showing vertebral artery (*arrow*), mastoid tip (*star*), cranial nerve XI (*arrowhead*), and internal jugular vein (*star*) with tumor inside.

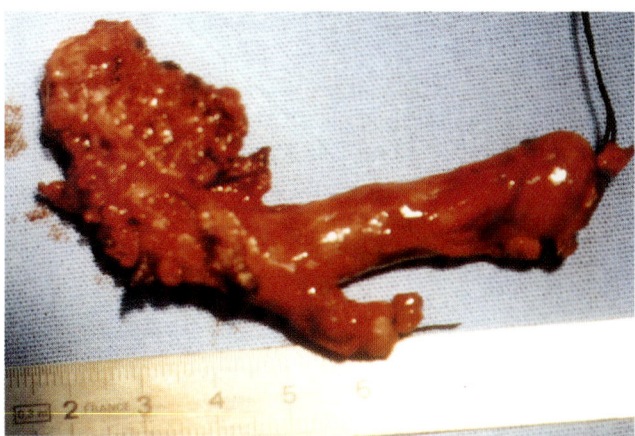

FIG. 28. Approach 5. Surgical specimen shows a ligated fenestrated internal jugular vein with tumor inside. On the left, the remaining extravascular portion of tumor removed from the jugular foramen.

pose the cranial nerves and be sure that no tumor was left behind.

The dura mater is opened in the medial wall of the ligated sigmoid sinus. This allows a good inspection of the intradural region with minimal retraction of the cerebellum (Fig. 29). The lesion usually penetrates the dura through the jugular foramen. This portion of the tumor usually covers cranial nerves IX, X, and XI. After identification of cranial nerves VII and VIII and the PICA and AICA, the bulbar cranial nerves are identified at the brain stem. These nerves are followed to the jugular foramen. In this way, a total removal of the lesion can be accomplished with bipolar coagulation and piecemeal removal. Very often, nerve fascicles are infiltrated by the lesion and must be sacrificed to assure total removal of the lesion. The connection between the intradural and extradural portions of the jugular foramen is clearly seen to be sure that no tumor is left behind. If the tumor involves the brain stem, it is initially debulked with bipolar and microsurgical techniques. This portion of the tumor is usually very adherent to the brain stem, which may share circulation with the tumor. If the facial nerve is involved intradurally, opening of the internal auditory canal is recommended. The nerve is identified within the canal and followed to the brainstem after piecemeal tumor removal.

If the lesion reaches the prepontine region and the inferior clivus, we prefer to remove a portion of the occipital condyle to approach it. In these cases, the basilar artery can be involved in the lesion.

After total tumor removal is carried out, nerve reconstruction is performed if necessary using as graft the greater auricular nerve or the sural nerve. The dura mater is closed in watertight fashion. The temporalis–periosteum flap is sutured over the dura suture. The eustachian tube and the jugular foramen are closed with a piece of muscle (digastric) to avoid CSF fistula. The temporal muscle is incised in "Z" fashion and sutured to the sternocleidomastoid muscle. A very satisfactory cosmetic result is obtained in this way, avoiding the use of abdominal fat.

The patient is extubated only after being responsive, to avoid aspiration. If needed a tarsorrhaphy may be done.

DISCUSSION

Tumors at the petrous apex region present special surgical problems and because of their deep-seated location permit no easy access (Table 1). The cranial nerves, the basilar artery and its branches, and the internal carotid artery are displaced by, adherent to, or embedded in the lesion. The brain stem may be involved. Tumor may invade the mastoid, middle ear, and cavernous sinus. These factors are the reason for subtotal removal and high surgical mortality. The development of microsurgical techniques and the cooperative work of otologists and neurosurgeons achieved significant improvement in total tumor resection and in avoiding complications. In this chapter we present our experience in the treatment of this kind of lesion using multidisciplinary approaches. Retraction of the brain is an important factor for a poor result. Removal of bone at the skull base permits better exposure and reduces the need for brain retraction. Identification of the internal carotid artery and the facial nerve in the petrous bone is mandatory for total removal

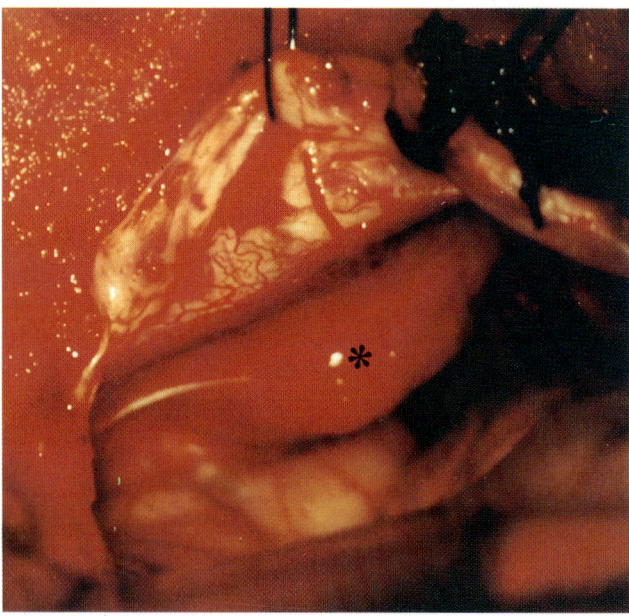

FIG. 29. Approach 5. Operative view of tumor (*star*) in jugular foramen, seen through a posterior fossa craniotomy. Vascularized dura mater is reflected by suture. Tumor appears as red mass.

TABLE 1. *Types of petrous apex lesions*

Acoustic neurinomas	16
Paragangliomas	14
Meningiomas	7
Cholesteatomas	4
Trigeminal neurinoma	3
Facial nerve neurinoma	3
Facial nerve trauma	3
CSF fistula (trauma)	1
Jugular foramen neurinoma	2
Teratoma	1
Pituitary adenoma (recurrence)	1
Total	55[a]

[a] During the period from January 1987 to September 1989, 55 patients with petrous apex lesions were operated on by the Curitiba Skull Base Group. Other lesions treated or isolated by neurosurgeons or otologists are not included in this series.

of large lesions and nerve reconstruction. Injury to Labbé's vein and other venous sinuses produces temporal lobe hemorrhage and edema. Preservation of the venous structures is therefore important. The risks of cerebrospinal fluid leak and meningitis associated with the surgical defect are reduced by planning muscle-fascia flaps and occluding the open pneumatized cells. Our surgical mortality was two patients. One 67-year-old woman died 6 weeks after uneventful removal of a very large paraganglioma of the jugular foramen due to pulmonary embolism. Another patient died because of myocardial infarction. She was a 64-year-old woman, who underwent an uneventful resection of a huge trigeminal neurinoma. Seven days later she died suddenly. After the operation she presented only trigeminal nerve paralysis.

Complications related to surgery included trigeminal nerve paralysis in two patients (trigeminal nerve neurinomas) and facial nerve paralysis requiring reconstruction in five patients (two jugular foramen paragangliomas and three acoustic neurinomas). In all cases, some function of facial nerve returned. One patient presented hydrocephalus requiring shunt and one patient developed meningitis after CSF leak but was treated successfully with antibiotics.

In our opinion, benign lesions at the petrous apex can be removed by a multidisciplinary approach with low mortality and morbidity.

FURTHER READINGS

Al-Mefty O, Fox JL, Smith RR. Petrosal approach for petroclival meningiomas. *Neurosurgery* 1988;22:510–517.

Brackmann DE, Hitselberger WE, Beneke JE, House WF. Acoustic neuromas: middle fossa and translabyrinthine removal. In: Rand RW, ed. *Micro neurosurgery*. St. Louis: Mosby, 1985;311–334.

Glasscock ME, Harris PF, Newsome G. Glomus tumors: diagnosis and treatment. *Laryngoscope* 1974;84:2006–2032.

Fisch U, Pillsbury HC. Infratemporal fossa approach to lesions in the temporal bone and base of the skull. *Arch Otolaryngol* 1979;105:99–107.

Rand RW, Kurze T. Micro neurosurgical resection of acoustic tumors by a transmeatal posterior fossa approach. *Bull Los Angeles Neurol Soc* 1965;30:17–20.

Sakaki S, Takeda S, Fujita H, Otita S. An extended middle fossa approach combined with a suboccipital craniectomy to the base of the skull in the posterior fossa. *Surg Neurol* 1987;28:245–252.

Samii M. Micro surgery of acoustic neurinomas with special emphasis on preservation of seventh and eighth cranial nerves and the scope of facial nerve grafting. In: Rand RW, ed. *Micro neurosurgery*. St. Louis: Mosby, 1985.

Sekhar LN, Estonillo R. Transtemporal approach to the skull base: an anatomical study. *Neurosurgery* 1986;19:799–808.

Sekhar LN, Jannetta PJ, Maroon JC. Tentorial meningiomas: surgical management and results. *Neurosurgery* 1984;14:268–275.

Yasargil MG, Mortara RW, Curcic M. Meningiomas of basal posterior cranial fosa. In: Krayen BH, ed. *Advances and technical standards in Neurosurgery* vol 7. Wien: Springer Verlag, 1980;1–115.

CHAPTER 20

Petrosal Approach to Clival Tumors

Ossama Al-Mefty

Tumors of the clival and petroclival area remain a formidable challenge. The number and diversity of approaches targeting this area testify to that challenge. This chapter presents the petrosal approach as has been refined and used by the author for intradural tumors located in the clival and petroclival areas. This approach is centered on the petrous ridge, analogous to the pterional approach, which is centered on the sphenoid ridge. It allows access to tumors extending from the suprasellar area and the cavernous sinus to as caudal as the foramen magnum. It provides the following advantages: (a) the cerebellum and temporal lobes are minimally retracted; (b) the operative distance to the clivus is shortened by 3 cm; (c) the surgeon has a direct line of sight to the lesion and the anterior and lateral aspects of the brain stem; (d) the neural and otologic structures, including the cochlea, labyrinth, and facial nerves, are preserved; (e) the transverse and sigmoid sinuses, as well as Labbé's vein and the basal and occipital veins are preserved; (f) the tumor's vascular supply is intercepted early in the procedure as the petrous bone is being drilled; and (g) multiple axes for dissection are provided. A detailed evolution of this approach is described elsewhere (1).

This approach stems from the Fraenkel and Hunt description in 1904 of a suboccipital–translabyrinthine approach (5). In 1939, Bailey described a combined supratentorial–infratentorial approach (4), incorporating incision of the tentorium and ligation of the sigmoid sinus. Morrison and King used a combined subtemporal and translabyrinthine approach for an acoustic tumor (9), while Hakuba et al. preserved the labyrinth and used this approach in removing a clival meningioma (6).

SPECIFIC DIAGNOSTIC CONSIDERATIONS

Detailed radiological studies are crucial for surgical planning. Contrast enhanced CT scans and MRI, in coronal, sagittal, and axial views, are obtained preoperatively for complete definition of the tumor: its location, extension, relation to the brain stem, encasement of cerebral vessels, and involvement of the cavernous sinus and the temporal bone. Angiography remains a necessary preoperative diagnostic study to identify a vascular lesion, to demonstrate cerebral vascular anatomy and displacement, to outline the tumor's blood supply, and to confirm patency and the connection between the two transverse sinuses. MRI angiography may soon replace conventional angiography in this role. An audiogram and baseline auditory and somatosensory evoked potentials are obtained preoperatively. In cases of cavernous sinus involvement, adequate cerebral collateral circulation is assessed through a carotid occlusion test with transcranial Doppler and SPECT scan studies.

PATIENT SELECTION

The petrosal approach is used for patients harboring intradural tumors located at the clivus or in the petroclival area, or tumors that extend into both the middle and posterior fossae. This approach is ideal for meningiomas of the clivus and the petrous apex with origins medial to the fifth nerve, fifth nerve schwannomas, giant acoustic tumors, and dermoid and epidermoid tumors (3). Since these lesions are benign, the objective of treatment is total resection, which is best achieved during the first operation when arachnoidal membranes are intact, facilitating dissection of neurovascular structures and resection of the tumor. Although surgeons should pursue total removal with skill and zeal, their judgment should not be skewed from the goal of preserving or improving neurologic function. This may, at times, require them to accept subtotal removal (10).

Since these tumors are slow growing and may be discovered accidentally on neuroradiological tests, a watchful waiting is justified in elderly patients who are asymptomatic, until evidence of brain stem compression is

---

O. Al-Mefty: Division of Neurological Surgery, Loyola University Medical Center, Maywood, Illinois 60153

evident. Stereotaxic radiosurgery has recently become an alternative treatment for small or residual tumors (13). The effectiveness and long-term results of this modality, however, await further reports.

OPERATIVE TECHNIQUE

Anesthesia and Monitoring

A flawless administration of anesthesia is crucial in the successful removal of clival tumors. The choice of anesthetic agents should be flexible and tailored to suit the circumstances of each case. Averting intracranial hypertension and maintaining adequate cerebral perfusion are mandates of anesthesia. The use of intraoperative monitoring for cranial nerve and brain stem evoked potentials necessitates the use of certain anesthetic agents or switching intraoperatively from one to another. Normotension is the goal, and hypotension should be avoided. Should temporary vascular occlusion be necessary during surgical resection of the tumor, a barbiturate is given for its known cerebral protective effect.

Electrophysiological monitoring is obtained by bilaterally recording brain stem auditory evoked potentials and median nerve somatosensory evoked potentials. Facial nerve function and localization are monitored by recording an EMG from several groups of facial muscles on the ipsilateral side. Other cranial nerves are similarly monitored as necessary.

Patient Position

The patient is placed supine with the head at the foot-end of the operating table, allowing space and ease of movement for the seated surgeon. The table is flexed to allow 20°–30° elevation of the head and trunk. The patient's ipsilateral shoulder is slightly elevated. The head is turned away from the side of the tumor, inclined toward the floor, and tilted toward the opposite side. The neck position is inspected to avoid compression of the contralateral jugular vein. The head is fixed in a three-point Mayfield head rest. During surgery, the surgeon's line of sight can be altered by rotating the table from side to side or up and down (Fig. 1).

Operative Procedure

Craniotomy Flap

A reverse question-mark incision is made starting at the zygoma in front of the ear, circling above the ear, and descending 1 cm medial to (behind) the mastoid process (Fig. 1). The skin flap is elevated and retracted anteriorly and inferiorly. A large triangular pericranial flap with an

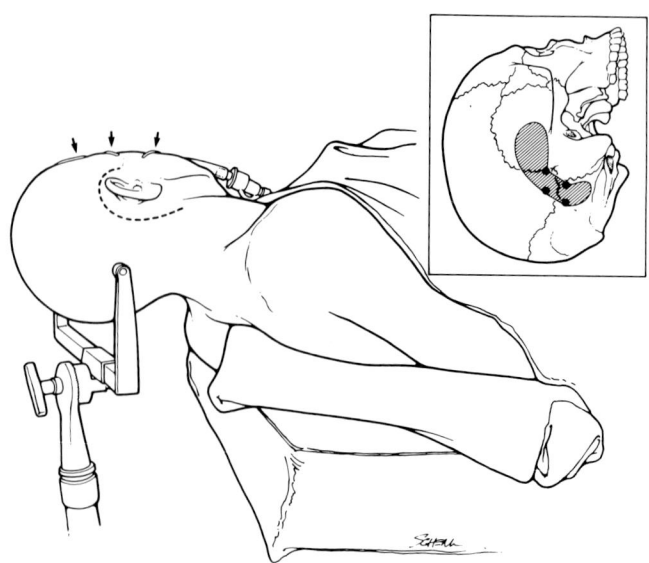

FIG. 1. Artist's illustration of patient's position and the skin incision for a right-sided petrosal approach. EMG needle electrodes (*arrows*) are inserted in muscle groups innervated by the facial nerve. **Inset:** Skull model depicting position of the burr holes and outlining the bone flap. (From ref. 16, with permission.)

intact vascular base is elevated and retracted over the skin flap to the level of the external ear canal. This flap is used to cover the drilled surface of the temporal bone at the time of closure. The temporal muscle then is retracted anteriorly while the sternomastoid insertion is detached and retracted posteriorly and inferiorly. The bony surface of the temporal fossa, mastoid, and lateral posterior fossa are thus exposed.

Four burr holes are made, two on each side of the transverse sinus. A hole made just medial and inferior to the asterion opens into the posterior fossa below the transverse sigmoid sinus junction, while a hole located at the squamal and mastoid junction of the temporal bone, along the projection of the superior temporal line, opens into the supratentorial compartment (Figs. 1 and 2). The burr hole at each of these points will exactly flank the sigmoid sinus. The temporal bone and a portion of the occipital bone above the tentorium, as well as the occipital bone below the tentorium, are incised between burr holes using the foot attachment of the Midas Rex drill (Midas Rex, Fort Worth, TX). The foot attachment is not used to cross over the sinus. The burr holes flanking the lateral sinus are then connected using a thin rongeur or are drilled with the B-1 attachment of the Midas Rex drill. Particular attention should be paid to avoid tearing the wall of the venous sinus, which domes into a bony impression on the inner surface of the skull.

The single bone flap is elevated, exposing the transverse and sigmoid sinuses. The bone adheres tightly to the dura at the junction of the sigmoid and transverse sinuses and requires careful dissection and elevation. An alternative to this method of skull-bone removal is to perform a temporal craniotomy, followed by a posterior fossa craniectomy extending over the transverse sinus.

Temporal Bone Drilling

A thorough knowledge of the anatomy of the petrous bone and surrounding structures is required to perform drilling of the temporal bone. The surgeon performs a complete mastoidectomy using a high-speed air drill. A diamond bit should be used when drilling is close to vital anatomical structures. The sigmoid sinus is skeletonized down to the jugular bulb. The sinodural angle, Citelli's angle, which identifies the position of the superior petrosal sinus, is exposed. The superficial mastoid air cells behind the posterior wall of the external ear canal, as well as the deep (retrofacial) air cells, are resected to identify the facial canal and the lateral and posterior semicircular canals. Drilling is continued along the pyramid to thin the petrous bone toward its apex. The facial canal as well as the middle and inner ear structures are kept intact, while opened air cells are obliterated with bone wax (Figs. 2 and 3).

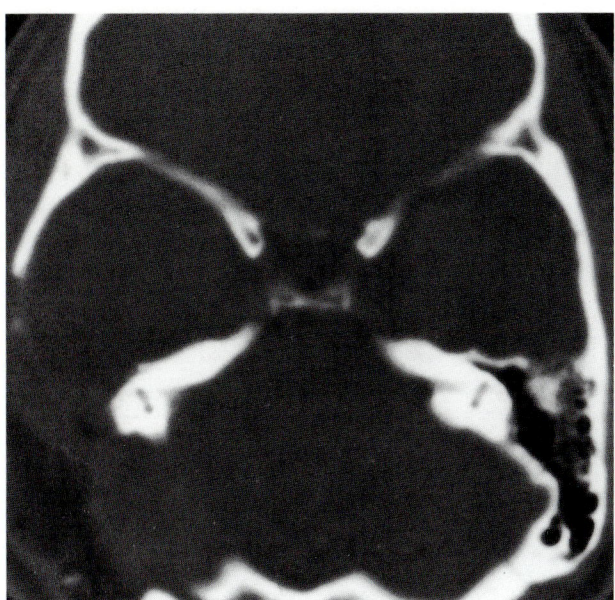

FIG. 3. Postoperative CT scan demonstrating the extent of temporal bone drilling with preservation of inner ear structures.

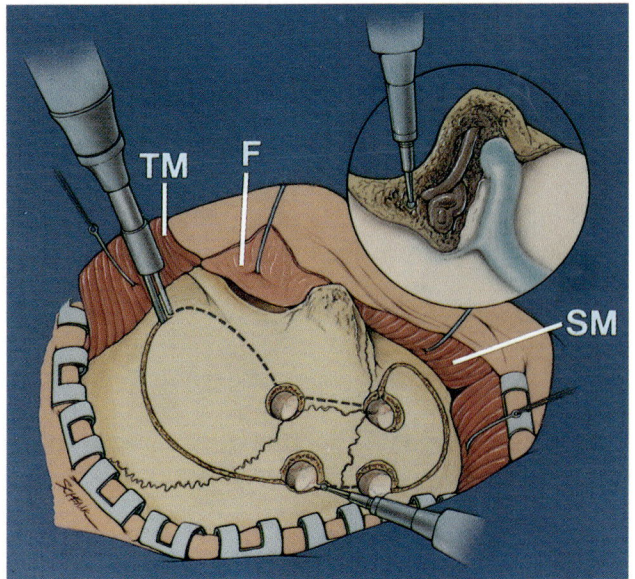

FIG. 2. Artist's illustration (right side) of the surgeon's view. The temporal muscle (TM) and sternomastoid muscle (SM) are elevated and retracted. A pericranial triangular flap (F) is elevated and saved for later covering of the drilled surface of the temporal bone. The position of the burr holes flanking the transverse sigmoid sinus is outlined. A craniotome with foot attachment is used to make the bony cut in the temporal and posterior fossae, while a drill is used to cross over the sinus. **Inset:** The bone flap has been removed, the dura of the temporal and posterior fossae are exposed, the right sigmoid sinus (SS) is skeletonized, and the petrous bone has been extensively drilled. The anatomical landmarks in the temporal bone (the facial canal and the semicircular canals) are demonstrated. (From ref. 16, with permission.)

Dural Opening, Sectioning of the Tentorium, and Tumor Exposure

The posterior fossa dura anterior to the sigmoid sinus is opened along the anterior margin of the sinus. The incision is then extended upward toward a supratentorial dural incision made on the floor of the temporal fossa. The temporal lobe is gently retracted. Labbé's vein is preserved by dissection from the cortical surface, allowing retraction of the temporal lobe without tension on the venous wall (Figs. 4 and 5). The superior petrosal sinus is clipped or coagulated and transected (Fig. 4A), and the incision is continued on the tentorium, parallel to the pyramid, and extended through the incisura. During this maneuver, the surgeon must make every effort to preserve the trochlear nerve by keeping the incision of the tentorial notch behind the area where the fourth nerve pierces the notch (Fig. 5 inset). Opening the tentorium allows excellent exposure of the upper pole of the tumor and the anterior and lateral aspects of the brain stem (Figs. 5 and 6). Trigeminal nerve rootlets, frequently stretched and separated by the tumor, are found under the tentorium (Fig. 7). The retractor is then placed anteriorly, holding medially the sigmoid sinus, the cerebellum, and the cut edge of the tentorium (Fig. 5).

Tumor Resection

Further relaxation is obtained by opening the arachnoid of the cerebellomedullary cistern and draining cerebrospinal fluid (CSF). The tumor is further devascular-

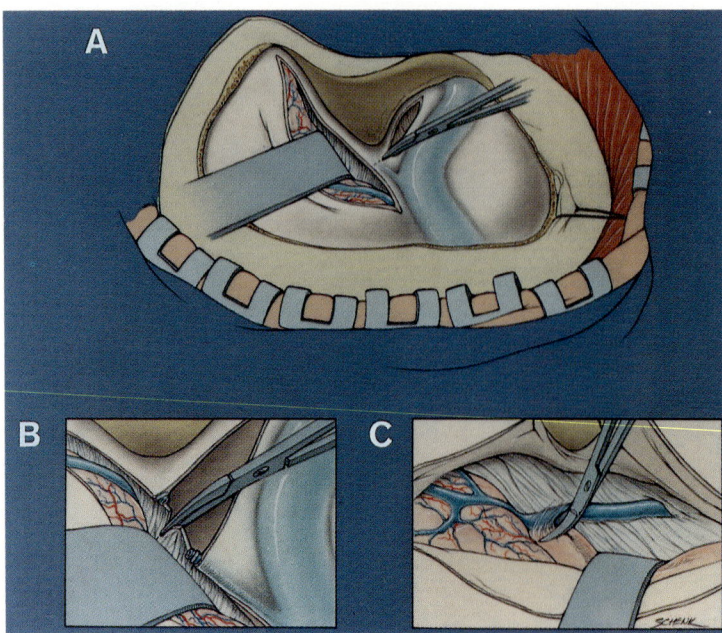

FIG. 4. A: Artist's illustration (right side) of the surgeon's view, demonstrating the initial exposure via a presigmoid (retrolabyrinthine) avenue. The temporal dura is incised along the floor of the temporal fossa. The posterior fossa dura anterior to the sigmoid sinus is incised toward the superior petrosal sinus. The sectioning of the petrosal sinus and the dissection of Labbé's vein are magnified in insets B and C. **B:** Clipping and sectioning of the superior petrosal sinus and the beginning of the tentorial incision. **C:** Dissection of Labbé's vein in order to retract the temporal lobe and preserve the vein. (From ref. 16, with permission.)

ized by coagulating its insertion on the pyramid and the meningeal feeders over the tentorium. When the tumor is small or moderate in size, the seventh and eighth cranial nerves are usually stretched posteriorly and thus are easily identified. When the tumor reaches a large size, however, these cranial nerves may well be engulfed in the tumor.

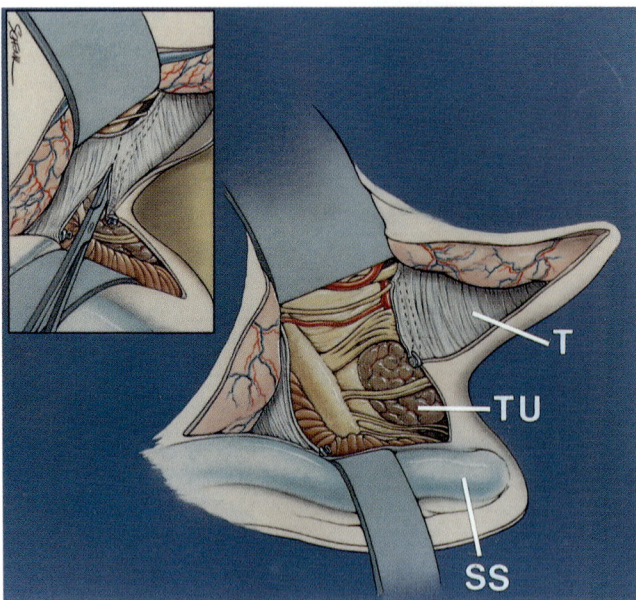

FIG. 5. Artist's illustration (right side) of the surgeon's view, demonstrating exposure of the tumor via a presigmoid sinus avenue. The sigmoid sinus (SS) and cerebellum are retracted medially while the temporal lobe is retracted superiorly. The tentorium (T) is incised along the pyramid through the incisura. The brain stem, cranial nerves, and tumor (Tu) are visualized. **Inset:** Demonstration of tentorial sectioning along the pyramid toward the incisura. (From ref. 16, with permission.)

A suitable area on the tumor surface is selected and the arachnoid over the tumor is opened. The tumor is then debulked with extreme caution since the posterior inferior cerebellar artery (PICA) and anterior inferior cerebellar artery (AICA), or the cranial nerves, may be embedded in the tumor. Debulking is performed using suction, laser, Cavitron ultrasonic surgical aspirator (CUSA; Cooper Medical Devices, Mountain View, CA), and/or bipolar coagulation and microscissors.

The tumor capsule is then dissected free from the surrounding structures. Maintaining dissection within the arachnoidal planes is crucial to preservation of the vital neural and vascular structures. Cranial nerves and the basilar artery and its branches may, however, be embedded in a large tumor, demanding meticulous and tedious dissection. A cut edge of the tumor should not be allowed to slip away lest the plane of cleavage be lost. Further hollowing of the tumor may be necessary before dissection of the thinned-out capsule can be continued.

The lower cranial nerves are dissected off the inferior pole of the tumor. Gentle dissection is required to avoid hypotension and bradycardia from vagal stimulation. The seventh and eighth cranial nerves are carefully dissected from the tumor. Stimulation and EMG recordings assist in localizing the facial nerve. The sixth nerve, stretched anteriorly and inferiorly, is dissected free from the tumor and followed distally (Fig. 6). Alternating the visual field between the supratentorial and infratentorial routes allows the tumor capsule to be dissected carefully from the brain stem. If it is not embedded in the tumor, the basilar artery is usually displaced to the opposite side (Fig. 8). The preservation and careful dissection of the main and small branches of the basilar artery cannot be overemphasized.

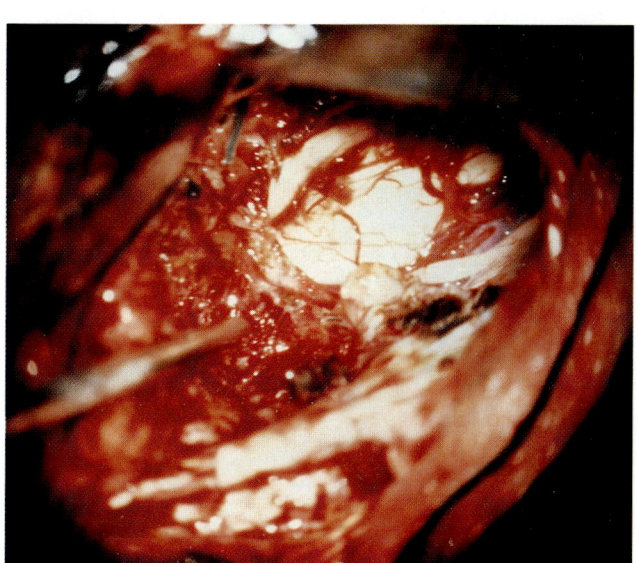 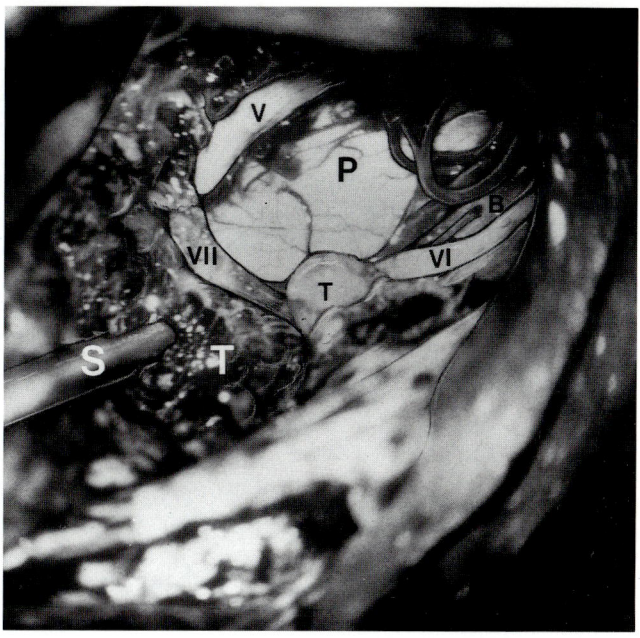

FIG. 6. A: Color operative photograph (right side) during the dissection of a meningioma: the upper portion of the tumor has been dissected from the brain stem and cranial nerves V, VI, and VII. The pons and basilar artery are clearly seen. The lower part of the tumor is still present. **B:** Artist's enhancement of the photograph in (**A**). P, pons; B, basilar artery; T, tumor; S, suction tool; V–VII, cranial nerves.

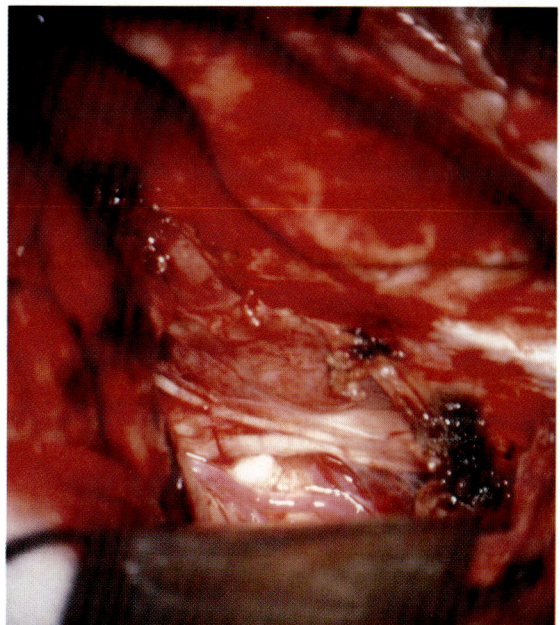 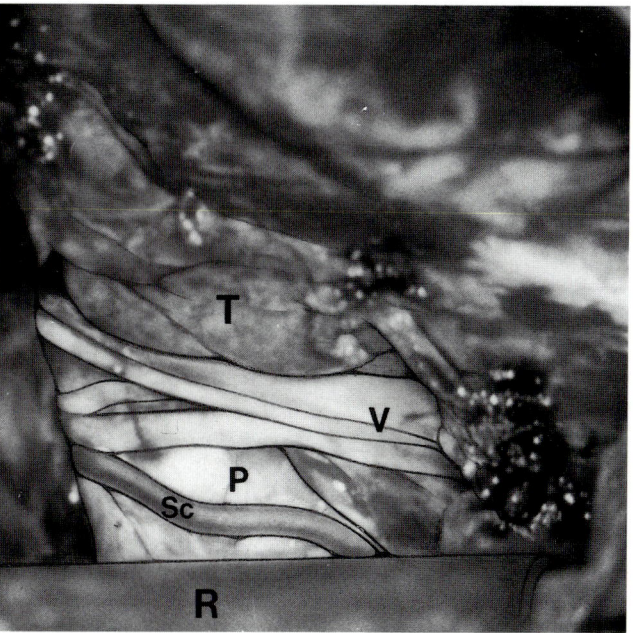

FIG. 7. A: Color operative photograph. Surgeon's view, demonstrating the trigeminal rootlets stretched by the tumor as viewed through the open tentorium. **B:** Artist's enhancement of the photograph in (**A**). P, pons; T, tumor; V, trigeminal rootlets; SC, superior cerebellar artery; R, retractor.

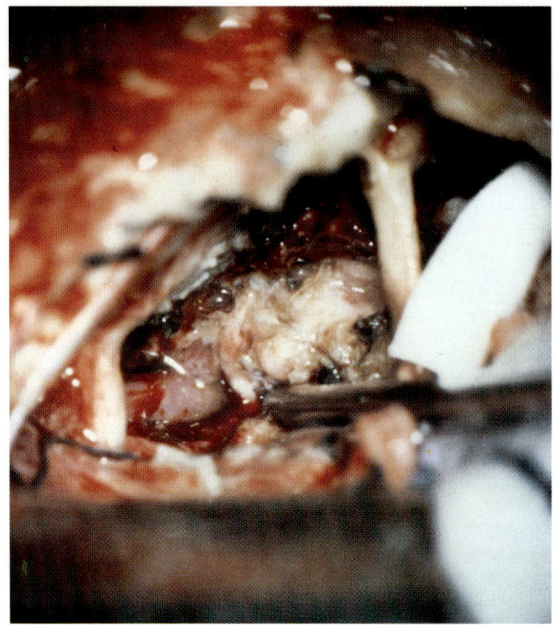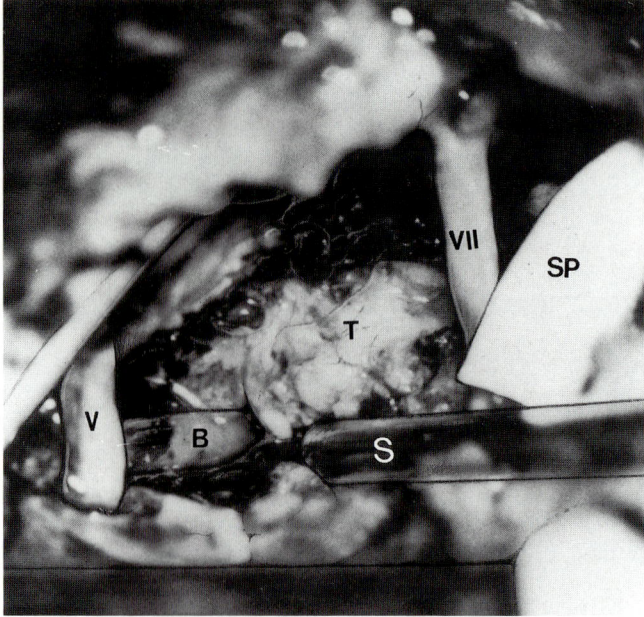

FIG. 8. A: Color operative photograph (right side): the basilar artery is displaced by the tumor to the opposite side. Cranial nerves V, VII, and VIII were displaced posteriorly and easily visualized. Note the tumor extension across the clivus. **B:** Artist's enhancement of the photograph in (**A**). B, basilar artery; T, tumor; S, suction tool; V and VII, cranial nerves; SP, surgical patty.

Once the tumor has been excised, all neurovascular structures in the posterior fossa are covered with wet surgical patties, and the area of tumor insertion is vaporized extensively with the laser. If the tumor has extended into the internal auditory meatus, the meatus wall is drilled and the tumor removed. Extension through the jugular foramen is likewise removed.

Closure

Both the temporal and presigmoid dura are closed watertight primarily, the periosteum is turned over the petrous bone to avoid CSF leak, the temporal muscle is rotated over the defect and sewed to the sternomastoid muscle, and the soft tissues are closed in multiple layers.

POSTOPERATIVE MANAGEMENT

We prefer the patient's prompt emergence from anesthesia and neurological evaluation. Fluid and electrolyte balance is monitored closely. Particular attention is paid to airway protection and pulmonary care, particularly in patients with lower cranial nerve paralysis. Steroids are tapered gradually in the postoperative period. In seizure-free patients, anticonvulsants are discontinued after 6 months.

COMPLICATIONS AND THEIR MANAGEMENT

Surgery of clival tumors highlights all potential complications of intracranial surgery. Surgical mortality, usually resulting from manipulation of or interference with the brain stem or its blood supply, is high, particularly in the premicroscopic area. Infarction of the lateral tegmental region of the pons results from an occluded AICA. This complication is magnified when collateral circulation is poor. Occasionally, the appearance of deficit may be delayed during the postoperative period.

Temporal lobe swelling and hemorrhage are grave potential consequences of the subtemporal exposure, particularly on the dominant hemisphere. It is precipitated by coagulation or tearing of Labbé's vein or the basilar occipital veins. Consequently, every effort should be made to preserve these veins and alleviate temporal lobe retraction (2,15). Likewise, cerebellar swelling and intracerebellar hematoma may follow excessive retraction of the cerebellum. The retrolabyrinthine presigmoid avenue alleviates cerebellar retraction and minimizes the risk of cerebellar swelling. Cerebellar resection is seldom needed today. Posterior fossa hematomas remain a frightening complication because of the resulting rapid and direct brain stem compression. Venous hemostasis is deceptive when the head is elevated and the veins are collapsed. Thus, a repeated Valsalva maneuver and jugular compression prior to closure are essential to assure meticulous hemostasis.

Ligation of the sigmoid sinus is a step incorporated into other surgeons' techniques. Although thought to be inconsequential, it has been associated with fatal complications (7,14). Assurance of the patency of the opposite sigmoid sinus and normal connection through the torcular Herophili is a prerequisite to ligation of the sigmoid sinus. The above described approach preserves the sinus and eliminates the risk associated with its ligation.

Any of the cranial nerves (III to XII) are at risk during surgery of clival tumors. Injury to the trochlear nerve is a frequent hazard during tentorial splitting because of its fineness, fragility, and close relation to the incisura. Morbidity resulting from its paralysis, however, is minimal compared to paralysis of other cranial nerves. Trigeminal nerve deficit is more morbid because of the resulting corneal anesthesia and subsequent keratitis, particularly if the facial nerve is also paralyzed. Protective measures should be taken promptly to avoid this serious complication. Trigeminal nerve trauma may result in facial pain, anesthesia dolorosa, and trigeminal neuralgia. Facial pain may develop months or years postoperatively (15).

Justifiable emphasis has been placed on facial nerve injury. Anatomical preservation, however, does not necessarily mean functional preservation. Tumor size is one of the most decisive factors in preserving facial nerve function. Removal of large tumors fares worse than small ones. The facial nerve is usually displaced posteriorly by petroclival meningiomas and may actually traverse the tumor. Intraoperative end-to-end direct anastomosis or graft offers the best results, with recovery in up to 80% of cases. Otherwise, a hypoglossal-to-facial anastomosis is the next preferred and most common procedure.

Although hearing loss usually exists preoperatively, normal hearing is not infrequent. In these instances, loss of hearing becomes a potential complication of surgery. Thus the eighth cranial nerve and the inner ear should be preserved, particularly since improvement in hypoacusis has been reported. Lateral-to-medial retraction of the cerebellum during posterior fossa surgery is more dangerous to hearing than retraction in a caudal-to-rostral direction. When preserving hearing, sparing the cochlear blood supply is as important as preserving the nerve itself.

While great emphasis is given to facial nerve preservation, a stronger one should be given to preservation of lower cranial nerves. Their deficit is a significant cause of morbidity and mortality (12). Injury to the lower cranial nerves may be troublesome both intraoperatively and postoperatively. Intraoperatively, dissection of these nerves may produce bradycardia and hypotension. Postoperatively, dysphagia, vocal cord paralysis, and a depressed cough and gag reflex may lead to grave pulmonary complications that could be fatal. Careful dissection of the inferior pole of the tumor and use of nonadherent patties help protect the nerves.

Complications related to CSF dynamic disturbance include CSF leak, hydrocephalus, and pseudomeningocele. Although hydrocephalus may be present prior to surgery and persist despite total removal of the mass, it may also develop postoperatively. Acute postoperative hydrocephalus is usually obstructive and related to mass effect (tumor, edema, hemorrhage), while delayed hydrocephalus is usually communicating and related to poor absorption of CSF or scarring of the basal cistern. A CT scan is diagnostic, and the treatment is shunting.

CSF leak is a significant risk in the petrosal approach, occurring via the skin or through the middle ear. The leak is best avoided with watertight closure of the dura, applying bone wax to the drilled surface of the temporal bone, and placing the pericranial flap over the drilled temporal bone surface.

When a CSF leak occurs, the incidence of meningitis is one in five (8). Initial management of CSF leak includes head elevation, repeated spinal tap, or continuous spinal drainage. If the leak does not cease in a few days, or the area has been previously heavily irradiated, a cisternography with water-soluble contrast can determine the leakage site and may be followed by watertight dural closure with a fascial graft. The use of fibrin glue might augment closure (11). If hydrocephalus is an underlying factor, shunting is required.

ILLUSTRATIVE CASES

Case 1

A 49-year-old female presented with a 1-year history of staggering and poor balance, a several year history of occasional nausea and vomiting, and a 10–15-year history of night terrors and sleep-walking. Several years prior to her admission, she was medically treated for trigeminal neuralgia on the left side, which has subsided without recurrence. Her neurological exam was significant for left cerebellar signs, as well as a positive Rhomberg with the patient falling to the left. An audiogram showed bilateral high-frequency hearing loss. Both CT and MRI demonstrated a large petroclival tumor with extensions through the tentorial hiatus (Fig. 9). A cerebral arteriogram showed that the sinuses were patent. Using the petrosal approach, we gained access to and totally removed the meningioma.

Her postoperative course was uneventful with the patient neurologically intact aside from the cerebellar signs present preoperatively, which gradually resolved over 1 month. On follow-up after 2 weeks, the patient demonstrated a large CSF collection under the skin flap. This was successfully treated with spinal drainage. There has been no sign of tumor recurrence after 4 years of follow-up.

Case 2

A 39-year-old female was referred with a history of several years of poor balance and right-hand tremor, as well as an occipital headache. She complained of numbness of the right tongue and face but had no nausea, vomiting, dizziness, or seizure.

The neurological exam revealed an alert and oriented

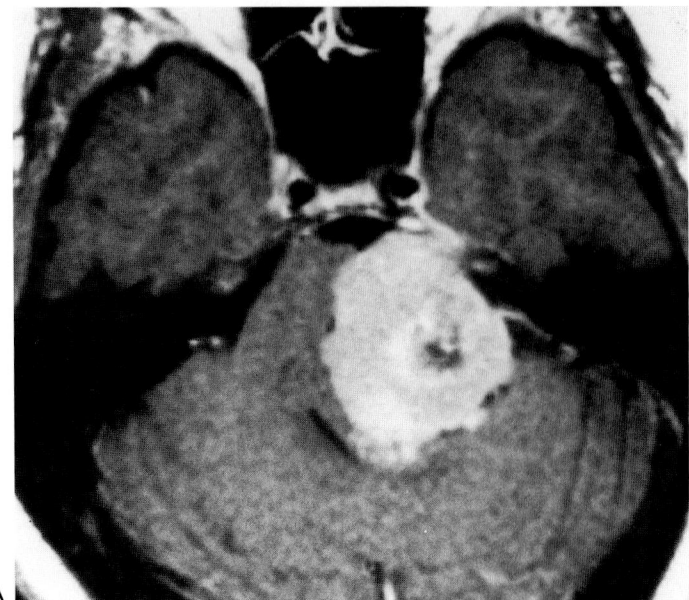 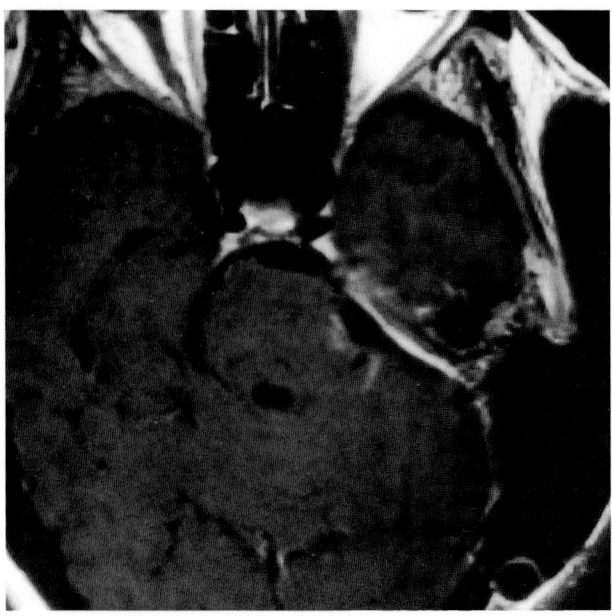

FIG. 9. MRI of large petroclival meningioma: various views assist in preoperative planning by delineating the tumor's relationship to the surrounding neura and vascular structures and confirming total removal. **A:** Contrast enhanced axial MRI of petroclival meningioma depicting distortion of the brain stem. **B:** Postoperative contrast enhanced MRI of the same patient, demonstrating total removal and the expansion of the previously compressed brain stem. Note CSF collection under the skin flap.

patient. Cranial nerve deficit included a decreased corneal reflex on the right as well as hypalgesia in the V-1 and V-2 distribution. Good functional hearing was present on both sides. A finger-to-nose test showed obvious dysmetria on the right. Her gait was unsteady, and she was noted to fall to either side. MRI showed a large right petroclival mass with brain stem compression and extension into Meckel's cave. She underwent total removal of the tumor, which proved to be a schwannoma.

Two days postoperatively, she developed delayed seventh cranial nerve palsy; subsequently, she developed corneal abrasion, which was treated immediately and a tarsorrhaphy was performed. She also suffered decreased hearing in the right ear but maintained functional hearing. Her seventh nerve palsy started to recover by the time of discharge 10 days postoperatively.

PATIENT SERIES

During the years 1984 through 1990, we operated on 31 patients using the approach described above: 19 meningiomas, 7 schwannomas, and 4 epidermoid tumors. There was no mortality in this series; total removal was achieved in all but three meningiomas. These three cases have demonstrated recurrence on follow-up scans; radiation therapy was administered to two of them. None of the totally removed tumors has demonstrated recurrence; however, the average follow-up period is only 2.5 years.

Complications included hemiparesis and dysphasia from temporal lobe venous infarction in one patient, and permanent facial nerve palsy in two patients, which required facial reanimation. Three patients had temporary facial nerve palsy, from which they have recovered. There were three incidences of other temporary cranial nerve palsies which recovered. One patient suffered the loss of preoperative functional hearing and another had a decrease in hearing. Hearing improved in only one patient. Facial pain has not been encountered in this series.

Pulmonary embolism was documented in five of these patients. CSF leak occurred in two patients; one subsided with spinal drainage and the other required operative closure. A pseudomeningocele, which occurred in one patient, also subsided with spinal drainage.

REFERENCES

1. Al-Mefty O. Petrosal approach for petroclival meningiomas. *Neurosurgery* 1988;22:510–517.
2. Al-Mefty O. *Surgery of the cranial base.* Boston: Kluwer, 1989;239–258.
3. Al-Mefty O. Surgical exposure of petroclival tumors. In: Wilkins RH, Rengachary SS, eds. *Neurosurgery update.* New York: McGraw-Hill, 1990.
4. Bailey P. Concerning the technique of operation for acoustic neurinoma. *Zentralbl Neurochir* 1939;4:1–5.
5. Fraenkel J, Hunt JR. Contribution to the surgery of neurofibroma of the acoustic nerve. *Ann Surg* 1904;40:293–319.
6. Hakuba A, Nishimura S, Tanaka K, Kishi H, Nakamura T. Clivus meningioma: six cases of total removal. *Neurol Med Chir (Tokyo)* 1977;17:63–77.

7. Hitselberger WE, House WF. A combined approach to the cerebellopontine angle. *Arch Otolaryngol* 1966;84:267–285.
8. House WF, Hitselberger WE. Monograph II: surgical complications of acoustic tumor surgery. *Arch Otolaryngol* 1968;88:659–667.
9. Morrison AW, King TT. Experiences with a translabyrinthine–transtentorial approach to the cerebellopontine angle: technical note. *J Neurosurg* 1973;38:382–390.
10. Ojemann RG. Meningiomas: clinical features and surgical management. In: Wilkins RH, Rengachary SS, eds. *Neurosurgery.* New York: McGraw-Hill, 1990;635–654.
11. Shaffrey CI, Spotnitz WD, Shaffrey ME, Jane JA. Neurosurgical applications of fibrin glue: augmentation of dural closure in 134 patients. *Neurosurgery* 1990;26:207–210.
12. Sekhar LN, Jannetta PJ, Burkhart LE, Janosky JE. Meningiomas involving the clivus: a 6-year experience with 38 patients. *Neurosurgery* 1992; *in press.*
13. Steiner L, Lindquist C. Meningiomas and gamma knife radiosurgery. In: Al-Mefty O, ed. *Meningiomas.* New York: Raven, 1991;263–272.
14. Symon L. Surgical approaches to the tentorial hiatus. In: Krayenbühl H, et al, eds. *Advances and technical standards in neurosurgery,* vol 9. New York: Springer-Verlag, 1982;69–112.
15. Yasargil MG, Mortara RW, Curcic M. Meningiomas of basal posterior cranial fossa. In: Krayenbühl H, et al, eds. *Advances and technical standards in neurosurgery,* vol 7. New York: Springer-Verlag, 1983;1–115.
16. Al-Mefty O, et al. Petroclival meningiomas. In: *Neurosurgical operative atlas.* Baltimore: Williams & Wilkins. 1992 (*in press*).

CHAPTER 21

Classification, Technique, and Results of Surgical Resection of Petrous Bone Tumors

Shlomo Pomeranz, Laligam N. Sekhar, Ivo P. Janecka,
Barry E. Hirsch, and Sai S. Ramasastry

Resection of the petrous bone for tumor has traditionally been a difficult operation (27). The surrounding critical structures, the difficulties in avoiding postoperative cerebrospinal fluid (CSF) leakage (30) and infection, the accompanying lower cranial nerve dysfunction (19), and the need for radical surgery to assure total tumor resection (3) are the central challenges with this surgery. Since the initial piecemeal resections in 1951 by Campbell et al. (6) and Ward et al. (39), many advances have evolved: precise preoperative imaging; balloon occlusion testing or permanent occlusion of the ICA and embolization of feeding vessels; intraoperative microtechniques; and cranial base repair with rotation or free flaps. Nevertheless, tumor-infiltrated petrous bone resection remains a major surgical challenge.

In this chapter, a technique of total petrous temporal bone resection is described, applicable with modifications to a spectrum of invasive tumors. For benign tumors, this is the definitive treatment; for low-grade malignancies, surgery and radiation are usually effective; and for high-grade malignancies, early diagnosis and effective adjuvant therapy will be required to attain adequate treatment outcomes. A system of classification of petrous region tumors based on their anatomical spread has been developed (27). This classification allows grouping of petrous tumors for comparison and may be of value when deciding on treatment modalities, alongside tumor histology and other criteria.

INDICATIONS FOR SURGERY

It is obvious that growing benign tumors should be resected; while, clearly, malignant tumors beyond resectable boundaries preclude a cure. Between these extremes lie the majority of petrous tumors. Though large malignant tumors have a poor prognosis (11,14,23,25,27,36,38), about one-quarter of the patients harboring large petrous malignancies can be expected to have long-term tumor-free survival following radical surgery with adjuvant therapy. Following radical surgery of low-grade malignancies, two-thirds of the patients can be expected to have long-term tumor-free survival. When a neoplasm involving the petrous bone and surrounding structures is felt to be totally resectable on the basis of preoperative radiological studies, operation is indicated. The patient's general health must be good. Most importantly, the patient and his/her family must have a clear understanding of the expected postoperative morbidity and potential for failure of the treatment modality.

Patient Population

Twenty patients with petrous bone neoplasms were treated surgically during the last 6 years in our institu-

---

S. Pomeranz: Department of Neurosurgery, Hadassah University Hospital and Hebrew University, Kiryat Hadassah, il-91 120 Jerusalem, Israel.

L. N. Sekhar: Department of Neurosurgery, Center for Cranial Base Surgery, University of Pittsburgh School of Medicine, Presbyterian University Hospital, Pittsburgh, Pennsylvania 15213.

I. P. Janecka: Center for Cranial Base Surgery, University of Pittsburgh School of Medicine, Presbyterian University Hospital, and Department of Otolaryngology, Eye and Ear Institute, Pittsburgh, Pennsylvania 15213.

B. E. Hirsch: University of Pittsburgh School of Medicine, and Department of Otolaryngology, Eye and Ear Institute, Pittsburgh, Pennsylvania 15213.

S. S. Ramasastry: Division of Plastic Surgery, University of Pittsburgh School of Medicine, Pittsburgh, Pennsylvania 15261.

tion. In this patient population, the presenting primary symptoms (in descending frequency) were drainage from the ear or localized pain, peripheral facial nerve paresis, decreased ipsilateral hearing, a parotid mass, and multiple lower cranial nerve dysfunction. Sixty-one percent of the patients were male, and the age range was 14–72 years, with a mean age of 46 years. The average duration of symptoms previous to our surgery was 7 years. These patients had an average of 1.2 previous operations per patient and 20% had undergone previous radiotherapy. The histological spectrum of our series is listed in Table 1. All these patients had recurrent or actively growing tumor on admission. One patient had increased intracranial pressure secondary to the tumor, and seven patients were debilitated due to tumor-related pain.

Preoperative Evaluation and Treatment

In addition to a careful medical history, neurological and general physical examination, the patients are evaluated according to a standard protocol. All patients with known or suspected malignancy undergo a skeletal survey and abdominal and thoracic imaging to evaluate for metastases. All patients undergo axial and coronal computerized tomography (CT), with soft tissue and osseous algorithms, and magnetic resonance imaging (MRI). All patients undergo four-vessel cerebral angiograms and balloon test occlusion (BTO) of the involved internal carotid artery (ICA) with follow-up stable xenon CT cerebral blood flow evaluation (33). Special attention is paid to the configuration of Labbé's vein and whether it is draining only to the sigmoid sinus or also to the anterior venous complex. The transverse and sigmoid sinuses are also noted as to dominance and cross-drainage. Tumor feeder arteries are routinely embolized, particularly from the external carotid arteries, and an ICA that is to be sacrificed may be permanently balloon occluded preoperatively.

In patients with highly malignant tumors, the necessity for sacrifice of a dominant or noncollateralized sigmoid sinus precludes the operation. Similarly, if the patient has clinically failed the BTO-ICA, and the ICA is involved by a highly malignant neoplasm, operation is not performed.

Somatosensory evoked responses (SSER) and contralateral brain stem evoked responses (BSER) are obtained preoperatively.

Anesthesia, Monitoring, and Positioning

General endotracheal anesthesia is administered without long-acting muscle paralysis to allow intraoperative neurophysiological monitoring. Bilateral SSEPs and the BSER from the contralateral ear are monitored. The

TABLE 1. Profile of 20 petrous bone tumors

Pathology	Classification grade[a]	Number of patients[b]	Resection: total/partial	Adjuvant therapy[c]	Outcome[d] NED	AWD	DOD
Squamous cell carcinoma	1	3	2/1	RT	1	—	2
	2	1	1/—	RT	—	—	1
	3a	3	1/2	RT	1	1	1
	3b	3	2/1	RT	1	1	1
	3c	2	—/2	RT	—	1	1
	3d	2	1/1	RT	—	1	1
	3e	1	—/1	RT	—	1	1
Osteogenic sarcoma	3b	2	—/1	Chemo	—	—	1
	3c	1	—/1	Chemo	—	—	1
Hemangiopericytoma	3a,b	1	1/—	—	1	—	—
	3b	1	1/—	—	1	—	—
Parotid acinar cell carcinoma	3b,c	1	1/—	RT	—	1	—
Parotid adenocystic cell carcinoma	3a,b	1	—/1	RT	—	—	1
Mixed myoepithelial carcinoma	3b	1	1/—	RT	1	—	—
Malignant choroid plexus papilloma	3a	1	1/—	—	1	—	—
Benign meningioma	3a	1	—/1	1	—	1	—
	3b	2	2/—	—	2	—	—

[a] See Table 2.
[b] Tumors may fit more than one category; therefore the total number is greater than 20.
[c] RT, radiotherapy; Chemo, chemotherapy.
[d] NED, no evidence of disease; AWD, alive with disease; DOD, dead of disease.

BSER is an indicator of excessive temporal lobe retraction, presumably due to brain stem compression or distortion. Facial nerve monitoring is used if an attempt is to be made to dissect and preserve the facial nerve (especially in benign tumors). An intraoperative electroencephalograph is monitored to follow burst suppression if barbiturate or etomidate coma may be induced. A lumbar subarachnoid drain is used for brain relaxation.

The patient is placed either in the lateral decubitus position with the head in neutral position, or in the supine position with the ipsilateral shoulder elevated and the head rotated 60° contralaterally. Tissue harvesting is done for the planned reconstruction: free myocutaneous graft, saphenous vein–ICA graft, and sural nerve for cranial nerve cable grafts play a role in determining the positioning of the patient. Sequential compression stockings are utilized intraoperatively as prophylaxis against deep vein thrombosis.

If the patient's head position may be changed during the operation, the endotracheal tube is secured to the teeth with 28-gauge stainless steel wire passed interdentally. If postoperative cranial nerve (CN) IX and X palsy is anticipated, a tracheostomy is performed at the beginning or at the end of the operation.

Incision and Exposure

A retroauricular incision, starting from the frontotemporal hairline and ending down onto the neck to provide exposure and control of the carotid and jugular vessels and lower cranial nerves, is used (29,31). This allows transection of the cartilaginous external auditory canal (EAC) and forward rotation of the large flap (Fig. 1). The external canal is sutured closed and covered with a periosteal flap. The incision is modified to resect tumor-infiltrated or infected skin and to accommodate previous incisions. The extracranial facial nerve is exposed from the stylomastoid foramen through its division into the two major branches (32). If the mastoid is uninvolved by tumor, a partial mastoidectomy is performed and the sigmoid sinus is skeletonized. The temporomandibular joint is opened, and the condyle and neck of the mandible are excised. The temporalis muscle is elevated from the temporal fossa, and a temporal craniotomy is performed. The transverse sinus is separated under direct vision, and then a suboccipital craniotomy is performed. A reciprocating saw is used to cut the zygomatic arch from just posterior to the glenoid fossa to the zygomatic–maxillary suture. The squamous temporal bone is rongeured to the level of the floor of the middle fossa. Extradural dissection of the middle fossa floor is done using the surgical microscope (32,33). The middle meningeal artery is coagulated and transected. The greater superficial petrosal nerve (GSPN) is transected. The lateral and anterior aspects of the foramen ovale are unroofed, and the mandibular nerve is mobilized (Fig. 2). Unroofing of the petrous ICA along its ascending and horizontal portions is done by a combination of drilling and rongeuring, and it is translocated anteriorly from the carotid canal (Fig. 3). If the preoperative BTO demonstrated ade-

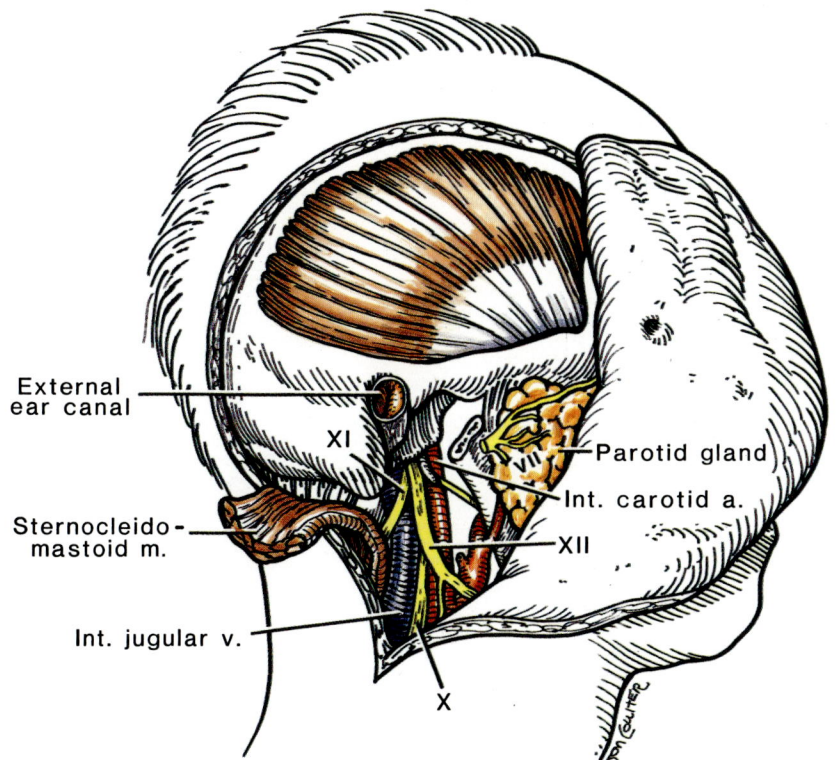

FIG. 1. Frontotemporo, retroauricular, cervical skin flap rotated forward. The external ear canal has been transected. The facial nerve has been transected just beyond the stylomastoid foramen. The temporomandibular joint has been opened and the mandibular ramus resected. Cranial nerves IX–XII and the jugular and carotid vessels are exposed in the neck.

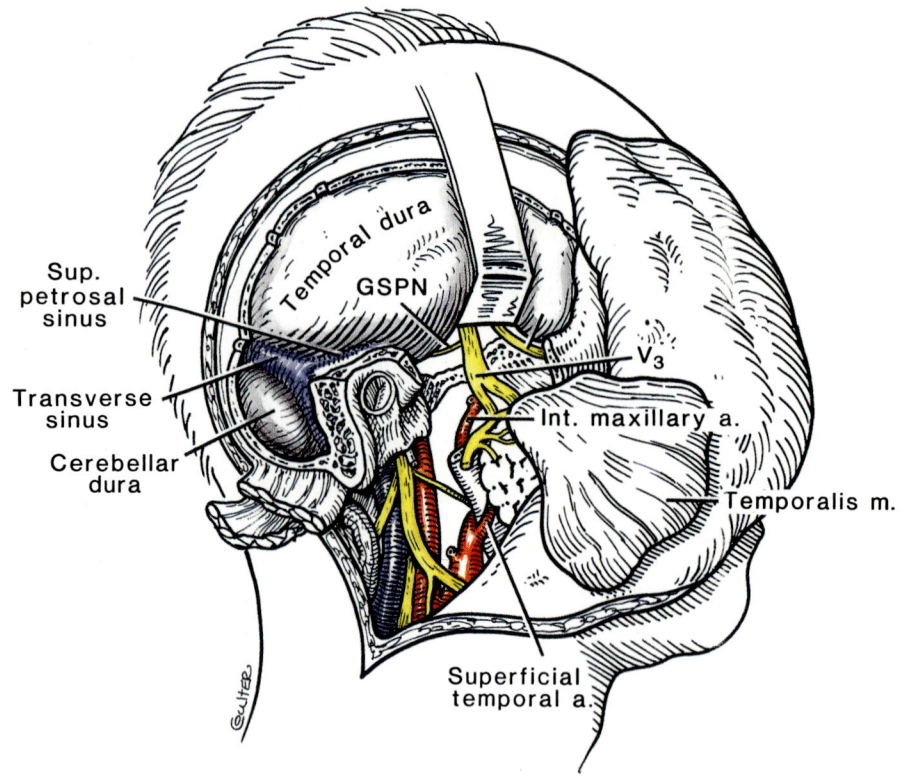

FIG. 2. A temporal and suboccipital craniotomy has been extended over the transverse sinus and lateral posterior fossa. A zygomatic osteotomy has been performed. A partial mastoidectomy has been performed. The osseous middle fossa floor has been partially resected to expose CNs V_3 and V_2 and the greater superficial petrosal nerve. The middle meningeal artery has been transected.

quate cerebral blood flow and the ICA is infiltrated by a malignant tumor, it may be ligated and resected. If required, a saphenous vein graft can be interposed for the resected segment of ICA (35). The eustachian tube is transected during the exposure of the petrous ICA. The cartilaginous end of the transected eustachian tube must be packed with fat and sutured shut just medial to V_3 to avoid a postoperative cerebral spinal fluid leakage. The petrous apex and clival bone located medial to the carotid canal are removed with drills and rongeurs.

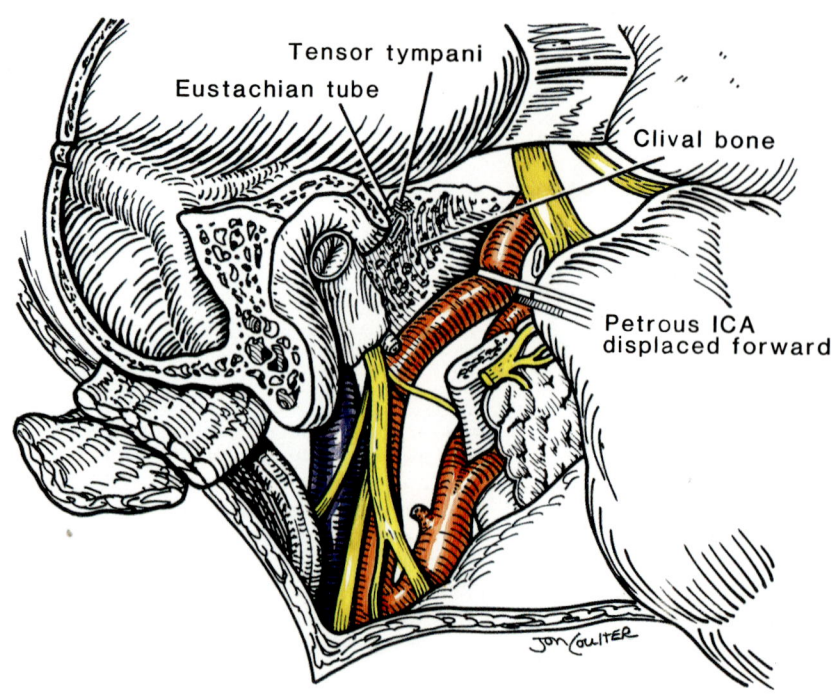

FIG. 3. Continuing resection of the osseous middle fossa floor; the eustachian tube and the tensor tympani muscle have been transected. The ascending and transverse segments of the petrous ICA have been unroofed and the ICA has been mobilized anteriorly.

In patients with highly malignant tumors, the sigmoid sinus is ligated and divided if adequate cross flow is present. In patients with benign tumors, the sigmoid sinus is preserved if it is not involved by tumor, if it is dominant, or has poor cross flow. The sinus may be ligated with 2-0 neurolon or the two walls sutured together using 4-0 neurolon and transected. The internal jugular vein is either ligated or, if it is to be used as the venous drainage of a myocutaneous free-flap, is temporarily clipped. Labbé's vein may be ligated and transected if this allows a completion of tumor resection and the preoperative angiogram demonstrates adequate collateral drainage to the sylvian venous system.

Benign and Low-Grade Malignancy Tumors: Piecemeal Resection

Benign and low-grade malignancy tumors can be removed piecemeal, following the initial approach. The facial nerve is mobilized from the meatal segment to the stylomastoid foramen. Tumor invasion may dictate opening of the nerve sheath and nerve segments may have to be resected and resutured or reconstructed with a graft. The jugular bulb is opened to remove the tumor and to dissect CNs IX, X, and XI. If necessary, the hypoglossal canal is opened to unroof CN XII. Tumor-free osseous and dural margins must be attained and vascular and neural structures inspected for tumor infiltration. Intraoperative histological inspection and the resection of questionable margins increase the chance of total resection. Even with benign tumors, sacrifice of tumor-involved CNs IX–XII may be necessary. In such cases, CNs IX, XI, and XII are reconstructed if possible.

Malignant Tumors: En Bloc Resection

Whenever possible, en bloc resection of petrous bone infiltrated by malignant tumor is performed. The dura is incised in the posterior fossa behind and parallel to the sigmoid sinus, and across the transverse sinus supratentorially. Over the temporal lobe, dural incision is made at the junction with the middle fossa. The dural incision is then continued medially along the middle fossa floor across Meckel's cave, the superior petrosal sinus, and the edge of the tentorium. The tentorium is then incised from the transverse sinus transection to the tentorial notch, posterior to the petrous edge and the superior petrosal sinus, to meet the middle fossa incision (Figs. 4

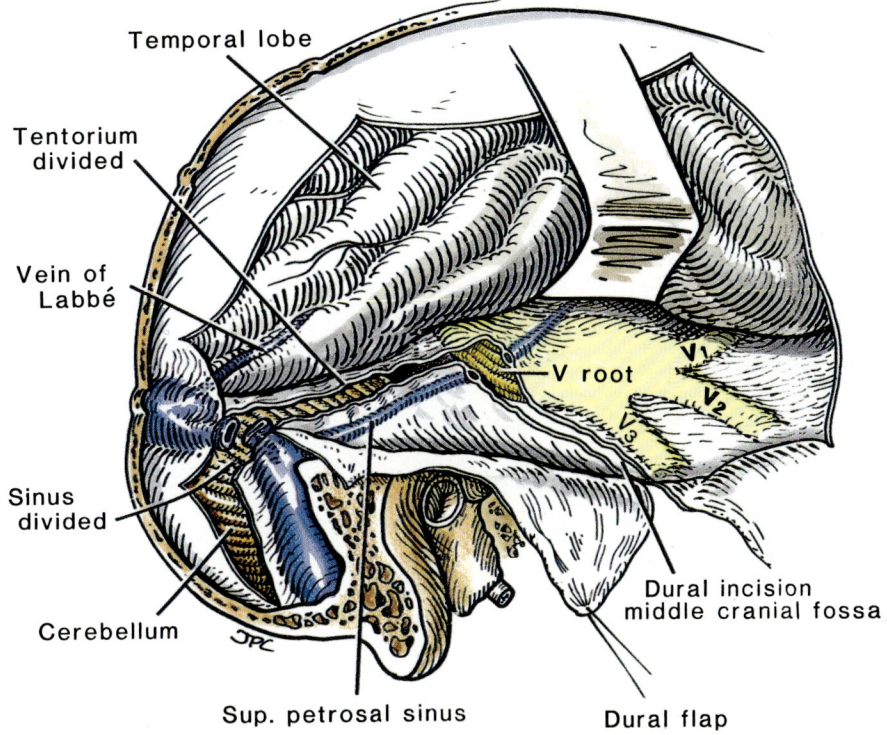

FIG. 4. The temporal dura and retrosigmoid dura have been opened. The lateral sinus has been ligated at its junction with the sigmoid. The tentorium has been opened along the inferior edge of the mandibular nerve, trigeminal ganglion, and roof, with the interruption of the superior petrosal sinus. If uninvolved, the superior petrosal sinus drainage into the transverse sinus may be preserved by changing the dura incision lines. The dura has been cut over the cerebellum, the transverse sinus ligated and transected, and a dural flap brought down from over the temporal lobe. The tentorium has been divided from the transverse sinus transection, alongside and behind the petrous ridge, and anteromedially across the superior petrosal sinus. This cut has been connected to a cut in the dura on the middle cranial fossa floor, anterior to the petrous base. The outline of the trigeminal ganglion and roots can be seen through the middle fossa dura.

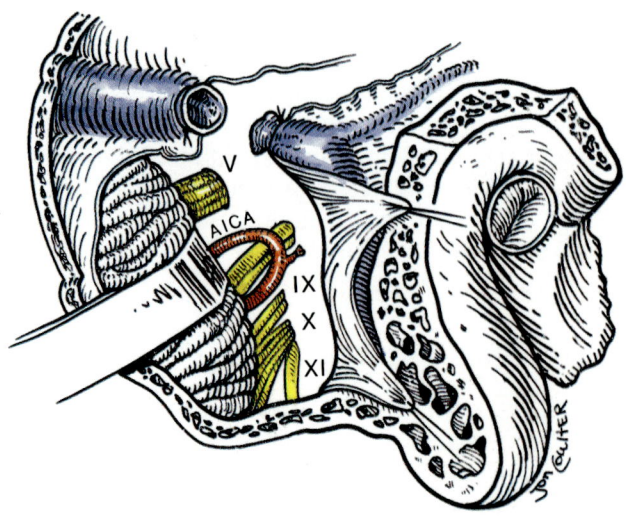

FIG. 5. With the cerebellum retracted medially, CNs V and VII–XI can be seen. The labyrinthine (internal auditory) artery has been transected at its origin from the anterior inferior cerebellar artery.

and 5). The trigeminal root and ganglion and V_3 are thus isolated from the surgical specimen. CSF is drained from the posterior fossa cisterns or via the spinal drain to decrease temporal lobe retraction. Tumor infiltrated dura and tentorium are incised well away from the tumor margins to be included in the resection. The petrosal vein is coagulated and divided. The facial nerve, CN VIII, and the labyrinthine artery are divided at the internal auditory meatus (IAM). The clival dura is divided medial to CNs VII and VIII and the petrous bone. The inferior petrosal sinus is divided in the process and packed with Surgicel. When the resection includes the jugular foramen, CNs IX–XI are transected intradurally (Fig. 6). If the jugular foramen is at the resection border, an attempt is made to dissect and preserve these nerves. The bone of the petrous apex and clivus are removed by drilling through the posterior fossa to connect to the extradural drilled groove posterior to the petrous ICA. Residual bone connections are resected under direct vision to complete the osseous mobilization of the petrous bone. The basilar venous plexus often requires extensive hemostasis by packing with Surgicel. The resection of the tumor-infiltrated petrous bone is completed with soft tissue dissection and transection on the inferior aspect of the petrous bone. Tumor-involved temporal lobe or cerebellum can be resected with adequate margins. Any residual tumor in the occipital condyle, clivus, ICA, or the cavernous sinus is removed to achieve tumor-free margins.

Reconstruction

As needed, petrous ICA reconstruction is performed with a saphenous vein graft (34). CNs VII and XI are cable grafted with the greater auricular nerve, segments of other resected cranial nerves, or the sural nerve. A hypoglossal–facial nerve anastomosis is usually not performed since the loss of CN XII function worsens the disability due to the loss of CNs IX and X. If resected,

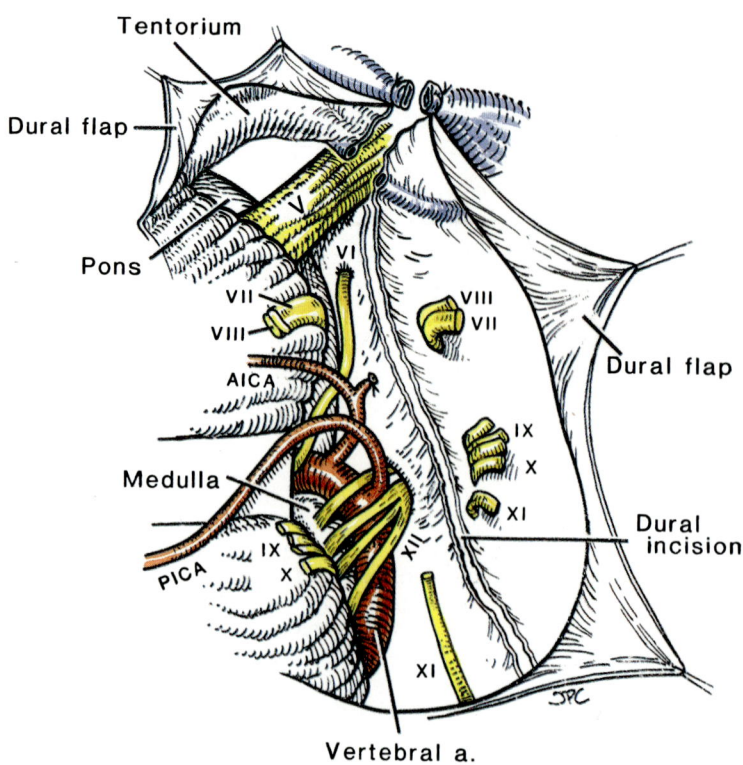

FIG. 6. CNs VII–XI have been transected and the underlying dura incised as the posterior border of the en bloc resection of the petrous bone.

CNs IX and XII can also be reconstructed with interposition grafts. A patch graft of autologous pericranium or fascia lata is used to close the dural defect. The graft is sutured to the dural edges under the calvarium, but, at the base, the dural patch is tucked inward, anchored with as many sutures to the clival dura as possible, and holes are plugged with autologous fat (Fig. 7). A watertight closure is usually not possible.

The temporalis muscle is rotated posteriorly and the edges of the temporalis, sternocleidomastoid, and semispinalis capitis muscles and the posterior aspect of the parotid gland are sutured together. The superior edge of the temporalis muscle is sewn onto the dura to provide an additional seal over the dural patch and provide bulk to fill the operative defect (Fig. 8). If the defect is large and these adjacent muscles are inadequate or devascularized, a trapezius or pectoralis rotation flap or a latissimus dorsi or rectus abdominis free flap may be placed (31). Free flaps may be muscular or myocutaneous and are attached by an arterial anastomosis to the external carotid system and venous anastomosis to the internal jugular system (Fig. 9). A closed system drain coming out superiorly is left under the skin flap for 2–4 days, to drain by gravity (Fig. 10). This drain removes blood and excess CSF until the wound is sufficiently healed. Lumbar CSF drainage is occasionally necessary to promote wound healing. If used, about 20–25 cc are removed every 4 hr. This prevents the problems associated with excessive CSF drainage and allows early ambulation.

If a facial palsy is expected at the end of the operation, a lateral tarsorrhaphy is performed.

Postoperative Care

Following surgery, the patient is closely observed in an intensive care unit for several days with the head raised 30°–45°. The patient is ambulated as early as possible. Sequential compression stockings are maintained until the patient is fully ambulatory, and subcutaneous heparin prophylaxis against deep vein thrombosis is utilized. Head CT is performed on the day following surgery and before discharge home. ICA angiography is done if the vessel was repaired or grafted, or there is suspicion of possible intraoperative damage to the vessel.

CN IX and X palsies require a prolonged tracheostomy and a gastrostomy, especially in older patients. Patients should be prepared for this preoperatively. Removal of the tracheostomy is aided by Teflon injection

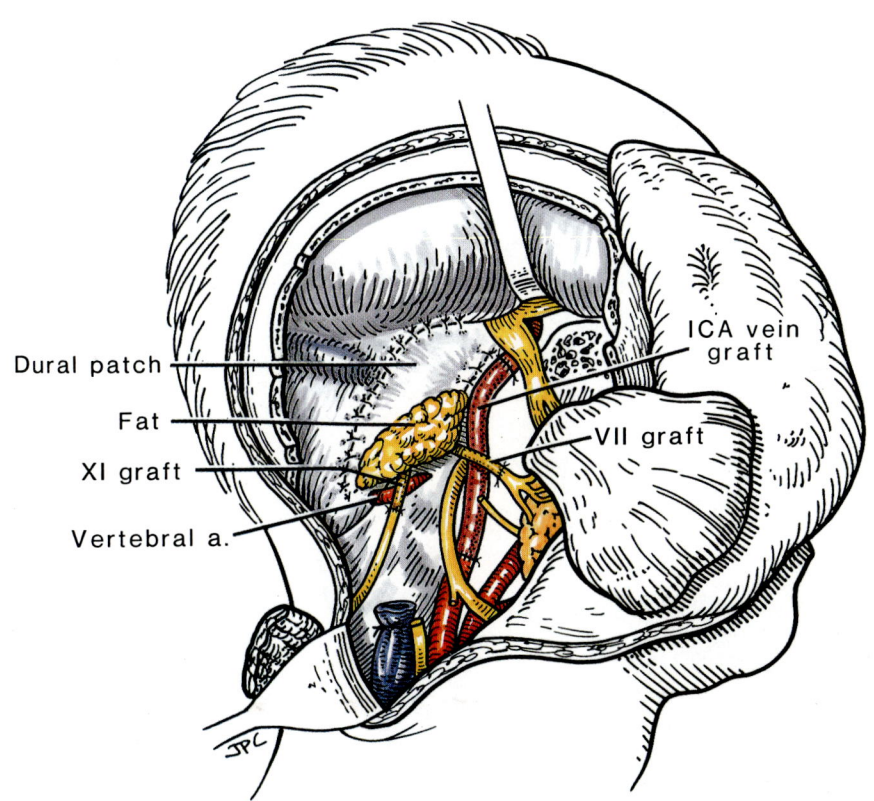

FIG. 7. Reconstruction: Following resection of the petrous bone and transection of the internal jugular vein, the petrous ICA has been resected and a saphenous vein graft interposed. CNs VII and XI, which had been resected, are cable grafted. The distal stumps of CNs IX and X are visualized. A patch graft is sewn into the temporal dural resection defect.

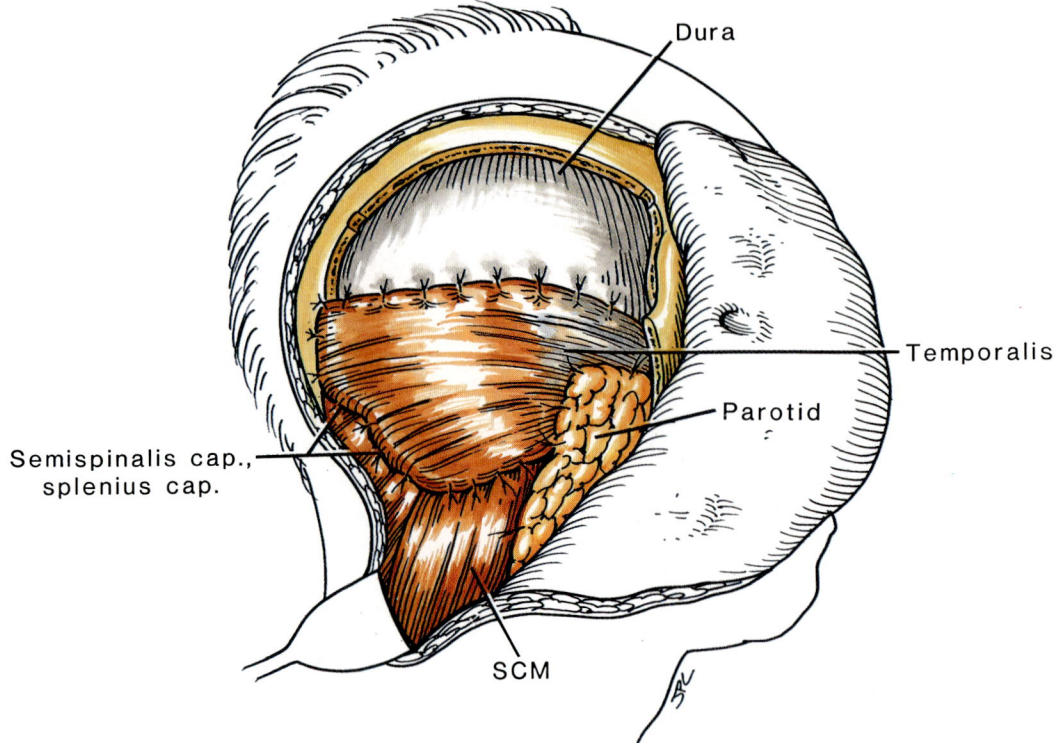

FIG. 8. Reconstruction: The temporalis, sternocleidomastoid, semispinalis, and splenius capitis muscles are sewn to each other and to the dura and beyond the dura patch to seal the dural defect.

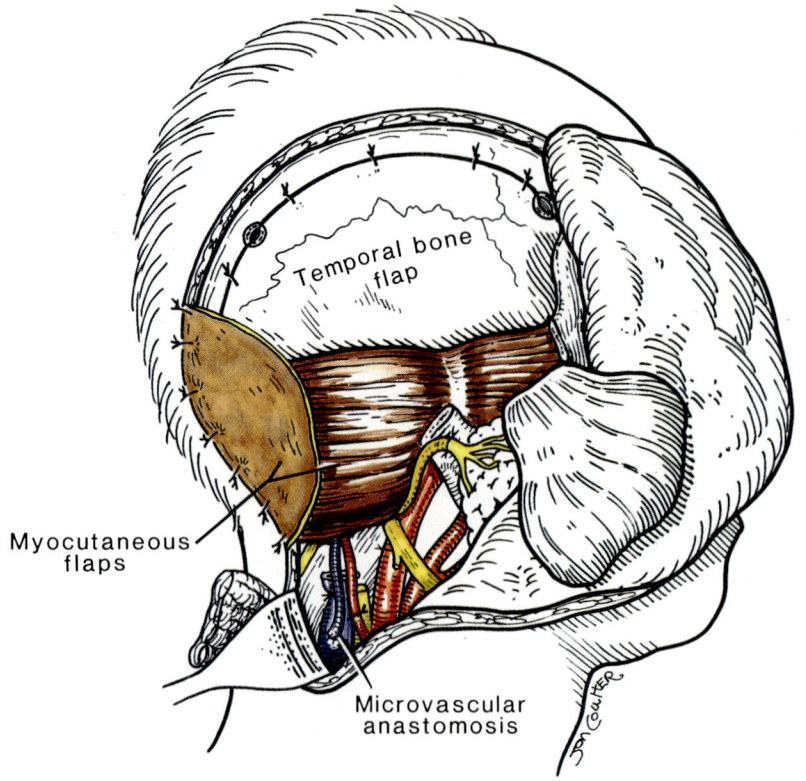

FIG. 9. Reconstruction: A free myocutaneous rectus abdominis graft has been anastomosed to a branch of the ECA with the draining vein to the IJV. The muscle overlies the dural repair to provide a mechanical barrier as well as bulk to fill the defect.

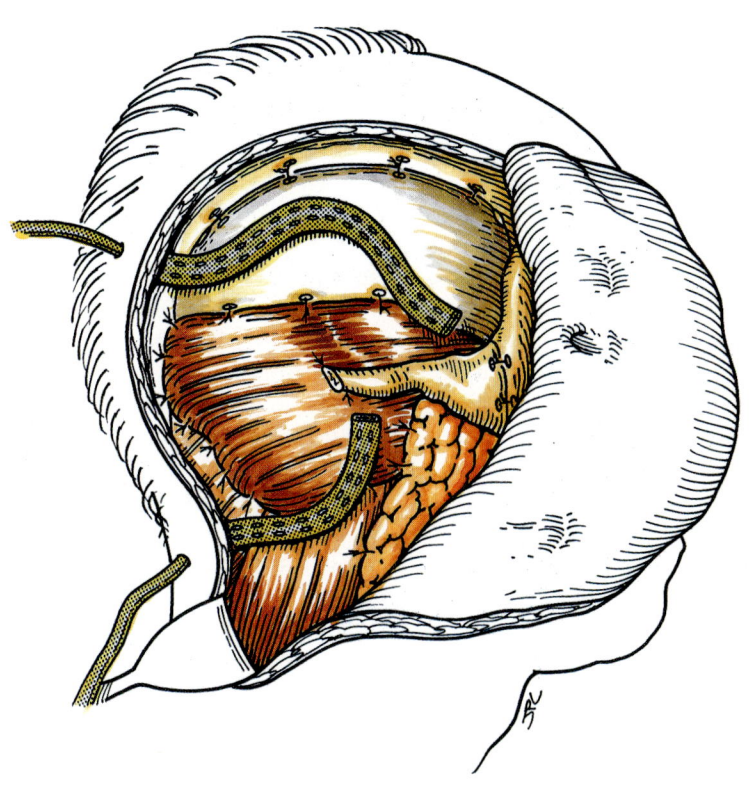

FIG. 10. Reconstruction: The zygoma has been replaced and anchored by sutures anteriorly to its transected facet and posteriorly to the rotated temporalis muscle to provide stability and an adequate facial contour. Two closed-system drains to gravity have been placed.

of the vocal cords. Removal of the gastrostomy requires the demonstration of adequate swallowing without aspiration by a modified barium swallow. The removal of the tracheostomy may take 1–2 months, and the gastrostomy removal may take up to 1 year in some patients. Recovery of adequate facial function (House grade III) after graft reconstruction usually occurs 12–18 months postoperatively.

After discharge, periodic clinic follow-ups are accompanied with CT and/or MRI studies every 3–12 months.

Adjuvant Treatment

Postoperative radiotherapy (typically for squamous cell and parotid carcinoma) and chemotherapy (sarcomas) are planned individually in conjunction with the radiation or medical oncologist.

Complications

In our series, there were no deaths within 6 months of surgery (28). Four patients had wound dehiscences that required wound revision, and four patients had minor dehiscences that healed spontaneously.

Two patients had CSF leaks from the operative wound with meningitis, one requiring an operative revision. One pseudomeningocele resolved spontaneously. Five patients developed pneumonia, one sepsis, and one a urinary tract infection. Three patients had dysphasia and confusion lasting several weeks, one following resection of Labbé's vein on the dominant hemisphere. Three patients had single bouts of seizures under appropriate anticonvulsive treatment. One patient had pulmonary emboli 2 days after surgery and one had minor myocardial ischemia. One patient had prolonged temporomandibular joint pain. Four patients had prolonged depression and anxiety following surgery.

Outcome

In our series, 44% of the patients with malignancies have died within 18 months of surgery due to the primary disease and 10% have recurrent tumor in the operative region an average of 28 months after surgery (Table 1). Twenty-five percent of the high-grade malignancies are tumor-free for an average of 29 months after surgery. Five of the seven patients with low-grade petrous bone malignancies are well and without evidence of tumor an average of 20 months following surgery. Obviously, in these patients, a longer follow-up will be required for formulation of long-term outcomes.

Classification of Tumor Spread and Petrous Resection

Based on our experience and a review of the literature (1,2,14,22), an anatomical classification of tumor spread

TABLE 2. *Classification of anatomical tumor spread in petrous bone tumors*

Grade	Area
1	Partial petrous bone (two of three of these areas: inner ear, middle ear, and about external canal)
2	Entire petrous bone (all three of above-mentioned areas)
2a	Petrous ICA infiltration
3	Entire petrous bone plus:
3a	Adjacent cranial base bone (i.e., middle fossa osseous floor, clivus, occipital condyle)
3b	Dural infiltration
3c	Infratemporal upper cervical soft tissue
3d	Cavernous sinus infiltration

in and about the petrous bone has been proposed, which can be evaluated by CT, MRI, and intraoperatively (Table 2, Fig. 11). This classification, alongside the tumor histology, should simplify comparison of cases and outcome and may help predict an outcome preoperatively. The basis of this classification is the degree of petrous bone involvement (grades 1 and 2), and adjacent cranial base bone, dural, infratemporal/cervical soft tissue, and cavernous sinus involvement (grades 3A to 3D). Obviously, some tumors will overlap more than one category. We classify to the highest pertinent grades; that is, a tumor involving the whole petrous bone, petrous ICA, clivus, and dura would be classified 2A, 3A,B.

ILLUSTRATIVE CASES

Benign Meningioma (Patient E.O.)

This 45-year-old woman was evaluated 8 years previously for Meniere's disease. She presented now with a complete hearing loss on the left and vertigo. CT and MRI scans revealed a tumor involving the petrous ridge, tentorium, and the middle cranial fossa on soft tissue windows, and the petrous bone (Fig. 12). During an initial operation (Fig. 13), meningioma was removed from the posterior and middle fossae. Residual tumor was present in the internal auditory canal, the petrous bone, Meckel's cave, and the clival dura around CN VI. During a second operation 9 days later, a subtotal piecemeal petrosectomy with the removal of all residual tumor was performed (Fig. 14). CN VII was tumor encased in the intracanalicular, labyrinthine, and tympanic segments. Resection of the epineurium allowed the nerve to be preserved. The patient sustained a temporary palsy of CNs VI and VII postoperatively.

The patient developed a necrosis of the posterior edge of the very thin scalp flap. This required debridement and a trapezius muscle rotation flap. The abducens palsy resolved quickly, and the facial nerve palsy improved over 5 months, eventually with House grade II function (Fig. 15). No tumor recurrence was noted a year later (Fig. 16).

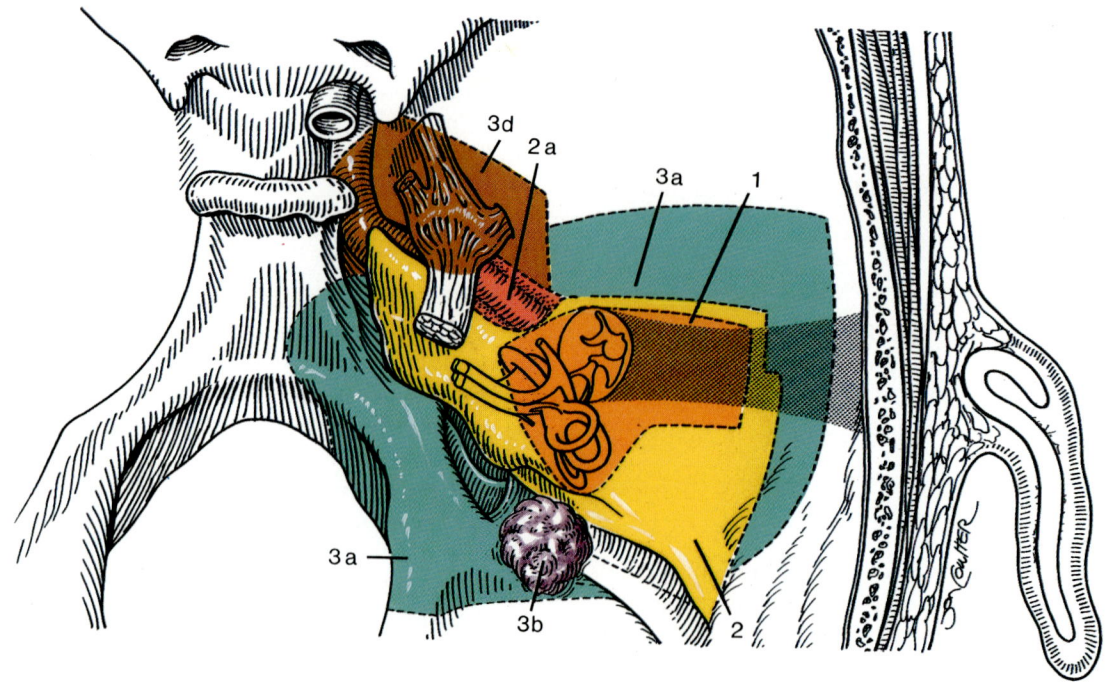

FIG. 11. Superior view of sketch of clivus and right middle fossa demonstrating grading classification of petrous tumors as delineated in Table 2. 1: Tumor infiltrating part of and contained within the petrous bone. 2: Tumor infiltrating entire petrous bone. 2a: Petrous ICA infiltration. 3b: Dural infiltration. 3d: Cavernous sinus infiltration. (3c: infratemporal upper cervical soft tissue infiltration.)

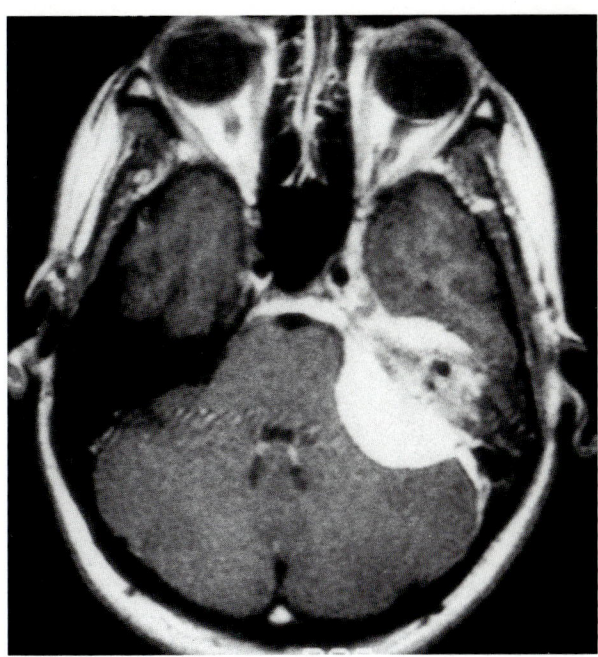

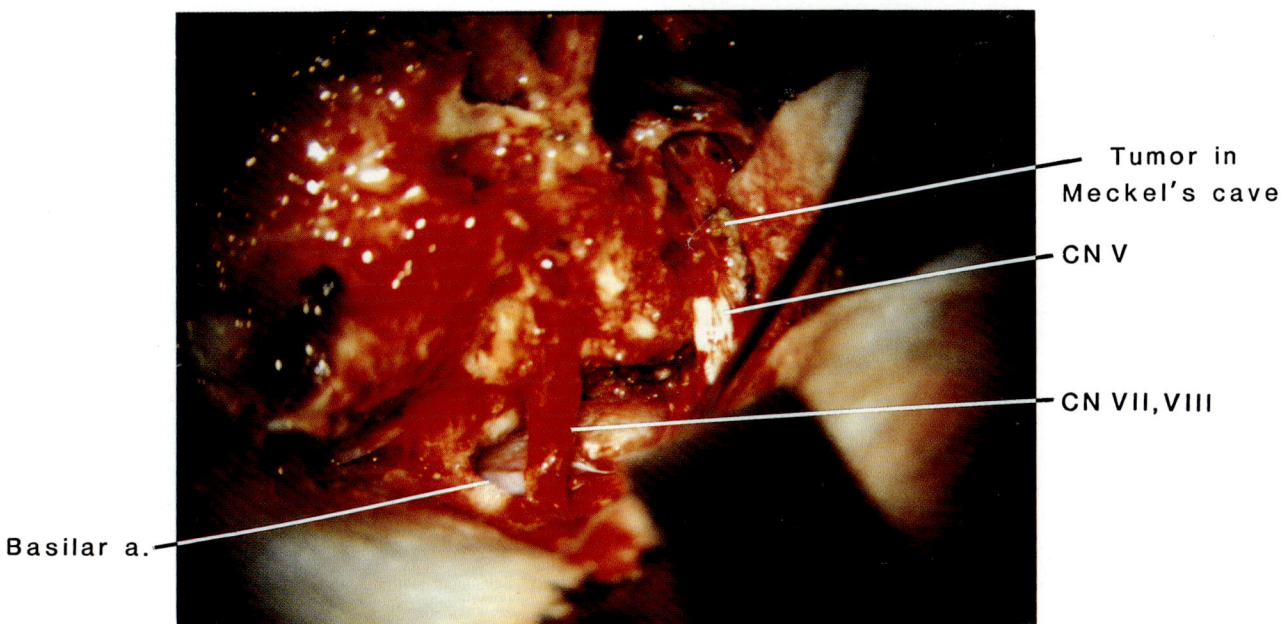

FIG. 12. Patient E.O.—Preoperative axial MRI with gadolinium, demonstrating infiltration of the left petrous bone, including apex and lateral clivus, cerebellopontine angle, and the posterior aspect of the middle fossa by the meningioma.

FIG. 13. Intraoperative microphotograph of patient E.O.

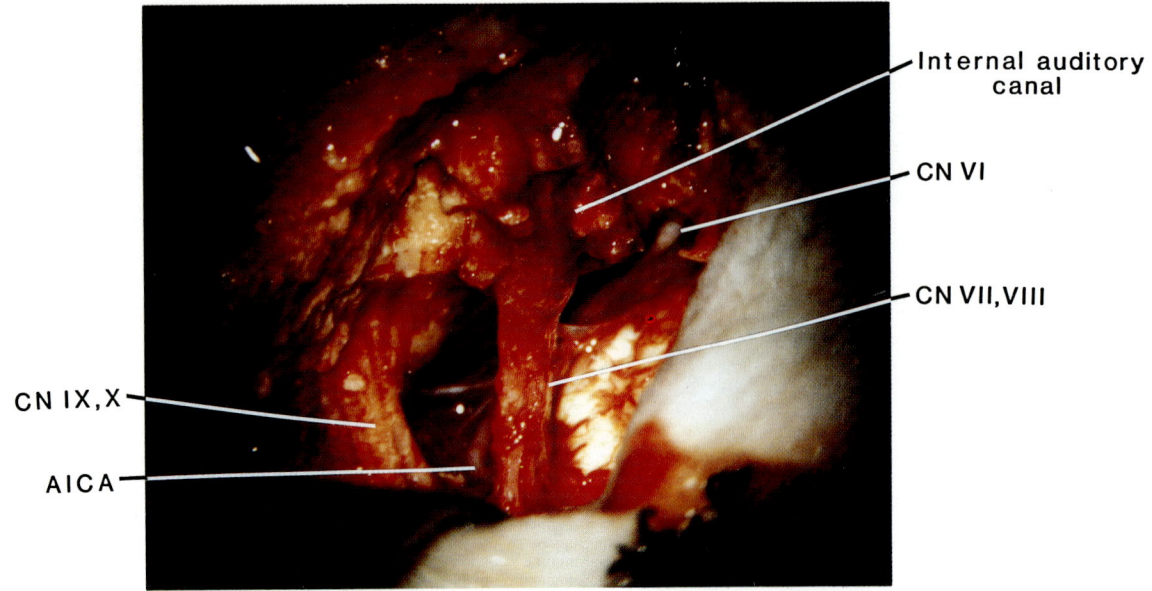

FIG. 14. Intraoperative microphotograph of patient E.O.

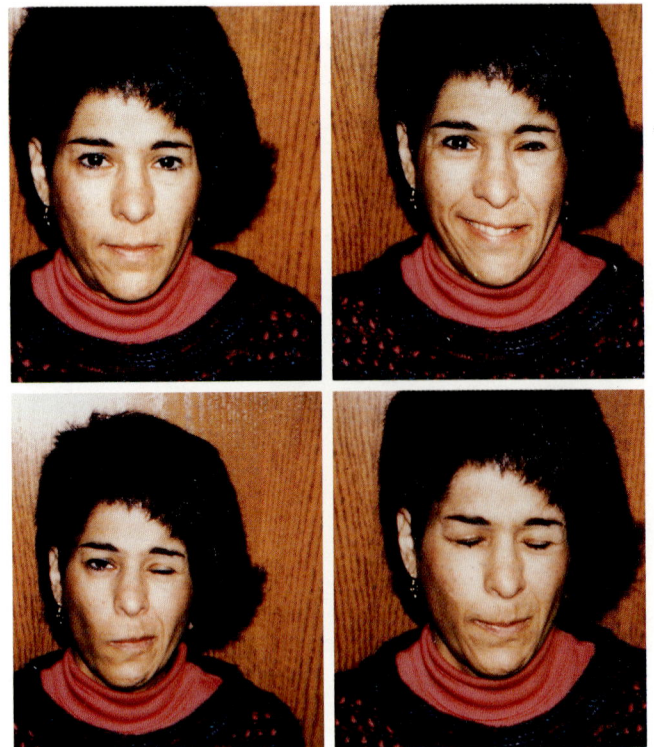

FIG. 15. Patient E.O.—One year following resection of the left petrous meningioma.

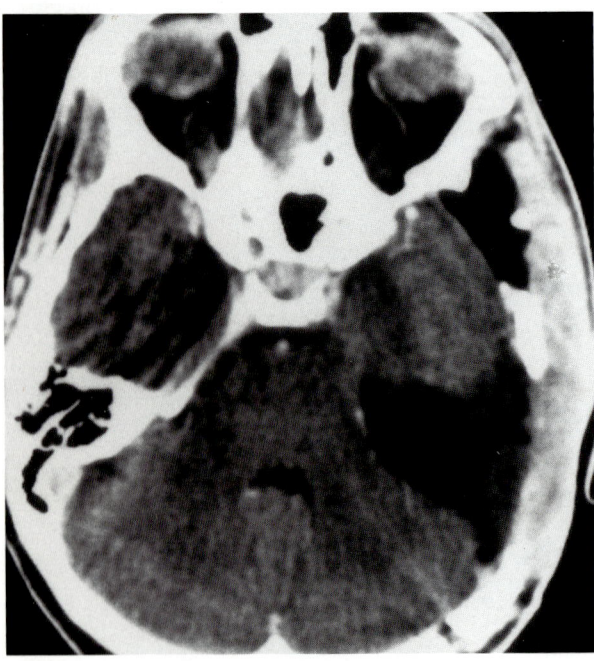

FIG. 16. Patient E.O.—Postoperative axial CT demonstrating complete resection of the left petrous bone. The extent of the convexity bone flap can be seen.

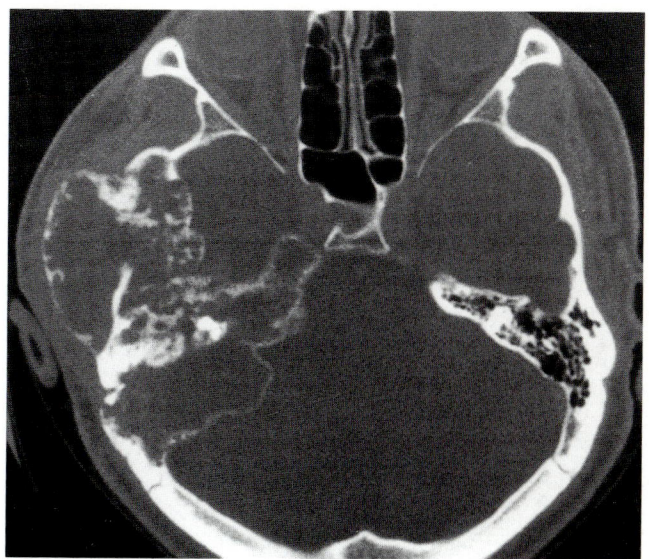 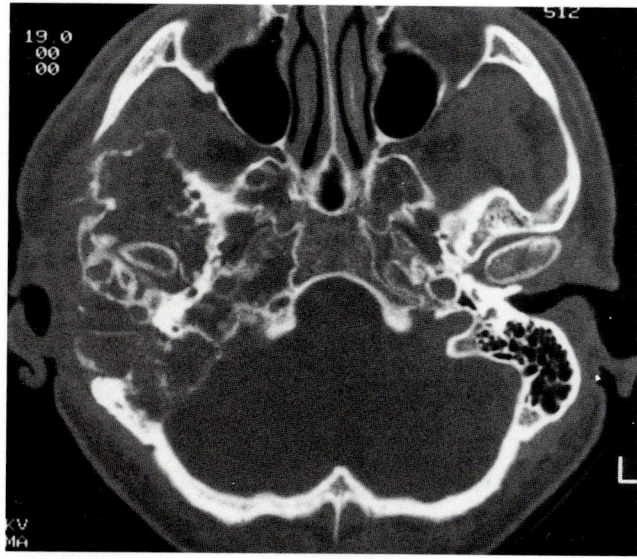

FIG. 17. Patient T.H.—**A, B:** Preoperative axial CT bone window algorithms, demonstrating widespread destruction of the right petrous and squamous temporal bone with myxoma invasion into the posterior and middle fossas.

Metastatic Atrial Myxoma (Patient T.H.)

This 34-year-old man presented with progressive right-sided hearing loss and swelling in the temple. Nine and three years previously he had undergone resection of osteomas from the mastoid area, and 4 years previously, resection of a left atrial myxoma. CT and MRI scans (Figs. 17 and 18) revealed a tumor involving the squamous and petrous temporal bone, encasing the petrous ICA. The jugular bulb and sigmoid sinus did not fill upon arteriography.

The tumor was removed completely in a piecemeal fashion during a single operation. It was vascular and cartilaginous in consistency (Fig. 19). The petrous ICA was injured and was repaired with a saphenous vein patch (Figs. 20 and 21). The ipsilateral CNs IX and X were resected, and a partially filling sigmoid sinus was occluded. CN VII was resected with tumor and was reconstructed with a 5-cm-long greater auricular nerve graft from the intracranial to the extracranial segment.

The patient developed a CSF leak from the cervical incision and meningitis with *E. coli.* He was successfully treated by wound reclosure, spinal drainage, and antibiotic therapy. A mild hemiparesis and ataxia resolved quickly. Swallowing difficulties required a temporary gastrostomy. The tumor was the solitary metastasis of the cardiac myxoma, presenting before the cardiac lesion. Twenty-eight months later, the patient had returned to his former occupation and had a House grade III facial function with no evidence of tumor recurrence (Figs. 22 and 23).

Osteogenic Sarcoma (Patient G.K.)

This 19-year-old woman was referred with a diagnosis of recurrent osteoblastoma of the temporal bone, having

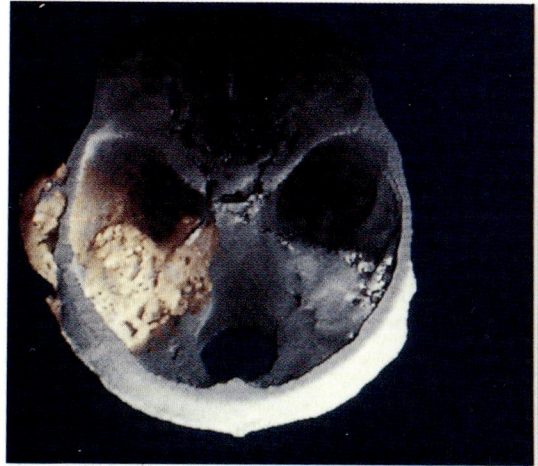 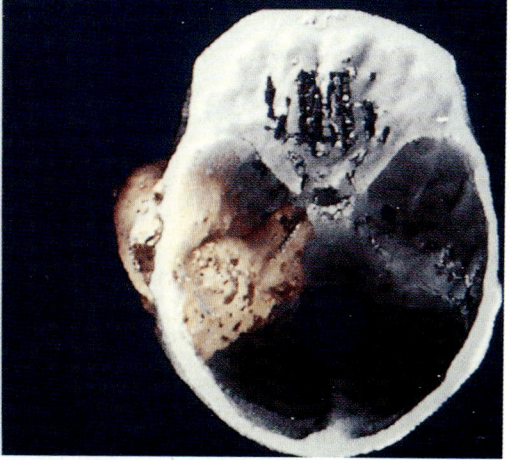

FIG. 18. Patient T.H.—Reconstructed three-dimensional CT looking from above, demonstrating the tumor in relation to the cranial anatomy.

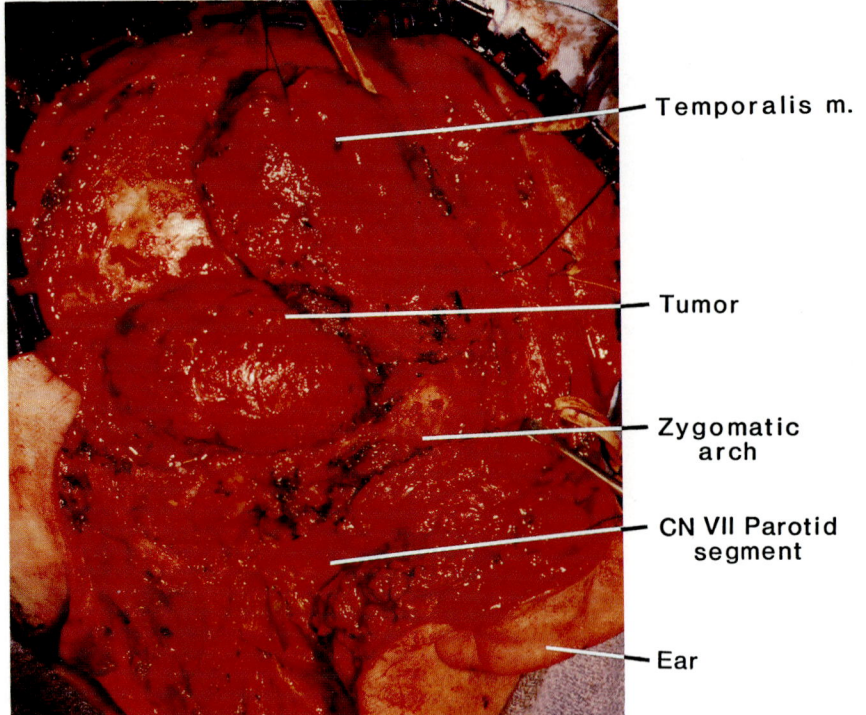

FIG. 19. Intraoperative microphotograph of patient T.H.

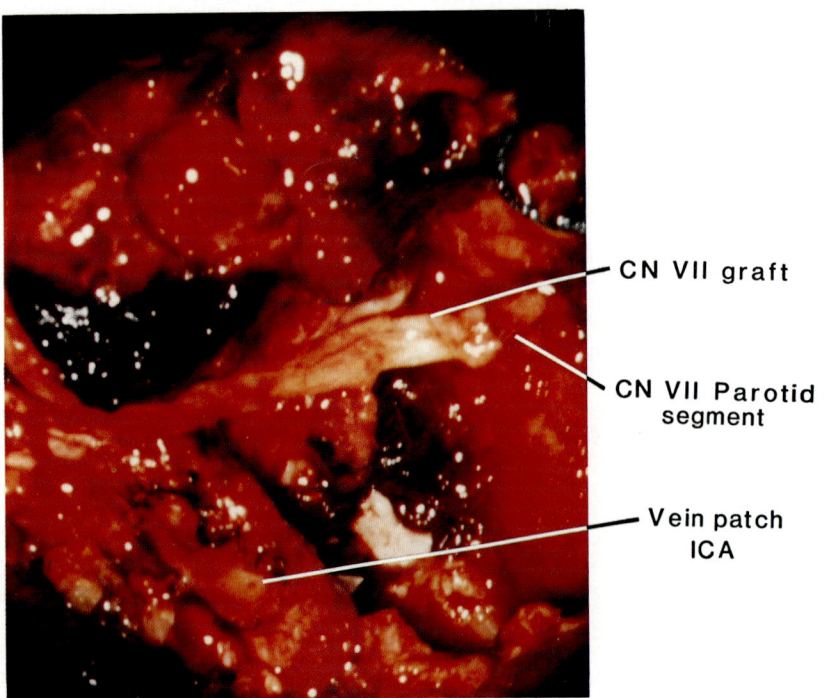

FIG. 20. Intraoperative microphotograph of patient T.H.

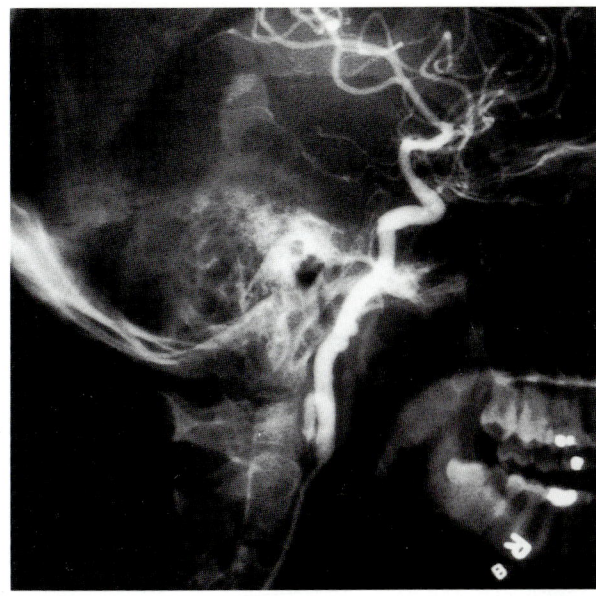

FIG. 21. Patient T.H.—Postoperatively, right ICA angiogram demonstrating smooth horizontal petrous segment contour following patch graft repair.

undergone two previous partial excisions and radiotherapy. CT and MRI scans revealed a large lesion of the petrous bone, mandibular condyle, sphenoid bone, and the middle cranial fossa (Fig. 24). The temporal lobe was edematous, with displacement of brain structures. Upon admission, the patient exhibited significant headaches and vomiting, a tender swelling of the temporal region, trismus, and deficits of CNs VIII, VII, V_2, and V_3. A metastatic workup was negative. She tolerated the BTO-ICA well and the ICA was occluded with a detachable balloon preoperatively.

The lesion was totally excised (Fig. 25) including a part of the cavernous sinus, the inferior temporal gyrus and CNs V_2, V_3, VII, and VIII. CN VII was reconstructed with a graft. The operative defect was repaired

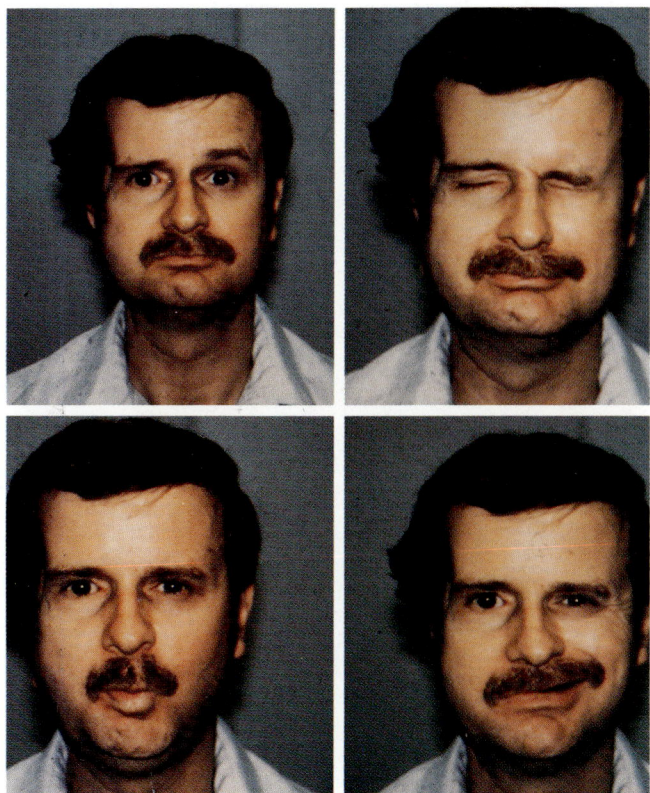

FIG. 22. Patient T.H. following the tumor resection.

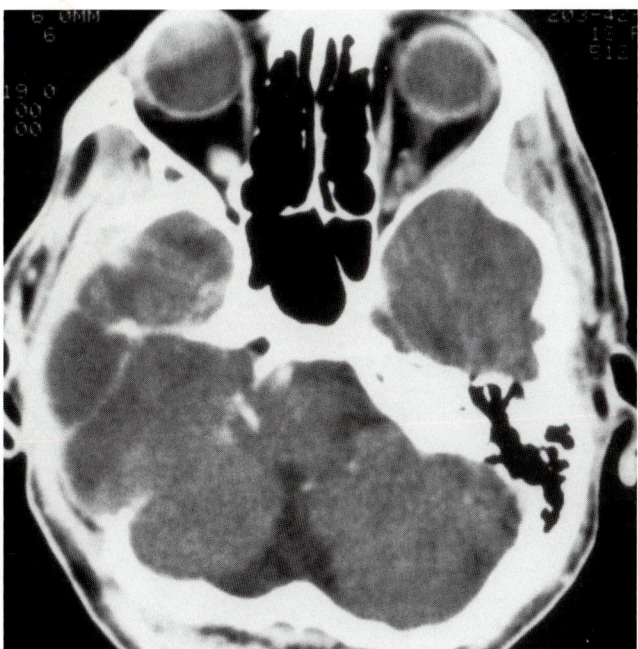

FIG. 23. Patient T.H.—Postoperative axial CT demonstrating petrous bone resection without evidence for tumor presence.

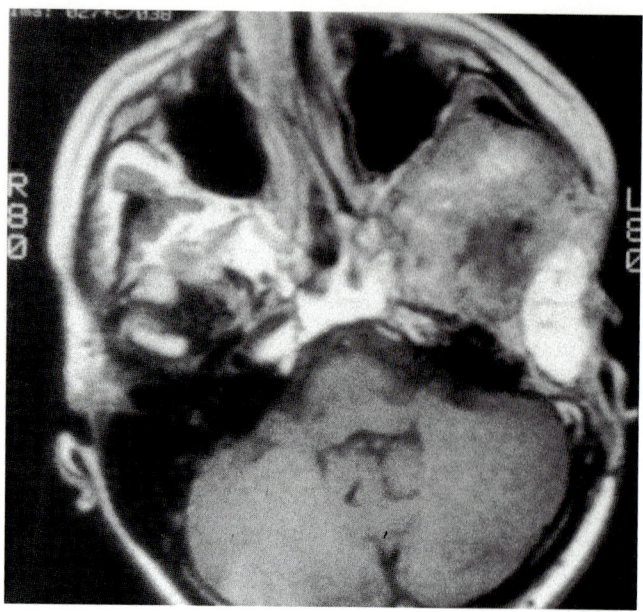

FIG. 24. Patient G.K.—Preoperative axial MRI demonstrating osteogenic sarcoma within petrous bone, middle fossa, and sphenoid wing.

with fascia lata, pericranium, and a rectus abdominis myocutaneous flap (Fig. 26). The final pathological diagnosis was osteogenic sarcoma, which corresponded to the biological behavior of the tumor.

Postoperative complications included a wound hematoma due to a fall while walking, staphylococcal septicemia, hepatitis, pneumonia, and depression. She was transferred back to her referring hospital (and country) 3 weeks postoperatively. At 7 months postoperatively, her facial function was improving and deficits of CNs VI, IX, and X were almost resolved.

Recommended chemotherapy was not initiated because of a disagreement about the pathological diagnosis. The disagreement resolved when pulmonary metastasis appeared 4 months later, but it was too late to treat the patient aggressively. One year later, the patient died, with tumor recurrence in the face and distant metastases.

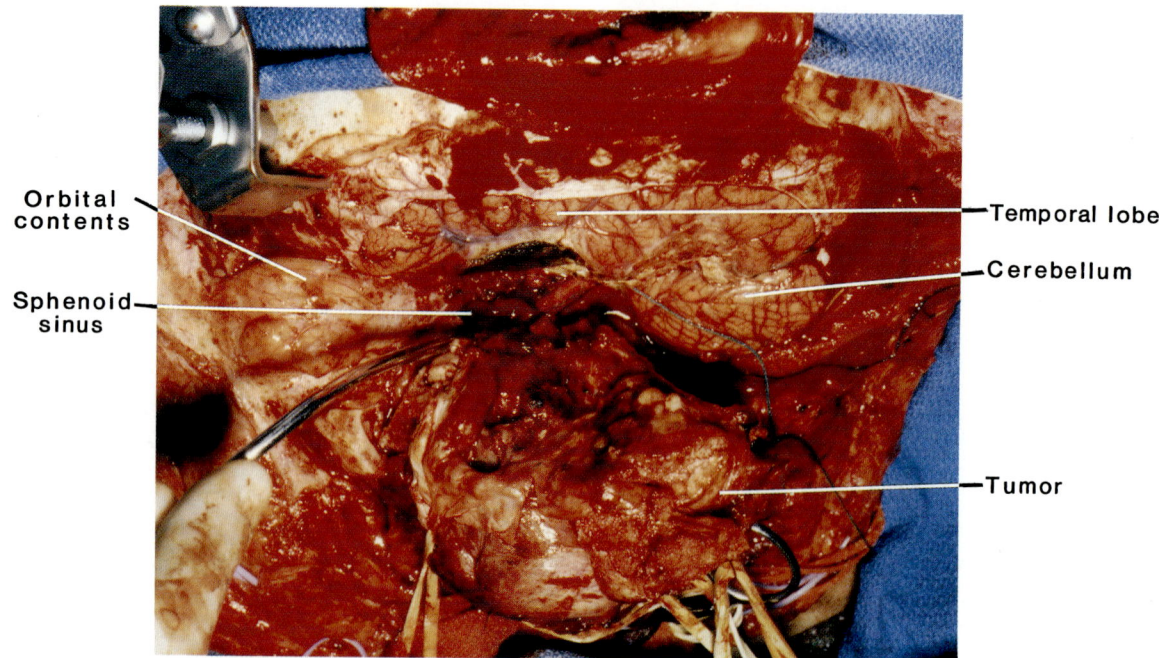

FIG. 25. Intraoperative microphotograph of patient G.K.

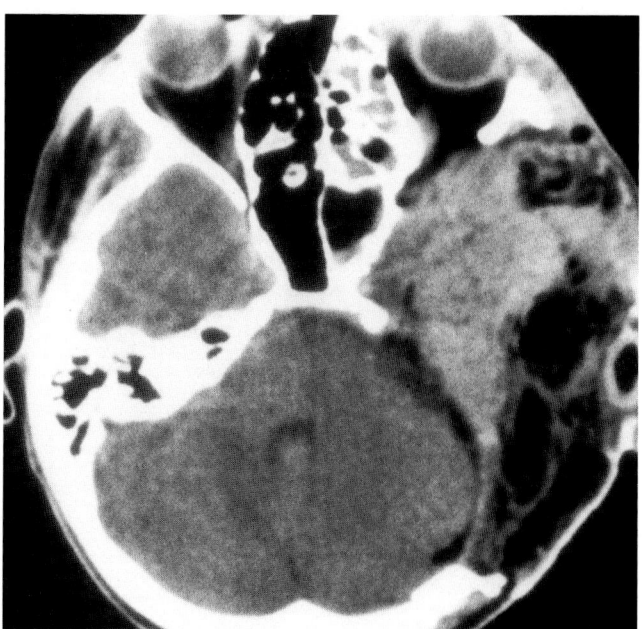

FIG. 26. Patient G.K.—Postoperative axial CT demonstrating resection of petrous bone with rectus abdominis muscle graft in middle fossa, petrous, and sphenoid wing area.

DISCUSSION

The prominent therapeutic limitations of nonsurgical treatment, with or without partial tumor resection of petrous bone tumors, have been demonstrated in squamous cell carcinoma (11,14,23,25,36), metastatic adenocarcinoma (27), salivary gland cancer (14), and benign glomus tumors (4,5,20,35,36). It has been shown in squamous cell carcinoma, the most common petrous bone tumor, that incomplete tumor resection is prognostic of a dismal outcome (40) with a 94% death or recurrence rate within 3 years. Therefore a major impetus exists for complete resection of petrous tumors, preferably with en bloc resection of malignant tumors in the Halstead tradition. Wagenfeld et al. (38), in a series of 25 primary petrous malignancies of various histologies and of limited spread, demonstrated that radical surgery with postoperative radiotherapy had the best outcome, with four of six patients alive at 4 years. Of their patients with primary radiotherapy and surgery for recurrence of residual disease, only 4 of 12 patients survived 4 years.

Historical Perspective

Parsons and Lewis (26), in 1954, pioneered en bloc tumor infiltrated petrous bone resection. Of their 11 resections, two patients died perioperatively and seven others had residual tumor. In 1966, Coleman (8) reported seven patients who underwent en bloc petrous bone malignancy resection with local rotation flap reconstruction. Massive blood loss was a central intraoperative problem; three patients died perioperatively, and one had recurrence of his tumor. Hilding and Selker (17), in 1969, reported a single case of well differentiated squamous cell carcinoma involving the external auditory canal and mastoid that underwent total en bloc petrous resection with a good long-term outcome. The authors attributed their success in complete tumor resection to prompt diagnosis following the appearance of symptoms, a multidisciplinary team approach, and adequate rotation flap reconstruction. In 1975, Lewis (23) reviewed 100 of his cases of limited en bloc petrous resection for cancer with a 5% perioperative mortality and 27% five-year cure rate. Ariyan et al. (2), in 1981, reported 9 patients who underwent petrous resections for squamous or basal cell carcinomas with no perioperative deaths, and five patients were free of disease at an average of 4 years postoperatively following "full course" postoperative irradiation. Graham et al. (15), in 1984, described two patients who underwent total en bloc resection of the temporal bone and carotid artery for cancer, following preoperative gradual occlusion of the ICA. In 1987, Schramm (28) and Sekhar et al. (31) presented overviews of the indications, technique, and complications of temporal bone resection, which have been developed and incorporated in the care of the present series of patients.

PRESENT SERIES: TECHNICAL LIMITATIONS

This present series includes 11 patients with total en bloc resection of the petrous bone, including wide resection of the involved and adjacent dura and brain, and all cranial nerves involved by the tumor. The infiltrated Labbé's vein was resected in three cases without any prolonged untoward results, and the transverse-sigmoid sinus complex was resected in 13 cases. The ICA was sacrificed in two cases and repaired in one. During these one-stage operations, the facial and accessory nerves were grafted and flap reconstructions were performed as needed.

The technical limits of surgery for petrous bone neoplasms are the danger of resecting an infiltrated dominant vertebral artery or sigmoid sinus (which could potentially be graft replaced) and, for malignancies, the inability to en bloc resect tumors extending multifocally or extensively unifocally beyond the petrous bone. More effective adjuvant therapy will be required to make substantial improvement in the outcome of patients with petrous bone malignancies. The greatest postoperative difficulty occurs when the function of CNs IX, X, and XII is lost, especially in older persons with decreased compensatory mechanisms.

Although these patients undergo extensive operations, evaluation of the functional status, using the Karnofsky scores, shows similar preoperative and postoperative lev-

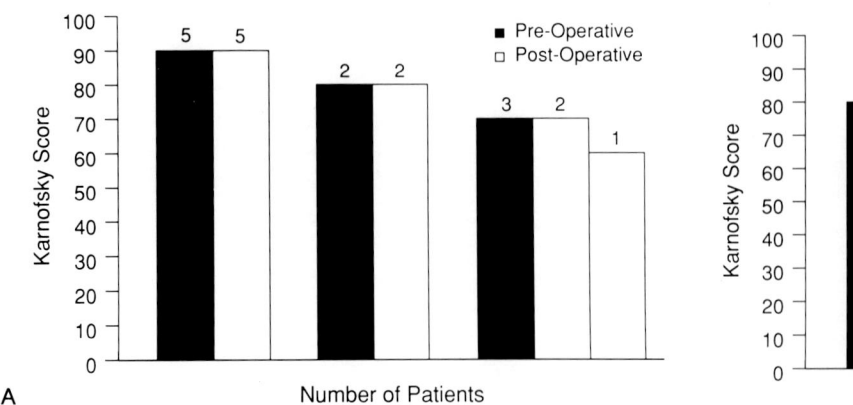
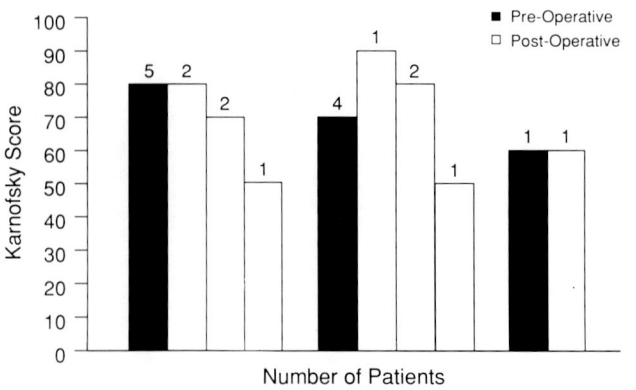

FIG. 27. Preoperative and postoperative Karnofsky functional scores. **A:** Benign and low-grade malignancies. **B:** High-grade malignancies.

els for patients with benign and low-grade malignant tumors. For high-grade malignancies, the postoperative Karnofsky scores vary with those scores that are relatively lower, due to a combination of perioperative complications and tumor recurrence (Fig. 27).

The Importance of Early Treatment

In our experience and in multiple publications (1,8–10,12,18,21,25,37), many patients with petrous bone tumors have had a long history of indicative symptoms. A negative correlation between the petrous bone region spread of malignancies and long-term outcome has been demonstrated (13,16,17). It is therefore imperative that the tumors be diagnosed and treated as early as possible.

A second aspect that may improve surgical outcome is meticulous evaluation of the thin-cut multiplane CT and MRI scans for tumor spread. In 1983, Lewis demonstrated that computerized tomography could help screen out those patients whose tumor was unresectable (24). Obviously, tumor beyond the resectable region precludes a surgical cure. We concur with Ariyan et al. (2) and Goodwin and Jesse (14) that following gross total resection, "full dose" appropriate adjuvant therapy is required.

CONCLUSION

Petrous bone resection, though a complicated procedure, can be safely performed today. A multidisciplinary approach and awareness of multiple possible postoperative difficulties are needed for optimal execution of this operation. Petrous bone resection is the definitive treatment of benign tumors and the effective mainstay of low-grade malignancies; its place for high-grade petrous malignancies is presently being defined.

REFERENCES

1. Arena S. Tumor surgery of the temporal bone. *Laryngoscope* 1974;84:645–670.
2. Ariyan S, Sasaki CT, Spencer D. Radical en bloc resection of the temporal bone. *Am J Surg* 1981;142:443–447.
3. Arriaga M, Hirsch BE, Kamerer DB. Squamous cell carcinoma of the external auditory meatus (canal). *Otolaryngol Head Neck Surg* 1989;101:330–337.
4. Belal A Jr, Sanna M. Pathology as it relates to ear surgery. I. Surgery of glomus tumours. *J Laryngol Otol* 1982;96:1079–1097.
5. Brammer RE, Graham MD, Kemink JL. Glomus tumors of the temporal bone: contemporary evaluation and therapy. *Otolaryngol Clin North Am* 1984;17:499–512.
6. Campbell E, Volk BM, Burklund CW. Total resection of temporal bone for malignancy of the middle ear. *Ann Surg* 1951;34:397–404.
7. Cannoni M, Pech A, Pellet W, et al. Techniques et indications des petrectomies reglees. Interet de l'association d'une voie transcochleaire et infra-temporale. *Ann Otolaryngol Chir Cervicofac* 1985;102:31–45.
8. Coleman CC Jr. Removal of the temporal bone for cancer. *Am J Surg* 1966;112:583–590.
9. Conley JJ, Novack AJ. The surgical treatment of malignant tumors of the ear and temporal bone. *Otolaryngol Head Neck Surg* 1960;71:635–651.
10. Fayemi OA, Toker C. Primary adenocarcinoma of the middle ear. *Otolaryngol Head Neck Surg* 1975;101:449–452.
11. Figi FA, Weisman PA. Cancer and chemodectoma in the middle ear and mastoid. *JAMA* 1954;156:1157–1162.
12. Fisch U, Fagan P, Valavanis A. The infratemporal fossa approach for the lateral skull base. *Otolaryngol Clin North Am* 1984;17:513–552.
13. Gacek RR, Goodman M. Management of malignancy of the temporal bone. *Laryngoscope* 1977;87:1622–1634.
14. Goodwin WJ, Jesse RH. Malignant neoplasms of the external auditory canal and temporal bone. *Otolaryngol Head Neck Surg* 1980;106:675–679.
15. Graham MD, Sataloff RT, Kemink JL, et al. Total en bloc resection of the temporal bone and carotid artery for malignant tumors of the ear and temporal bone. *Laryngoscope* 1984;94:528–533.
16. Hanna DC, Richardson GS, Gaisford JC. A suggested technic for resection of the temporal bone. *Am J Surg* 1967;114:553–558.
17. Hilding DA, Selker R. Total resection of the temporal bone for carcinoma. *Otolaryngol Head Neck Surg* 1969;89:636–645.
18. House WF, Hitselberger WE. The transcochlear approach to the skull base. *Otolaryngol Head Neck Surg* 1976;102:334–342.
19. Kaye AH, Hahn JF, Kinney SE, et al. Jugular foramen schwannomas. *J Neurosurg* 1984;60:1045–1053.
20. Kinney SE. Glomus jugulare tumor surgery with intracranial extension. *Otolaryngol Head Neck Surg* 1980;88:531–535.

21. Kumar A, Mafee M, Vassalli L, et al. Intracranial and intratemporal meningiomas with primary otologic symptoms. *Otolaryngol Head Neck Surg* 1988;99:444–454.
22. Lederman M. Malignant tumours of the ear. *Laryngol Otol* 1965;79:85–119.
23. Lewis JS. Temporal bone resection. Review of 100 cases. *Arch Otolaryngol* 1975;101:23–25.
24. Lewis JS. Surgical management of tumors of the middle ear and mastoid. *Laryngol Otol* 1983;97:299–311.
25. Lewis JS, Page R. Radical surgery for malignant tumors of the ear. *Otolaryngol Head Neck Surg* 1966;83:114–119.
26. Parsons H, Lewis JS. Subtotal resection of the temporal bone for cancer of the ear. *Cancer* 1954;5:995–1001.
27. Sekhar LN, Pomeranz S, Janecka IP, Hirsch B, Ramastry S. Temporal bone neoplasms: A report on 20 surgically treated cases. *J Neurosurg* (in press).
28. Schramm VL Jr. Temporal bone resection. In: Sekhar LN, Schramm VL Jr, eds. *Tumors of the cranial base: diagnosis and treatment.* Mount Kisco, NY: Futura Publishing 1987;683–698.
29. Sekhar LN, Estonillo R. Transtemporal approach to the skull base: an anatomical study. *Neurosurgery* 1986;19:799–808.
30. Sekhar LN, Schramm VL Jr, Jones NF. Operative management of large neoplasms of the lateral and posterior cranial base. In: Sekhar LN, Schramm VL Jr, eds. *Tumors of the cranial base: diagnosis and treatment.* Mount Kisco, NY: Futura Publishing, 1987; 655–682.
31. Sekhar LN, Schramm VL Jr, Jones NF. Subtemporal–preauricular–infratemporal fossa approach to large lateral and posterior cranial base neoplasms. *J Neurosurg* 1987;67:488–499.
32. Sekhar LN, Schramm VL Jr, Jones NF, et al. Operative exposure and management of the petrous and upper cervical internal carotid artery. *Neurosurgery* 1986;19:967–982.
33. Sekhar LN, Janecka IP, Jones NF. Subtemporal–infratemporal and basal subfrontal approach to extensive cranial base tumours. *Acta Neurochir* 1988;92:83–92.
34. Sekhar LN, Sen CN, Jho HD. Saphenous vein graft bypass of the cavernous internal carotid artery. *Neurosurgery* 1990;72:35–41.
35. Spector GJ, Fierstein J, Ocura JH. A comparison of therapeutic modalities of glomus tumors in the temporal bone. *Laryngoscope* 1976;86:690–696.
36. Spector GJ, Sobol S. Surgery for glomus tumors at the skull base. *Otolaryngol Head Neck Surg* 1980;88:524–530.
37. Tucker WN. Cancer of the middle ear. A review of 89 cases. *Cancer* 1965;18:642–650.
38. Wagenfeld DJH, Keane T, Van Nostrand AWP, et al. Primary carcinoma involving the temporal bone: analysis of twenty-five cases. *Laryngoscope* 1980;90:912–919.
39. Ward GE, Loch WE, Lawrence W Jr. Radical operation for carcinoma of the external auditory canal and middle ear. *Am J Surg* 1951;82:169–178.
40. Zieske LA, Johnson JT, Myers EN, et al. Squamous cell carcinoma with positive margins. *Otolaryngol Head Neck Surg* 1986; 112:863–866.

CHAPTER 22

The Transsphenoidal Approach to Invasive Sellar and Clival Lesions

Rudolf Fahlbusch and Michael Buchfelder

The principles of modern transsphenoidal microsurgery of the sellar and clival region are based on the early operative techniques of the surgeons Schloffer, from Innsbruck (1906), and Hirsch, from Vienna (1910). Harvey Cushing and Norman Dott pioneered and refined the sublabial–transseptal approach and established its routine use in the 1930s. A renaissance of the technique occurred following the introduction of intraoperative fluoroscopy, the use of the operating microscope, and the development of a selective operative procedure for the removal of pituitary adenomas by Gerard Guiot and Jules Hardy.

SPECIFIC DIAGNOSTIC CONSIDERATIONS

Magnetic resonance imaging (MRI) of the sellar region and sphenoid sinus is the most helpful test in the neuroradiological workup of patients with invasive sellar and clival tumors. MRI not only depicts tumor size, extension, and tumor characteristics such as hemorrhagic and cystic changes, but it also helps to delineate the tumor from the surrounding anatomical structures. Even if MR angiography is not available, the position of the carotid artery is in most instances sufficiently depicted by the coronal MRI so that no carotid angiography is required. The relationship of the tumor to the osseous structures is best depicted, however, by computed tomography (CT). Conventional x-rays of the skull document the size and shape of the sella and provide information about the structure of the nasal and sphenoidal septae.

Visual compromise develops only if the suprasellar tumor extension is more than 15 mm above the plane of the diaphragma sellae. Assessment of visual fields and visual acuity are only useful in cases with suprasellar tumor extension. Parasellar tumor extension sometimes leads to palsies of cranial nerves (CNs) III, IV, and VI. However, acutely developing intrasellar lesions with only minor parasellar extension such as pituitary adenoma hemorrhage and infarction may also provoke palsies of CNs III, IV, and VI. The trigeminal nerve is rarely involved in parasellar tumors, which are amenable to surgery via the transsphenoidal route.

Endocrine workup is mandatory as soon as the pituitary fossa or gland is involved in the pathological process. Anterior pituitary function and a possible hormonal activity of the pituitary adenoma are assessed by separate dynamic tests. The authors have routinely used a combined pituitary stimulation test consisting of bolus injection of LRH, TRH, and ACTH to rule out or document hypopituitarism necessitating hormonal replacement therapy. While prolactin secreting tumors are identified by the determination of basal serum prolactin levels, a battery of tests is required to better define other hypersecretory states, such as acromegaly and Cushing's disease. Glycoprotein-hormone secreting adenomas are extremely rare and their preoperative endocrine workup has not yet been standardized.

PATIENT SELECTION

The transsphenoidal operation is preferentially used for the operative resection of pituitary adenomas. About 90% of all pituitary adenomas in the author's department, namely, all intrasellar tumors and those with symmetrical suprasellar extension, were operated via this ap-

R. Fahlbusch and M. Buchfelder: Neurosurgical Department, University of Erlangen–Nürnberg, D 8520 Erlangen, Germany.

proach. However, asymmetrically growing tumors are also amenable to this operative technique, provided that the sella is large enough to enable proper access to the lesion. Generally, invasive tumors and those cases with tumors primarily developed outside the sella should be treated via a transcranial–intradural approach. Transsphenoidal surgery is strictly contraindicated in those suprasellar tumors that lack a proper "tumor capsule" and those growing diffusely into the cranial cavity. These tumors may be preoperatively recognized as large suprasellar lesions that lack a correspondingly adequate visual compromise and do not exhibit an elevation of the A1 segment of the anterior cerebral arteries on MR or conventional angiography. Transsphenoidal operations are also contraindicated in patients with acute inflammations of the nasal sinuses. For large tumors extending into the cranial cavity and/or cranial base, the combination of a transsphenoidal and transcranial operation may be necessary to achieve the most radical resection possible. Both operations may be performed within 2–3 weeks of each other, preferably starting with the transsphenoidal operation. Transsphenoidal surgery for pituitary adenomas is still indicated in most of the symptomatic and asymptomatic lesions although prolactinomas may alternatively undergo a trial of medical therapy with dopamine agonists. The transsphenoidal operation is also a suitable approach for lesions arising from the sphenoidal sinus or upper clivus, irrespective of whether they are invasive into the sphenoid sinus or not.

OPERATIVE TECHNIQUE

Anesthetic Considerations

Transsphenoidal surgery is routinely carried out under general anesthesia and oral endotracheal intubation. Controlled ventilation is required for ideal operating conditions. The endotracheal tube is fixed in the (left) lateral corner of the mouth and a gauze pack is inserted between the teeth to protect the tube. A gauze tampon is inserted into the pharynx. Hypertension should be avoided to reduce bleeding from the oral and nasal mucosa. Arterial blood pressure and electrocardiogram are monitored.

Patient Position

We prefer Cushing's original method, where the patient is placed in the supine position and the surgeon is standing behind the patient's head, to the semisitting position used by Guiot and Hardy. The patient's neck is extended slightly 10°–15° but initially not rotated (Fig. 1). We do not employ fixation of the head at any stage of the operation so that the head may easily be rotated whenever required. If excessive venous bleeding occurs,

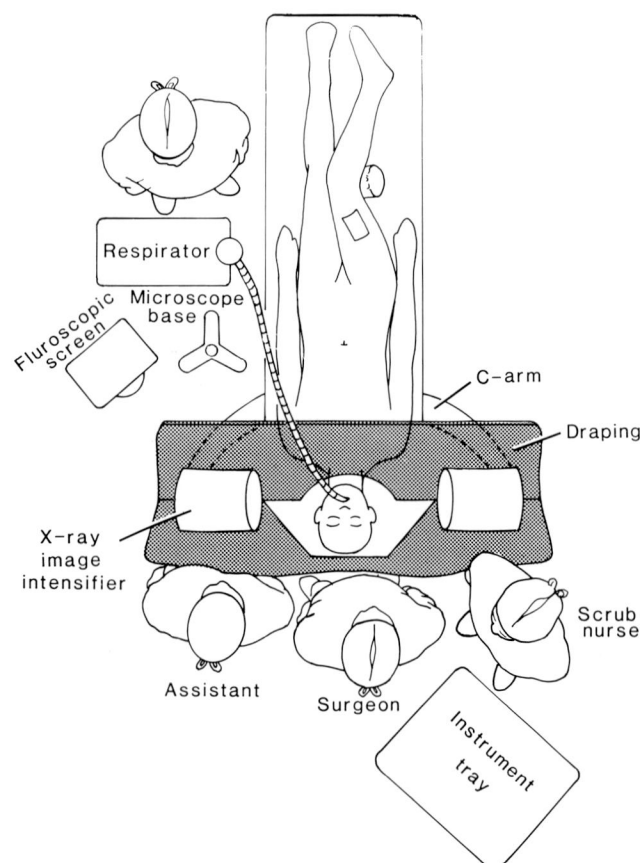

FIG. 1. Diagram of operation room arrangement for transsphenoidal surgery (modified Cushing approach).

the head may be slightly elevated. Draping is performed by using three towels, corresponding to a craniotomy. One towel is placed around the head and the others above and below this plane. Finally, only a small quadratic field above the upper lip and below the nose is exposed (Fig. 2). Michel clips are used for fixation in each corner. The assistant stands to the surgeon's left and the scrub nurse to the surgeon's right. The C-arm of the x-ray image-intensifier is placed below the operating table (Fig. 1). Care is taken to obtain a strictly lateral projection. The patient's right leg is slightly flexed at the hip and knee and is rotated internally to enable access to the lateral thigh for the simultaneous removal of a fascia lata graft. Draping of this operative field is performed separately from the nasal area. The operating microscope comes into place from the left side of the surgeon.

Surgery

Prior to the operation, the mucosa of the vestibulum oris and the nasal mucosa on both sides of the cartilaginous nasal septum are infiltrated with a ornipressin solution diluted in saline in order to lessen bleeding and to facilitate dissection of the mucosa from the septum.

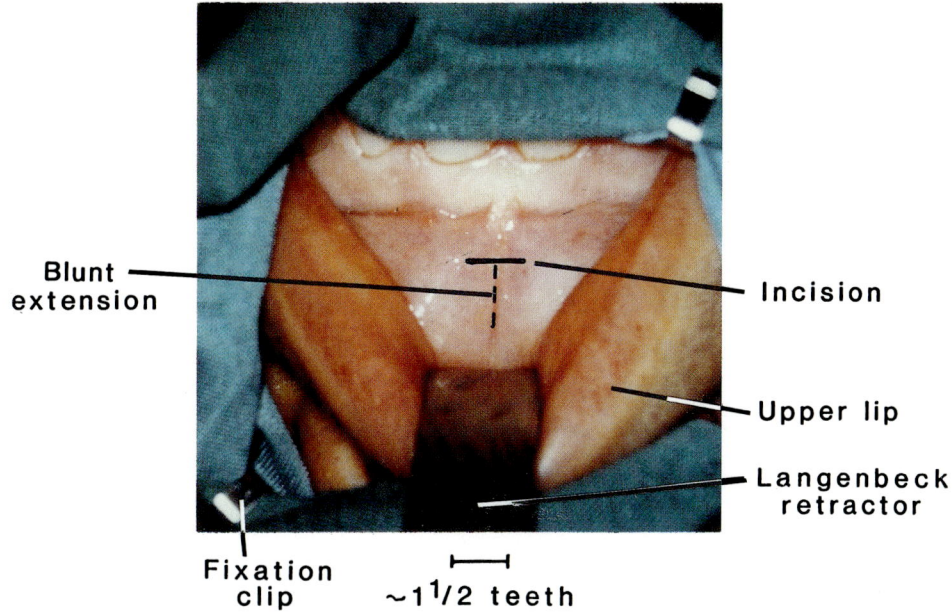

FIG. 2. Sublabial–paraseptal approach: incision of the mucosa.

The operation may start with either a sublabial or a medial nasal mucosal incision. The latter should be restricted to patients with large nostrils and small or medium-sized tumors.

When the sublabial incision is chosen (Fig. 2), the upper lip is retracted by the assistant using a small Langenbeck retractor. The horizontal incision is only 3–4 mm long and is bluntly extended in the form of a T (dotted line). The upper margin of the nasal cartilage is identified and mucosa and perichondrium are bluntly detached from the cartilaginous nasal septum until a pouch has been created (Fig. 3). The cartilaginous septum is then incised parallel to the nasal floor just at the border of the osseous nasal septum or the osseous basal rim. Basally, the mucosa is usually very adherent to the maxilla, and careful, blunt, and sometimes sharp dissection are needed to avoid tears of the basal mucosa.

In the perinasal approach (Fig. 4), the medial nasal mucosa is incised about 10 mm below the opening of the nasal orifice until the nasal cartilage is exposed. The mu-

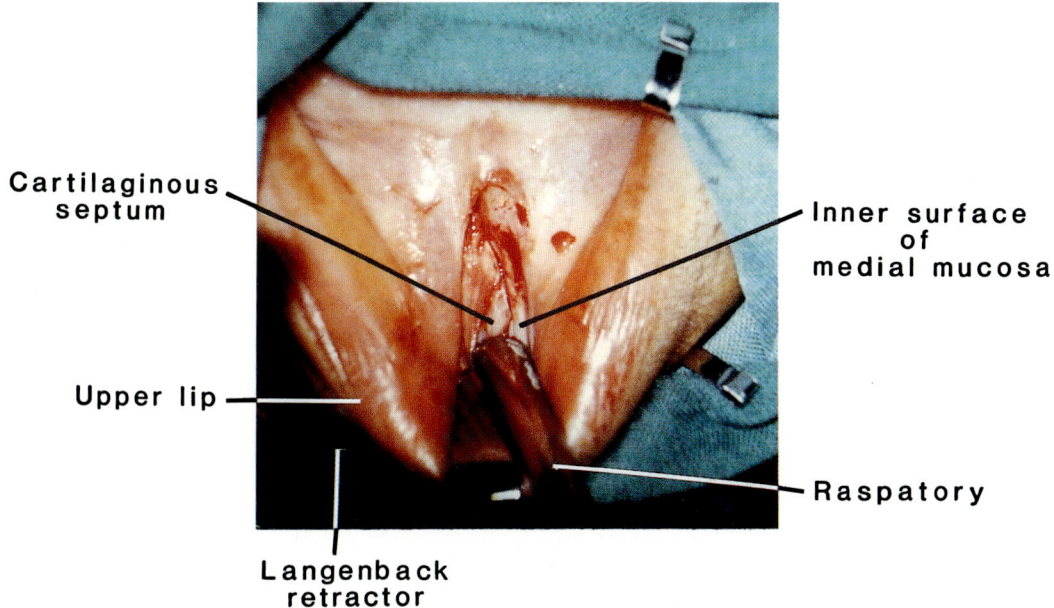

FIG. 3. Sublabial–paraseptal approach: dissection of a mucocartilaginous tunnel.

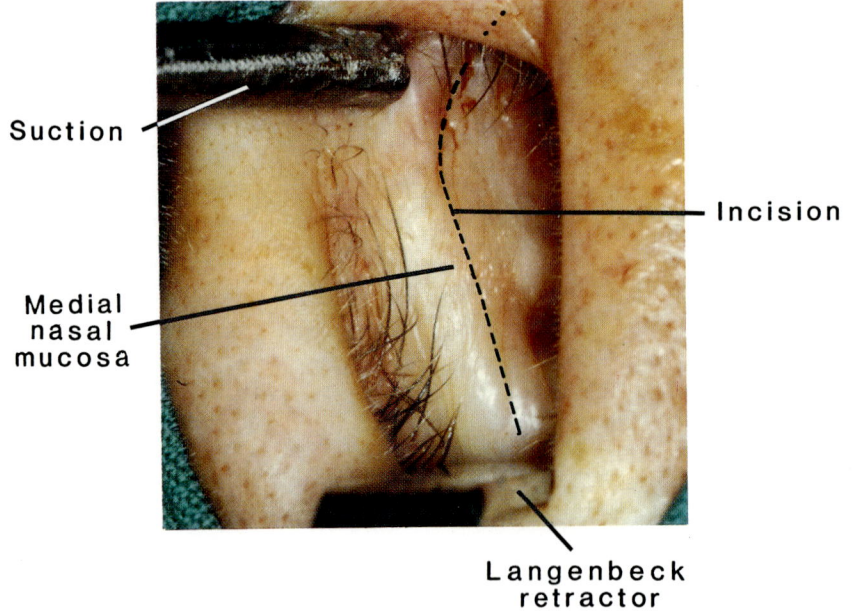

FIG. 4. Pernasal paraseptal approach: incision of the mucosa.

cosa is separated from the nasal cartilage in the subperichondral cleavage plane by blunt dissection until a pouch is created.

Beyond this stage, the operative technique is identical for both the sublabial and perinasal approach. The mucosa and perichondrium are gently detached from the cartilaginous and osseous nasal septum. To avoid tears in the nasal mucosa, attention should be paid to a septal deviation, which must be expected in almost all individuals.

The cartilaginous septum is separated from the osseous nasal septum and the mucosa is also gently detached from the contralateral side of the septum. The osseous septum is partly resected. In cases with a thin bony septum, this may be broken basally just below the floor of the sphenoid sinus. At this stage, the blunt, slender, conical nasal speculum is inserted into the muco-osseous tunnel (Fig. 5). It is cautiously opened above the base of the nasal septum, which appears "keel-shaped" (Fig. 6). Midline orientation is provided by an imaginary line drawn between the anterior nasal spine and the base of the osseous nasal septum (vomer). The anterior nasal spine is resected in order to enable better visualization of the dorsal sphenoidal sinus, clivus, and posterior sella floor. Bleeding from vessels of the mucosa is mostly encountered basally close to the vomer and necessitates coagulation of the arteries. Bleeding from bone is controlled by slight pressure of a fast rotating diamond burr or by applying bone wax.

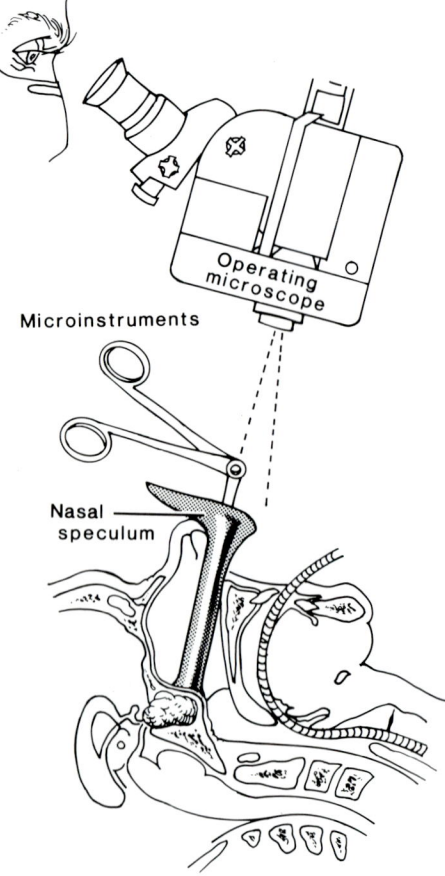

FIG. 5. Insertion of the nasal speculum.

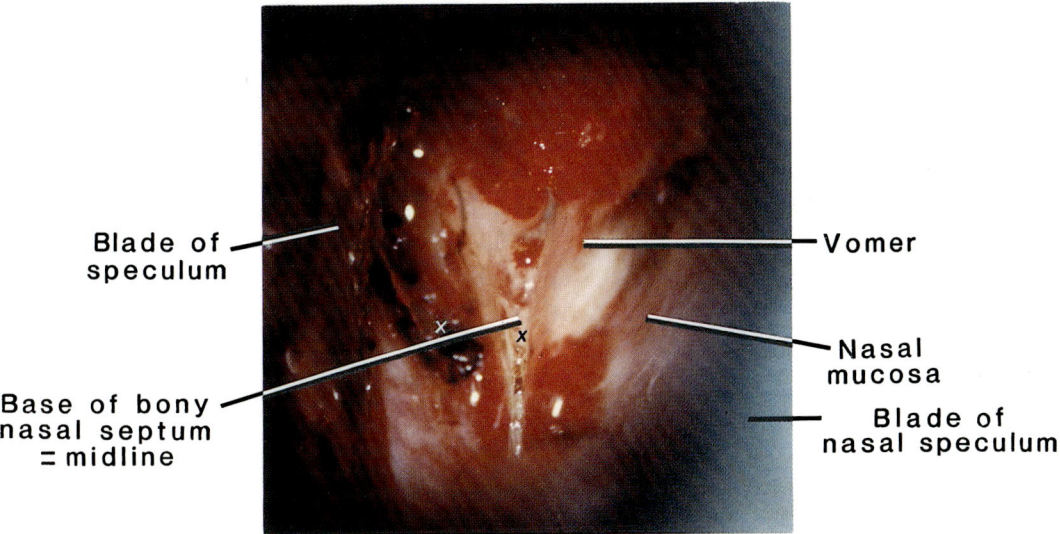

FIG. 6. Typical appearance of the vomer.

In patients who have had ENT operations for nasal septum deviation or previous transsphenoidal surgery, a considerable nasal septum defect may have resulted, which makes a strictly paraseptal approach impossible. In such cases, it is usually easier to initially insert the nasal speculum deep into one nasal cavity up to the vomer under fluoroscopic control. The speculum is opened and the medial nasal mucosa is incised at the level of the sphenoid sinus floor. The operating microscope is used. Since the remnants of the bony nasal septum are usually fragile, the perpendicular lamina of the vomer is easily fractured and thus the nasal speculum is brought into a midline position.

If the floor of the sphenoid sinus is thin, it can be opened by gripping the vomer with a robust forceps and fracturing by rotation of the instrument, preferably in the region of the anterior ostium (Fig. 7). This opening is enlarged by a rongeur or a drill. In patients with a thick

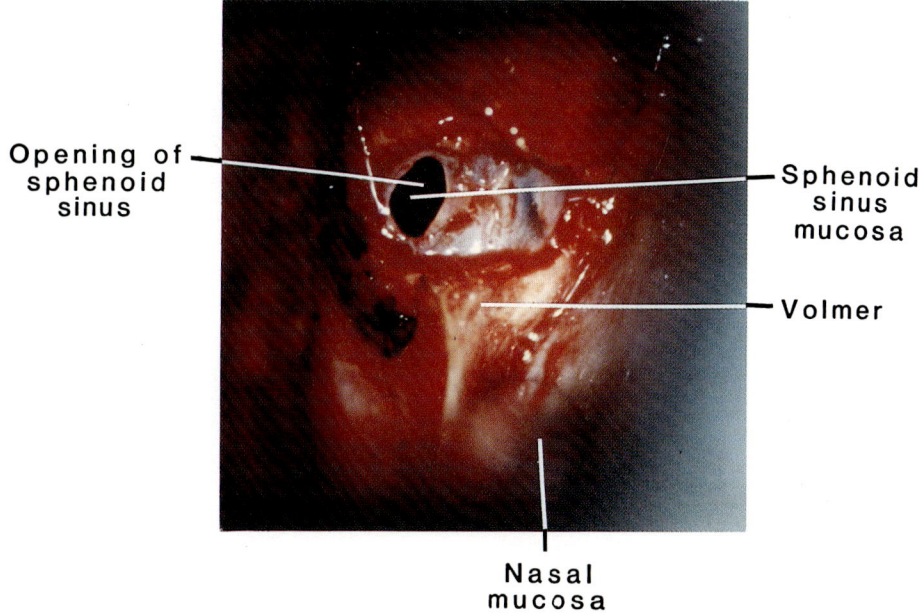

FIG. 7. Opening of the sphenoid sinus.

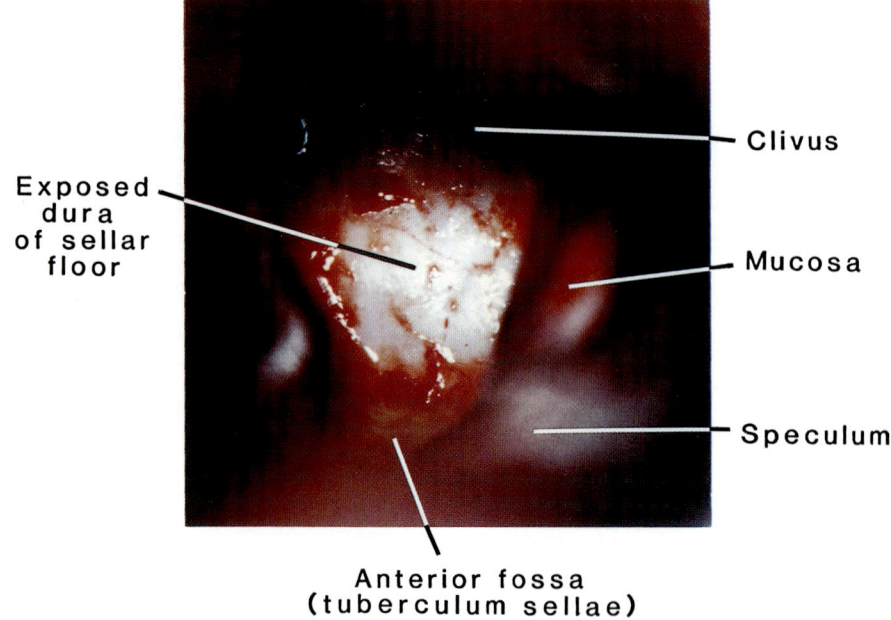

FIG. 8. The endosteum before incision.

floor of the sphenoid sinus, the bone is eroded away by using a cutting drill. As soon as the sphenoid sinus is opened, the operating microscope is brought into use. Septae of the sphenoid sinus are frequently found and are usually asymmetrically developed. They are resected with a rongeur or a diamond burr. The mucosa is also carefully and completely resected so as to prevent a sphenoid sinus mucocele. The sphenoid sinus is then packed with cotton patties soaked in hydrogen peroxide for a few minutes (hemostasis and disinfection). Adequate exposure of an enlarged sella by a sufficient opening of the sphenoid sinus is considered mandatory for a safe surgical procedure. Attention should be paid to the carotid artery canal, which may protrude into the posterior sphenoid sinus. In most cases of pituitary adenomas with an enlarged sella, the sella floor is thinned out and very fragile so that it can easily be removed with a bone rongeur. The white endosteum comes into view (Fig. 8). It should not be opened until complete resection of the bony sellar floor has been accomplished. In cases with a

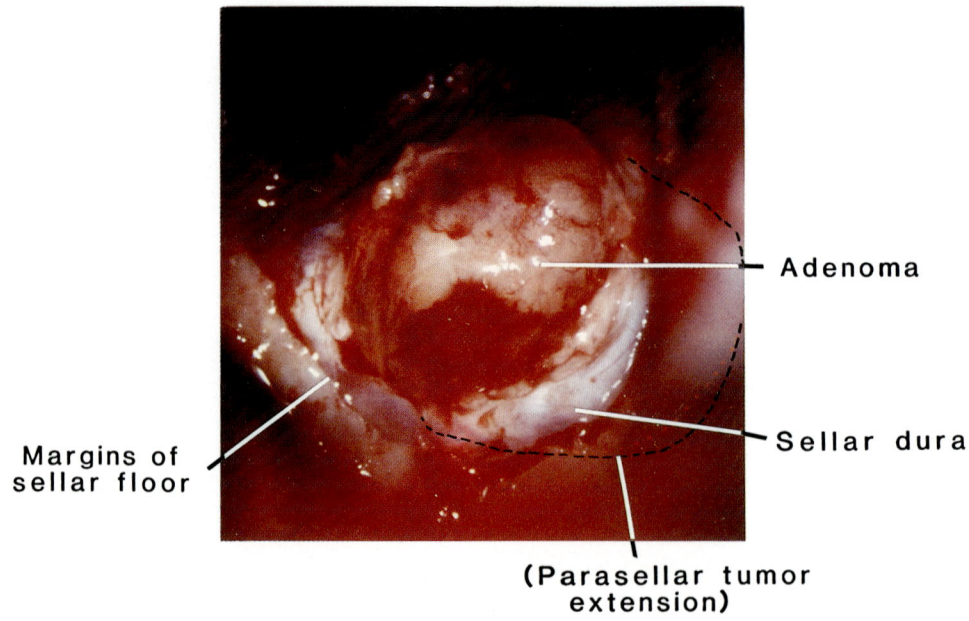

FIG. 9. Typical appearance of a pituitary macroadenoma just after cruciate incision of the endosteum.

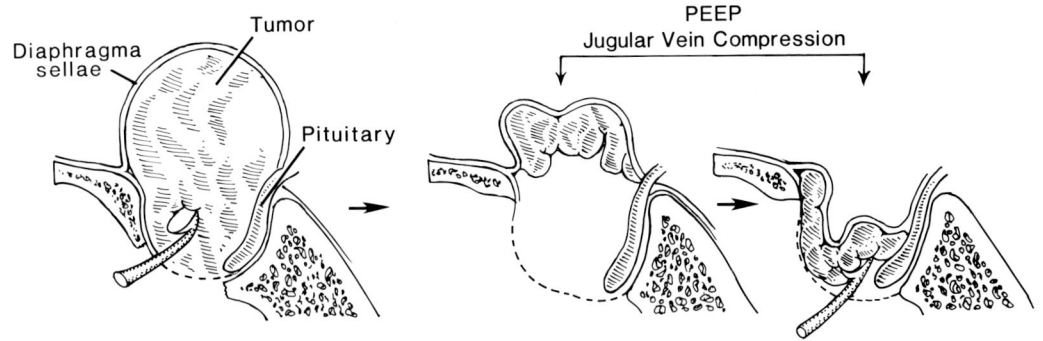

FIG. 10. Removal of a suprasellar adenoma by resection of the intrasellar portion and increase of intracranial pressure.

normal pituitary fossa, which is only 12 mm wide in the coronal plane, a diamond burr is preferred to remove the anterior wall of the sella. The diamond burr is particularly useful to generously extend the opening of the fossa toward the sphenoid sinus. The sellar dura (endosteum) is opened in a cruciate fashion. Transverse intercavernous sinuses may cause bleeding, particularly in a normal-sized sella, but this is usually controlled by extensive bipolar coagulation. Venous bleeding after incision of the sellar dura may also be stopped by coagulation or may require compression by Gelfoam. In macroadenomas, soft tumor material extrudes spontaneously through the opening of the endosteum (Fig. 9). The adenoma is then removed by systematic, stepwise curettage from all parts of the sella. Tumors perforating the sellar floor and invading the sphenoid sinus are removed in the same manner. However, one should always attempt to identify remnants of the sellar floor and intact residual sellar dura. Tumor removal should be done after this plane of cleavage has been located. In suprasellar extending adenomas, curettage is also performed within and lateral to the sella in order to allow the suprasellar portion to descend. The residual pituitary tissue is usually identified in the posterior aspect of the sella or preserved as a thin layer below the diaphragma sellae but may also be displaced laterally adjacent to the wall of the cavernous sinus. In most instances, suprasellar tumor portions automatically descend into the sella after removal of the sellar contents (Fig. 10). This process may be accelerated by an increase of the intracranial pressure mediated by bilateral jugular vein compression and PEEP ventilation (8–12 cm H_2O).

Adenomas with extensive lateral displacement of the cavernous sinus require a lateral curettage, which, in the author's series, was commonly extended as far as 2–3 cm from the midline (Fig. 11) and occasionally even further. Bleeding from lacerations of the medial wall is commonly encountered in parasellar adenomas but generally does not present a serious surgical problem. In most cases, bleeding is easily controlled by gentle compression with Gelfoam. In cases of parasellar invasion, the tumor resection may be extended into the cavernous sinus. Suction and curettage are applied to remove tumor tissue from the trabecular system, which can be visualized if the sella turcica is sufficiently enlarged. Care must be taken not to injure the carotid artery, which is sometimes in contact with the intrasellar dura and may be felt to pulsate. After satisfactory removal of the tumor, complete hemostasis is achieved by coagulation, and compression by Gelfoam, and with cotton patties soaked in hydrogen peroxide.

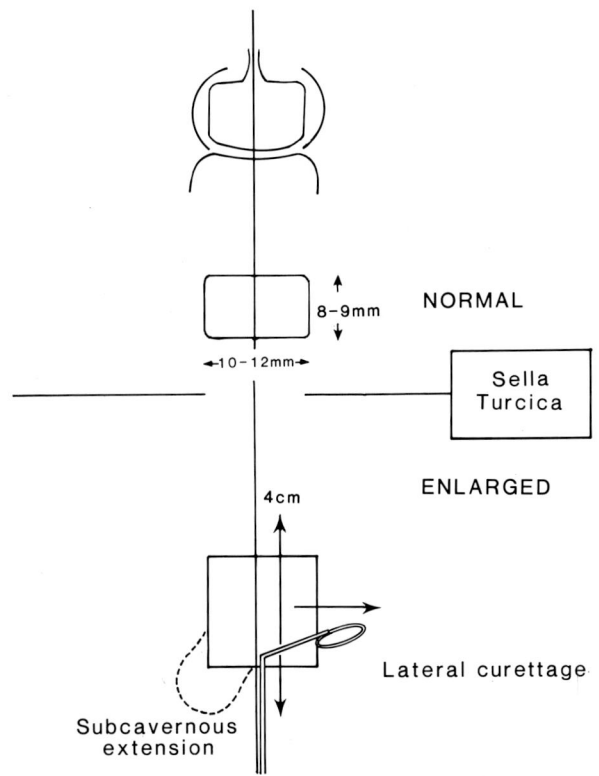

FIG. 11. Removal of a parasellar adenoma by lateral curettage and size relation of a normal and enlarged sella.

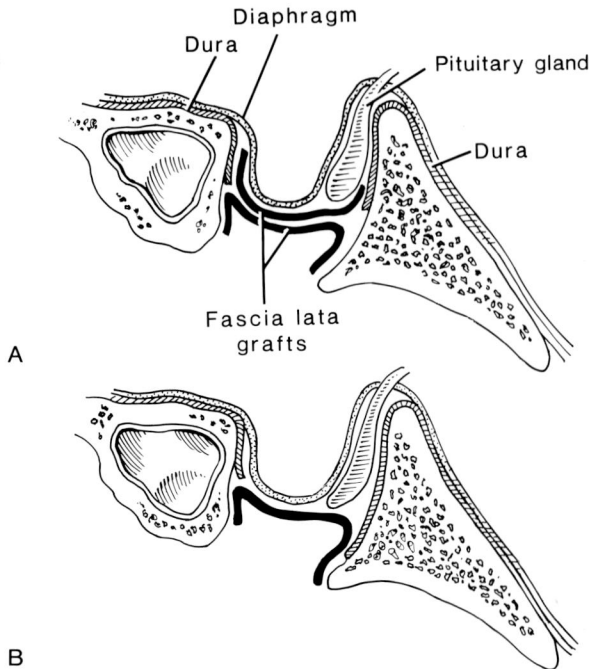

FIG. 12. Closure of the operative field by a fascia lata graft. **A:** In the event of intraoperative CSF leakage fascia lata is inserted in two layers: below and above the level of the endosteal margins. **B:** Closure by a single layer graft.

In cases with a thin diaphragma sellae, and whenever intraoperative cerebrospinal fluid (CSF) leakage was observed, a small piece of fascia lata from the lateral thigh is used to cover the diaphragm in two layers (Fig. 12). The fascia should be about twice the size of the operative field. It is gently placed onto the diaphragm and is not used to raise the herniated arachnoid membrane since any foreign tissue within the sella will render the interpretation of a postoperative CT or MRI examination more difficult. In cases where the remaining bony structures do not provide adequate support for the descended diaphragm (e.g., in giant invasive adenomas), fat and/or muscle may be inserted into the sphenoid sinus to prevent rebleeding.

The incision in the vestibulum oris is sutured with resorbable sutures (Dexon 3-0). For suturing the incision in the medial nasal mucosa or any mucosal tears, Vicryl 4-0 is used. A tampon consisting of vaseline impregnated gauze is inserted into both nasal cavities and left for 24 hr.

POSTOPERATIVE MANAGEMENT

The patients routinely go to the recovery room for 2–4 hr. Intensive care is usually not necessary after transsphenoidal surgery and is reserved for severely ill patients with increased risk factors, for example, those suffering from Cushing's disease. The nasal tampon is removed 24 hr after the end of the operation. Rarely, bleeding from the nose after removal of the tampon requires retamponing. Spontaneous rebleeds originating from larger branches of the ethmoidal arteries are extremely rare but may in some instances require reopening of the wound and coagulation of the respective artery.

In order to reduce swelling of the nasal mucosa, vasoconstrictory agents ("nose drops") are applied 7 times a day for 5 days. Subsequently, a nasal fatty emulsion is used for 1–2 weeks to prevent atrophic rhinitis.

In the case of a perioperative CSF leakage, drainage of 15–20 ml of CSF three times daily, via an intrathecally implanted lumbar catheter or via repeat lumbar punctures for three days, is performed to reduce intracranial CSF pressure. Patients who are found to have secondary adrenocortical failure prior to surgery routinely receive substitution therapy with hydrocortisone intraoperatively and postoperatively, starting with a dose of 100 mg hydrocortisone over 24 hr administered via a perfusor during the day of surgery. The daily dose is then gradually reduced to 80 mg (1st postoperative day), 70 mg (2nd day), 60 mg (3rd day), 50 mg (4th day), 40 mg (5th day), 30 mg (6th day), and finally to the maintenance dose of 25 mg (10-5-5-5) from the 7th postoperative day. Perioperative substitution therapy with thyroid hormones was not found to be necessary. However, substitution therapy with thyroid hormones and sex steroids was started as soon as a deficiency was documented by dynamic endocrine testing and continued from the first postoperative day. Routine postoperative endocrine testing was repeated 1 week and 2–3 months after surgery, during normal patient follow-up.

Diabetes insipidus may become evident within 2 days after transsphenoidal surgery. A total urine output up to 3000 ml/24 hr may be tolerated on the day of surgery or the first postoperative day. DDAVP (desmopressin acetate) requires intramuscular administration in cases where the urinary output is greater than 2500 ml/24 hr after the first postoperative day and when the specific gravity is below 1005. The nasal mucosa will usually have recovered sufficiently for the nasal administration of DDAVP from the 5th or 6th postoperative day.

The authors have not routinely used antibiotics except for patients with acute inflammatory disorders who need to have surgery urgently, and for patients with a deficient immune system, such as those with Cushing's disease. In cases of febrile sinusitis, usually tetracyclines were given, even if no abnormality was observed on the x-ray views of the nasal sinuses.

The patients can usually be mobilized within a few hours after surgery and may soon get up for a few minutes. They are practically fully mobilized as of the 1st or 2nd postoperative day so that low-dose heparinization need only be employed in patients with Cushing's disease.

COMPLICATIONS AND MANAGEMENT

The most important complications of transsphenoidal surgery, namely, meningitis and CSF fistula, occur in less than 1% of the patients operated on for pituitary adenomas. Early postoperative rhinorrhea is usually stopped by a lumbar drainage of 45–60 ml for 3–4 days but requires reoperation if it does persist. The mucous channel is reopened and the previous operative field displayed. An attempt is made to visualize the fistula. The defect is covered by a fresh fascia lata graft and thereafter lumbar CSF is routinely drained as described previously. If no distinct fistula is identified, the whole region of exposure is covered by a fascia lata graft and the sphenoid sinus is additionally packed with fat or muscle. Meningitis requires antibiotic treatment. A rebleeding must be suspected if severe headache associated with deterioration of vision occurs postoperatively. It requires evacuation of the hematoma by reusing the transsphenoidal approach and careful hemostasis. Ocular nerve palsies occurring after transsphenoidal resection of parasellar pituitary adenomas have, in our experience, been rare and always transient. Diabetes insipidus is usually transient and, after 3 months following the operation, less than 1.5% of the patients had a daily urine output exceeding 2500 ml. A detailed survey of the complications of transsphenoidal surgery is presented in Table 1.

TABLE 1. *Transsphenoidal surgery: a survey of complications*

A. *Complications from the nasal approach*
   More frequent:
      Asymptomatic septum perforation
      Fluid retention
      Sinusitis
   Rare:
      Denervation of teeth
      Septum deviation
      Nasal deformity
      Mucocele
      Maxilla fracture
      Epistaxis
B. *Complications in the sellar region*
   Rhinorrhea
   Rebleed
   Lesion of carotid artery
      Hemorrhage
      Aneurysm
      AV fistula
   Lesion of cavernous sinus
      CN III palsy
      CN VI palsy
   Lesion of optic nerves or chiasma
   Infection
      Meningitis
      Sellar abscess
   Secondary empty-sella syndrome
   Deterioration of pituitary function

ILLUSTRATIVE CASES

Case 1: Chordoma of the Clivus

This patient is a 60-year-old man presenting with acute left abducent nerve palsy. The sella turcica was not found to be enlarged and there was no evidence of neuroendocrine dysfunction. MRI demonstrated an invasive clival lesion (Fig. 13). The sphenoid sinus was exposed via a standard sublabial–transsphenoidal approach. In order to achieve ready access to the inferior posterior aspects of the sphenoid sinus, generous amounts of the inferior nasal septum and spine were removed with a diamond burr. Highly vascularized tumor tissue was encountered in the posterior half of the sphenoid sinus. Since its consistency was firm, the tissue could only be partly removed by curettage (Fig. 14). Large parts were removed in small portions by use of the microforceps. Profuse bleeding from the lesion necessitated extensive coagulation and repeated tamponing of the sphenoid sinus by Gelfoam. The posterior part of the sellar floor was infiltrated by the tumor, but the sellar dura was found to be intact, and tumor tissue was detached from it. This cleavage plane finally led to the descending clival dura, where the tumor was dissected and subsequently removed downward along the midline (Fig. 15). The clival dura was finally exposed over a vertical distance of 3.5 cm. At this stage, removal of the lateral tumor portions was aimed at and readily achieved. While total resection of the right side was easy, the tumor tissue adjacent to the left cavernous sinus was most highly vascularized and extremely adherent so that extensive coagulation was needed. Complete hemostasis was finally achieved and the whole region of exposure was cov-

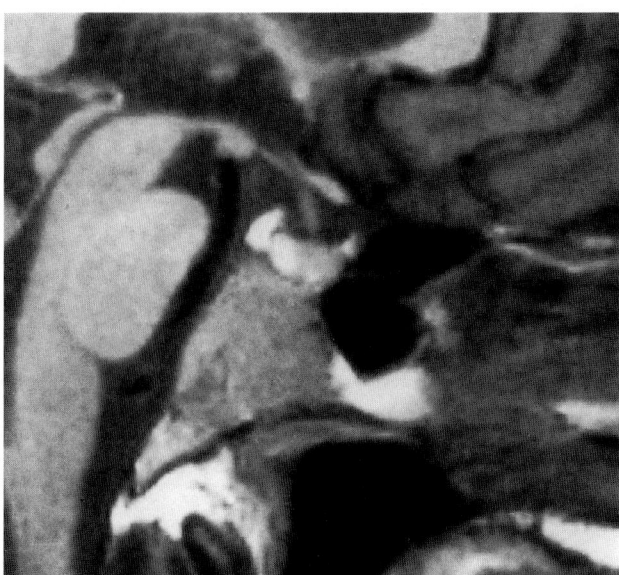

FIG. 13. Case 1—preoperative MRI scan demonstrating a large chordoma of the clivus.

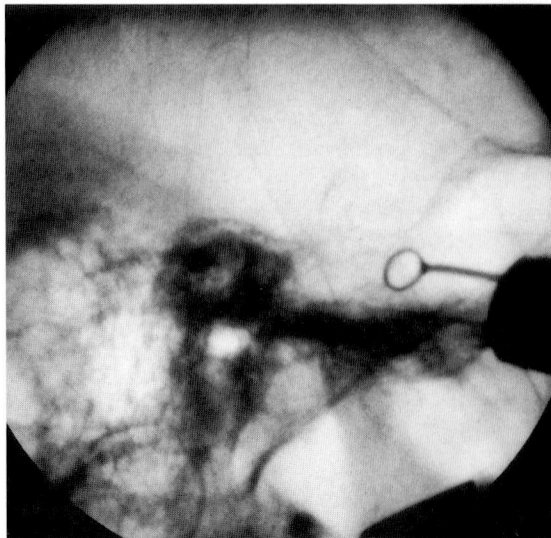

FIG. 14. Case 1—intraoperative fluoroscopy at the stage of dissection and curettage of the anterior tumor margin.

ered by fibrin glue-coated Gelfoam. Histologically, the diagnosis of a chordoma was confirmed. The postoperative course was uneventful and the abducent nerve showed some recovery within 2 weeks following surgery.

Case 2: Pituitary Macroadenoma in Acromegaly

This patient is a 40-year-old woman presenting with a 1-year history of acromegaly. Before therapy, basal growth hormone levels were elevated (25 ng/ml) and could not be suppressed by an oral glucose load. MRI showed an intrasellar, parasellar, and slightly suprasellar pituitary adenoma (Fig. 16). She was initially started on subcutaneous injections of octreotide (Sandostatin) for 6

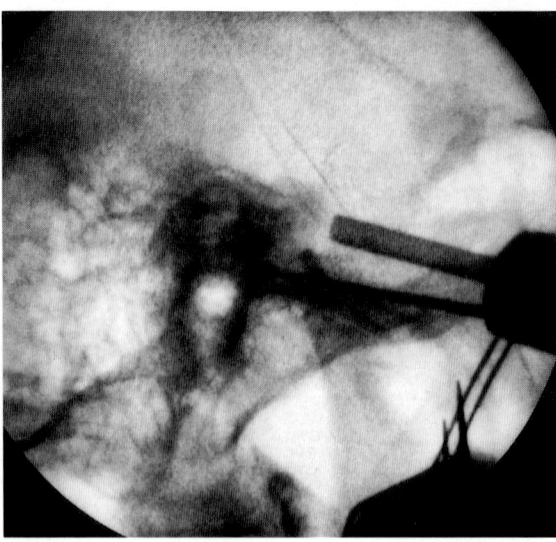

FIG. 15. Case 1—intraoperative fluoroscopy during removal of the dorsobasal portions.

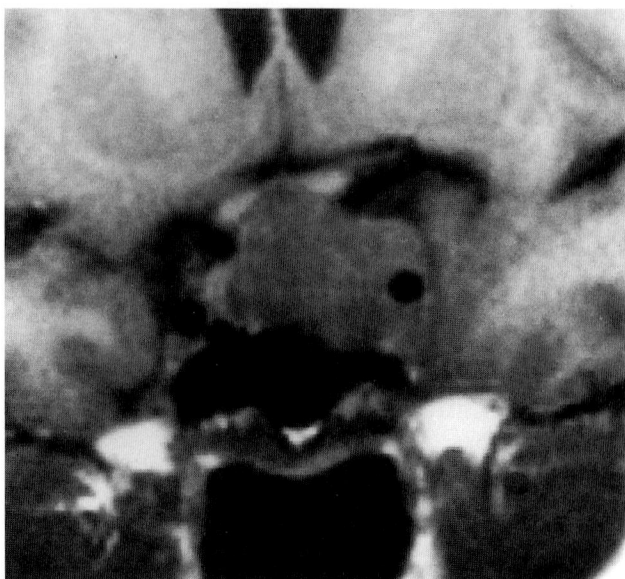

FIG. 16. Case 2—preoperative coronal MRI scan showing a large intrasellar and parasellar pituitary adenoma surrounding the carotid artery.

weeks and had received increasing daily doses ranging up to 300 µg. Neither basal serum growth hormone nor somatomedin C levels were significantly decreased and there was no change in tumor size and extension as documented by repeat MRI scanning. Figure 16 shows a section through the midsellar portion of the tumor just prior to surgery. Since the patient had previously undergone surgery for a nasal septum deviation resulting in a septum perforation, a direct pernasal transsphenoidal route was chosen. The nasal speculum was inserted into the right nostril up to the floor of the sphenoid sinus. The medial nasal mucosa was then incised and the vomer exposed and opened widely. The sellar floor was found to protrude into the sphenoid sinus right dorsolaterally. There was a circumscribed invasion of the sellar floor in a region 4 mm in diameter approximately in the midline. The sella floor was removed and the sellar dura resected. The intrasellar tumor portion could easily be removed by curettage. The medial aspect of the right cavernous sinus was then visualized (Fig. 17) and was found to be invaded by the adenoma. This could be removed by curettes and microforceps, resulting in an exposure of the right carotid artery over a distance of about 10 mm. The trabecular structure of the medial cavernous sinus was clearly visible by higher magnification (Fig. 18). Normal pituitary tissue was identified and preserved in the left lateral and dorsal parts of the sella. The exposed region was covered with fibrin glue-coated fascia lata and a nasal tampon was inserted bilaterally without any suturing of the nasal mucosa. The postoperative course was uneventful. Postoperatively, basal growth hormone levels decreased to 6.1 ng/ml and could be suppressed to 3.9 ng/ml after an oral glucose load.

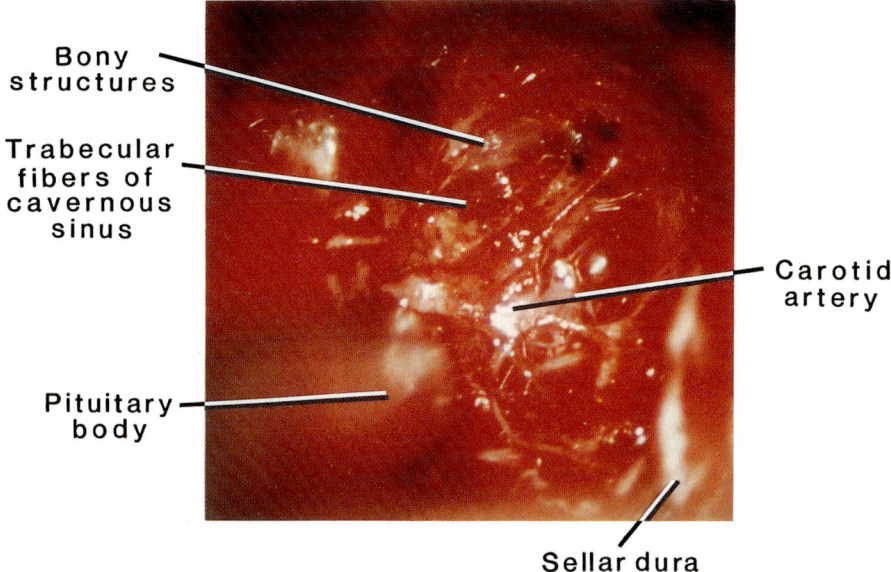

FIG. 17. Case 2—intraoperative appearance of exposed right cavernous sinus and carotid artery. The tumor was already removed by suction and curettage at this stage.

Case 3: Pituitary Macroadenoma in Acromegaly

This patient is a 51-year-old woman with a 5-year history of acromegaly. The sella turcica was moderately enlarged and the floor was double contoured. Thin collimation CT reconstructions depicted an intrasellar and right parasellar tumor (Fig. 19). Carotid angiography demonstrated that the right carotid artery was not significantly laterally displaced but was bulging slightly into the sella. Basal growth hormone levels were markedly elevated (32.3 ng/ml) and were not significantly suppressed (28.2 ng/ml) during an oral glucose load. The sella turcica was exposed via a standard sublabial–paraseptal–transsphenoidal approach. The sellar floor was found bulging into the right side of the sphenoid sinus and was locally perforated by invasive adenoma tissue, which had also invaded the mucosa of the sphenoid sinus. The sellar floor was completely removed and the intrasellar parts of the adenoma were resected. The adenoma had a medium to firm consistency. Following re-

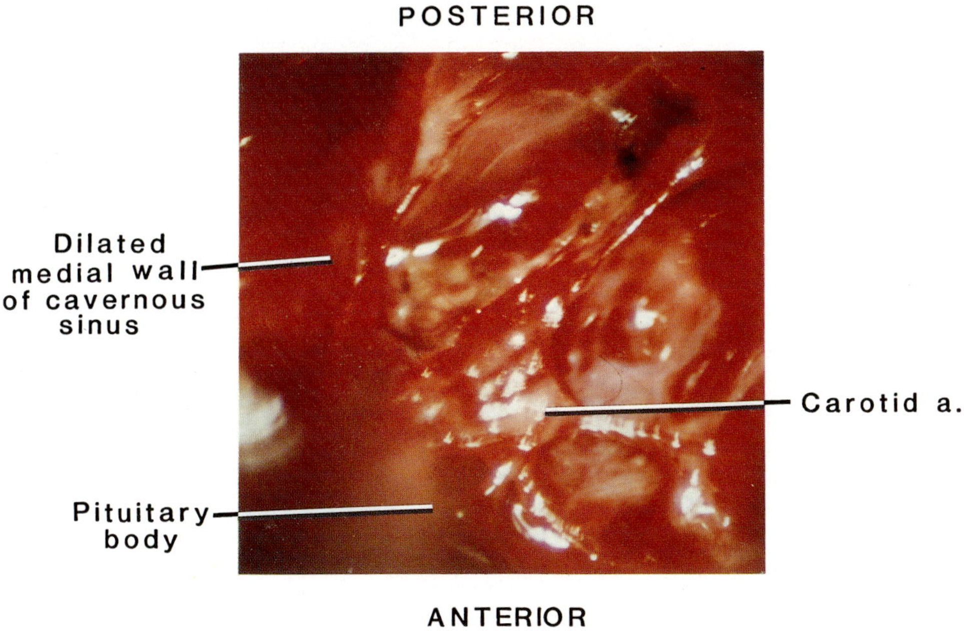

FIG. 18. Case 2—same sites as Fig. 17 but at a higher magnification.

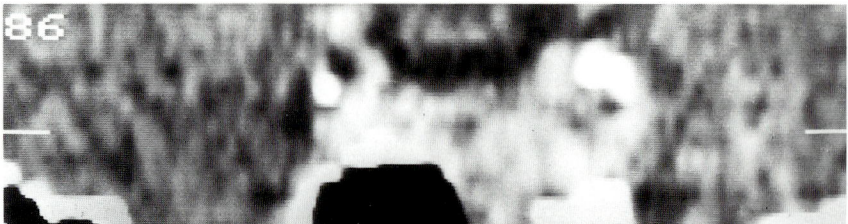

FIG. 19. Case 3—coronal CT reformations displaying the intrasellar and parasellar adenoma.

moval of the intrasellar tumor portions, the right cavernous sinus gradually shifted into the midline and could be inspected from below. It was found to be invaded by tumor tissue, which was removed from around the carotid artery and could then be visualized. Following removal of the invasive tumor, the cavernous sinus laterally showed a perforation (Fig. 20). The diaphragma sellae had not been elevated by the tumor and consequently did not descend markedly into the sella following tumor removal. Normal pituitary tissue was identified in the left and posterior aspect of the sella and was preserved. The area of exposure was covered by fibrin glue-coated fascia lata. Following surgery, growth hormone levels decreased to 8.5 ng/ml and could readily be suppressed to below 2 ng/ml during an oral glucose load. Since basal growth hormone levels remained slightly, but persistently, elevated on repeat follow-up determinations, the patient was submitted for external megavoltage radiotherapy.

AUTHORS' EXPERIENCE

The authors have performed 941 transsphenoidal operations for tumors of the sella turcica, sphenoid sinus, and clivus in a 7-year interval between December 1982 and December 1989. The vast majority of these were pituitary adenomas ($n = 887$). In the authors' service, the corresponding number of transcranial operations for pituitary tumors in the respective time interval was 90 (9.2%). Of the adenomatous lesions treated by transsphenoidal surgery, 166 (18.7%) were found to have an invasive character. Table 2 gives an overview of the relation between invasive and noninvasive adenomas and the endocrinological classification, as well as figures on nonadenomatous lesions operated on via the transsphenoidal route in the same period. The overall mortality in our whole series of 941 transsphenoidal operations was 2/941 (0.21%). After transsphenoidal surgery, major complications such as meningitis or CSF fistula occurred

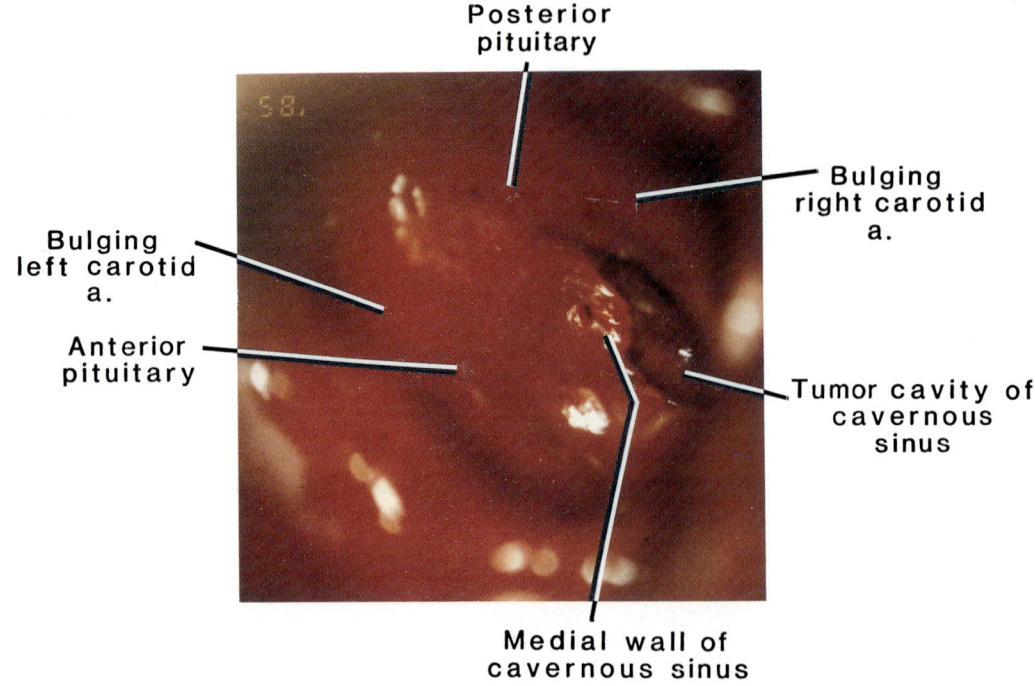

FIG. 20. Case 3—perforation in the medial wall of the cavernous sinus after tumor removal from the region the carotid artery.

TABLE 2. *Authors' experience of transsphenoidal surgery: 941 lesions (December 1982 to December 1989)*

Type of lesion	Number	Invasive
Pituitary adenomas		
Hormonally inactive	293	69
Prolactinomas	192	29
Acromegaly	241	54
Cushing's disease	140	5
Nelson's syndrome	17	5
Others	4	2
Total	887	164
Dysembryonic tumors		
Craniopharyngiomas	22	5
Rathke's pouch cysts	3	—
Chordoma	8	8
Teratoma	1	—
Total	34	13
Other lesions		
Metastases	2	2
Carcinoma	2	2
Esthesioneuroblastoma	2	2
Meningioma	5	4
Hemangiopericytoma	1	—
Sellar abscess	2	—
Granulomas	2	1
Colloid cyst	2	—
Arachnoid cyst	2	—
Total	20	11

in about 1% of cases. Deterioration of anterior pituitary function and a persistent diabetes insipidus are rare if a selective technique is applied. Acquired ocular nerve palsies and a deterioration of vision were always transient in the authors' series and their incidence was less than 1%. Since intrasellar and suprasellar tumors can be approached by the transsphenoidal route with low morbidity and mortality, this method should be primarily considered. In a considerable proportion of hormonally active adenomas, the total removal of invasive parasellar and sphenoidal tumors by transsphenoidal microsurgery has been documented by both postoperative neuroradiology and dynamic endocrine testing.

BIBLIOGRAPHY

1. Cushing H. The Weir Mitchell lecture: surgical experiences with pituitary disorders. *JAMA* 1914;63:1515–1525.
2. Dott NM, Bailey P. A consideration of the hypophyseal adenomata. *Br J Surg* 1925;13:314–366.
3. Fahlbusch R. Surgical treatment of pituitary adenomas. In: Beardwell C, Robertson GL, eds. *Clinical endocrinology* 1: *the pituitary.* London: Butterworths, 1981;76–105.
4. Fahlbusch R, Buchfelder M. Transsphenoidal surgery of parasellar pituitary adenomas. *Acta Neurochir* 1988;92:93–99.
5. Guiot G, Derome P. Surgical problems of pituitary adenomas. In: Krayenbühl H, et al, eds. *Advances and technical standards in neurosurgery,* vol 3. New York: Springer-Verlag, 1976;7–33.
6. Hardy J. Transsphenoidal microsurgery of the normal and pathological pituitary. *Clin Neurosurg* 1969;16:185–216.
7. Landolt AM, Strebel P. Techniques of transsphenoidal operations for pituitary adenomas. In: Krayenbühl H, et al, eds. *Advances and technical standards in neurosurgery,* vol 7. New York: Springer-Verlag, 1980;119–177.
8. Laws ER. Transsphenoidal approach to lesions in and about the sella turcica. In: Schmidek HH, Sweet WH, eds. *Operative neurosurgical techniques, indications, methods and results.* New York: Grune & Stratton, 1982;327–341.
9. Laws ER, Kern EB. Complications of transsphenoidal microsurgery. *Clin Neurosurg* 1976;23:401–416.
10. Tindall GT, Barrow DL. Pituitary surgery. In: *Disorders of the pituitary.* St Louis, Mosby, 1986;349–400.

CHAPTER 23

Translabyrinthine/Transcochlear Approaches

Derald E. Brackmann

TRANSLABYRINTHINE APPROACH

The translabyrinthine approach is the most direct route to the cerebellopontine angle. As of June 1989 this approach has been used to remove over 2500 acoustic tumors at the Otologic Medical Group, Inc. In addition to acoustic tumor removal, the translabyrinthine approach is used for total cochleovestibular nerve section for disabling vertigo when no useful hearing remains. It is also used for facial nerve decompression and repair following temporal bone fractures and for removal of facial nerve neuromas when hearing is lost.

We believe that the translabyrinthine approach offers many advantages. It requires a minimum of cerebellar retraction. Exposure and dissection of the lateral end of the internal auditory canal ensure complete tumor removal from that area and also allow positive identification of the facial nerve in a consistent anatomic location (1).

If the facial nerve is lost during acoustic tumor removal, the translabyrinthine approach offers the best opportunity for immediate repair by end-to-end anastomosis or interposition of a nerve graft (2).

Finally, and most importantly, this approach carries the lowest morbidity and mortality rates. The mortality rate for this approach is 4/10 of 1% for the last 2300 cases.

The obvious disadvantage of the translabyrinthine approach is the sacrifice of any residual hearing in the operated ear. It is therefore reserved for patients whose hearing is poor or for large tumors when the possibility of hearing preservation is slight.

In this chapter the translabyrinthine approach for removal of acoustic tumors is detailed. Modifications of the approach for other indications are also described.

D. E. Brackmann: Department of Otolaryngology, University of Southern California, and Otologic Medical Group, Inc., and House Ear Clinic and Institute, Los Angeles, California 90057.

Indications and Patient Selection

Small tumors that extend no further than 1 cm into the cerebellopontine angle in patients with good hearing are usually approached via the middle fossa. (See Brackmann, The Middle Fossa Approach.) Larger tumors where good hearing remains are approached via the retrosigmoid route. This route is ideal when the tumor arises more medially and is not impacted into the fundus of the internal auditory canal and does not expand the internal auditory canal.

In general, the outlook for hearing preservation for tumors with greater than 2-cm extension into the cerebellopontine angle is very poor. These tumors and all tumors with poor hearing are removed via the translabyrinthine approach.

There is no tumor too large to be approached via the translabyrinthine route. For large tumors, more bone removal is accomplished posterior to the sigmoid sinus to gain access.

Operative Technique

Anesthesia

General endotracheal anesthesia with inhalation agents is used. Muscle relaxants are only used for induction of anesthesia since intraoperative monitoring of facial nerve activity is routinely used. Prophylactic antibiotics or steroids are not routinely used. Occasionally, with very large tumors, these measures are employed.

Positioning

In the translabyrinthine approach the patient is placed supine on the operating table with the head at the foot of the table. This allows the anesthesiologist, who is seated at the patient's feet, easy access to the controls for moving the table. The patient's head is turned toward the

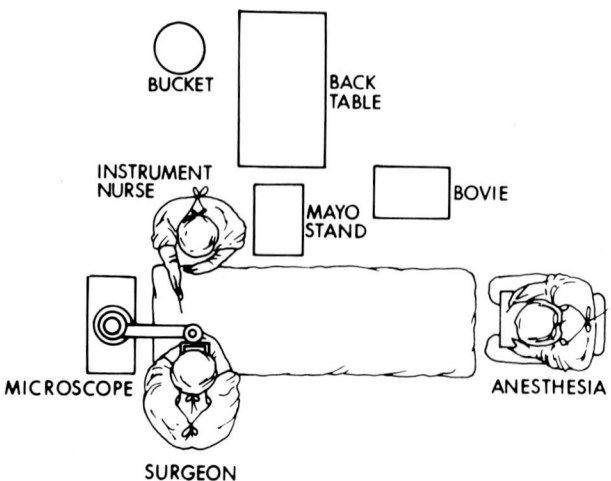

FIG. 1. Room arrangement for translabyrinthine approach. Note positions of surgeon, anesthesiologist, and nurse.

opposite side and maintained in a natural position without fixation. The ear is prepared with povidone-iodine (Betadine solution) and plastic drapes are applied.

The surgeon is then seated at the patient's side. This position minimizes fatigue and allows stabilization of the arms and hands during the exacting microsurgical procedures (Fig. 1).

A postauricular incision is made approximately 2 cm behind the postauricular crease (Fig. 2). The incision is curved anteriorly to allow anterior retraction of the pinna. The posterior curve of the incision allows access to the area behind the sigmoid sinus. Because most of the surgical view of the cerebellopontine angle is along the plane of the posterior fossa dura, posterior access is important.

The incision first extends to the fascia temporalis, and the dissection is carried to the linea temporalis, lateral to the fascia temporalis. Incision is then made through the fascia and periosteum along the linea temporalis posteriorly to the sinodural angle and then inferiorly on the mastoid bone to the mastoid tip. The Lempert periosteal elevator is used to free the postauricular tissues from the underlying cortex, posterior to the sinodural angle and forward until the spine of Henle and the external auditory canal are identified. Care must be taken not to tear into the external auditory canal, since this would introduce a possible route for infection.

Self-retaining retractors are placed to maintain the ear forward and also to elevate the temporalis muscle superiorly. Suction on the posterior blade of the retractor removes excess irrigation fluid and blood from the wound.

Cortical Mastoidectomy

After adequate exposure of the cortex has been obtained, bone removal is carried out with continuous suction-irrigation and a large cutting burr. Bone removal is started along the external auditory canal, and then a horizontal incision is made along the temporal line. The junction of these incisions will lie over the mastoid antrum. Identification of the mastoid antrum and the lateral semicircular canal therein is the key to the beginning dissection of the temporal bone.

Bone removal continues with care taken not to undercut the mastoid cortex. The external opening must be as

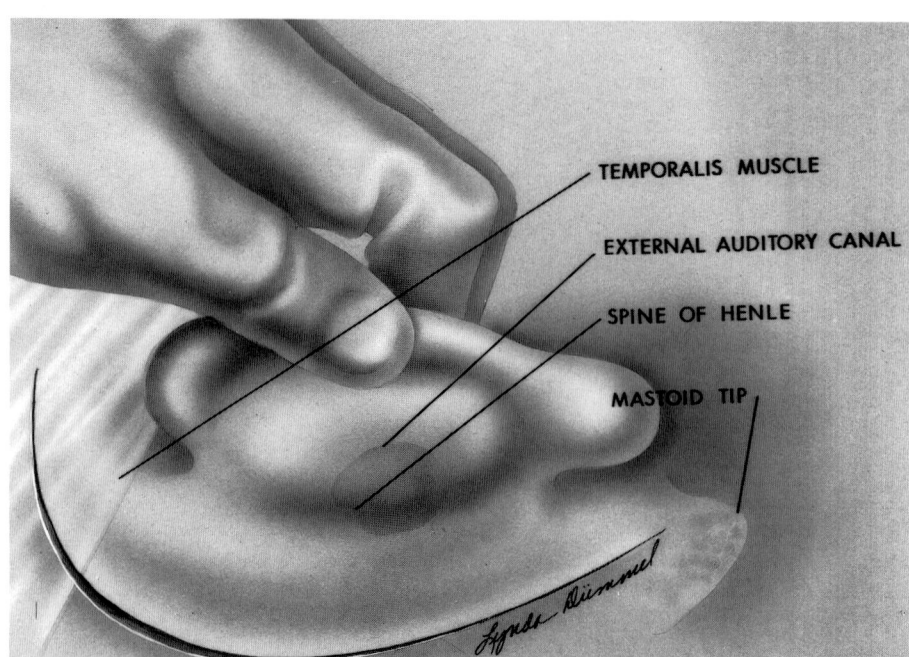

FIG. 2. Skin incision 2 cm behind the postauricular suicus.

large as possible. The middle fossa plate is identified superiorly and the sigmoid sinus posteriorly. Removal of bone is then continued over the sigmoid sinus to the area of the posterior fossa dura.

In large tumors bone removal is carried out far behind the sigmoid sinus. In some cases the bone is removed with a rongeur or drill as far as 2 or 3 cm posterior to the sigmoid sinus and inferiorly beneath the cerebellar hemisphere. This gives more decompression of the posterior fossa and allows room for retraction of the dura posteriorly. Care must be taken, however, not to injure the dura. Dural tears allow the cerebellum to herniate into the defect, which may result in infarction of that portion of the cerebellum.

Removal of bone over the sigmoid must be done carefully. If the cutting burr tears the sigmoid sinus, profuse bleeding will ensue and will require packing with oxidized regenerated cellulose (Surgicel). Large emissary veins often arise from the posterior aspect of the sigmoid sinus. They can be identified through the bone as it is removed, since the suction-irrigation keeps the bone clean. If the emissary vein is injured, bleeding must be controlled with bone wax, cautery, Surgicel packing, or in some cases suture of the emissary.

Complete, Simple Mastoidectomy

As soon as the mastoid cortex has been removed and the sigmoid sinus has been outlined, the operating microscope is brought into place. Magnification allows more accurate bone removal and exposure of all the structures of the temporal bone. A thin layer of bone is left over the sigmoid sinus and around the emissary veins, and a complete, simple mastoidectomy is performed down to the level of the horizontal semicircular canal (Fig. 3). It is important that the antrum be opened and the horizontal semicircular canal be identified. This canal is the basic landmark in temporal bone surgery. Once the position of this canal is known, the depth and three-dimensional relationship of the facial nerve and posterior and superior semicircular canals can be viewed. Expertise in temporal bone surgery depends on a thorough knowledge of the anatomy of the temporal bone and the ability to identify the structures as they are encountered. This appreciation of the anatomy comes only after many hours of diligent temporal bone dissection.

Labyrinthectomy

After the mastoid air cells have been removed to the level of the horizontal semicircular canal, labyrinthectomy is begun. Bone is removed in the sinodural angle along the superior petrosal sinus. This area, which is farthest from the facial nerve, is the key to this step in the dissection. The opening along the superior petrosal sinus is gradually deepened and widened until the labyrinthine bone is encountered. The lateral and posterior semicircular canals are then progressively removed, and the facial nerve, which lies anteriorly (Fig. 4), is carefully approached. The lateral semicircular canal is opened, and the common crus of the superior and posterior semicircular canals is identified deep in the dissection. The superior semicircular canal is followed to its ampulla. The vestibule is then opened, and the facial nerve is skeleton-

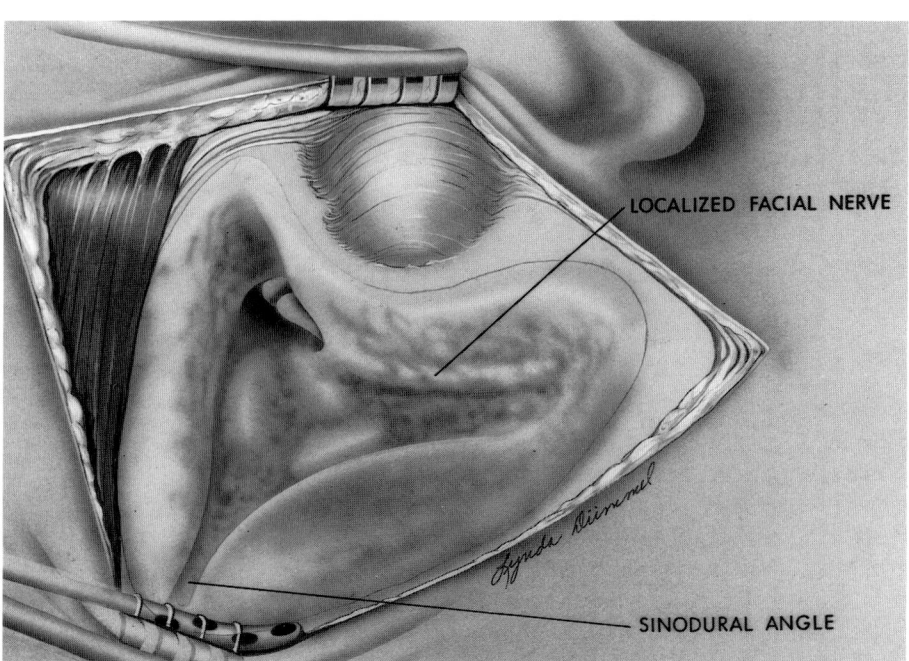

FIG. 3. Mastoidectomy is completed. Facial nerve is localized and sigmoid sinus skeletonized.

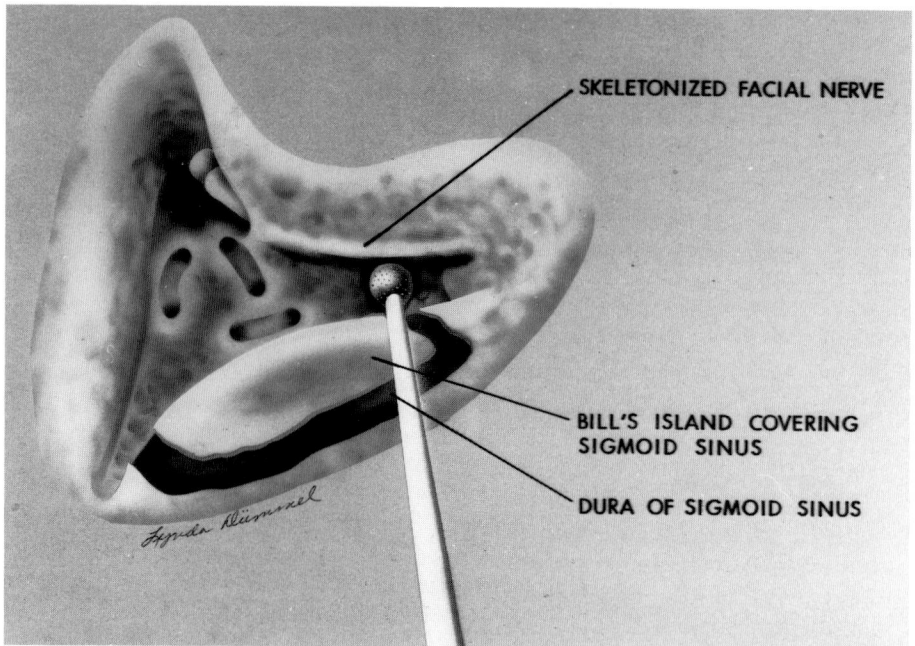

FIG. 4. Semicircular canals are opened. An island of bone over the sigmoid sinus is created.

ized from the genu inferiorly to near the stylomastoid foramen. It is not necessary to remove bone lateral to the facial nerve; rather, the facial nerve is skeletonized from a posterior direction, where access is needed to approach the cerebellopontine angle.

The final removal of bone along the facial nerve is accomplished with a diamond burr. Having removed the labyrinthine bone from posterior to the nerve, the surgeon may then use the side of the diamond burr rather than the end and at all times view the plane between the side of the burr and the facial nerve. This reduces the hazard of injury to the facial nerve, which is very slight with this technique. As the facial nerve is skeletonized, the cribriform area of the superior vestibular nerve entering the vestibule will be seen. It is important to skeletonize the facial nerve adequately so that the vestibule can be seen in this area (Fig. 5).

Internal Auditory Canal Dissection

After the labyrinthine bone has been removed to the level of the vestibule, dissection of the bone surrounding the internal auditory canal is started (Fig. 6). This dissection is started along the superior petrosal sinus and then is gradually enlarged in all directions toward the internal auditory canal. The dura of the internal auditory canal is identified posteriorly, as is the dura of the posterior fossa. This bone is gently removed, with care taken to leave an eggshell thickness of bone over the dura of the internal auditory canal and the posterior fossa to prevent injury to the soft tissue. Dissection is carried inferior to the labyrinth, with removal of the retrofacial air cells, until the blueness of the dome of the jugular bulb is seen through the overlying bone.

As the bone posterior to the internal auditory canal is removed, the vestibular aqueduct and the beginning of the endolymphatic sac will be removed. Bone is further removed along the posterior fossa dura beneath the sigmoid sinus. If the sigmoid sinus is overhanging into the mastoid cavity, which makes the dissection difficult, the eggshell covering of bone over the sinus may be removed so that the sinus can be retracted posteriorly. It is good to leave an island of bone (Bill's island) over the dome of the sigmoid sinus to protect it from the rotating burr and retraction of the suction-irrigation at this point.

We complete the dissection around the inferior portion of the internal auditory canal first. This is the area that is farthest from the facial nerve, and we find that completing the dissection here makes orientation to the superior portion of the internal auditory canal easier. Bone removal is continued medially and anteriorly between the dome of the jugular bulb and the internal auditory canal until the cochlear aqueduct is identified.

The cochlear aqueduct is not always readily identifiable. In large tumors it will be occluded at its medial orifice, and spinal fluid is not likely to escape. The cochlear aqueduct enters the posterior fossa directly inferior to the midportion of the internal auditory canal above the jugular bulb. It is an important landmark because it identifies the location of the ninth, tenth, and eleventh cranial nerves in the neural compartment of the jugular foramen anterior to the jugular bulb. If the dissection is confined to the area superior to the cochlear aqueduct, these nerves will not be injured.

After the cochlear aqueduct has been identified, bone

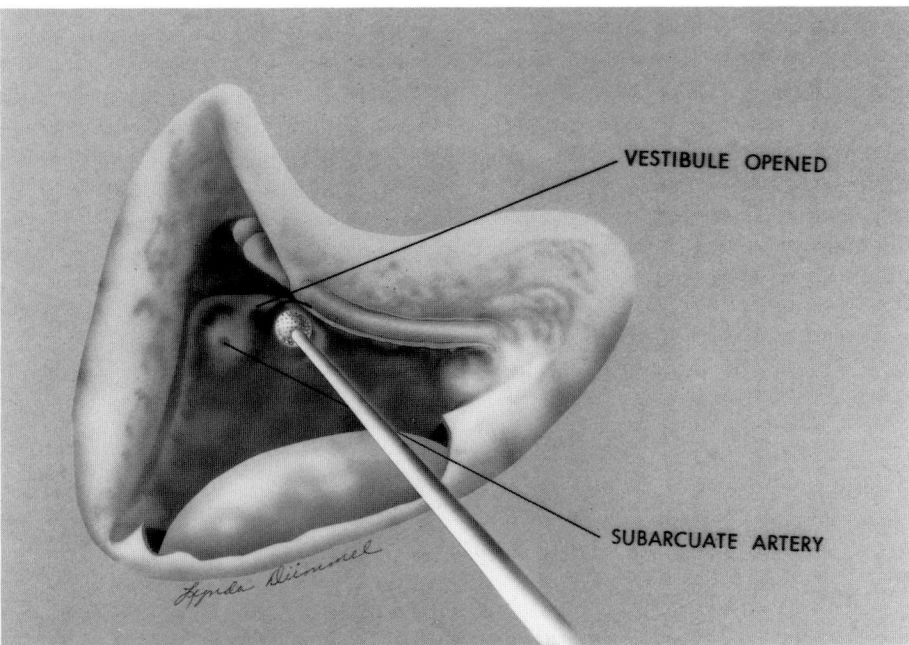

FIG. 5. Lateral and posterior semicircular canals are removed, vestibule is opened, and facial nerve is skeletonized in its tympanic segment.

removal is continued around the internal auditory canal to the porus acusticus until the entire inferior lip of the internal auditory canal is removed. The diamond burr is used for these later parts of the dissection. The bone of the posterior fossa dura is then removed inferiorly until the sigmoid sinus is skeletonized. This completes the dissection inferiorly.

Dissection is then carried superiorly and anteriorly around the internal auditory canal. This bone removal is tedious because the facial nerve often underlies the dura along the anterosuperior aspect of the internal auditory canal. The surgeon must be very careful not to allow the burr to slip into the internal auditory canal. We prefer to remove the entire porus and the medial portion of the internal auditory canal first, leaving the dissection of the lateral end of the internal auditory canal until last. In this way the facial nerve is not exposed until most of the bone removal is completed.

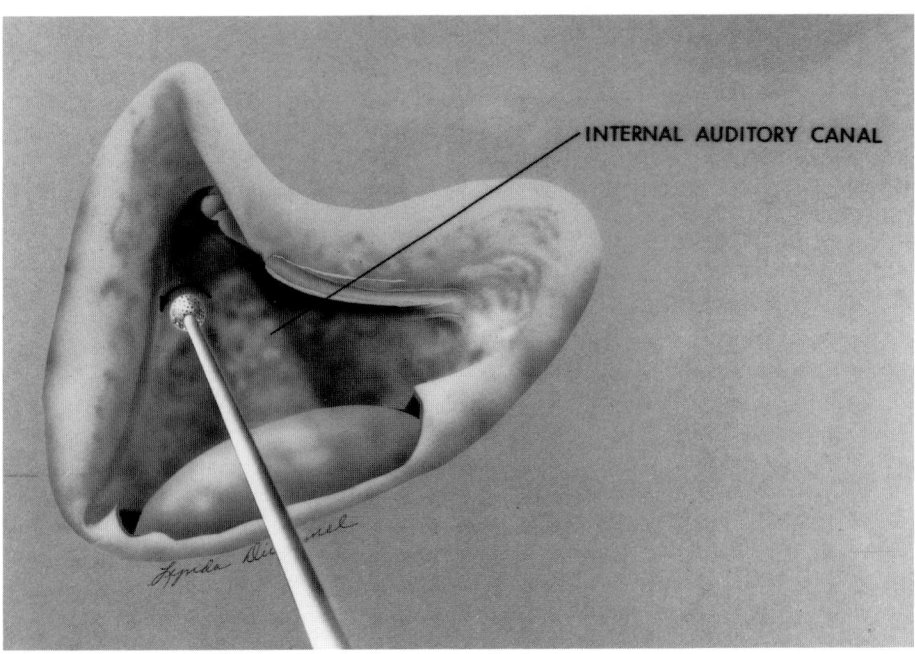

FIG. 6. Internal auditory canal is skeletonized. Note direction of rotation of burr.

Removal of the superior lip of the porus acusticus is tedious, but it is one of the most important parts of the dissection. If this is not entirely removed, the facial nerve will underlie the ridge of bone at the porus and will make identification and removal of the tumor from the nerve in this area very difficult. Diamond burrs are used to continue the dissection until two-thirds of the porus acusticus is removed. Bone removal is then carried laterally, and the end of the internal auditory canal is exposed.

Dissection of the lateral end of the internal auditory canal begins inferiorly. The singular nerve is first identified, and bone removal done inferiorly then exposes the inferior vestibular nerve. As dissection proceeds superiorly, the transverse crest is identified. The superior aspect of the internal auditory canal is then dissected, and the facial nerve is identified as it exits the internal auditory canal and begins its labyrinthine segment. Finally, the bar of bone (Bill's bar) separating the superior vestibular nerve from the facial nerve is identified. This completes the dissection around the internal auditory canal.

During the dissection of the internal auditory canal, an eggshell thickness of bone was left on the sigmoid sinus and the posterior and middle fossa dura. At this stage this is removed completely, and the surgeon is ready to open the posterior fossa dura to expose the cerebellopontine angle (Fig. 7). It is noteworthy that until this point all the dissection has been extradural and the morbidity of the approach has been minimal.

Venous Bleeding

A rare problem that can occur during the translabyrinthine approach is inadvertent tearing of the jugular bulb or the sigmoid sinus. In most cases this can be readily controlled by careful Surgicel packing. Care must be taken not to pack Surgicel into the lumen of the sinus or a portion of it may embolize to the lung. Because of the recumbent position of the patient, air embolism is not a problem. Blood loss, however, can be rapid.

If bleeding continues despite careful placement of Surgicel packs (this usually occurs only if a tear in the sinus is large), it may need to be controlled by occluding the sinus with extraluminal packing at the sinodural angle and by tying the jugular vein in the neck. Tying this vein prevents embolization of the Surgicel. Bleeding may still occur from the inferior petrosal sinus, however, and care must be taken not to pack the area of the inferior petrosal sinus too firmly or paralysis of the ninth, tenth, and eleventh cranial nerves can result.

Dural Incision

The dura of the posterior fossa is then incised over the midportion of the internal auditory canal. The incision then extends around the porus acusticus superiorly and inferiorly. Care is taken to avoid vessels on the surface of the tumor and anteriorly/superiorly care is exercised to avoid injury to the facial nerve, which lies directly be-

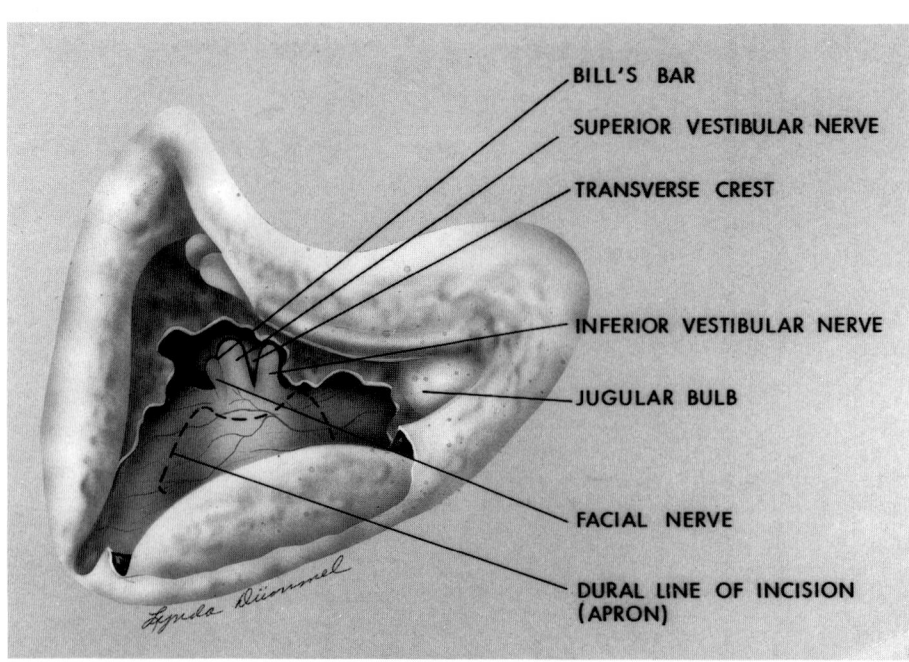

FIG. 7. Superior and inferior vestibular nerves are identified in the internal auditory canal. Note transverse crest between the nerves.

neath the dura in this area. Posteriorly the petrosal vein lies just beneath the dura and insertion of a Rosen elevator will separate underlying blood vessels from the dura prior to incision. Keeping the deep blade of the scissors just beneath the dura prevents injury to underlying blood vessels as the incision progresses. The dural flaps are then retracted superiorly and inferiorly and cottonoids are placed between the tumor and the cerebellum posteriorly.

An arachnoid cyst is often encountered around the posterior aspect of the tumor. The cyst is opened and the plane of the tumor and cerebellum is further developed around the posterior aspects of the tumor. Cottonoids are advanced into this plane. It is extremely important to accurately develop this plane, since doing so will separate the major vessels of the cerebellopontine angle from the tumor. The operating microscope makes it possible to follow this proper plane and to a large extent has eliminated the major bleeding often associated with cerebellopontine angle tumor removal.

Petrosal Vein

As the dura is retracted posteriorly, it will lie over the petrosal vein, which originates in the cerebellum and drains into the superior petrosal sinus near the level of the internal auditory canal. At times this vein will be torn near its entry into the superior petrosal sinus as it is retraced posteriorly.

Bleeding from the proximal portion of the vein can be controlled by a clip. However, bleeding from the superior petrosal sinus is often much more difficult to manage. One means of controlling this bleeding is to fill the superior petrosal sinus with Surgicel. Another technique is to pack Surgicel extradurally over the petrous ridge at the anterior limit of the dissection. This produces extradural compression of the superior petrosal sinus and thus controls proximal bleeding. Distal back-bleeding from the sinus is controlled by placing a clip on the sinus between the sinodural angle, where it enters the sigmoid sinus, and the petrosal vein.

Partial Tumor Removal

In the case of a small tumor the surgeon can begin development of the inferior and superior planes of the tumor. With a medium or large tumor it is better to begin intracapsular removal of the tumor to reduce its size before developing the other planes.

The posterior surface of the tumor is first carefully inspected for nerve bundles. On rare occasions the facial nerve may lie on the posterior surface of a tumor. After it has been determined that no nerve bundles are present on the posterior surface of the tumor, the capsule of the tumor is incised and intracapsular removal of the tumor is begun with the House/Urban dissector (Figs. 8–10). During intracapsular removal of the tumor it is important to avoid excessive movement and pressure on the tumor because this may stretch and injure the facial nerve.

Isolating the Tumor

Once the interior of the tumor has been extensively gutted, the development of the tumor plane is carried

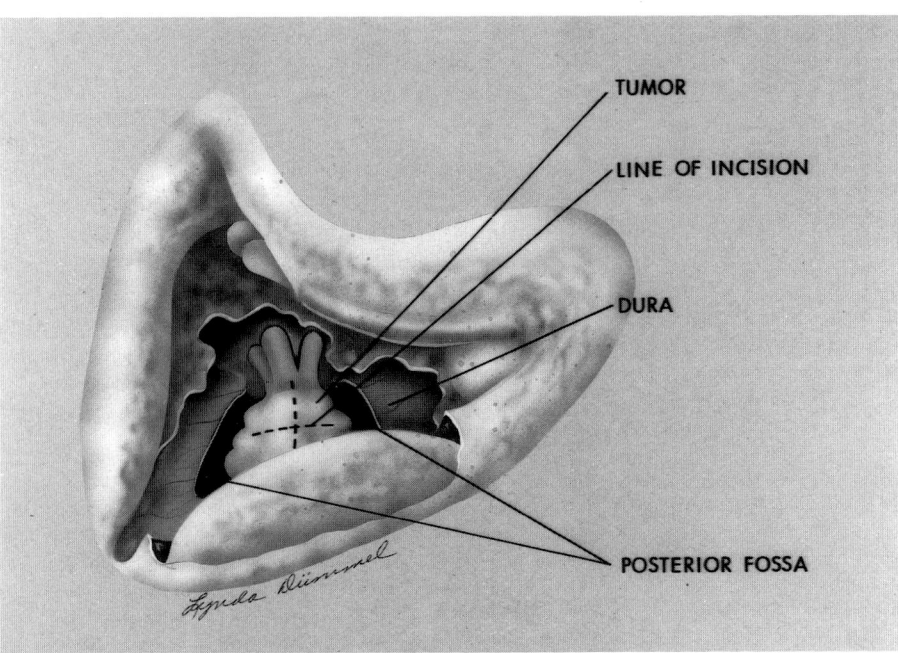

FIG. 8. Tumor is exposed by incising the dura covering the internal auditory canal and posterior fossa.

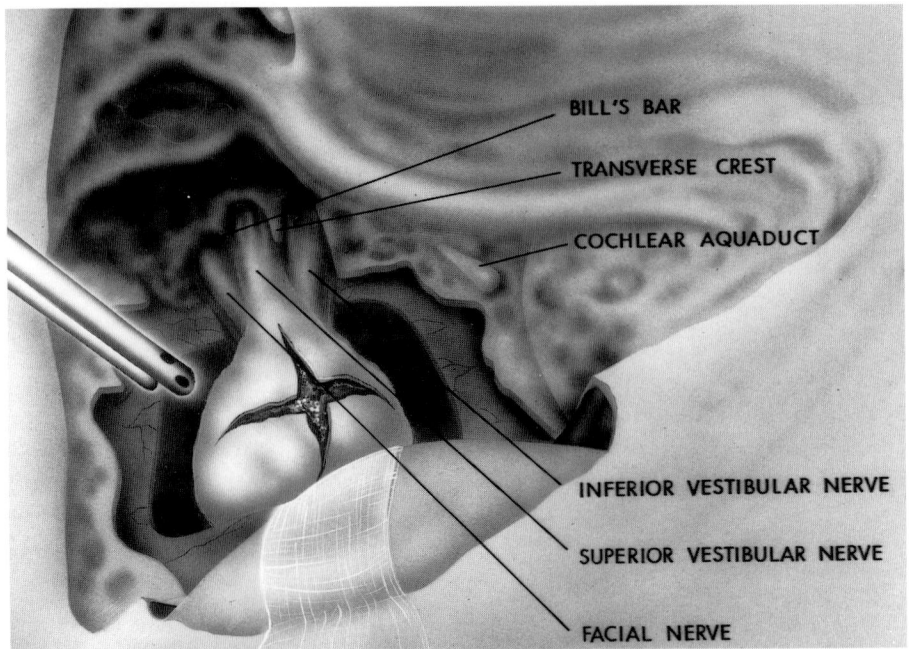

FIG. 9. Facial nerve is identified by localizing Bill's bar. Tumor capsule is incised.

out further inferiorly and superiorly. Small cottonoids are used to develop the plane of the tumor and to separate surrounding structures. Avoidance of injury to surrounding structures is greatly facilitated by use of the fenestrated neurotologic suction tip. Since the tumor has been extensively gutted, the capsule is displaced into the interior of the tumor. The surface of the capsule is then followed to the brain stem. We attempt to develop the posterior aspect of the tumor to the point where it can be seen at the brain stem, and cottonoids are placed into this plane.

Inferiorly, an attempt is made to localize the ninth cranial nerve, which can best be identified near its exit medial to the jugular bulb. In larger tumors the ninth cranial nerve may be stretched over the surface of the tumor. This plane is carefully developed, and the ninth cranial nerve is isolated from the field with cottonoids. During manipulation of the ninth and tenth cranial

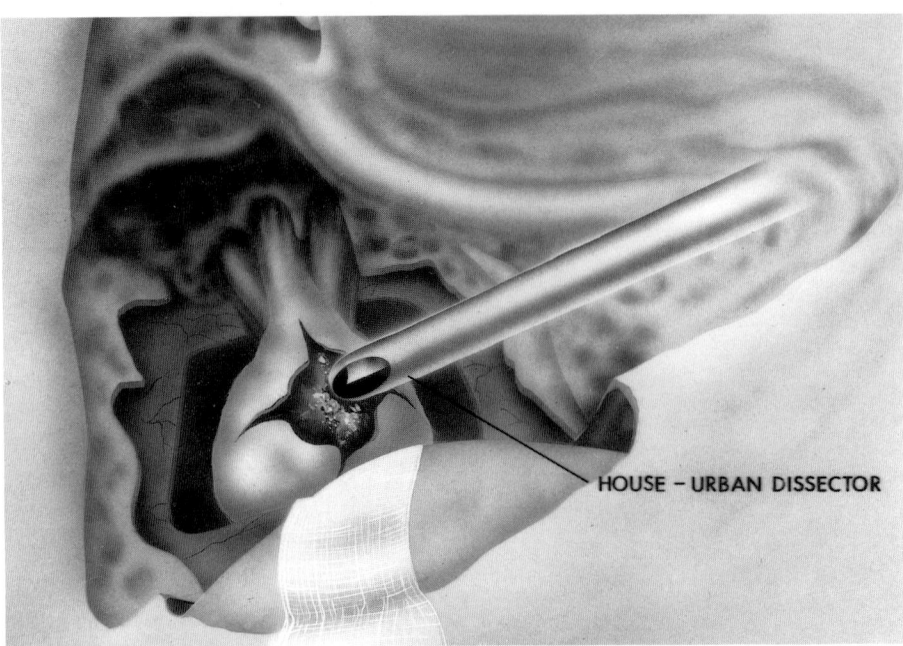

FIG. 10. House/Urban rotating vacuum dissector starts gutting the tumor within its capsule.

nerves there are often changes in the pulse rate. If these occur, we stop manipulation of the nerves and allow the vital signs to stabilize.

Often large vessels are located around the inferior aspect of the tumor, and these must be carefully separated from the tumor capsule and preserved. After the inferior aspect of the tumor has been developed down to the brain stem, additional debulking of the tumor and removal of a portion of the capsule can be completed.

The superior aspect of the tumor capsule is next developed. The petrosal vein will be encountered in this location and must be carefully separated from the tumor. The facial nerve usually lies more anteriorly, but it is not unusual for it to come over the top of the tumor. The fifth cranial nerve is identified at the medial superior aspect of the tumor, and all these structures are carefully separated from the capsule and packed away from the field with cottonoids (Fig. 11).

Identification of the Facial Nerve

The lateral end of the internal auditory canal is dissected, and the plane of the facial nerve is established. During bone removal the vertical crest of bone (Bill's bar) separating the facial nerve from the superior vestibular nerve has been clearly identified. A long fine hook is then inserted lateral to Bill's bar to identify the superior vestibular nerve. The hook is gently passed medially and slightly anteriorly until it falls over Bill's bar into the facial nerve canal, which positively identifies the facial nerve. The hook is then withdrawn and placed beneath the superior vestibular nerve, turned inferiorly, and the superior vestibular nerve is pulled out from its canal (Fig. 12). At this point the underlying facial nerve is seen, and the plane of the facial nerve from the tumor is definitely identified. Positive identification of the facial nerve at the lateral end of the internal auditory canal is one of the principal advantages of the translabyrinthine approach. Continuous intraoperative facial nerve monitoring is routinely used.

Next the hook is used to remove the inferior vestibular nerve, and the dura of the internal auditory canal is opened along the inferior aspect of the tumor. The dura is also opened superiorly, with great care taken to avoid the facial nerve. Incision of the dura of the internal auditory canal frees the tumor so that it can be gently retracted posteriorly away from the facial nerve. The Rosen separator and hooks are used to carefully develop the plane between the facial nerve and the tumor. The tumor is gently retracted posteriorly to bring this plane into relief. After the lateral end of the facial nerve has been definitely identified and separated from the tumor, all tumor remnants are removed from the lateral end of the internal auditory canal. The cochlear nerve is usually removed along with the tumor and the vestibular nerve.

Facial Nerve Dissection

Usually it is relatively easy to develop the plane along the facial nerve within the internal auditory canal, but considerable difficulty often arises when the porus acusticus is reached. Dural adhesions to the surface of the

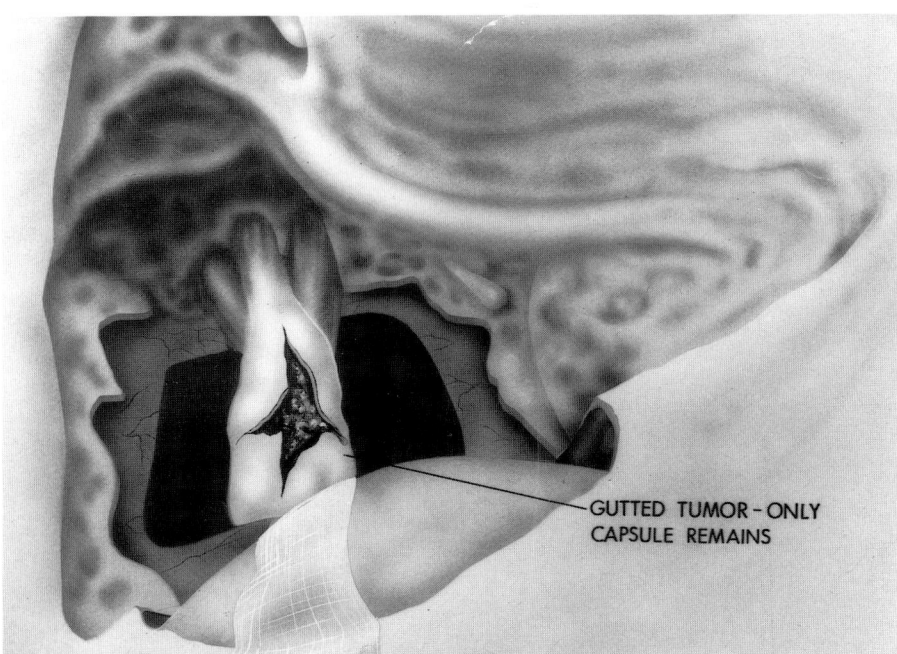

FIG. 11. Tumor is gutted, and only the capsule remains. Note the size of the tumor as compared to Fig. 8.

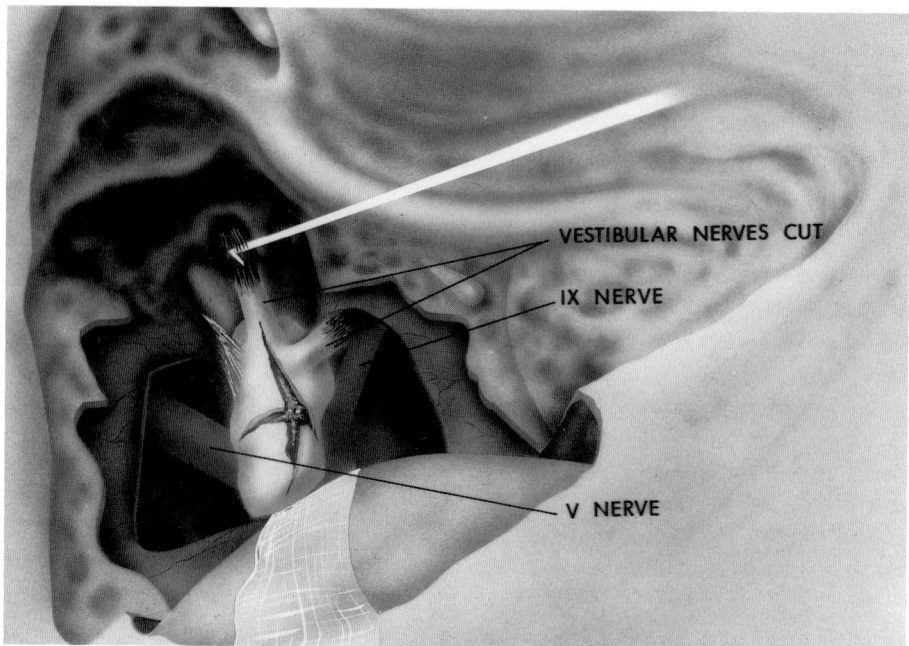

FIG. 12. Superior and inferior vestibular nerves are cut above the level of the transverse crest. Note the ninth nerve and the fifth nerve in the posterior fossa.

tumor at the porus acusticus invariably make dissection of the facial nerve from the tumor very difficult in this area. The facial nerve usually can be followed past the area of adhesions without undue difficulty. At times, however, this plane becomes very difficult, and we rotate the tumor posteriorly to identify the facial nerve on the tumor medially nearer the brain stem. The facial nerve is then followed medially to laterally until the plane becomes apparent, and tumor removal can be completed at the porus acusticus (Fig. 13). During this entire dissection the surgeon must be careful not to push the tumor forward or medially, which would stretch the facial nerve. It is better to gently retract the tumor posteriorly and laterally, removing the stretch from the facial nerve.

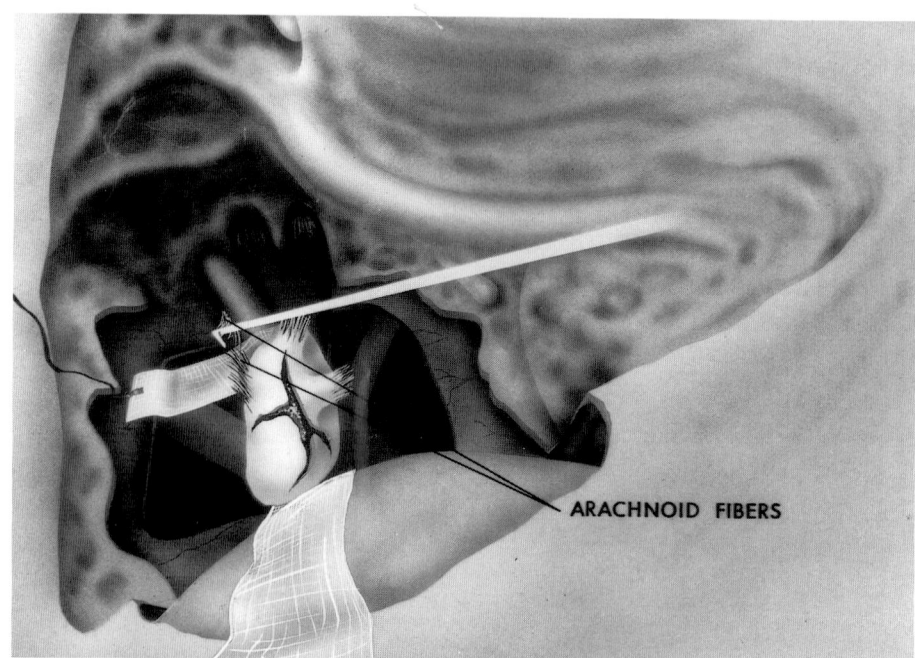

FIG. 13. Tumor capsule is separated from the facial nerve by careful cutting of the arachnoid sheath.

Completion of Tumor Removal

Once the facial nerve has been separated from the tumor to the brain stem, the bulk of the tumor is removed with the House/Urban dissector, leaving only a small portion of tumor attached to the brain stem (Fig. 14). Removing the bulk of the tumor allows greater visibility of the tumor–brain stem plane. The last bit of tumor is then removed from the brain stem under direct vision. The adhesions between the tumor and the brain stem are usually not dense and can easily be separated. Bleeding in this area is controlled with bipolar cautery. Only those vessels that actually enter the tumor capsule are coagulated; the others are carefully freed from the tumor capsule. Often a small artery accompanies the eighth cranial nerve into the tumor. Bleeding from this artery is controlled by placing a clip on the eighth nerve and contained artery or by bipolar coagulation.

Hemostasis and Closure

After total tumor removal, the wound is profusely irrigated with Ringer's solution to remove any blood clots. The cottonoids are then removed, and all bleeding points are controlled with either clips or bipolar cautery. Absolute hemostasis must be obtained, and this may require considerable time and effort. It is best to control bleeding with clipping or cautery rather than Surgicel packing. Using large amounts of Surgicel must be avoided because this substance expands considerably with fluid absorption and can consequently cause pressure on surrounding vessels or the brain stem.

After hemostasis is complete, the dura is sutured and the area of the mastoidectomy obliterated with strips of fat taken from the abdomen. A small piece of muscle is used to obliterate the additus. The mastoid cavity is then filled to the surface of the cortex with strips of abdominal fat, and the postauricular incision is closed in layers. The skin is closed with interrupted subcuticular sutures. The patient is kept on the operating table until responding well and then is transferred directly to the intensive care unit.

Postoperative Management

The patient is observed in the intensive care unit for a period of 36 hr. Steroids or antibiotics are not routinely used. In some patients with very large tumors that exhibit signs of cerebellar swelling, we do use steroids. The mastoid dressing remains in place 4 days and the patient is instructed not to lift or strain during the early postoperative period.

Complications and Management

Although rare, the most common early postoperative complication is a hematoma in the cerebellopontine angle. This is manifested by signs of cerebellopontine angle pressure and is managed by immediate opening of the wound and removal of the fat in the intensive care unit. This is a further advantage of the translabyrinthine approach in that the angle may be rapidly decompressed for this uncommon complication. The patient is then

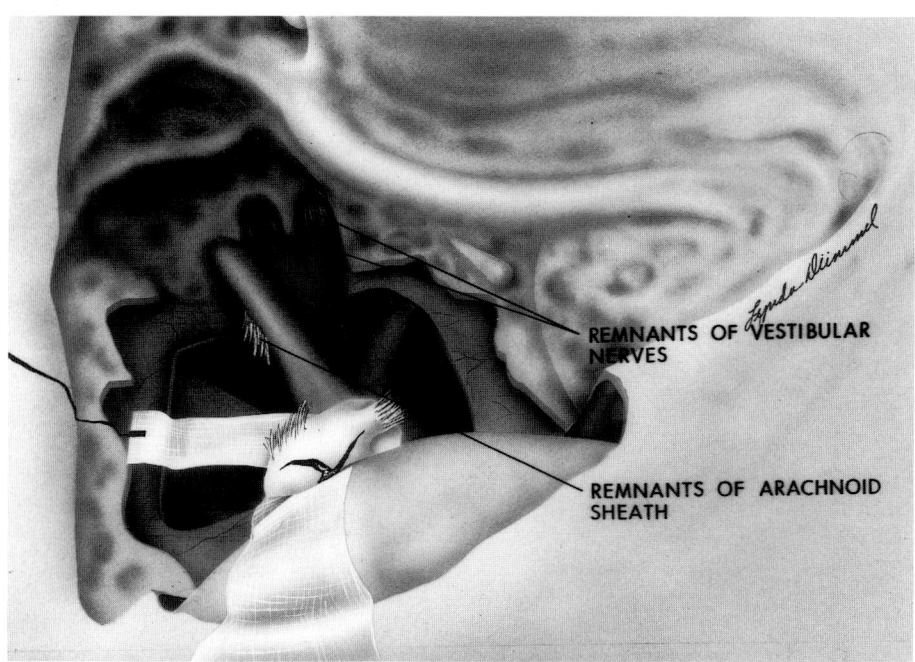

FIG. 14. Tumor capsule is carefully separated from the facial nerve.

taken to surgery, where complete hemostasis is obtained and the wound again closed with abdominal fat.

Meningitis is an uncommon complication and is managed in the usual manner with appropriate antibiotics following culture and identification of the offending organism.

If facial weakness occurs, eye care is provided by a consulting ophthalmologist. Conservative measures are first used including artificial tears, moisture chambers, and soft contact lens. If these measures fail to provide adequate corneal protection, a palpebral spring is inserted. The latter procedure is more commonly necessary when there is a concomitant fifth nerve deficit with corneal anesthesia. The average hospitalization is 7–8 days. The patient is advised to avoid heavy lifting or strenuous activity for approximately 3 weeks.

Modifications of Approach

Total Cochleovestibular Nerve Section

To section the eighth nerve for vertigo when hearing is absent requires less bone removal than for acoustic tumor removal. It is not necessary to remove bone behind the sigmoid sinus or to remove bone extensively from the posterior fossa dura. One-half of the circumference of the bony internal auditory canal is removed rather than two-thirds as in acoustic tumor surgery.

Total Facial Nerve Decompression or Repair

The facial nerve is exposed throughout its course in the temporal bone for decompression in transverse temporal bone fractures or for removal of facial nerve tumors when hearing is absent. The labyrinthine segment of the nerve is followed distally to the geniculate ganglion and then the entire tympanic and descending portion of the nerve is exposed. The nerve sheath is opened for decompression.

If the nerve is transected by trauma it may be rerouted into the angle and a primary anastomosis accomplished with a single 9-0 or 10-0 monofilament suture.

After resection of a facial nerve neuroma, a greater auricular nerve graft is inserted from the brain stem segment to the descending segment. Several epineural sutures are placed in the distal anastomosis (9-0 or 10-0 monofilament), which is accomplished first. A single suture of the same material stabilizes the proximal anastomosis.

Discussion of Series

The Otologic Medical Group series numbers over 2500 acoustic tumors as of June 1989. The results in the first 700 patients have been published previously (3). With experience and refinements in technique the results have improved throughout the years.

We have studied the results in 216 patients who underwent surgery for acoustic tumor in 1980 and 1981. The average age of these patients was 47.3 years, and the group was equally divided as male and female.

Tumor size, measured on cranial CT, has been reported as extension into the cerebellopontine angle. Small tumors are those that extend less than 0.5 cm into the cerebellopontine angle; 20 of the 216 (9%) fit this category. Medium tumors, which are considered those that extend from 0.5 to 2.0 cm into the cerebellopontine angle, numbered 110 (51%). Large tumors are those extending from 2 to 4 cm into the cerebellopontine angle; this group included 67 (31%) of the tumors. Tumors that extend more than 4 cm into the cerebellopontine angle are considered giant tumors; 19 patients (9%) had tumors of this size.

The average length of surgery was 3 hr and 12 min. There was one death in this series (0.4%). The patient had a postoperative hemorrhage and, despite early evacuation of the clot, sustained brain stem infarction and died.

Facial nerve function was studied 1 year after surgery. At that time 180 patients (83%) had normal facial function. There was a partial paralysis in 34 patients (16%). In four of these patients the facial nerve had been divided during tumor removal; they underwent immediate facial anastomosis in the cerebellopontine angle and had satisfactory recovery of facial function. Two patients had total facial paralysis 1 year after surgery; they then underwent hypoglossal facial anastomosis and had satisfactory recovery of facial function.

There was a direct correlation between preservation of normal facial nerve function and size of tumor. All 20 patients with small tumors had normal facial function at 1 year. Of the patients with medium-sized tumors, 85% had normal facial function. In the group with large tumors, 81% of the patients had normal facial function. Of those patients with giant tumors, 63% had normal facial function 1 year after surgery. Despite this correlation, it must be noted that some patients with relatively small tumors may have invasion of the facial nerve and thus incomplete recovery. Therefore the surgeon must be careful not to be overly optimistic in patient discussion even when the tumor is a small one.

Conclusion

The translabyrinthine approach is the preferred method for removal of all sizes of acoustic tumors when there is nonserviceable hearing. This approach is also used for vestibular nerve section and facial nerve decompression and repair when there is total loss of hearing.

TRANSCOCHLEAR APPROACH

The transcochlear approach is described for resection of lesions arising on the petrous bone anterior to the internal auditory canal as well as for those arising directly from the clivus.

Indications

Meningiomas arising from the petrous ridge and primary cholesteatomas centered anterior to the internal auditory canal are the most common indications for this approach. This approach is used when there is nonserviceable hearing in the involved ear. When hearing remains good, an extended middle fossa approach is used.

Total removal of these lesions through a conventional suboccipital approach is often not possible because of the interposition of the cerebellum, facial nerve, and brain stem. With the translabyrinthine approach the facial nerve limits the anterior dissection and prevents removal of the origin of the tumor along the petrous ridge or anterior to the brain stem. This approach, which involves rerouting the facial nerve posteriorly, allows removal of the petrous bone to the internal carotid artery and a wide exposure of the anterior cerebellopontine angle. The fifth, seventh, ninth, tenth, and eleventh cranial nerves, the clivus, both vertebral arteries, and the basilar artery are routinely seen. One added advantage of the approach is that during the bony dissection to obtain exposure the blood supply and the tumor base are removed, which is particularly important in petrous ridge meningiomas.

Operative Technique

With the same preparation, draping, and positioning as for the translabyrinthine approach, that exposure is first accomplished. When first described by House and Hitselberger (4), the tympanic ring was not removed but I have modified the approach to include removal of the entire tympanic bone, malleus, and incus, with blind sac closure of the external auditory canal as in the infratemporal fossa approach (Fig. 15). Two-thirds of the circumference of the entire fallopian canal is then removed from the geniculate ganglion through the stylomastoid foramen. Continuous intraoperative facial nerve monitoring is routinely used during this dissection. Bone is then removed from about the labyrinthine segment of the facial nerve. The greater superficial petrosal nerve is transected. The eggshell of bone remaining on the fallopian canal is removed and the facial nerve is mobilized from the entire fallopian canal and displaced posteriorly from the cerebellopontine angle through the stylomastoid foramen. A large piece of Gelfoam is placed over the nerve to protect it during the remainder of the bone removal.

Using a diamond burr, the cochlea is then removed and the carotid artery is skeletonized anteriorly (Fig. 16). The entire petrous apex is removed with diamond burrs following the internal carotid artery throughout its intra-

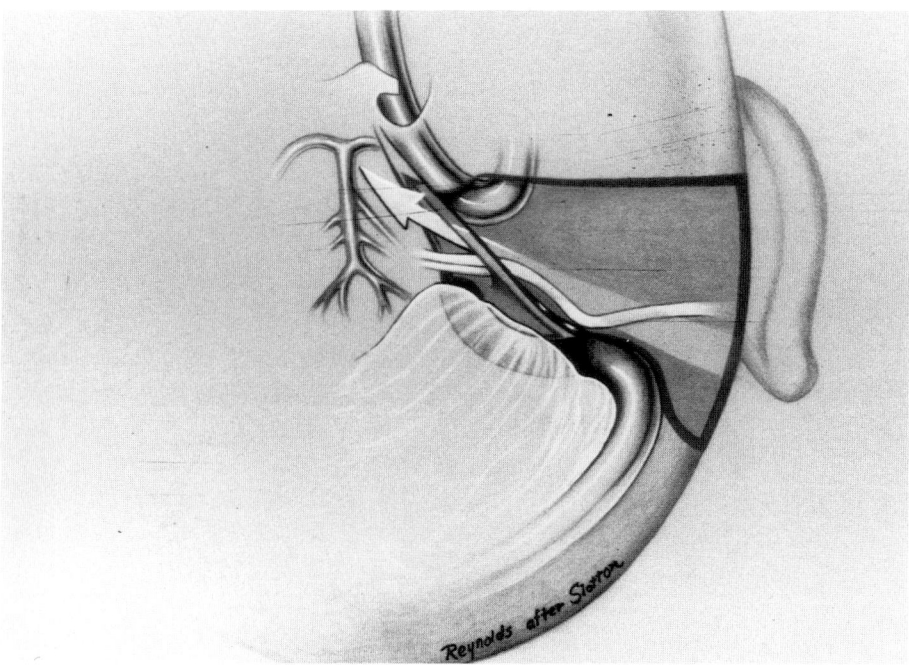

FIG. 15. Extent of bone removal for the transcochlear approach. The entire tympanic bone, labyrinth, and cochlea are removed.

temporal course to the area of the cavernous sinus. The entire petrous ridge is removed as well as the entire internal auditory canal and the bone anterior to it.

The dural incision is extended along the superior petrosal sinus until the tumor is widely exposed. In the case of a meningioma, the tumor is gutted with the House/Urban dissector and separated carefully from surrounding structures. The origin of the tumor along the petrous ridge is resected along with the superior petrosal sinus. Bleeding from the superior petrosal sinus near the cavernous sinus is controlled with light Surgicel packing. The sixth cranial nerve is identified at the petrous apex. All the structures of the posterior fossa are identified and the tumor is carefully removed from them. If the tumor extends across the midline, lifting the basilar artery and its branches will bring the cranial nerves in the opposite cerebellopontine angle into view. After completion of tumor removal, hemostasis is secured and the defect is obliterated with strips of abdominal fat taken from the abdomen. The facial nerve is supported on either side by these strips of fat.

Postoperative Management

The postoperative management of these patients is the same as for the translabyrinthine approach.

Complications

In addition to the complications inherit to all intracranial procedures, temporary facial nerve weakness occurs in all these patients because of the extensive rerouting of the facial nerve with its attendant devascularization. Since using intraoperative facial nerve monitoring, recovery of function has been good but most patients do have minor sequelae of reinnervation.

Discussion of Series

The transcochlear approach has been used in 24 patients—19 meningiomas and 5 primary cholesteatomas. Total tumor removal was accomplished in all but five patients, all of whom had extensive involvement of the basilar artery or cavernous carotid artery by meningioma. There were two deaths early in the series: one was the result of toxic shock in a diabetic patient. There was no evidence of residual tumor at the time of autopsy. The other patient had an early postoperative bleed from the vertebral artery that required clipping for control of the hemorrhage. Infarction of the brain stem occurred with death 1 week postoperatively.

Conclusion

Tumors arising from the petrous bone anterior to the porus acusticus and those arising directly from the clivus present difficult surgical problems. The transcochlear approach exposes these extensive tumors in cases where there is nonserviceable hearing. This approach allows complete tumor removal with acceptable morbidity and mortality in lesions at times previously considered unresectable.

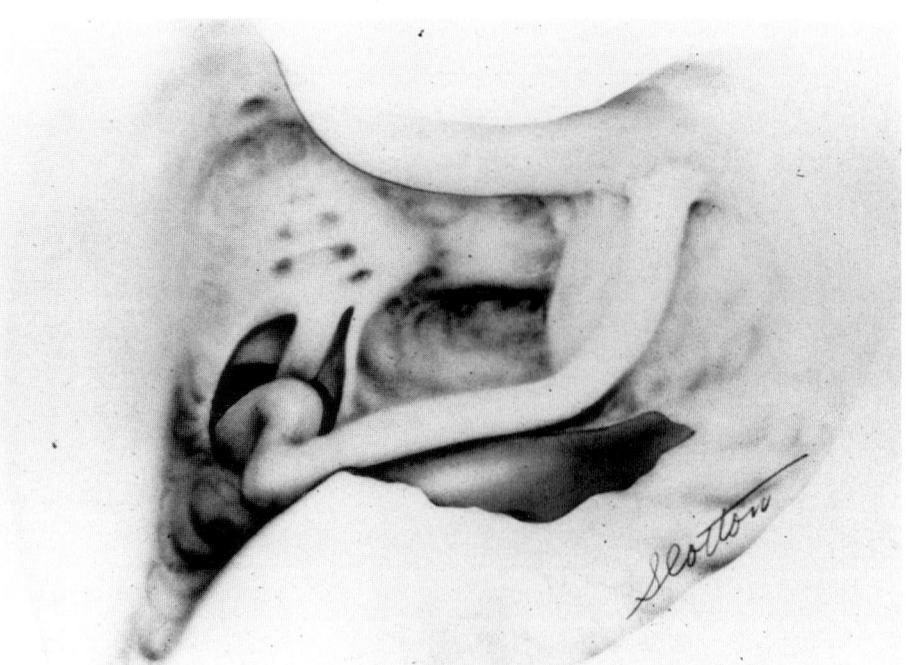

FIG. 16. The facial nerve has been rerouted posteriorly. Removal of the cochlea has begun.

REFERENCES

1. Brackmann DE, Hitselberger WE, Beneche JE, House WF. Acoustic neuromas: middle fossa and translabyrinthine removal. In: Rand RW, ed. *Microneurosurgery.* St Louis: Mosby, 1985.
2. Brackmann DE, Hitselberger WE, Robinson JV. Facial nerve repair in cerebellopontine angle surgery. *Ann Otol Rhinol Laryngol* 1978;87:772–777.
3. House WF, Luetge CM, eds. *Acoustic tumors,* vol 1, *Management.* Baltimore: University Park Press, 1979.
4. House WF, Hitselberger WE. The transcochlear approach to the skull base arch. *Otolaryngology* 1976;102:334–342.

CHAPTER 24

The Middle Fossa Approach

Derald E. Brackmann

The middle fossa approach for the removal of acoustic tumors was developed by William F. House in the early 1960s (1). It has been used in many thousands of cases for a variety of conditions. It has been shown to be a safe approach with a minimum of mortality and morbidity. In this chapter, the approach for removal of an acoustic tumor is described. Other indications for the approach are also noted and the modifications for each described.

INDICATIONS AND PATIENT SELECTION

The indications for the middle fossa approach are (a) removal of small laterally placed acoustic tumors; (b) exposure of the labyrinthine and upper tympanic segment of the facial nerve for idiopathic facial palsy, temporal bone fractures, or removal of tumors affecting the facial nerve; (c) selective vestibular nerve section; and (d) decompression of the internal auditory canal for bilateral acoustic neuromas.

The middle fossa approach offers several advantages for the removal of small, laterally placed acoustic tumors. First, the majority of the dissection is extradural, thereby lowering morbidity. Second, the lateral end of the internal auditory canal is exposed, which assures removal of all tumor. With the retrosigmoid approach, the most lateral end of the internal auditory canal cannot be exposed safely without entering the labyrinth. Third, positive identification of the facial nerve is possible at the lateral end of the internal auditory canal. This facilitates tumor dissection from the facial nerve in this area (2).

The middle fossa approach allows exposure of the labyrinthine and upper tympanic segments of the facial nerve while preserving hearing and balance function.

D. E. Brackmann: Department of Otolaryngology, University of Southern California, and Otologic Medical Group, Inc., and House Ear Clinic and Institute, Los Angeles, California 90057.

The nerve may be safely decompressed in idiopathic facial palsy or in longitudinal temporal bone fractures. Tumors of the facial nerve, both neuromas and hemangiomas, typically arise in the area of the geniculate ganglion. The middle fossa approach is used to remove these tumors and repair the facial nerve while preserving auditory and vestibular function.

Selective vestibular nerve section for disabling vertigo may be performed through the middle fossa, retrolabyrinthine, or retrosigmoid approaches. The middle fossa approach offers the advantage of more distal exposure of the eighth nerve where it has divided into its vestibular and cochlear branches.

The middle fossa approach has been used in a small group of patients with bilateral acoustic neuromas to decompress the internal auditory canal. The principle of this is to allow the tumor to expand superiorly, thereby decreasing pressure on the blood supply to the cochlea and also on the cochlear nerve. Several patients have had prolonged preservation of hearing using this technique (3).

For acoustic tumor removal, we select patients who have tumors that extend no further than 1 cm into the cerebellopontine angle. If the tumors are medially placed and do not extend to the fundus of the internal auditory canal, the retrosigmoid approach is preferred. Tumors that involve the distal end of the internal auditory canal are better approached via the middle fossa.

Candidates for hearing preservation surgery are those that have serviceable hearing, usually no greater than a 40-dB pure tone loss with speech discrimination of at least 80%. Preservation of wave form with only a slight increase of latencies on ABR is a favorable prognostic sign. Loss of function of the superior vestibular nerve as indicated by a reduced vestibular response on electronystagmography is also a favorable sign, indicating a tumor in the superior compartment of the internal auditory canal. Tumors in the superior compartment are less likely to intimately involve the cochlear nerve and are also more likely to displace the facial nerve anteriorly rather than be located beneath the facial nerve.

There are also disadvantages to the middle fossa approach. The first is that with this approach, the surgeon must work past the facial nerve to remove tumor. This subjects the facial nerve to more manipulation than does the translabyrinthine approach. A second problem sometimes encountered is postoperative unsteadiness resulting from partial preservation of vestibular function. This problem also occurs with the retrosigmoid approach, but it rarely occurs with total vestibular denervation with the translabyrinthine approach. Careful section of the remaining vestibular nerve fibers reduces the incidence of postoperative unsteadiness but also increases the risk of hearing loss.

The final potential problem with the middle fossa approach is limited access to the posterior fossa in the event of bleeding either at surgery or postoperatively. Although this has not occurred in our series, a problem could arise if significant bleeding occurred from the anterior–inferior cerebellar artery.

OPERATIVE MANAGEMENT

Anesthesia

This operation is performed under general endotracheal anesthesia using inhalation agents. Facial nerve monitoring is routinely used so that relaxation is not used except for the initial induction of anesthesia. Diuretics and mannitol are usually used to promote diuresis.

Positioning

The patient is placed supine on the operating table with the head turned so that the operated ear is upmost. No external fixation is used. The surgeon is seated at the head of the table. The remainder of the operating room setup is shown in Fig. 1.

A large area of hair removal is required because the incision extends far superiorly. The area of preparation extends nearly to the top of the head and far anteriorly and posteriorly. The skin is prepared by Betadine scrub and self-adhering plastic drapes are applied.

Incision

The middle fossa incision begins in the natural hairline just anterior to the base of the helix and extends superiorly approximately 7–8 cm, curving first anteriorly and then posteriorly (Fig. 2). Curving the incision allows the surgeon to spread soft tissue widely to gain

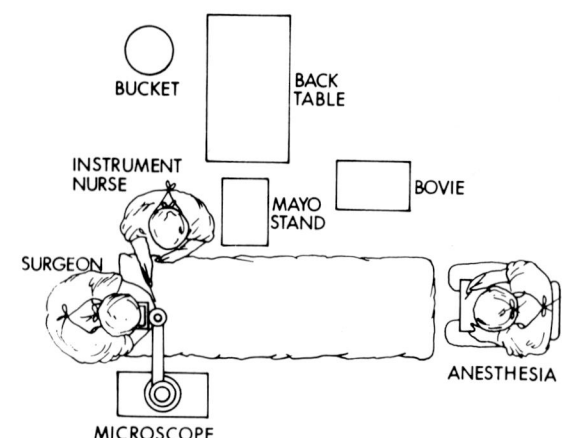

FIG. 1. Operating room arrangement. The surgeon is seated at the head of the table.

more access anteriorly. Bleeding vessels are controlled with cautery. The surgeon often encounters a branch of the superficial temporal artery, which is ligated with nonabsorbable suture to avoid late postoperative bleeding and hematoma.

The initial incision extends to the level of the temporalis fascia. Finger dissection develops the plane of the temporalis fascia along the temporal line. An incision is then made posteriorly/superiorly along the insertion of the temporalis muscle onto the squamous portion of the temporal bone. The temporalis muscle is freed from the temporal bone and retracted anteriorly/inferiorly. Elevation of the temporalis muscle in this fashion preserves its nerve and blood supply so that it could later be used for a temporalis muscle transfer to the lower face in case of persistent facial paralysis. The temporalis muscle is elevated to the temporal line and held in place with self-retaining retractors.

Elevation of the Bone Flap

A craniotomy opening is made in the squamous portion of the temporal bone (Fig. 3). The opening is approximately 4.0 cm^2 and is located two-thirds anterior and one-third posterior to the external auditory canal. It is important to place the craniotomy opening as near as possible to the floor of the middle fossa. This usually requires hand retraction of soft tissue by an assistant.

A medium cutting burr and continuous suction-irrigation are used. The bone flap is thicker superiorly as the squamoparietal suture is approached. It is important not to lacerate the dura during the bone removal for this could allow herniation of the temporal lobe. Herniation can best be avoided by leaving a thin plate of bone over the dura. The bone can then easily be fractured and removed. We prefer to make a bone flap rather than a burr hole and rongeur enlargement so that the temporal bone

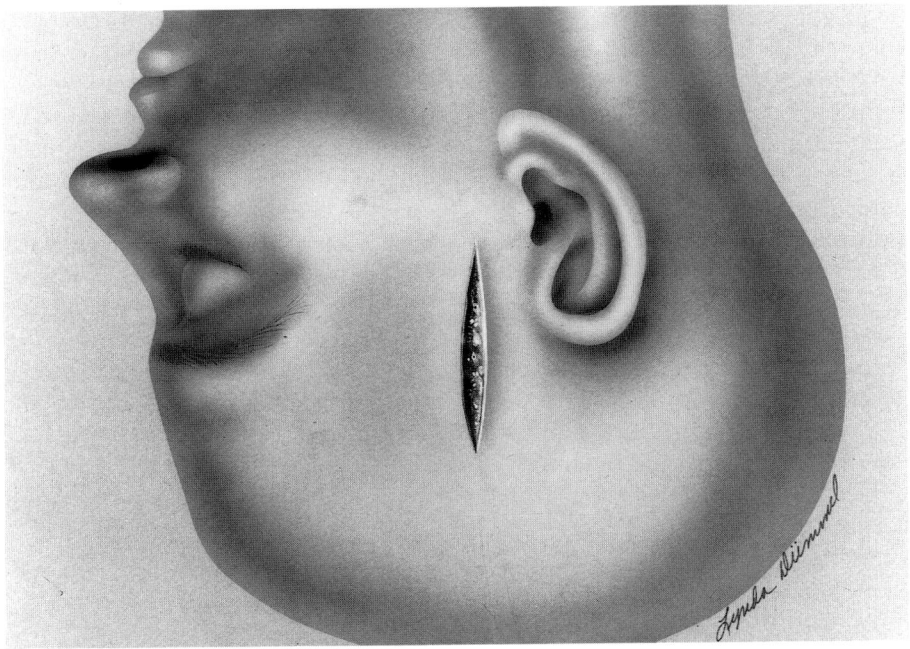

FIG. 2. Incision extends 7–8 cm superiorly from the natural hairline and is 0.5 cm anterior to the helix.

flap can be replaced at the end of the procedure. This results in less retraction in the area of the incision, thus improving the cosmetic appearance. Replacement of the bone flap also reduces the possibility of transmission of brain pulsations to the skin, which is cosmetically undesirable.

Bone bleeders are commonly encountered and are controlled with bone wax. It is important to keep the edges of the bone flap parallel. This facilitates placement of the middle fossa retractor.

Once the surgeon has drilled nearly through the temporal bone flap, a joker elevator is used to separate the underlying dura and the bone flap is removed. Sharp edges are trimmed from the bone and it is placed in normal saline solution during the operation.

Elevation of the Dura

The dura is separated from the margin of the craniotomy defect with the joker elevator. Any sharp edges are

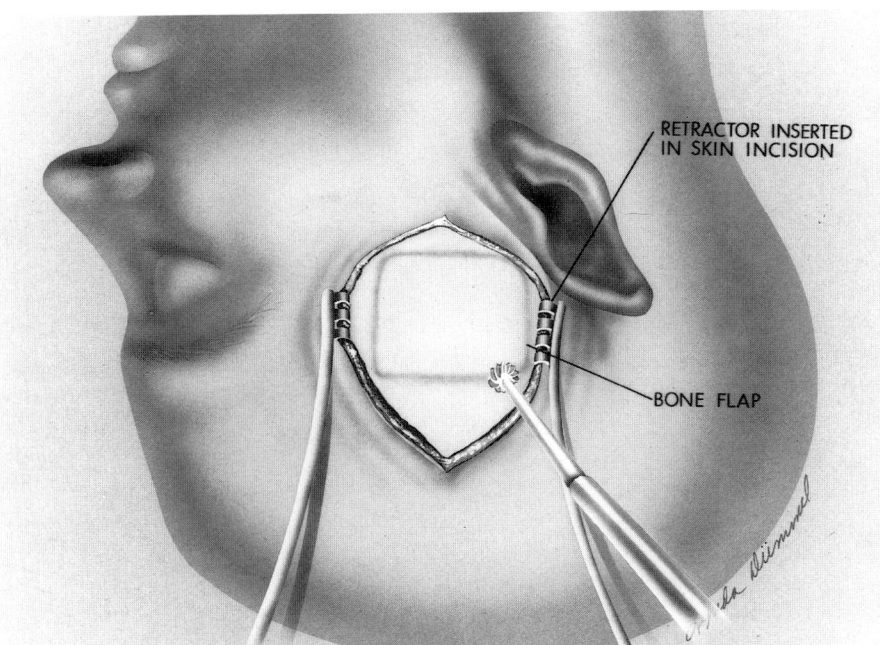

FIG. 3. Bone flap is made two-thirds anterior and one-third posterior to the external auditory canal.

removed with the rongeur. Occasionally, the inferior bone cut is above the floor of the middle fossa. This excess bone is removed with the rongeur. At times, there will be bleeding from the branches of the middle meningeal artery on the surface of the dura. This is best controlled with bipolar cautery with care being taken not to burn a hole in the middle fossa dura. The level of cautery must be reduced to the minimum necessary to coagulate the vessel. It is important to maintain the integrity of the dura since any defect may allow herniation of the temporal lobe. If a small tear is produced, it should be closed with dural silk suture to prevent extension and herniation. After separation of the dura from the edges of the craniotomy defect, the House/Urban retractor is put in place and firmly locked. The blade of the retractor is then set in place and gentle elevation of the dura from the floor of the middle cranial fossa is begun (Fig. 4).

The House/Urban retractor contains three adjustments, allowing for the desired placement of the retractor. The first adjustment affords movement of the entire blade mechanism in an inferior/superior direction. Once the blade is properly centered at the depth of the middle fossa dissection, this adjustment is secured at a position that gives maximum exposure but does not impinge on the superior edge of the craniotomy opening.

Dural elevation is carefully begun from posterior to anterior. As the dura is elevated, the tip of the blade is advanced. The two other adjustments are arranged appropriately. One adjustment allows for anterior to posterior movement of the tip of the retractor blade. The other adjusts the placement of the tip of the blade in a superior/inferior direction.

The structures within the temporal bone as viewed from above are shown diagrammatically in Fig. 5. The first landmark to be identified is the cranial entrance of the middle meningeal artery at the foramen spinosum. This marks the anterior limit of the dural elevation. Frequently, venous bleeding is encountered in this area. It may be necessary to control this bleeding by placing a firm pack of Surgicel into the foramen spinosum.

The surgeon's attention is then directed posteriorly and the medial elevation of the dura is accomplished from posterior to anterior. First, the petrous ridge is identified posteriorly. Care is taken in this area because the petrous ridge is grooved by the superior petrosal sinus, which the surgeon must avoid entering. If the sinus is inadvertently entered, bleeding can usually be controlled by extraluminal packing with Surgicel. However, small pieces of Surgicel must not be placed in the lumen of the sinus because they can produce a pulmonary embolus.

The dura is then elevated from the floor of the middle fossa medially from posterior to anterior. In approximately 5% of cases, the geniculate ganglion of the facial nerve will not be covered by bone. Blind or rough elevation of the dura in such cases can result in damage to the facial nerve. It is best to gently elevate the dura from the temporal bone rather than to scrape the elevator along the bone of the middle fossa.

The posterior to anterior elevation avoids raising the greater superficial petrosal nerve. If this nerve were elevated and the dissection carried posteriorly, the geniculate ganglion and facial nerve would again be subject to injury. In the literature on the middle fossa approach to

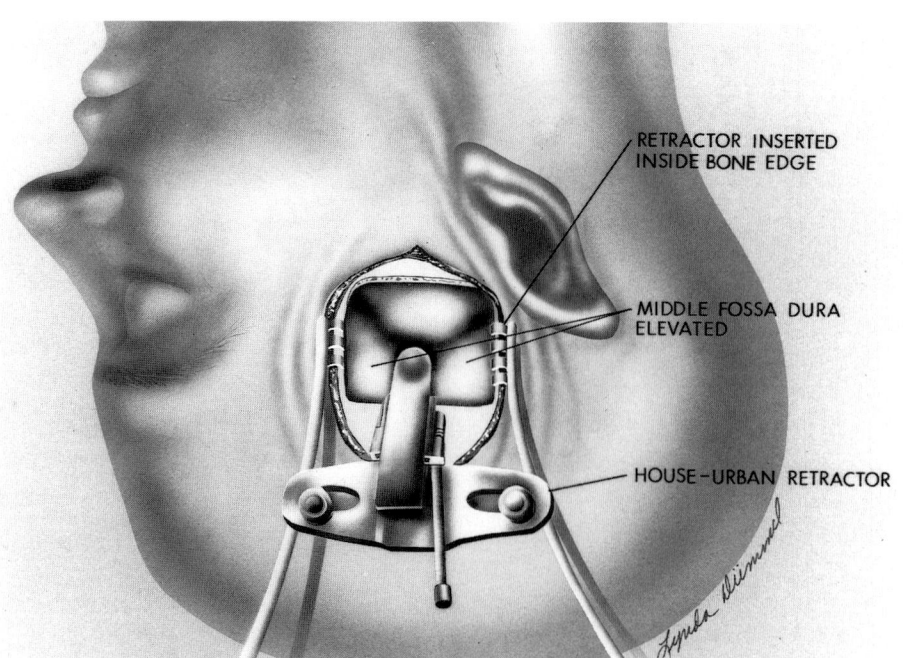

FIG. 4. Middle fossa retractor is firmly locked in place, and dural elevation is begun.

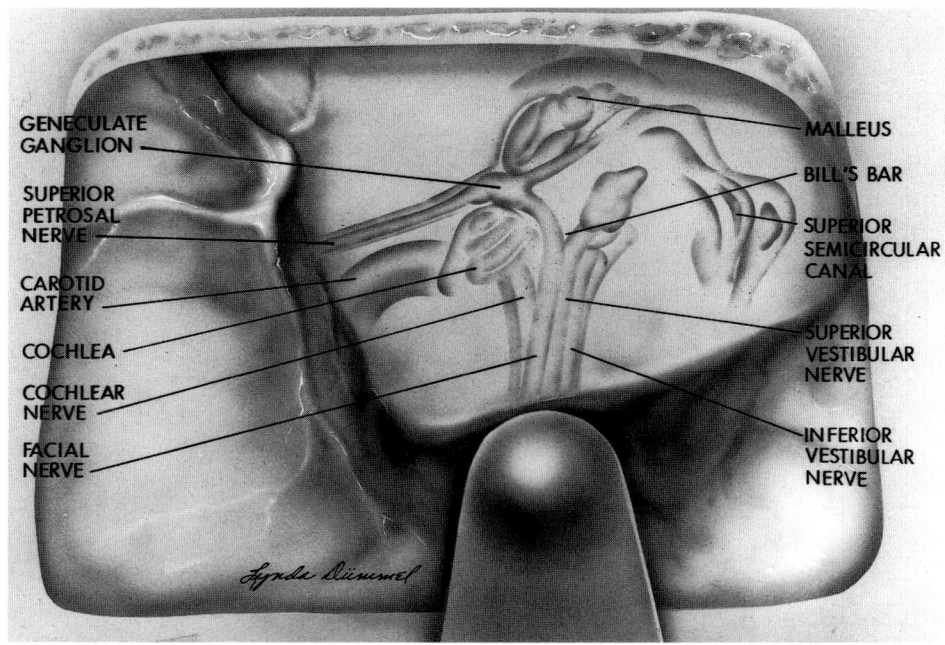

FIG. 5. Relationship of structures within the temporal bone as viewed from the middle fossa.

the gasserian ganglion, an up to 5% incidence of facial paralysis has been reported. With careful dural elevation performed with the aid of the surgical microscope, this complication can be avoided in all cases.

As dural elevation proceeds, the arcuate eminence is encountered. At times, this is an obvious landmark but sometimes it is indistinct. The positive landmark is the greater superficial petrosal nerve, which passes parallel to the petrous ridge from the geniculate ganglion anteri-

orly. This nerve lies medial to the middle meningeal artery. Once the greater superficial petrosal nerve has been identified, it is carefully followed to the hiatus of the facial nerve and the blade of the middle fossa retractor is readjusted (Fig. 6).

A word of caution is necessary regarding pressure on the bone of the floor of the middle fossa. Both in the area of the tegmen and over the internal carotid artery the bone may be very thin and rarely even dehiscent. Al-

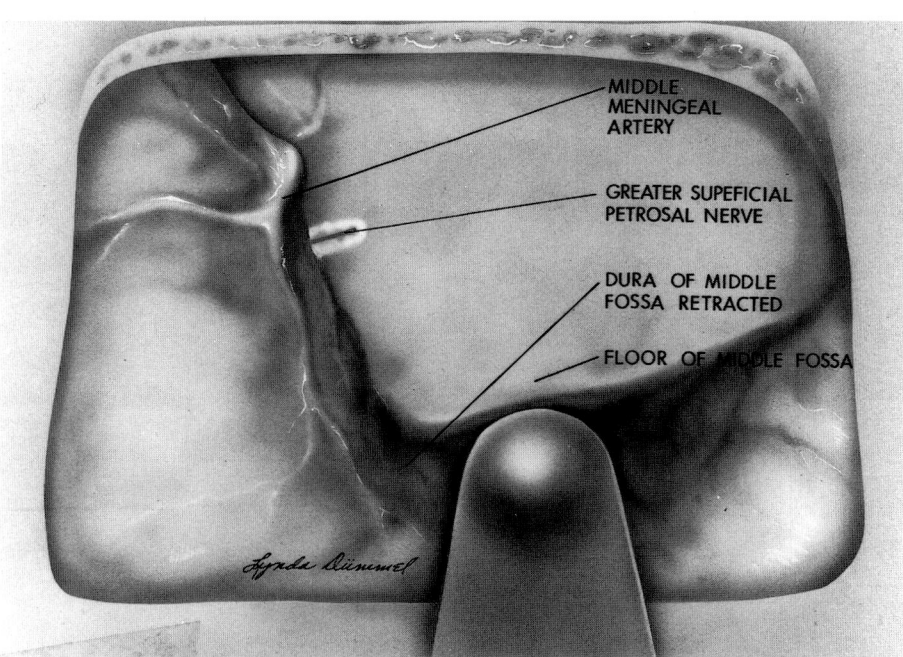

FIG. 6. Dura is elevated and the greater superficial petrosal nerve is identified medial to the middle meningeal artery.

though injury to the internal carotid artery has not occurred in our cases, care must be taken to avoid this complication. At this point the major landmarks of the middle fossa approach have been identified. These are the middle meningeal artery, arcuate eminence, and the greater superficial petrosal nerve and facial hiatus. Therefore the surgeon is ready to begin bone removal over the internal auditory canal. There is often considerable bleeding from small vessels on the surface of the dura and the floor of the middle fossa. This bleeding is particularly troublesome since it pools into the most dependent portion of the wound where the bone removal is to begin. Considerable bleeding from any one vessel must be controlled. It is usual, however, for oozing to occur from multiple sites. We have found that such bleeding will stop spontaneously and it is best to proceed with the operation at this point.

Exposure of the Internal Auditory Canal

A large diamond burr and continuous suction-irrigation are brought in and careful removal of bone to identify landmarks of the temporal bone is begun. It is important to use the largest burr early in the bone removal since it offers the most protection against accidental injury to the geniculate ganglion, facial nerve, or superior semicircular canal. Attention is directed to the greater superficial petrosal nerve and bone is gently removed from the area of the hiatus until the geniculate ganglion is identified. A thin shell of bone is usually left over the geniculate ganglion but the ganglion itself is readily apparent through the bone (Fig. 7). By this time, bleeding has usually subsided. If not, it is advisable to spend the time necessary to control the bleeding before proceeding.

The labyrinthine portion of the facial nerve is then followed from the geniculate ganglion to the internal auditory canal (Fig. 8). The labyrinthine portion of the facial nerve courses parallel to the plane of the superior semicircular canal. A smaller diamond burr is necessary for this bone removal since the ampullated end of the superior semicircular canal lies only a few millimeters posterior to the facial nerve at this point and the cochlea lies only a few millimeters anteriorly.

Some surgeons prefer to proceed with removal of bone over the internal auditory canal following the identification of the superior semicircular canal. The internal auditory canal makes an angle of 45°–60° with the superior semicircular canal. We have found it easier to positively identify the internal auditory canal by following the facial nerve. We have not experienced problems with facial nerve paralysis by using this technique. Continuous monitoring of the facial nerve alerts the surgeon when the facial nerve is exposed.

Once the internal auditory canal has been identified, bone removal is continued medially until the entire superior surface of the internal auditory canal is exposed. As the surgeon proceeds medially it is possible to enlarge the exposure because the superior semicircular canal courses posteriorly and the dissection is medial to the cochlea (Fig. 9). Bone removal is continued until the porus acusticus is removed. The superior petrosal sinus grooves the

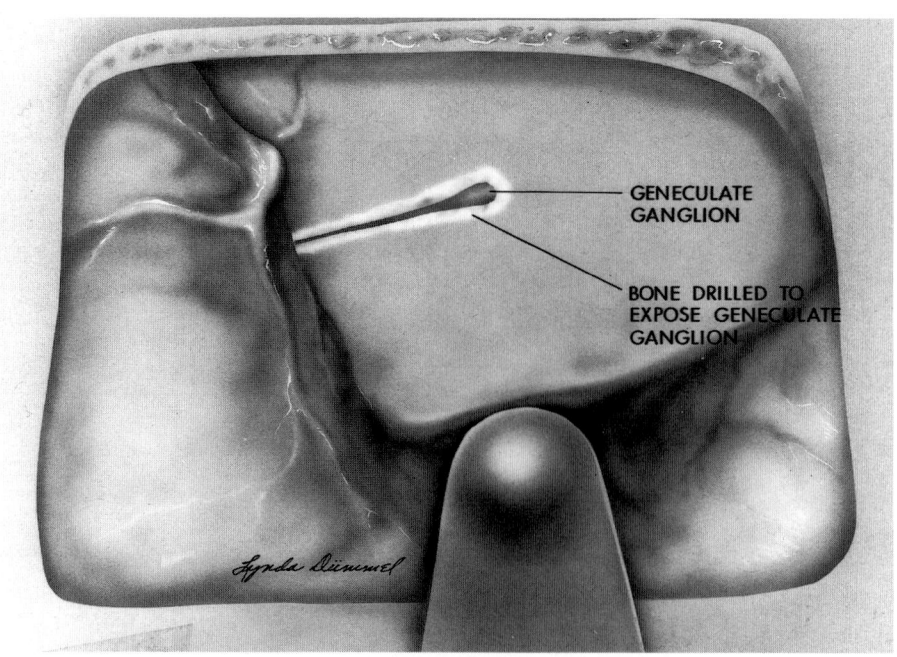

FIG. 7. Bone is removed from the greater superficial petrosal nerve until the geniculate ganglion is identified.

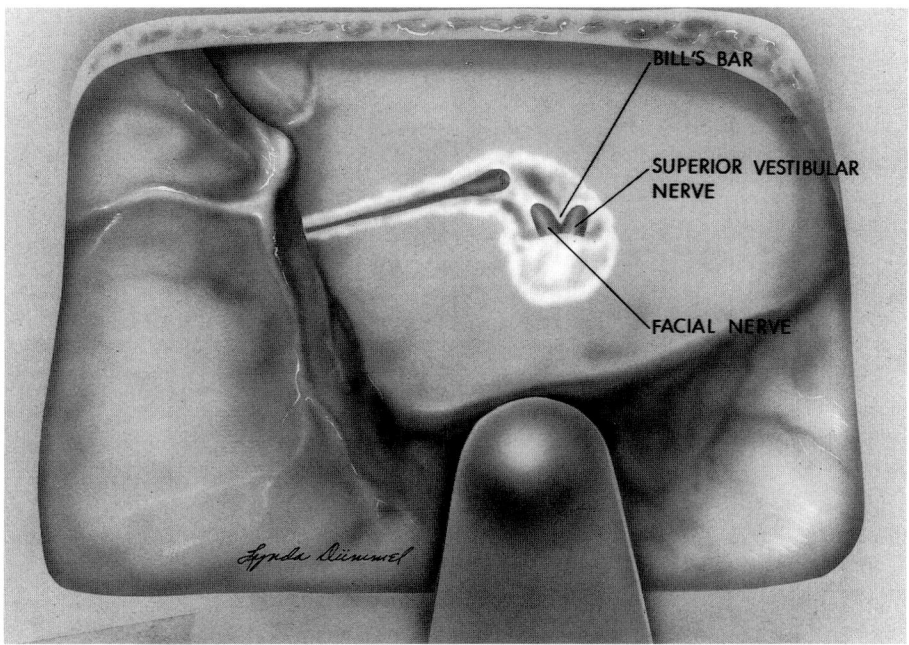

FIG. 8. Labyrinthine portion of the facial nerve is uncovered from the geniculate ganglion to the internal auditory canal.

petrous ridge and care is taken not to enter the superior petrosal sinus.

Great care must be taken to remove the bone without entering the dura because the facial nerve lies directly against the dura. It is best to leave an eggshell thickness of bone over the entire surface of the internal auditory canal until all the bone removal has been completed.

Bone removal must be extensive for middle fossa acoustic tumor surgery. Medially, bone removal is carried far anterior and posterior to the internal auditory canal. The superior petrosal sinus will be lying free in the dura following removal of the petrous ridge. Care must be taken to avoid bleeding but should it occur it may be controlled with extraluminal packing of Surgicel or with clips.

The dissection is limited posteriorly by the superior semicircular canal. Bone is carefully removed from the entire extent of the internal auditory canal, which allows

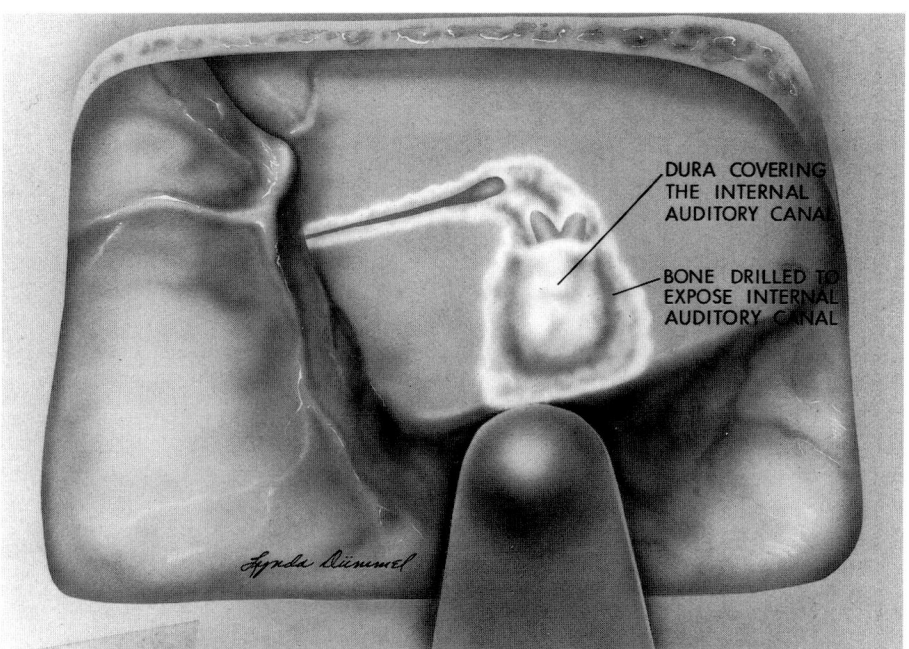

FIG. 9. Bone is removed from the entire length of the internal auditory canal, including the porus acusticus.

exposure of approximately three-quarters of the circumference of the canal at the porus. It is not possible to achieve this degree of exposure in the lateral portion of the internal auditory canal because of the restricting position of the ampulla of the superior semicircular canal and the cochlea.

When bone removal has been completed medially, the lateral end of the internal auditory canal is dissected and the vertical crust of bone separating the facial nerve from the superior vestibular nerve (Bill's bar) is identified.

This completes the bone removal. The fine eggshell layer of bone is then removed and the dura is open along the posterior aspects of the internal auditory canal (Fig. 10). The facial nerve lies anteriorly and the first exposure of the internal auditory canal should be away from the facial nerve. The dural flap is carefully elevated from the underlying tumor and the facial nerve is identified at the lateral end of the internal auditory canal where the vertical crest of bone (Bill's bar) allows positive identification (Fig. 11). The superior vestibular nerve lies posteriorly at this point and a fine hook is used to begin the separation of the superior vestibular nerve and tumor from the facial nerve.

Tumor Removal

The vestibulofacial anastomotic fibers are cut and the superior vestibular nerve is cut at the end of the internal auditory canal. Separation of the tumor from the end of the internal auditory canal and the facial nerve is next begun. The principle of the tumor removal is that the tumor is freed from the facial nerve and the internal auditory canal and is delivered posteriorly out from under the facial nerve. For this reason, it is most important to remove all the bone from the posterior aspect of the internal auditory canal (Fig. 12).

Freeing of the lateral end of the tumor, particularly in the inferior compartment of the internal auditory canal, is one of the most difficult parts of the dissection. This difficulty is attributable to the poor view of the most lateral aspect of the inferior compartment of the internal auditory canal. The removal is accomplished with a long hook that is used to palpate the end of the internal auditory canal. It is best to totally section both the superior and inferior vestibular nerves to prevent postoperative unsteadiness. A partial vestibular denervation is more likely to result in unsteadiness than is total removal of both vestibular nerves.

The tumor is gently teased out of the lateral end of the internal auditory canal. The blood supply to the cochlea usually runs between the facial and cochlear nerves and in most cases is preserved with those nerves. At times, however, the arterial supply to the cochlea is interrupted, resulting in hearing impairment even though preservation of the cochlear nerve was achieved.

Once the lateral end of the tumor has been freed, the plane between the cochlear and facial nerves and tumor becomes apparent. This plane is then carefully developed through the use of fine hooks and the Rosen separator. Tumor dissection is continued medially and a search for the anterior/inferior cerebellar artery is begun. The

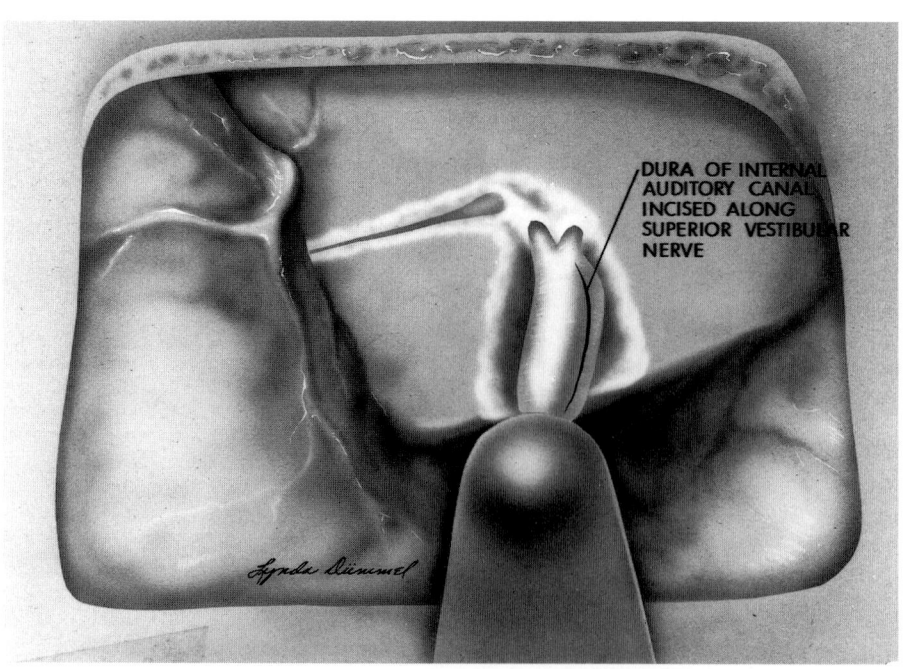

FIG. 10. Lateral end of the internal auditory canal has been dissected and the vertical crest (Bill's bar) identified. The dura is then incised at the posterior margin of the internal auditory canal.

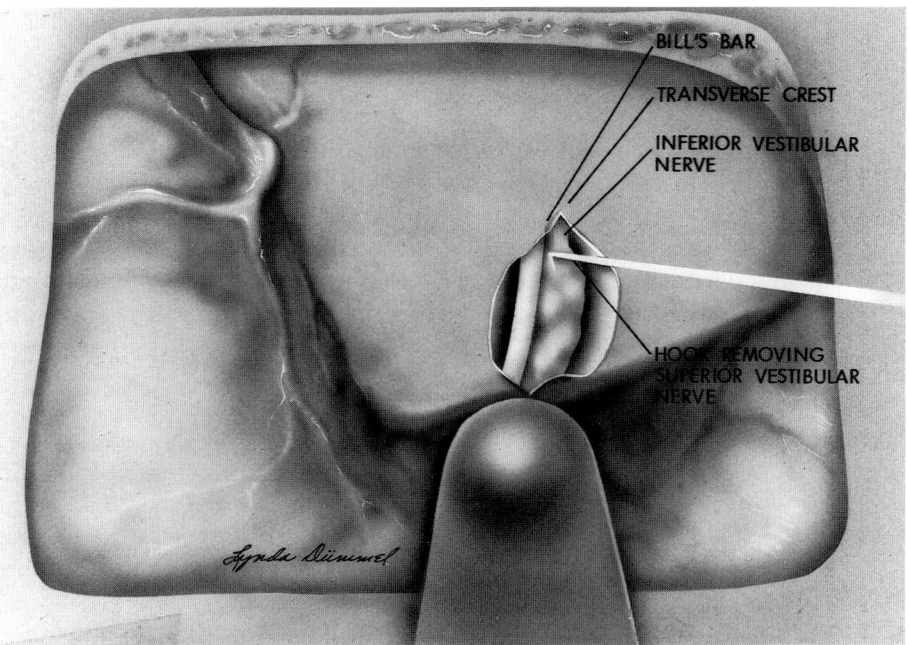

FIG. 11. Tumor is separated from the facial nerve at the end of the internal auditory canal. It is carefully freed from the facial and cochlear nerves and delivered posteriorly.

artery may loop up into the internal auditory canal inferior to the cochlear nerve or the tumor may displace it into the cerebellopontine angle. Great care must be taken to identify and not injure this most important artery.

After the anterior/inferior cerebellar artery has been identified, it is freed from the surface of the tumor by careful blunt dissection with the Rosen elevator. The final problem is freeing the most medial aspect of the tumor. Before this, it is often necessary to partially remove the tumor with small cup forceps. This prevents stretching of the facial nerve. During the course of the dissection the surgeon must be careful not to injure the facial nerve with the suction. This possibility is reduced by the use of fenestrated neurotologic suction (4). Freeing of the medial end of the tumor with small hooks

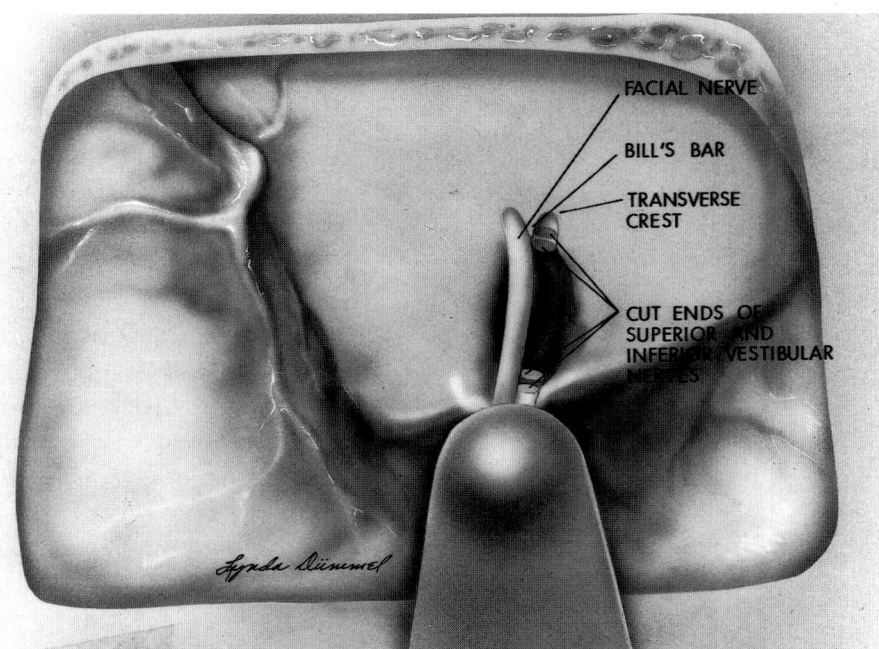

FIG. 12. Tumor has been removed. It is best to section the inferior vestibular nerve to minimize the risk of postoperative unsteadiness.

allows its removal (Fig. 12). Continuous intraoperative monitoring of facial nerve activity greatly facilitates dissection of the tumor from the facial nerve and is routinely used.

After total tumor removal, the tumor bed is irrigated profusely. Bleeding from small vessels usually subsides during the irrigation. At times larger vessels will require bipolar cautery for control of bleeding.

Inadvertent injury to the anterior/inferior cerebellar artery is always a possibility during removal of the medial aspect of the tumor. Control of bleeding would be extremely difficult in this situation because of limited access. Fortunately, this has not occurred in our experience: but if it should, it might be necessary to remove more bone in the area of the superior semicircular canal to expose more of the posterior fossa dura in order to gain access for the application of a clip. If bleeding should still not be controlled, it might be necessary to perform a postauricular approach and translabyrinthine exposure of the cerebellopontine angle to achieve this control.

Wound Closure

Closure of the defect in the internal auditory canal is accomplished with a free graft of temporalis muscle. The temporal bone flap is then replaced and the temporalis muscle resutured to its insertion. The subcutaneous tissue and skin are closed in layers and a sterile dressing is applied. If there is excessive oozing, a Penrose drain is used.

COMPLICATIONS AND MANAGEMENT

An epidural hematoma is an uncommon early postoperative complication. The incidence of this may be reduced by use of a Penrose drain where there is excessive oozing. Meticulous attention to hemostasis is a necessity. Patients with this complication will exhibit signs of increasing intracranial pressure. Treatment is immediate evacuation of the hematoma in the intensive care unit. The patient is then taken to surgery where more definitive control of the bleeding is accomplished.

Other complications are those that are common to any intracranial procedure, such as meningitis. Temporal lobe injury from retraction on the temporal lobe was an early concern but has not been a problem in our series. We have had no patients who have had signs of cortical injury such as hemiparesis or aphasia. Hearing loss and facial paralysis are expected complications in some of these patients as with any acoustic tumor removal.

DISCUSSION OF SERIES

The middle fossa approach has been used to remove 106 acoustic neuromas at the Otologic Medical Group as of December 1986 (5). The size of these tumors has varied from 0.4 to 2 cm. Hearing was preserved in 63 patients (59%). In 37 patients (35%), hearing was the same as before surgery. There was a partial loss of hearing in 26 patients (25%). In the remainder a total sensorineural hearing loss occurred despite preservation of the cochlear nerve in 89% of patients. Hearing roughly correlated with tumor size: hearing preservation is better for smaller tumors.

Eighty percent of patients had normal facial nerve function 1 year after middle fossa surgery for removal of acoustic tumors. Another 9% had Grade II function and the remainder a greater degree of weakness. No patient had a total facial nerve paralysis. These statistics demonstrate the increased risk to the facial nerve in the middle fossa approach. In the translabyrinthine approach, with tumors of this size, 88% have normal facial function. The attempt at hearing preservation offered by the middle fossa approach does increase the risk to the facial nerve.

Other than hearing loss and facial weakness, there were no other serious complications or deaths in this series.

MODIFICATIONS OF THE MIDDLE FOSSA APPROACH

Facial Nerve Decompression and Repair

The middle fossa approach is modified for exposure of the facial nerve for decompression in idiopathic facial palsy or temporal bone trauma and for the removal of tumors affecting the facial nerve. For these conditions, exposure of the facial nerve is continued distal from the geniculate ganglion into the upper tympanic segment of the nerve to the area of the cochleariform process. This requires removal of the tegmen. Great care is taken to avoid injury to the head of the malleus, which lies just beneath the tegmen slightly laterally.

For facial nerve decompression it is not necessary to expose the medial aspect of the internal auditory canal. Only the distal aspect of the canal is exposed so that there is adequate decompression of the labyrinthine segment of the nerve with free flow of cerebrospinal fluid after the dura is incised.

Selective Vestibular Nerve Section

Exposure of the internal auditory canal for selective vestibular nerve section is similar to that for acoustic tumor removal except that it need not be as extensive, particularly medially in the area of the porus acusticus. The entire roof of the internal auditory canal is removed, however, to allow careful identification and section of the vestibular nerves while preserving the cochlear nerve, facial nerve, and the blood supply to the inner ear.

Decompression of the Internal Auditory Canal for Bilateral Acoustic Tumors

The exposure for this procedure is very similar to that for acoustic tumor removal. The entire roof of the internal auditory canal is removed and the dura opened to allow superior expansion of the tumor within the internal auditory canal. Great care is taken to avoid the cochlea and superior semicircular canal as the lateral end of the internal auditory canal is dissected.

CONCLUSION

The middle fossa approach is the preferred method for removal of small, laterally placed acoustic neuromas. It also offers the possibility of treatment of facial nerve disorders and selective vestibular neurectomy with preservation of hearing and balance function.

REFERENCES

1. House WF, Luetje CM, eds. *Acoustic tumors,* vol 1, *Management.* Baltimore: University Park Press, 1979.
2. Brackmann DE, Hitselberger WE, Benecke JE, House WF. Acoustic neuromas: middle fossa and translabyrinthine removal. In: Rand RW, ed. *Microneurosurgery.* St Louis: Mosby, 1985.
3. Gadre AK, Kwartler JA, Brackmann DE, House WF, Hitselberger WE. Middle fossa decompression of the internal auditory canal in acoustic neuroma surgery: a therapeutic alternative. *Laryngoscope,* 1990;100:948–952.
4. Brackmann DE. Fenestrated suction for neuro-otologic surgery. *Trans Am Acad Ophthalmol Otolaryngol* 1977;84:975.
5. Shelton MF, Brackmann DE, House WF, Hitselberger WE. Middle fossa acoustic tumor surgery: results in 106 cases. *Laryngoscope* 1989;99:405–408.

CHAPTER 25

Surgical Strategy for Jugular Foramen Tumors

Madjid Samii and Walter Bini

A rarity among skull base tumors are those involving the jugular foramen. Due to the location and its role as neurovascular pathway, the diagnosis and management of lesions involving this area remain a challenge to neuroradiologists, ENT, and neurosurgeons. Interdisciplinary cooperation is needed to achieve an optimal therapeutic outcome.

With the sophistication of microsurgical techniques and technical progress in diagnostic methodology, decisive advances have been made in the treatment of this type of pathology. Using angiography, high-resolution computed tomography (CT), and magnetic resonance imaging (MRI), the neuroradiologist and surgeon are able to completely evaluate the pathological process, obtaining detailed data concerning the vascularization of the lesion and of the adjacent normal tissue with its possible variations, information about the osseous anatomy of the cranial base, and the relationship between lesion and neighboring neurovascular structures.

Using the clinical evaluation along with the topographic diagnostic details, the optimal treatment plan can be formulated (1,4).

In our experience over the past decade with 1029 skull base interventions, we treated 55 tumors involving the jugular foramen (Table 1). The experience gained has led to a well defined preoperative diagnostic workup protocol, an interdisciplinary team evaluation, and a modifiable microsurgical approach.

SPECIAL DIAGNOSTIC CONSIDERATIONS

Our preoperative diagnostic protocol begins with a high-resolution CT study without and with intravenous contrast medium in axial and coronal projections. Dynamic studies may also be performed if highly vascularized lesions are suspected. Special attention is given to the skull base. An area extending from the craniocervical junction up to the tentorial notch is examined in 1.5-mm slices. CT of the osseous skull base (bone window) is extremely important. The simple enlargement or a destruction/erosion of the foramen and nearby area has a decisive differential diagnostic value (Figs. 1 and 2). It is possible to document the important neurovascular structures that are affected by the process, that is, carotid, hypoglossal, and facial nerve canal, as well as the petrous bone and clivus. By localizing the process and its relation to the bony skull base, possible approaches can be considered and discussed.

To further form a three-dimensional surgical representation, the next step is a MRI study including administration of paramagnetic contrast medium. Of special value are the sagittal and coronal projections (Figs. 3 and 4)

TABLE 1. *Distribution of the 55 cases in our series with involvement of the jugular foramen considering pathological entities*

Tumors in jugular foramen N = 25	
Neurinomas	13
Chemodectomas	10
Paraganglioma	1
Vascular tumor	1
Tumors affecting the jugular foramen N = 30	
Meningiomas	20
CPA (11)	
Petroclival (6)	
Craniocervical (2)	
Intraosseous (1)	
Epidermoids	4
Clivus chordoma	5
Carcinomas (mastoid)	1

M. Samii: Department of Neurosurgery, Hannover Medical School, and Neurosurgical Clinic, Nordstadt Hospital, 3000 Hannover, Germany.
W. Bini: Neurosurgical Clinic, Nordstadt Hospital, 3000 Hannover 1, Germany.

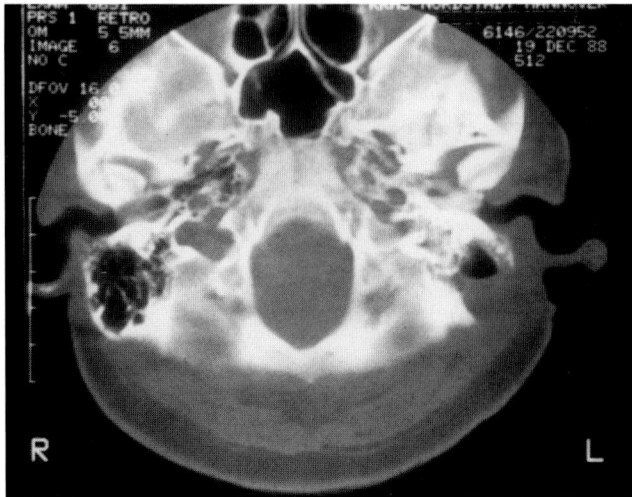

FIG. 1. Axial CT slices of the skull base (bone window) showing an enlarged jugular foramen characteristic for a neurinoma (*left* in photograph).

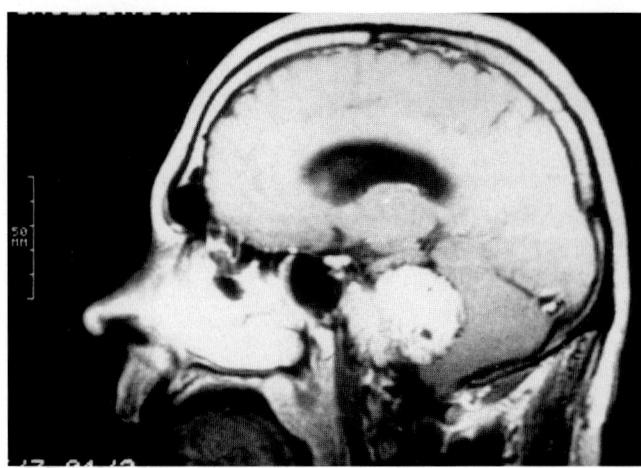

FIG. 3. Sagittal MRI slices after administration of paramagnetic contrast medium, demonstrating an extensive glomus jugulare tumor. The actual surgical anatomy can be better analyzed as osseous superimposition is excluded.

with enlargement of the region of interest. The tumor size can be sharply delimitated, and by exclusion of the osseous skull base, we obtain the intrinsic relationship of the lesion to the brain stem and medulla oblongata, as well as the exact intracranial and extracranial extension. Mass displacement and the actual surgical anatomy are seen. In recent cases, we perform MR angiography as a screening test to evaluate blood vessel involvement and to exclude an early invasion of a venous sinus (Figs. 5 and 6). MRI is also highly sensitive in delimiting the area of peritumoral edema.

Next, an angiogram is carried out with modifications depending on the mass and extension of the lesion as demonstrated by the noninvasive procedures. A detailed angiographical examination is essential for evaluation of the following:

1. Type, number, and size of the feeding vessels.
2. Angio architecture and vascular composition, as well as the relationship with adjacent tissue vascularization.
3. Venous drainage and patency or invasion of dural sinuses.
4. Circulation time through the vascular bed.

Lateral and anteroposterior projections are mandatory. Only by analyzing both can we detect contralateral supply, assess collateral circulation, evaluate the position of dural sinuses and the jugular bulb in the venous angiogram, and detect intracranial intradural extensions. All four vessels are studied, and the internal–external carotid arteries are studied selectively.

With the angiographic information, fundamental de-

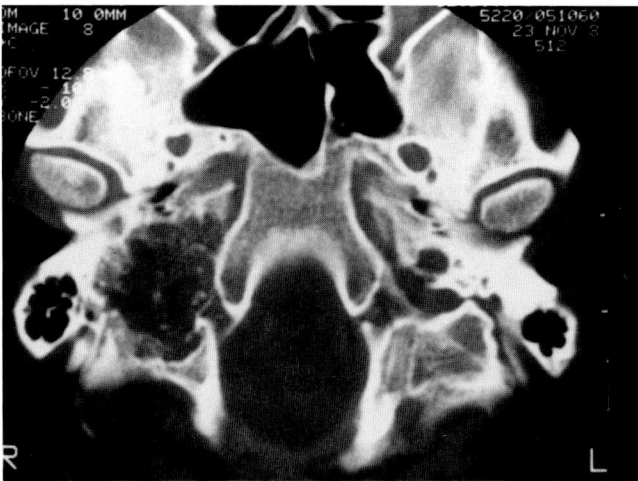

FIG. 2. An example of erosion/destruction of the foramen pathognomonic of a chemodectoma (*left* in photograph).

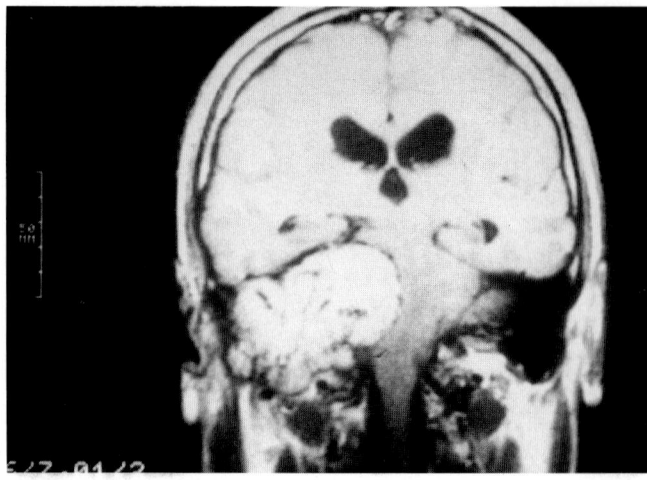

FIG. 4. Coronal MRI slices, for area and conditions as in Fig. 3.

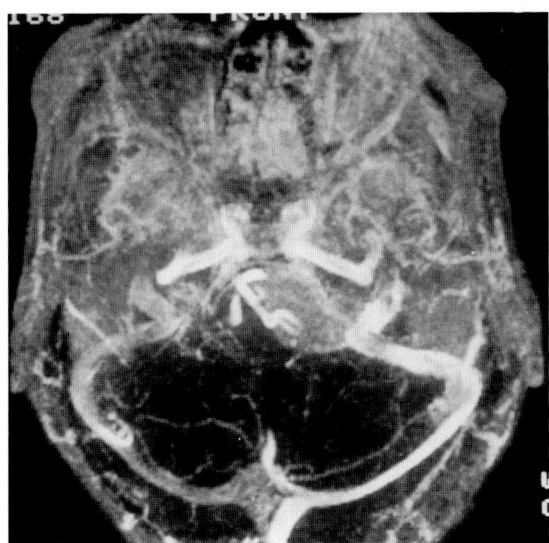

FIG. 5. MR angiography in axial projections (front view). A noninvasive vascular study or screening is possible.

cisions about tumor management can be made. The combination of surgical neuroangiography followed by microsurgical exposure has clearly reduced intraoperative complications, permitting a more complete tumor excision (1,13).

SURGICAL STRATEGY

The choice of the surgical approach is determined by the location, extension, and nature of the lesion. Tumors arising from the jugular foramen, which extend intracranially to the cerebellopontine angle, are approached via a lateral suboccipital route, whereas those extending extracranially into the neck are removed through a cervical exposure. More difficult and controversial are those tumors that are located within the jugular foramen and extend both intracranially and extracranially. In the 1970s, based on pioneering work (Shapiro, Neuss, House, Dennecke, Kempe, Fisch, Glasscock, Jackson, Gardner, Hakuba, Samii, and Draf), the combined otoneurosurgical approach was introduced. Our modification of the combined lateral suboccipital–infralabyrinthine approach has proved advantageous and has contributed to better surgical results with radical tumor removal (2,3,5–12,16,17).

We operate on patients in the supine position with the head turned 50° to the opposite side, elevated 10° from the horizontal plane, and flexed 15° after fixation in the Mayfield pins and head rest. A retroauricular skin incision is extended along the anterior border of the sternocleidomastoid muscle up to the level of the hyoid bone (Fig. 7). The mastoid bone is exposed after mobilizing the origin of the sternocleidomastoid muscle and the posterior belly of the digastric muscle, the latter one being detached from the digastric groove. The caudal cranial nerves are identified in the neck along with the internal jugular vein and followed cranially to the skull base. Above and anterior to the origin of the digastric muscle, in the depth of the tympanomastoidal fissure, we find the main stem of the facial nerve, inferior to the stylomastoid foramen.

Then the otological approach to the superior aspect of the jugular foramen is performed. First, we perform a cortical mastoidectomy exposing the antrum, the lateral semicircular canal, and the vertical portion of the facial nerve. Rerouting cranial nerve VII is only necessary if the tumor extends to the middle ear cavity or to the carotid canal, as in cases of extensive glomus jugular tumors. For the whole procedure, we use a diamond drill under constant irrigation suction.

Lateral to the occipitomastoidal suture, we remove a part of the occipital squama, performing a lateral suboccipital osteoclastic craniotomy, exposing both the trans-

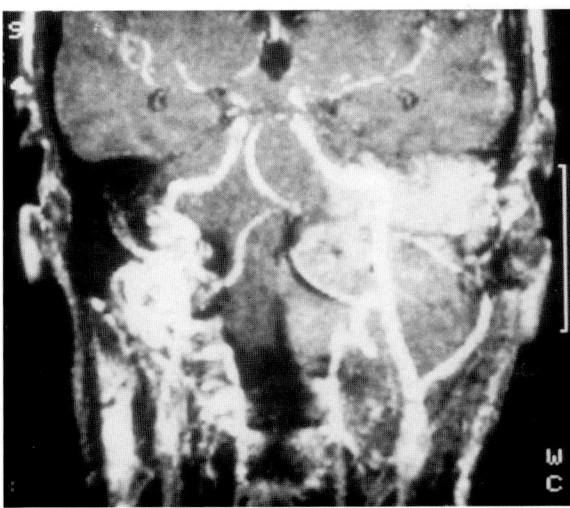

FIG. 6. MR angiography in coronal projections.

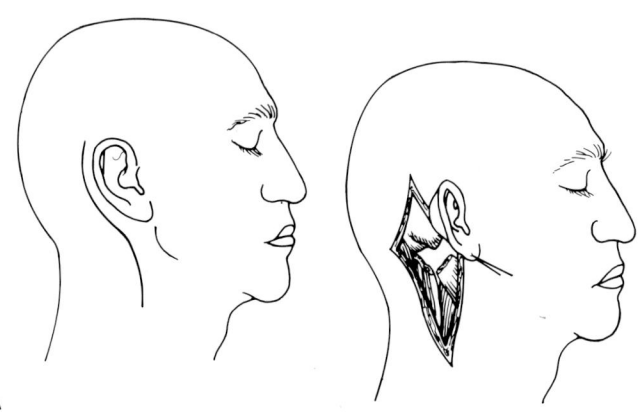

FIG. 7. Illustrations showing the skin incision (**A**) and the exposure (**B**) for the modified combined otoneurosurgical approach to the jugular foramen.

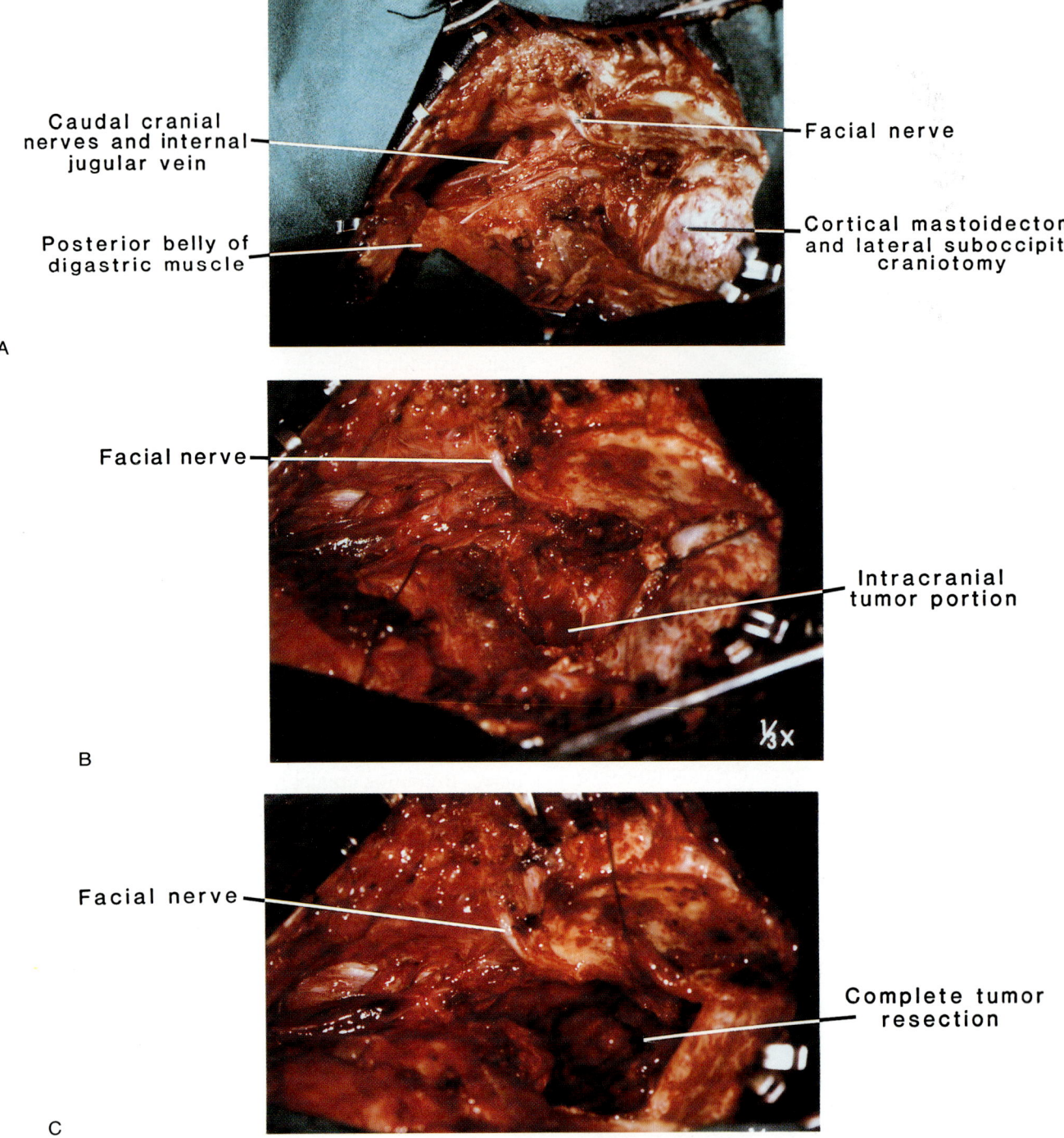

FIG. 8. The four steps shown here illustrate the step-wise surgical resection of a tumor involving the jugular foramen. **A:** Left retroauricular exposure (patient is in supine position with the head turned 50° to the opposite side and elevated approximately 10° from the horizontal plane and flexed 15°). Exposure of mastoid is achieved after mobilizing the origin of both sternocleidomastoid and posterior belly of the digastric muscles. Caudal cranial nerves are identified in the neck and prepared in cranial direction. Main stem of the facial nerve is under view. Cortical mastoidectomy and lateral suboccipital craniotomy expose the transverse and sigmoid sinuses. **B:** Dura is incised ventral to the sigmoid sinus, extending the incision to the jugular foramen and shifting the sinus medially. Exposure of intracranial tumor portion is achieved. **C:** After the extracranial portion is removed, the intracranial extension is resected through the widened jugular foramen. In cases of chemodectomas, the sigmoid sinus is ligated and packed as well as the IJV. After intracranial enucleation, an en bloc resection is performed. In neurinoma surgery, the sinus is left intact. **D:** Dural closure using lyophilized patch and fibrin glue. The muscles are then returned to their site of insertion.

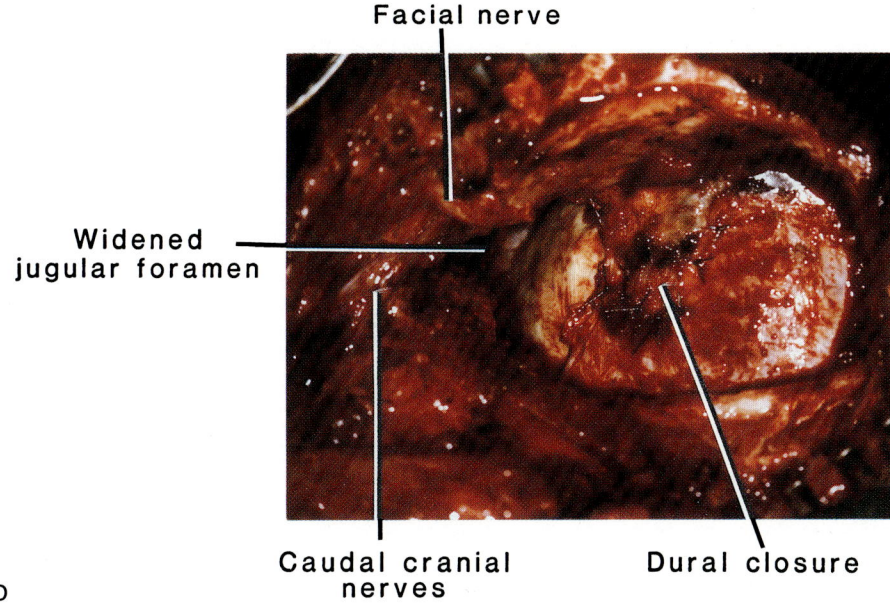

FIG. 8. Continued.

verse and sigmoid sinuses. The sigmoid sinus is mobilized from its bony groove caudally down to the jugular foramen. The temporal bone is further drilled away anteromedial to the fallopian canal to the styloid process, and inferior to the labyrinth, and the mastoid tip is removed. Extending the exposure, the posterior part of the occipital condyle is removed, thus opening the jugular foramen dorsolaterally. Medial to the junction of the jugular bulb and internal jugular vein, the lateral process of the atlas with the origin of the oblique atlantis muscle is to be identified. Through this exposure, the lesion, the sigmoid sinus, the jugular bulb, and the internal jugular vein come into view. Neurinomas displace the jugular bulb dorsally, whereas chemodectomas arise from the dome of the jugular bulb extending intraluminally to the sigmoid sinus and internal jugular vein, causing erosion of the skull base.

The dura of the posterior cranial fossa is incised anterior to the sigmoid sinus, extending the incision to the jugular foramen and moving the sinus medially. In case of extensive intracranial extension, the dura is opened cranial to the transverse sinus, with transection of the tentorium.

After retraction of the dura, transverse and sigmoid sinuses, and the jugular bulb medially, the cerebellum is retracted, gently opening the cerebellopontine cistern, and thus releasing CSF. The intracranial tumor portion is thus exposed.

We start by resecting the extracranial portion of the lesion so that the caudal cranial nerves remain under vision. The piecemeal enucleation is performed microsurgically. The intracranial portion is then resected through the widened jugular foramen, taking care not to injure the neural structures (nerves IX–XII) ventral to the tumor mass. In cases of chemodectomas, the sigmoid sinus is ligated and packed as well as the internal jugular vein. After enucleating the tumor intraluminally, an "en bloc" resection follows. With neurinomas and other nonvascular lesions, we leave the sinus intact (Fig. 8).

After meticulous hemostasis, we return the jugular bulb to its site and then close the dura. The defect at the jugular foramen is covered with a cone-shaped piece of lyophilized dura, fat, or fascia lata and packed with the posterior belly of the digastric muscle. Fibrin glue is also used during the closure procedure. The mastoid antrum and mastoid air cells are also sealed with muscle and fibrin glue. Finally, the sternocleidomastoid muscle is resutured to its site of origin.

To avoid a postoperative CSF fistula, we place a lumbar drainage under antibiotic coverage for 10 days (Table 2). It is important for the patients to be informed carefully about the risks of additional impairment of the

TABLE 2. *Main surgical steps*

1. Skin incision (modifiable depending on extent of tumors)
2. Identification of parotid gland and ventral border of sternocleidomastoid muscle preparation of vessels and caudal cranial nerves, exposure of VIIth nerve
3. Ligation of ECA and pharyngeal branch, when preoperative embolization not performed; when embolization required this will be performed 3–5 days prior to surgery using PVA particles and Gelfoam.
4. Lateral suboccipital craniotomy, exposure of sigmoid sinus and jugular bulb
5. Partial/total petrosectomy
6. Ligation of IJV and sigmoid sinus; this latter one can be resected when tumor extends extradurally
7. Microsurgical piecemeal tumor debulking
8. Closure of dural gap
9. Sealing of eustachian tube using digastric muscle
10. Resuture sternocleidomastoid muscle, closure of neck cavity; lumbar drainage for 10–14 days.

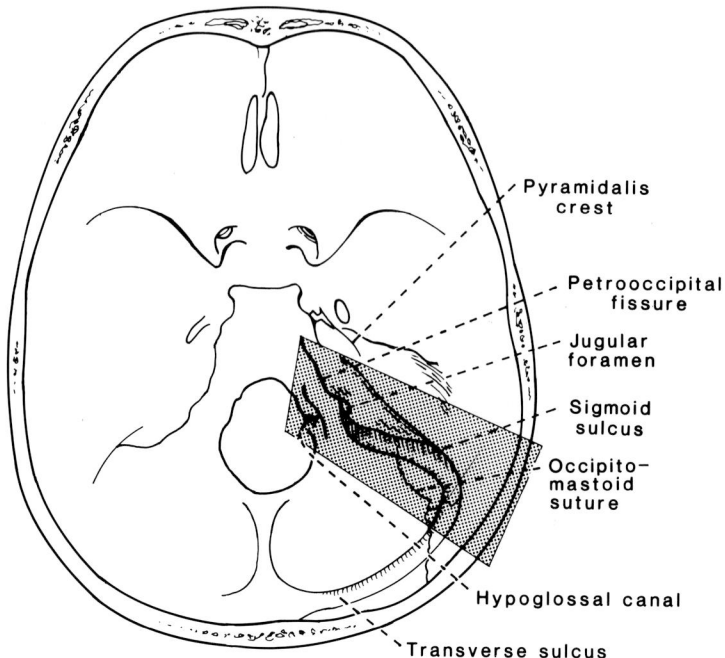

FIG. 9. Illustration of the route opened through our exposure and the relationship of the main anatomical landmarks of the region.

caudal cranial nerves, as well as the significant risk of postoperative aspiration. A second surgical procedure might be necessary for repair of the pharyngeal paresis. In our experience, we have observed that if the paresis of nerves IX, X, and XII has been slowly progressive, the altered mechanism of swallowing has been compensated. Greater problems occur in those patients who have normal caudal cranial nerve function preoperatively. Intensive patient observation and care must be stressed in the immediate postoperative phase. The moment of extubation is a critical instant, at which time a thorough neurological evaluation must be made.

RESULTS AND DISCUSSION

After introduction and standardization of the combined approach for jugular foramen surgery, total tumor removal with low morbidity in one stage is possible (15). Our modification to the surgical technique has shown very satisfactory results in varied pathology (Fig. 9) (17). The overall results are summarized in Table 3.

There was no operative mortality and total tumor excision was achieved in all but two cases. The subtotal or partial removals were a case of clivus chordoma and an extensive infiltrative petroclival meningioma that also affected the cavernous sinus. The surgical morbidity was 34.5%. Regarding postoperative cranial nerve affection, Tables 4 and 5 document the new deficits and the total number of permanent new cranial nerve palsies. The danger of aspiration pneumonia is considerably high.

Even though several approaches exist and can be used to excise lesions with intracranial and extracranial por-

tions, we believe that for a one-stage removal, the modified combined otoneurosurgical approach is the method of choice (Fig. 8). The infralabyrinthine approach is indicated in cases with intact hearing, where the upper tumor limit does not involve the internal auditory meatus. This method is a modification of the operative technique described by Fisch and Jenkins for excising chemodectomas arising within the jugular foramen. Often, to allow for lower morbidity and greater radicality, a posterior fossa craniectomy approach must be performed as a second-stage operation. The translabyrinthine or transcochlear approach may be selected for those cases with poor hearing, or where the lesion's upper limit reaches the internal auditory meatus but does not extend considerably intracranially nor downward into the neck. For these cases also, a posterior fossa approach is necessary to remove tumor safely at the level of the cerebellopontine angle. Facial and cochlear nerve morbidity is considerable via this route.

The extended facial recess approach was used in addition to the above-mentioned techniques by Horn,

TABLE 3. *Overall results in 55 cases of lesions involving the jugular foramen*

Number of patients	55
Total removal	53
Subtotal resection, including clivus chordoma and petroclival meningioma	2
Operative mortality	0
Surgical morbidity	19 (34.5%)
Cranial nerve lesions	19
Aspiration pneumonia	8
CSF leak	6

TABLE 4. *Preoperative and postoperative cranial nerve affection*

Nerve	Preoperative	Postoperative
V	1	3
VI	—	1
VII	4	11
VIII	17	20
IX	8	11
X	12	13
XI	6	8
XII	10	10

TABLE 5. *Temporary versus permanent new cranial deficits (N = 19)*

Nerve	Temporary	Permanent
V	1	1
VI	1	—
VII	5	2
VIII	—	3
IX	—	3
X	—	1
XI	2	—
XII	—	—
		10

House, and Hitselberger, providing an improved exposure of the hypotympanum. On removal of the mastoid tip, a complete exposure of the sigmoid sinus, jugular bulb, and internal jugular vein can be achieved.

In the retrolabyrinthine approach, a total mastoidectomy is first done followed by a posterior fossa exposure over and behind the sigmoid sinus. The jugular bulb is exposed and the bone between the bulb and the posterior semicircular canal is removed to expose the facial and vestibulocochlear nerve complex over the superior aspect of the tumor. Marked postoperative CSF leak and a higher morbidity for both the abducens and facial nerves have been reported.

Our modification of the combined lateral suboccipital–infralabyrinthine approach has the following advantages:

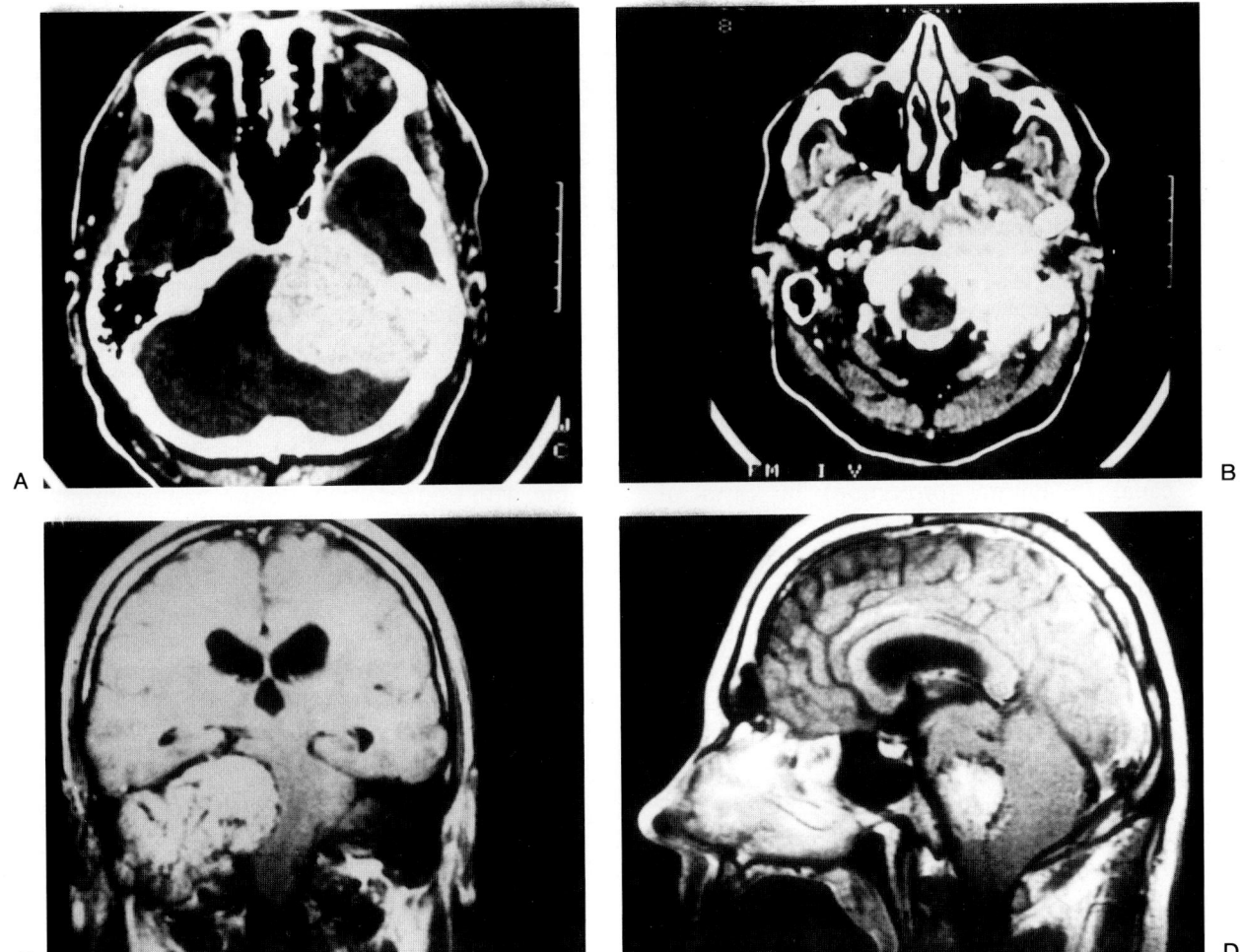

FIG. 10. Preoperative enhanced axial CT scans (**A, B**), demonstrating an extensive skull base process with involvement of the petrous bone and cerebellopontine angle. The MRI study with gadolinium (**C, D**) better delimits the tumor and its intrinsic relationship to the brain stem.

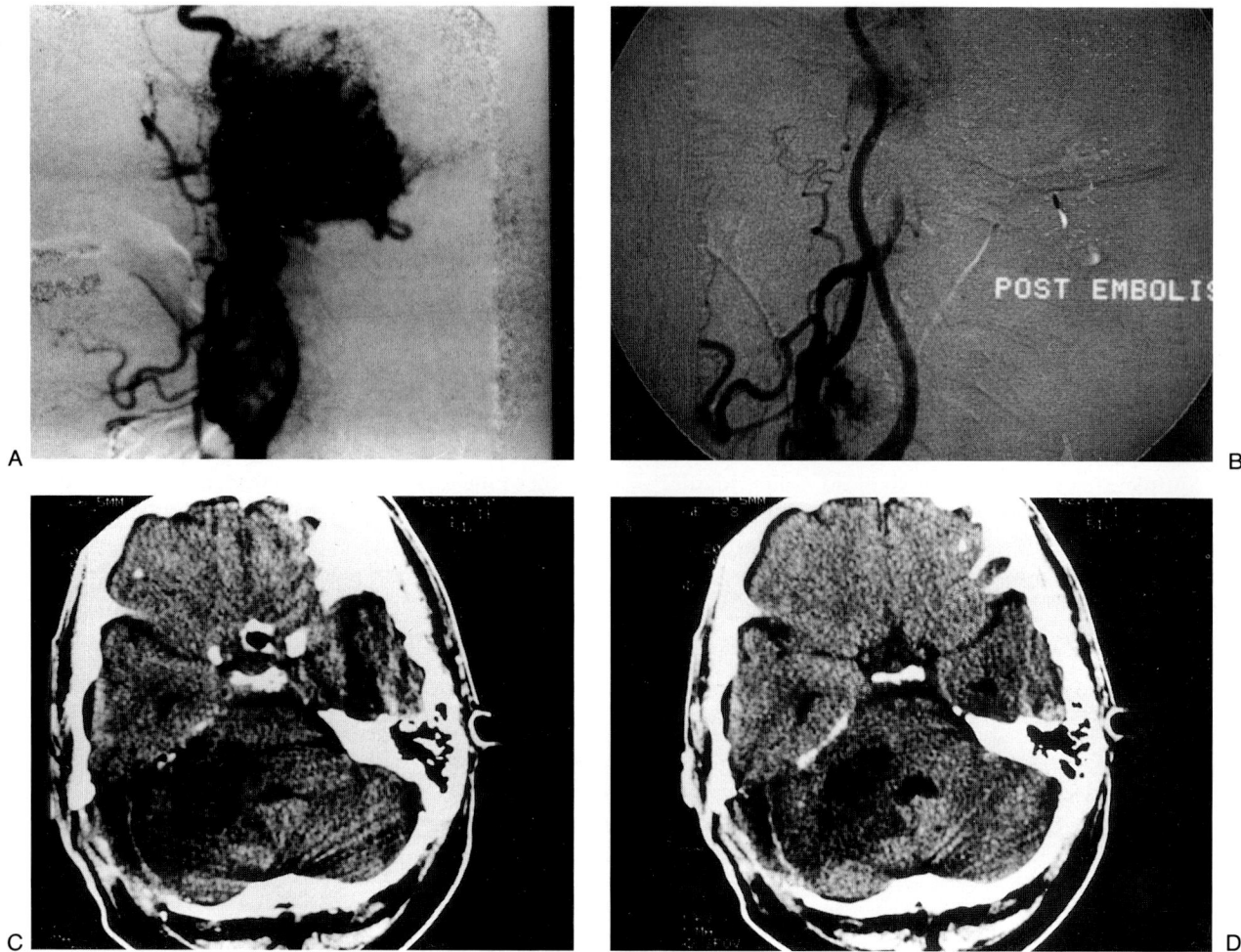

FIG. 11. A, B: Pre-embolization and postembolization (selective angiographical protocol). **C, D:** Immediate postoperative control CT after total tumor removal (please take note that the control study was performed with a different scanner and therefore the inversion of the side).

1. The facial nerve is left untouched in the bony fallopian canal (a natural protection) in cases of neurinomas.
2. Drilling the temporal bone inferior to the labyrinth and cochlea allows hearing preservation and vestibular function.
3. In case of injury of the spinal accessory nerve during resection of a neurinoma, reconstruction can be performed using the greater auricular nerve as an interposition graft.
4. Mobilizing the sigmoid sinus and the transverse sinus, until the jugular bulb, has the advantage of better exposure and, in cases of neurinomas, avoids the ligation of the sigmoid sinus.
5. Our closure technique and placement of a lumbar drainage for 10 days can avoid or manage successfully the hazard of CSF leak.

Through a detailed neuroradiological evaluation, adjuvant treatment and interdisciplinary team effort based on microsurgical techniques, an optimal surgical outcome, with a one-stage procedure, can be ensured (Figs. 10 and 11).

REFERENCES

1. Bini W, Samii M, Lasjaunias P, Sepehrnia A, Prawitz RH. Neuroradiological–neurosurgical treatment of jugular foramen tumors. Sixth Radiological Symposium, Graz, Austria, 1989.
2. Crumley RL, Wilson C. Schwannomas of the jugular foramen. *Laryngoscope* 1984;94:772–777.
3. Denecke HJ. Die chirurgie ausdedehnter tumoren des felsenbeines und der otobasis. *Laryngol Rhinol Otol (Stuttg)* 1978;57:287–190.
4. Draf W, Samii M. *Diagnostik und operative strategie bei großen glomustumoren der lateralen schädelbasis. Aktuelles in den oto-rhinolaryngologie.* Stuttgart: Thieme-Verlag, 1982.
5. Fisch U, Pillsbury C. Infratemporal fossa approach to lesions in the temporal bone and base of the skull. *Arch Otolaryngol* 1979;105:99–107.
6. Gardner G, Cocke EW, Robertson JT, et al. Combined approach surgery for removal of glomus jugular tumors. *Laryngoscope* 1977;87:665–688.
7. Glasscock ME, Jackson CG, Dickins IR, Wiet RJ. Surgical man-

agement of glomus tumors. Panel discussion. *Laryngoscope* 1979;89:1640–1653.
8. Hakuba A, Greenberg A. Surgery for large glomus jugular tumors: the combined suboccipital transtemporal approach. *Arch Otolaryngol* 1971;93:227–231.
9. Hakuba A, Hashi H, Fujitanietal K. Jugular foramen neurinomas. *Surg Neurol* 1979;11:83–94.
10. Horn K, House WF, Hitselberger WE. Schwannomas of the jugular foramen. *Laryngoscope* 1985;95:761–765.
11. Kaye AH, Hahn I, et al. Jugular foramen schwannomas. *J Neurosurg* 1984;60:1045–1053.
12. Kempe LG. Glomus jugular tumors. In: Youmans, ed. *Text book of neurological surgery,* vol. 5. Philadelphia: Saunders, 3285–3298.
13. Lasjaunias P, Berenstein A. Temporal and cervical tumors. In: *Surgical neuroangiography,* vol. 2. New York: Springer-Verlag, 127–162.
14. Menzel J. Neurochirurgische therapie extensiver glomus jugular tumoren. *Laryngol Rhinol Otol (Stuttg)* 57:281–286.
15. Samii M, Draf W. The diagnosis and operative strategy of large glomus tumors. In: Scheunemann H, Schürmann K, Helms J, eds. *Tumors of the skull base.* Hawthorne, NY: de Gruyter, 1986;237–244.
16. Samii M, Draf W. *Surgery of the skull base.* Heidelberg: Springer-Verlag, 1988.
17. Samii M, Sepehrnia A, Mahran A, Bini W. Surgery of the jugular foramen. In: Frowein RA, Brock M, Klinger M, eds. *Advances in neurosurgery,* vol 17. New York: Springer-Verlag, 140–152.

CHAPTER 26

Extreme Lateral Transcondylar and Transjugular Approaches

Chandranath Sen and Laligam N. Sekhar

The inferior clivus is defined as that portion of the clivus extending from the level of the jugular bulb to the foramen magnum. Chordomas, chondrosarcomas, metastases, and glomus jugulare tumors are the most common extradural tumors encountered here, while meningiomas and neurilemomas comprise the majority of intradural neoplasms. A significant proportion of these tumors are situated ventrally or ventrolaterally to the brain stem (1). Aneurysms arising from the vertebral artery and vertebrobasilar junction may also be found in this location. Intimate involvement of the vertebral artery and the caudal cranial nerves at least on one side is a common occurrence with these tumors. Such a ventral or ventrolateral predominance of meningiomas and neurofibromas also occurs in the cervical spine (2).

The area of the lower clivus and upper cervical spine, ventral to the brain stem and spinal cord, is difficult to access. This is because of the location of the jugular bulbs, occipital condyles, and vertebral arteries that impede the lateral extent of exposure through a transoral approach and medial exposure through a posterolateral route (3). Safe and total removal of these tumors necessitates adequate control of the ipsilateral vertebral artery and the ability to mobilize it completely in its entire extradural course from C2 through its dural entry and being able to follow the caudal cranial nerves from their origin to their extradural portion without manipulation of the neuraxis. The principal features of the present approach that allow the surgeon to attain such a goal are a laterally placed incision, isolation and mobilization of

the vertebral artery from C2 to its dural entry, and partial or complete resection of the occipital condyle. Occasionally, the jugular bulb may be obliterated and opened to remove tumor from this area (4,5). This maneuver extends the approach more medially in the clivus. The combination of this approach with the subtemporal and infratemporal approach allows the resection of the majority of extradural tumors in the middle and lower clivus.

PREOPERATIVE EVALUATION

The initial neurological examination must focus on the function of cranial nerves VII through XII. Impairment of the glossopharyngeal, vagus, and hypoglossal nerves must be noted, including their duration, completeness, and laterality. The approach is usually selected through the impaired side. The possibility of a tracheostomy in the perioperative period should be discussed with the patient in advance.

As in other tumors at the cranial base radiographic imaging includes high resolution CT scanning before and after intravenous contrast. These studies must include bone and soft tissue algorithms. The extent of the bony involvement especially in the region of the condyles and hypoglossal and jugular foramina is important to note so that this may be dealt with adequately. The soft tissue relations and the location of the vertebral arteries are further defined with the MRI scans without and with gadolinium. Angiography is performed to evaluate the caliber of the vertebral arteries and the status of the vessel wall when a segment of the artery is encased within tumor. Depending on the tumor vascularity, preoperative embolization if possible is carried out. The status of the jugular bulb and communication of the transverse sinuses at the torcular is determined. In the absence

---

C. Sen: Department of Neurosurgery, Mt. Sinai Medical Center, New York, New York 10029.
L. N. Sekhar: Department of Neurosurgery, Center for Cranial Base Surgery, University of Pittsburgh School of Medicine, Presbyterian University Hospital, Pittsburgh, Pennsylvania 15213.

of communication between the two sides or when dealing with the dominant sigmoid sinus, its integrity must be maintained.

OPERATIVE TECHNIQUE

Anesthesia

The anesthetic technique must permit the electrophysiological monitoring of multiple modalities. Somatosensory evoked responses, brain stem auditory responses, and evoked as well as spontaneous electromyographic (EMG) activity from the muscles innervated by the caudal cranial nerves are monitored during these operations. Electrodes for the purpose of EMG monitoring are inserted into the appropriate muscles after the patient is anesthetized. Other monitoring modalities include an intra-arterial catheter, a central venous catheter, and precordial Doppler probe. Due to the lengthy nature of these operations, sequential pneumatic compression stockings are used throughout the operation to reduce the incidence of deep venous thrombosis in the lower limbs. Steroids are administered preoperatively and continued intraoperatively in the case of intradural tumors. Intraoperative antibiotic coverage consists of ceftriaxone, which is continued for 48 hr after the operation.

Operative Procedure

The following description is a general one for intradural and extradural lesions including subsequent stabilization. The operation should be tailored to the particular case at hand. The patient is positioned in the lateral decubitus with the head in a three-point head rest. The posterolateral aspect of the head, neck, ear, and ipsilateral thigh and iliac crest region are prepared in the usual manner. The incision is made about 1 cm medial to the mastoid process and extended down the side of the neck. The cephalic end is extended anteriorly over the temporal area or posteriorly as an inverted "U" into the occipital region (Fig. 1). Muscle dissection in the neck is carried out in anatomic layers. The sternomastoid and the splenius capitis muscles are detached from their cranial attachment, and the splenius cervicis as well as the upper fibers of the levator scapulae are divided close to their anterior attachments (Figs. 2–4). The area of dissection is modified according to the location of the pathology. This manner of dissection not only facilitates closure but also reduces the postoperative pain and promotes retention of good range of neck motion. The vertebral artery can be identified between C1 and C2 by following the caudal border of the inferior oblique muscle and the ventral ramus of the C2 nerve root (Fig. 4). The lateral mass of C1 also serves as a landmark for the vertebral artery and can be easily felt once the sternomastoid muscle has been reflected from the mastoid process. If the lesion is at or above the level of the foramen magnum, the artery is isolated at the foramen transversarium of C1 by dividing the attachment of the oblique muscles to the transverse process of C1 under which it is located. The artery is completely isolated up to its dural entry. If the lateral mass of C1 is also involved by the tumor, the foramen transversarium of C1 is opened and the artery displaced laterally to permit resection of this bone.

Bony exposure is dictated by the longitudinal extent of the tumor and consists of the mastoid process (up to the external ear canal), suboccipital area, articular condyles of occiput-C1, and the entire articular facets and adja-

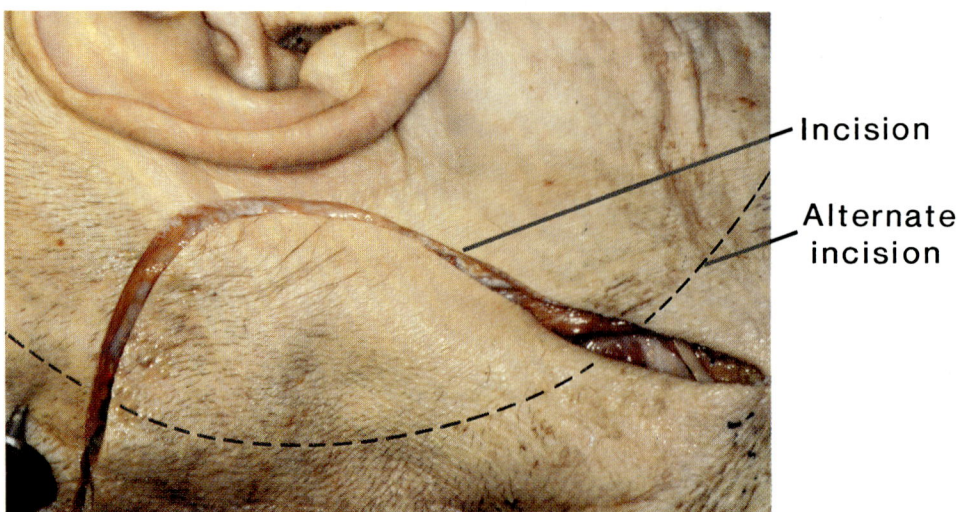

FIG. 1. An inverted "U" incision about 1 cm medial to the mastoid tip is usually used or sometimes a "C" shaped retroauricular incision (*dotted line*) can be used.

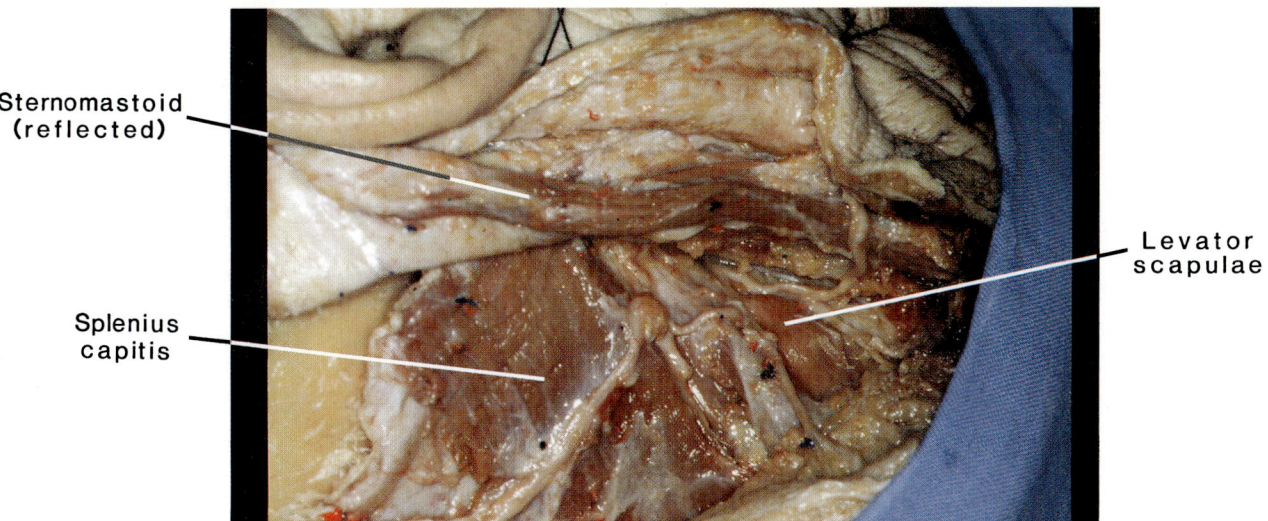

FIG. 2. The superior attachment of the sternomastoid muscle has been reflected to expose the splenius capitis, levator scapulae, and C2 branches.

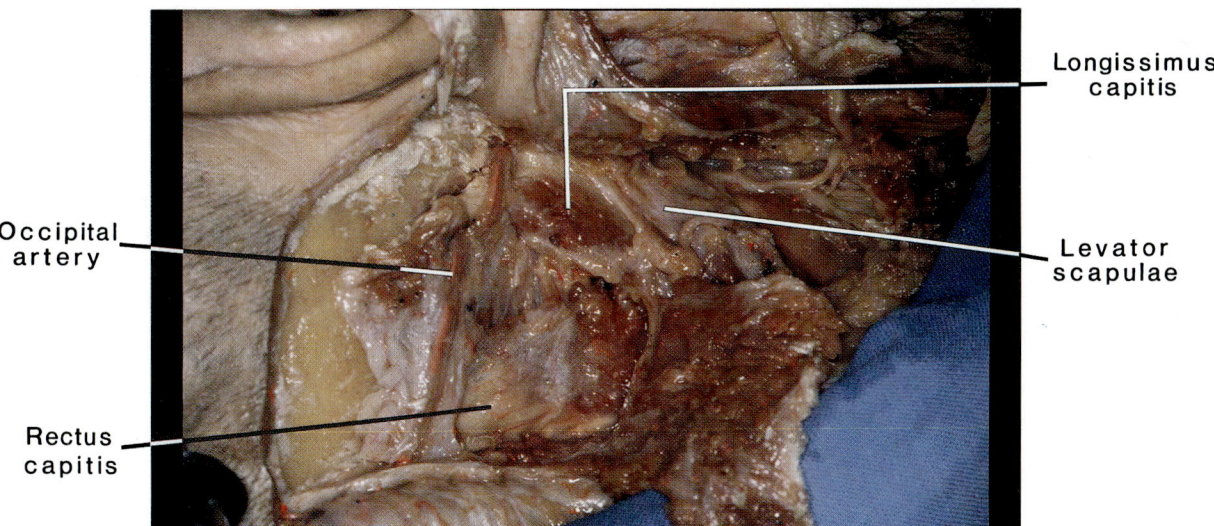

FIG. 3. After reflection of the splenius capitis, the next layer of muscles is seen.

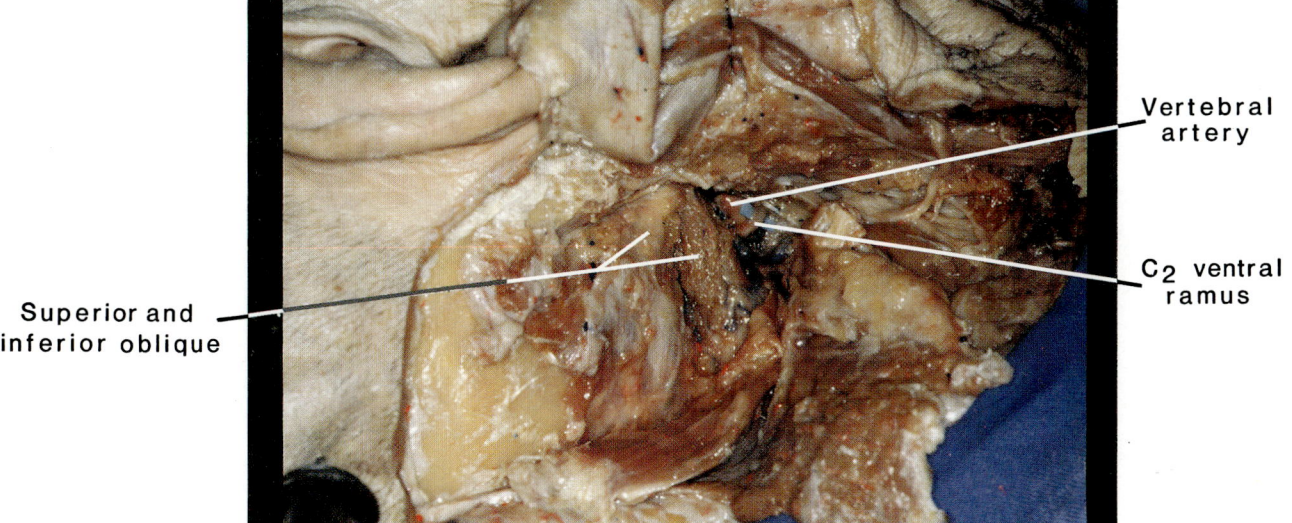

FIG. 4. The deepest muscle layer consisting of the superior and inferior oblique muscles attaching laterally to the transverse process of C1. The vertebral artery between C1 and C2 is seen caudal to the inferior oblique crossed by the ventral ramus of C2 root.

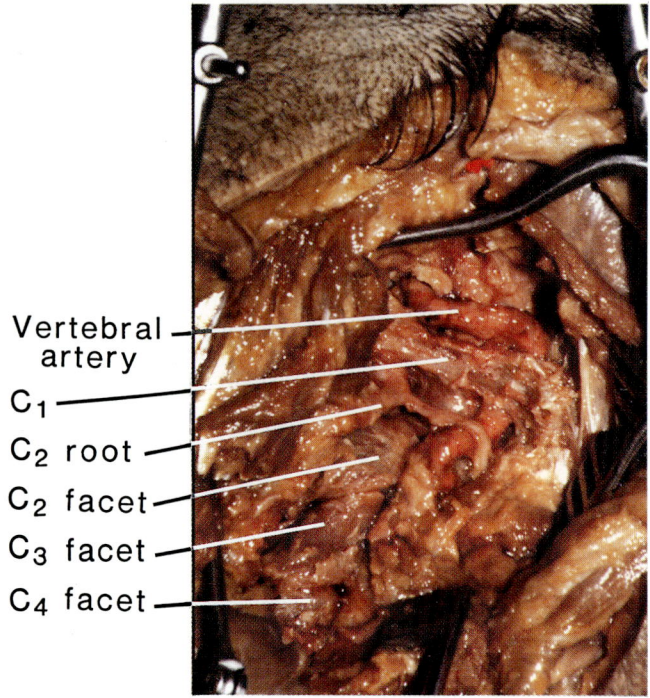

FIG. 5. Exposure of the lateral aspect of the cervical spine up to the craniocervical junction. The vertebral artery is seen up to its entry into the dura.

cent laminae on one side of the vertebrae from C1 caudally as required (Fig. 5). Vigorous venous bleeding is usually encountered while working around the vertebral artery as it turns around the occipital condyle and is controlled with the bipolar cautery or packing with Surgicel and elevation of the head.

Bone removal for foramen magnum lesions consists of a mastoidectomy, which is carried forward up to the vertical segment of the facial nerve (not unroofed); the middle ear is not entered (Fig. 6). The sigmoid sinus and jugular bulb are fully unroofed. In older patients this poses a problem because of the dense adhesion of the thin sinus wall to the bone. All the rents in the sinus are repaired to maintain patency unless it is deliberately sacrificed. Unroofing the sigmoid sinus permits access up to the level of the internal acoustic meatus and can be avoided for lesions that do not extend that high. Craniectomy is extended into the retrosigmoid area and caudally to include the foramen magnum. The posterior half to two-thirds of the occipital condyle is removed with a high-speed drill after excising the joint capsule, which is closely related to the vertebral artery (Fig. 7). The internal jugular vein is located immediately anterior to the condyle and the facial nerve exits the stylomastoid foramen lateral to the vein. For predominantly cervical lesions extending up to the foramen magnum, mastoidectomy is not necessary and bone removal is confined to the posterior two-thirds of the articular facets and adjacent laminae (Fig. 8). The entire facet joints may be removed if the neural foramen needs to be completely exposed, as in the case of dumbbell neurofibromas. The vertebral artery is anterior to the facet joints and the nerve roots and hence is not in the way of the surgeon.

The dura is opened posterior to the sigmoid sinus and is carried down and completely around the vertebral artery so that it is completely freed up at its dural entry and can be sufficiently mobilized to be moved anteriorly and posteriorly during dissection from the tumor (Fig. 9). If the jugular bulb is patent, the entire sigmoid sinus can be retracted anteriorly along with the dura. However, if the bulb is occluded by the tumor, the sigmoid sinus can be ligated further cephalad and the area of the bulb opened to allow an even better access to the jugular and hypoglossal foramina.

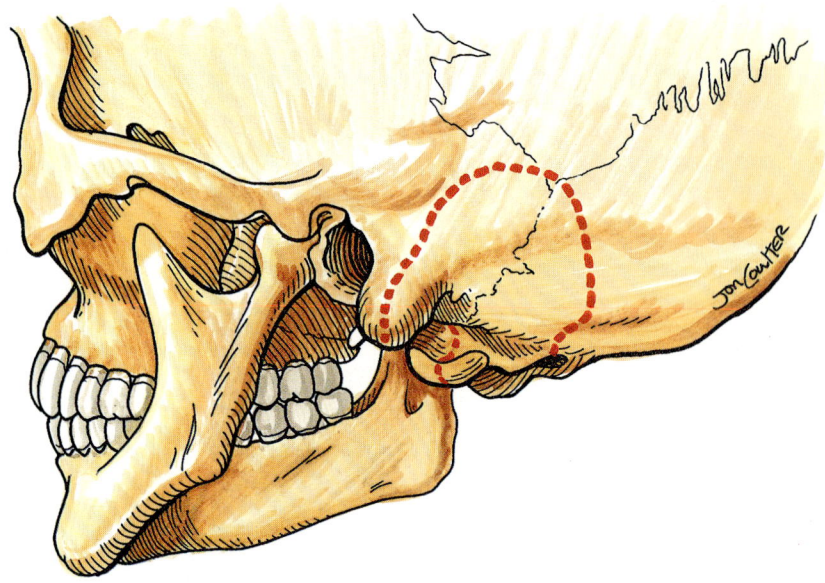

FIG. 6. The area of bone removal for posterior fossa lesions extending down to the foramen magnum. Note the inclusion of the posterior half of the occipital condyle.

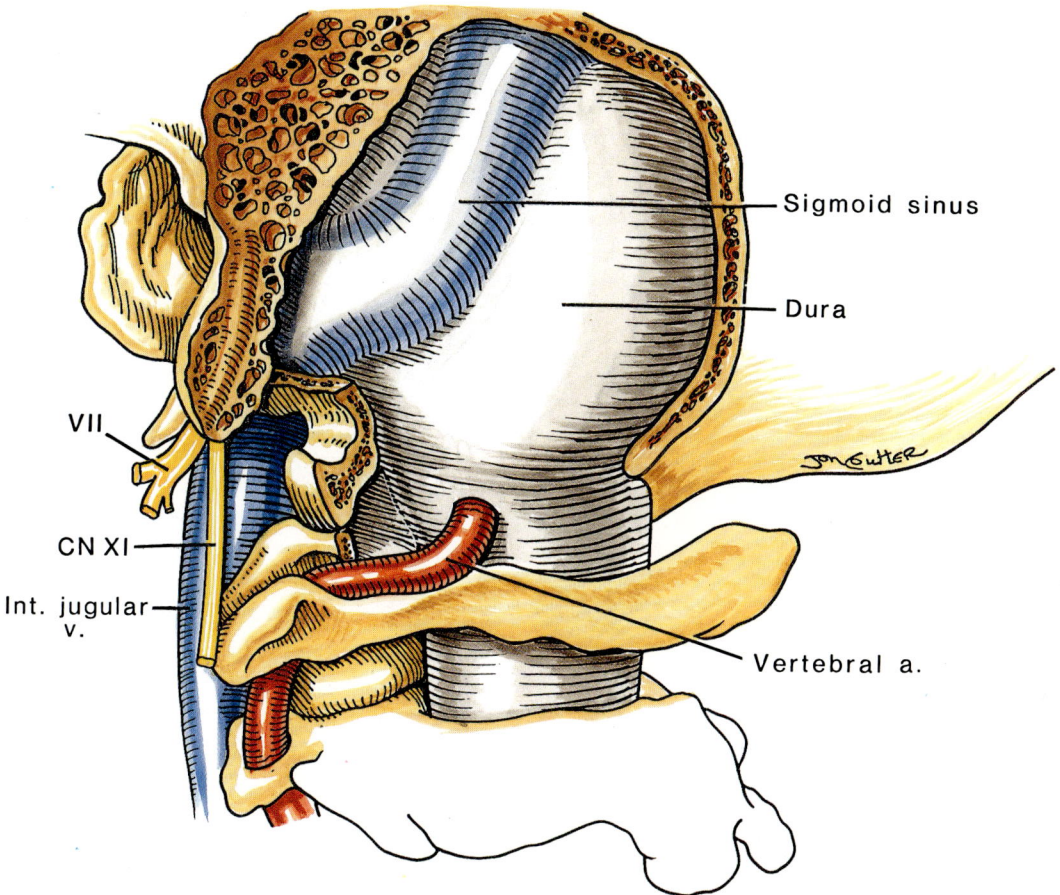

FIG. 7. The dural exposure after bone removal. Note that the area in front of the vertebral artery entry into the dura is exposed in preparation for complete mobilization of the vessel upon opening the dura.

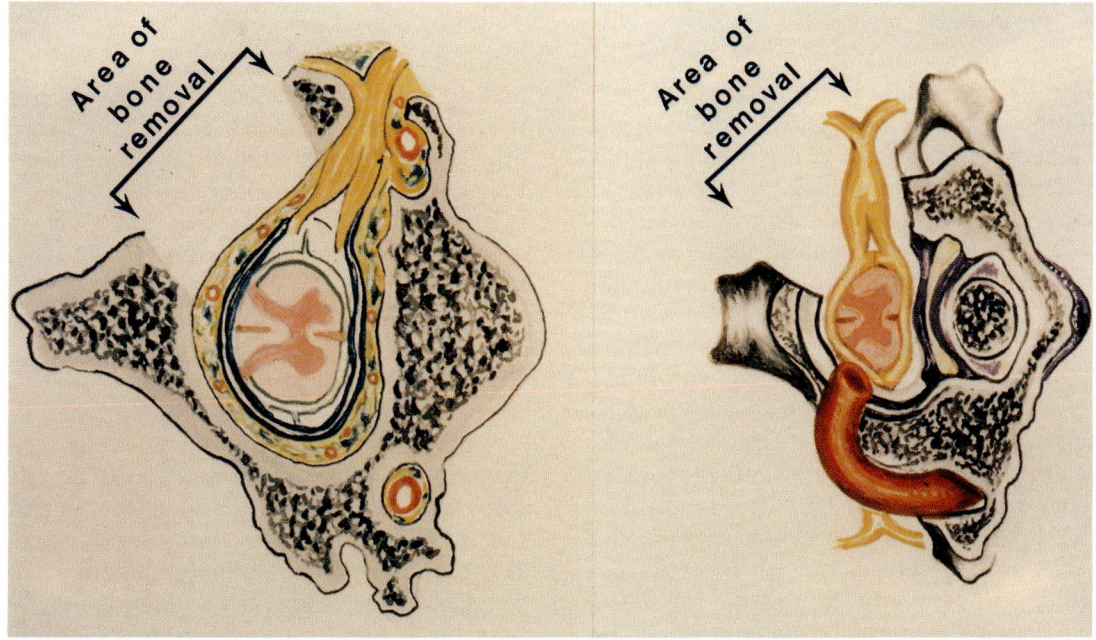

FIG. 8. Cross-section diagrams of the cervical spine to show the area of bone removal. The *arrows* show the surgeon's line of sight.

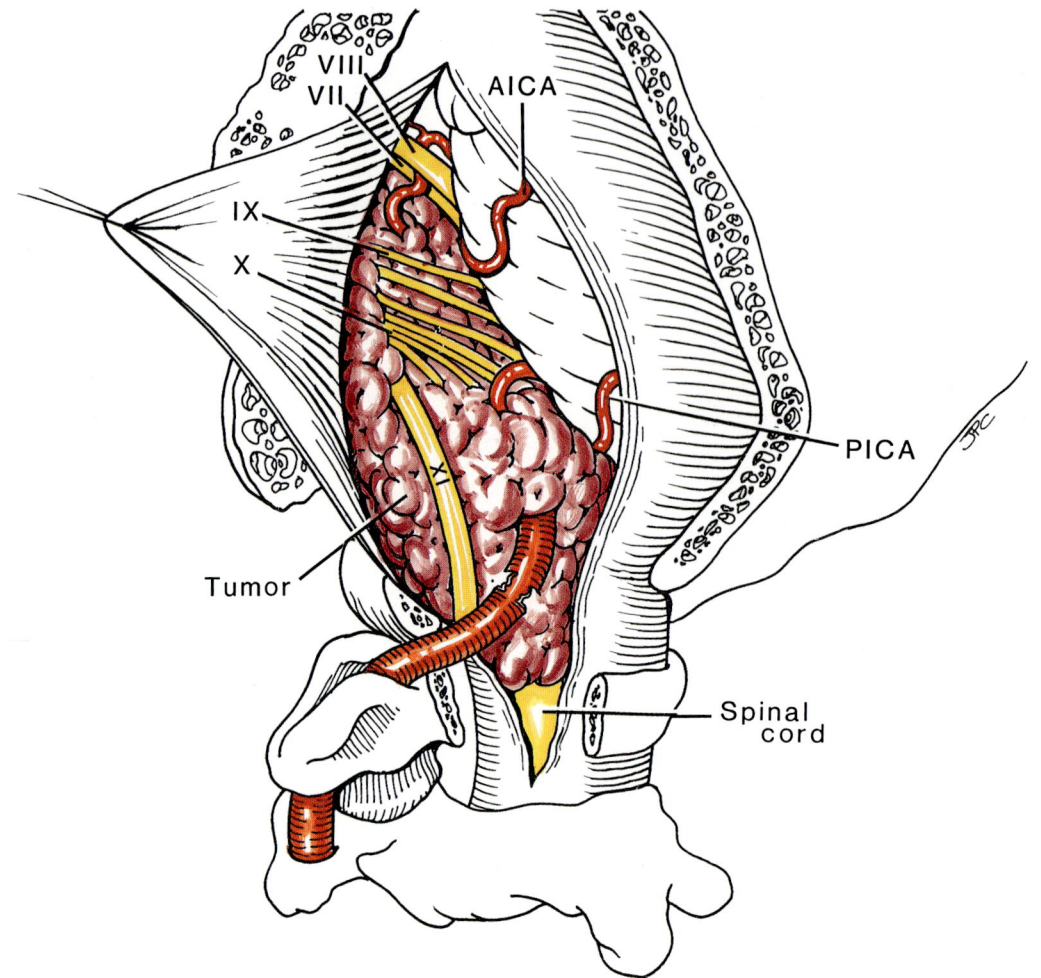

FIG. 9. Diagram of the cranial nerves, tumor, and vertebral artery from the surgeon's perspective. Note the dural opening in front of and behind the vertebral artery to permit complete mobilization of the vessel at its dural entry point.

In the cervical area the dura is opened on the lateral aspect of the thecal sac immediately posterior to the nerve roots. In most cases only the tumor is visible at this point, since the spinal cord is displaced posteriorly, out of the surgeon's view. Because of the narrow area of access, the core of the tumor is debulked using the CO_2 laser or the bipolar cautery prior to any further manipulation. Dissection of the tumor capsule from the ventral aspect of the medulla and spinal cord needs to be done under direct vision especially when dealing with broad based and recurrent meningiomas. This is well accomplished by this approach because of its true lateral perspective that allows the surgeon to see along the tumor/brain stem interface (Figs. 5 and 10). After removal of the tumor the dural base can be coagulated or excised and a dural graft used for repair.

When dealing with extradural tumors the infiltrated bone of the clivus and the occipital condyle must also be removed. Aggressive tumor and bone removal here requires ligation of the sigmoid sinus and the jugular vein and the jugular bulb is opened for unimpeded access to the pars nervosa. The area of bone removal is shown in Fig. 11. The caudal cranial nerves are skeletonized in their extradural course. Electrophysiological monitoring is a helpful adjunct to identify and isolate the nerves. After tumor removal the cavity is filled with autologous fat.

Stability

When only a portion of the occipital condyle or the posterior two-thirds of the articular facets of the cervical spine have been removed and all the other elements of the spine are intact, instability is not a consequence. However, if the occipital condyle is completely removed, stability of the craniocervical junction may be impaired. A fusion is then performed using a titanium plate and autologous bone after the tumor has been removed. If such a procedure is planned the skin incision is an in-

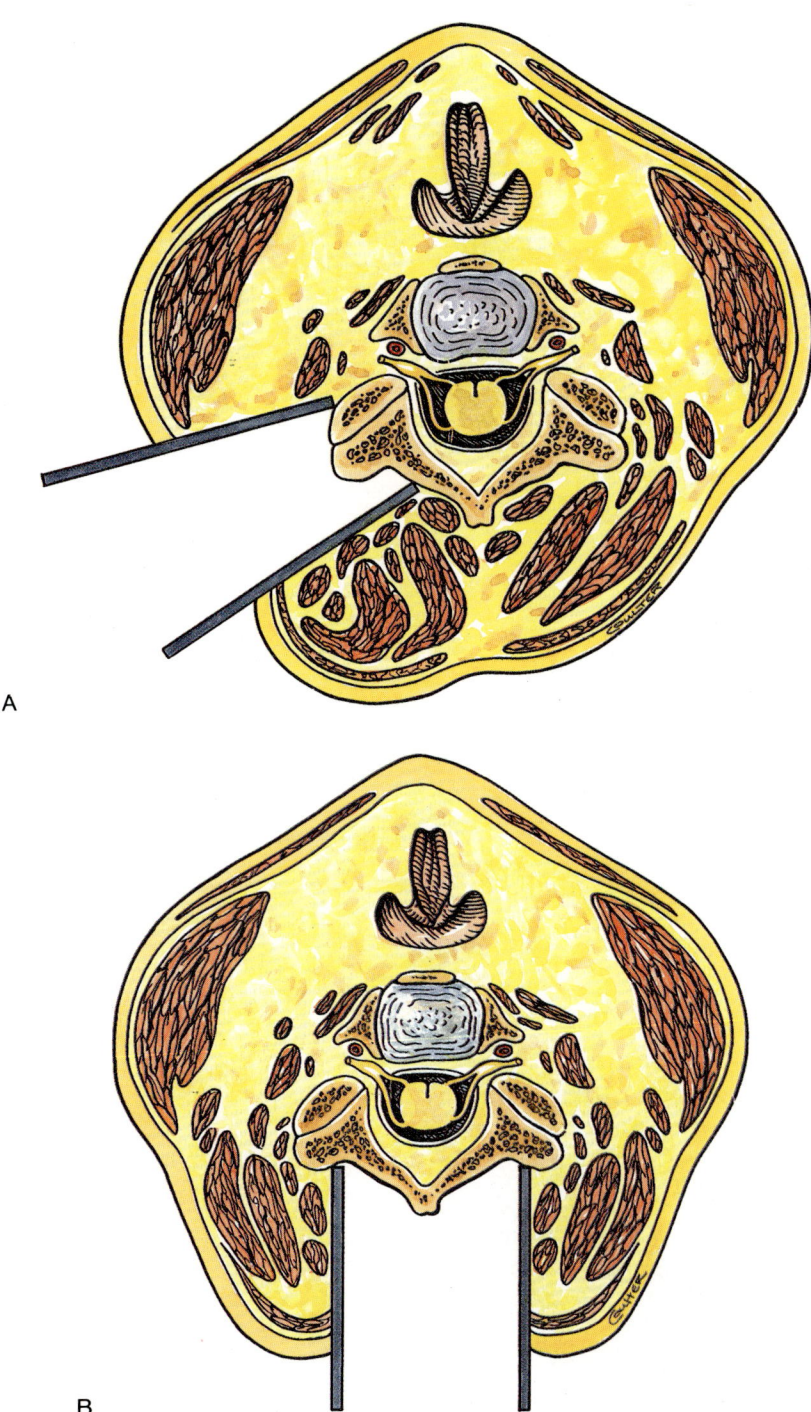

FIG. 10. Comparison of the direction of viewing by the lateral approach (A) and the posterior approach (B). Even when the articular facet and pedicle are drilled down by the posterior approach, it is difficult to visualize the ventral aspect of the canal, which can easily be accomplished by the lateral approach.

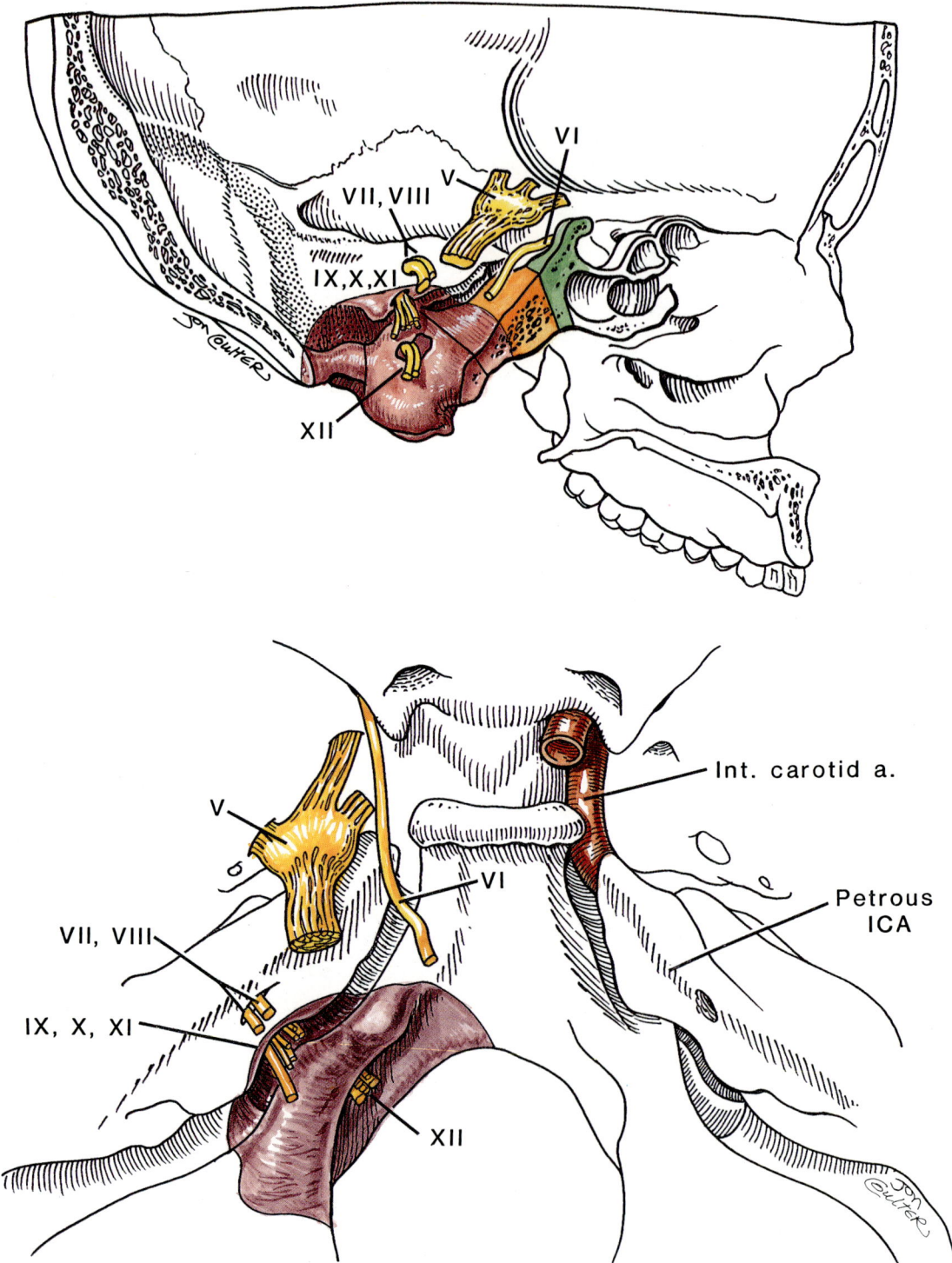

FIG. 11. Area of bone removal and extradural tumor accessibility by the extreme lateral transcondylar approach. Note its relationship with the cranial nerves and the ventral midline.

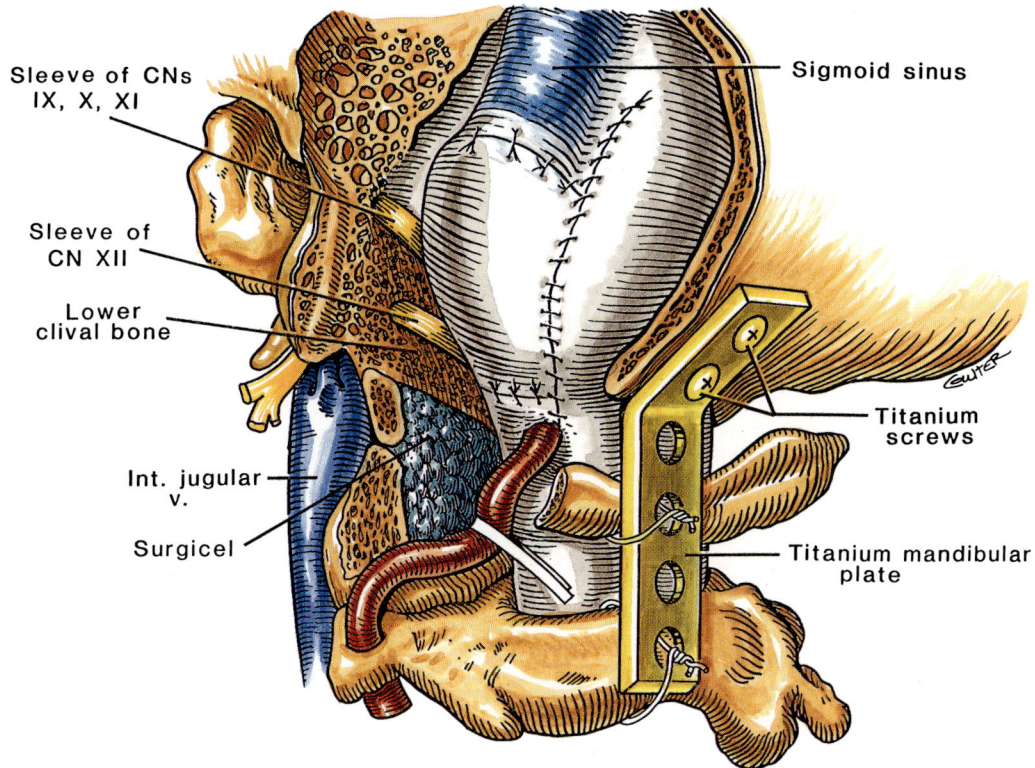

FIG. 12. Following extradural tumor removal, note the skeletonized hypoglossal and jugular foramen nerves, occluded jugular bulb, and titanium plate fixation after complete removal of the occipital condyle. This fixation allows relatively artifact-free imaging and maintains the normal distance between occiput-C1-C2.

verted "U" and the posterior arm of the incision is made in the midline. A titanium plate (6 or 7 hole mini AO plate, Synthes Co., Paoli, PA) is bent to conform to the occiput-C1-C2 region and is secured with sublaminar 24 gauge steel wire twisted on itself to the laminae of C1 and C2 and to the occiput posterior to the craniectomy with titanium screws (Fig. 12). The bone around the plate is decorticated and autologous iliac crest bone is laid over it.

POSTOPERATIVE CARE

Extubation of the patient in the postoperative period is carefully assessed depending on the function of the lower cranial nerves. If dysfunction of the cranial nerves IX to XII preexisted or was caused during the surgical procedure, a tracheostomy should be considered early in the course and is left in until recovery of airway protection and normal swallowing function is documented. A feeding gastrostomy or jejunostomy is preferable to nasogastric tube feeding to avoid aspiration and is also more comfortable for the patient. Dysfunction of these cranial nerves is the greatest cause of morbidity from such operations and the tracheostomy and gastrostomy should be done prior to the onset of complications.

If a fusion procedure is performed the patient is immobilized in a hard collar or a halo device depending on the security of the fusion assembly. The length of immobilization is determined by follow-up radiographic studies.

If a satisfactory dural closure has not been accomplished, a lumbar subarachnoid drain may be left in place for 48 hr after the operation. If postoperative spinal fluid drainage is used, it must be carefully regulated to drain no more than 30 cc every 8 hr.

Prophylaxis against pulmonary embolism, including sequential compression stockings and subcutaneous heparin, is instituted until the patient is ambulatory. Vigorous pulmonary toilet is necessary to avoid pneumonia. For these reasons the patient should be cared for in an intensive care environment until stable.

A high-resolution CT scan and MRI scan are done early without and with contrast to obtain a "baseline" examination to evaluate the extent of tumor resection and for future comparison.

RESULTS

This approach has been used in 13 posterior fossa lesions extending down to the foramen magnum (Table 1). Six extramedullary spinal tumors have also been managed by this approach (Table 2). The results with respect

TABLE 1. Summary of clival tumors

Number	Type of lesion	Extent of tumor	Vertebral arteries Left	Vertebral arteries Right	Occipital condyle involvement Left	Occipital condyle involvement Right	Comment
1	Meningioma	Lower clivus to base of dens	Displaced	Encased	—	—	Partial resection of condyle
2	Meningioma	Lower clivus to tip of dens	—	Encased	—	—	Partial resection of condyle, right VA occluded
3	Meningioma	Midclivus to C1	Displaced	Encased	—	—	Transcondyle approach combined with petrosectomy approach
4	Meningioma	Lower clivus to base of dens	—	Displaced	—	—	Partial resection of condyle
5	Meningioma	Lower clivus to base of dens	—	Displaced	—	—	Partial resection of condyle
6	Meningioma	Lower clivus to base of dens	Encased along with PICA	—	—	—	Partial resection of condyle
7	Chordoma	Petrous apex to foramen magnum	Displaced	—	—	+	Transcondyle approach combined with ST-ITF
8	Chordoma	Pontomedullary junction to base	Displaced	Encased	—	—	Transcondyle approach combined with ST-ITF
9	Chondrosarcoma	Middle fossa to foramen magnum	—	—	+	—	Combined operation with ST-ITF and total resection of condyle; titanium plate fusion
10	Chordoma	Internal auditory canal to C1 lateral mass	—	Displaced	—	+	Combined operation ST-ITF and resection of occipital condyle and C1 lateral mass; posterior occipitocervical fusion
11	Chordoma	Petrous apex to foramen magnum	—	—	+	—	Combined ST-ITF and resection of condyle; titanium plate fusion
12	Chordoma	Middle fossa to foramen magnum	—	—	+	—	Combined ST-ITF and resection of condyle; titanium plate fixation
13	Glomus jugulare	Mid clivus to C1	—	—	+	—	Combined ST-ITF, partial resection of condyle
14	Plasmacytoma	Internal auditory canal to C1	—	—	—	—	Partial resection of condyle
15	PICA aneurysm	—	—	—	—	—	Partial resection of condyle

Abbreviations: VA, vertebral artery; PICA, posterior inferior cerebellar artery; ST-ITF, subtemporal–infratemporal approach.

to tumor resection and complications are described below.

Extent of Tumor Resection

Posterior Fossa Lesions

In the six patients with meningiomas, gross total excision of the tumor was achieved in all. Four of these were recurrent or residual tumors. The vertebral artery was encased in tumor at its dural entry in five cases and could be preserved in four of them. The dural base of the tumor was excised in one patient.

Four of the chordomas were recurrent tumors, while for the fifth patient this was the first operation. Radiographic gross total excision was achieved in four while in one patient the fibrous and invasive nature of the tumor prevented aggressive resection. The patients with extradural tumors required the combination of other approaches (subtemporal and infratemporal) to remove

TABLE 2. *Summary of spinal tumors*

Histology	Location of tumor	Operation	Tumor resection	Neurological outcome
Meningioma	Foramen magnum to C2 body; lateral	Extreme lateral approach[a]	Total removal; base coagulated	Complete resolution of deficits
Meningioma	C1 and C2; ventral	(1)1981 C2 laminectomy[b]	Total removal	Normal
		(2)1988 Laminectomy[b]	Partial removal	Hemiplegia
		(3)1989 Extreme lateral approach[a]	Subtotal removal	Unchanged
Meningioma	C1 to C5; ventral	(1)1970 Laminectomy[b]	NA[c]	Normal
		(2)1985 Laminectomy[b]	Partial removal	Normal
		(3)1988 Laminectomy[b]	Partial removal	Quadriparesis
		(4)1989 Extreme lateral approach[a]	Subtotal removal	Quadriplegic; expired
Neurofibroma	C1 to C3; ventrolateral	1989 Extreme lateral approach[a]	Total removal	Normal pain resolved
Meningioma	C5 and C6; ventrolateral	1990 Extreme lateral approach[a]	Total removal; base excised	Complete resolution of deficits
Chordoma	C2 and C3; ventrolateral intradural and extradural	7/90 Anterior corpectomy and fibular strut graft[a]		
		7/90 Laminectomy and iliac crest graft[a]		
		11/90 Extreme lateral approach[a]	Total removal including involved bone	Complete resolution of deficits

[a] Operation performed at the University of Pittsburgh School of Medicine.
[b] Operation performed elsewhere.
[c] NA, not available.

tumor from other areas. The patients with the plasmacytoma and glomus tumor have also had gross total excision.

Spinal Lesions

In the two patients with previously unoperated meningiomas, gross total removal of the tumor was achieved with excision of the dural base in one. Complete removal of the intra- and extracanalicular portion of the neurofibroma was accomplished in a single operation in the patient with neurofibromatosis. The two patients with recurrent meningiomas presented a difficult problem. Only partial tumor removal was possible despite an adequate exposure in both these cases. The operation was hampered by the extensive scarring, which obscured the planes of dissection between the spinal cord and the tumor. In the patient with residual chordoma, gross total removal of the intradural and extradural tumor was accomplished and the entire vertebral artery was dissected free from the tumor.

Complications

Posterior Fossa Lesions

Cranial Nerves. Of the 13 patients operated on by this approach, those that had preexisting complete paralysis of the cranial nerves failed to regain their function. Partial dysfunction was usually reversible. Seven patients sustained new cranial nerve deficits, all of whom except for three have regained function. Two of the three are less than 1 year since the surgery while the patient with the glomus tumor continues to have partial deficits of nerves VII, IX, and X, 3 years since his operation. None of the patients have a permanent tracheostomy or gastrostomy or suffered cerebrospinal fluid leakage.

Instability. Two patients required a fusion performed after resection of the entire occipital condyle on one side. The others in whom a partial resection of the condyle was carried out have not had any evidence of instability.

Spinal Lesions

Neurological Deficits. One patient with a third time recurrent meningioma suffered further deterioration of the already compromised spinal cord function after the operation, which ultimately led to her demise. This resulted from inadvertent ischemic injury to the spinal cord, probably due to the extensive scarring.

Cerebrospinal Fluid Leakage. CSF leak through the incision occurred in four of the patients with cervical region tumors, two of whom had recurrent meningiomas. One of the patients had to be reexplored for this problem while the rest were treated with temporary lumbar spinal drainage. Dural closure is usually difficult in

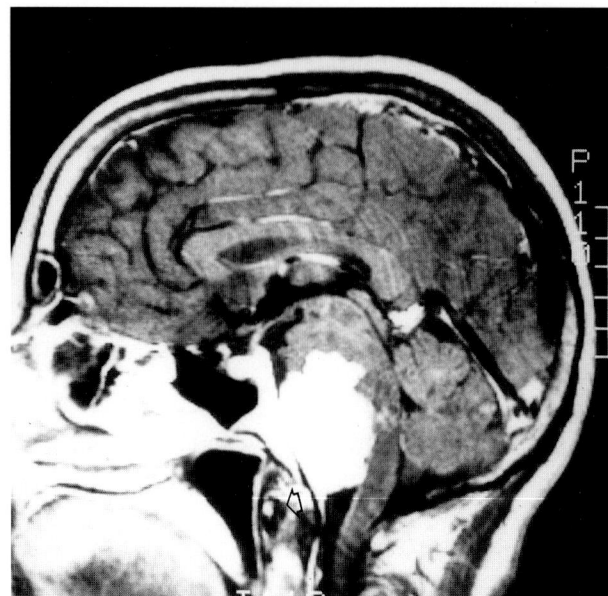

FIG. 13. Extensive recurrent meningioma indenting the brain stem. Note the caudal limit of the tumor at C1 (*arrow*).

these patients from the extensive coagulation required to control the epidural bleeding. Use of a dural graft should be considered and this is best sutured under the microscope.

Illustrative Cases

Case 1

PB is a patient who had a cerebellopontine angle meningioma that was subtotally resected in 1978. Because of further tumor growth she subsequently underwent proton beam irradiation on two occasions, which failed to arrest progression. At the time of her admission at this institution she had neurological deficits of several months duration, which included a dense left hemiparesis and hemianalgesia, palsy of nerves VIII, IX, and X on the right, and a paresis of the right VIth and VIIth nerves. MRI scans showed the mass significantly indenting the brain stem and extending from the midclivus to C1 (Fig. 13). The vertebral artery on the right was encased and narrowed.

The operative resection was performed in two stages. The first operation consisted of a total petrosectomy on the right side and displacement of the petrous ICA. Only the portion of the tumor above the level of the jugular bulb could be removed by this route (Fig. 14). About 2 weeks later the remaining tumor was removed by an extreme lateral approach on the same side (Fig. 15). The ipsilateral vertebral artery that was encased was followed from its extradural to the intradural course up to the vertebrobasilar junction and the opposite one followed down the other side. The ipsilateral and contralateral cranial nerves were also identified and traced through the tumor. Postoperatively, she had additional paresis of the left VIth, IXth, and Xth nerves, which was improving at 4 months follow-up.

Case 2

DL, a 43-year-old woman, underwent a retrosigmoid approach with partial resection of a foramen magnum meningioma in 1988. Tumor was left behind at the site where the vertebral artery entered the dura and at the jugular foramen. In the 2 years of follow-up there was progression of the tumor (Fig. 16).

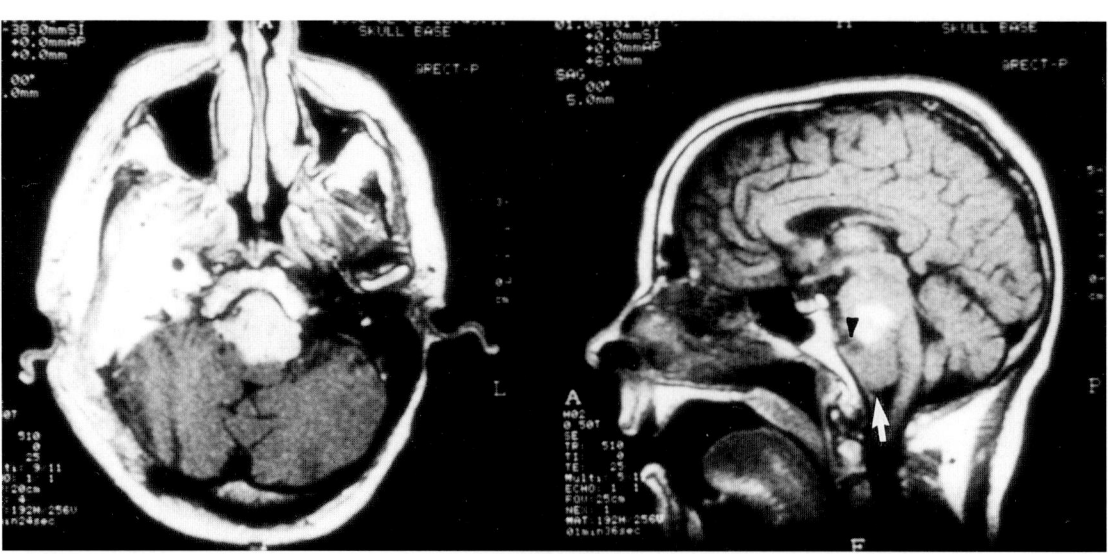

FIG. 14. Residual tumor in the lower clivus delineated by the *arrows* in the sagittal scan. There is also a contusion in the brain stem; the high signal in the temporal region is from the fat and temporalis muscle used to fill the petrosectomy defect.

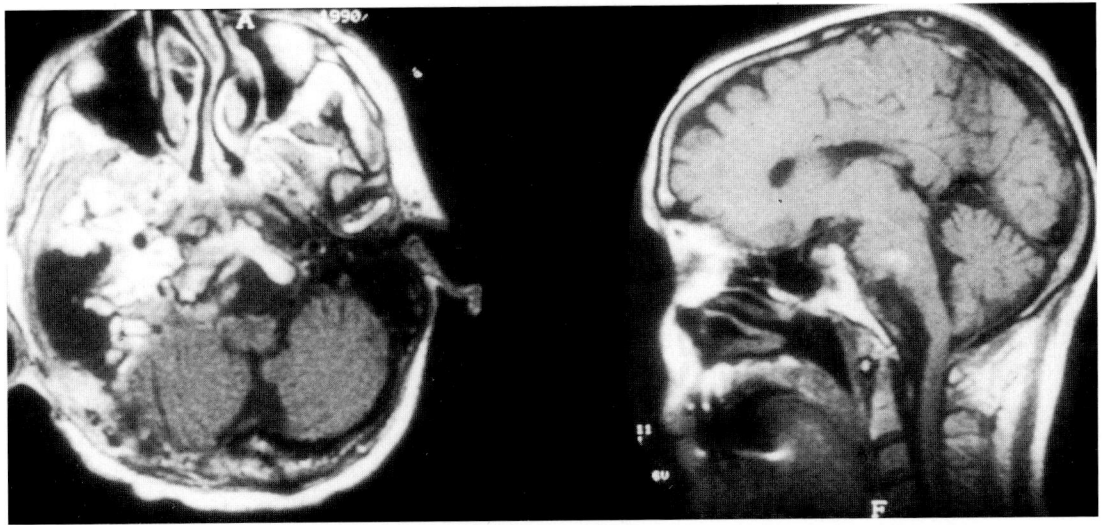

FIG. 15. MRI scans following the second operation showing removal of the remaining tumor.

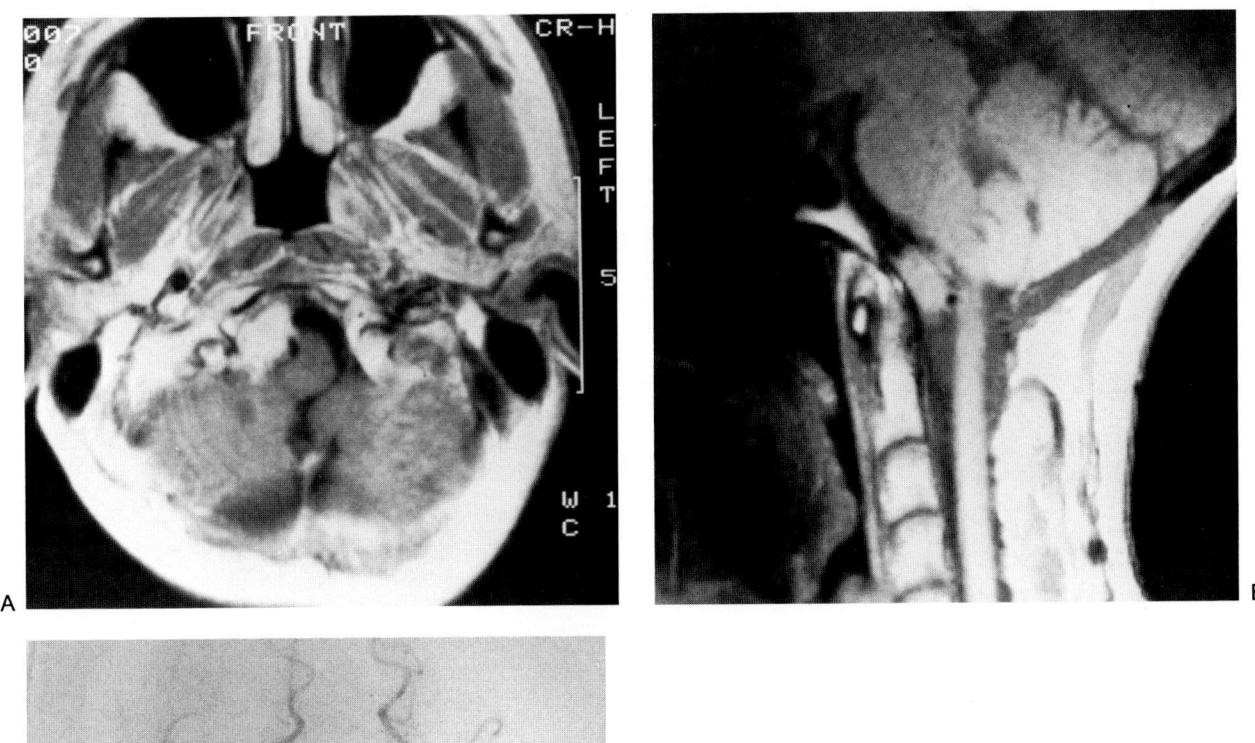

FIG. 16. A, B: Residual meningioma at the foramen magnum anterolateral to the cervicomedullary junction. C: Vertebral arteriogram showing the narrowing of the vessel on the right at its entry into the dura.

The operation was performed by extending the retrosigmoid craniectomy and unroofing the sigmoid sinus completely down to the jugular bulb. The posterior one-third of the occipital condyle was drilled away to facilitate mobilization of the extradural vertebral artery, which was followed from its extradural portion through its dural entry into the tumor where it was encased. The artery was lacerated during its dissection from the tumor (Fig. 17). This could be adequately repaired since proximal control of the vessel had been secured. The cranial nerves were also followed through the tumor. The dural base of the tumor was partially excised and that in the region of the jugular bulb was coagulated. Her postoperative follow-up 2 months hence showed persistent deficits of cranial nerves XI and XII.

Case 3

EW is a patient who presented with headaches and a left VIth nerve paresis. The lesion, which was found to be a low-grade chondrosarcoma, extended from the middle fossa down to the foramen magnum (Fig. 18). It surrounded the left internal carotid artery.

At the first operation the main bulk of the extradural tumor in the petrous bone and clivus was removed. Six weeks later, through an intradural transsylvian approach, the remnant in the cavernous sinus was removed. One month after this the portion of the tumor in the bone of the anterior foramen magnum and left occipital condyle was removed by an extreme lateral approach (Figs. 19 and 20). Since the condyle was completely re-

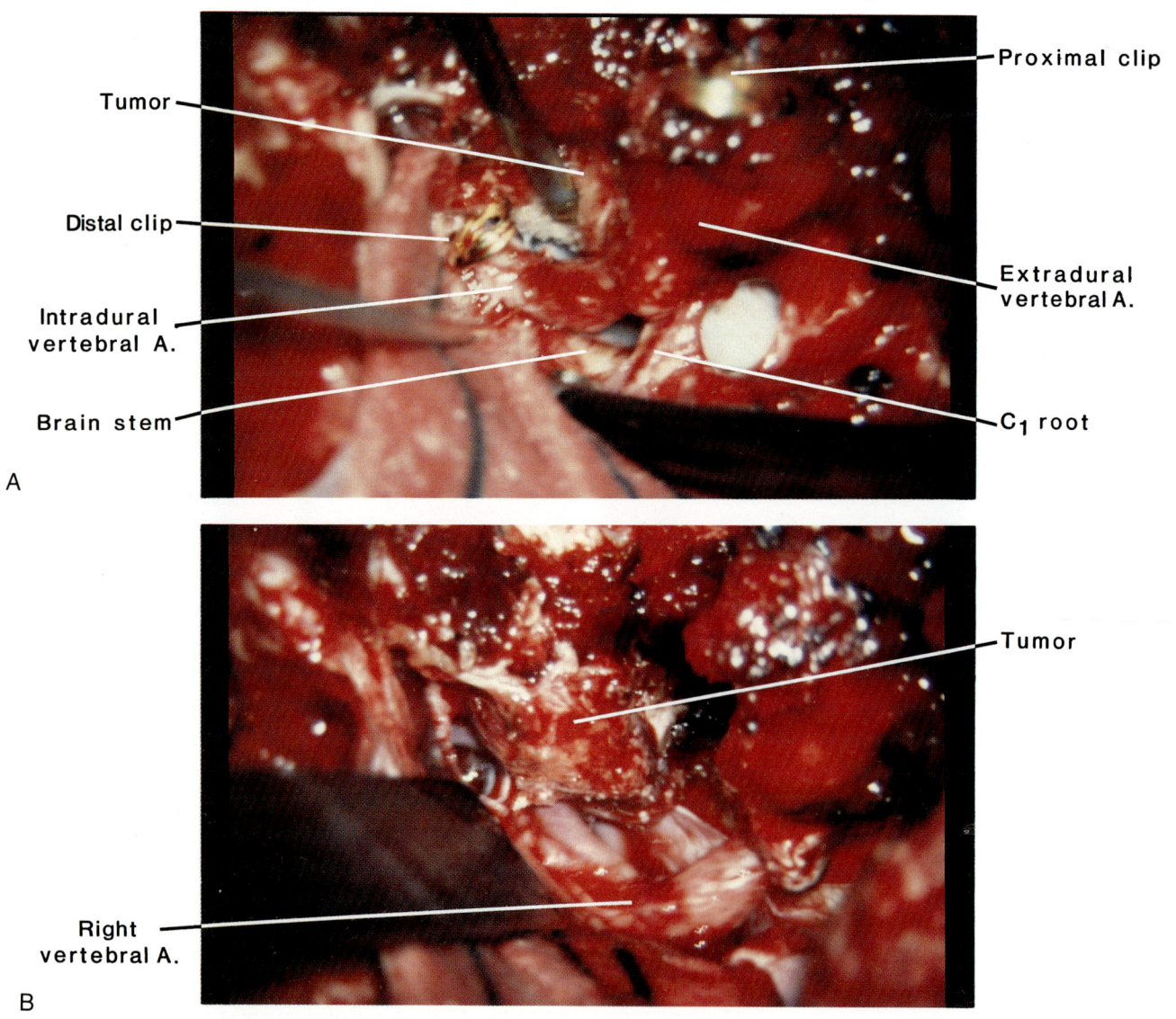

FIG. 17. The right vertebral artery has been completely exposed in its extradural (**A**) and intradural (**B**) course. The ensuing laceration on the ventral aspect of the artery during dissection from the tumor was repaired between temporary clips.

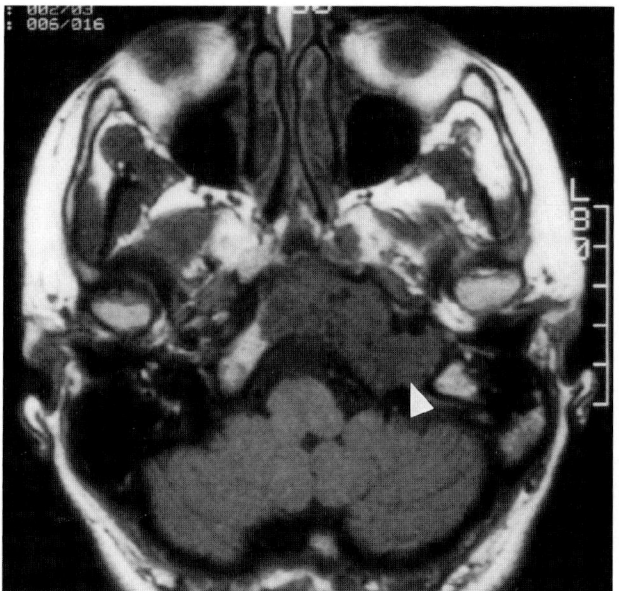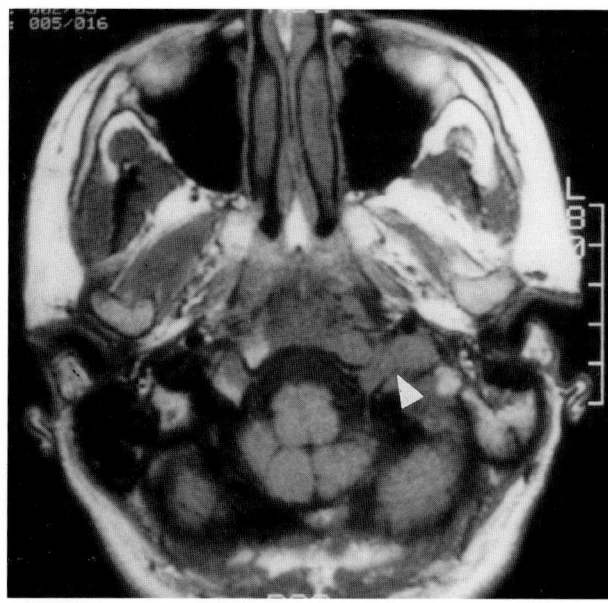

FIG. 18. Large chondrosarcoma involving the left petrous bone, with clivus extending across the midline. Note the left jugular bulb and hypoglossal foramen (*arrows*) occupied by tumor.

sected, an immediate fusion was done as described previously (Fig. 21). A gross total excision of the tumor has been achieved on the basis of high-resolution magnetic resonance imaging studies and she remains neurologically normal.

Case 4

AJ, a 60-year-old woman, presented with several years' history of bioccipital headaches, 4 months of temperature sense disturbance on the left side of the body, and, more recently, clumsiness of the right hand. MRI scans revealed a foramen magnum lesion situated ventrally and to the right (Fig. 22). The vertebral artery on the right was partially encased immediately at its entry into the dura.

The operation was carried out with the patient in a left lateral decubitus position and using an inverted "U" incision. The vertebral artery was completely isolated from the foramen transversarium of C1 up to its dural entry and a partial mastoidectomy, retrosigmoid craniectomy, C1 hemilaminectomy, and partial resection of the occipital condyle were carried out. The vertebral artery was freed up completely at its dural entry and followed into the tumor intradurally (Fig. 23). The tumor was re-

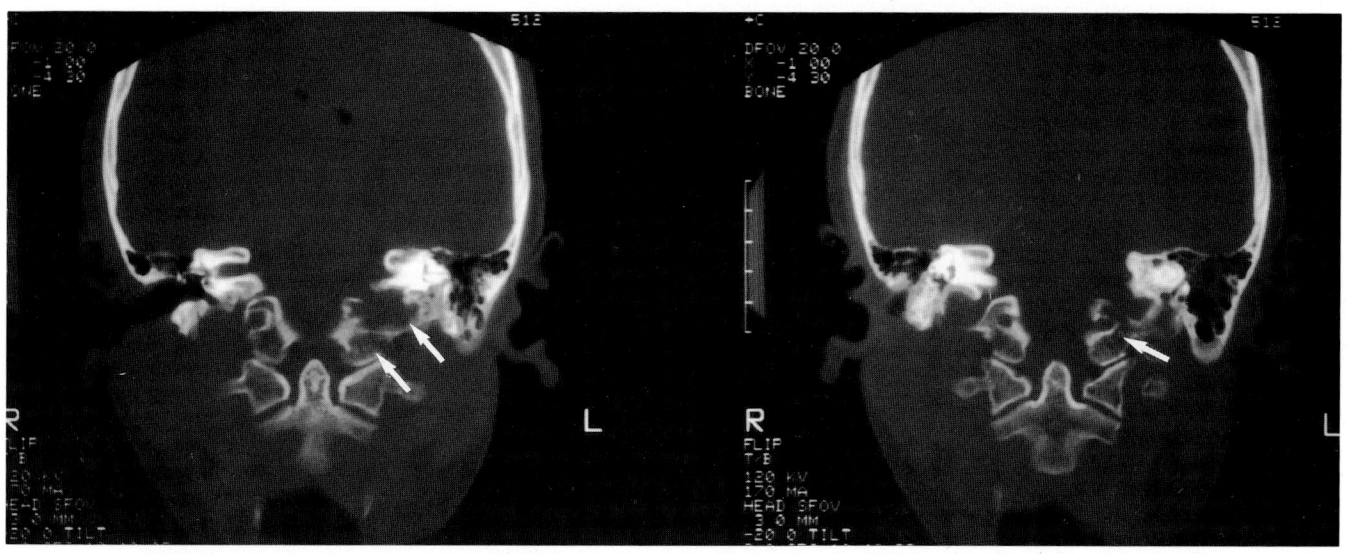

FIG. 19. Coronal CT scan with bone algorithms showing the bony erosion of the occipital condyle and hypoglossal and jugular foramina (*arrows*).

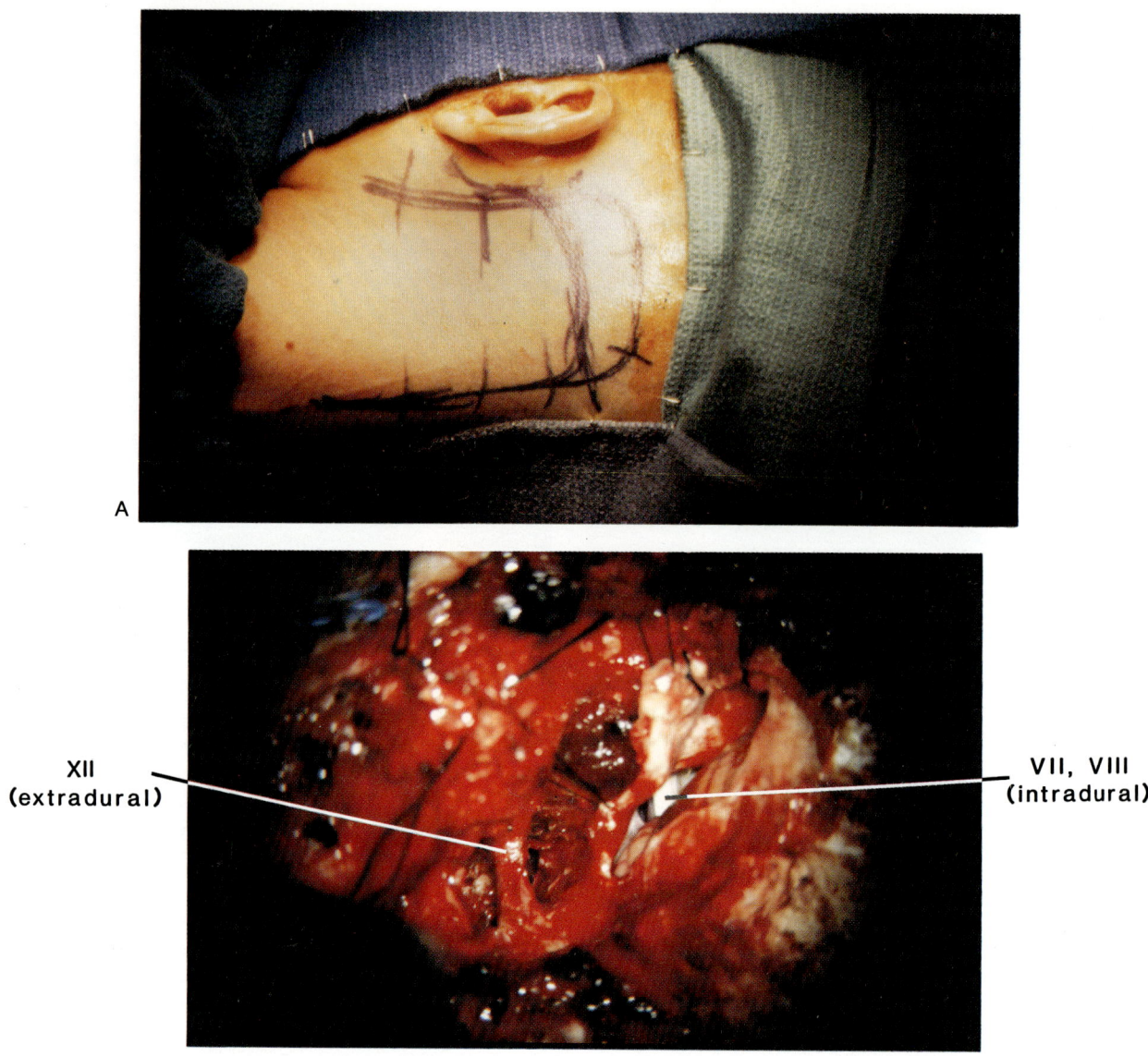

FIG. 20. Incision used for the removal of the condyle and tumor in jugular and hypoglossal areas. The skeletonized extradural portions of the cranial nerves are seen after removal of the jugular bulb.

moved after debulking it with the aid of the bipolar cautery and the dural base was coagulated. The ipsilateral hypoglossal nerve was monitored electrophysiologically during the operation to facilitate its identification and dissection from the tumor (Fig. 24). The dural closure was incomplete in the region of the vertebral artery.

Postoperatively, she had no additional deficits and her upper extremity weakness rapidly resolved.

Case 5

MP, 62 years old, presented with several months of progressive stiffness and loss of use of her left hand. More recently, she had become unsteady on her feet. Neurological examination revealed her to have a Brown-Séquard syndrome with spastic hemiparesis on her left side most pronounced in her left hand. Preoperative MRI scans and computed myelotomography revealed a ventrolateral intradural tumor at C5–C6 with the spinal cord distorted in a crescentic manner posteriorly (Fig. 25).

During the operation the tumor was approached through an extreme lateral approach on the left side. The skin incision was made in a vertical linear fashion between the posterior border of the sternomastoid and anterior border of the trapezius muscles. The accessory nerve was at the upper end of the incision and was protected. The tumor was exposed by drilling away the posterior two-thirds of the articular facets of C5 and C6 along with the adjacent laminae (Fig. 26). Epidural bleeding was controlled with Surgicel packing. The tumor was debulked with the CO_2 laser and removed. The dural base of the tumor ventral to the cord was excised and repaired with a cadaver dural graft (Fig. 27).

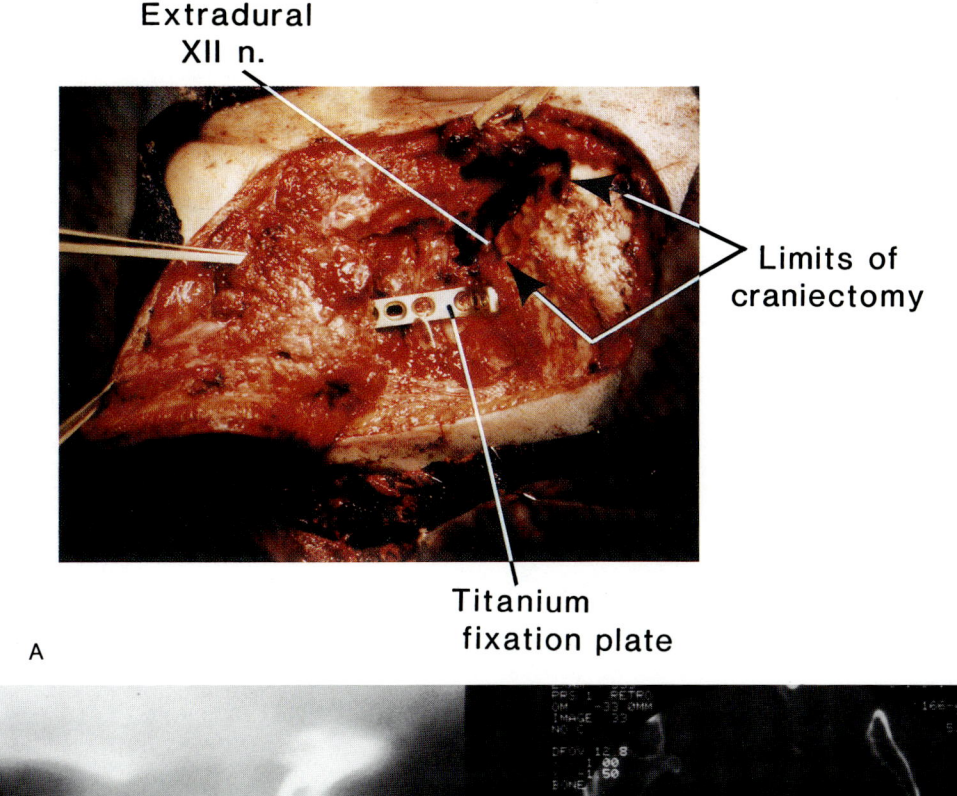

FIG. 21. A: *Arrows* delineating the area of tumor and bone removal and the titanium plate fusion in place. **B:** Postoperative radiographs showing the symmetric relation of the occiput to C1 and C2 maintained by the plate. The *arrow* indicates the area of the excised condyle.

The patient's neurological deficits resolved completely within 1 month after the operation.

Case 6

SV, a 14-year-old girl with neurofibromatosis, presented with neck pain and was found to have a normal neurological examination. MRI scans revealed a high cervical tumor ventrolateral to the spinal cord and a small component of the tumor in the intervertebral foramen (Fig. 28).

During the operation the lesion was approached through an incision on the left side of the neck (Fig. 29). The adjacent facets at C2 and C3 were drilled away along with the adjacent laminae. On opening the dura only the tumor was seen since the spinal cord had been displaced posteriorly. The tumor was debulked with the use of the ultrasonic aspirator and subsequently delivered out. The dura was approximated primarily.

Postoperatively, the patient remained normal except for a subcutaneous cerebrospinal fluid collection. This was treated with temporary lumbar spinal drainage. CT scans confirmed total tumor removal (Fig. 30).

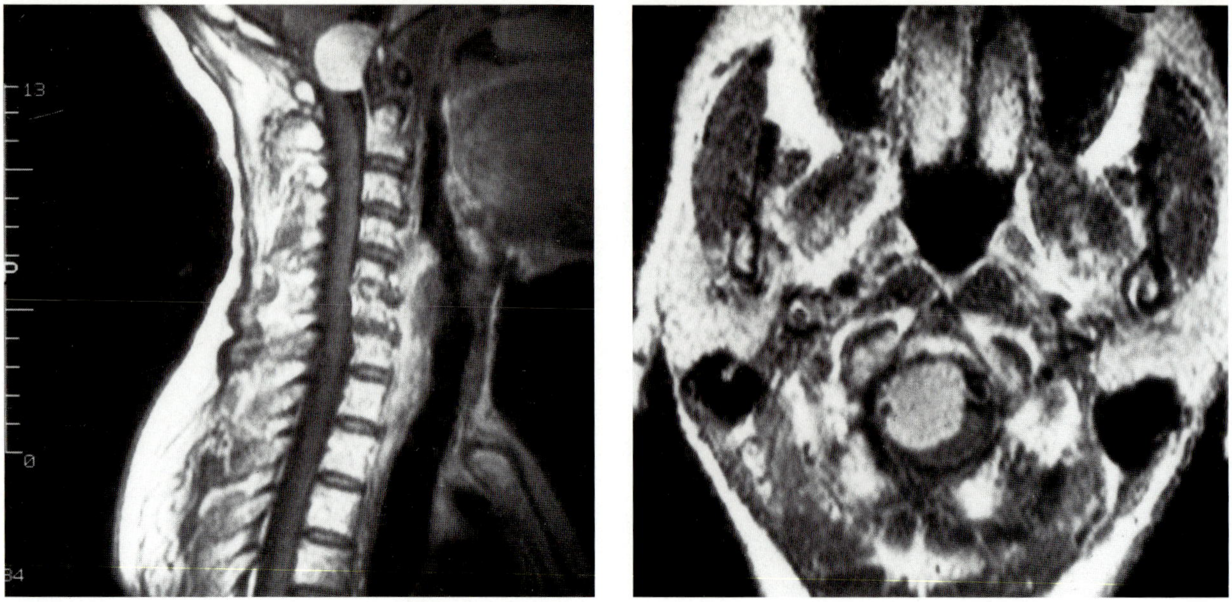

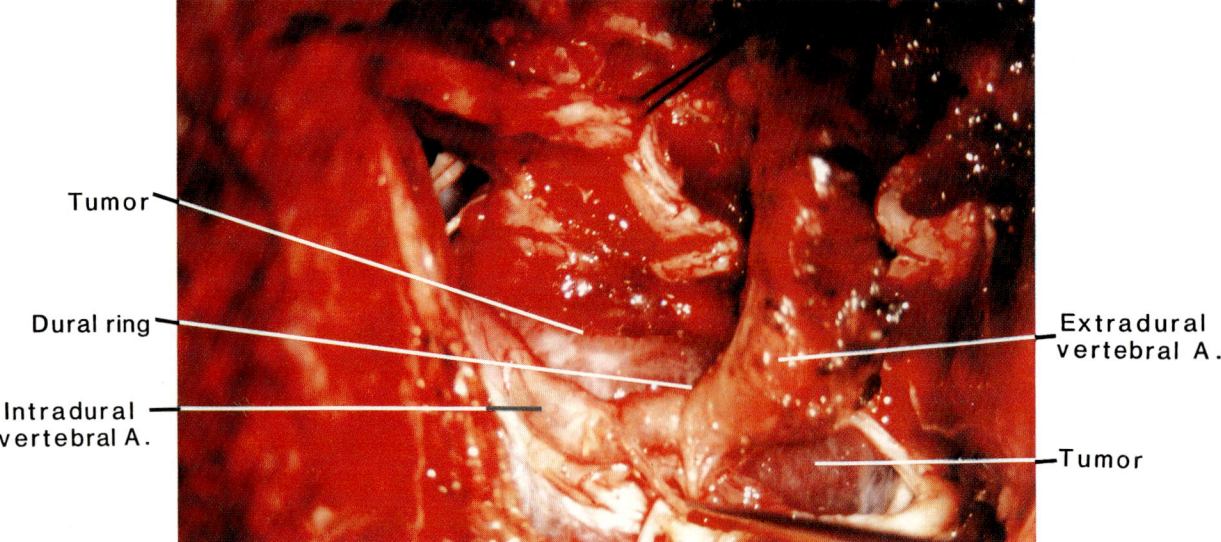

FIG. 22. A, B: Sagittal and axial MR scans showing the relation of the tumor to the cervicomedullary junction and the right vertebral artery. **C:** Vertebral arteriogram on the same patient.

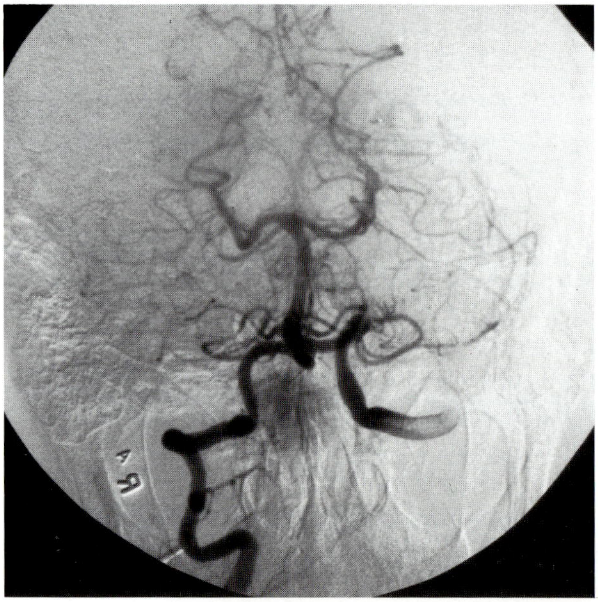

FIG. 23. Vertebral artery completely mobilized extradurally and intradurally. Note the tumor medial to the artery as indicated on the arteriogram.

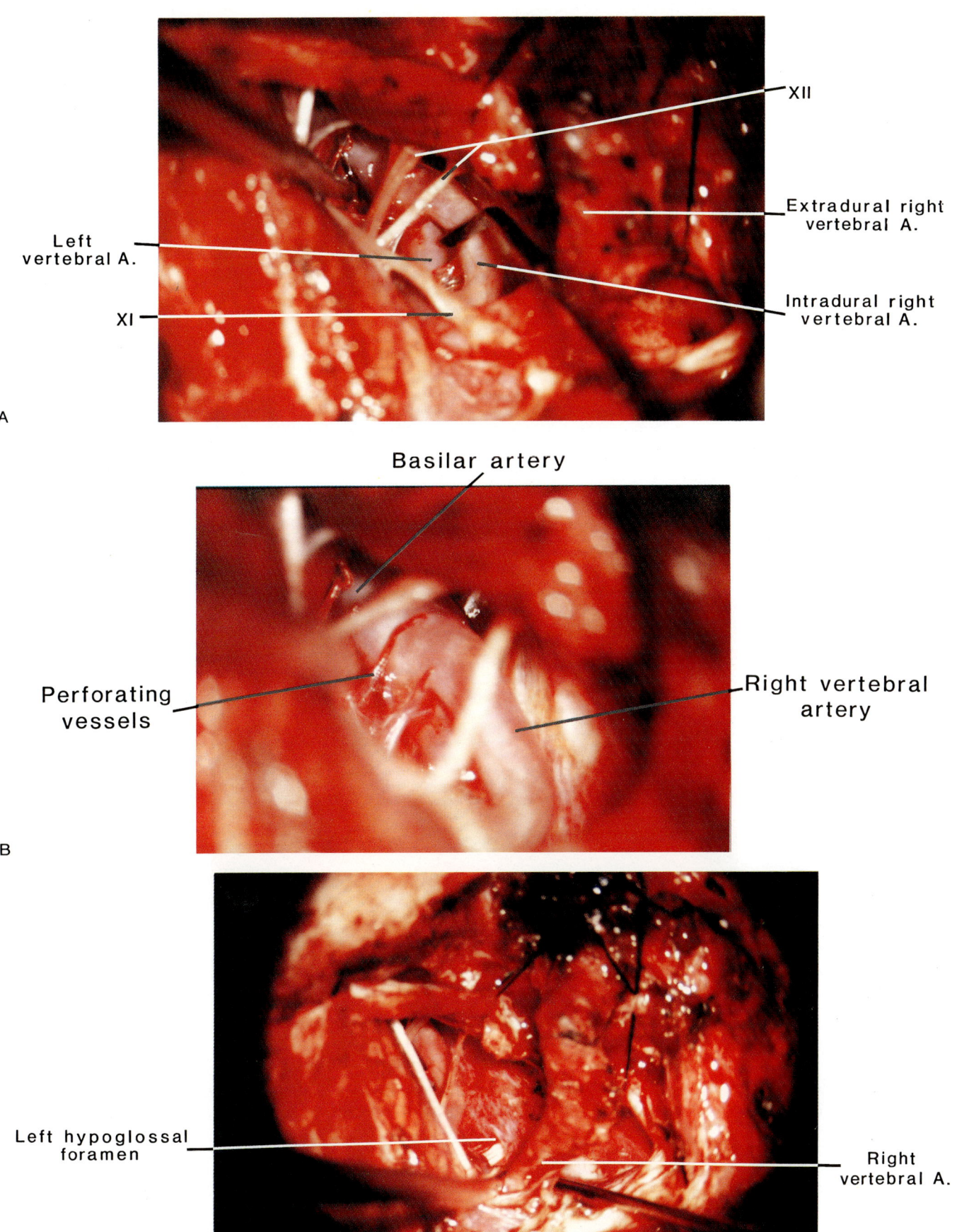

FIG. 24. Anatomy of the vertebral artery, vertebrobasilar junction, and the caudal cranial nerves seen after tumor removal.

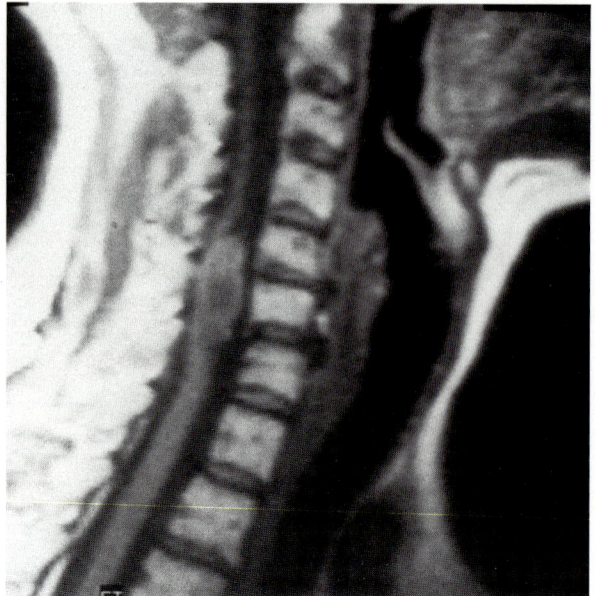

FIG. 25. Sagittal MRI scan showing the ventrolateral intradural tumor at C5–C6.

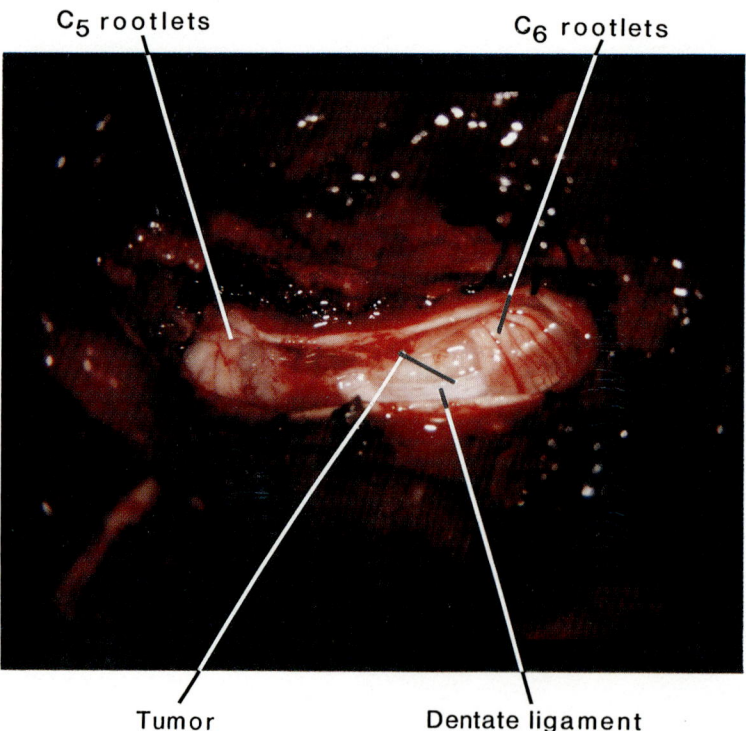

FIG. 26. View of the tumor on opening the dura. Note that only the tumor and the nerve roots are seen; the spinal cord does not herniate out, thus avoiding the risk of further neurological injury.

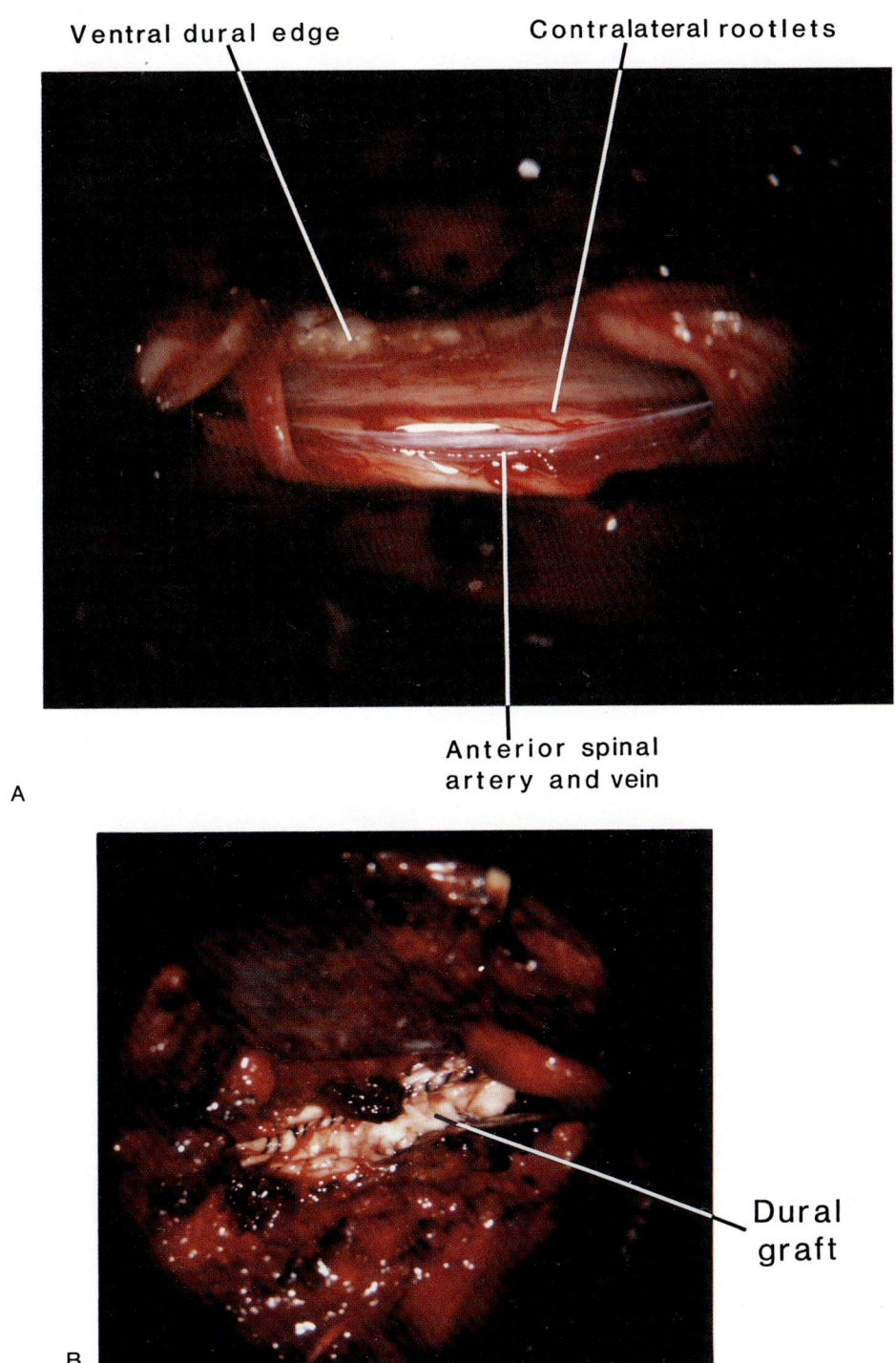

FIG. 27. A: View after removal of the tumor and excision of the ventral dural base. **B:** Dural graft sutured in under the microscope.

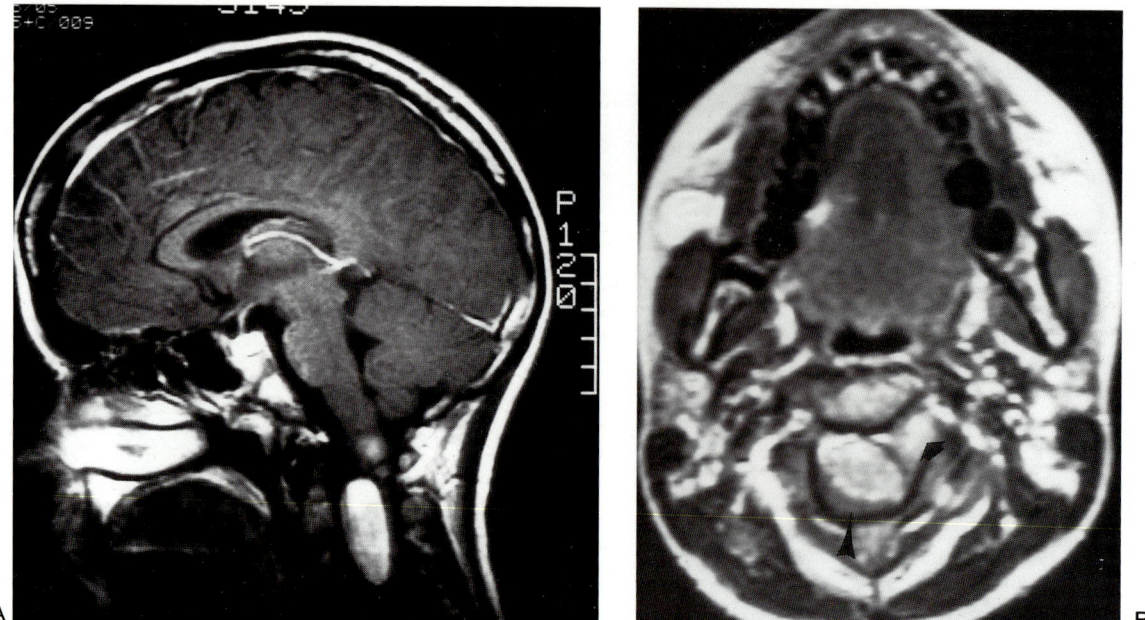

FIG. 28. A: Sagittal MRI scan of the upper spinal neurilemoma occupying three segments. **B:** Axial MRI scan showing the crescentic deformed spinal cord (*arrowhead*) and portion of the tumor extending into the neural foramen (*arrow*).

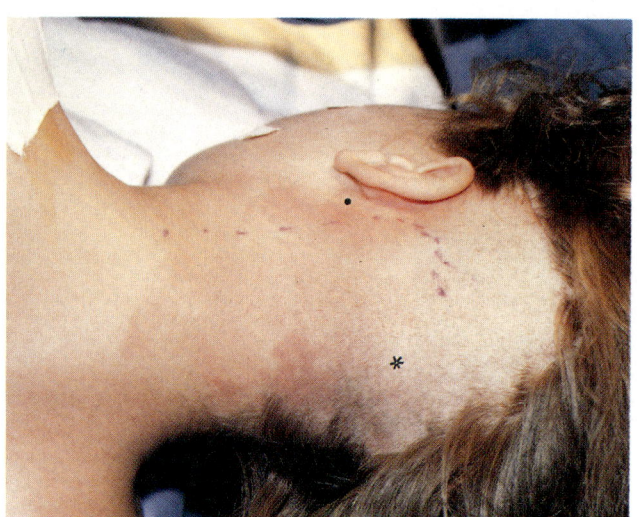

FIG. 29. The patient is in a lateral decubitus position with the incision marked; the *dot* is on the mastoid tip and the *asterisk* is on the inion.

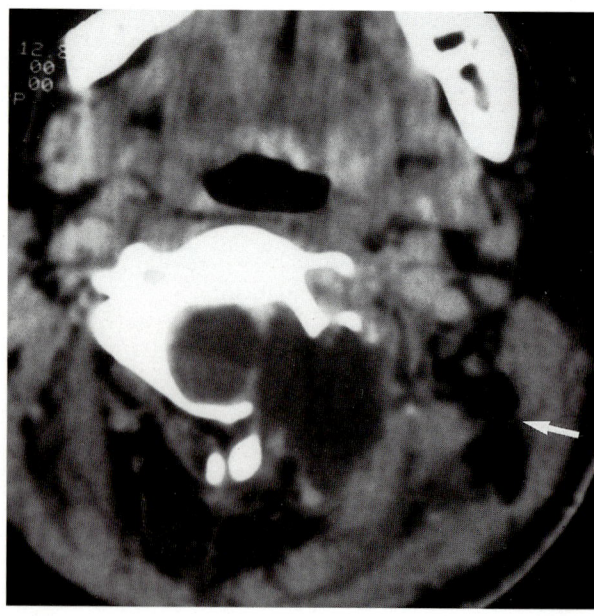

FIG. 30. Postoperative CT scan showing the area of bone removal; the air bubbles (*arrow*) indicate the direction of the operative approach.

DISCUSSION

The main difficulty with the surgical management of intradural tumors situated ventrally at the craniocervical junction seems to be related to access. Visualizing the midline and the area across on the other side of the midline without significantly manipulating the neuraxis is usually not possible unless the tumor has so deformed the brain stem or spinal cord to make this possible. The other issue involves the vertebral artery, which is frequently adherent to or surrounded by the tumor at least on one side along with cranial nerves IX through XII. When dealing with extradural tumors in this area, a problem arises with removal of the diseased bone of the lower clivus and occipital condyles. Although the retrosigmoid approach permits the removal of most of these intradural lesions, some tumor may be left behind and in some instances morbidity may result from manipulation of the brain stem or injury to the vertebral artery.

The transoral approach and its modifications provide a direct route to this area and avoid any manipulation of the neuraxis. These are most frequently used for extradural lesions (6–9). Although some surgeons have successfully used this for management of purely intradural pathology, its use here is limited (3). The limitations of the transoral route involve the lateral margins of the exposure, which is restricted by the occipital condyles and the jugular and hypoglossal foramina. The great depth of the working area is also a hindrance to lateral visualization. Lack of proximal control of the vertebral artery precludes significant manipulation of the vessel. Infection and cerebrospinal fluid leakage are other problems that can be prevented to some extent.

The present series, as well as others, demonstrates that the extreme lateral approach with partial or complete resection of the occipital condyle or the spinal articular facets successfully circumvents the difficulties of operating in this region (4, 5, 10). The approach permits the management of both extradural and intradural tumor with excellent control and complete mobilization of the vertebral artery. This is a very important feature of this exposure. Complete mobilization of the artery at its dural entry is not possible without partial resection of the condyle because the artery closely hugs the occipitoatlantal joint capsule as it comes around to enter the dura. Full mobilization of the artery is essential so that the surgeon may work anterior and posterior to the vessel to remove a lesion that surrounds it. The brain stem/spinal cord/tumor interface is directly visualized since the surgeon's line of vision is along this plane, thus permitting safe dissection. For extradural tumors the involved bone on one side can be removed safely by working around the jugular bulb and additional use of the preauricular infratemporal approach to the anterior aspect of the jugular bulb after displacement of the petrous ICA may be combined. This is, however, much more facilitated when the bulb is occluded. If an unstable situation is created, a fusion can also be done at the same sitting as described. Use of the titanium construct for stabilization permits artifact-free imaging to follow the tumor in the future.

REFERENCES

1. Meyer FB, Ebersold MJ, Reese DF. Benign tumors of the foramen magnum. *J Neurosurg* 1984;61:136–142.
2. Levy WJ, Bay J, Dohn D. Spinal cord meningioma. *J Neurosurg* 1982;57:804–812.
3. Crockard HA, Sen CN. The transoral approach for the management of intradural lesions at the craniovertebral junction: a review of 7 cases. *Neurosurgery* 1991;28:88–98.
4. Sen CN, Sekhar LN. An extreme lateral approach to intradural lesions of the cervical spine and foramen magnum. *Neurosurgery* 1990;27:197–204.
5. Sen CN, Sekhar LN. Surgical management of anteriorly placed lesions at the craniocervical junction—an alternative approach. *Acta Neurochir (Wien)* 1991;108(122, Feb).
6. Menezes AH, VanGilder JC. Transoral transpharyngeal approach to the anterior craniocervical junction. *J Neurosurg* 1988;69:895–903.
7. Pasztor E, Vajda J, Piffes P, Horvath M, Horvath M, Gadon I. Transoral surgery for craniocervical space occupying processes. *J Neurosurg* 1984;60:276–281.
8. Delgado TE, Garrido E, Harwick RD. Labiomandibular transoral approach to chordomas in the clivus and upper cervical spine. *Neurosurgery* 1981;8:675–679.
9. Uttley D, Moore A, Archer DJ. Surgical management of midline skull base tumors: a new approach. *J Neurosurg* 1989;71:705–710.
10. George B, Dematon SC, Cophignon C. Lateral approach to the anterior portion of the foramen magnum. *Surg Neurol* 1988;29:484–490.

CHAPTER 27

Regional Flaps and Craniofacial Skeleton

Ivo P. Janecka and Carl H. Snyderman

Reconstruction constitutes an integral part of cranial base surgery. Predictable repair is a primary requirement of uncomplicated healing and has a profoundly positive effect on our overall therapeutic result.

Careful planning of the surgical approach as well as tumor removal can frequently permit reconstruction of the surgical defect with regional tissue without compromising oncological principles.

In oncological surgery only the nontumor-involved tissues can be preserved. These can serve as invaluable sources of reconstructive material, affording us a unique opportunity to achieve optimal tissue replacement in an expedient way. The impact of our reconstructive steps on our patient must be kept in mind—from the expendability of the donor tissue to its ultimate functional potential. The direction of our planning should be from the simplest to the most complex methodology appropriate, not only as to the defect to be reconstructed but also as to the general status of the patient.

The most frequently used flaps in cranial base surgery are the pericranial and temporalis muscle flaps. Often enough they are used in combination. When these flaps are not available, microvascular free-flaps provide an excellent substitute.

The craniofacial skeleton, often disassembled to some extent for exposure purposes, is replaced in its original site during reconstruction, augmented with split cranial bone grafts. The overall stability of the craniofacial skeleton and its soft tissue coverage are the primary determinants of its survival and tolerance to adjuvant treatment.

PLANNING

Close integration of the approach and the reconstructive phase of cranial base surgery assures the greatest potential regional function for the patient without any compromise of oncological principles. The goals are as follows:

1. Reestablishment of extracranial and intracranial separation; CSF containment and protection of key anatomical structures from extracranial environment.
2. Functional preservation of independent craniofacial units (orbit, nasopharynx).
3. Reestablishment of three-dimensional craniofacial skeletal framework and its soft tissue envelope.
4. Minimization of donor site morbidity.

Detailed evaluation of the placement and extent of the patient's old scars gives us clues as to the extent of previous surgery that potentially might compromise our reconstructive plans (Fig. 1). For example, an anteriorly

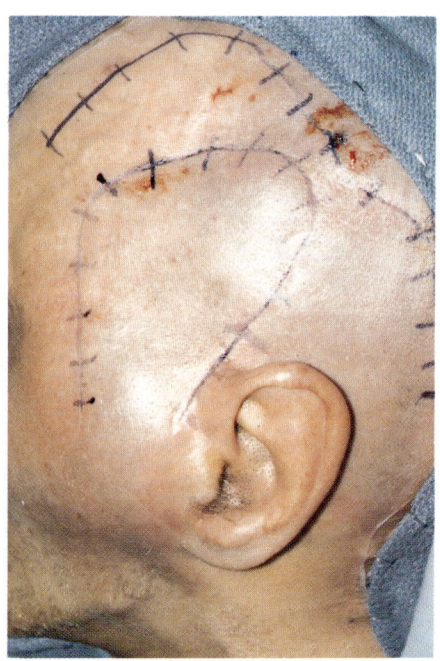

FIG. 1. Multiple scalp scars.

I. P. Janecka and C. H. Snyderman: Center for Cranial Base Surgery, University of Pittsburgh School of Medicine, Presbyterian University Hospital, and Department of Otolaryngology, Eye and Ear Institute, Pittsburgh, Pennsylvania 15213.

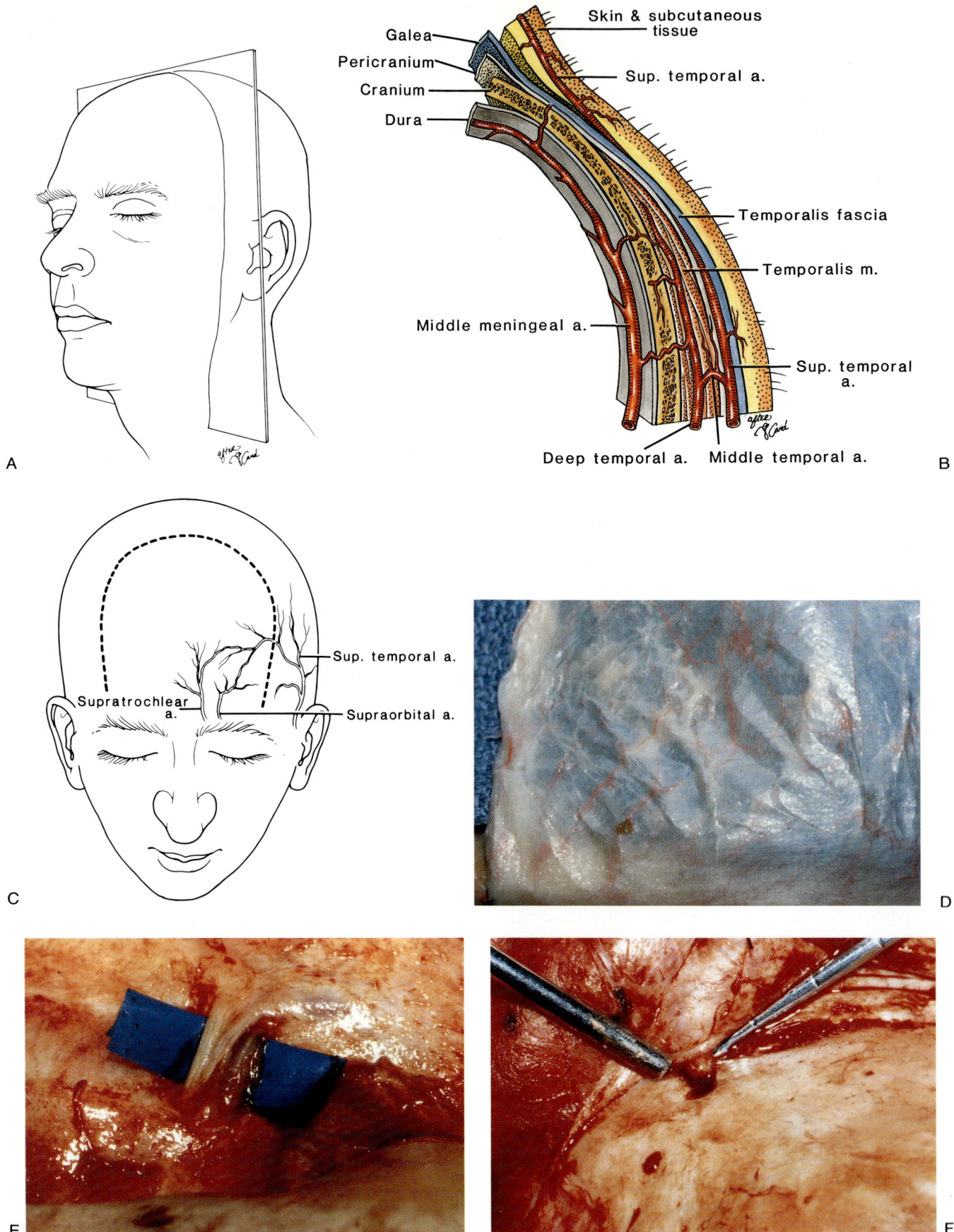

FIG. 2. A: Orientation, coronal plane. **B:** Anatomic layers of left parietotemporal region. **C:** Schematic outline of blood supply to a pericranial flap. **D:** Fine network of vessels in a pericranial flap following arterial latex (*red*) injection in a cadaver. **E:** Supraorbital neurovascular pedicle exiting from orbital soft tissue and entering forehead scalp. **F:** Freed (with mini-osteotomies) neurovascular pedicle from left supraorbital foramen.

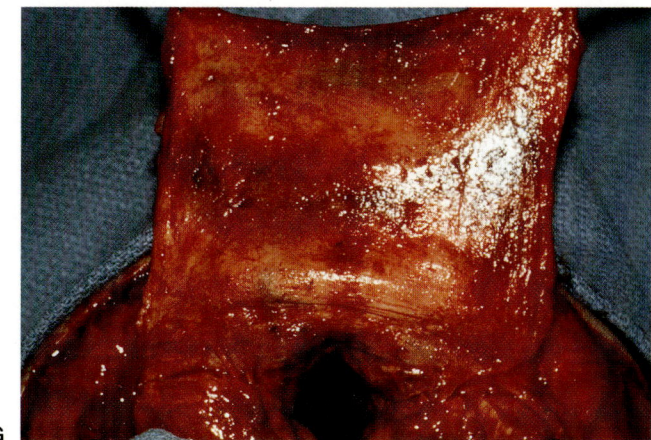

FIG. 2. *Continued.* **G:** Pericranial flap.

placed (at the hairline) bicoronal scar would indicate a significant limitation of our potential to develop an adequate pericranial flap. Similarly, previous temporal fossa dissection with elevation of temporalis muscle would also suggest likely foreshortening of the temporalis muscle. Any evidence of denervation of this muscle would strongly indicate the need for selection of an alternate muscle flap (e.g., microvascular).

SURGICAL STEPS

Pericranial Flap

This flap is developed from the pericranium as well as the loose areolar tissue, which lies between the pericranium and the galea. It receives its primary blood supply from the branches of the supraorbital and supratrochlear vessels bilaterally. This flap is usually designed in rectangular fashion with the base in the supraorbital area and its tip at the level of the bicoronal scalp incision. Its length is approximately 10 cm from the supraorbital level. Laterally, it extends to the level of the temporal line, where it merges with the origin of the temporalis muscle. Initially, the pericranium is elevated with the entire bicoronal scalp flap to the level of the supraorbital rims. The supraorbital neurovascular pedicle is preserved. If it enters the supraorbital region through a separate foramen, it should be freed from it. This then permits an easy dissection over the supraorbital rim into the orbit (Fig. 2).

At the completion of oncological surgery, the pericranial flap is raised sharply from the galea. When the dissection is nearing the region of the blood supply, it is possible to incorporate a portion of the frontalis muscle fibers with the pericranium in order to prevent injury to the vessels. This by itself does not compromise the function of the frontalis muscle. The placement of the pericranial flap into the cranial cavity can be done above or below the supraorbital skeleton (an area often disassembled during the approach phase of cranial base surgery). The inferior placement of the pericranial flap intracranially, along the roof of the orbit, increases its reach. The flap itself is secured to the basal dura while it provides coverage for the anterior cranial fossa. It is possible to use fibrin glue along the flap for additional seal. The dura of the frontal lobe is permitted to come into direct contact with the pericranial flap (Fig. 3).

Occasionally, additional lateral rotation of the pericranial flap is necessary in order to reach into the cavernous sinus region. In such an instance, sacrifice of the contralateral supraorbital vascular pedicle permits further rotation of the pericranial flap in the anterolateral plane centered at the ipsilateral vascular pedicle (Fig. 4). The donor site morbidity from raising the pericranial flap is minimal. The inclusion of the galea to form a galeopericranial flap provides additional bulk to the flap as well as increases its vascularity (if the superficial temporal arterial tree is incorporated in the flap), but it simultaneously devascularizes the forehead skin to a great extent. This could have a potentially detrimental effect on the final healing of the forehead especially in patients previously operated on or who received radiotherapy.

The pericranial flap is an excellent reconstructive material but seldom can be reused. It is important that the bicoronal incision in "standard" frontal craniotomy does extend beyond the hairline in order to protect the length of the frontal pericranium, which is potentially usable as a flap.

Temporalis Muscle Flap

The true versatility of this flap has not yet been fully explored. The origin from the temporal fossa and the insertion on the coronoid process provide a fan-shaped muscle with its rotational point optimally located to cover most of anterolateral skull base (Fig. 5). The pri-

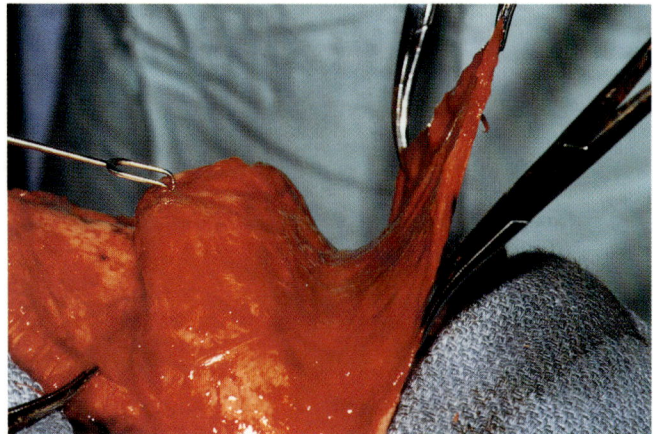

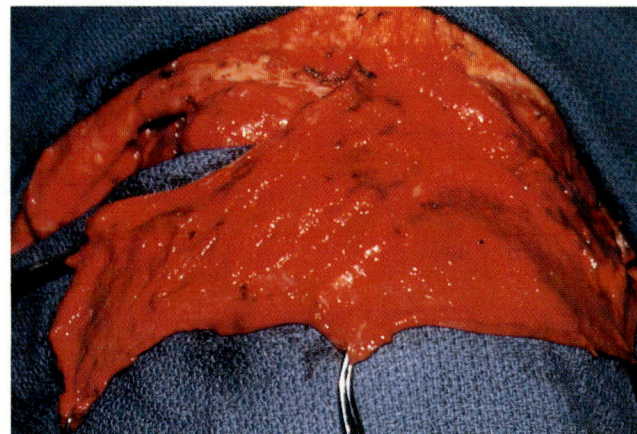

FIG. 4. Lengthening of the rotational arc of the pericranial flap by left supraorbital release.

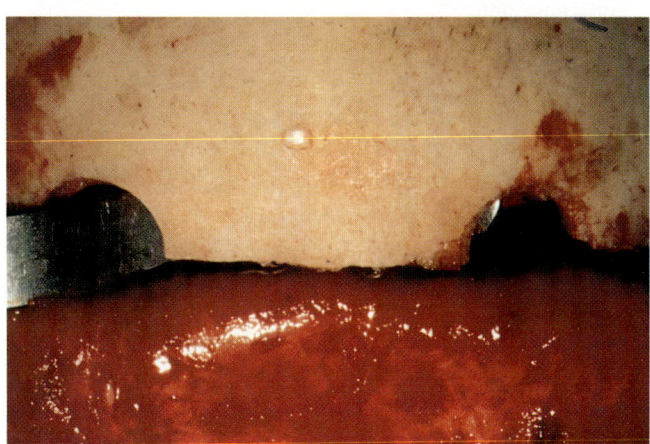

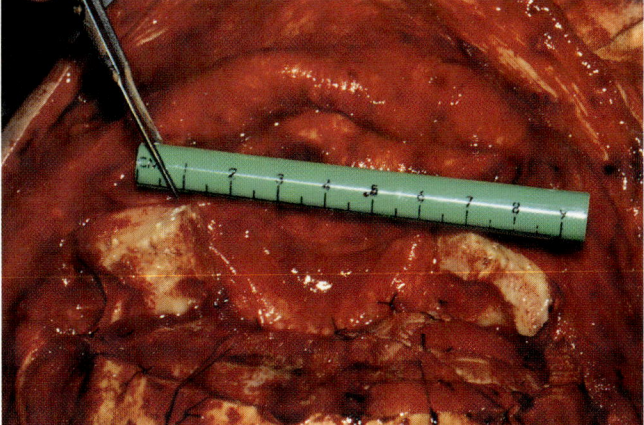

FIG. 3. A: Raising of pericranial flap from galea. **B:** Pericranial flap inserted intracranially between the supraorbital bone (covered by flap) and bifrontal craniotomy. **C:** Pericranial flap introduced intracranially below the level of supraorbital bone.

mary blood supply of this muscle comes from the internal maxillary artery through several branches (anterior and posterior deep temporal arteries) (Fig. 2B). The superficial temporal artery does have one communication with this muscle and its deep arterial system through the middle temporal branch. It is a constant branch that enters the muscle just above the posterior aspect of the zygomatic arch (Fig. 6). With the internal maxillary ar-

tery and its branches to the temporalis muscle preserved, it is relatively safe to free the entire temporalis muscle down to the coronoid process (Fig. 7). This achieves maximum rotational capability of this muscle flap. The soft tissue attachment to the coronoid process is preserved to assure adequate venous return. For increase of the rotational arc of the muscle, it is possible to fracture the coronoid process following subperiosteal undermining. The variable course of the internal maxillary artery could bring it just posterior to the coronoid process and it can be easily injured here. A strictly subperiosteal osteotomy of the coronoid process must be performed.

It is also feasible to base the temporalis muscle on its distal internal maxillary arterial network, providing no surgery has been done in the vicinity of the pterygopalatine vessels. Following transection of the proximal course of the internal maxillary vessel, a reversal of blood flow takes place (through the pterygopalatine vessels), which seems to provide adequate vascularity to the muscle. This permits the use of the temporalis muscle for reconstruction even in cases where the infratemporal fossa is involved with a tumor and the resection of the internal maxillary vessel is carried out.

The temporalis muscle can be used in its entirety or it may be segmented through a vertical split where only the anterior or posterior half of the muscle is used. The remaining portion of the muscle can be replaced into the temporal fossa (Fig. 8). Another way to maximize the use of the temporalis muscle is to develop separate flaps from the deep temporal fascia and the muscle in their distal two-thirds. This then allows additional flexibility of placement of the muscle and the fascia. If only a relatively small but vascularized flap is necessary, the temporalis fascia can be developed as an arterialized flap based on the superficial temporal arterial pedicle. It has an adequate reach for the lateral skull base and provides an excellent seal for defects in the floor of the middle cranial fossa (Fig. 9).

Transfer of the entire temporalis muscle creates a con-

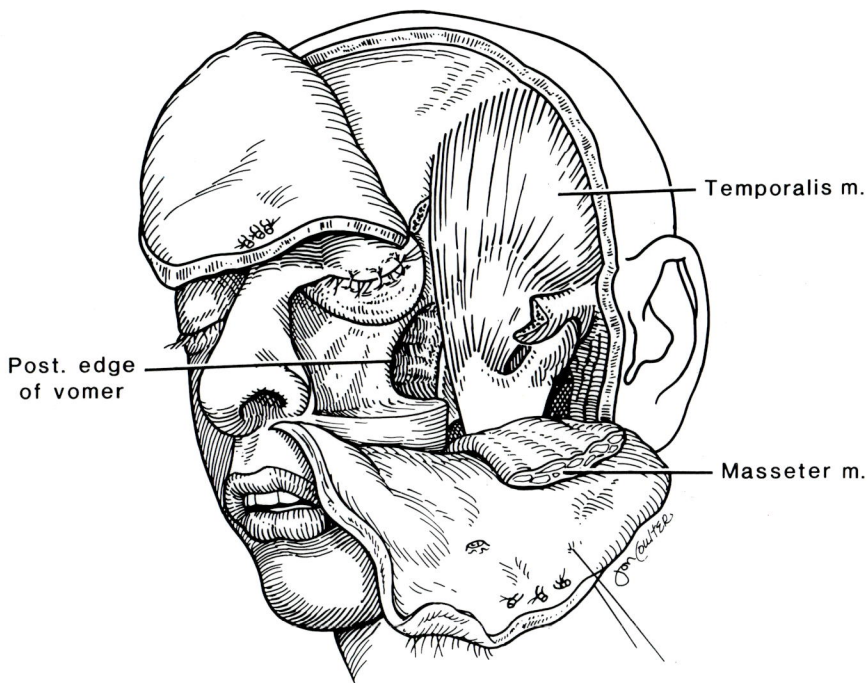

FIG. 5. Anatomic location of temporalis muscle.

cavity of the temporal fossa. This can be minimized to some extent with placement of a free-fat graft (from the abdomen) in the temporal fossa. Even after some atrophy of the fat graft, the depression of the temporal fossa is lessened (Fig. 10).

Scalp Flaps

Because of the richness of its blood supply, the scalp is an excellent donor site for soft tissue flaps. These flaps can be used for coverage of scalp defects or may reach fronto-orbital as well as midfacial regions. The selective utilization of the hair-bearing or hairless scalp may provide an excellent substitution for soft tissue defects. The eventual donor site may be covered with a skin graft (Fig. 11).

Pectoralis and Trapezius Muscle Flaps

The pectoralis muscle or myocutaneous flap, supplied by the acromiothoracic vessels, will reach the upper cervical and lower mastoid region and may be used for reconstruction of these areas (Figs. 12 and 13). Full cranial base, however, cannot be reconstructed with this flap.

Trapezius muscle flap, however, can reach the poste-

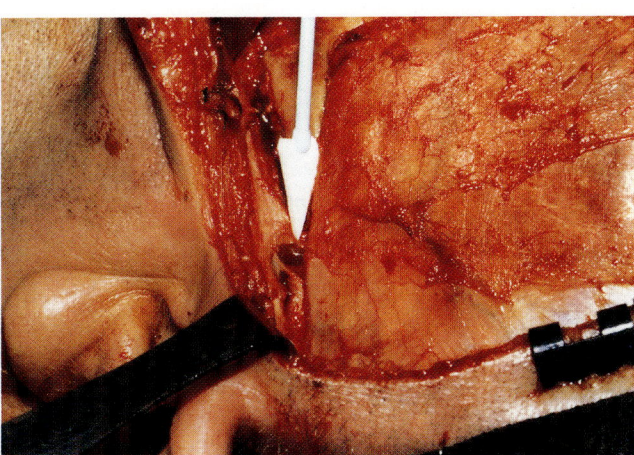

FIG. 6. Middle temporal branch of left superficial temporal artery entering temporalis muscle.

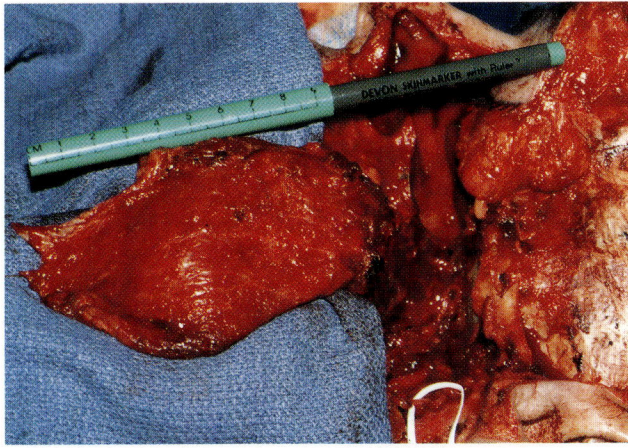

FIG. 7. Inferiorly dissected left temporalis muscle to achieve maximum of rotational arc for reconstruction.

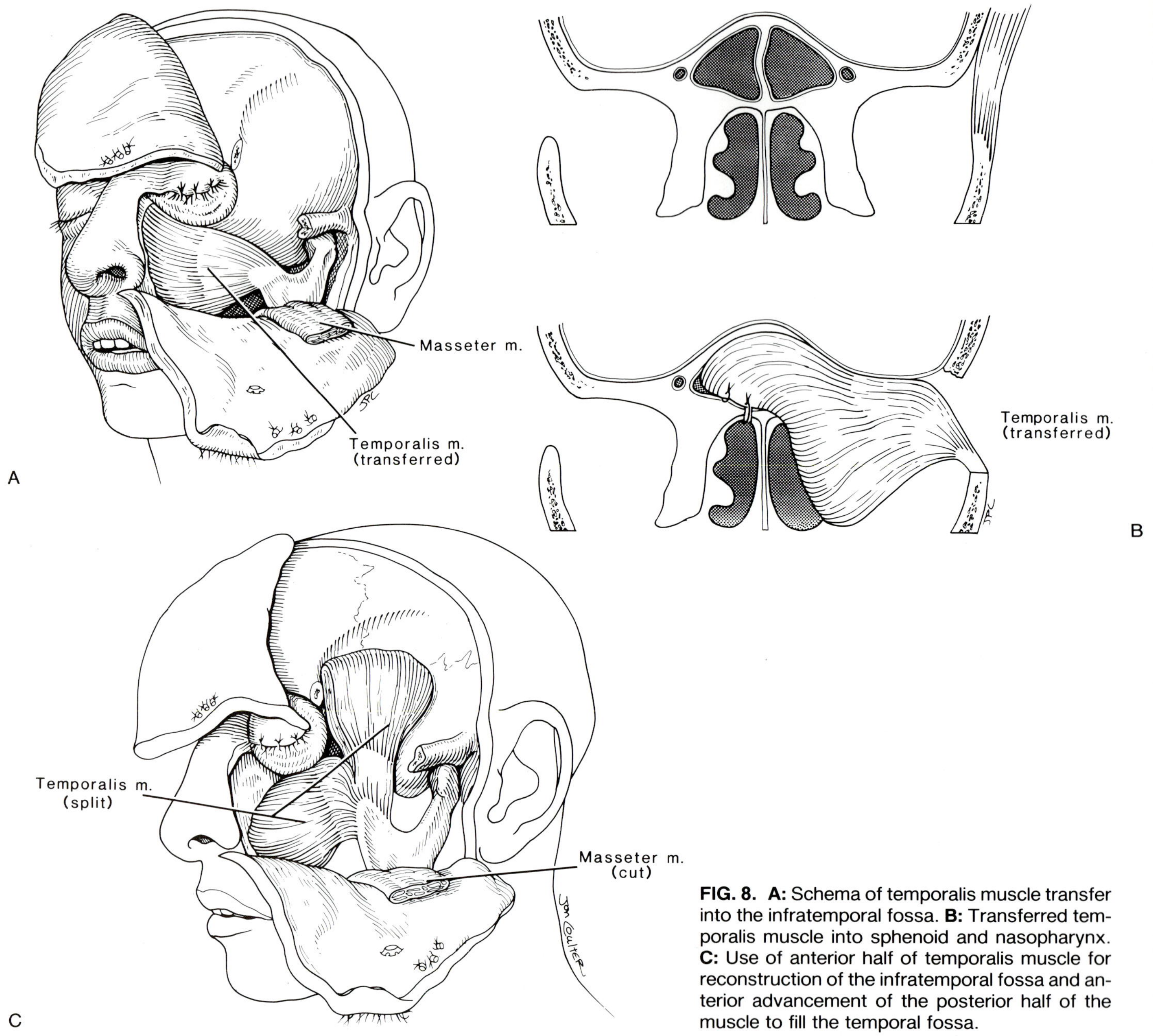

FIG. 8. A: Schema of temporalis muscle transfer into the infratemporal fossa. **B:** Transferred temporalis muscle into sphenoid and nasopharynx. **C:** Use of anterior half of temporalis muscle for reconstruction of the infratemporal fossa and anterior advancement of the posterior half of the muscle to fill the temporal fossa.

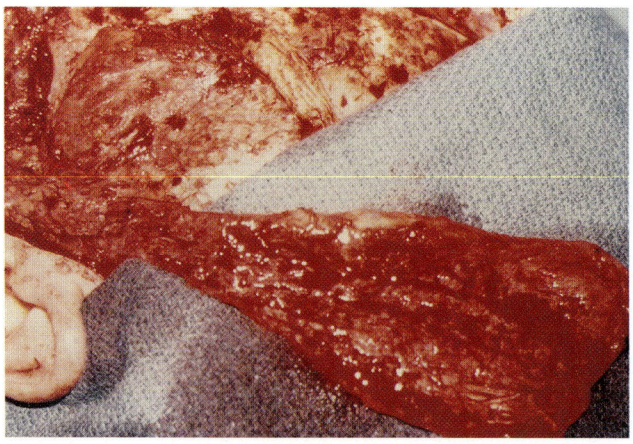

FIG. 9. Arterialized left temporalis fascial flap.

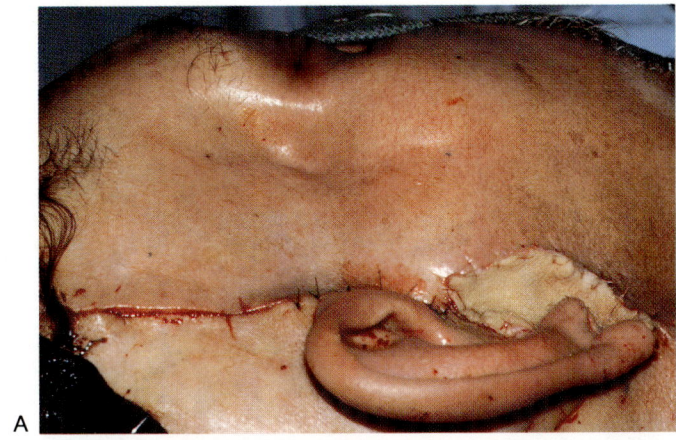
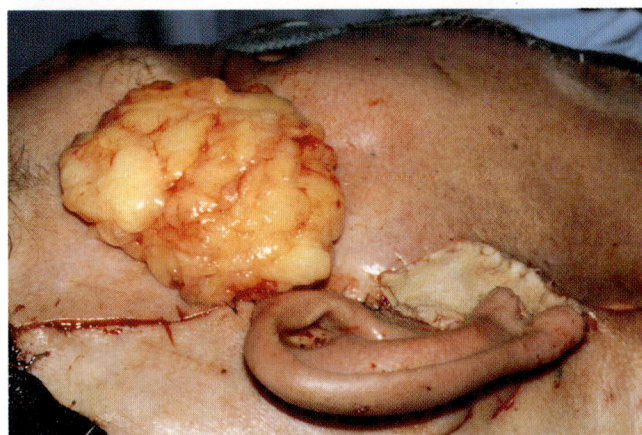
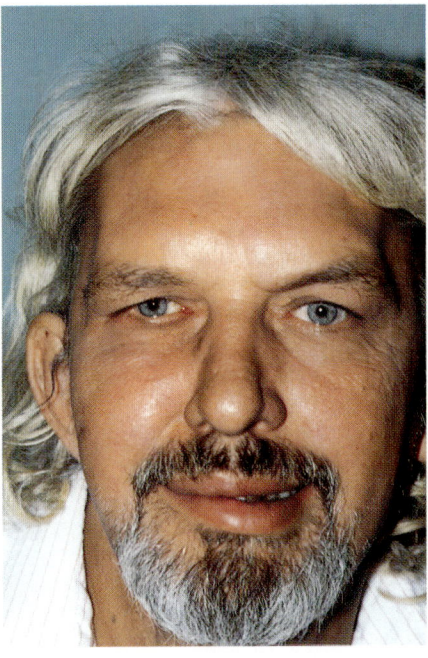

FIG. 10. A: Intraoperative appearance (depression) of right temporal fossa following temporalis muscle transfer. **B:** Free abdominal fat (placed externally for demonstration) to be used in augmentation of temporal fossa depression. **C:** Appearance of both temporal fossae 1.5 years following free-fat graft placement into right temporal fossa.

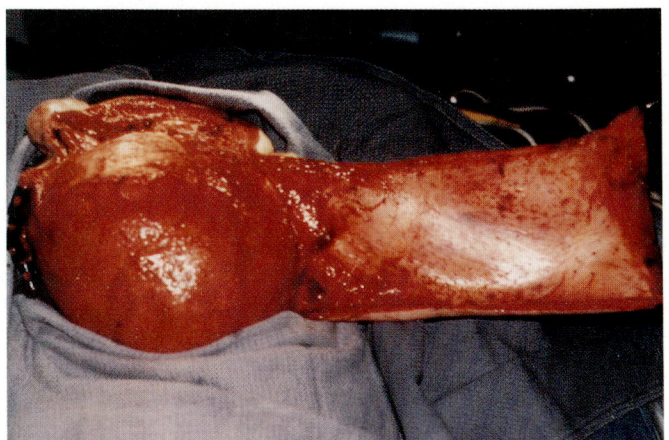
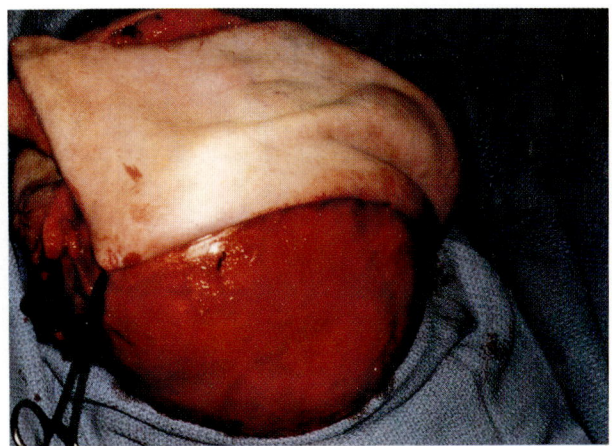

FIG. 11. A: Raised scalp flap based on right temporo-occipital blood supply. **B:** Transferred scalp flap over right fronto-orbital region.

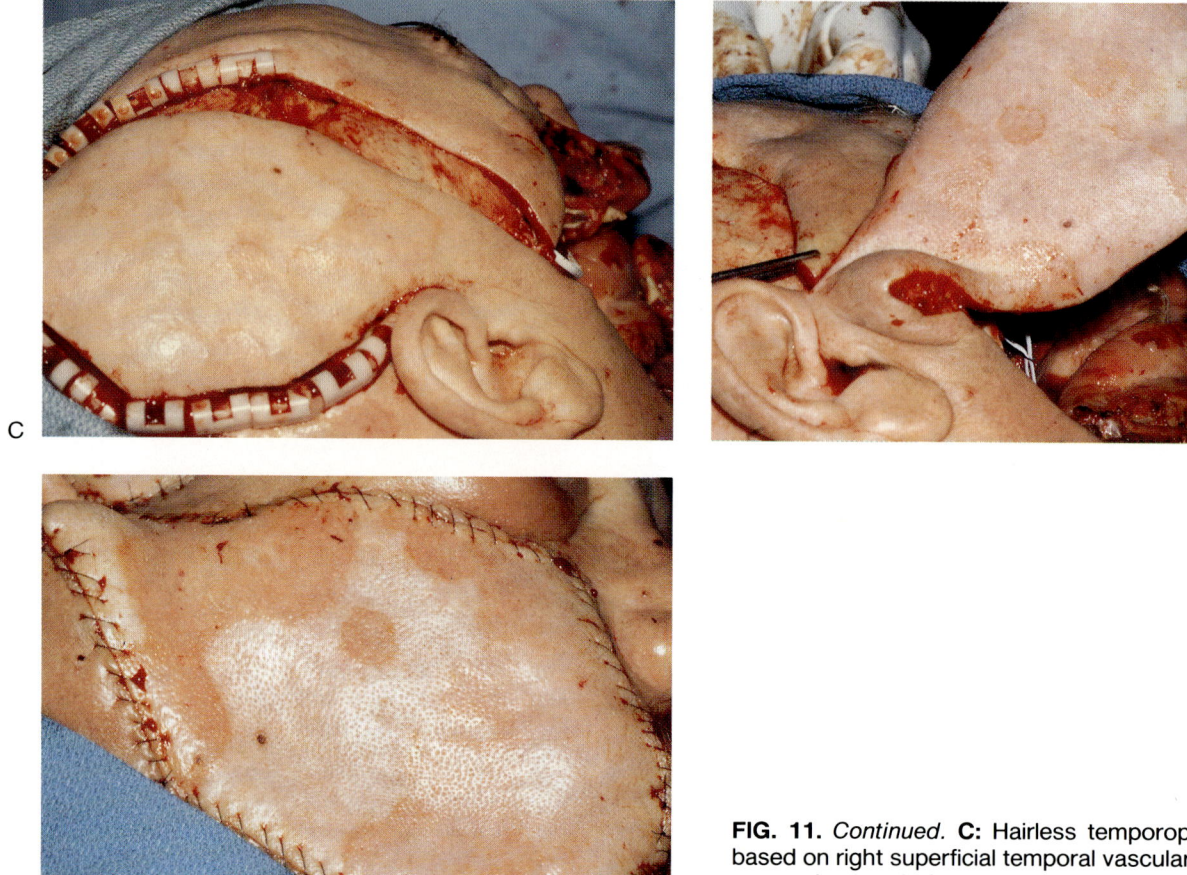

FIG. 11. *Continued.* **C:** Hairless temporoparietal scalp flap based on right superficial temporal vascular pedicle. **D:** Temporoparietal scalp flap is being transferred to facial region. **E:** Inset of temporoparietal scalp flap into right facial region.

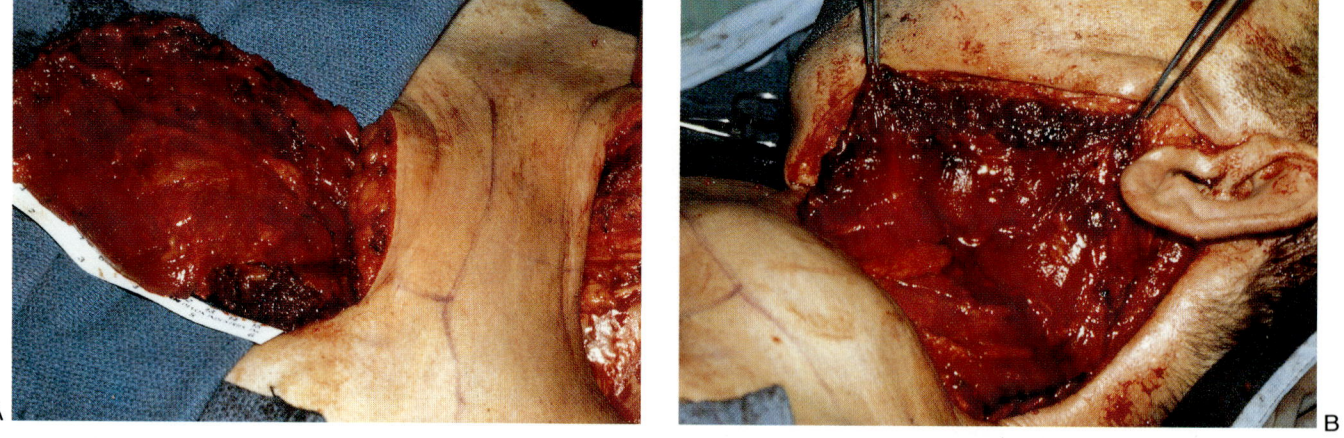

FIG. 12. A: Left pectoralis muscle is raised. **B:** Pectoralis muscle is brought into the left neck and suboccipital defect demonstrating the level of an average reach of this muscle flap.

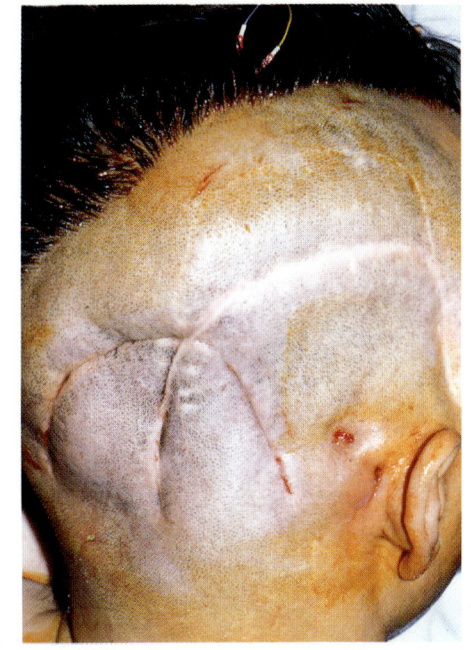
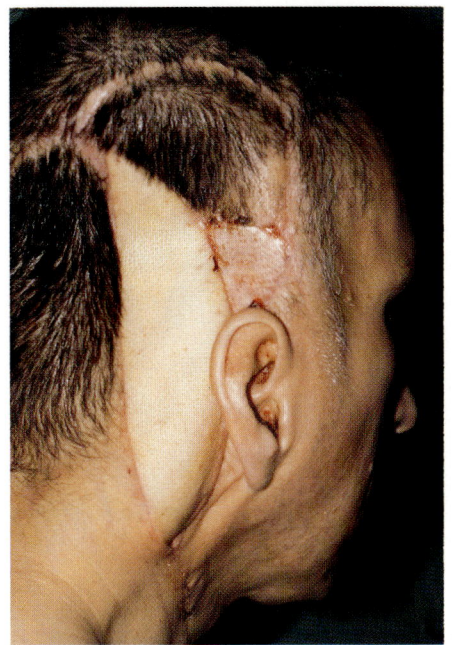
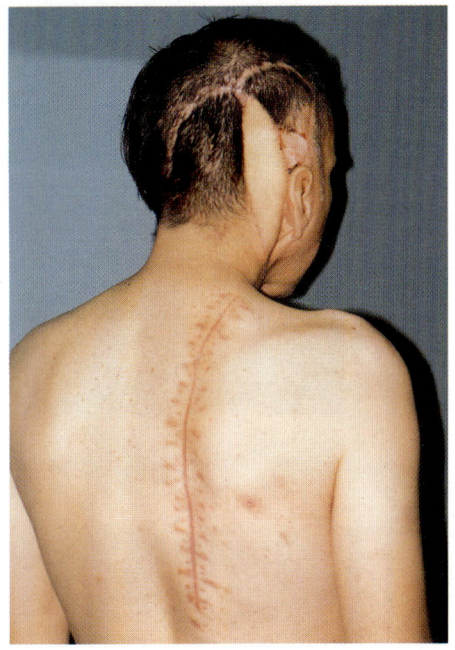

FIG. 13. A: Multiple scars in parieto-occipital scalp. **B:** Following tumor resection (including some scalp) trapezius myocutaneous flap was inset. (Courtesy of Dr. Ramasastry). **C:** Trapezius myocutaneous flap in occipital scalp and flap donor site.

rior cranial base, with or without its cutaneous island. Its primary blood supply is from the transverse cervical artery. The secondary blood supply comes from paravertebral vessels, which permit greater superior rotation and thus an adequate reach of the posterior skull base. Designing the flap axis in a vertical direction uses this secondary blood supply and also permits preservation of function in the lateral portion of this muscle.

Craniofacial Skeleton

Various forms of craniofacial disassembly are used in most cranial base procedures (Fig. 14). This reflects our ability to temporarily remove craniofacial skeleton (noninvolved with tumor), which, however, would otherwise prevent us from reaching the tumor at the cranial base.

Various osteotomies free the skeletal units. The extent of craniofacial disassembly varies from limited removal of the supraorbital bar to bilateral removal of orbitofacial skeleton (Fig. 15). The direction of the osteotomies is designed in such a way as to provide the greatest stability of the reassembled skeleton. This is accomplished with a "key/keyhole" pattern of osteotomies (Fig. 16). The ultimate bony fixation, enhanced by this pattern of osteotomy, is assured with miniplate fixation. We have used

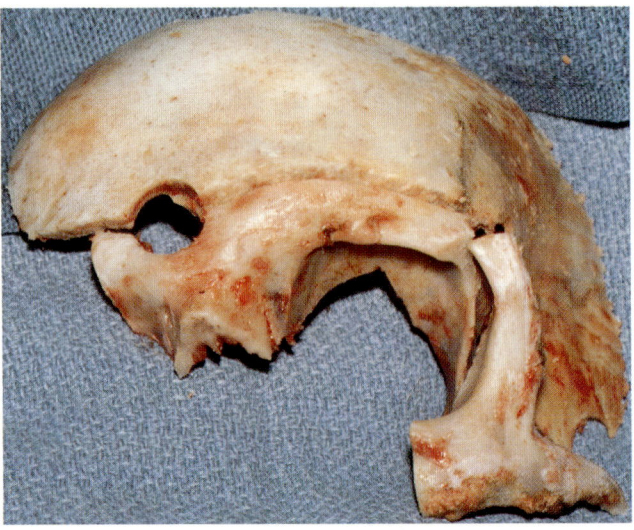

FIG. 14. Craniofacial and frontotemporal bony disassembly for exposure of cranial base.

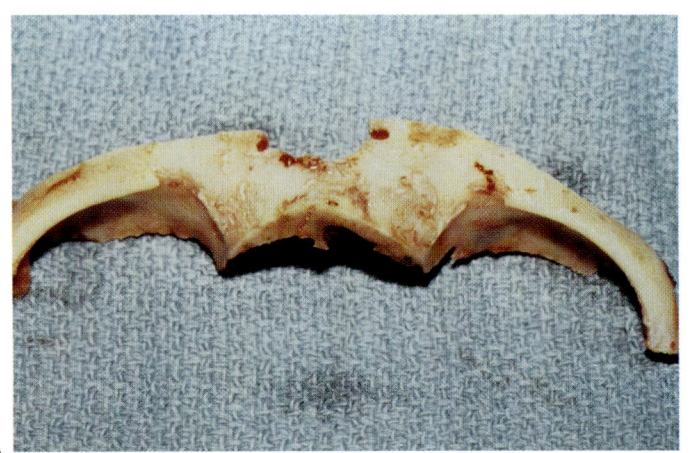

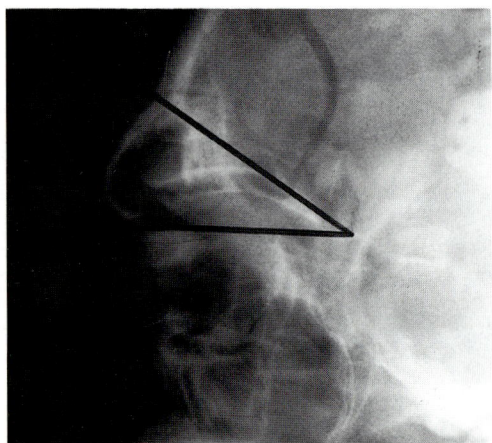

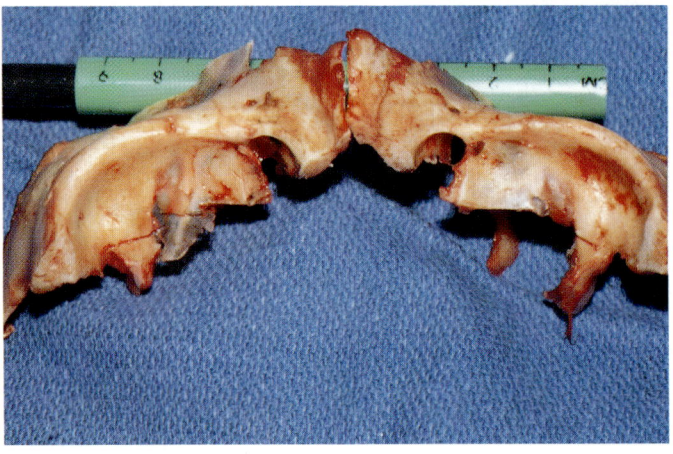

FIG. 15. A: Removed supraorbital bone (with orbital roofs) for exposure of anterior cranial fossa. **B:** Lateral skull radiograph demonstrating an improved angle of visualization of anterior cranial fossa following supraorbital bone removal. **C:** Removed bilateral facial skeleton; a view from above demonstrates nasal bones, naso–maxillary processes, inferior halves of both orbits, and malar bones.

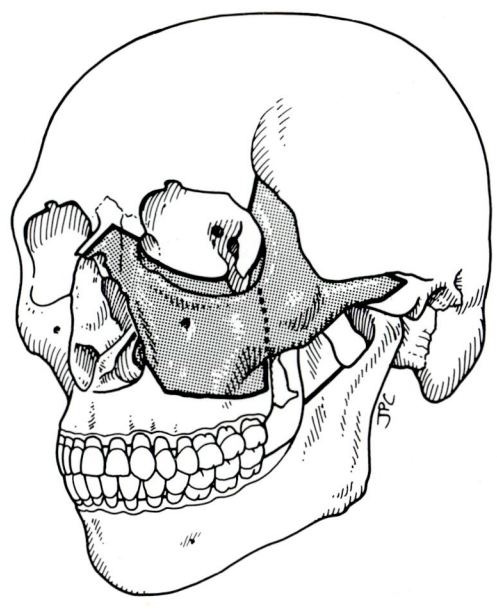

FIG. 16. Key/keyhole pattern of bony osteotomies.

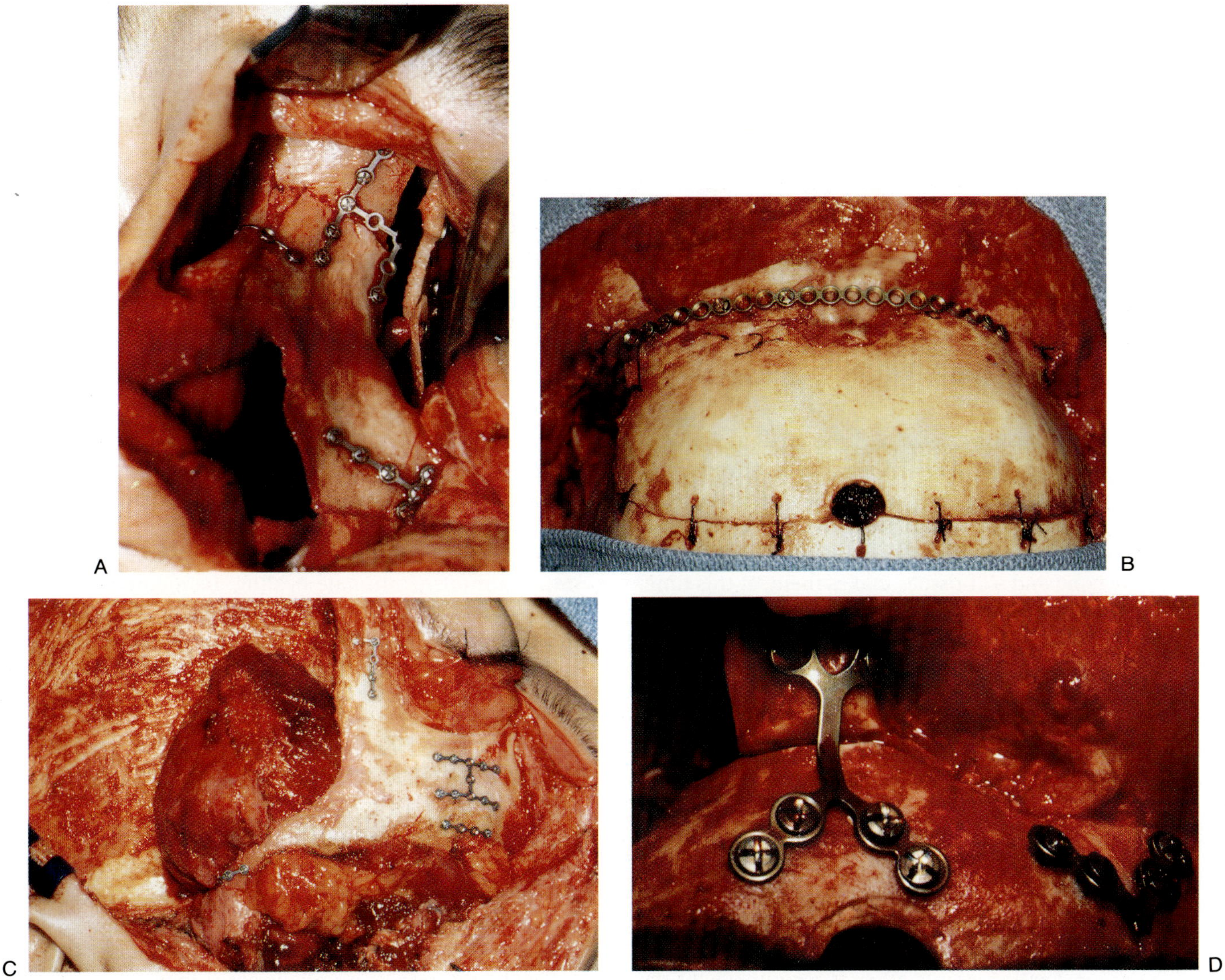

FIG. 17. A: Nasofrontal and maxillary bony fixation (with vitallium microplates) following bony reassembly; cranial bone graft, reconstructing medial wall of left orbit, is also visible. **B:** Superior (frontal) fixation of craniofacial bony segment. **C:** Microplate fixation of right orbitomaxillary bony segments over transferred temporalis muscle. **D:** Titanium miniplate fixation of nasofrontal osseous segments.

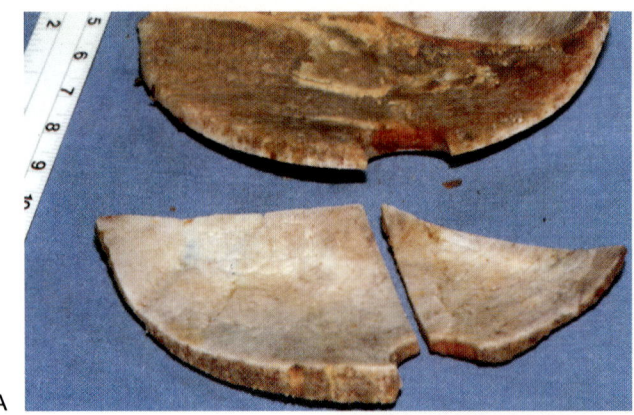
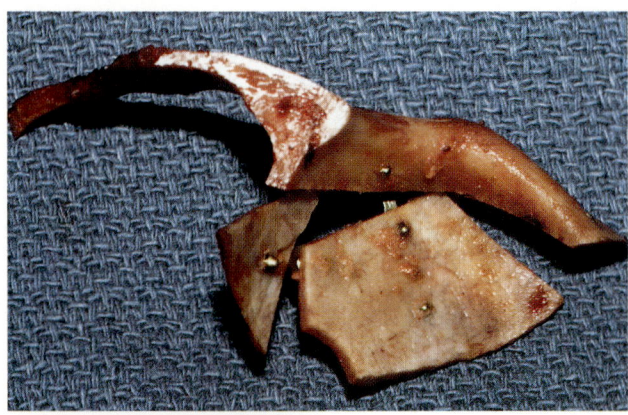
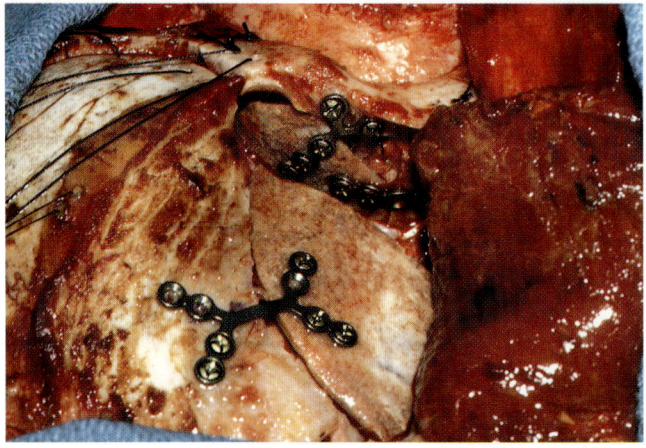

FIG. 18. **A:** Split cranial bone graft obtained from bifrontal craniotomy. **B:** Reconstruction of right lateral bony orbit attached with miniplates. **C:** Multiple cranial bone grafts affixed with titanium miniplates used for reconstruction of right orbit and temporal fossa.

both the titanium miniplates and the vitallium microplates. For thin midfacial bones, the microplating system is quite satisfactory. When greater stability is required (e.g., pterygoid plates, zygomatic arches) stronger miniplates might be used. The excellent tolerance of these plates by bone and soft tissues makes them, at this time, the fixation modality of choice. Also, in the postoperative period these plates provide only a minimal interference with CT and MRI scanning, important for oncological follow-up (Fig. 17). Other fixation modalities have been used, for example, wire or even braided nylon. The steel wire is a time-tested method. However, it creates a great degree of interference with CT. Titanium wire, giving minimum CT interference, is, however, not readily available and it is quite brittle. Also, the biomechanics of wire fixation versus plate fixation clearly favors the plating systems. The braided nylon fixation can be used in areas that are totally without internal stress (e.g., craniotomy). However, regardless of the frequency of the nylon fixation points along the perimeter of the replaced skeleton, this method of fixation must be considered only fair.

Any important defect of the craniofacial skeleton created for oncological purposes can be substituted with split cranial bone graft, properly afixed to the remaining skeleton. This is especially important in reconstruction of the orbit. The source of the split cranial bone grafts is usually the bifrontal craniotomy (Fig. 18).

Primary soft tissue coverage of craniofacial skeleton is important for its ultimate healing. Its membranous nature, however, permits healing even if a small segment of the bone may be exposed (primarily in the paranasal sinus regions). Rapid overgrowth by mucosa is often seen in such cases.

PREOPERATIVE CARE

It is important to ascertain the extent of scarring from previous surgical procedures. This may limit the availability of regional reconstructive soft tissue flaps. Occasionally, the true extent of scalp scarring is not appreciated until the head is fully shaved (Figs. 1 and 13A). As far as the temporalis muscle is concerned, preoperative assessment of the function of the muscle can be judged by bilateral palpation of the muscles and comparing the degree of prominence during teeth clenching. This demonstrates grossly the potential bulk of the temporalis muscle available for reconstruction as well as confirms its innervation. Denervated muscle (e.g., in trigeminal neurilemomas) is seldom suitable for transfer. Also, in patients who have had prolonged trismus or have been malnourished for other reasons, the bulk of the temporalis muscle may be surprisingly small and other alternatives for reconstruction should be planned.

The craniofacial osteotomies and subsequent stability of the skeleton may be altered by previous surgery on the skeleton (e.g., orthognathic, sinus surgery).

POSTOPERATIVE CARE

The stability of the craniofacial (craniomaxillary) skeleton is maintained by its original fixation method (miniplates). Additional fixation (e.g., intermaxillary) is seldom indicated. Occasionally, in bilateral craniofacial procedures, the instability of the hard palate and its effect on occlusion have to be kept in mind. In such cases temporary postoperative intermaxillary banding can be used. Effective maintenance of intranasal hygiene is a prerequisite to uneventful secondary healing of the interorbital and paranasal sinus space.

The transferred regional soft tissue flaps maintain their original position following intraoperative suspension. The critical placement of suction drains permits adequate coaptation of the flaps with the underlying tissues contouring appropriately to the defect. Also, in the temporal fossa following transfer of a free-fat graft, it is important to maintain, with a closed suction system, contact of the scalp to the underlying graft. Even in cases where dural repair was required (potential CSF leak), vacuum drains may be placed at a distance from the dural repair, providing the overlying soft tissue is permitted to come into direct apposition with the dura. Maintaining this contact, with moderate suction (90 mm Hg), permits rapid healing at the site of dural repair. On the contrary, if no adequate drainage is provided, blood is permitted to accumulate and thus separate the overlining soft tissue from the underlining dura. This may actually delay healing at that site and potentially create space for CSF leak.

COMPLICATIONS

The ultimate failure of a soft tissue flap is the demise of its circulation. This is reflected in soft tissue necrosis. The consequences then depend on the location of the flap as well as the extent of the necrosis. It is therefore essential that the vascularity of the flap is protected throughout the procedure. This means not only protecting the actual blood supply to the flap but also maintaining the capillary perfusion at the periphery. Retraction of a flap for many hours, as well as allowing it to dry with direct operating room lights, is very detrimental to the capillary perfusion of the flap. Intraoperative attention to these factors (by periodic release of the flap permitting reflow through its main blood supply as well as maintenance of moisture over the entire surface of the flap) will encourage postoperative primary healing.

The treatment of complications depends primarily on the extent as well as the site of the tissue necrosis. Small areas of necrosis over nonessential sites may be allowed to separate spontaneously and be permitted to head by secondary intention. However, tissue necrosis over essential areas (e.g., carotid artery, dura) requires surgical intervention to avoid the ultimate reconstructive failure, a demise of an essential structure originally designed to be protected by our reconstructive measures.

As far as the craniofacial skeleton is concerned, the key elements in prevention of complications is the skeletal stability and its soft tissue coverage. Any exposed bone that is unstable should be removed or restabilized and covered with soft tissue.

FOLLOW-UP

Once primary healing takes place, no specific care is required for soft tissue flaps or craniofacial skeleton. However, it is important to obtain baseline imaging with MRI and/or CT scans at approximately 6–12 weeks postoperatively to ascertain the radiologic appearance of the site of reconstruction. This helps immeasurably in subsequent oncologic follow-up. Any tumor recurrence is suspected when a noticeable change develops in the contour lines of the soft tissue flaps. These subsequent scans also show progressive atrophy of transferred muscles. This is pronounced with microvascular (denervated) free-flaps where the muscle bulk almost disappears.

DISCUSSION

There are almost always several ways of reconstructing a surgical defect. The selected procedure is a reflection of the available soft tissues, the extent of the surgical defect, as well as the skills of the surgeon. As long as the primary goals of reconstruction are achieved, the preference for a reconstructive choice is usually individual. However, regional reconstructive tissues are our preferred choice. Also, the degree of craniofacial disassembly and therefore the potential amount of skeleton "at risk" vary from procedure to procedure as well as from surgeon to surgeon. In our hands the wide exposure achieved by significant craniofacial disassembly is well rewarded by improved visualization, safety of the procedure, and better control of the oncological perimeter.

CONCLUSIONS

Reconstructive techniques with regional flaps and craniofacial skeleton manipulation are integral parts of cranial base surgery. Their displacement during the approach phase of surgery is essential for adequate exposure and oncological therapy of cranial base tumors. Their subsequent replacement, rotation, or adjustment during reconstruction enhances the esthetic as well as functional rehabilitation of our patients.

SUGGESTED READINGS

1. Abul-Hassan HS, von Drasek Ascher G, Acland RD. Surgical anatomy and blood supply to the fascial layers of the temporal region. *Plast Reconstr Surg* 1986;77:17.
2. Antonyshyn O, Gruss JS, Birt BD. Versatility of temporal muscle and fascial flaps. *Br J Plast Surg* 1988;41:118.
3. Argenta LC, Friedman RJ, Dingman RO, Duus EC. The versatility of pericranial flaps. *Plast Reconstr Surg* 1985;76:695.
4. Casanova R, Cavalcante D, Grotting JC, et al. Anatomic basis for vascularized outer-table calvarial bone flaps. *Plast Reconstr Surg* 1986;78:300.
5. Cutting CB, McCarthy JG, Berenstein A. Blood supply of the upper craniofacial skeleton: the search for composite calvarial bone flaps. *Plast Reconstr Surg* 1984;74:603.
6. Jackson IT, Adham MN, March R. Use of the galeal frontalis myofascial flap in craniofacial surgery. *Plast Reconstr Surg* 1986;77:905.
7. Johns ME, Winn HR, McLean WC, Cantrell RW. Pericranial flap for the closure of defects of craniofacial resection. *Laryngoscope* 1981;91:952.
8. Matsuba HM, Hakki AR, Little JW, Spear SL. The temporal fossa in head and neck reconstruction: twenty-two flaps of scalp, fascia, and full-thickness cranial bone. *Laryngoscope* 1988;98:444.
9. Salyer KE, Taylor DP. Bone grafts in craniofacial surgery. *Clin Plast Surg* 1987;14:27.
10. Stiernberg CM, Bailey BJ, Weiner RL, et al. Reconstruction of the anterior skull base following craniofacial resection. *Arch Otolaryngol Head Neck Surg* 1987;113:710.
11. Stock AL, Collins HP, Davidson TM. Anatomy of the superficial temporal artery. *Head Neck Surg* 1980;2:466.
12. Janecka IP, Sekhar LN. Reconstruction of base of skull surgical defects. In: Jackson CG, ed. *Surgery of skull base tumors.* New York: Churchill Livingstone, 1991;251–272.

CHAPTER 28

Microvascular Reconstruction of the Cranial Base

Kenneth C. Shestak, Neil Ford Jones, and Sai S. Ramasastry

Local and regional flap reconstruction is suitable for many smaller defects in the cranial base region. However, as the surgical defect becomes more medial and more extensive, free tissue transfer assumes a greater role in the reconstructive hierarchy. This method requires experience in microvascular surgery, but such expertise is becoming common in most centers throughout the world. Available free-flap donor sites for reconstruction of the cranial base include the greater omentum, the scapular flap, the latissimus dorsi muscle and its musculocutaneous flap, and the rectus abdominis muscle flap.

Following appropriate diagnostic workup, tumor localization, and routine medical evaluation, the operative treatment is carried out. In our institution this is most often performed by a multidisciplinary team consisting of a neurosurgeon, ENT surgeon, and plastic surgeon.

The primary objective in cranial base reconstruction is to ensure separation of the oral cavity from the intracranial space following tumor ablation. As defects become extensive, local flaps become less reliable and therefore microvascular free-flap transfer is needed. Most often this is the transfer of a muscle free-flap that has the ability to conform to almost any defect. Muscle tissue can be precisely inset to margins of the defect to provide a reliable, watertight seal. Due to their accessibility and vascular anatomy, the rectus abdominis and latissimus dorsi flaps have proved to be most useful for free-flap reconstruction of the cranial base.

K. C. Shestak: Division of Plastic Surgery, University of Pittsburgh School of Medicine, and University Surgical Associates, Inc., Magee-Womens' Hospital, Pittsburgh, Pennsylvania 15213.

N. F. Jones and S. S. Ramasastry: Division of Plastic Surgery, University of Pittsburgh School of Medicine, Pittsburgh, Pennsylvania 15261.

RECTUS ABDOMINIS FLAP

Surgical Steps

The anterior truncal location of this muscle makes it *the* most useful free-flap donor tissue for cranial base reconstruction, since this eliminates the need for changing the patient's position on the operating room table during flap elevation. Another major advantage is this muscle's remote location from the cranial area, which allows the extirpation and free-flap harvest to proceed simultaneously, thus minimizing total operating time.

The rectus abdominis muscle spans the abdomen longitudinally, arising from the pubis and inserting on a costal cartilage syncytium of ribs 8–11. It has dual arterial blood supply with contributions from the superior and deep inferior epigastric arteries. The deep inferior epigastric artery and its venae commitantes make the microvascular transfer of the lower half or even the entire muscle very reliable. This artery and the accompanying two veins are large diameter vessels that provide a pedicle of 8–10 cm in length.

Although the long-term morbidity of rectus abdominis muscle transfer is not precisely known, sacrifice of the muscle is normally well tolerated by most patients. Caution is needed when planning rectus flap transfer in the setting of previous abdominal or pelvic surgery. Also, the removal of this muscle in the young growing child should probably be done only if other donor sites, such as the scapular or groin flap, are unavailable.

Preoperatively, the patients are vigorously hydrated with balanced salt solutions beginning the night before surgery. Patients who smoke are asked to stop smoking 2 weeks prior to surgery. During the operation all fluids are warmed and blood pressure should be maintained without the use of pressors. It is our custom to administer low molecular weight dextran

—dextran 40 at 25 cc/hr—during surgery and this continues for 5 days following the operation.

The flap is usually harvested using either a midline or a paramedian incision; however, it can be raised through a suprapubic incision and the concealed scar is often preferable in the female patient. The anterior rectus fascia is opened longitudinally and the muscle is dissected free from the fascia by carefully dividing the tendinous inscriptions of the rectus muscle. There are usually three inscriptions within the rectus muscle and the lower two are most often divided. The deep inferior epigastric vascular pedicle enters the posterior surface of the muscle laterally, below the arcuate line. It is easily located at the lateral margin of the muscle and then can be dissected to its origin from the external iliac artery by retracting the tissues of the retroperitoneum (Fig. 1). It is possible to develop a pedicle length between 8.0 and 10.0 cm. The artery is interrupted first by placing a double ligature or clip at its junction with the external iliac artery. Next, the veins are divided and the muscle is ready for transfer. As mentioned, flap elevation can often be accomplished simultaneously with the ablative surgery.

Most often the prospective surgical defect is analyzed prior to flap elevation and after suitable recipient vessels for the flap have been selected and prepared. There are a plethora of blood vessels in the head and neck region but the most commonly used recipient vessels are branches of the external carotid system, with the facial artery and vein most often utilized. The superficial temporal, the occipital, and superior thyroid vessels are also useful as recipient vessels. Next, the borders of the defect in the nasopharynx are carefully studied as it is extremely important to accurately suture the flap to the margins of the defect. The flap is first inset to the posterior and lateral aspects of the defect and the anterior inset is completed following revascularization. The internal surface of the muscle within the nasopharynx has not required skin grafting as it becomes "mucosalized" within several days. Separate tongues of muscle may be used to obliterate open sinuses (sphenoid and ethmoid) and to drape over exposed dural repairs or dural grafts (Fig. 2–5). Part of the muscle may be used to cover an exposed saphenous vein graft should reconstruction of the internal carotid artery be required because of involvement with tu-

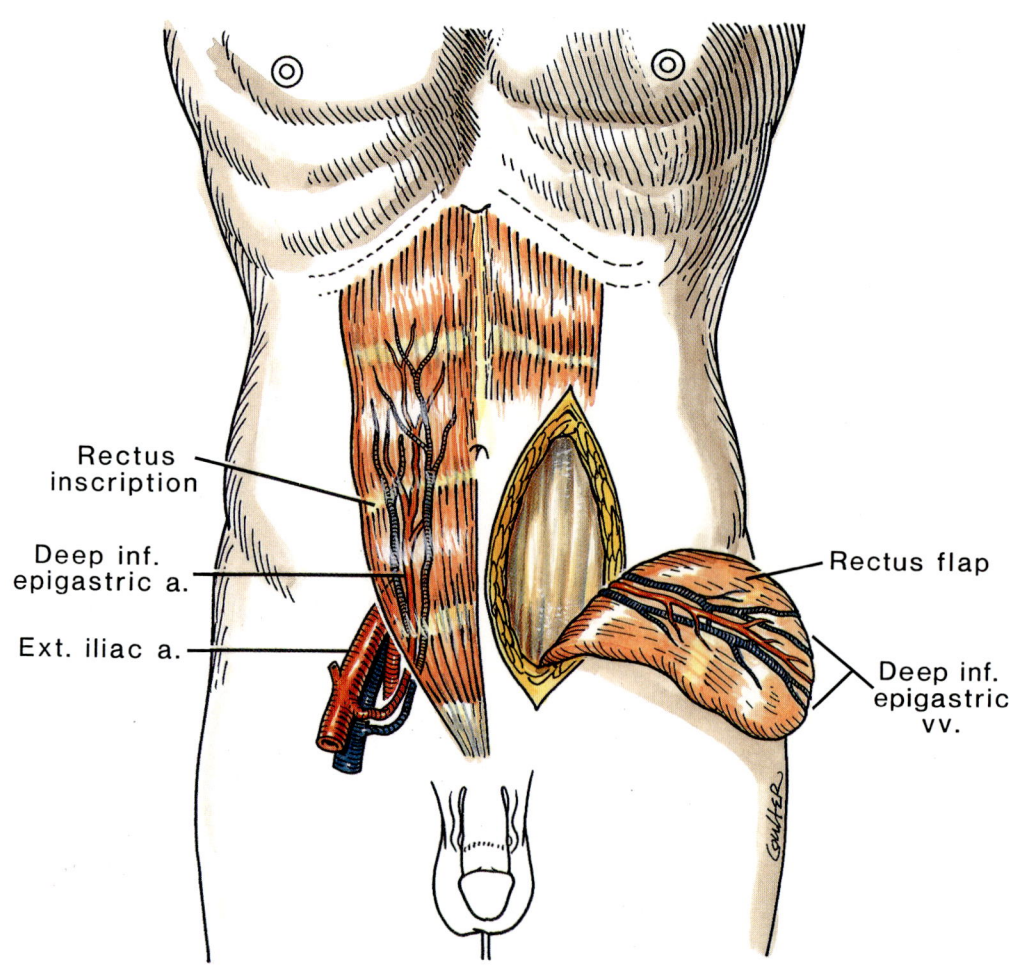

FIG. 1. Vascular anatomy of rectus abdominis muscle.

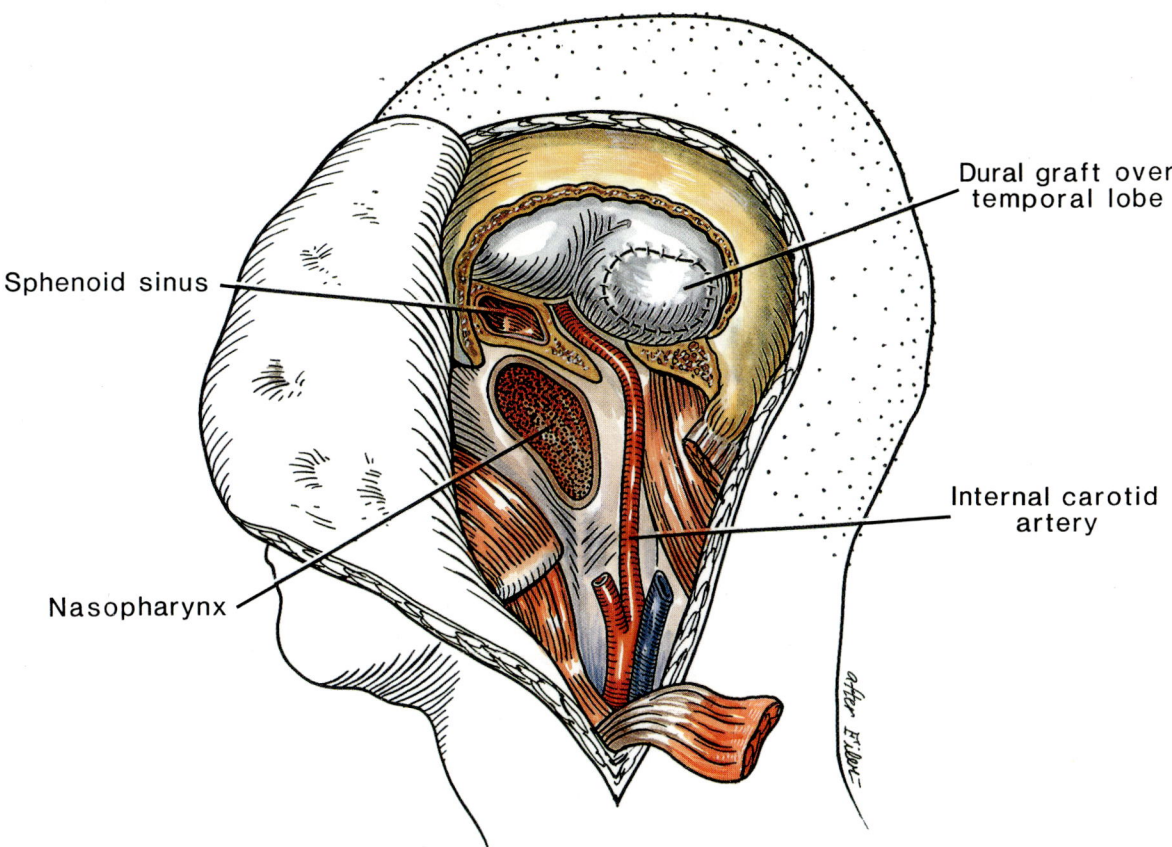

FIG. 2. Defect of lateral cranial base with placement of fascia lata graft to reconstruct dural defect.

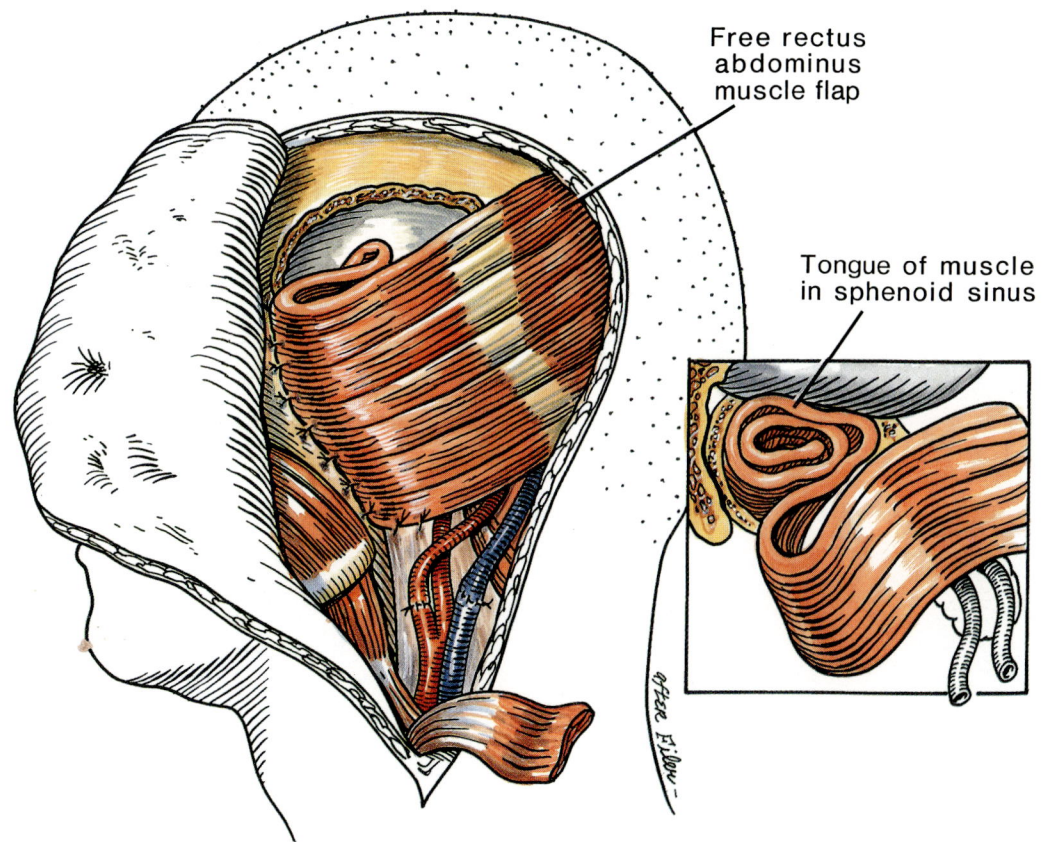

FIG. 3. Revascularization and inset of rectus abdominis muscle flap.

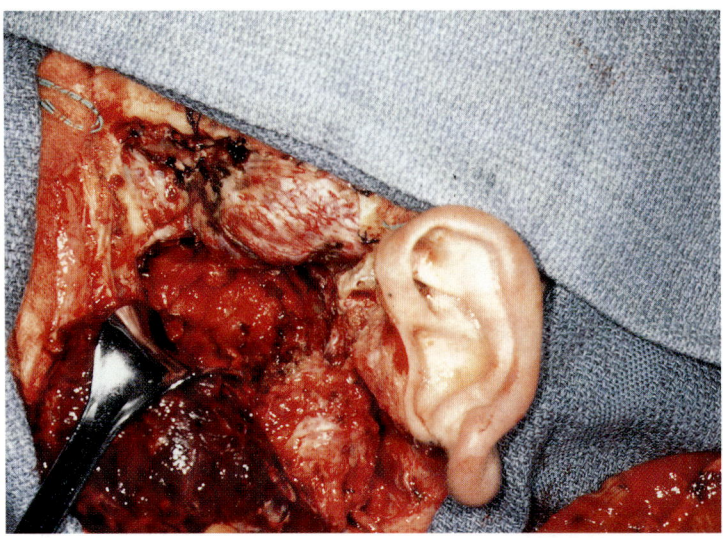

FIG. 4. Defect of left cranial base and infratemporal fossa following resection of cranial base tumor.

mor. The flap is then revascularized by anastomosing the flap vessels to the recipient vessels using the operating microscope. Vascular anastomoses can be done by either the end-to-end or end-to-side anastomotic technique depending on vessel position and size match. The veins are customarily repaired first followed by the repair of the artery; however, if the artery is located deep to the veins the order may be reversed. The abdominal wound is closed by repair of the anterior rectus fascia. Careful hemostasis must be obtained at both cut muscle ends. Usually one drain is placed above the anterior rectus fascia and brought out through the skin. It is removed within the first three postoperative days. The skin is apposed in customary fashion with either a sutured or stapled skin closure.

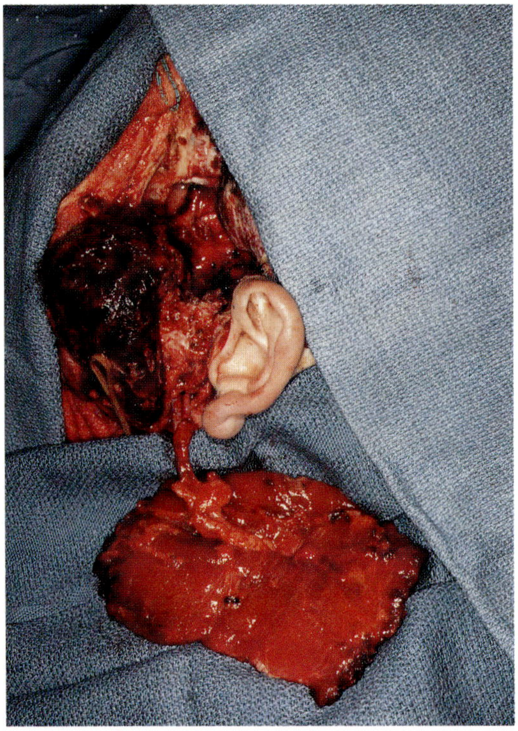

Patients are kept at bed rest for the first day but thereafter they are allowed out of bed. They are maintained on dextran for 5 days and appropriate antibiotics for 48 hr. Aspirin, 325 mg/day, is begun when the patients are able to tolerate oral feedings. Skin sutures are removed between 7 and 10 days following surgery.

Follow-up

It is very unusual for a patient to complain of decreased abdominal muscle strength for routine activities of daily living. In fact, a patient who has had one rectus muscle transferred can undergo the transfer of the opposite rectus muscle should this be necessary without significant decrease in abdominal wall muscle strength. The incidence of hernia formation following rectus abdominis free-flap transfer has been very low in our hands.

LATISSIMUS DORSI FLAP

Planning

For very large defects or those where considerable soft tissue bulk is needed, the latissimus dorsi flap is the free flap of choice (Figs. 6–10). The main advantages of this flap are that it can supply a large amount of muscle or a composite of skin and muscle (musculocutaneous flap) with the longest possible vascular pedicle of any free flap in the body. Multiple musculocutaneous skin paddles can be designed and spatially separated on the flap, allowing reconstruction of multiple tissue surfaces. Since the intramuscular arterial pattern and nerve supply are

FIG. 5. Revascularized rectus abdominis muscle free flap.

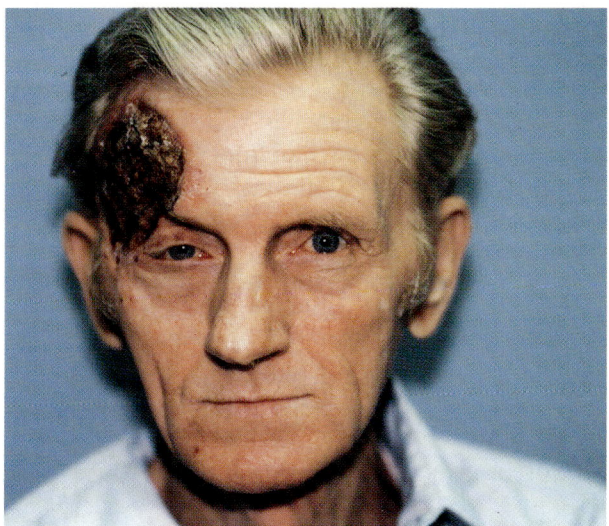

FIG. 6. Squamous cell carcinoma of temporal scalp with invasion of frontal sinus and orbit.

segmental, the muscle may be "split" with the lateral portion used for transfer and an innervated and functional medial segment remaining behind.

Surgical Steps

The latissimus dorsi is a broad flat muscle that arises through the thoracolumbar fascia from the lower six tho-

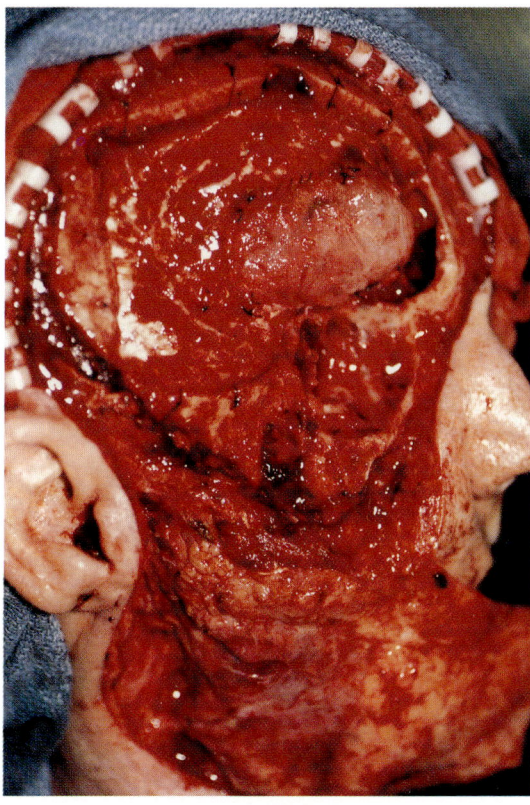

FIG. 7. Surgical defect.

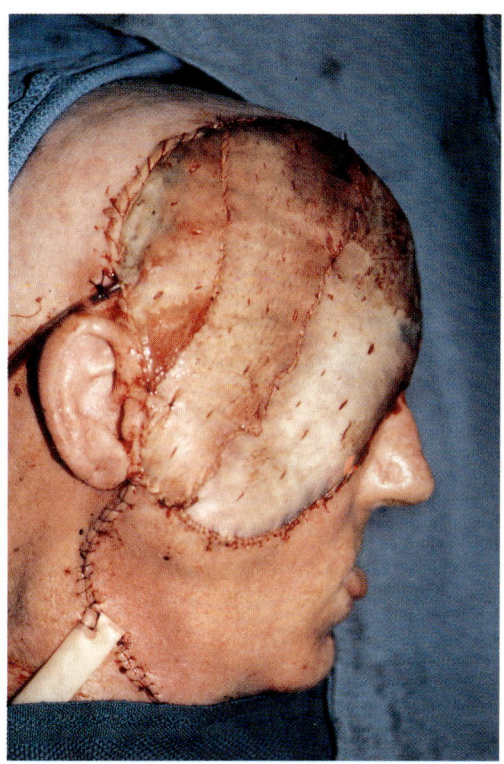

FIG. 8. Latissimus dorsi muscle free flap revascularized and covered with split thickness skin graft.

racic and lumbar vertebrae, spans the upper back, and inserts into the bicipital groove of the humerus. The dominant blood supply is from the thoracodorsal artery, a branch of the subscapular artery that arises from the axillary artery (Fig. 11). This pedicle has a large cross-sectional diameter and can be made quite lengthy with a relatively straightforward intramuscular dissection de-

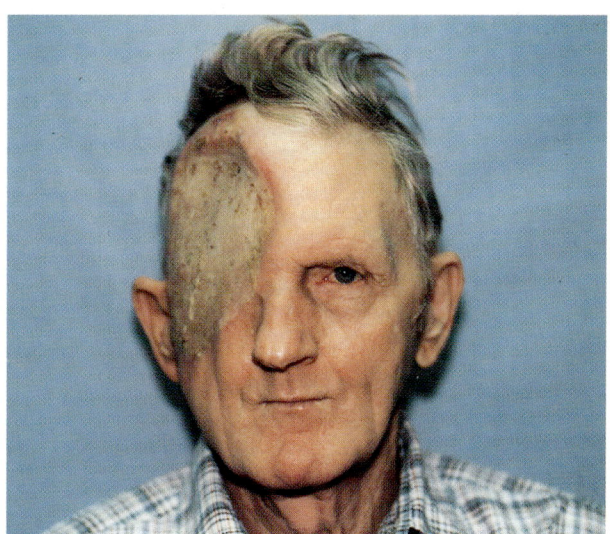

FIG. 9. Two-year follow-up demonstrating healed flap and contour defect, which allows use of prosthesis.

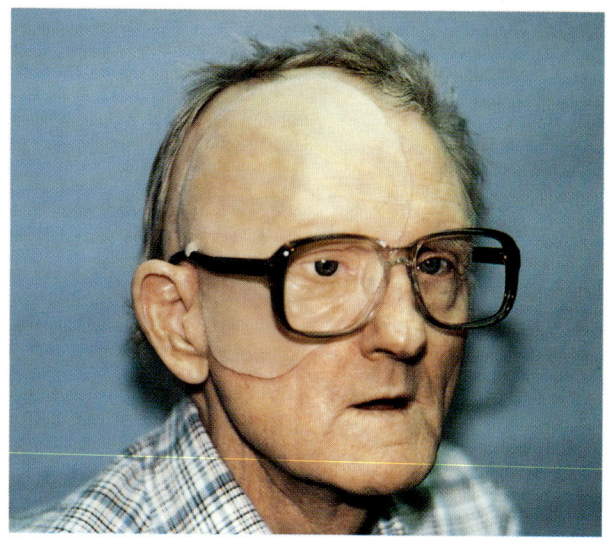

FIG. 10. Same patient with an external prosthesis.

signed to separate the thoracodorsal pedicle from the latissimus dorsi at its point of entry into the muscle.

The muscle is harvested using an incision along its anterior edge on the lateral chest wall. It can be elevated from lateral to medial and then from inferior to superior with a dissection of the dominant pedicle usually proceeding all the way to the axillary vessels. The only major distal branch of the thoracodorsal system is the branch to the serratus anterior muscle, and after this is divided just above the tip of the scapula (Fig. 11), the dissection of the proximal pedicle is greatly facilitated. The patient is normally placed in a lateral decubitus or oblique position with the arm surgically prepped so it can be moved freely throughout the course of dissection. This facilitates exposure of the pedicle and allows improved pedicle visualization deep into the axilla. Once again the artery is interrupted first and secured with double sutures, and subsequently the veins are divided. The back wound is

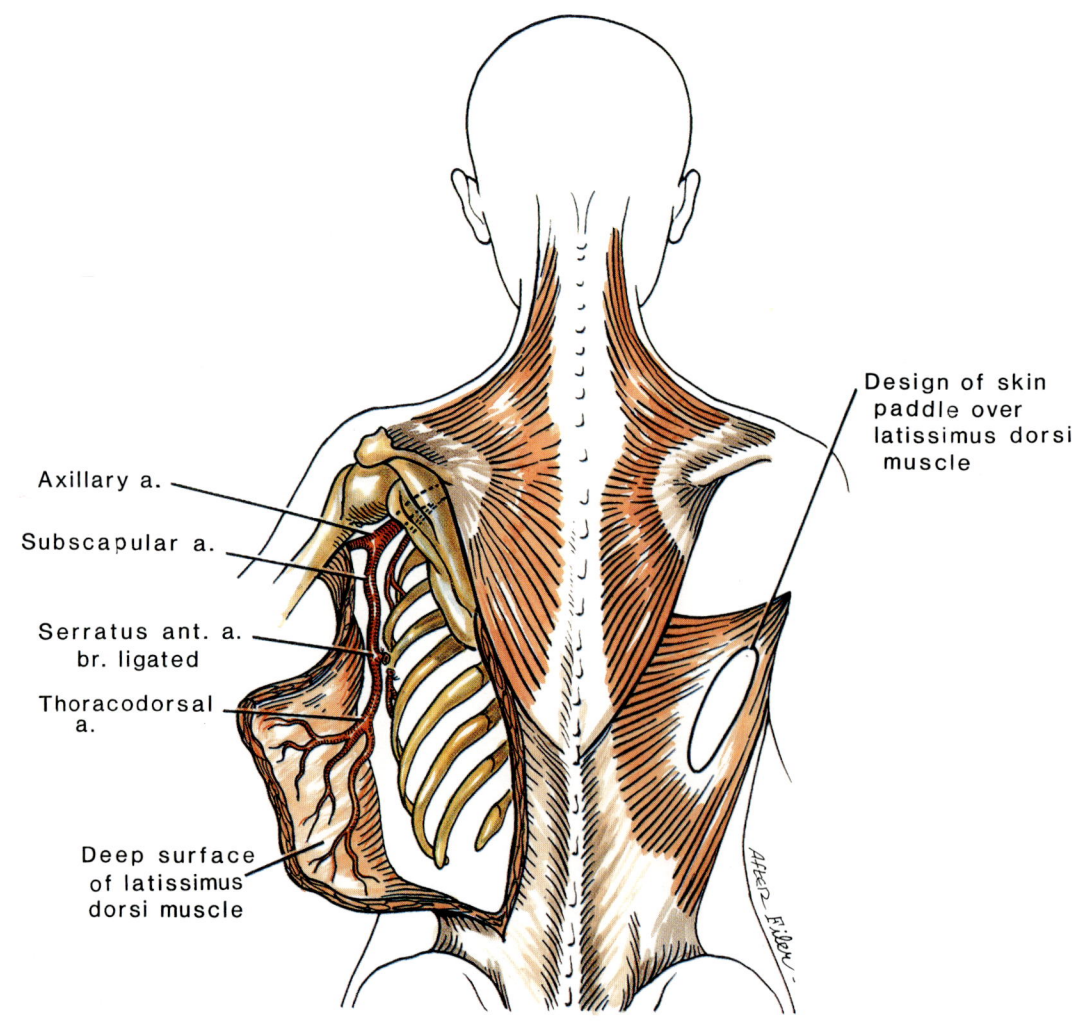

FIG. 11. Muscle and vascular anatomy of latissimus dorsi.

closed in layers using an absorbable polyglycolic acid suture for the deep subcutaneous tissue and a removable monofilament intradermal suture for the skin. Two suction drains are placed and brought out the lateral aspect of the chest wall. They are removed only when drainage is less than 30 cc per 24 hr (5–10 days postoperative) to minimize the chance of seroma formation. The major disadvantage is that the patient must be placed in the lateral or oblique position for flap harvest and this often necessitates two position changes on the operating table.

Follow-up

There is normally no significant contour deficit noted on the back. In children, the "split" muscle transfer is preferred since innervated and functional latissimus muscle remains in the back and theoretically this will minimize muscle imbalance across the spine. The morbidity of muscle sacrifice is minimal and wound seroma is largely preventable with the use of these suction drains. Skin sutures are removed from the back between 10 and 14 days following surgery.

DISCUSSION

Patency of the microvascular anastomosis between the recipient artery and vein and the flap vessels is paramount to ensure survival of these transfers. Since anastomotic difficulties are most likely to occur within the first 72 hr, it is important to monitor the flaps every hour for the first 3 days. If a portion of the flap is external or if the pedicle is immediately beneath the skin, monitoring can be accomplished with an external hand-held Doppler. However, if the transfer is entirely buried, this is not possible, and an internal Doppler probe may be placed directly on the artery or vein. To accomplish this we have used a 20-MHz implantable ultrasonic Doppler. Any change in the arterial signal mandates an immediate return to the operating room for reexploration. The majority of flaps that get into difficulty because of anastomotic problems may be salvaged if these problems are detected promptly and corrected.

We have had extensive experience using microvascular free-tissue reconstruction of cranial base defects over the past 5 years. This experience has revealed them to be quite reliable, with the success rate exceeding 95%. Appropriate flap selection and experience with flap design, elevation, and inset have proved to be very important in the success of these procedures.

BIBLIOGRAPHY

1. Jones NF, Sekhar LN, Schramm VL. Free rectus abdominis muscle flap reconstruction of the middle and posterior cranial base. *Plast Reconstr Surg* 1986;78:471–477.
2. Mathes SJ, Nahai F. *Clinical applications for muscle and musculocutaneous flaps.* St Louis: Mosby, 1982.
3. *Gray's anatomy,* 28th ed. Philadelphia: Lea & Febiger, 1971.
4. Shestak KC, Schusterman MA, Jones NF, Janecka IP, Johnson JT, Sekhar LN. Immediate microvascular reconstruction of combined palateal and midfacial defects. *Am J Surg* 1988;156:252–255.

CHAPTER 29

Facial Nerve Management and Reconstructive Techniques

Ivo P. Janecka, Laligam N. Sekhar, and Erick Stephanian

The facial nerve is one of the key cranial nerves. Its lengthy course from the posterior fossa through the temporal bone into the parotid region is subject to numerous pathological processes, which may interfere with its function on a temporary or a permanent basis (Fig. 1). The rigid boundaries of the nerve in the temporal bone and the horizontal extracranial direction cause frequent technical difficulties in handling the facial nerve during surgery for tumors of the temporal bone and the infratemporal fossa.

The overall management of the facial nerve in cranial base surgery falls into two basic categories. One is *nerve protection* during the approach and the oncological phase of cranial base surgery. This in principle requires nerve isolation, manipulation, or full transposition. With these measures, the continuity of the facial nerve is protected. The nerve manipulation frequently results in temporary (often prolonged) facial nerve malfunction. The second basic category of facial nerve management in cranial base surgery involves *nerve resection* as part of an oncological procedure. This is followed by nerve reconstruction or rehabilitation of the paralyzed face.

The disability of a facial nerve deficit justifiably creates a high degree of the patient's as well as surgeon's concern when facial nerve malfunction is anticipated preoperatively. However, it is important to keep in mind the goals of oncological surgery. The primary goal is an adequate tumor extirpation, which offers the best chance for control of the disease, and not necessarily preservation of a single cranial nerve. In spite of its importance, if the oncologic procedure fails, the facial nerve function almost always succumbs to the ongoing neoplastic process.

At the present time facial nerve reconstruction, in conjunction with other methods available to rehabilitate a paralyzed face, cannot fully eliminate sequelae of facial paralysis. It can, however, offer substantial improvement.

PLANNING

Under optimal circumstances, lateral skull base surgery is performed with total preservation of the facial nerve and at the same time with accomplishment of all oncologic goals. If those two goals are mutually exclusive, one should give priority to the oncologic concerns and plan on subsequent reconstitution of the continuity of the facial nerve. In such cases, a nerve graft (greater auricular or sural) is used (Fig. 2A, B). The donor site morbidity is quite acceptable and nerve graft harvesting usually does not compromise oncologic concerns. In patients who previously underwent parotid or upper neck surgery, the greater auricular nerve may not be available.

SURGICAL STEPS

The anatomy of the facial nerve (Fig. 1) reflects its complex function as well as its unusual course. The presence or absence of a true nerve sheath at different levels of the facial nerve is important in terms of the nerve's functional resiliency to our surgical manipulation. For example, the same degree of manipulation done to the

---

I. P. Janecka: Center for Cranial Base Surgery, University of Pittsburgh School of Medicine, and Department of Otolaryngology, Presbyterian University Hospital, and Eye and Ear Institute, Pittsburgh, Pennsylvania 15213.

L. N. Sekhar: Department of Neurosurgery, Center for Cranial Base Surgery, University of Pittsburgh School of Medicine, and Presbyterian University Hospital, Pittsburgh, Pennsylvania 15213.

E. Stephanian: Department of Neurosurgery, Presbyterian University Hospital, Pittsburgh, Pennsylvania 15213.

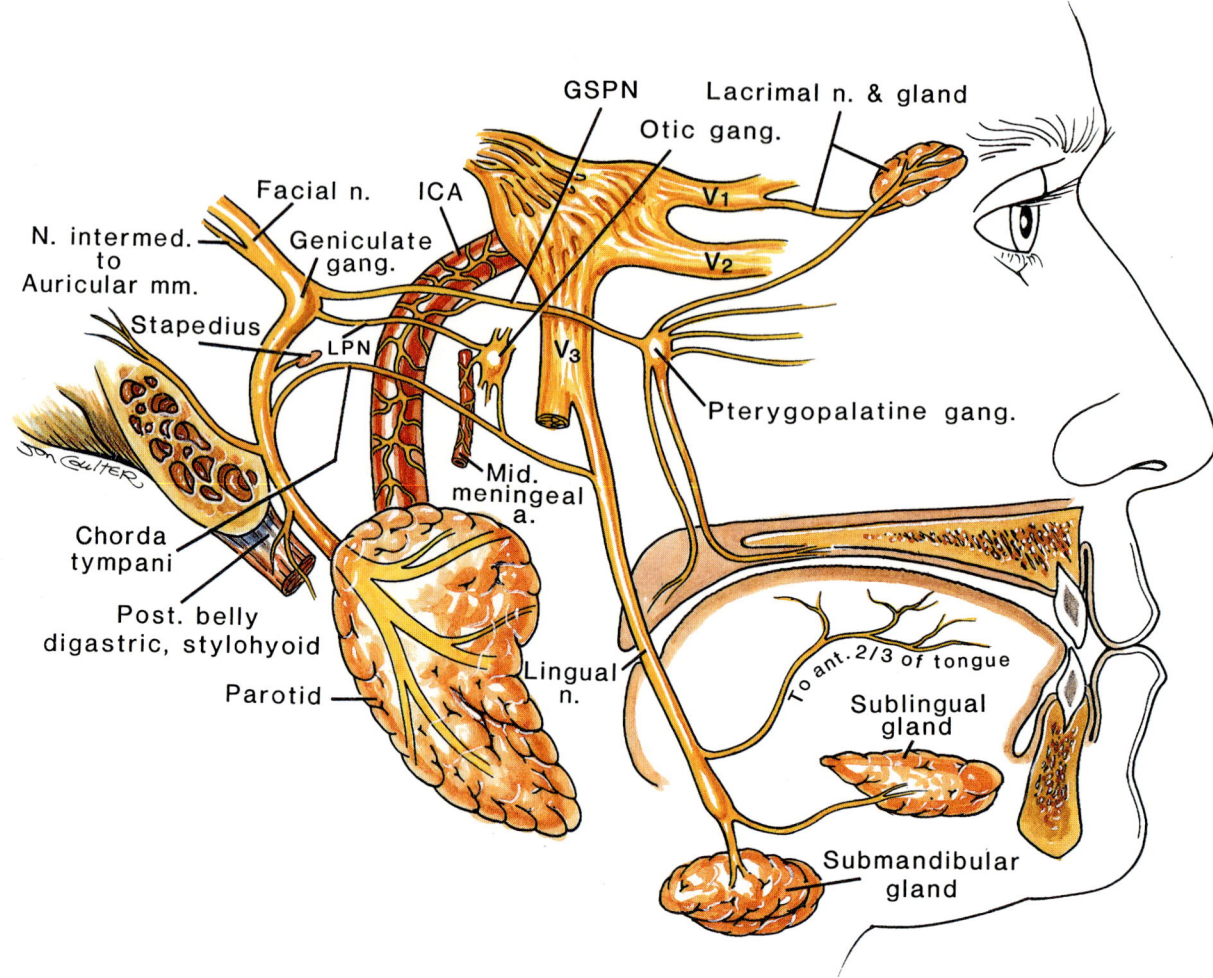

FIG. 1. Anatomic course of the facial nerve, its branches and target organs.

facial nerve in the posterior fossa or the internal auditory canal produces greater functional deficit than if the nerve is manipulated in its extracranial segment. The well-developed nerve sheath extracranially affords the nerve much greater protection of its structure as well as its blood supply. Within the temporal bone (lateral to the geniculate ganglion), the nerve sheath progressively thickens within the fallopian canal encasement. If the nerve has to be transposed from its normal course in the temporal bone, preservation of a thin layer of bone around the facial nerve seems to limit the extent of surgical trauma to this nerve. Extracranially, the fan-shaped branching of the facial nerve (Fig. 3) complicates the surgeon's attempt to reach the inferior aspects of the infratemporal fossa. This is balanced, to some extent, by the multiple connections between the major divisions of the facial nerve in the periphery, which offer extra functional tolerance to manipulation.

The peripheral facial nerve course can be graded in terms of functional importance of individual branches. For example, the ophthalmic division is considered functionally the most important because of its integration into the blink reflex, offering protection to the cornea. Other branches have less functional importance but assume a great esthetic importance. The degree of acceptance of postoperative facial nerve deficit varies from patient to patient as well as from surgeon to surgeon. For example, in the past, the deficit resulting from the sacrifice of the mandibular branch of the facial nerve, as part of radical neck surgery, was an expected consequence to surgeons and acceptable to most patients.

The key to intraoperative protection of the facial nerve is its isolation (which may be assisted by monitoring, Fig. 4) and visibility during surgery. This is frequently accomplished through the identification of the facial nerve trunk at the stylomastoid foramen and then tracing off the peripheral branches for a variable distance depending on the needed access to the infratemporal fossa or upper neck. Circumferential freeing of the facial nerve from its bed permits maximal mobilization (Fig. 5). There is, however, a definite limit on the available surgical space gained by dissection of the peripheral facial nerve. The nerve movement is restricted by its fixed attachment to the stylomastoid foramen and its termina-

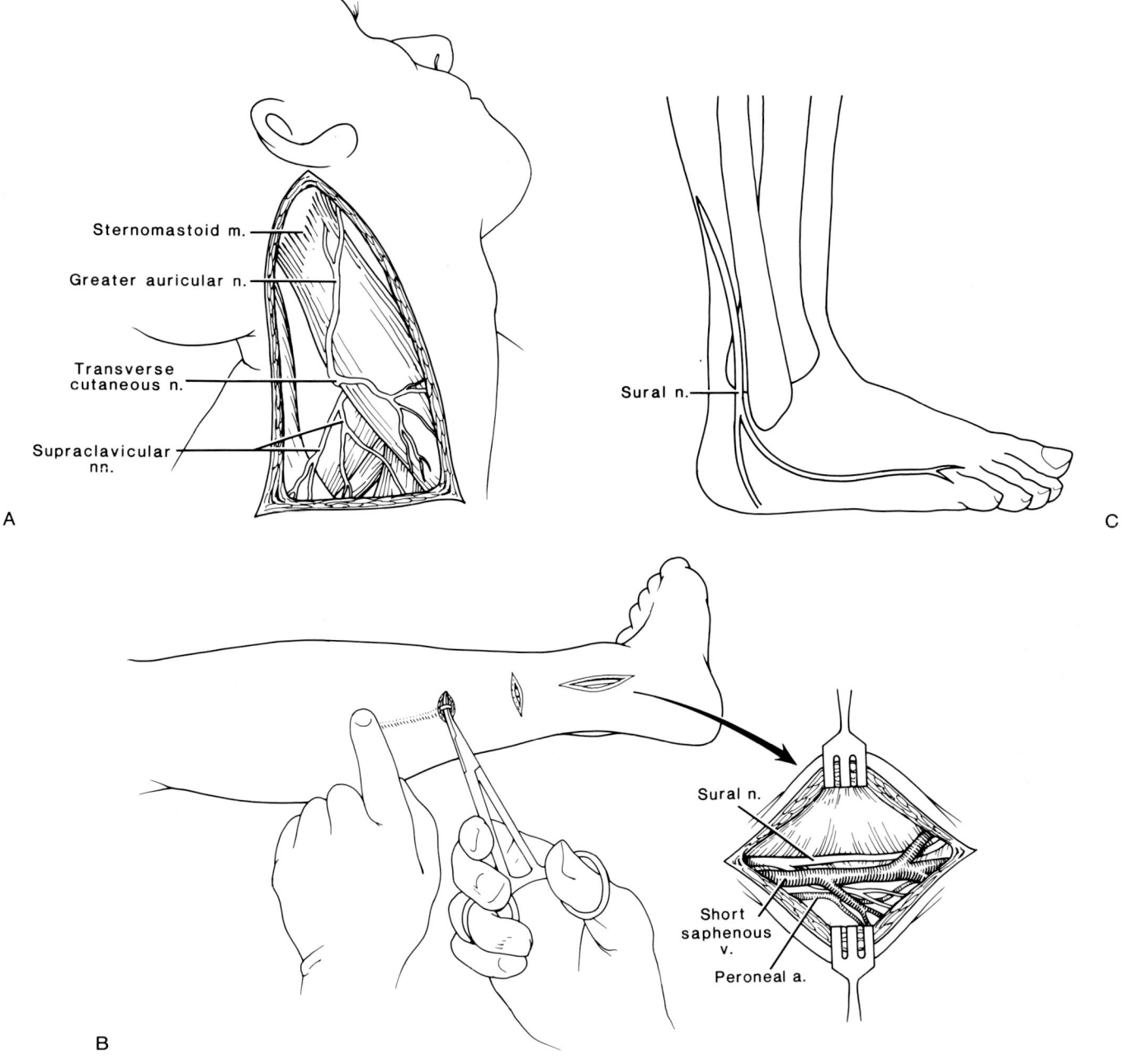

FIG. 2. A-C: Normal course of greater auricular and sural nerves.

tion in the facial muscles. The frontal and mandibular branches of the facial nerve form the superior and the inferior most branches of the peripheral facial nerve distribution. Their transection increases the surgical space available to surgeons in order to better reach the infratemporal fossa while still preserving the buccal and ophthalmic branches (Fig. 6A, D). The transected branches may be reconstituted at the completion of the surgical procedure.

In more extensive lateral skull base surgery, which, for example, requires lateral or posterior access to the jugular foramen, further (infratemporal) facial nerve mobilization is necessary. This then leaves the facial nerve attached at the geniculate ganglion/internal auditory canal and the peripheral connections to the facial muscles. The surgical space is greatly enhanced by this maneuver, but the resultant long, tenuous course of the facial nerve is now more vulnerable to trauma and significant devascularization (Fig. 7).

In cases requiring access only to the temporal fossa, the peripheral facial nerve may not have to be directly exposed if one enters the fascial layer under the superficial musculoaponeurotic system (SMAS) in the temporal fossa and along the deep temporalis muscle fascia (Fig. 8). Further dissection under the periosteum of the zygomatic arch brings us to the attachment of the mas-

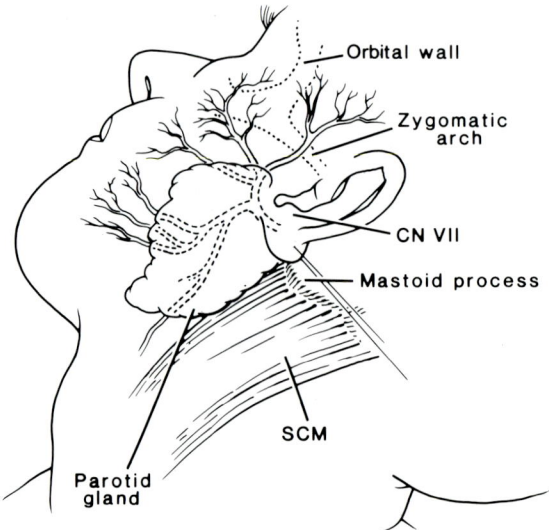

FIG. 3. Peripheral branching of the facial nerve.

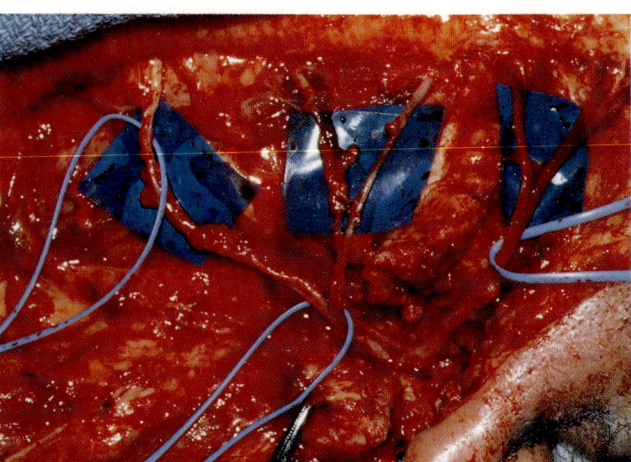

FIG. 5. Circumferentially dissected left facial nerve from stylomastoid foramen to facial muscles.

seter muscle. Transection of the masseteric fascia below the zygomatic arch leads us further inferiorly (in the space between the masseter fascia and the muscle itself). Blunt dissection at this plane is an easy one with the facial nerve well protected in the soft tissue above this layer. In most cases, this maneuver permits surgical access to the base of the temporal fossa and has an excellent chance for preserving the function of the facial nerve.

In the facial translocation procedure, an elective transection of the frontal branches of the facial nerve is carried out. The branches of the temporal division of the facial nerve are identified under magnification above the level of the zygomatic arch with the aid of an electric nerve stimulator and EMG. The nerve branches (up to six have been identified in some patients) can be electively transected and at the completion of the procedure reapproximated. This provides an excellent exposure to the infratemporal fossa and, concomitantly, the lateral facial and even nasopharyngeal area with preservation of the remaining major branches of the facial nerve (Fig. 9). In order to increase the functional regrowth of the frontal branches following neurorrhaphies, a methodology for rapid neurorrhaphy was developed at our institution. It involves the EMG assisted location of the branches, then placing a thin silicone tubing (8 mm in length) around them prior to their transection. The silicone tubings are secured with 7-0 nylon at each end, and the transection is done through the midportion of the tubing. Following completion of the oncological surgery, these two ends are approximated (with slight telescoping of one end into the other) and another 7-0 stitch is placed between them. This method has the following advantages: it helps to identify numerous branches; it protects the transected ends; and it provides for adequate support of the ends following repair so they are in a close end-to-end opposition. This methodology usually results in recovery of the frontalis muscle within 6–9 months (Fig. 10). A similar procedure may be applied to the mandibular branch of the facial nerve in selected cases.

Facial Neurorrhaphy

Primary repair of the facial nerve is the preferred choice for reestablishment of the nerve continuity. The basic principles of facial nerve microsurgery are fully applicable to the repair of this cranial nerve. An epineural repair, with interrupted 10-0 monofilament nylon done under magnification, is standard. The neurorrhaphy has to be absolutely tension free. At the level of the main trunk of the facial nerve, six to eight epineural sutures should accomplish a satisfactory neurorrhaphy (Fig. 11).

Two to three stay sutures are placed in the facial nerve within the temporal bone if replacement of the nerve into its original bony canal is anticipated. Further strength of the reapproximated nerve site may be ob-

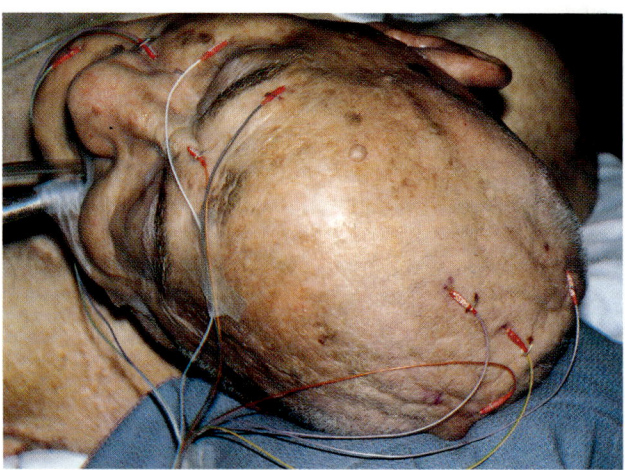

FIG. 4. Needle electrodes used in monitoring facial nerve function and somatosensory evoked potentials (SSEP).

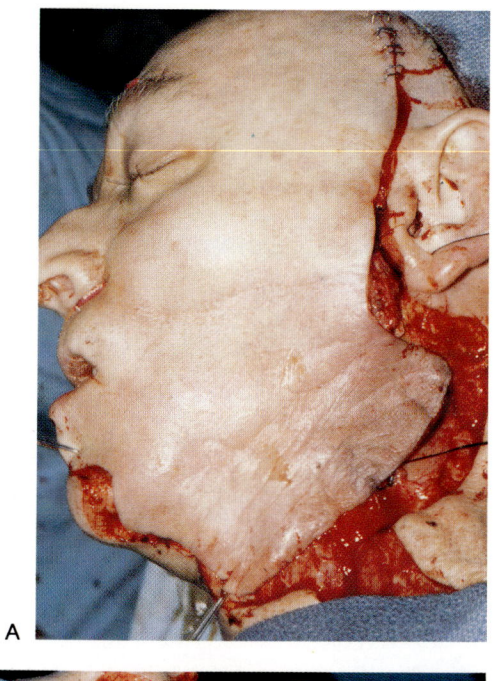
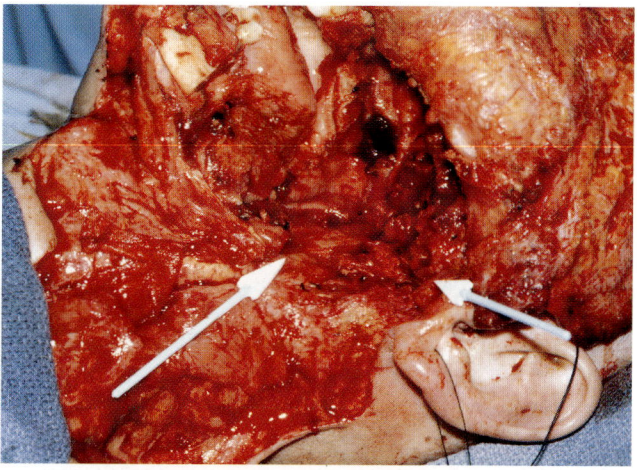
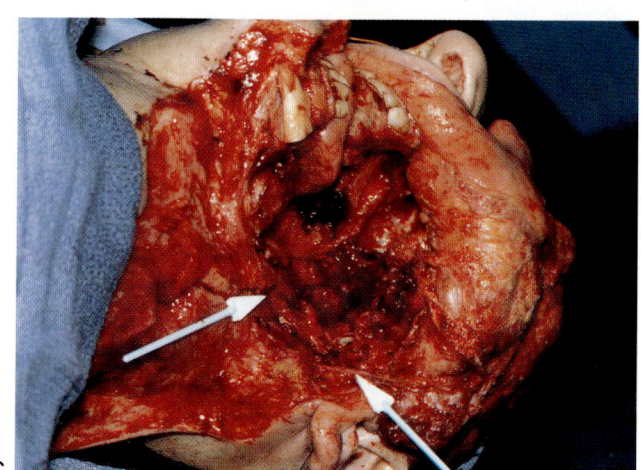
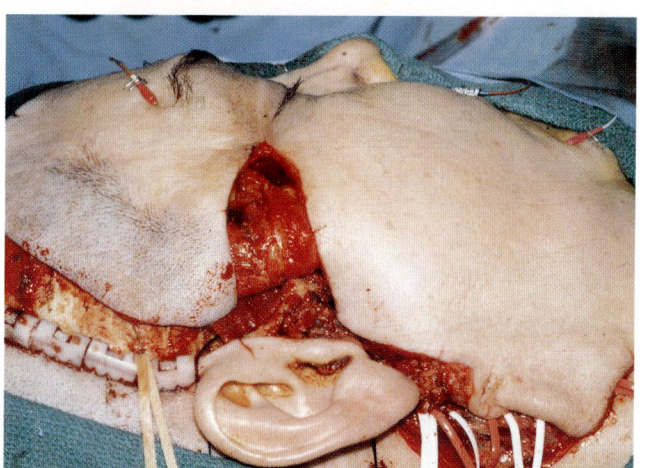
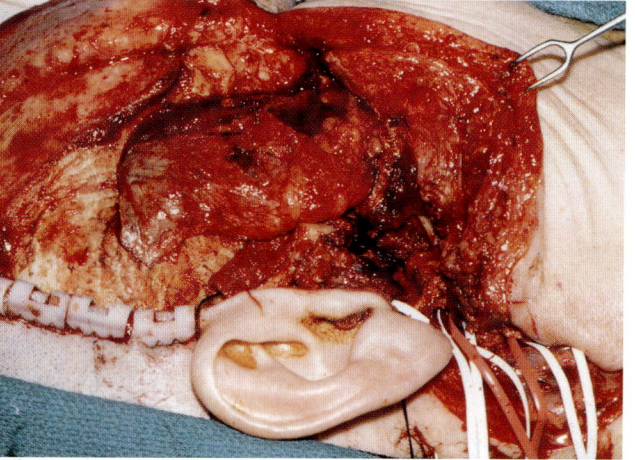

FIG. 6. Increased access to infratemporal fossa following transection of the mandibular branch (**A–C**) of the facial nerve. **A:** Cervicofacial skin flap. **B:** Infratemporal fossa, lateral view (ICA and main trunk of facial nerve marked with *arrows*). **C:** Inferior view. After transection of the frontal branches (**D, E**) of the facial nerve. **D:** Skin flaps. **E:** Superior–lateral view of the infratemporal fossa.

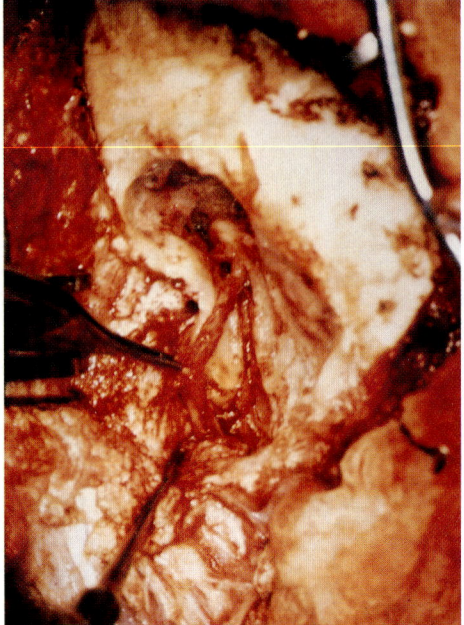

FIG. 7. Left facial nerve is being removed from the fallopian canal.

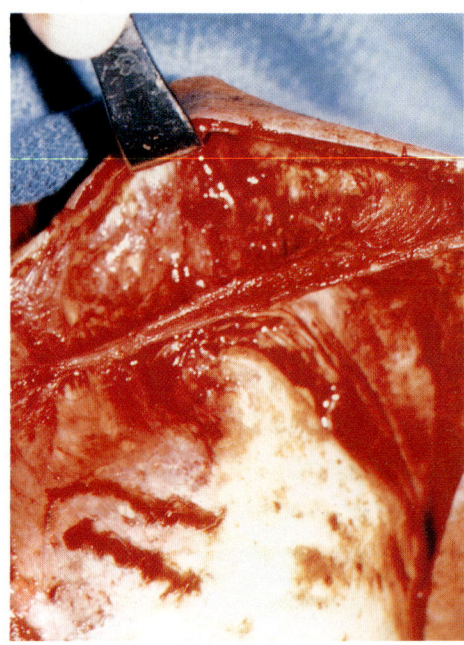

FIG. 8. Left temporal fossa with dissected superficial musculoaponeurotic system (SMAS) containing the frontal branches of the facial nerve.

tained with the use of fibrin glue. A similar methodology may be used for repair of the facial nerve within the posterior fossa.

Facial Nerve Graft

In principle, the ultimate degree of function of the facial nerve repaired with a nerve graft depends on several factors: (a) The proximal and distal nerve segments must be available. This requires viable axons in a proximal segment which are tumor-free. In the distal nerve segment, healthy appearing axons visible during surgery provide reasonable assurance that following denervation new axons will regrow through their paths. (b) The selected nerve graft should be long enough to assure a tension-free neurorrhaphy. The length of the nerve graft at harvesting must take into account the final position of

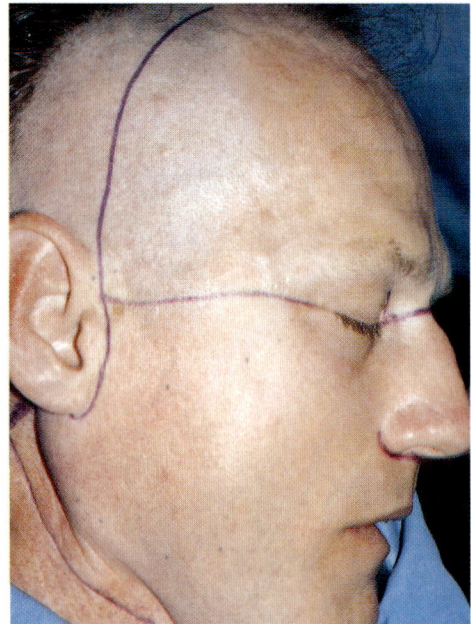
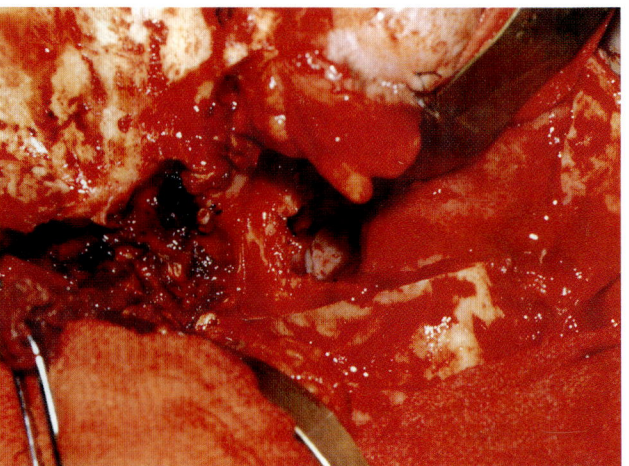

FIG. 9. A: Incisions used in facial translocation procedure. **B:** Exposure of right infratemporal fossa and nasopharynx; maleable retractor (*upper*) supports right orbital content.

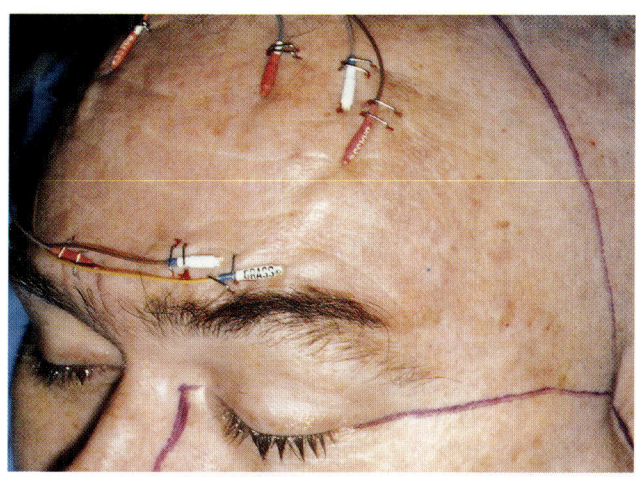
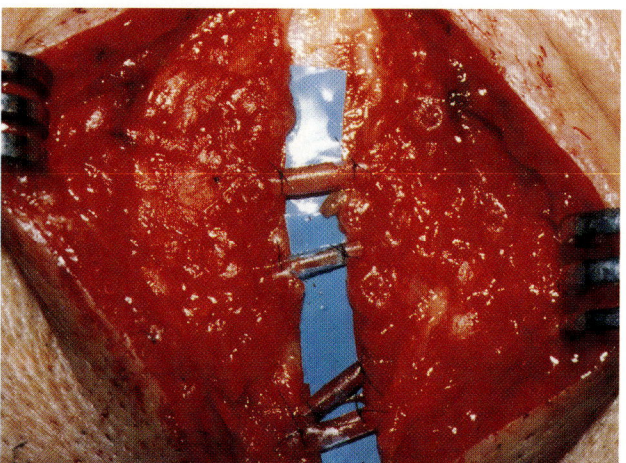
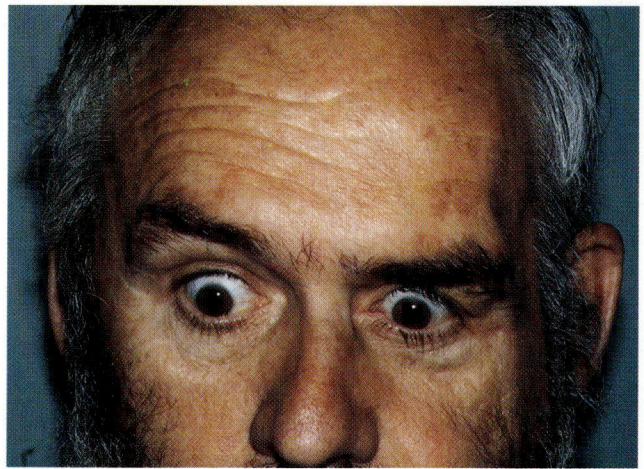

FIG. 10. Skin incision and needle electrodes. **A:** Isolation of frontal branches of the facial nerve. **B:** Four frontal branches of the facial nerve in silicone tubing ready for transection. **C:** Postoperative absence of left frontalis muscle function. **D:** Three months later, early return of left frontalis muscle function is visible.

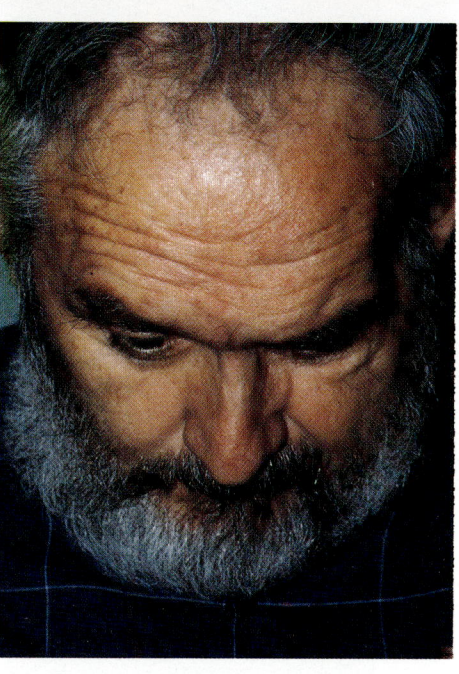

FIG. 11. Schema of epineural repair.

the nerve graft within the surgical defect. This often means a longer nerve graft than the resected nerve segment. If a muscle transfer is contemplated for the surgical defect, the nerve graft may then lay within or on top of the muscle flap and thus increase its potential for rapid revascularization. (c) The diameter of the nerve graft should correspond to the outer diameter of the facial nerve at the proximal and distal end. The greater auricular nerve provides an excellent donor nerve for a nerve graft because of its similar diameter and, in most cases, adequate length. Also, the natural branching of the greater auricular nerve is similar to the distribution of the peripheral segments of the facial nerve. Therefore multiple direct neurorrhaphies with facial nerve graft can be performed (Fig. 12).

In patients with anticipated prolonged or permanent

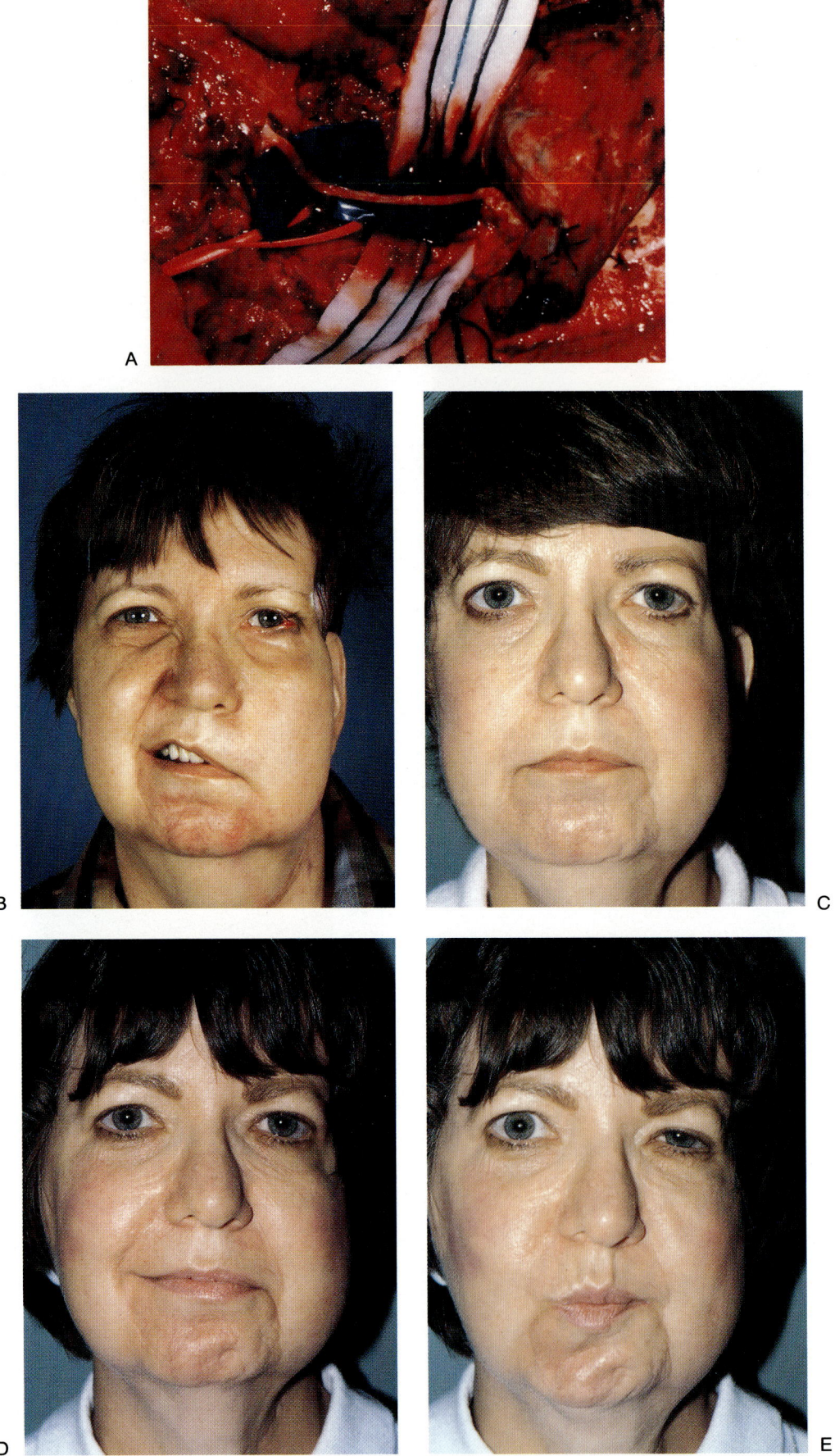

FIG. 12. A: Greater auricular nerve graft from left internal auditory canal to facial nerve periphery. **B:** Patient's postoperative appearance, demonstrating left facial paralysis. **C–F:** Patient's static and functional appearance 2 years following facial nerve graft.

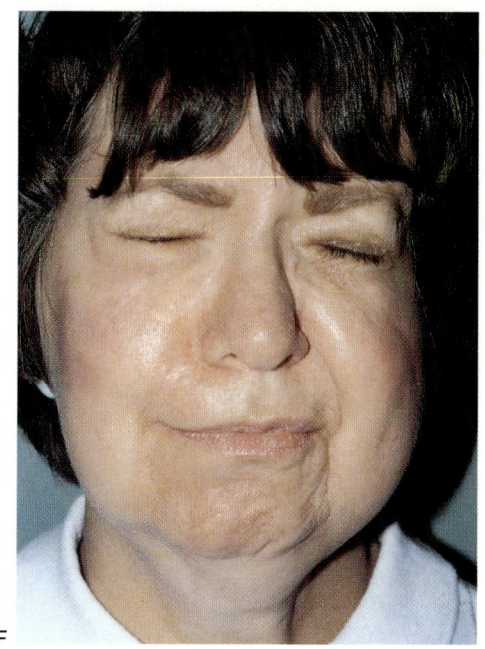

FIG. 12. Continued.

postoperative facial paralysis, it is feasible to provide immediate improvement in facial symmetry with static procedures (fascia lata slings, Fig. 13) as well as eyelid rehabilitation (gold weight for the upper eyelid and a cartilage graft for the lower eyelid, Fig. 14). This gives the patient immediate improvement of the facial appearance as well as eye protection. As the anticipated facial nerve recovery takes place, some of the temporary measures may be discontinued (gold weight and cartilage grafts may be removed from lids and fascia lata slings may be disconnected). There may be another potential benefit of immediate facial rehabilitation in patients with an anticipated long (12 months) facial nerve functional recovery period. It involves the possible prevention (with facial suspension) of elongation (by gravitational cheek pull) of the paralyzed facial muscles during the period of facial inactivity.

Specific Concerns

As with any peripheral nerve that needs to be surgically manipulated, we have to be concerned with traction on the nerve and protection of its vascularity (Fig. 15). Aggressive traction on the nerve, even if it does not result in interruption of its external continuity, may create internal axonotmesis with a resultant poor recovery potential. In cases where a great degree of traction is anticipated, it may be better functionally to electively transect the nerve than subject it to internal disruption with subsequent scarring. In general, nerve vascularity is protected by limiting nerve mobilization and, for exposed branches, providing a moist environment during surgery. Any nerve desiccation is extremely detrimental to its subsequent function. If a long nerve mobilization is required, subsequent placement on a vascularized bed (e.g., transferred temporalis muscle) will enhance revascularization of the nerve (Fig. 16).

In patients who were previously operated on, the identification of the facial nerve may be extremely difficult. In such instances, a combination of anatomic isolation with magnification and electrical isolation with EMG assisted nerve stimulation is of great help. However, there are limitations in terms of our ability to recognize a nerve surrounded by heavy scar and its response to electrical stimulation. A useful method is to find the nerve at a site previously not touched by surgery and then retrace the nerve. However, this is not always feasible.

SURGICAL CARE

Preoperative Care

Clinical assessment of the facial nerve function should be carefully evaluated and documented preoperatively. Any asymmetry should be pointed out to the patient. Preoperative facial nerve paresis is strongly suggestive of nerve involvement by the tumor. In such cases, advanced planning for a nerve graft and eye protection are the best options in most instances.

The determination of the extent and direction of old scars will give us potential clues for sites of "virginal" facial nerve branches and thus areas that would offer us the greatest potential for accurate facial nerve isolation. In patients where the CT or MRI scan suggests tumor

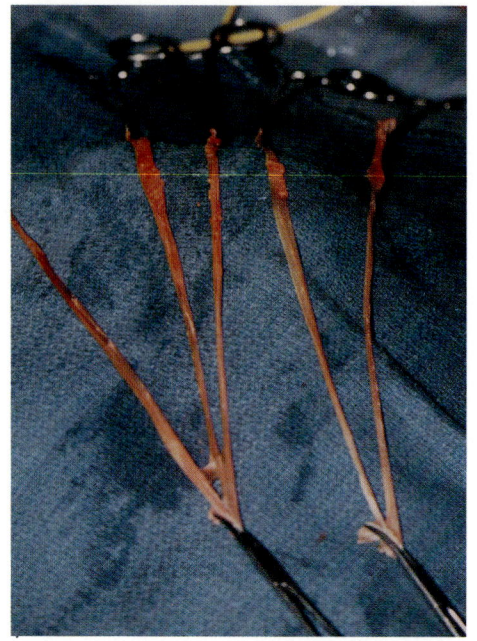
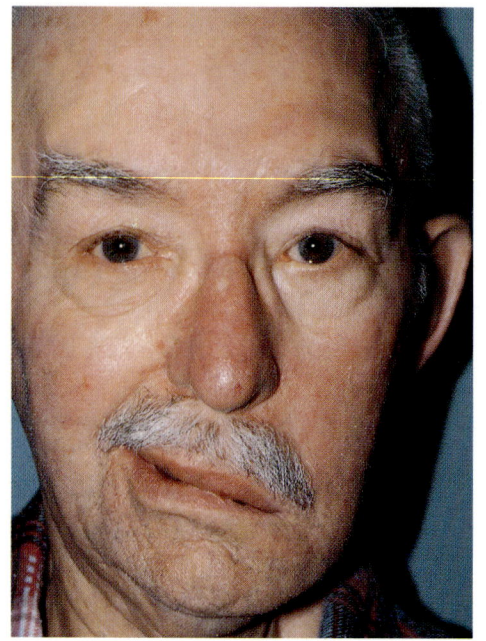
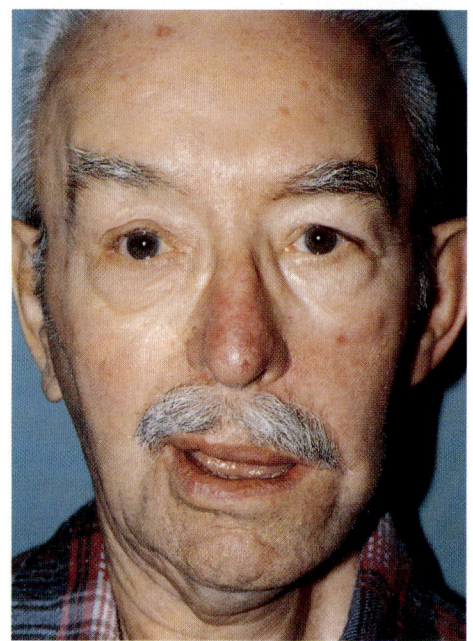

FIG. 13. A: Fascia lata strips used for facial static suspension following facial paralysis. **B:** Preoperative facial appearance. **C:** Postoperative facial appearance.

proximity to the facial nerve, but our clinical examination does not show involvement, preoperative nerve conduction studies and facial EMGs may uncover substantially reduced electrical function of the clinically normal appearing facial nerve.

Postoperative Care

Facial nerve malfunction is manifested in several ways postoperatively. The most significant is lagophthalmos, resulting in diminished eye protection. This can be remedied by using artificial eye lubrication. The overall postoperative eye care is enhanced in patients who have a gold weight inserted into the upper eyelid. This assists in better eye closure by increased gravitational pull.

In addition to the obvious unesthetic facial asymmetry following nerve malfunction, the clarity of speech and ease of intraoral food manipulation on the ipsilateral side are also affected.

Loss of facial nerve function in combination with other cranial nerve deficits compounds its significance. For example, absent trigeminal nerve function in its first division and facial paralysis are a grave combination in terms of the potentially detrimental effect on the eye. In such cases, the dryness of the eye, lack of blink reflex,

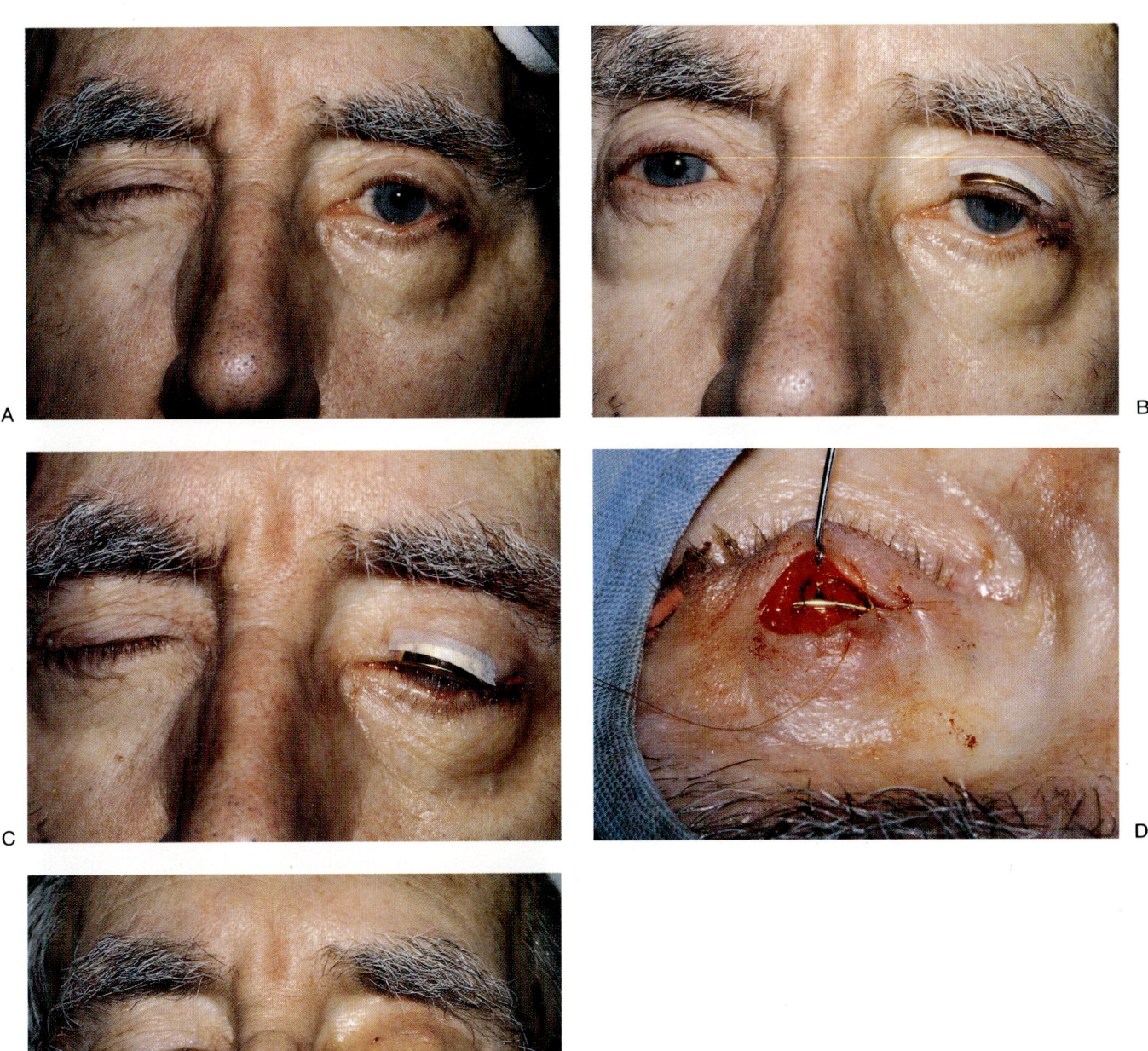

FIG. 14. A: Lagophthalmos accompanying left facial paralysis. **B:** Estimation of proper gold weight preoperatively in a sitting patient, open eyelid position. **C:** Closed eyelid position. **D:** Intraoperative placement of gold weight over tarsal plate, superior view. **E:** Postoperative result with gold weight implantation eliminating lagophthalmos.

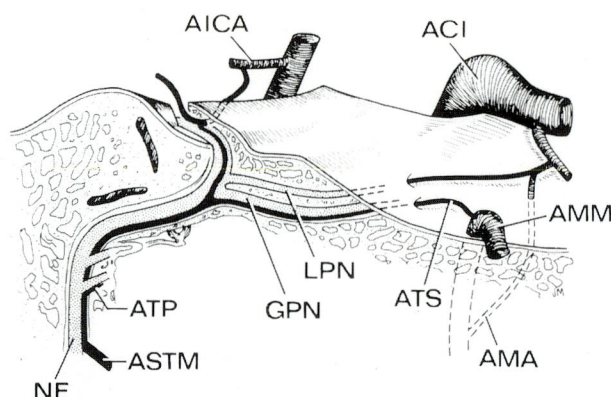

FIG. 15. Schema of blood supply to the facial nerve. AICA, anteroinferior cerebellar artery; ACI, internal carotid artery; AMM, middle meningeal artery; AMA, anastomosis of middle meningeal artery; ATS, superior temporal artery; LPN, lesser petrosal nerve; GPN, greater petrosal nerve; ATP, posterior temporal artery; NF, facial nerve.

and lack of protective corneal sensation often lead to a devastating loss of sight.

Follow-up

Our clinical assessment of facial nerve recovery begins at the time of reestablishment of neuromuscular junctions and its reflection in either facial movement or muscle contraction on EMG. Depending on the level of nerve injury and repair, the subsequent recovery may be either slow or rapid. In principle, the more proximal the lesion, the slower and poorer the recovery. It is important to follow our patients with recovering facial nerve function to determine the plateau and quality of recovery achieved. If any further spontaneous functional recovery is judged to be limited, additional rehabilitative steps might be taken (gold weight implantation, muscle transfer, fascia lata suspension, etc.).

Once clear movement in the face is detected following facial nerve reconstruction, the patient is instructed to strengthen the functioning muscles by exercises for a period of several months. After adequate muscle strength is achieved, a second phase of rehabilitation begins. This focuses on facial symmetry and is best accomplished through the performance of facial exercises in front of a mirror. A patient who is now able to move the previously paralyzed face practices the addition of normal opposite facial expression to achieve a greater degree of symmetry. Often a quite harmonious facial movement can be achieved even if some modification of the normal (presurgery) facial expression is necessary. The third phase of rehabilitation may involve EMG assisted biofeedback. This further enhances the quality of facial movement and symmetry.

COMPLICATIONS

The ultimate complication of facial nerve rehabilitation is the failure to regain its function. Also, the direct effect of the paralyzed facial nerve on the patient's eye status, speech, and swallowing as well as the interference with normal social functioning (due to its esthetic deficiency) must be seriously considered. In planning facial nerve reconstructions, it is important to focus on the total time of afunctionality of the face with anticipated progressive muscle atrophy. Following complete facial nerve mobilization or a facial nerve graft, it is anticipated that the recovery of facial function may take place over a period of 12 months. We must therefore use some of the immediate options available for rehabilitation of the face.

CONCLUSION

Management of the facial nerve in cranial base surgery assumes great significance because of the functional and esthetic disability facial paralysis creates for our patients. Detailed knowledge of facial nerve anatomy as well as functional microsurgery can indeed significantly lessen surgical morbidity in the vicinity of a facial nerve.

A great variety of options for facial nerve rehabilitation exist today. None of them, however, restores normal facial function. Therefore surgical preservation of the facial nerve should be a primary aim but should not override oncological concerns.

SUGGESTED READING

1. Chiu C, Janecka IP, Krizek TJ, Wolff M, Lovelace RD. Autogenous vein graft as a conduit for nerve regeneration. *Surgery* 1982;91:226.

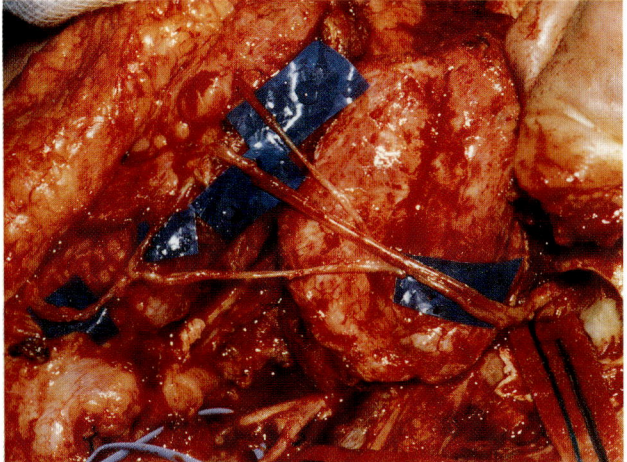

FIG. 16. Left facial nerve graft from internal auditory canal to peripheral branches of the facial nerve, supported by a transferred temporalis muscle.

2. Chiu D, Lovelace R, Yu L, Wolff M, Stergel S, Middeltown L, Janecka IP, Krizek T. Comparative electrophysiologic evaluation of the nerve grafts and vein grafts as nerve conduits—an experimental study. *Surg Forum* 1983;34:601.
3. Cosman B, Janecka I. *Facial palsy. Plastic surgery of the head and neck.* New York: Churchill Livingstone, 1987;839–873.
4. Janecka IP. Integrity of facial function: its preservation and repair. *Crit Rev Neurosurg* 1991;1.
5. Freed WJ, Medinacelli L, Wyatt RJ. Promoting functional plasticity in the damaged nervous system. *Science* 1985;227:1544–1552.
6. Samii M, Jannetta PJ, eds. *The cranial nerves.* New York: Springer-Verlag, 1981;649.

CHAPTER 30

Reanimation of the Paralyzed Face Without the Facial Nerve

Mark May and Steven M. Sobol

Over the past 15 years, 1635 reanimation procedures have been performed on 551 patients. Using this experience, combined with well-established principles of applied neuroscience, we have established a total approach to the rehabilitation of facial paralysis, which emphasizes restoration of facial symmetry and function (1). A variety of factors are key in determining the most appropriate rehabilitative technique(s) chosen, including (a) cause of paralysis, (b) extent of paralysis, (c) duration of paralysis, (d) likelihood of recovery, (e) extent of functional deficits, (f) presence of other cranial nerve deficits, (g) life expectancy, and (h) psychological status and perceived needs and expectations.

In choosing a rehabilitative approach, it is axiomatic that restoration of facial nerve continuity (i.e., grafting) is the procedure of choice when possible, assuming it can be performed within 24 months from the date of injury. When the central stump of the facial nerve is unavailable, and the mimetic muscles are still viable, hypoglossal–facial crossover is the favored technique, although it is not without its drawbacks. When the facial nerve is unavailable, or the mimetic muscles are absent, deficient, or fibrotic, alternatives to nerve grafting and crossover techniques must be utilized (2).

Techniques for rehabilitating the paralyzed face in the absence of the facial nerve include both dynamic and static procedures. Dynamic procedures include regional muscle transposition, that is, temporalis, masseter, and various eyelid reanimating procedures including gold weight lid loading, eyelid spring implantation, and silastic encircling prosthesis implantation, all of which are aimed at the restoration of eyelid closure. Static procedures include fascial or alloplastic slings, brow lift, rhytidoplasty, canthoplasty, and lid-tightening. Clearly, different surgeons favor different combinations of these procedures. Our experience with these procedures suggests that an approach that divides the face into upper and lower segments (i.e., looks at the eye and mouth separately) provides the best results in terms of regional reanimation.

EYE REANIMATION

Ideally, any method for correcting paralytic lagophthalmus should (a) provide adequate corneal protection, (b) avoid visual field restriction, (c) be cosmetically acceptable, (d) be dynamically reanimating, (e) be reversible in the event of recovery, and (f) be technically possible. While tarsorrhaphy has been the classical method of providing corneal protection in patients with eyelid paralysis, its drawbacks include that it is cosmetically unappealing, it may restrict the visual field, and it fails to dynamically reanimate. Moreover, in patients with reversible facial paralysis, lysis of the tarsorrhaphy may produce trichiosis and notching along the lid margin. Implantation of a gold weight or eyelid spring eliminates these shortcomings and is a functionally and cosmetically superior alternative in most patients.

Our experience with over 280 gold weights and over 250 eyelid springs has allowed us to establish criteria for patient selection and develop methods that afford reproducible results (3). The gold weight implantation works best for patients with (a) reversible or partial paralysis and (b) paralysis associated with minimal lid retraction. Eyelid closure is enhanced by the force of gravity after gold weight insertion, and, as such, works best in patients

---

M. May: Department of Otolaryngology, Head and Neck Surgery, University of Pittsburgh, Pittsburgh, Pennsylvania 15232.
S. M. Sobol, Head and Neck Surgery, Decatur, Illinois 62526.

whose upper lid tends to drop somewhat with blinking. Eyelid closure during sleep may be improved by elevating the head. Implant extrusion is extremely rare provided it is properly placed beneath the orbicularis oculi and levator aponeurosis. Likewise, implant migration is rare if the pocket created is of proper size and the weight is sutured securely. Our failure rate for the gold implant was less than 10% and primarily related to patient dissatisfaction with ptosis associated with lid-loading or the cosmetic bulge. A particular advantage of the gold is its ease of reversibility. Removal of the implant in a patient with a recovered facial palsy or a dissatisfied patient can be performed as an outpatient under local anesthesia.

GOLD WEIGHT IMPLANTATION TECHNIQUE

The patient is prepped and draped in the usual manner, topical anesthetic is placed in the eye, and a scleral shield for protection is placed over the cornea. One percent xylocaine with 1:100,000 of epinephrine is injected into the tarsal supratarsal fold as indicated along the dotted line. An incision is made with a razor blade knife in the fold about 1 cm in length (Fig. 1A). The incision is extended through skin, subcutaneous tissue, and orbicularis oculi muscle through the levator superiorus down to and on top of the tarsus. The pocket is elevated to accommodate the gold weight (Fig. 1B, C). Usually a 1-g weight is sufficient for the majority of patients. At times a lighter weight, 0.75 g, or a heavier one, 1.2 g is used. This is determined prior to surgery by pasting the gold weight on the eyelid and by trial and error the proper weight is selected. The gold weight is approximately 1 mm thick, 5 mm high, and 1 cm long with three holes made in it. The gold is 24 carat and polished so that there are no rough edges. The gold weight is placed in the pocket and held in place with 8-0 permanent monofilament suture that is placed through each of the three holes in the gold (Fig. 1D). Two upper openings are sutured to the orbital septum while the lower one is sutured to the tissue just lateral to the tarsus. It should be noted that the suture is not passed through the tarsus. Figure 1E demonstrates the gold in its position about 3 mm from the lash line and camouflaged under the supratarsal fold when the eyelid is in the opened position (Fig. 1F).

The eyelid spring was most effective for patients with complete and/or permanent facial paralysis, particularly when associated with strong lid retraction and/or poor Bell's phenomenon. Compared to the gold weight, the spring offers the potential for the best degree of restoration of normalcy to rapid, spontaneous, and voluntary blink in all patients. The potential drawbacks of the eyelid spring include (a) the difficulty in mastering the surgical technique, (b) ptosis if the spring is open too much, (c) the bulge created by the Dacron cuff in thin-skinned patients, (d) the need to adjust spring tension in some patients, (e) the increased difficulty with removal compared to the gold, and (f) the increased extrusion rate in inexperienced hands. Despite these potential problems, failure or dissatisfaction occurred in less than 15% of patients.

OPEN EYELID SPRING IMPLANTATION TECHNIQUE

The patient is prepped and draped in the usual manner and 1% xylocaine with 1:100,000 of epinephrine is infiltrated along the supratarsal–tarsal upper lid fold. The injection is extended along the lateral orbital rim to the periosteum. A razor blade knife is used to make an incision through the skin, subcutaneous tissue, and orbicularis oculi muscle to the tarsus (Fig. 2A). Bleeding is controlled with bipolar forceps and the tarsus is uncovered with double action scissors. The periosteum over the lateral orbital rim is exposed next through a separate incision (Fig. 2B). The spring is fabricated during the time that the patient is evaluated in the office setting. The spring is made with 0.01-in. round orthodontic wire and it is formed as illustrated in Fig. 2C–F using orthodontic instruments. The final configuration is determined by making the spring conform to the natural curvature of the patient's orbit (Fig. 2G). The proper tension is adjusted in order to provide adequate opening and closing of the eyelid. A number 19 spinal needle is passed just lateral to the tarsus under the tunnel of soft tissue and out the lateral orbital rim pocket just lateral to the periosteum (Fig. 2H). The obturator from the spinal needle is then removed (Fig. 2I). The wire is then placed through the spinal needle and the spinal needle is then removed (Fig. 2J, K). The lower limb of the spring now in place is sutured using 5-0 supramid to secure the spring to the periosteum (Fig. 2L). Two or three sutures are placed around the fulcrum to the periosteum in the area of the lateral canthus. This fixes the fulcrum to the periosteum just above and lateral to the lateral canthus. The upper limb of the wire is looped and sutured with two 5-0 supramid sutures along its shaft (Fig. 2M), then the lower limb is looped (Fig. 2N) and enveloped in Dacron as noted in Fig. 2O. The Dacron is closed over the loop with 8-0 monofilament suture. The wound is closed in layers using 5-0 vicryl for the deep layer and 6-0 chromic for the skin (Fig. 2P).

Temporalis muscle transposition has been used by Rubin, Tucker, and others for eyelid reanimation (4,5). Our experience with this approach, even with attention to the details stressed by Rubin, has been less satisfactory for several reasons. Eye closure appeared unnatural, as the lateral canthus was pulled laterally by the muscle's vector forces. Eyelid movement only occurred with chewing, and most patients could not separate eyelid closure and mouth movement. In addition, the cheek bulge

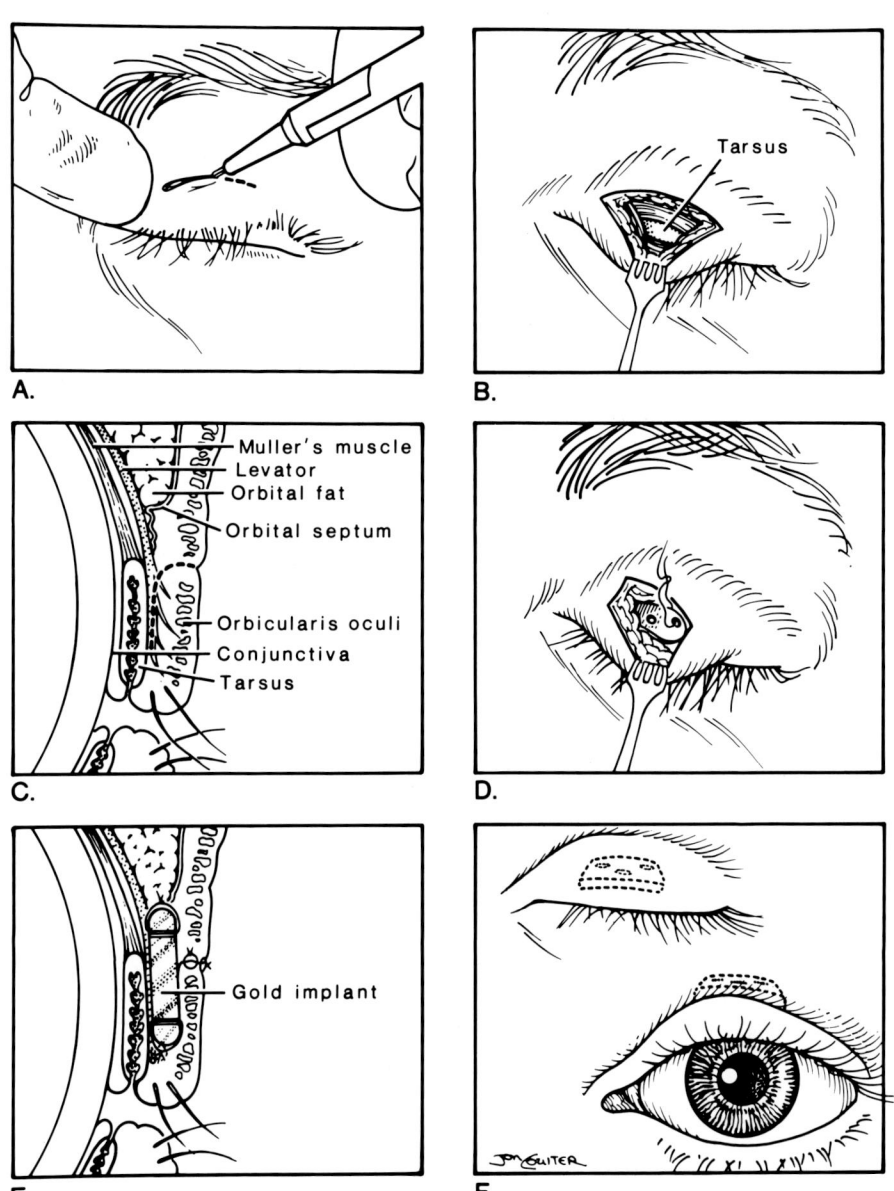

FIG. 1. A–F: Gold weight implantation technique. See text for details. (Adapted from ref. 1.)

produced by the transposed muscle was increased by the additional muscle used for both the mouth and eyelid reanimation.

For these reasons, we favor the gold weight or spring implantation for eye reanimation. Both techniques allow for eyelid closure independent of mouth movement. Since neither the gold nor the spring relieve the lack of lower lid tone, ectropion, and brow ptosis associated with the paralysis, they are often combined with static procedures aimed at correcting these defects. Our preferred method of lower-lid tightening has been the Bick procedure (1). It is not difficult and does not cause the eyelashes to invert and irritate the cornea as occasionally occurs with the Kuhnt–Szymanowsky technique. Care must be taken not to remove too much tissue since this can result in pulling the puncta away from the globe, resulting in increased epiphora. The Bick procedure may be combined with a medial canthoplasty if there is a prominent gap medially with unsightly exposure of the caruncle. Another useful technique, not yet published, for improving paralytic ectropion and epiphora in selected cases is the implantation of autogenous auricular cartilage to the lower lid. In a soon to be presented series, we illustrate the value of this technique as an adjunct to eye reanimation. Brow lift with or without blepharoplasty may be used to correct brow ptosis and supratarsal fold hooding, in an effort to improve symmetry. Caution must be exercised not to overexercise suprabrow tissue,

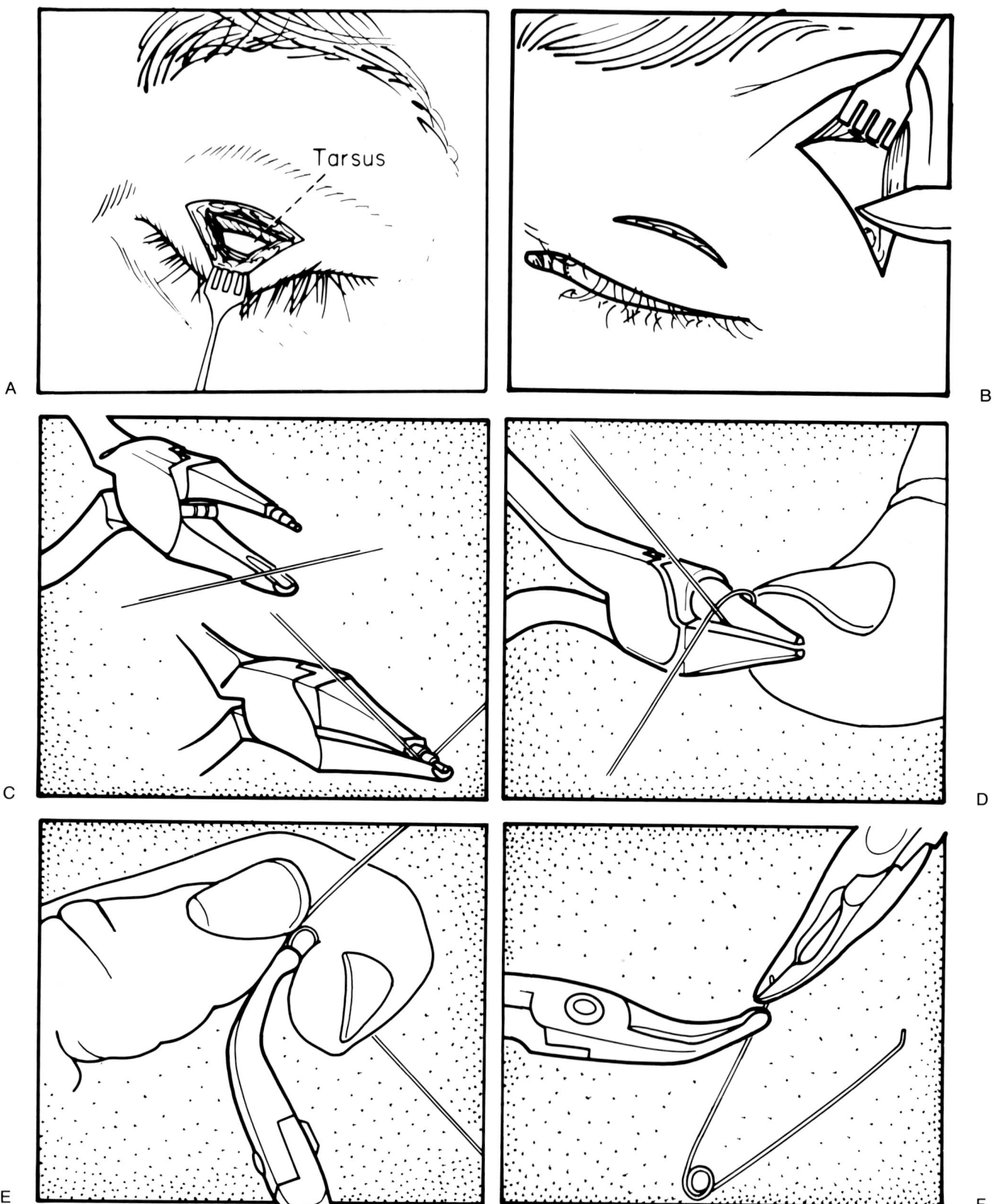

FIG. 2. A–P: Open eyelid spring technique. See text for details. (Adapted from ref. 1.)

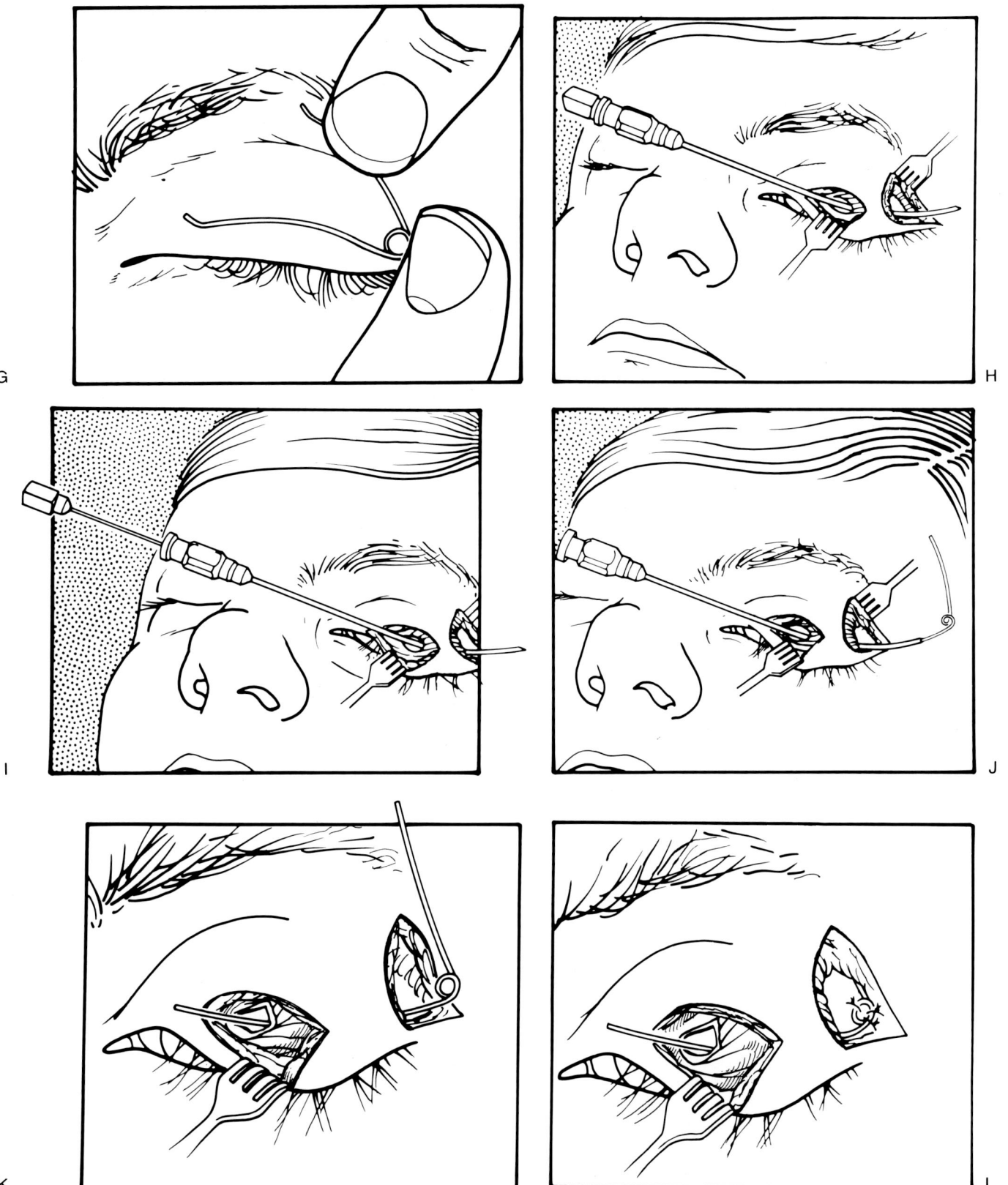

FIG. 2. *Continued.*

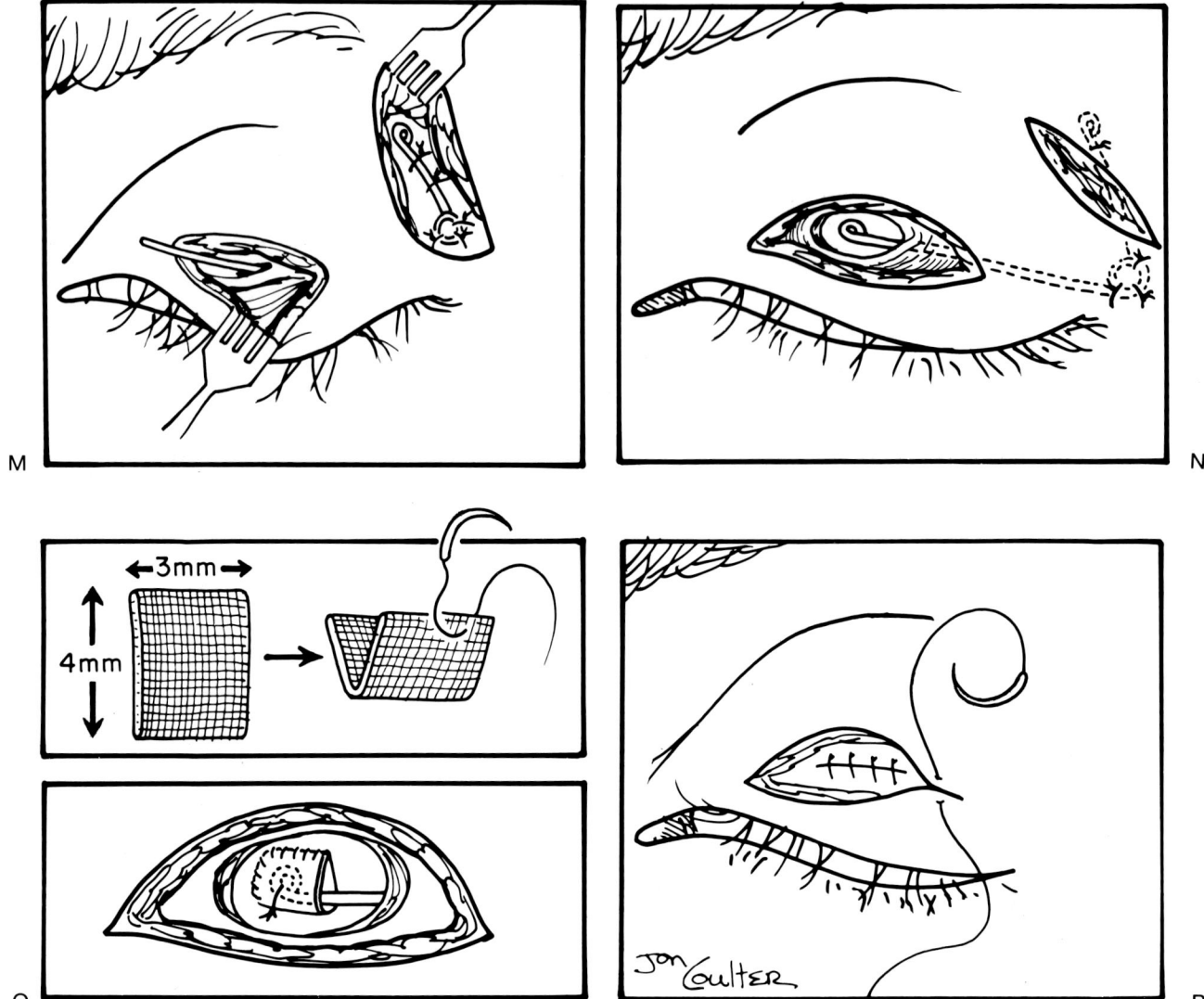

FIG. 2. Continued.

however, since the patient's ability to close the eye may be impaired.

In a small number of patients, persistent drooping of the lower lid and inadequate upper lid closure persist despite use of the above techniques. At the suggestion of Dr. John Conley, a closed eyelid spring technique was developed and used in 27 patients (6). Success was achieved in over 90% of patients. The spring functions in a reciprocal fashion to that of the open spring, in that the spring tends to return to a closed rather than open position during levator relaxation. Problems are similar to that for the open spring.

MOUTH (LOWER FACIAL) REANIMATION

Reanimation of the mouth has been most rewarding using the temporalis muscle transposition. It is useful for longstanding facial paralysis and has been employed in selected cases to augment results with nerve grafts or XII–VII crossover. To date, over 200 procedures have been performed. The majority of patients had longstanding facial paralysis following acoustic tumor removal. Satisfactory results have been reproducible in 90% of cases. Symmetry and voluntary smile are achieved in 3–6 weeks and improve over a period of 1 year. Results are best in motivated patients and may be enhanced through motor–sensory reeducation techniques. Spontaneous movement in response to emotional stimuli has been observed in roughly 10%, while only symmetry was achieved in less than 10%.

As our experience with the temporalis muscle transposition increased, a number of modifications have been introduced to eliminate many of the problems noted by ourselves and others contributing to the lack of uniformity or high quality results. The muscle is used exclusively for the mouth and not the eye region, thus separating eye and mouth functions. The unsightly bulge in the cheek has been reduced by creating an adequate tunnel to allow the transposed muscle to lie flat. Only the middle one-third of the temporalis muscle is used, thus reducing the bulge and the temporal depression. The depression is remedied with a soft silastic implant placed at the time of transposition. Proper preoperative smile analysis and attention to correct positioning and suturing of the muscle slips to the mouth in an effort to achieve the mirror image of muscle pull seen on the normal side are emphasized. Using Conley's modification of raising periosteum attached to the temporalis muscle fascia, rather than repositioning and sewing the temporalis fascia to the muscle as proposed by Rubin, has given better results. Access to the oral area is through a vermilion–cutaneous incision along the oral commissure, which further reduces the visible scar. Multiple sutures placed in the muscle–submucosal layer at the level of the superolateral and inferolateral aspects of the orbicularis oris, creating an overcorrected smile, have afforded the most consistent results. The importance of overcorrection cannot be overemphasized (1).

DESCRIPTION OF PROCEDURE

The patient is prepared and draped in the usual fashion. The hair is parted and, using scissors, the hair is removed through a narrow path over the region of the proposed incision in the scalp line (Fig. 3A). The areas of incision in the vermilion and in the scalp are infiltrated with 1% xylocaine and 1:100,000 of epinephrine for hemostasis. After waiting 5–10 min, the incision in the scalp was made with a cutting cautery down to the superficial musculoaponeurotic system (SMAS). The SMAS is divided with scissors, exposing the fascia over the temporalis muscle. The temporalis muscle is elevated in its midportion approximately 4 cm wide, extending above the fascia periosteal attachment superiorly to the level of the zygomatic arch inferiorly (Fig. 3B). The cutting cautery outlines the flap and an elevator lifts the muscle periosteum from the skull (Fig. 3C, D). The layer between the subcutaneous tissue and SMAS is identified and a pocket is made between the two with scissors (Fig. 3E). This ensures that any residual function that might be present via the facial nerve will be preserved since the facial nerve fibers lie in or deep to the SMAS. Then an incision is made in the vermilion and the orbicularis oris muscle is elevated off the submucosa superiorly to about the level of the lip cheek crease (Fig. 3F). Again the layer just deep to the subcutaneous tissue and lateral to the SMAS is established using scissors (Fig. 3G). The pocket started in the scalp lateral to the SMAS and that in the vermilion region are connected with scissors and then enlarged to accommodate two fingers (Fig. 3H). The temporalis muscle that was elevated is bisected and 2-0 supramid sutures in a figure-eight fashion are passed through each of the pedicles (Fig. 3I). The sutures are then brought through the tunnel using Kelly clamps (Fig. 3J). Now that the muscle is pulled down through the pocket (Fig. 3K), it is sutured to the submucosa (Fig. 3L) and to the subcutaneous layer (Fig. 3M). This double closure sandwiches the muscle between the submucosa and the subcutaneous layers. The corner of the mouth is overcorrected in order to ensure a pleasing result (Fig. 3N). The overcorrection will begin to come down over a period of 3–6 weeks. Following this the defect left by rotating the muscle out of the temporal region may be filled in by placing a soft silastic implant. A drain is placed through the scalp into the cheek and hooked to wall suction for 2 days.

While the masseter has been used alone or in combination with the temporalis muscle by some surgeons, our experience has been less satisfactory. We have found it less optimal in terms of vector forces and less easy to suture into optimal position. Moreover, it adds little to the effect of the temporalis muscle.

Complications of the temporalis muscle transposition have included hematomas, seromas, infection, and suture granulomas. Experience has shown that placing a separate lip–cheek drain plus a temporal–facial drain reduces the incidence of blood and serum collection. The use of highly nonreactive suture material and the strict avoidance of penetrating the mucosa with the suspension sutures reduce the likelihood of suture reaction. Prophylactic antibiotics are routinely given. Use of the soft Mentor prefabricated temporal implant has reduced the early experience with implant extrusion seen with the hard silastic carved implants.

ADJUNCTIVE STATIC TECHNIQUES

A variety of adjunctive static suspension techniques may be used to enhance facial symmetry in repose (1). The temporalis muscle itself creates a moderate degree of static suspension in addition to providing dynamic reanimation to the mouth area. The temporalis muscle may be tightened or augmented with the use of fascia (i.e., fascia lata), palmaris longus, or alloplastic material (i.e., Gortex) (*unpublished data*). These same materials may be used to provide static suspension alone in patients whose temporalis muscle is unusable. Our experience has been more favorable with palmaris longus when using autogenous tissue rather than fascia. Its tendon is long and thin and easily wraps around the zygomatic arch, which acts as a pulley. Attachment to the midface and oral region is similar to that for the temporalis muscle with overcorrection again being key to long-term success.

A face-lift may be combined with any of the reanimating techniques discussed and is quite useful for longstanding facial paralysis accompanied by loss of skin tone and sagging. Its effects, however, may be relatively short-lived, necessitating tuck-up revisions periodically. Blepharoplasty and brow lift have already been discussed

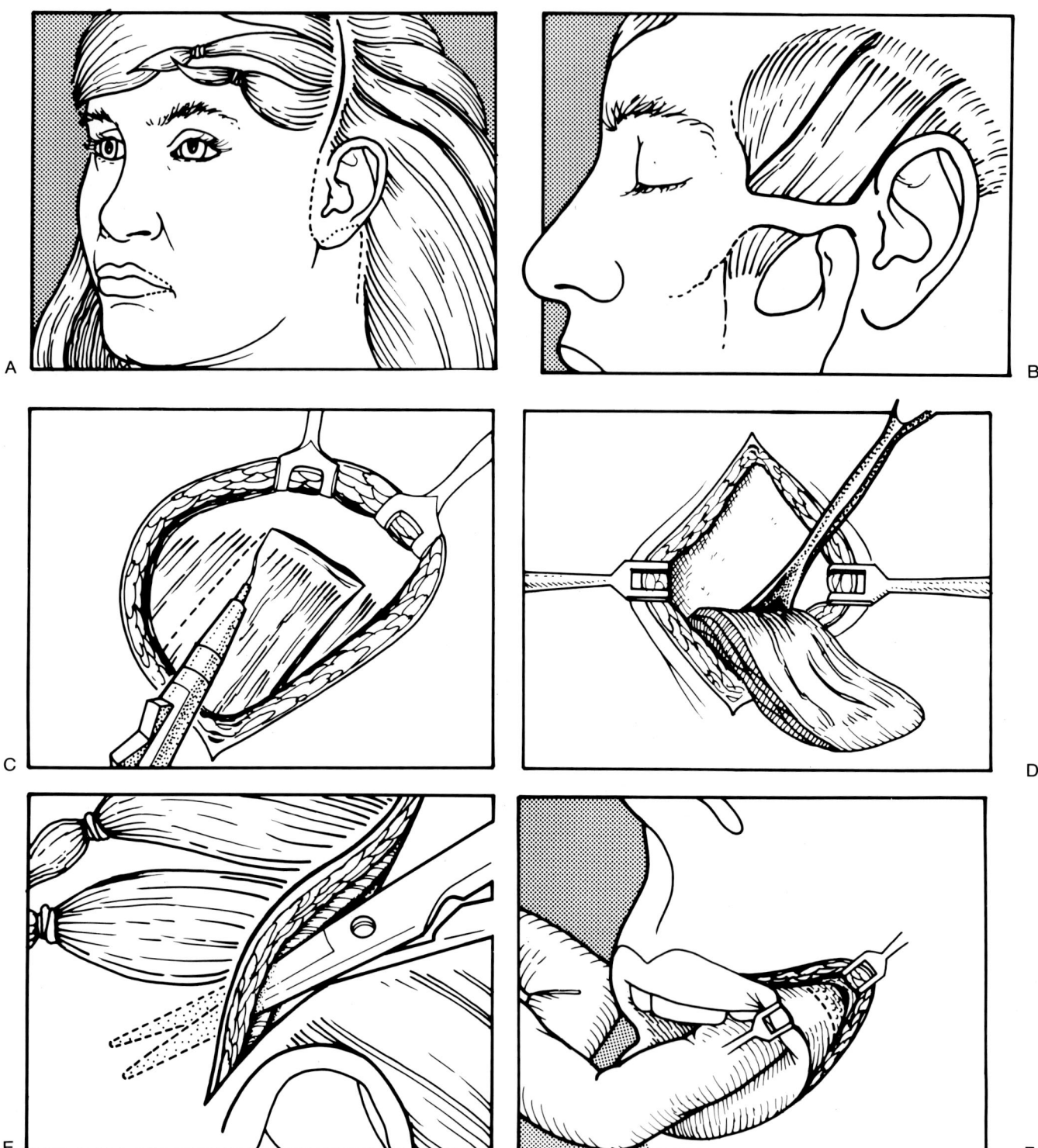

FIG. 3. A–N: Temporalis muscle transposition technique. See text for details. (Adapted from ref. 1.)

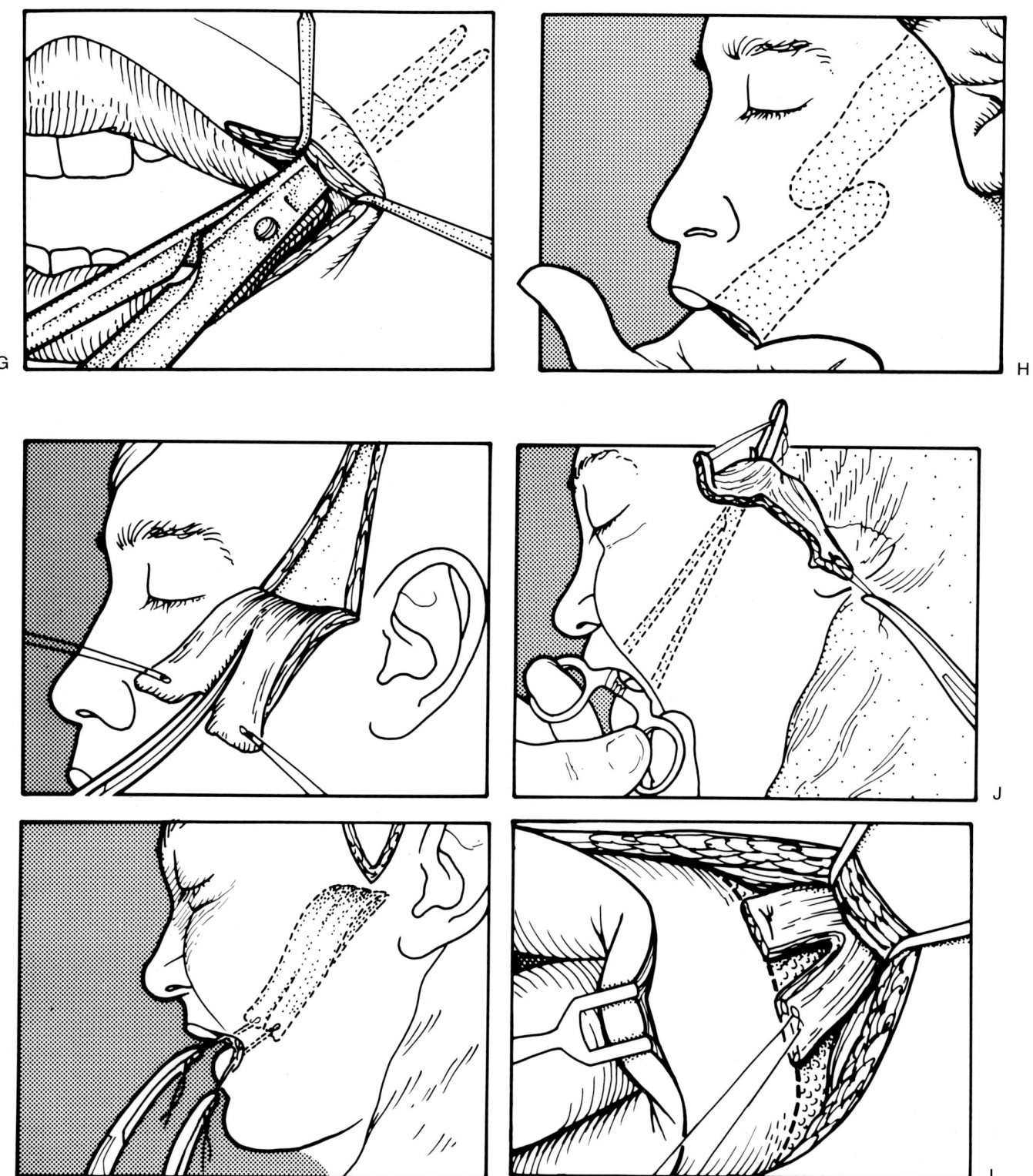

FIG. 3. Continued.

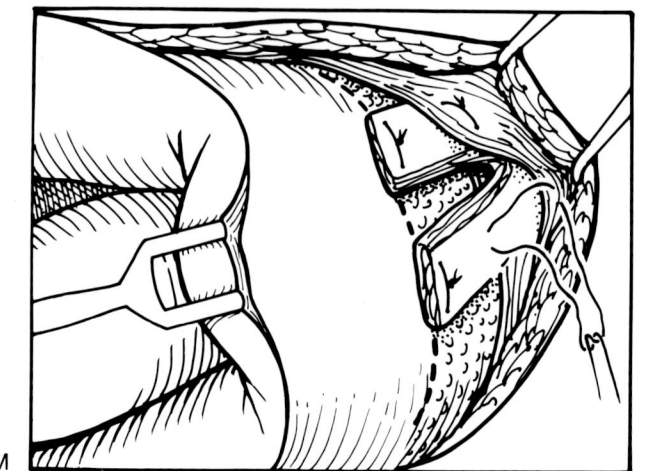 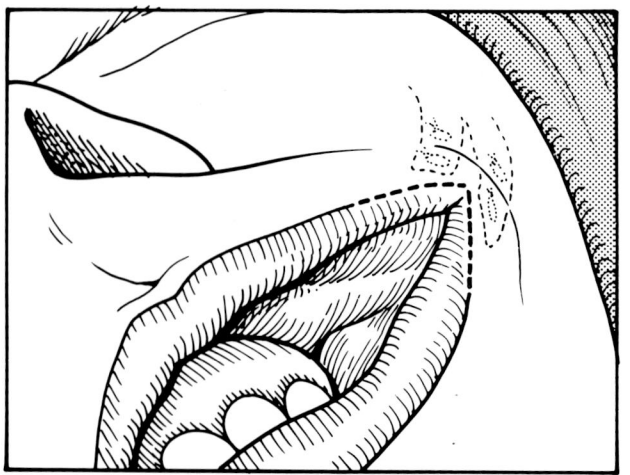

FIG. 3. *Continued.*

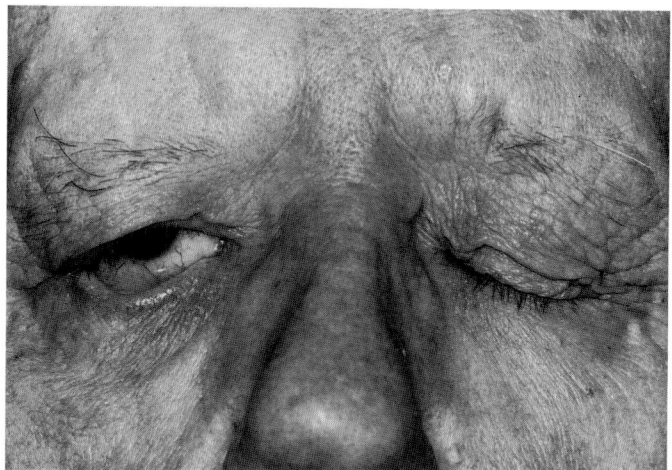 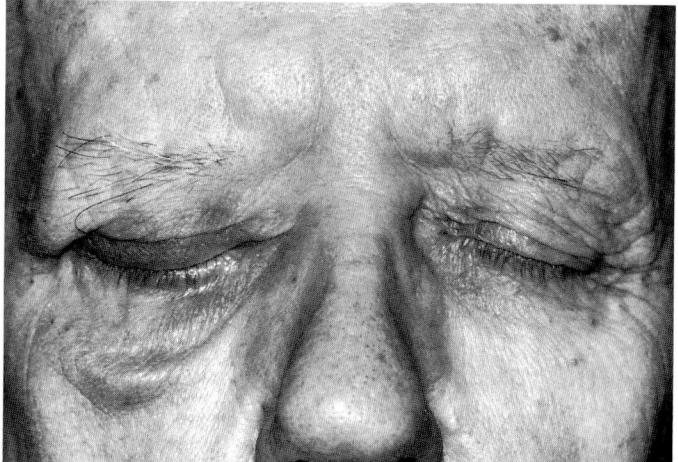

FIG. 4. A: Patient with right facial paralysis showing lack of eyelid closure and paralytic ectropion. **B:** After gold weight implantation and Bick lid-tightening procedure.

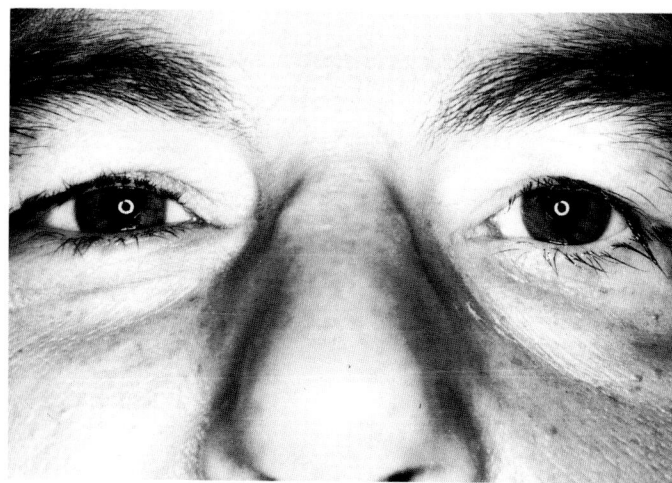 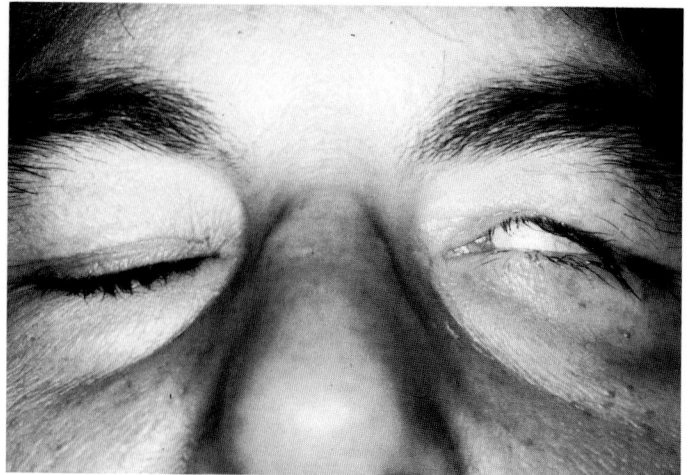

FIG. 5. Patient with left facial paralysis shown with eyes open (**A**) and closed (**B**) prior to eye spring implantation. After eye spring implantation, complete eyelid closure (**C**) is seen and without significant ptosis with eyes open (**D**).

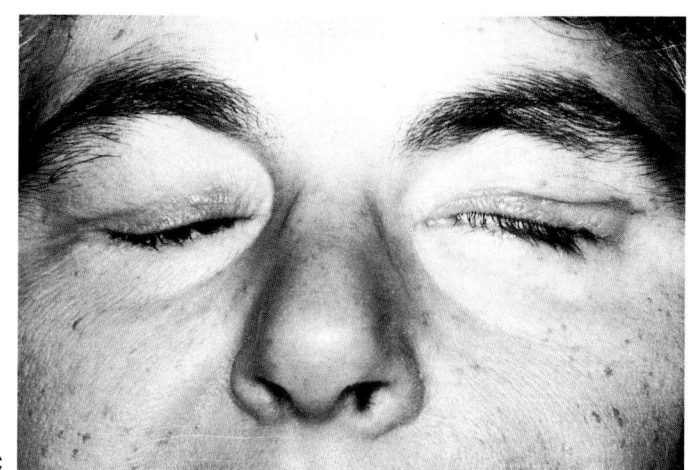
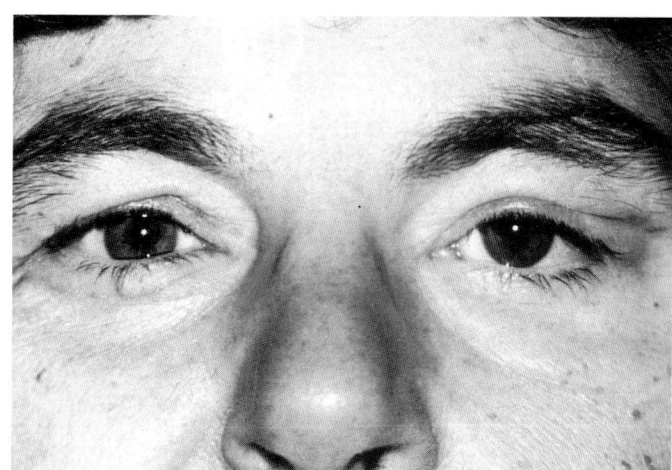

FIG. 5. *Continued.*

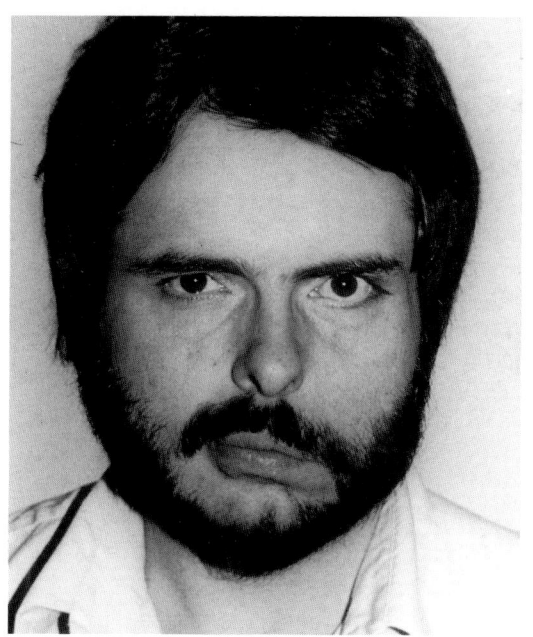
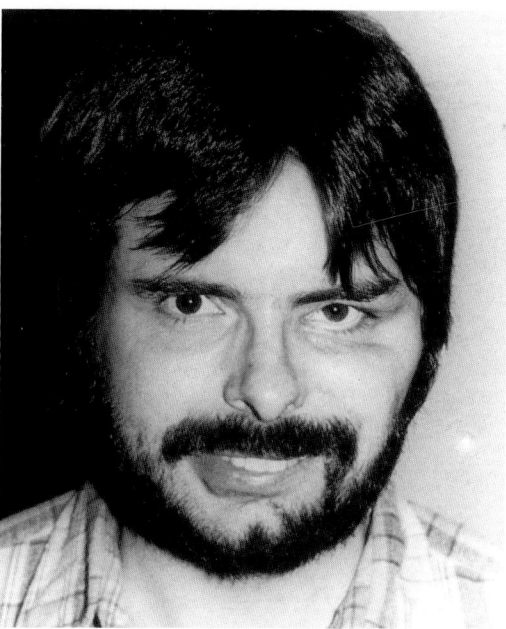

FIG. 6. Patient with left facial paralysis after acoustic tumor surgery before (**A**) and after (**B**) temporalis muscle transposition.

as adjuncts to eye reanimation procedures, as have canthoplasty and lid-tightening procedures.

CONCLUSIONS

Without a useful facial nerve, facial reanimation can only be achieved using methods other than nerve grafting and nerve crossover techniques. Separate eyelid reanimation using gold weight and spring implantation, combined with regional temporalis muscle transposition to the mouth, provides the best opportunity for independent eye and mouth movement (see Figs. 4–6 for patient examples). When combined with appropriate static procedures aimed at correcting brow ptosis, lower lid ectropion, and facial sagging, facial symmetry and function are improved dramatically in most patients. Although these approaches represent progress and an improvement, methods for facial reanimation continue to evolve as the innovative surgeon strives for perfection.

REFERENCES

1. May M. Surgical rehabilitation of facial palsy. In: May M, ed. *The facial nerve.* New York: Thieme-Stratton, 1986;695–777.
2. Conley J. Perspectives in facial reanimation. In: May M, ed. *The facial nerve.* New York: Thieme-Stratton, 1986;645–663.
3. May M. Gold weight and wire spring implant as alternatives to tarsorrhaphy. *Arch Otolaryngol* 1987;13(6):656–660.
4. Rubin LR. Temporalis and masseter muscle transposition. In: May M, ed. *The facial nerve.* New York: Thieme-Stratton, 1986; 665–679.
5. Tucker HM. Restoration of selective facial nerve function with the nerve muscle pedicle technique. *Clin Plast Surg* 1979; July:293–300.
6. May M. Paralyzed eyelid reanimated with a closed eyelid spring. *Laryngoscope* 1988;98(4):382–385.

CHAPTER 31

Alloplastic Materials in Skull Base Reconstruction

Jan Helms and Götz Geyer

For closure of perforating skull base defects it is essential that the site of repair is impervious to cerebrospinal fluid (CSF) and bacteria. This will preclude the risk of an ascending infection with subsequent endocranial complications (13,14).

For smaller and medium-sized defects (up to approximately 1.5 cm in diameter), the extradural placement of galea/periosteum, fascia, or lyophilized dura has proved to be of value (1,2,8). The use of muscle tissue or abdominal fat in combination with fibrin tissue adhesive has been recommended to cover defects in regions that do not allow easy access or are difficult to visualize, such as the roof of the sphenoid sinus or when the tympanic roof requires support (3,9).

Use of xenogenic (bovine) bone chips has been abandoned because of implant intolerance (7). Satisfactory results have been reported, however, on the use of Ceravital plates (4) or Frialit plates (5) (Fa. Friedrichsfeld, D-6800 Mannheim, Germany) for defects of 1–3 cm diameter. Following grinding to the required size and shape, these plates were additionally fitted to the undersurface of lyophilized dura.

Glass-ionomer cement (Ionos bone cement, Fa. Ionos, Medizinische Produkte GmbH & Co. KG, D-8031 Seefeld, Germany) should hold great promise for covering larger lesions or skull base defects. In addition to providing mechanical stabilization, the material is safely resistant to water and cerebrospinal fluid owing to its firm bonding to bone.

This bone replacement material is obtained by the reaction of a glass powder with a polycarboxylic acid (15). In contrast to polymerization, there is no release of monomers. The cement, after setting, is well tolerated by tissue and has the additional advantage of being biocompatible and permanently stable in a biological environment (primate bone and soft tissue) (6).

SPECIFIC DIAGNOSTIC CONSIDERATIONS

Preoperative identification of a defect is accomplished by computer tomography (CT). However, when lesions are tumor induced, the actual spread of the defect can be verified only intraoperatively because even sensitive imaging techniques do not allow identification of the full extent of bone destruction.

The diagnosis of cerebrospinal fluid fistulas escaping radiological localization rests on the detection of a specific protein (β-transferrin) in nasal secretions (11).

At 1 hr after intrathecal administration of 2 ml of 5% sodium fluorescein (Merck, D-6100 Darmstadt, Germany), endoscopy of the nose performed in a darkened room with a blue-light filter and a barrier filter at the optical equipment will reveal the precise localization of a fistula (10,12).

PATIENT SELECTION

The selection of surgical candidates is dictated by their general condition, the particular anesthetic risk, operability, diagnosis, and economic factors. The use of expensive bone replacement materials should thus be reserved to defects of more than 0.5–1 cm in size if adequate coverage with soft tissue cannot be achieved.

By using alloplastic materials such as ceramics, which are premolded outside the body, pericranial coverage of even larger defects has come within the surgeon's reach (4,14). The easily handled biocompatible glass-ionomer cement displays strong adhesive bonding to the bone and

---

J. Helms and G. Geyer: Universitäts Hals-Nasen-Ohren-Klinik, 8700 Würzberg, Germany.

provides stable bridging of even very extensive bony defects, which, after tumor resection, may exceed 10 cm in size.

OPERATIVE TECHNIQUE

Anesthesiological Considerations

Neuroleptanesthesia is preferentially used if the duration of anesthesia exceeds 4 hr; it is invariably given in all operative procedures involving opening of the dura. The intracranial pressure may be reduced by hyperventilation or by use of a Trapanal perfuser when dural and pericranial closure is undertaken. Tension-free placement of the lyophilized dura and the ceramic material can be obtained. Postoperative lumbar drainage for reduction of the cerebrospinal fluid pressure or cranial pressure can be omitted if a stable closure of the cranium or the skull base is ensured.

Patient Position

The decision concerning how to position the patient's head is dependent on the localization of the skull lesion. Thus, when using the frontoethmoid route, the head will be slightly extended, thereby permitting the operating microscope to move at a highly obtuse angle to the skull base. If a joint rhino/neurosurgical procedure is chosen (e.g., coverage of a defect in the anterior cranial fossa), elevation of the frontal lobe and its dura is followed by insertion of the alloplastic material from the cranial end.

To cover defects in the lateral skull base, the patient's head is rotated away from the operator with slight dorsal flexion. This position of the head is the same as that employed in otological operations.

For the transtemporal approach, the patient's head is turned to the side, the operating surgeon inspecting the middle cranial fossa from the cranial end.

Operative Technique

The use of alloplastic materials in reconstruction of the skull, and specifically the skull base, is based on the requirement that the bone at the borders of the defect, serving as contact surface or supporting structure for the bone replacement material, is basically stable and strong. It is recommended that in all procedures involving coverage of a bony skull lesion, the residual dura is lined with lyophilized dura, autogenic or dehydrated fascia lata, and galea/periosteum in combination with a fibrin tissue adhesive. This combined procedure, taken by itself, may already lead to a reduction or even cessation of liquorrhea (Fig. 1A). With bone defects exceeding 1 cm in size, the stabilizing effect of the lyophilized dura will usually not suffice. In such instances, premolded ceramic plates can be inserted between the lyophilized dura and the margins of the bone. Such stabilizing measures will effectively prevent dural extrusion or the development of a meningoencephalocele (Fig. 1B).

Glass-ionomer cement also lends itself to closing small and medium-sized defects. After mixing outside the body, the bone replacement material is transferred to the site of operation on a siliconized spatula while still being viscous. It forms contact at its margins with the adjacent bone and will harden. The operation site should be kept as dry as possible in order to ensure proper hardening of the cement. Humid zones of contact prolong the setting process but do not detract from the final quality. The additional time required is 5–20 min. A layer of cement, which is forced into position between the lyophilized dura and the bone, exerts an additional stabilizing effect (Fig. 1C).

After approximately 15 min, the surface of the cement can be smoothed, when indicated, with a diamond burr to remove any residual dehiscences; this surface conditioning will promote jointless union with the adjacent bone.

In our experience, the bone cement bonding is impervious to water and cerebrospinal fluid and acts as a bacterial barrier at the bone–cement interface (Fig. 1C). Thus the material is particularly useful in cases when, after a preceding interposition of lyophilized dura, a cerebrospinal fluid leak could not be completely prevented.

A pedicled flap of skin or mucosa from the neighboring region is used to cover the alloplastic material from the outside. It is essential that this flap cover be well vascularized.

Technical Problems

Technical problems are related to the size and localization of the bone defect to be covered.

A hemicoronal incision permits a fronto-orbital or transfrontal access and inspection of the anterior and posterior wall of the frontal sinus and the anterior and middle roof of the ethmoid bone with cribriform plate. If smaller defects (less than 1 cm in size) must be repaired, support is provided either by the exclusive interposition of lyophilized dura or by the supplementary insertion of a ceramic plate (Figs. 1B and 2). In a number of cases, use of the microscope alone does not permit a comprehensive visualization of defects involving the posterior ethmoid bone and sphenoid sinus. Angular endoscopes, however, allow inspection of the entire defective region, particularly when the extradural route is taken. Glass-ionomer cement is the preferred material if coverage with lyophilized dura and sealing with fibrin adhesive

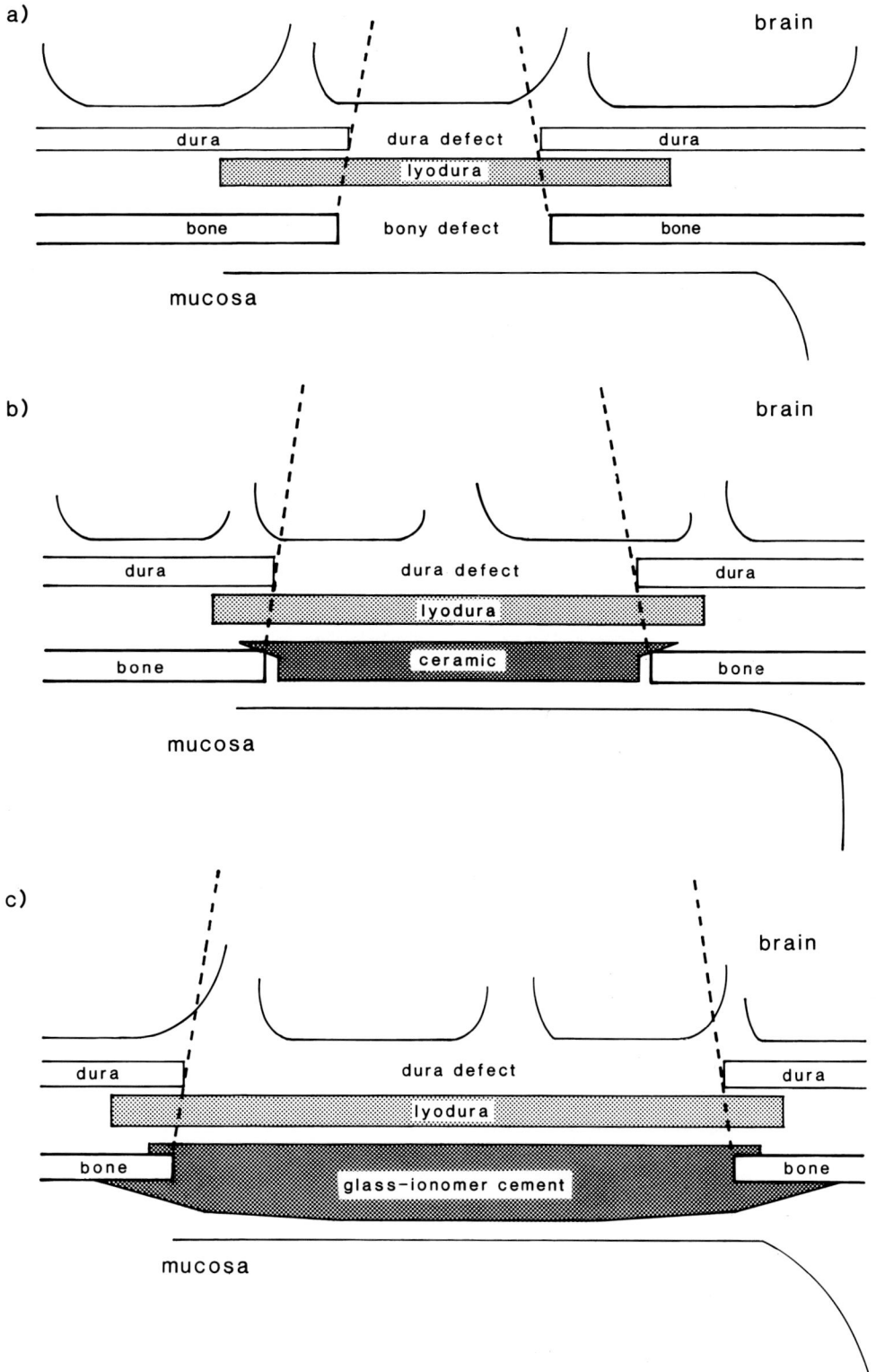

FIG. 1. Techniques for reconstruction of skull defects. **A:** Insertion of lyophilized dura. **B:** Stabilization with a ceramic plate. **C:** Watertight sealing with glass-ionomer cement.

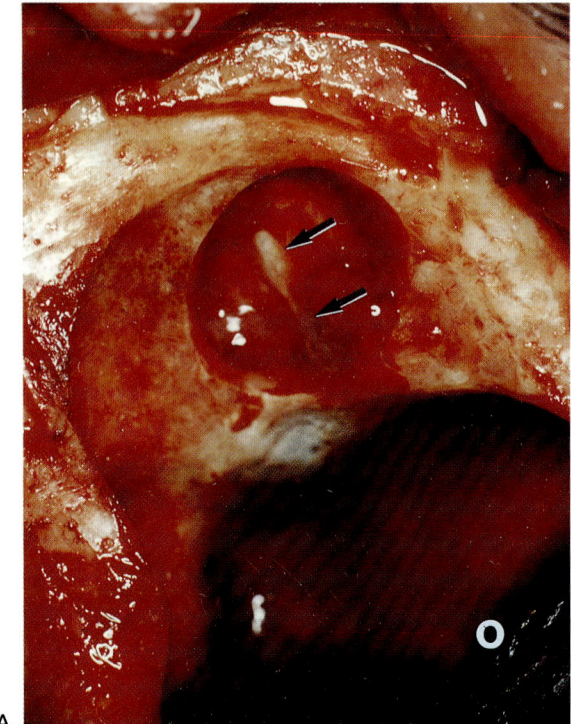 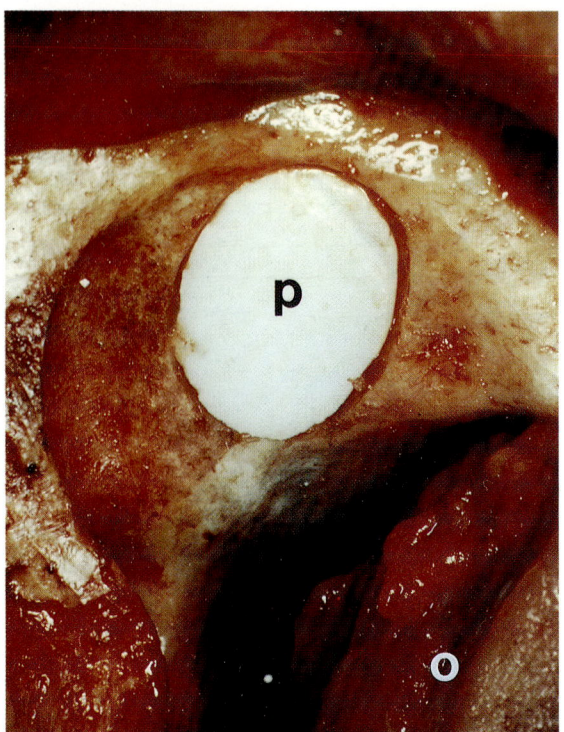

FIG. 2. A: Bone dura lesion at the posterior wall of the left frontal sinus. *Arrows,* dural lesion; o, orbital contents. **B:** Reconstruction of the posterior wall of left frontal sinus with a Ceravital plate (p). o, orbital contents.

prove to be insufficient. In such cases, the cement is placed while still viscous and allowed to harden *in situ.* If there are residual defects, another layer of cement can be placed after 10–15 min, thereby ensuring a watertight closure of the defect (Fig. 3).

A combined neurorhinosurgical operation, as used in reconstruction of the anterior cranial fossa with alloplastic material (Figs. 1C and 4), requires the stable bridging of large bone substance losses. During the hardening phase, displacement at the cement–bone interface should be avoided so as not to compromise a stable cement–bone union.

At the border of bony defects in the region of the middle cranial fossa (laterobasal fractures), reossification is observed at the floor of the middle cranial fossa particularly in patients having suffered trauma years ago. The resulting unevenness adversely affects the interposition of lyophilized dura between the bone and dura. A watertight closure cannot be guaranteed, nor is it possible to fit a ceramic prosthesis for support of the skull contents. In such cases, closure of the bony defect near the middle cranial fossa with glass-ionomer cement has proved to be of value (Figs. 1C and 5). Closure of these defects could be achieved, albeit liquorrhea could not be completely stopped. The phase of material hardening was correspondingly prolonged.

POSTOPERATIVE MANAGEMENT

Anesthesia

As operations, particularly those involving tumor resection, usually extend over prolonged periods, assisted breathing is instituted in patients under neurolept anesthesia until the onset of spontaneous breathing.

Antibiotics

Antibiotics (e.g., sulfamethoxazole-trimethoprim) are given prophylactically at the time of operation. They may be supplemented by cortisone medication (e.g., dexamethasone-21-acetate), depending on the extent of endocranial trauma. For long-term prophylaxis, this treatment is usually administered for 3 days postoperatively. Lumbar drainage is only instituted when, because of adverse localization of the defect, reconstructive procedures failed to produce sufficient stability.

COMPLICATIONS AND MANAGEMENT

Endocranial bacterial invasion calls for institution of specific chemotherapy, which may have to be revised

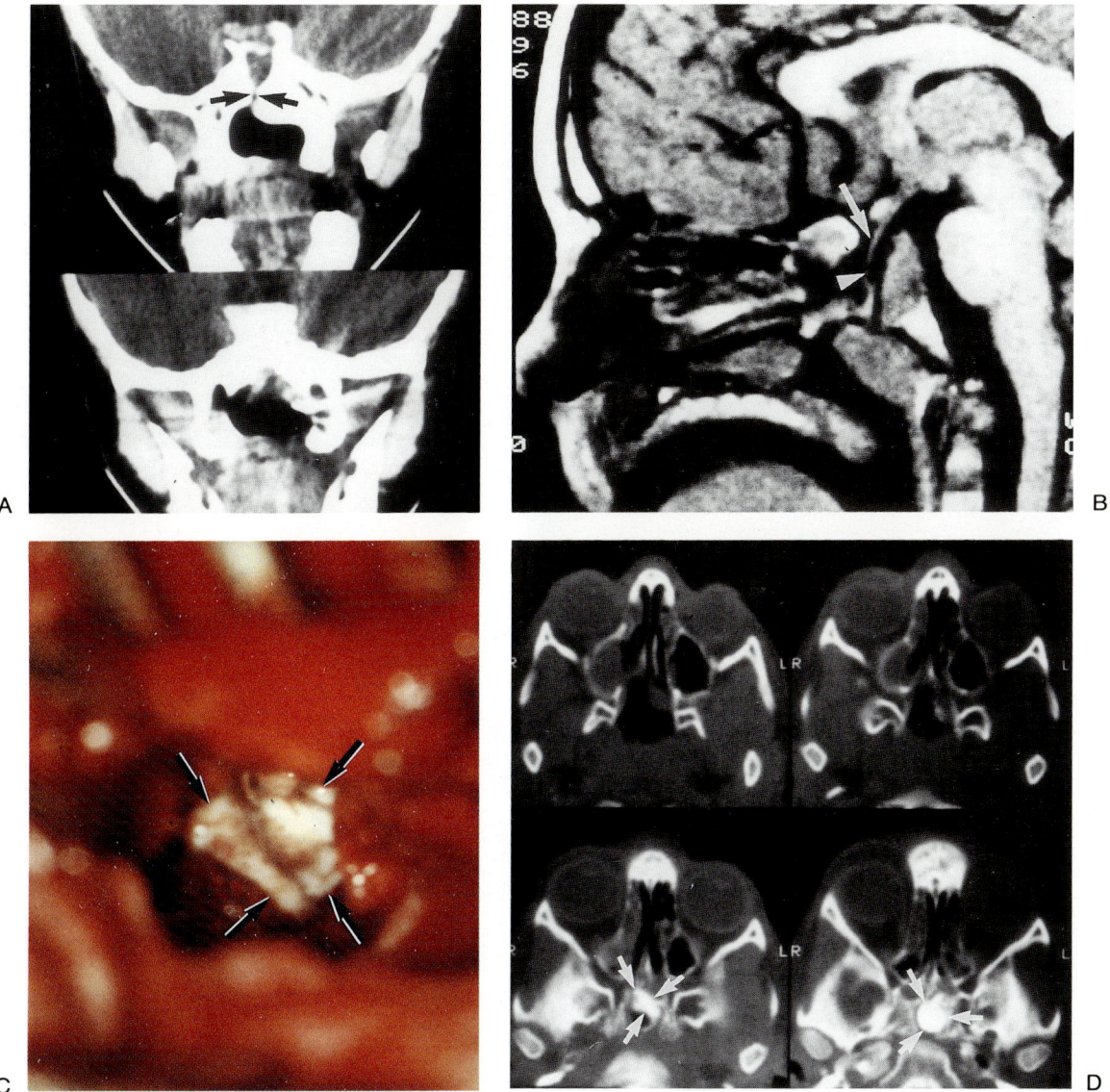

FIG. 3. A: Congenital defect between the sella floor and the sphenoid sinus (*arrows*), coronal section. **B:** Congenital defect of the sella floor. *Arrow*, pedicle of the pituitary gland; *arrowhead*, bony defect of the sella floor. **C:** Defect at the roof of the sphenoid sinus sealed with Ionos bone cement (*arrows*). Transmaxillary–transethmoid approach was modified according to Denker. **D:** Congenital defect of the sella floor after sealing with Ionos bone cement (*arrows*), 3 weeks postoperatively, axial section.

once the results of bacterial cultures are known. If liquorrhea develops postoperatively, surgical repair is required.

ILLUSTRATIVE CASES

Frontobasal Fracture

This patient is a 34-year-old female (Fig. 2) with recurrent meningitis following craniocerebral trauma 10 years earlier. There was formation of a mucopyocele due to stenosis of the aperture of the left frontal sinus. Upon examination we found a bony defect (1–2 cm in diameter) at the posterior wall of the frontal sinus, with a slit-like dural lesion. We treated the condition by lining the defect with lyophilized dura and fitting a Ceravital plate (Fig. 1B).

Congenital Fistula Involving Floor of Sella Turcica and Sphenoid Sinus

This patient is a 5-year-old male (Fig. 3) with recurrent meningitis of initially unknown etiology. There was visualization of the lesion by CT scan. We achieved closure of

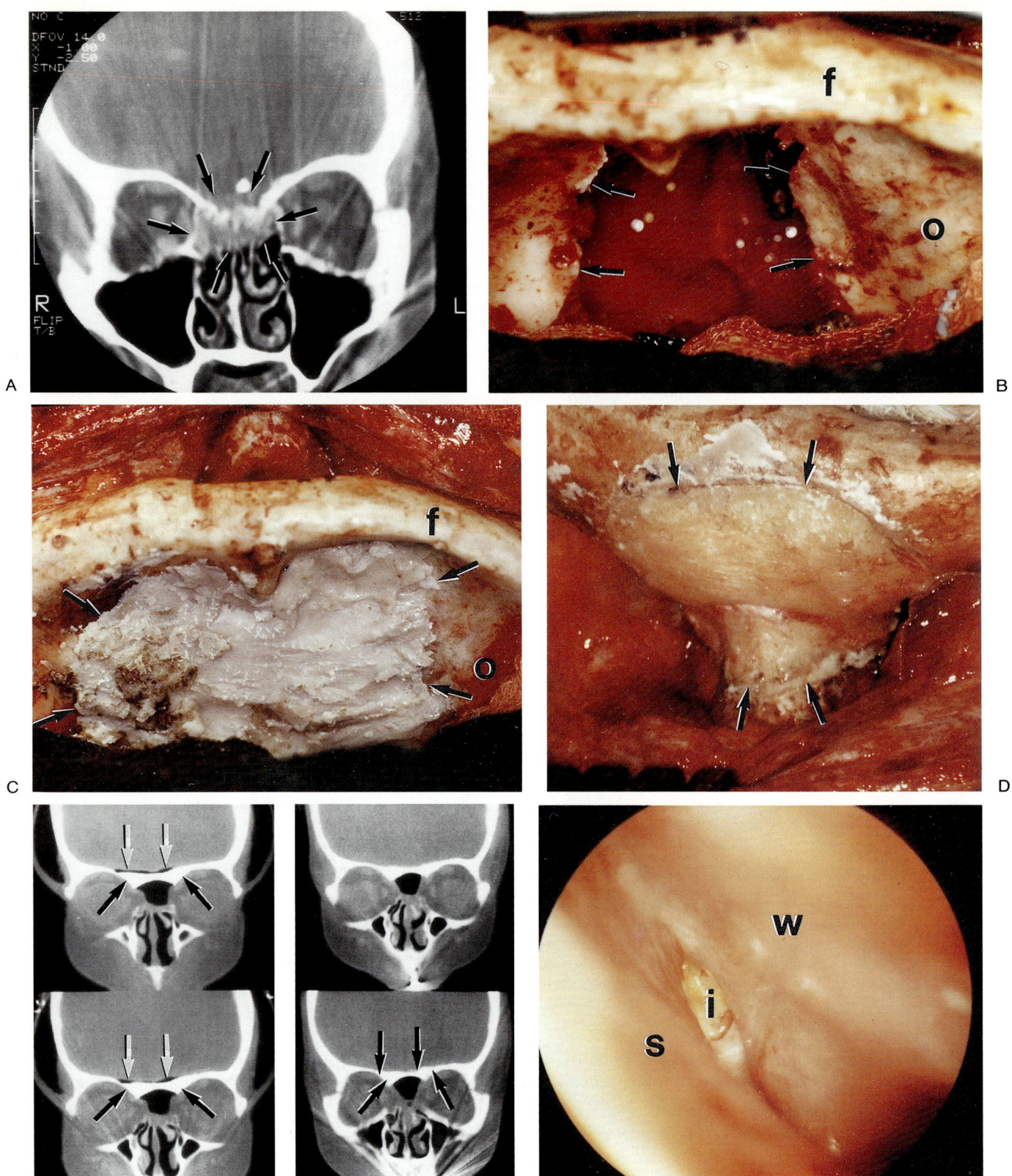

FIG. 4. A: Recurrence of a meningioma of the anterior skull base involving the frontal lobe, paranasal sinuses, and the orbit (*arrows*), coronal section. **B:** Anterior cranial fossa after resection of the ethmoid bone and parts of the orbital roof. *Arrows,* lip of defect; f, frontal bone; o, orbital roof. **C:** Defect of the anterior cranial fossa reconstructed with Ionos bone cement. *Arrows,* bone restorative cement; f, frontal bone; o, orbital roof. **D:** Temporarily removed nasal and frontal bones fixed with Ionos bone cement. *Arrows,* luting lines with cement excess. **E:** Ethmoid roof and (part of) orbit reconstructed with Ionos bone cement (*black arrows*). Air-filled space between dura and Ionos bone cement plate (*white arrows*), 2 weeks postoperatively, coronal section. **F:** Ethmoid roof and (parts of) orbit reconstructed with Ionos bone cement (*arrows*), 6 weeks postoperatively, coronal section. **G:** Transnasal endoscopic view of the ethmoid roof, 3 months after sealing with Ionos bone cement (i). Partial cover with mucosa. s, septum; w, lateral nasal wall.

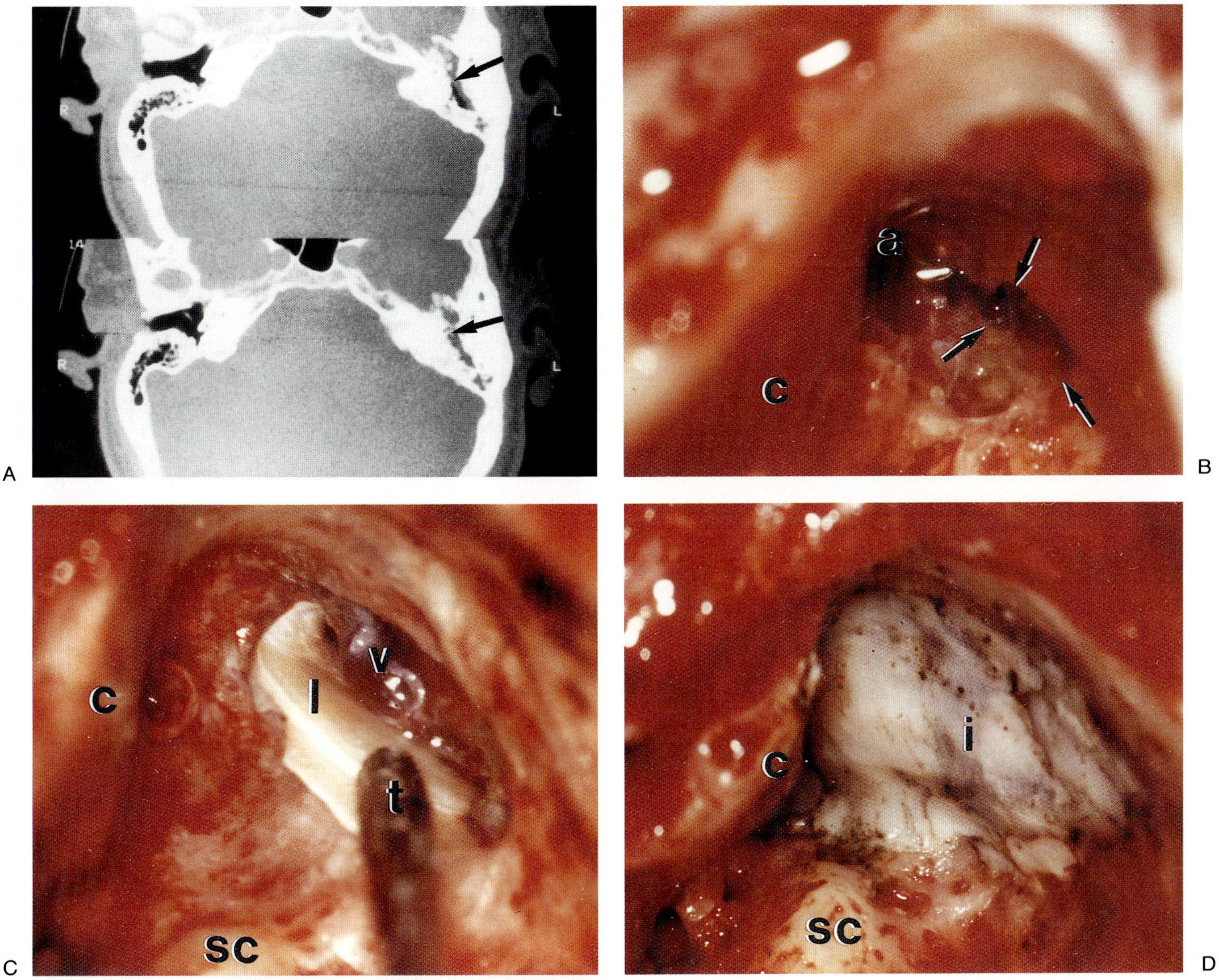

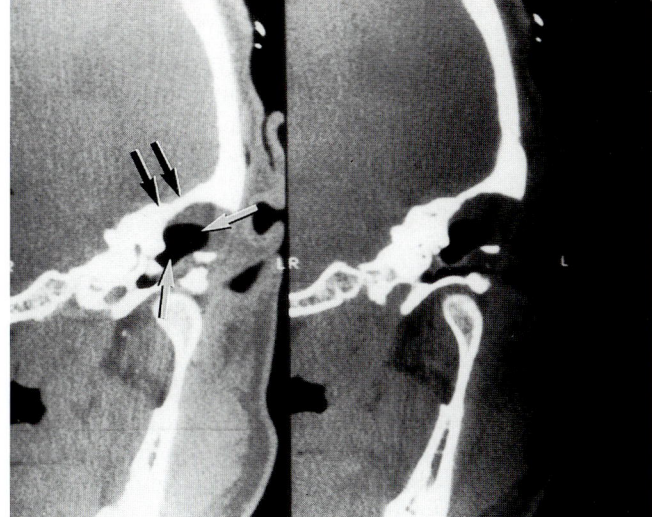

FIG. 5. A: CSF-filled spaces of the left middle ear (*arrows*), right side showing normal air-filling (axial section). **B:** Bony and dural lesion at the floor of the left middle cranial fossa, transmastoid approach. *Arrows,* margin of defect; c, bony wall of the external auditory canal; a, antral region. **C:** Insertion of lyophilized dura (l) at the floor of the left middle cranial fossa, transmastoid approach. c, bony wall of the external auditory canal; sc, horizontal semicircular canal; t, tip of suction; v, vessel at brain surface. **D:** Floor of left middle cranial fossa reconstructed with Ionos bone cement (i), transmastoid approach, c, bony wall of the external auditory canal; sc, horizontal semicircular canal. **E:** Floor of middle cranial fossa reconstructed with Ionos bone cement (*black arrows*), 1 week postoperatively, mastoid bowl partially filled with air (*white arrows*), coronal section.

the defect with Ionos bone cement using a transmaxillary–transethmoid approach (Fig. 1C).

Recurrent Meningioma

This patient is a 40-year-old female (Fig. 4) with a third recurrence of an extensive meningioma involving the frontal lobe and anterior cranial fossa; infiltrative growth was accompanied by increasing bilateral loss of vision. We performed a bifrontal craniotomy through a hemicoronal incision. We resected the infiltrated frontal lobe segments and reconstructed the dural lesion with lyophilized dura (neurosurgeon). The roof of the ethmoid bone and parts of the orbital margins were rebuilt using Ionos bone cement (Fig. 1C).

Fracture of Petrosal Bone

This patient is a 30-year-old male (Fig. 5) with recurrent meningitis following craniocerebral trauma 3 years earlier. CT scan showed CSF-filled cavities of the left middle ear, leading us to suspect a lesion at the floor of the middle cranial fossa. Our treatment consisted of a transmastoid approach, with visualization of the defect immediately adjacent to the geniculate ganglion, and resection of the head of the malleus and transposition of the incus (type III tympanoplasty according to Wullstein). The defect was lined with lyophilized dura and a CSF-resistant closure of the defect was achieved with Ionos bone cement (Fig. 1C).

PERSONAL EXPERIENCE AND DISCUSSION OF AUTHORS' SERIES

Anterior Base of Skull

Coverage of a defect at the roof of the sphenoid sinus involves complete removal of the mucosa, followed by application of lyophilized dura and filling in the defect with abdominal fat or muscle flaps. Fibrin tissue adhesive fixes the newly placed tissue in position. This procedure has been performed in 15 patients with favorable results. In the poorly accessible region and particularly when complete mucosal removal cannot be reliably undertaken, the use of glass-ionomer cement (Ionos bone cement) has proved to be of value. It can be placed conveniently, and firm bonding with the bone after hardening, thus preventing leakage of cerebrospinal fluid, is ensured.

The sphenoid sinus retains its lumen and continues to drain into the nose.

Roof of Ethmoid Bone/Olfactory Fissure

After visualization of the roof of the ethmoid bone and the olfactory fissure in 43 patients, the defect was closed with lyophilized dura, the site of repair thus becoming watertight. In 10 patients, the endocranium received additional support by insertion of ceramic plates. A regional pedicled mucosal flap was obtained either from the contralateral septal mucosa or from the deossified middle nasal concha for additional support.

When dealing with more extensive defects, experience has shown that sufficient stabilization of the anterior skull base using the described techniques could not be expected; these defects were closed extradurally or intradurally by neurosurgery using bifrontal craniotomy and insertion of a galea periosteum flap. It was possible to close even larger frontobasal lesions with glass-ionomer cement using the less aggressive extradural, fronto-orbital approach.

Posterior Wall of Frontal Sinus

In the presence of dural lesions, the readily accessible posterior wall of the frontal sinus was reconstructed in 35 patients by interposition of lyophilized dura and occasional stabilization with premolded ceramic plates. In the majority of cases, fibrin adhesive was employed for additional fixation of the lyophilized dura. In patients with extensive defects of substance, particularly lesions involving a cranialized frontal sinus (Riedel's operation), substantial crush fractures, or tumor-induced destruction, the use of glass-ionomer cement has made it possible to create a true replica of the defective bone segments. At this time, experience on reconstruction of bone defects in the anterior cranial fossa and frontal bone, and in the anterior wall of the frontal sinus, is limited to five patients; reconstruction yielded an invariably lasting sealing effect without leakage of cerebrospinal fluid.

Lateral Skull Base

In 37 patients with dural extrusion (some of them displaying dural defects and/or cerebral extrusion) the lateral skull base was closed. Lining the defect with lyophilized dura and fixation with fibrin tissue adhesive proved sufficient when defects were small. In a few cases, ceramic prostheses were positioned between the lyophilized dura and the exposed bone margins to improve stabilization. The additional placement of bone pâté promoted the incorporation and conversion of the surface-active glass-ceramic (Ceravital).

Glass-ionomer cement (Ionos bone cement) has been used with success in five cases for stable and watertight closure of defects involving dislocation of bone and extensive loss of bone substance.

The procedure of lining the defect with lyophilized dura should be limited to coverage of small lesions so as not to prepare the ground for an expanding fracture in a mechanically weakened region of the skull. This would give rise to cerebral extrusion, requiring reduction, or produce encephalocele with the need for resection. Support of the cerebral contents with premolded ceramic plates affords a substantial stabilization of the site of injury but carries the concomitant risk of a cerebrospinal fluid fistula developing later. Sharp edges may cause dural atrophy and leakage of cerebrospinal fluid (*unpublished observation*).

Cerebrospinal fluid leaks can immediately be prevented by placement of glass-ionomer cement. The firm bonding of the cement to bone promotes the stable bridging of large skull lesions, the bony skull becoming impervious to cerebrospinal fluid immediately after placement.

ACKNOWLEDGMENT

Thanks are due to Professor Dr. Nadjmi, Director of the Department of Neuroradiology at the Otolaryngological Clinic, Würzburg, who kindly provided x-ray films and CT scans.

REFERENCES

1. Boenninghaus H-G. *Die Behandlung der Schädelbasisbrüche.* Stuttgart: Thieme Verlag, 1960.
2. Boenninghaus H-G. Traumatologie der Rhinobasis und endokranielle Komplikationen. In: Naumann HH, ed. *Kopf-und Halschirurgie, Teil 2: Gesicht und Gesichtsschädel.* Stuttgart: Thieme Verlag, 1974.
3. Fisch U, Mattox D. *Microsurgery of the skull base.* Stuttgart: Thieme Verlag, 1988.
4. Geyer G. Proceedings in surgery of the anterior skull base with respect to microsurgical procedures. In: Krajina Z, ed. *Advances in nose and sinus surgery.* Zagreb: Dubrovnik, 1984.
5. Jahnke K, Plester D, Hennike G. Aluminiumoxid-Keramik, ein bioinertes Material für die Mittelohrchirurgie. *Arch Otorhinolaryngol* 1979;223.
6. Jonck LM, Grobbelaar C, Stratling H. The biocompatibility of glass-ionomer cement in joint replacement—bulk testing. *Clin Mater* 1989;4:85–107.
7. Katthagen B-D. *Knochenregeneration mit Knochenersatz-raterialien.* Berlin: Springer Verlag, 1986.
8. Kley W. Die Unfallchirurgie der Schädelbasis und der pneumatischen Räume. *Arch Klin Exp Ohren-Nasen-Kehlkopfheilk* 1968;191:1–216.
9. Kley W. Operationen bei Verletzungen der Ohrregion. In: Naumann HH, ed. *Kopf-und Halschirurgie, Band 3: Ohrregion.* Stuttgart: Thieme Verlag, 1976.
10. Messerklinger W. Nasenendoskopie: Nachweis, Lokalisation und Differentialdiagnose der nasalen Liquorrhoe. *HNO* 1972;20:268.
11. Oberascher G. Otoliquorrhoe-Rhinoliquorrhoe. *Laryngol Rhinol Otol (Stuttg)* 1988;67:375–381.
12. Reck R, Wissen-Siegert J. Ergebnisse der Fluoreszein-Nasenendoskopie bei der Diagnostik der Rhinoliquorrhoe. *Laryngol Rhinol Otol (Stuttg)* 1984;63:353–355.
13. Samii M, Draf W. *Surgery of the skull base.* New York: Springer-Verlag, 1989.
14. Thumfart W, Stennert E. Verletzungen und Frakturen des Felsenbeines und der angrenzenden Schädelbasis. *Arch Otorhinolaryngol [Suppl]* 1988;1:81–166.
15. Wilson AD, McLean JW. Glass-ionomer cement. *Quintessence* 1988.

CHAPTER 32

Esthesioneuroblastoma

Robert W. Cantrell

Esthesioneuroblastoma is a rare, malignant neoplasm originating from the olfactory epithelium. Less than 300 cases have been reported since it was first described by Berger and co-workers (1) in 1924 in the French medical literature. More reports appearing in the last 20 years reflect an increased awareness of the tumor by otolaryngologists–head and neck surgeons and increased diagnostic ability of pathologists rather than an increased incidence of the tumor.

The tumor is usually located in a relatively inaccessible site, high in the nose, grows slowly, gives few symptoms until quite large, then presents a formidable diagnostic challenge to both the clinician and the pathologist. Worse, owing to its rarity, few practitioners have an opportunity to treat many of these tumors and develop a comprehensive treatment regimen.

PATHOGENESIS

No specific etiologic agent has been identified. The known carcinogens for nasal and paranasal sinus cancer have not been shown to be related to these tumors.

Berger (1) originally termed the tumor l'esthesioneuroepitheliome olfactif, and it has been called olfactory neuroblastoma, olfactory neural neoplasm, olfactory esthesioneuroblastoma, and neuroendocrine carcinoma. Esthesioneuroblastoma is the term used most commonly today (2).

Arising from olfactory neuroepithelium high in the nasal cavity in close proximity to the cribriform plate, these tumors grow slowly and are asymptomatic until they produce nasal obstruction and epistaxis, invade the cranial cavity to produce headaches, or invade the orbit resulting in proptosis or visual defects.

R. W. Cantrell: Department of Otolaryngology and Head and Neck Surgery, University of Virginia School of Medicine, Charlottesville, Virginia 22908.

DIAGNOSIS

When a patient presents with nasal obstruction, epistaxis, or proptosis, and inspection of the nasal cavity reveals a fleshy, polypoid mass, appropriate radiological studies should be obtained prior to biopsy. If a paranasal sinus series shows a large tumor mass or bony erosion, high-resolution computerized tomographic (CT) scanning or magnetic resonance imaging (MRI) is ordered. CT scanning shows bony defects best, while MRI is better for delineating soft tissue planes, for example, determining whether tumor has invaded brain or the cavernous sinus.

Once these studies have been accomplished, a biopsy of the tumor mass is required. Depending on location and accessibility, this may be accomplished in the clinic, with prior preparation to stop bleeding, which occasionally can be profuse, or in the operating room in those cases where inaccessibility, patient comfort, or lack of cooperation necessitates this.

The pathologist should be notified in advance of the biopsy that this is a tumor requiring special handling and consideration. The tissue is usually sent fresh, that is, not in formalin, which allows touch preps to be made to evaluate the tissue for lymphoma. Some tissue is placed in glutaraldehyde to allow for electron microscopy if necessary, and the remainder is sent for the usual processing for light microscopy. The two findings on hematoxylin-eosin stained sections most diagnostic of esthesioneuroblastoma are intercellular fibrils and Home–Wright rosettes (Fig. 1). No clinical correlation with the histopathologic appearance has been demonstrated.

Electron microscopy and immunoperoxidase studies may be required for the diagnosis of poorly differentiated sinonasal tumors. Ultrastructurally, esthesioneuroblastoma contains dense-core neurosecretory granules, dendritic cell processes, filaments, and microtubules. Many immunohistochemical staining techniques are available to aid in identification of the various

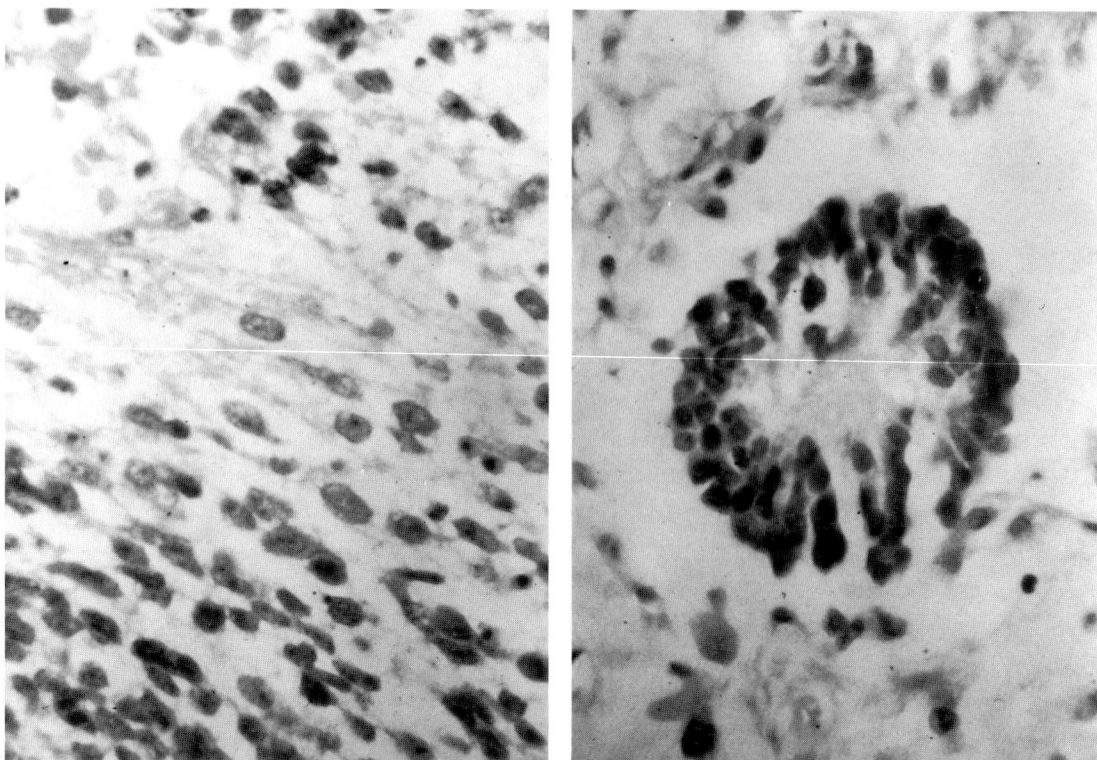

FIG. 1. Hematoxylin–eosin preparation of esthesioneuroblastoma showing intercellular fibrils (**left**) and Homer–Wright rosettes (**right**).

nasal tumors. These include leukocyte common antigen, neuron specific enolase, epithelial membrane antigens, S-100 protein, and cytokeratine. Esthesioneuroblastoma shows antibodies to neuron specific enolase and often to S-100 protein (3).

DIFFERENTIAL DIAGNOSIS

Owing to the varied tissue elements in the nose and paranasal sinuses, a number of nasal tumors may arise, and some of these are very difficult to diagnose. The list includes amelanotic malignant melanoma, embryonal rhabdomyosarcoma, hemangiopericytoma, lymphoma, plasmacytoma, and undifferentiated squamous cell carcinoma. Location, color, and patient category (i.e., young males) help to differentiate angiofibroma from these tumors.

A very highly malignant nasal tumor, termed sinonasal undifferentiated carcinoma (SNUC), has been delineated at the University of Virginia (4,5). This tumor is much more aggressive than esthesioneuroblastoma and the two are sometimes confused by pathologists. It is possible that highly malignant, rapidly growing tumors diagnosed in the past as esthesioneuroblastoma were actually SNUC. Rapidly growing nasal tumors which lead to early proptosis are probably SNUC.

Esthesioneuroblastomas are seen as rarely by the pathologist as by the clinician, and a second opinion from another pathologist is appropriate. The proper diagnosis is crucial to initiating the proper treatment. Even in centers where a relatively large number of nasal malignancies are seen and superbly qualified pathologists are available, mistaken diagnoses can occur.

STAGING

It is very important to stage the tumors as both treatment and prognosis depend on staging. The staging system proposed by Kadish and co-workers (6) is appropriate:

Stage A: tumor confined to the nasal cavity.
Stage B: tumor confined to the nasal cavity and one or more paranasal sinuses.
Stage C: tumor extending beyond the nasal cavity, including involvement of the orbit, base of skull or intracranial cavity, cervical lymph nodes, or distant metastatic sites.

Both clinical evaluation and radiological findings are used to determine the stage.

CLINICAL PRESENTATION

The age distribution of our patients with esthesioneuroblastoma is from 9 to 83 years with the median being

48. Most patients are between 40 and 60 years of age. All patients reported in the literature (7,8) have been white, but there have been anecdotal reports of the tumor occurring in three blacks. The male to female ratio is 1:1.7.

Nasal obstruction is the most common presenting symptom (65%), followed by epistaxis (55%) and orbital symptoms to include proptosis, partial or complete blindness, epiphora, and pain (50%). Headache is a complaint in one-quarter of the patients but only 15% complain of anosmia. Most patients experience these symptoms for an average of 12 months with a range of 1 month to 5 years.

The stage at presentation is roughly as follows: Stage A—4%, Stage B—40%, and Stage C—56%.

TREATMENT

Since 1976, all patients diagnosed as having esthesioneuroblastoma presenting to the University of Virginia for therapy receive the following regimen (8):

Stage A and B: Preoperative irradiation (50 Gy) in 5 weeks, followed in 4–6 weeks by a craniofacial resection by a team consisting of neurosurgeons, otolaryngologist–head and neck surgeons, and when the orbit or optic nerves were involved, a neuro-ophthalmologist.

Stage C: As above but with the addition of chemotherapy both preoperatively and postoperatively in the form of intravenous cyclophosphamide (650 mg/m^2) and vincristine (2 mg/m^2) intravenously on days 1 and 8 each month for 2 months. The response is evaluated and if no response is noted, irradiation therapy is started. If a response measurable by CT scan is present after 2 months, a third month of therapy is given plus the same regimen beginning 1 month postoperatively and continuing for 6 months. Most tumors respond to this therapy.

Nearly all tumors are responsive to irradiation. Even though gross tumor may disappear by radiological examination after irradiation or chemotherapy, this treatment does not always sterilize the tumor locus either intranasally or intracranially, and this cannot be determined preoperatively. Although several patients have shown complete resolution of tumor as determined by radiologic findings, 60% have tumor in the resected specimen. Craniofacial resection is therefore strongly recommended in all cases.

TECHNIQUE

General endotracheal anesthesia is induced following placement of arterial, central venous, and venous catheters plus a urinary catheter, and the usual anesthesia monitoring equipment. A neurosurgeon inserts two lumbar catheters to drain cerebrospinal fluid (CSF). This fluid is collected only for measurement purposes and is not replaced. It is important during the case and postoperatively to measure the amount of CSF to prevent excessive drainage, resulting in too much cerebral decompression. Postoperatively, after removal of the drains, CSF will occasionally leak into the soft tissues of the back, resulting in cerebral decompression and unconsciousness. Additionally, this negative intracranial pressure created may cause air to be drawn into the cranial cavity with the attendant risk of infection.

The patient is placed supine on the table with the head in a head holder. The neurosurgical team, through a bicoronal skin incision, raises an anterior scalp and forehead flap, leaving the periosteum and loose connective tissue on the frontal bone. This will serve as a pericranial flap (9) to be used later intracranially to traverse the defect created by removing the cribriform.

The various incisions used in combination are shown in Fig. 2.

After raising the frontal scalp flap and the pericranial flap, a piece of frontal bone is removed. Depending on the amount of access needed, this may be a triangular piece of bone that may also include the supraorbital rim (10) (Fig. 3). More recently, we have been traversing the frontal sinus via the traditional frontal osteoplastic flap when the frontal sinus is sufficiently pneumatized to permit this approach. The posterior wall of the frontal sinus is removed and discarded. The decompressed brain is carefully allowed to retract posteriorly as the dural attachments surrounding the olfactory bulb are severed. Careful repair of these dural defects as this area is elevated eliminates one of the major causes of postoperative CSF leak.

The goal of the neurosurgeon is to ensure that the tumor that originated in the nose has not invaded the dura or the brain and, after this has been determined, to free the cribriform plate (Fig. 4) to allow en bloc removal of the tumor from below.

After any intracranial tumor extensions have been removed and all CSF leaks are stopped, osteotomies around the cribriform plate are made from above. The neurosurgeon then yields the case to the otolaryngologist–head and neck surgeon.

Approximately 75% of these patients have some ophthalmologic complications due either to the tumor, irradiation, or surgery, thus a neuro-ophthalmologist should be a member of the operating team. When the tumor surrounds the optic nerves or invades the orbit, or ophthalmic decisions are necessary, the services of a neuro-ophthalmologist are invaluable. At the University of Virginia, such service is available, and of the last 25 patients treated for esthesioneuroblastoma only one has required orbital exenteration. In that case of recurrent intracranial tumor invading the right orbit and the cavernous sinus, preservation of the eye was not possible. In all other cases, the orbital contents plus serviceable vision were maintained.

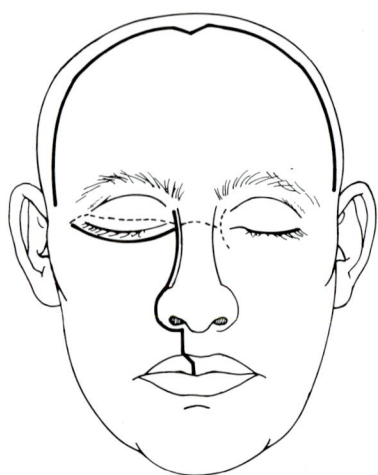

FIG. 2. Facial and scalp incisions for craniofacial resection of esthesioneuroblastomas. (From ref. 9, with permission.)

The otolaryngologist–head and neck surgeon usually approaches the tumor via a lateral rhinotomy incision extended across the root of the nose (Fig. 2). The classical Weber–Ferguson incision can be used in those cases requiring greater exposure or maxillectomy but is usually not necessary. Facial degloving has been utilized but tends to restrict access to the skull base and therefore is rarely used. All skin incisions on the face are made with a portion of a broken razor blade held in a razor blade breaker, and careful tissue handling is used in all cases to ensure optimum cosmetic results.

A chisel is used to perform a lateral osteotomy of the nasal (superior) process of the maxilla on the side of the lesion and is extended across the root of the nose. The bony septum and the posterior portion of the quadrangu-

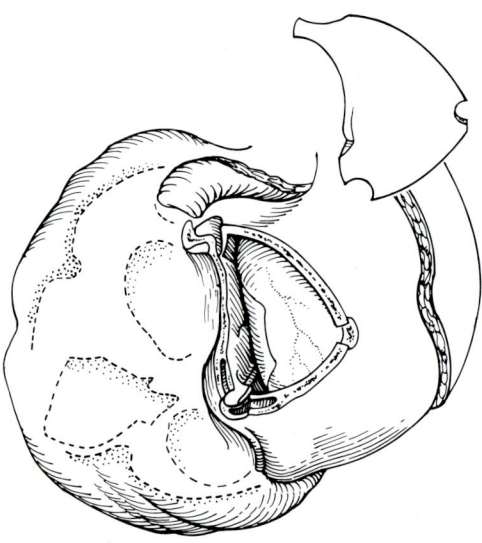

FIG. 3. Frontal bone flap (including supraorbital rim) for approaching anterior skull base tumors. (From ref. 10, with permission.)

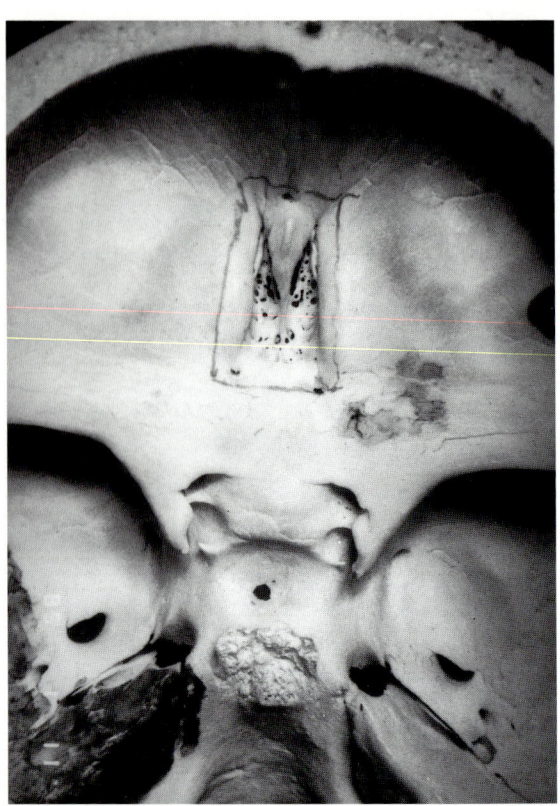

FIG. 4. Anterior (frontal) fossa of dry skull with cribriform plate and chisel cuts outlined.

lar cartilage are separated from the external nose using both scalpel and heavy scissors. The entire external nose is then reflected to the side away from the lesion (Fig. 5).

The lateral wall of the nose (medial maxilla) is removed, as is the entire ethmoid complex on the side of the lesion (bilaterally if there is any question about tumor extent). The lamina papyracea is removed but the medial periorbita is perserved intact. The cribriform

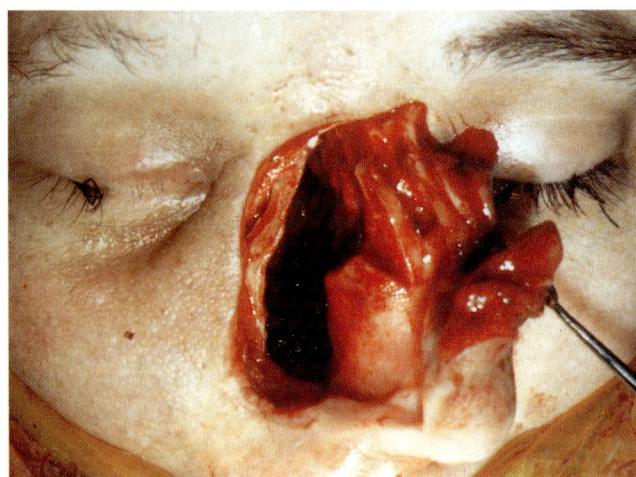

FIG. 5. Facial approach to an esthesioneuroblastoma via right lateral rhinotomy.

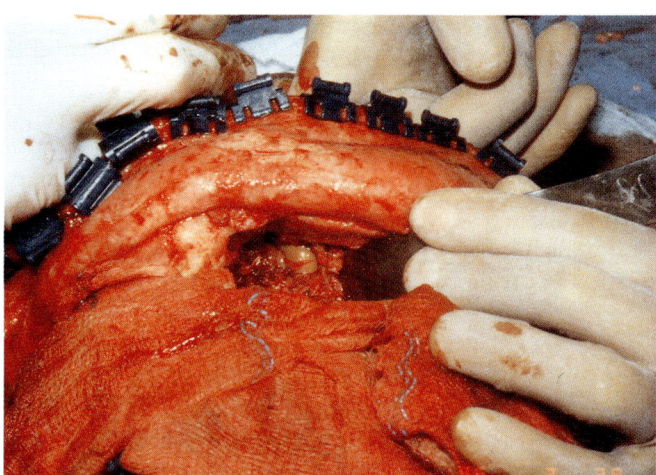

FIG. 6. View through the craniotomy with a gloved finger into the cribriform defect from below.

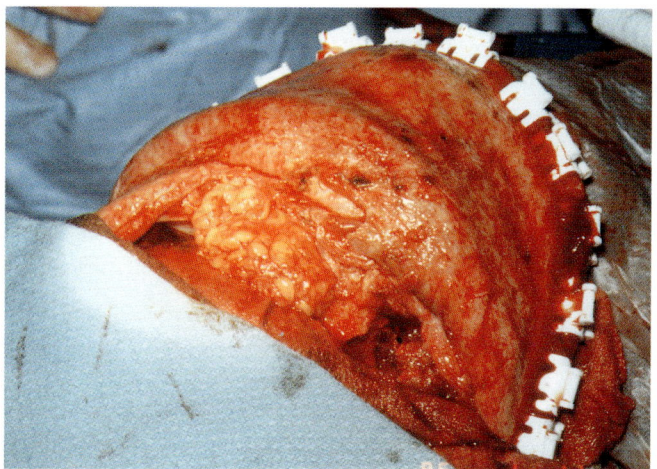

FIG. 8. Abdominal fat packed into the frontal sinus after removing the frontal sinus mucosa.

plate with attached nasal structures is pulled down into the nasal cavity, the anterior wall of the sphenoid is removed, the base of the septum is severed from the floor of the nose, and the specimen and surrounding structures are delivered from the nose. All bleeding is stopped with electrocautery and any additional suspicious tissue is removed. Frozen section biopsies should be sent from various areas to ensure complete tumor removal.

This approach offers excellent visibility while protecting the brain, orbital contents, optic nerves, and cavernous sinuses (Fig. 6).

After all tumor has been removed, an elliptical skin incision, measuring 3 by 6 cm depending on the size of the bony defect in the floor of the frontal fossa, is made in the previously prepped left lower quadrant of the abdomen. Full thickness skin and subcutaneous fat are harvested. The skin, trimmed of all subcutaneous tissue and cut to the size of the bony defect, is placed on a large piece of gelatin sponge (Fig. 7). This is placed from below upward, raw surface superior, into the bony defect created by removing the cribriform plate. Iodoform gauze impregnated with bacitracin ointment is then packed into the large nasal cavity created by removal of the tumor. The nose is replaced in its normal position; the skin is carefully approximated and held in place by fine sutures. All mucous membrane is removed from the frontal sinus, and it is packed with the abdominal fat previously removed (Fig. 8).

The neurosurgeons resume control of the case, laying the pericranial flap into the floor of the frontal fossa. The pericranial flap is thus in contact with the raw surface of the abdominal skin previously placed in the bony defect in the cribriform area.

The brain is allowed to expand and the dura is in-

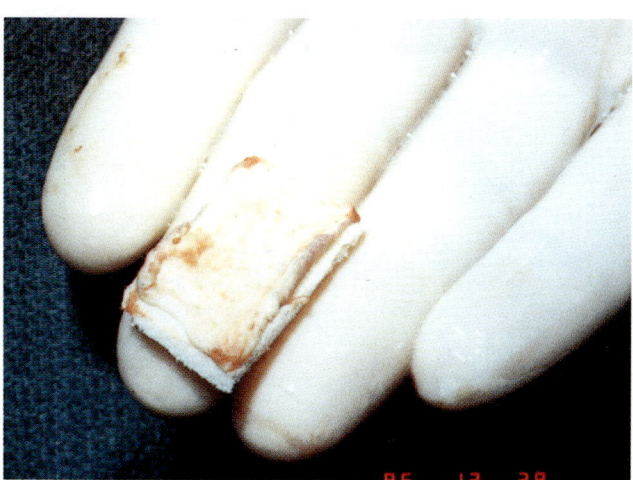

FIG. 7. Full thickness skin graft on gelatin sponge.

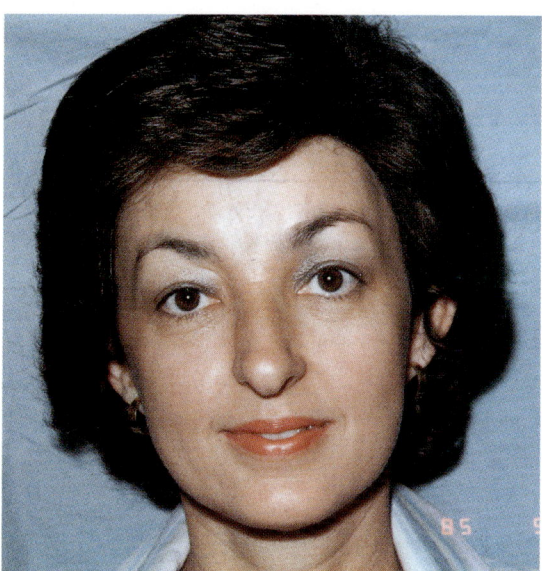

FIG. 9. Postoperative appearance of patient 4 months after undergoing a craniofacial resection (via right lateral rhinotomy) for esthesioneuroblastoma. Scar under right brow resulted from frontal sinus trephine for biopsy pretreatment.

spected for CSF leaks. If no leaks are found, the bone flap is wired in place, the skin flap replaced, and the bicoronal incision closed.

The patient is monitored in the intensive care unit for 24 hr or until stable, then moved to the neurosurgical step-down unit or the otolaryngology–head and neck surgery ward. Usual length of hospitalization is 7–10 days.

The cosmetic result of this can and should be quite good (Fig. 9).

PROGNOSIS

Applying the treatment regimen outlined here should result in 5-year survival rates approaching 100% in Stage A, and 60–75% in Stage B. Overall 5-year survival rates in the 60% range should be expected when treated as outlined here.

Five-year survivals are not the final word on this tumor, however, since it may recur 10 or 15 years after treatment. Obviously, prolonged follow-up care is necessary.

Recurrent disease should not be cause for despair since recurrences can be successfully controlled. Approximately 25% of these tumors may recur, and when they do, treatment with chemotherapy, radiation if feasible, and operation is usually successful.

COMPLICATIONS

When undertaking therapy of this magnitude, complications occur. Irradiation can cause hair loss, skin damage, or serous otitis, and blindness and cataract formation are potential problems.

Chemotherapy can result in hair loss, nausea and vomiting, and myelosuppression with the possibility of overwhelming sepsis.

Surgery results in anosmia in all cases and can result in infected bone flaps, transient coma secondary to CSF leaks through the spinal drain sites, CSF rhinorrhea, and subgaleal or epidural abscesses.

OBSERVATION

As can be seen by the foregoing, esthesioneuroblastoma is a rare, malignant nasal tumor arising from the olfactory epithelium. It is slow growing and asymptomatic until fairly large. It usually causes nasal obstruction or epistaxis as first symptoms, and histopathological diagnosis is frequently difficult, requiring a pathologist with experience in diagnosing this tumor. It may require electron microscopy or immunohistochemical staining to establish the diagnosis with certainty.

Evaluation and staging require CT scanning and MRI if the tumor is intracranial. These studies aid in staging, which is crucial to the proper treatment.

This tumor is best managed by a team consisting of a pathologist, a neuroradiologist, a chemotherapist, a radiation therapist, a neurosurgeon, a neuro-ophthalmologist, and an otolaryngologist–head and neck surgeon as coordinator for the team (8). Since this latter individual is the person whom the patient first sees and returns to for follow-up, the otolaryngologist–head and neck surgeon should be the contact. Teams bring together the expertise of the individual members, but this array of talent is sometimes confusing to patients or their families, and one person should be designated as the contact person.

Using irradiation and craniofacial resection in *all* cases and adding chemotherapy in those patients with Stage C disease result in decreased early recurrence and probably improves survival.

The disturbing aspect of this tumor to recur locally requires persistence on the part of the surgeons, radiotherapists, and chemotherapists as well as the patients. Salvage therapy can eradicate many of these recurrences, and the patients and the physicians must avoid discouragement.

REFERENCES

1. Berger L, Luc G, Richard D. L'esthesioneuroepithliome olfactif. *Bull Assoc Franc Etude Cancer* 1924;13:410–421.
2. Newbill ET, Johns ME, Cantrell RW. Esthesioneuroblastoma: diagnosis and management. *South Med J* 1985;78:275–282.
3. Taxy JB, Bharani NK, Mills SE, Frierson HF Jr, Gould VE. The spectrum of olfactory neural tumors. A light-microscopic immunohistochemical and ultrastructural analysis. *Am J Surg Pathol* 1986;10:687–695.
4. Frierson HF Jr, Mills SE, Fechner RE, Taxy JB, Levine PA. Sinonasal undifferentiated carcinoma. An aggressive neoplasm derived from Schneiderian epithelium and distinct from olfactory neuroblastoma. *Am J Surg Pathol* 1986;10:771–779.
5. Levine PA, Frierson HF Jr, Mills SE, Stewart FM, Fechner RE, Cantrell RW. Sinonasal undifferentiated carcinoma: a distinctive and highly aggressive neoplasm. *Laryngoscope* 1987;97:905–908.
6. Kadish S, Goodman M, Wang CC. Olfactory neuroblastoma. *Cancer* 1976;35:1571–1576.
7. Cantrell RW, Chorayeb BY, Fitz-Hugh GS. Esthesioneuroblastoma: diagnosis and treatment. *Ann Otol Rhinol Laryngol* 1977;86:760–765.
8. Levine PA, McLean WC, Cantrell RW. Esthesioneuroblastoma: The University of Virginia experience 1960–1985. *Laryngoscope* 1986;96:742–746.
9. Johns ME, Winn MR, McLean WC, Cantrell RW. Pericranial flap for the closure of defects of craniofacial resections. *Laryngoscope* 1981;91:952–959.
10. Johns ME, Kaplan MJ, Jane JA, Park TS, Cantrell RW. Supraorbital rim approach to the anterior skull base. *Laryngoscope* 1984;94:1137–1139.

CHAPTER 33

Transzygomatic and Transpalatal Excision of Juvenile Nasopharyngeal Angiofibroma with Intracranial Extension

The Surgical Procedure

Stephen J. Haines and Arndt J. Duvall III

Juvenile nasopharyngeal angiofibroma is a benign tumor of adolescent men, which occasionally extends intracranially. Until recently, such tumors with intracranial extension were considered unresectable. Advances in skull base surgery with cooperation between neurological surgeons and otolaryngologists have led to the development of techniques that allow complete excision of such tumors. These operations, often involving both intracranial and extracranial exposures, can be formidable. While intracranial exposure is necessary for large tumors that have violated the dura, there is a group of such tumors with limited intracranial but extradural extension that can safely be removed by combining a lateral transzygomatic completely extracranial approach with a transoral extended transpalatal tripartite exposure.

PATIENT SELECTION

It must be emphasized that this procedure is proposed for a restricted group of patients in whom there is no preoperative evidence of dural penetration or significant supply from the internal carotid artery. The preoperative evaluation will include thin section computerized tomography (CT) to define bony erosion, magnetic resonance imaging (MRI) to delineate the structures of the cavernous sinus and assess the integrity of the dura, and angiography for complete definition of the vascular supply and for preoperative embolization.

OPERATIVE TECHNIQUE

Preoperative Preparation

We have treated our patients preoperatively with diethylstilbestrol 5 mg t.i.d. for approximately 4 weeks. It is our clinical impression that this has made tumors less vascular and friable. Angiographic embolization of prominent arterial feeders is carried out 1 day preoperatively. We do not use additional preoperative steroids. Antibiotics are not routinely administered.

Anesthetic Considerations

As the intracranial space is not violated and the intracranial pressure is not increased in this category of patients, no special neuroanesthetic preparations are required. The orotracheal tube is located so as to interfere as little as possible with surgery.

S. J. Haines: Departments of Neurosurgery and Otolaryngology, University Hospital, University of Minnesota Center for Craniofacial and Skull Base Surgery, Minneapolis, Minnesota 55455.
A. J. Duvall III: Department of Otolaryngology, Head and Neck Surgery, University Hospital, University of Minnesota Center for Craniofacial and Skull Base Surgery, Minneapolis, Minnesota 55455.

Positioning

The transzygomatic stage of the operation is carried out first. The patient is positioned supine with the head turned approximately 45° away from the lesion and supported on a foam donut. For the transpalatal stage, maximal cervical extension in the Rose position with exposure utilizing the Dingman oral retractor is used. This has proved to be very satisfactory for most tumors. In the largest tumor we have treated in this way, we felt that simultaneous transzygomatic and transpalatal exposure would be prudent, and thus the entire procedure was carried out in the Rose position. This is uncomfortable, but not impossible, during the transzygomatic portion of the operation.

OPERATIVE TECHNIQUE

Figures 1–3 demonstrate a typical lesion seen through the intact skull. Figures 4–6 show the surgical approaches described next.

Transzygomatic Stage

The transzygomatic portion (Fig. 4) of the operation is carried out through a bicoronal incision behind the hairline from in front of the ear 1 cm below the root of the zygoma to the opposite temporal line. The scalp is reflected in the areolar layer, leaving pericranium and temporalis fascia intact. We have not experienced permanent frontalis palsy. This dissection is carried forward to expose the lateral orbital rim and the zygomatic maxillary suture. The periosteum along the lateral orbital rim and zygomatic arch is incised. Subperiosteal dissection frees the zygomatic bone from its surrounding soft tis-

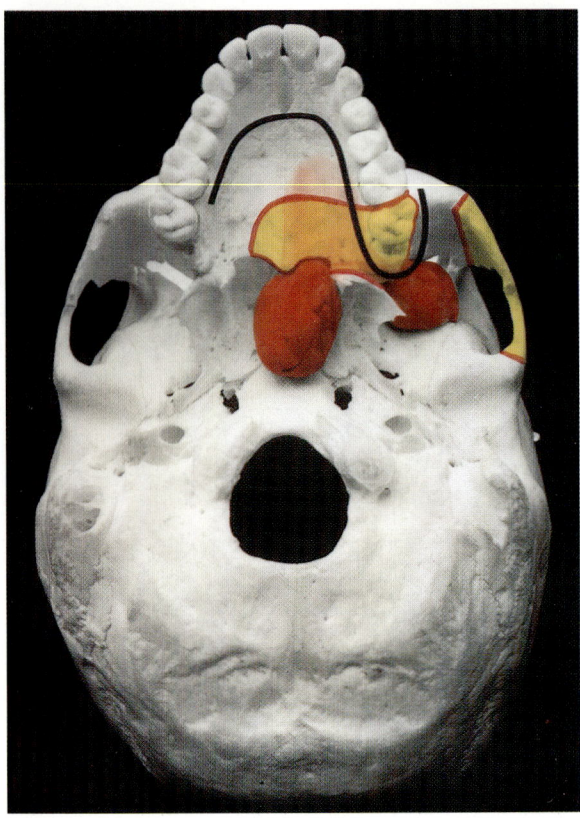

FIG. 2. Submentovertex view of same lesion shown in Fig. 1. The *black line* indicates the palatal incision.

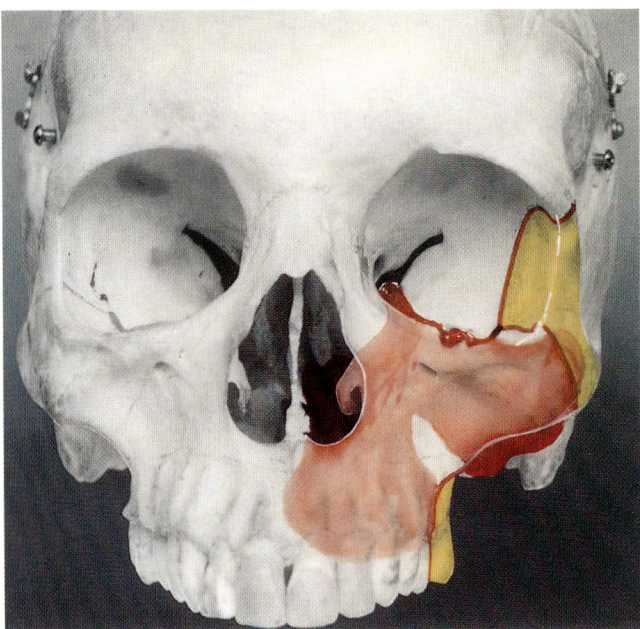

FIG. 1. Artist's concept of a typical lesion treated by combined transzygomatic–transpalatal approach. The tumor is shown in *red*, the areas of bone removal in *yellow*.

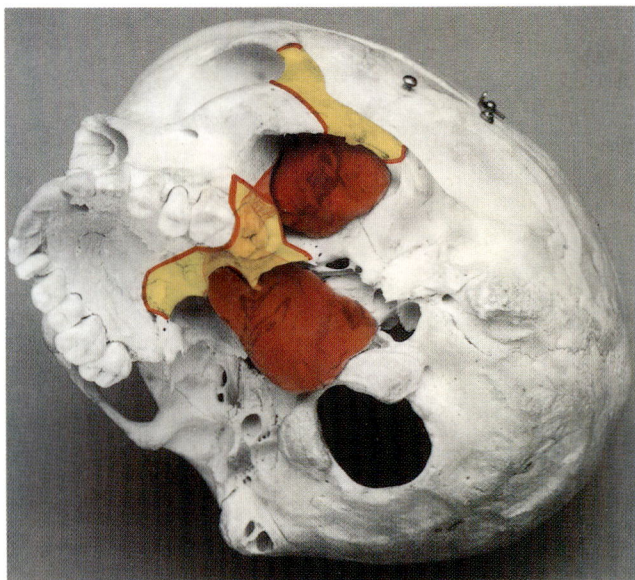

FIG. 3. The lesion seen in Figs. 1 and 2 viewed from the same angle as drawing in Fig. 6.

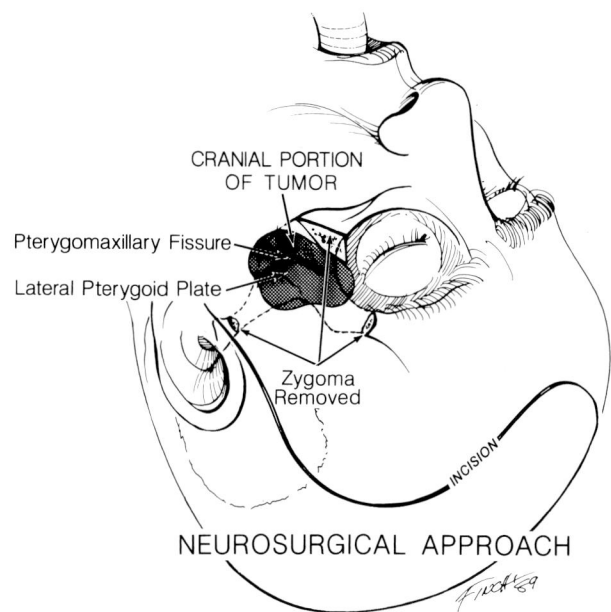

FIG. 4. Drawing from the surgeon's perspective showing the transzygomatic exposure of the superior pole of the tumor.

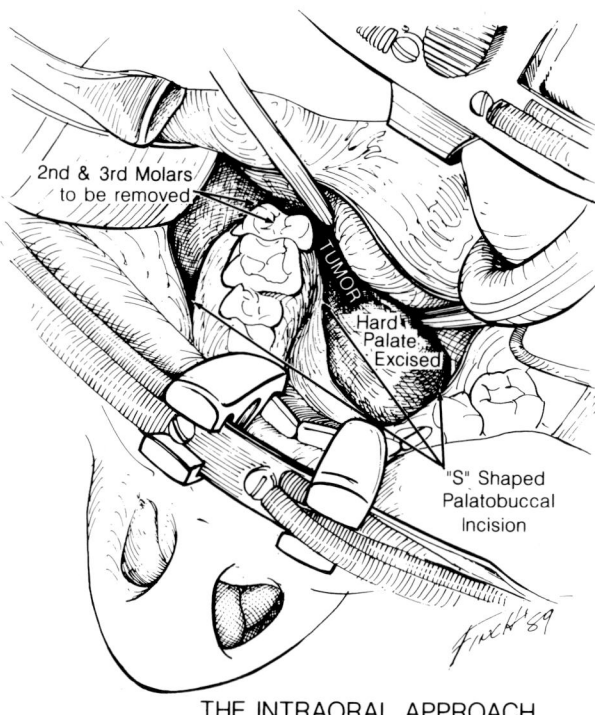

FIG. 5. Drawing from the surgeon's perspective showing the transpalatal exposure of the tumor.

sue. Osteotomies are made through the zygomatic arch, the frontozygomatic suture into the thin portion of the lateral orbital wall, and the zygomaticomaxillary suture back to the most anterior aspect of the inferior orbital fissure. Care is taken to protect the orbital contents with malleable retractors. The zygomatic bone can then be removed by fracturing through the thin orbital wall and floor. This exposes the superior pole of the tumor, which has usually widened the inferior orbital fissure. Bone of the lateral orbital wall can be resected with rongeurs or high-speed drill to allow dissection of the tumor along its superior pole separating it from the adjacent dura. Tumors appropriately selected for this operation will have elevated the dura away from the sphenoid bone from which it can be safely separated. No attempt at resection of tumor is made. A layer of Gelfoam is placed between the tumor and dura in the dissection bed after hemostasis is assured. The zygoma is then replaced and held with three wires. The periosteum is reapproximated particularly behind the frontozygomatic suture and the scalp replaced and closed with a layer of galeal suture and skin staples.

Transpalatal Stage

Excellent exposure is obtained transorally through an extended palatobuccal incision (Figs. 2 and 5). The Dingman self-retaining retractor was designed for children and the blades for the tongue are too small and one from a McIvor self-retaining retractor must be substituted. A continuous S-shaped incision is made just lateral to the vascular pedicle of the greater palatine foramen on one side swinging up forward on the palate to follow the curve of the alveolar ridge, then coursing behind the alveolar ridge on the other side and into the buccoalveolar gutter as far forward as necessary. The mucoperiosteum is elevated off the hard palate. The greater palatine artery is cauterized as it exits its canal on the side of the buccoalveolar gutter incision. The nasopharynx is entered at the junction of the hard and soft palates. The bone of the hard palate is removed as necessary to give exposure to the nasal fossae and the ethmoids. The muscles are then removed from the pterygoid plates by blunt dissection as would occur in a maxillectomy and the pterygoid plates are removed. This wide exposure laterally allows blunt dissection of the lateral extension, after the deep portion of that lateral extension has been freed from the cranial cavity via the transzygomatic approach. The lateral extension now having been delivered into the wound at its bottleneck at the pterygomaxillary fissure, an incision is made down through the periosteum surrounding the whole attachment of the tumor on the basiocciput (Fig. 6). The tumor attachment is then scraped off the basiocciput with a periosteal elevator. There is invariably a thumb-sized extension of the tumor into the sphenoid sinus, which easily is pulled from it as the tumor is dissected off the basiocciput. After removal of the tumor, biopsies are taken in any suspected areas of the basiocciput and more tumor is removed if frozen sections demonstrate its presence. Occasionally, there are bits of tumor in the basioc-

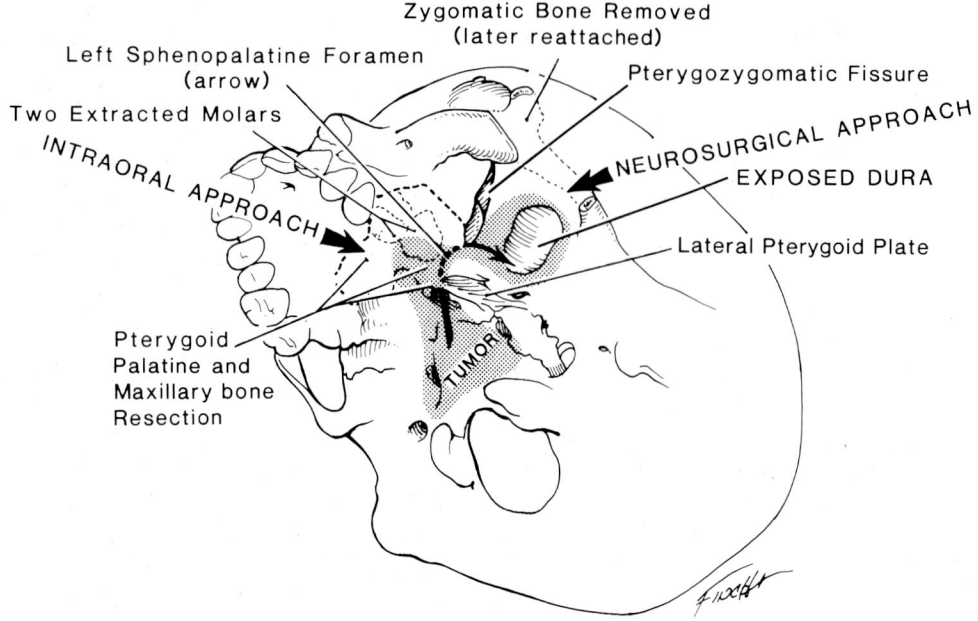

FIG. 6. Drawing showing combined transzygomatic–transpalatal approach. See text for details.

ciput in small crevices. The carbon dioxide laser facilitates removal of such small extensions.

The entire cavity is then lined with Gelfoam. A posterior pack smeared with bacitracin is placed. Anterior packing is usually necessary to prevent cutting of the anterior nares by the strings from the posterior pack. The incision is closed with interrupted sutures of vicryl.

POSTOPERATIVE MANAGEMENT

One week following the definitive surgery, the packing is removed in the operating room for comfort and to be in a position to repack if bleeding occurs.

COMPLICATIONS IN MANAGEMENT

Hemorrhage can occur, almost invariably at the site of excision from the basiocciput. Although blood can readily be replaced, visualization is made difficult, thus reducing confidence in total tumor extirpation. Surgical dissection of the nasopharynx results in eustachian tube dysfunction in a small percentage of cases. We have not encountered nasopharyngeal stenosis, hemorrhage at the time of removal of the nasopharyngeal packs, trigeminal facial nerve dysfunction, or jaw movement disturbances.

TECHNICAL PROBLEMS

The zygomatic approach offers limited exposure of the middle cranial fossa and thus this stage of the operation simply facilitates the safe excision of the tumor from the transpalatal approach. Attempt at tumor resection in this exposure is not recommended. Resection of small intraorbital extension should be possible from this exposure, although we have not encountered such a case.

ILLUSTRATIVE CASES

Case 1

An 11-year-old boy presented to his physician with recurrent epistaxis and nasal obsduntia. A CT scan diagnosed a large nasopharyngeal mass with minimal intracranial extension in the right parasellar region (Fig. 7A). Angiography showed no supply from intracranial vessels. He was otherwise healthy and had a normal neurologic examination.

After 4 weeks of preoperative diethylstilbestrol therapy and embolization of the internal maxillary feeding vessels on the day prior to surgery, the tumor was excised with a combined transzygomatic and transpalatal approach. There were no postoperative complications or neurologic deficits and 2 years postoperatively there was no clinical or radiographic evidence of recurrence (Fig. 7B).

Case 2

This 18-year-old boy was first diagnosed as having a juvenile nasopharyngeal angiofibroma at age 14. The tu-

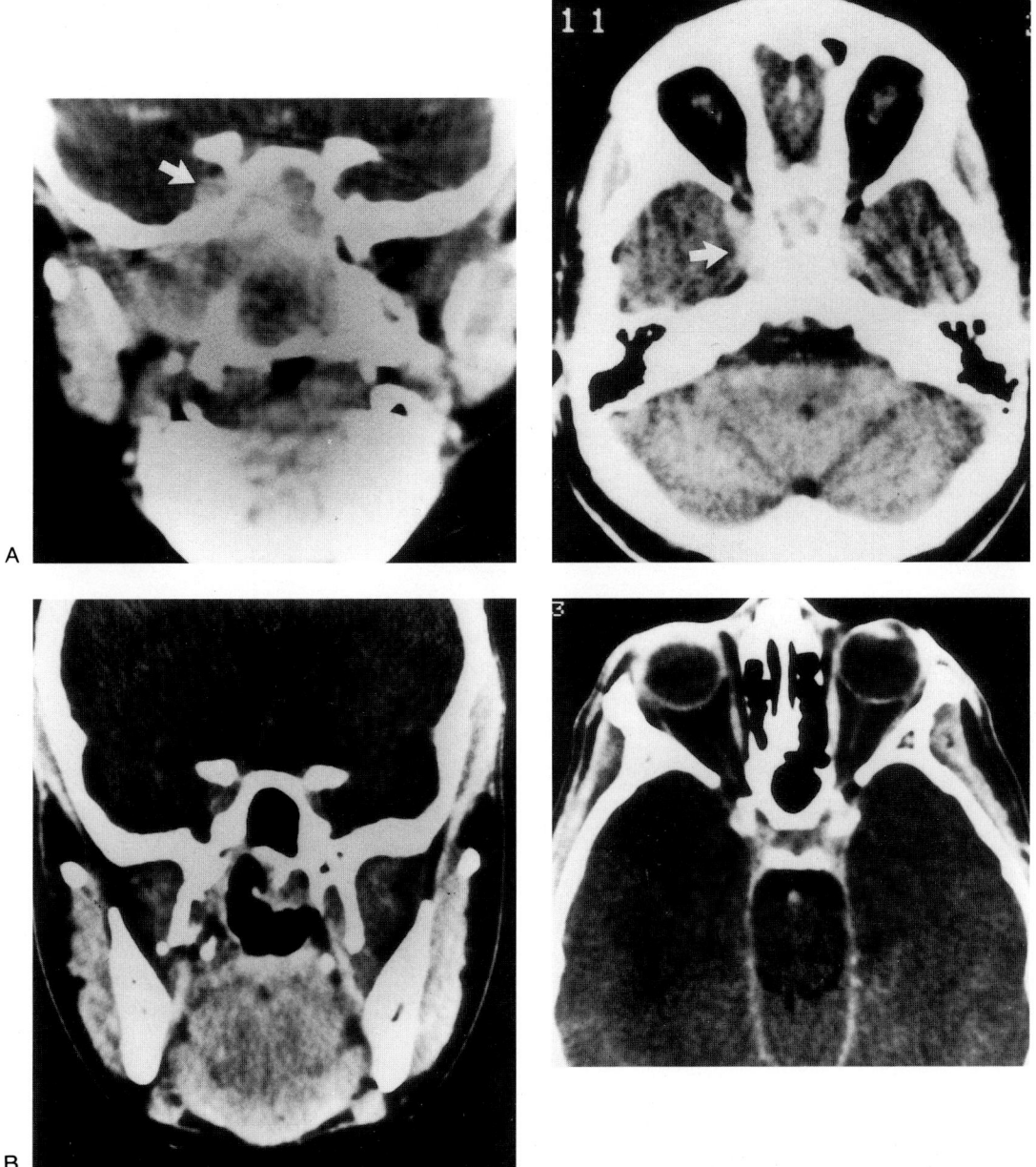

FIG. 7. A: Preoperative coronal and axial CT scans of Case 1. The *arrow* points to the small intracranial extension of the tumor. **B:** Scans of Case 1 taken 2 years postoperatively.

mor was removed but recurred and was operated again at age 16. At the time of his second recurrence, at age 18, there was evidence of intracranial extension in the parasellar region. Angiography did not show significant supply from the internal carotid artery and the transzygomatic and transpalatal approach was selected (Fig. 8A).

After 1 month of diethylstilbestrol therapy and preoperative embolization of major feeding vessels, the tumor was excised. There were no neurologic deficits postoperatively and $2\frac{1}{2}$ years later there was no clinical or radiologic evidence of recurrence (Fig. 8B).

Case 3

This 17-year-old boy presented to his physician with epistaxis and nasal obstruction. On examination there was a mass in the temporal fossa on the left. CT scan

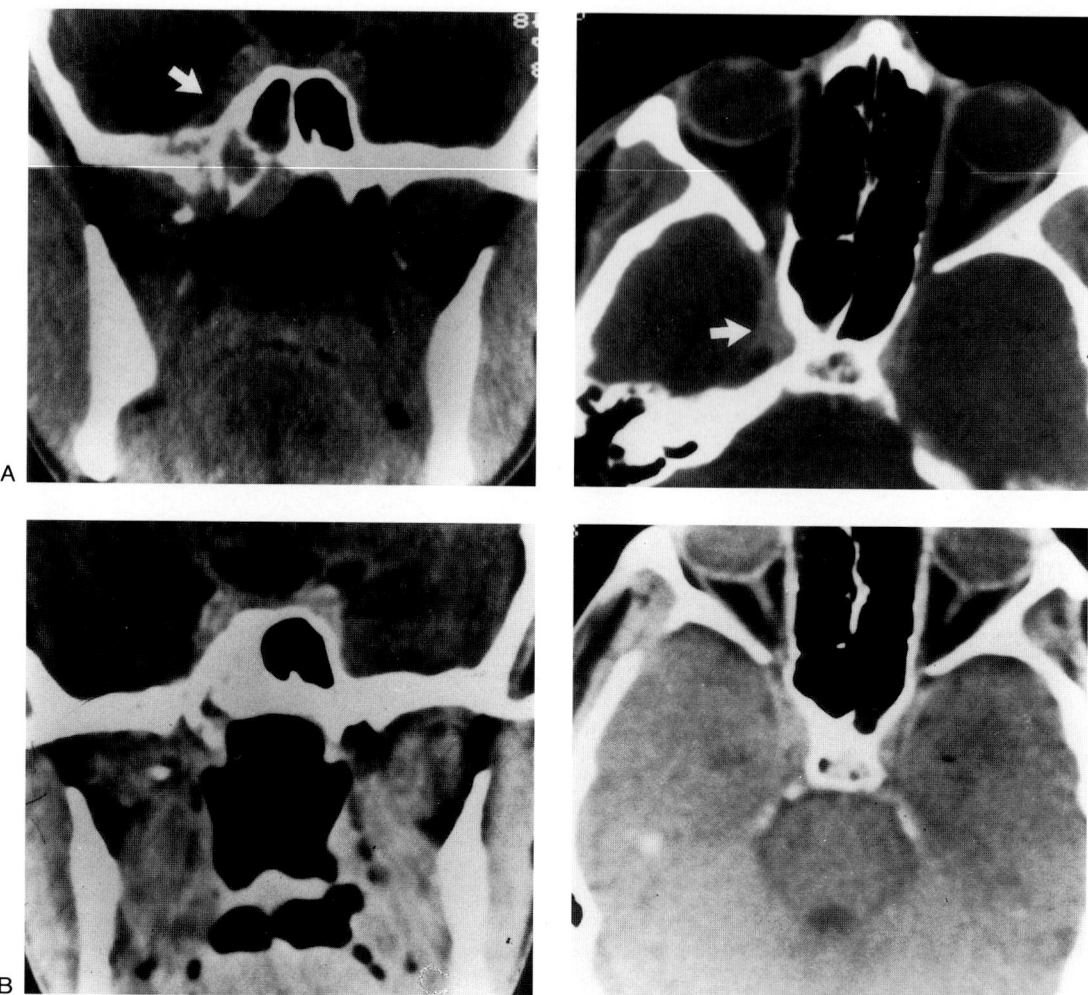

FIG. 8. A: Preoperative coronal and axial CT scans of Case 2. **B:** Scans of Case 2 taken 2 years postoperatively.

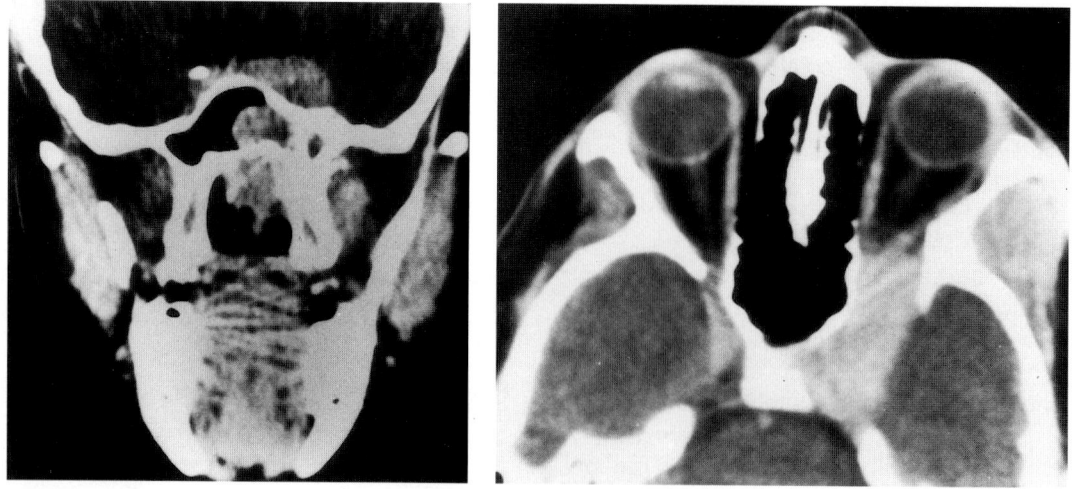

FIG. 9. A: Preoperative coronal and axial CT scans of Case 3. **B:** Preoperative carotid angiogram of Case 3 showing a small branch of the internal carotid artery feeding the tumor. **C:** Scans of Case 3 taken 4 years postoperatively.

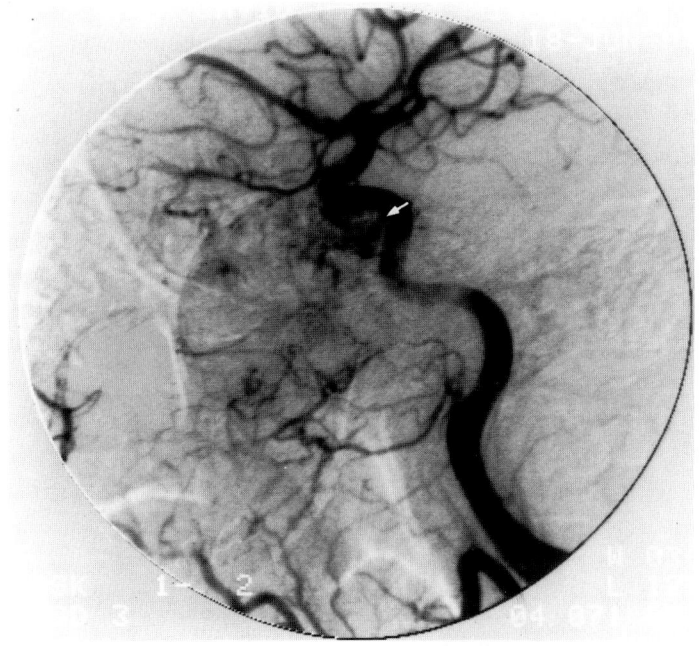

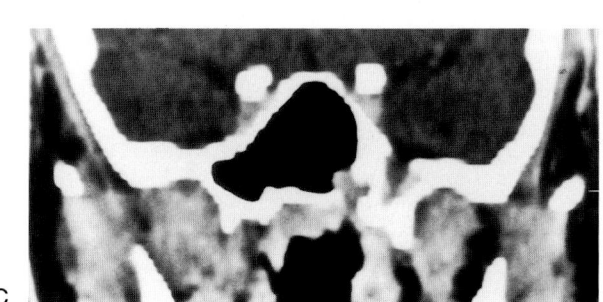
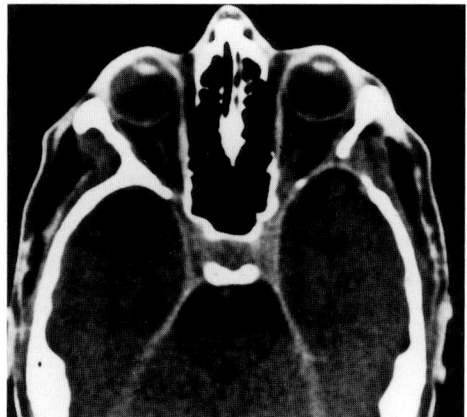

FIG. 9. Continued.

demonstrated significant intracranial extension in the left parasellar region with some erosion of the inferior orbital fissure (Fig. 9A). Angiography demonstrated one small feeding vessel from the internal carotid artery (Fig. 9B). He had no neurologic deficits.

The intracranial extension was delivered into the pharyngomaxillary space using an extended transzygomatic approach. Essentially, the entire sphenoid wing was removed, exposing the dura anterior to the temporal lobe. It was possible to develop a plane between the superior of the tumor and the dura and to displace the intracranial portion of the tumor into the pharyngomaxillary space. The tumor was then removed via the extended transpalatal tripartite approach.

Postoperatively there was a transient left VI nerve palsy. Four-year postoperative follow-up shows no clinical or radiographic evidence of tumor recurrence (Fig. 9C).

BIBLIOGRAPHY

1. Andrews JC, Fisch V, Valavanis A, Aeppli U, Makek MS. The surgical management of extensive nasopharyngeal angiofibromas with the infratemporal fossa approach. *Laryngoscope* 1989; 99:429–437.
2. Christiansen TA, Duvall AJ, Rosenberg A. Juvenile nasopharyngeal angiofibroma. *Trans AAOO* 1974;78:140–147.
3. Duvall AJ, Moreano AE. Juvenile nasopharyngeal angiofibroma: diagnosis and treatment. *Otolaryngol Head Neck Surg* 1987; 97:534–540.
4. Gill G, Rice DH, Ritter FN, Kindt G, Russo HR. Intracranial and extracranial nasopharyngeal angiofibroma. *Arch Otolaryngol* 1976;102:371–373.
5. Haughey BH, Wilson JS, Barber CS. Massive angiofibroma: a surgical approach and adjunctive therapy. *Otolaryngol Head Neck Surg* 1988;98:618–624.
6. Iyer GV, Vaishya ND, Bhaktaviziam A, Taori GM, Abraham J. Angiofibroma of the middle cranial fossa. *J Neurosurg* 1971; 35:90–94.
7. Jafek BW, Krekkorian EA, Kirsch WM, Wood RP. Juvenile nasopharyngeal angiofibroma: management of intracranial extension. *Otolaryngol Head Neck Surg* 1979;2:119–128.

8. Krekorian EA, Kato RH. Surgical management of nasopharyngeal angiofibroma with intracranial extension. *Laryngoscope* 1977;87:154–164.
9. Krekorian EA, Kempe LG. The combined otolaryngology. Neurosurgery approach to extensive benign tumors. *Laryngoscope* 1969;79:2086–2103.
10. Mickey B, Close L, Schaefer S, Samson D. A combined frontotemporal and lateral infratemporal fossa approach to the skull base. *J Neurosurg* 1988;68:678–683.
11. Standefer J, Holt GR, Brown WE Jr, Gates GA. Combined intracranial and extracranial excision of nasopharyngeal angiofibroma. *Laryngoscope* 1983;93:772–779.

CHAPTER 34

Juvenile Angiofibroma

Wolfgang Draf

Juvenile nasopharyngeal angiofibroma (JNA) is a benign, slowly growing, very vascular, locally invasive, cone-shaped tumor. JNA has no true capsule and spreads beneath the mucosa (19). The tumor is covered by a pseudocapsule. Dissection of the tumor rarely causes severe bleeding as long as the pseudocapsule remains intact (14). Variation in the vascularity can occur in the same tumor (12). JNA is a rare tumor in Europe and the United States but is very common in Oriental countries, the Near and Far East. JNA occurs almost exclusively in adolescent males. Ward et al. (18), in 1974, reported 35 cases, and only 3 of them were females. The highest prevalence of JNA is between the ages of 14 and 25 years (8). The youngest patient reported to date is a 5-week-old child (11). The site of origin of JNA still remains unclear (16). In our opinion, two points ought to be emphasized:

1. JNA originates most frequently in the sphenopalatine foramen area.
2. Spread of the tumor occurs through the sphenopalatine foramen toward the pterygomaxillary fissure, pterygoid, and infratemporal fossae. This histologically benign, but clinically malignant tumor can grow into the nasal cavity, paranasal sinuses, nasopharynx, sphenoid sinus, and the clivus. Finger-shaped extensions may invade the orbit and middle cranial fossa (parasellar) and compress the cavernous sinus. We have not seen penetration of the wall and complete obliteration of the cavernous sinus by this tumor.

W. Draf: Department of Ear, Nose, and Throat Diseases, Head, Neck, and Facial Plastic Surgery, Communication Disorders, Klinikum Fulda, Teaching Hospital, University of Marburg, D6400 Fulda, Germany.

SPECIFIC DIAGNOSTIC CONSIDERATIONS AND PREOPERATIVE PLANNING

The diagnosis of JNA can be made on the basis of symptoms and radiological findings. The symptoms depend on the size of the tumor (Table 1). Nasal obstruction, nasal speech, cheek swelling, displacement of orbital contents, recurrent middle ear effusion, and headache have been the most frequent findings in our 11 cases operated from 1980 to 1991. Recurrent epistaxis was not as frequent as is stated in the textbooks. In 8 out of the 11 cases, the tumor was very extensive. Four of these patients showed intracranial extension. Three of them had cranial nerve deficits (deterioration of vision).

Preoperative planning should involve a head and neck surgeon, a neuroradiologist, a neurosurgeon (if needed), an anesthesiologist, and other specialties as needed.

Successful surgical strategy requires, preoperatively, (a) precise delineation of the tumor, (b) determination of the vascular supply, (c) relation to the neighboring structures, (d) correction of medical conditions (e.g., anemia, hypoglobulinemia), and (e) embolization (except in very small tumors) of all the feeding blood vessels. Therefore a high-resolution computerized tomography (CT) with multiplanar reconstruction and magnetic resonance imaging (MRI) are mandatory. Superselective digital substraction arteriography is indispensable. Following diagnostic angiography, embolization of tumor feeders from the external and even the internal carotid artery is done. Embolization reduces the blood loss during surgery and shrinks the tumor (9). The clinical and radiological findings of JNA are so characteristic that one can usually perform definitive surgery without a diagnostic biopsy. In the differential diagnosis, cavernomas, hemangiopericytoma, and very vascular malignant tumors,

TABLE 1. *Juvenile angiofibroma symptoms*

Main symptoms
    Nasal obstruction
    Nasal speech
    Cheek swelling
    Dislocation of orbital content
    Middle ear problems
    Headache
Other symptoms
    Recurrent bleeding
    Cranial nerve palsy

especially rhabdomyosarcoma, have to be kept in mind. If biopsy is done, it must be in the operating room rather than in the office, and one has to be prepared for transfusion.

PATIENT SELECTION

Opinions are divided concerning the potential for spontaneous remission of JNA during puberty (14). We have never observed this phenomenon. There are well-documented cases of regression of residual tumor following incomplete excision. We agree with many other authors that the treatment of choice is radical surgical removal (14,17–19). Patients are young and usually in good general condition. The tumor is slowly growing, leaving time for precise surgical planning. Visual impairment necessitates urgent surgery. In our opinion, contraindications for surgery are very rare, for example, medical contraindications for general anesthesia or too extensive intracranial spread (2,15). In the "giant-size" tumors, the life threatening complications can be reduced significantly by embolization of the feeding blood vessels, balloon occlusion of vessels, and use of the cell-saver machine (immediate retransfusion of the patient's blood).

The role of radiotherapy is controversial. There have been reports that radiotherapy can control JNA in 80–95% of cases. These results are similar to those achieved with surgery (5,15). Goepfert et al. (7) reported five cases of successful treatment with chemotherapy in recurrent and in inoperable tumors with a follow-up between 3 and 10 years. We feel that radiotherapy and chemotherapy should be considered only in inoperable cases, because of the young age of the patients and the possibility of carcinogenic effects of radiation 20–30 years later.

OPERATIVE TECHNIQUES

Anesthetic Considerations

A thorough discussion of the patient and the radiological findings with the anesthesiologist preoperatively is a must. It is ideal for the same anesthesiologist to be with the patient during the whole operation. In addition to general anesthesia, infiltration of local anesthetics mixed with suprarenin and topical decongestion with 10% cocaine solution help to reduce blood loss and keep the surgical field relatively clear. In JNA with cavernous sinus involvement, major blood loss during surgery is expected. The anesthesiologist has to prepare the cell-saver machine in every patient. This allows immediate transfusion of patient's blood (after filtration and washing) and enables the surgeon to continue tumor dissection in spite of major bleeding.

Positioning of the Patient

The patient is placed in the supine position and is intubated transorally. The face should be uncovered up to the hairline. Depending on the size of the tumor, we use five different operative techniques, divided into two groups: extracranial and extracranial–intracranial approaches (Table 2).

Extracranial Approach

Endonasal Micro-endoscopic Approach Without External Incision

This approach is used for extracranial tumors at an early stage, restricted to the nasal cavity, the ethmoid cell system, the nasopharyngeal roof, and the sphenoid sinus. Preoperative embolization is performed 2 days prior to surgery. The lacrimal sac is identified after removal of the lacrimal bone microsurgically. This is the anterior margin of the surgical field. To gain access to the frontal sinus infundibulum and the skull base, the lacrimal bone and part of the frontal process of the maxilla are removed by a diamond drill. The lamina papyracea is identified, which is the lateral margin of the surgical field. The mucosa around the tumor is incised. One should always try to perform an "en bloc" resection, which means ethmoidectomy along the skull base including resection of middle turbinate, and complete removal of the anterior wall of the sphenoid sinus. Finally, the nasal cavity is packed with "rubber-finger" tamponades. They should be fixed to the nasal dorsum to prevent aspiration.

TABLE 2. *Juvenile angiofibroma operative techniques*

Extracranial
    Endonasal Micro-endoscopic approach
    Midfacial degloving approach
    Transfacial approach through an extended Moure incision
Combined extracranial–intracranial
    Transfacial–anterior fossa approach
    Transfacial–transzygomatic approach

Midfacial Degloving Technique

Midfacial degloving (1,3,4) permits good unilateral or bilateral access to the nasal cavity and paranasal sinuses, the anterior base of the skull, and the clivus. The incisions in the nasal and oral vestibules do not leave visible scars (Fig. 1). This approach is suitable for angiofibromas that do not extend intracranially.

In the midfacial degloving approach, the four incisions have to be combined (Fig. 1): the intercartilaginous incision, the transfixion incision of the nasal septum, the circumvestibular incision, and the transoral sublabial incision. The midfacial skin and soft tissue are elevated subperiostally until the glabella, the infraorbital rim, and the tuber maxillare. Through the sublabial subperiosteal elevation, the nasal incisions are reached, allowing the nasal soft tissue to be lifted up leaving the upper lateral cartilages in place. The infraorbital nerves are preserved. With a saw, osteoplastic bone grafts are made from the frontal process of the maxilla and the anterior wall of the maxillary sinus. This gives sufficient exposure of the nasal cavity, paranasal sinuses, clivus, and the pterygopalatine as well as the infratemporal fossae. The resection of tumor is followed by replacement and fixing of the osteoplastic bone grafts with microplates (10), which guarantees maximal stability with minimal foreign material. The most recent advance in this technique is the use of glass-ionomer bone cement. This material bonds bone grafts chemically and is extremely stable. Any metal is avoided. There is no need for secondary surgical removal of plates. Before fixation of the bone grafts, the surgical cavity is lined with a larger piece of silicone film to promote mucosal epithelialization. The sheet is held in place for about 3 weeks by gauze, moistened with antibiotic ointment.

Transfacial Technique Through an Extended Moure Incision

This technique (13,16) is suitable for most of the large JNAs extending into all paranasal sinuses, pterygopalatine, pterygoid and infratemporal fossae, the orbit, and the parasphenoidal and parasellar regions. The tumor must be extradural and must not extend deep into the anterior and middle cranial fossae or the clivus. The lateral rhinotomy technique enables access to tumor that is parallel to the skull base. This means better control of bleeding and better visualization of the tumor and its relation to the dura, enabling safer dissection. In our experience, this is the most versatile technique for nearly all major lesions. It allows excellent exposure of the tumor and the possibility of dissecting around it under optimal vision.

The outer incision starts beneath the eyebrow and extends paranasally toward the upper lip. Its length depends on the extent of the tumor. If the JNA has grown deep into the infratemporal fossa, Moure's lateral rhinotomy incision should be lengthened with a steplike lip incision, creating a large cheek flap. The soft tissue and the periosteum including the periorbit have to be stripped off from the bone as far lateral as the tumor exposure demands. The lacrimal sac is freed. One or two osteoplastic bone grafts of the frontal process of maxilla and the anterior maxillary sinus wall, similar to the degloving technique, are prepared. The infraorbital foramen and the infraorbital nerve are preserved during dissection of the cheek flap and anterior maxillary sinus wall bone graft. After that, the inferior border of the infraorbital canal is drilled off with a diamond burr, allowing lateral displacement and preservation of the infraorbital nerve during further surgery.

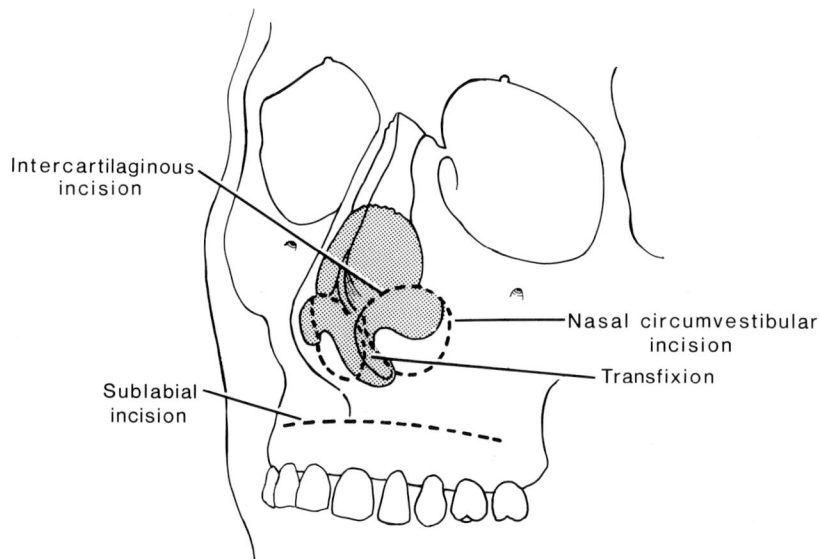

FIG. 1. Incisions for midfacial degloving approach (1).

For optimal functional lacrimal drainage, we have developed a special technique (Fig. 2) (6). After removal of the osteoplastic bone graft, the nasolacrimal drainage system is dissected until the nasal mucosa. The orifice of the nasolacrimal duct in the inferior nasal meatus can be outlined in the nasal mucosa with a scalpel. The duct and lacrimal sac are temporarily retracted out of the surgical field. The microscope is essential for tumor dissection from the nasopharyngeal roof, out of the orbit, the sphenoid sinus, the parasellar region, and the clivus. The diamond burr helps to smooth out the rough edges of the bone. Bleeding stops after the tumor has been resected in total. Frozen sections from suspicious margins will ensure complete resection. After completion of tumor resection, the funnel-shaped stump with the orifice of the nasolacrimal duct is sutured onto the nasal mucosa. At the end of the procedure, the cavity is lined with a silicone film as previously described. The bone grafts are fixed as mentioned in the degloving technique. For the skin, 6-0 monofilament material is preferred. After a few months, the scar is almost invisible.

Combined Extracranial–Intracranial Approach

In very rare cases with tremendous intracranial extension, the transfacial approach alone may be too danger-

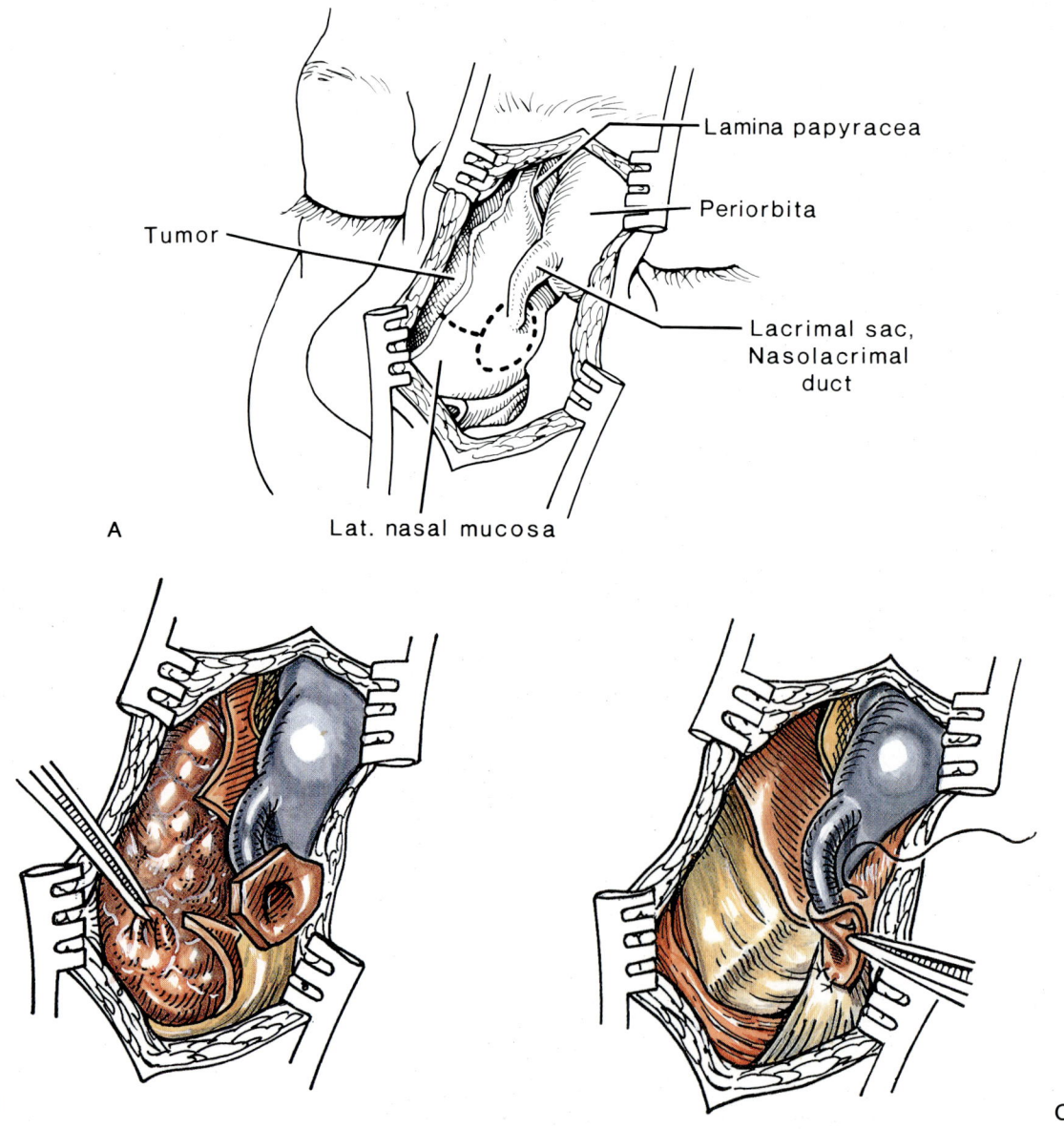

FIG. 2. Preservation of lacrimal drainage in the resection of nasal and paranasal sinus tumors (16). **A:** The orifice of the nasolacrimal duct is outlined with a scalpel in the nasal mucosa. **B:** The mobilized ductal orifice is retracted to the side. The nasal cavity tumor is removed with the adjacent mucosa. **C:** At the end of the operation, the stump of the nasolacrimal duct is sutured into the cheek flap with the opening directed nasally. Care is taken to avoid kinking of the duct.

ous. Under those circumstances, it may be combined with the transfrontal–intradural approach to the anterior fossa (for details see ref. 16) or with the direct lateral (transzygomatic) intradural or extradural approach. It has to be pointed out that these combined procedures are necessary only in those rare exceptions where a single tumor approach does not guarantee sufficient visualization of tumor and the surrounding tissue.

The microsurgical technique prevents injury to the infraorbital nerve. The biggest challenge to the surgeon is bleeding from the cavernous sinus. Before an attempt is made to dissect the tumor from the cavernous sinus, the blood volume should be balanced or even overcorrected if major blood loss is expected. Another problem could be to remove the intraorbital part of the tumor. The microscope is indispensable for atraumatic dissection in this delicate region.

POSTOPERATIVE MANAGEMENT

Lining of the postsurgical cavity with silastic film promotes mucosal re-epithelialization and reduces the frequency and duration of postoperative care. After removal of packing and silastic sheet, saline irrigations of the cavity are to be done daily by the patient. Periodic crust removal and cleaning of the cavity is to be done by the physician.

A follow-up CT is to be done 6 weeks postoperatively. This is an important baseline for follow-up. If there is residual tumor, plans for additional treatment should be made as soon as possible.

COMPLICATIONS AND MANAGEMENT

Proper preoperative workup, proper embolization, and proper and precise surgery done by an experienced surgeon drastically reduce the complication rate. Complications may arise preoperatively during angiography and embolization (e.g., spasm, embolization or thrombosis of cerebral vessels). Fortunately, those complications are rare in skilled hands. Their management falls under the responsibility of the interventional radiologist.

Severe intraoperative complications (e.g., bleeding and subsequent hypoxia) are the most serious ones. This can be prevented by:

1. Proper preoperative embolization.
2. "Cell-saver" during surgery.
3. General anesthesia with hypotension.
4. Additional local anesthesia.
5. Combination of macrosurgery and microsurgery.

Infiltration of the dura by tumor requires resection of invaded dura and immediate reconstruction to prevent CSF leak. Fortunately, JNA infiltrates the dura very rarely.

Postoperatively, delayed CSF leak may stop spontaneously, if duraplasty has been performed after tumor excision. If CSF leak persists after 8 days, lumbar drainage is advised. If the cavernous sinus is packed, a paresis of the oculomotor and/or abducens nerve may occur. This paresis may improve after a few days or weeks. One may avoid this sequela by gentle packing and the use of fibrin glue.

Another postoperative complication is impaired lacrimal drainage. We feel that the treatment of choice is endonasal microsurgical dacryocystorhinotomy. Using our technique of dissection of the lacrimal duct, we have never encountered this complication.

Crusting is another postoperative sequela. This occurs whenever there is a large cavity not lined by mucosa. Crusting can be diminished to a significant degree if the cavity is not lined with split thickness skin grafts, but rather with a silicone sheet, as described previously. Regular endoscopic guided cleaning of the cavity and application of antibiotic ointment will shorten the duration of crusting.

Long-term follow-up is important to prevent late complications. Facial deformity and eye displacement may occur some years after extensive resection of facial and orbital bone during tumor removal. To prevent this disfigurement, the osteoplastic bone graft technique should be used. Another long-term "complication" is tumor recurrence. This has been reduced in the last decade because of the following factors:

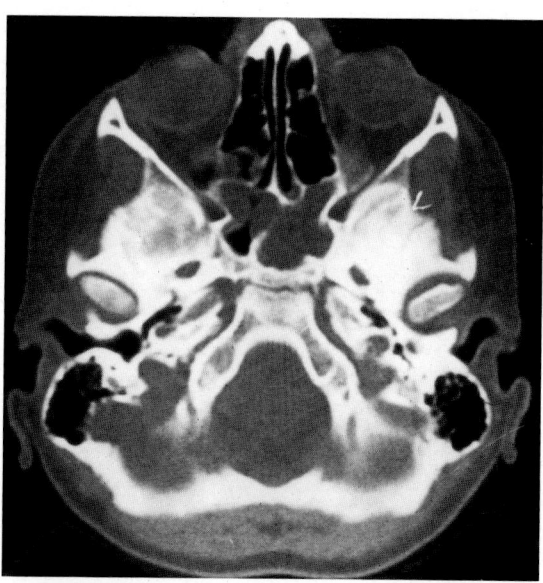

FIG. 3. Six-year-old boy with a small, early stage of juvenile angiofibroma in the right sphenoid sinus. Axial CT scan showing ethmoid cell system free of tumor. There was opacification of the right sphenoid sinus and thickening of mucosal lining in the left sphenoid sinus. No major bone destruction was noted.

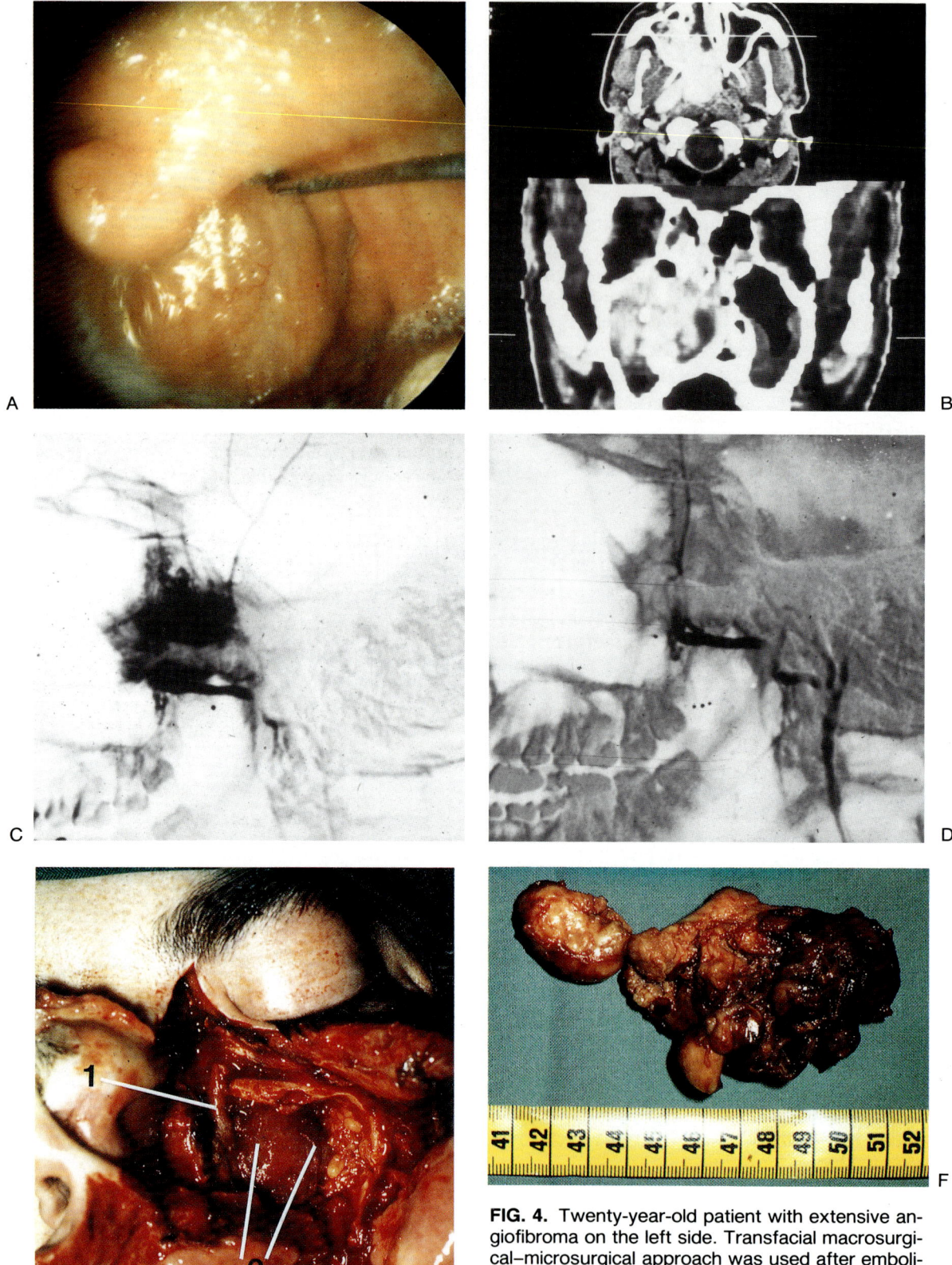

FIG. 4. Twenty-year-old patient with extensive angiofibroma on the left side. Transfacial macrosurgical–microsurgical approach was used after embolization. Reconstruction of facial skeleton was done. **A:** Transoral view of a large tumor behind the uvula. **B:** Axial CT scan and frontal reconstruction showing tumor extension. **C:** Superselective angiography: very vascular tumor seen before embolization. **D:** After embolization, no feeding blood vessels to the tumor are seen. **E:** Exposure of the nasolacrimal duct (1); the tumor (2) is seen in the infratemporal fossa. **F:** Tumor specimen.

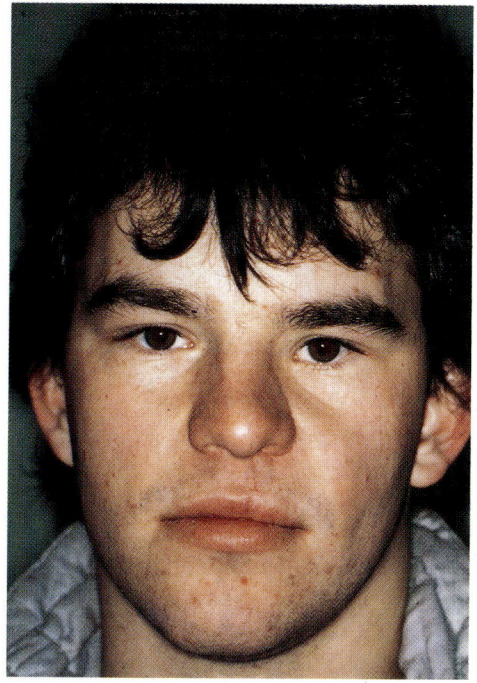
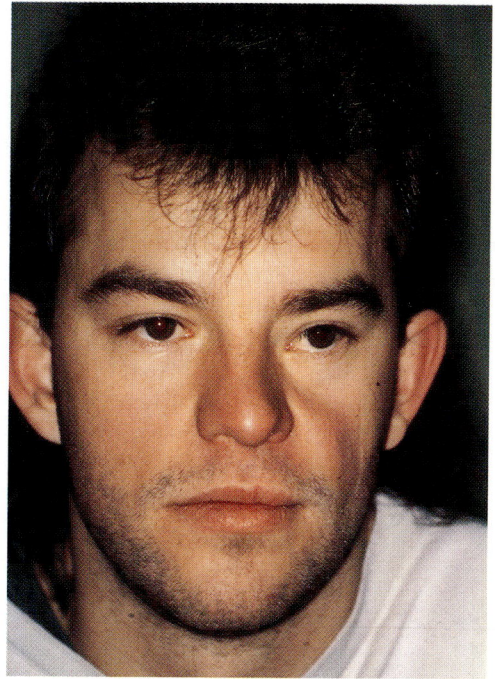

FIG. 4. *Continued.* **G:** Patient, 1 year after surgery, with slight facial deformity. **H:** Patient, 3 years after surgery, with more obvious facial disfigurement and displacement of the left eye.

1. Precise preoperative determination of tumor extension and its blood supply.
2. Preoperative embolization.
3. Macrosurgical and microsurgical tumor resection.
4. Interdisciplinary approach, when necessary.

If tumor recurs, surgery is to be repeated as soon as possible. Only patients that are not suitable for surgery should be treated with chemotherapy or radiotherapy.

ILLUSTRATIVE CASES

The different surgical approaches that can be used are demonstrated in the following cases.

Case 1

This 6-year-old boy suffered from nasal obstruction (Fig. 3). CT scans showed normal ethmoidal cells on both sides, complete opacification of the right sphenoid sinus, and some mucosal swelling in the inferior part of the left sphenoid. Biopsy from the right sphenoid sinus (done in another hospital) revealed juvenile angiofibroma.

The patient was referred to us for further treatment. He underwent endonasal micro-endoscopic surgery and removal of the tumor, including the mucosa of the right sphenoid sinus and the nasopharyngeal roof. Histopathology revealed remnants of tumor in the right sphenoid sinus. The nasopharyngeal roof and the left sphenoid sinus have been free of tumor. The postoperative course was uneventful. The boy is free of disease since surgery 2 years ago.

Comment. This was a small early-stage juvenile angiofibroma with atypical localization in the right sphenoid sinus. The endonasal micro-endoscopic approach was sufficient for complete resection.

Case 2

This 20-year-old male had nasal blockage secondary to a nasopharyngeal tumor seen on CT scan (Fig. 4). The tumor involved the left paranasal sinuses and the pterygopalatine and pterygoid fossae. Angiography confirmed an extremely vascular lesion. The diagnosis of juvenile angiofibroma seemed to be justified without biopsy. Complete embolization of all feeding vessels originating from the external carotid artery was done. The macrosurgical and microsurgical en bloc resection of tumor was achieved via a transfacial approach through an extended Moure incision with upper lip splitting and temporary lateral displacement of the nasolacrimal drainage system from the surgical field. No reconstruction of the facial skeleton was done. Total blood loss was only about 300 cc because of embolization. The postoperative cavity was temporarily lined with a silicone sheet. Healing was uneventful. Three months after surgery, an excellent mucosal lining was present. One year after surgery, the esthetic appearance was satisfying. Three years postoperatively, one can see some disfigurement of the left face, with displacement of the eye and loss of facial bone, because of scar retraction. The skin incision is almost invisible. Seven years after surgery, the patient remains free of recurrence and shows normal lacrimal drainage.

Comment. After embolization, through a transfacial approach, using macrosurgical and microsurgical techniques, en bloc resection of an extensive angiofibroma was done. The blood loss was minimal. The nasolacrimal drainage has been preserved. No crusting of the cavity occurred after 3 months because of sufficient mucosal lining. Because of a partial unilateral resection of maxilla without facial reconstruction, the esthetic result was not perfect. There was no recurrence 7 years after operation.

Case 3

A 12-year-old boy was referred to us because of swelling of the left cheek (Fig. 5). A large angiofibroma on the left side was found, involving nasal cavity, all sinuses, nasopharynx, pterygopalatine, pterygoid and infratemporal fossae, as well as the orbit and the clivus with intracranial extension, compressing the left cavernous sinus. After embolization, a macrosurgical and microsurgical transfacial approach with extended Moure incision was chosen. The anterior walls of the maxillary, ethmoid, and frontal sinus have been temporarily removed as bone grafts. The nasolacrimal duct and the infraorbital nerve were dissected and preserved by swinging them out of the surgical field. There was minimal bleeding during dissection of the tumor. However, major bleeding did occur when the tumor was dissected from the cavernous sinus. This was expected, and therefore the cell-saver was used. About 2000 cc of filtrated blood were autotransfused. The lesion was removed in one piece. The mucosa of the frontal sinus including part of the inner table was drilled out. The small frontal sinus was obliterated with orbital contents. Bone grafts have been bonded with a new bone cement (Ionos glass-ionomer, under clinical study), which connects chemically with bone. Therefore miniplates have been avoided. Before closing, the cavity was lined with a silicone sheet. Three months after surgery, no more crusting occurred, and a nice mucosal lining was endoscopically confirmed. Postoperative CT scan showed complete tumor removal. The esthetic appearance is satisfying.

Comment. This is an extremely large juvenile angiofibroma in a 12-year-old boy with compression of the cavernous sinus. In spite of complete occlusion of tumor feeding vessels, major blood loss from the cavernous sinus occurred as expected. The cell-saver allowed autotransfusion of almost 2000 cc. The tumor was removed completely and in one piece. Preservation of the lacrimal drainage system and infraorbital nerve was achieved.

The facial skeleton has been reconstructed with osteoplastic bone grafts and bone cement. The postoperative course was uneventful. Minimal crusting occurred after re-epithelialization of the cavity with mucous membrane under a silicone sheet.

Case 4

This 16-year-old boy suffered from a very extensive and fast growing tumor in the left nasal cavity, ethmoidal cell system, frontal sinus, both sphenoid sinuses, pterygopalatine, pterygoid, and infratemporal fossae, and left orbit, with extensive involvement of the anterior and middle cranial fossae with compression of the cavernous sinus and invasion of the clivus (Fig. 6). Clinically, swelling of the cheek and a left exophthalmos have been noted. The parents refused surgery, which was advised 2 years ago. In an attempt to diminish the growth, embolization was made elsewhere without success. Because of rapid growth of the tumor, headache, and increasing facial deformity, the parents agreed to our plan of treatment:

1. Embolization to be done in our hospital, which was performed successfully in spite of the many feeding blood vessels (both external and internal carotid arteries and left vertebral artery).
2. Extensive surgery. Because of tumor extension into the cavernous sinus and clivus, a severe blood loss during surgery was expected. Therefore the cell-saver machine was used. The tumor was excised through a combination of extracranial–intracranial technique via transfacial and direct lateral (16), transzygomatic, and osteoplastic approaches. The dissection of the huge tumor was extremely difficult because of extensive adhesions to the dura and cavernous sinus. The blood loss was severe. Several surgical interruptions were necessary during the 15 hr of surgery. With the cell-saver, 9000 cc of blood were autotransfused. Finally, the tumor was microscopically excised in one piece. A small dural leak at the cavernous sinus was closed with a preserved dural graft and fibrin glue. The lacrimal drainage and the infraorbital nerve were preserved. The infraorbital rim was destroyed by the tumor and was reconstructed with stored cartilage and miniplates. The osteoplastic bone graft was reinserted and fixed with vicryl sutures. The cavity was covered with a large piece of silicone sheet. The only postoperative complication was the transient abducens nerve paresis. CT scan performed 3 months postoperatively showed a nice smooth cavity without tumor. The patient is free of recurrence for 4 years. The facial appearance is acceptable.

Comment. This was an extremely large tumor with blood supply from all major blood vessels except the

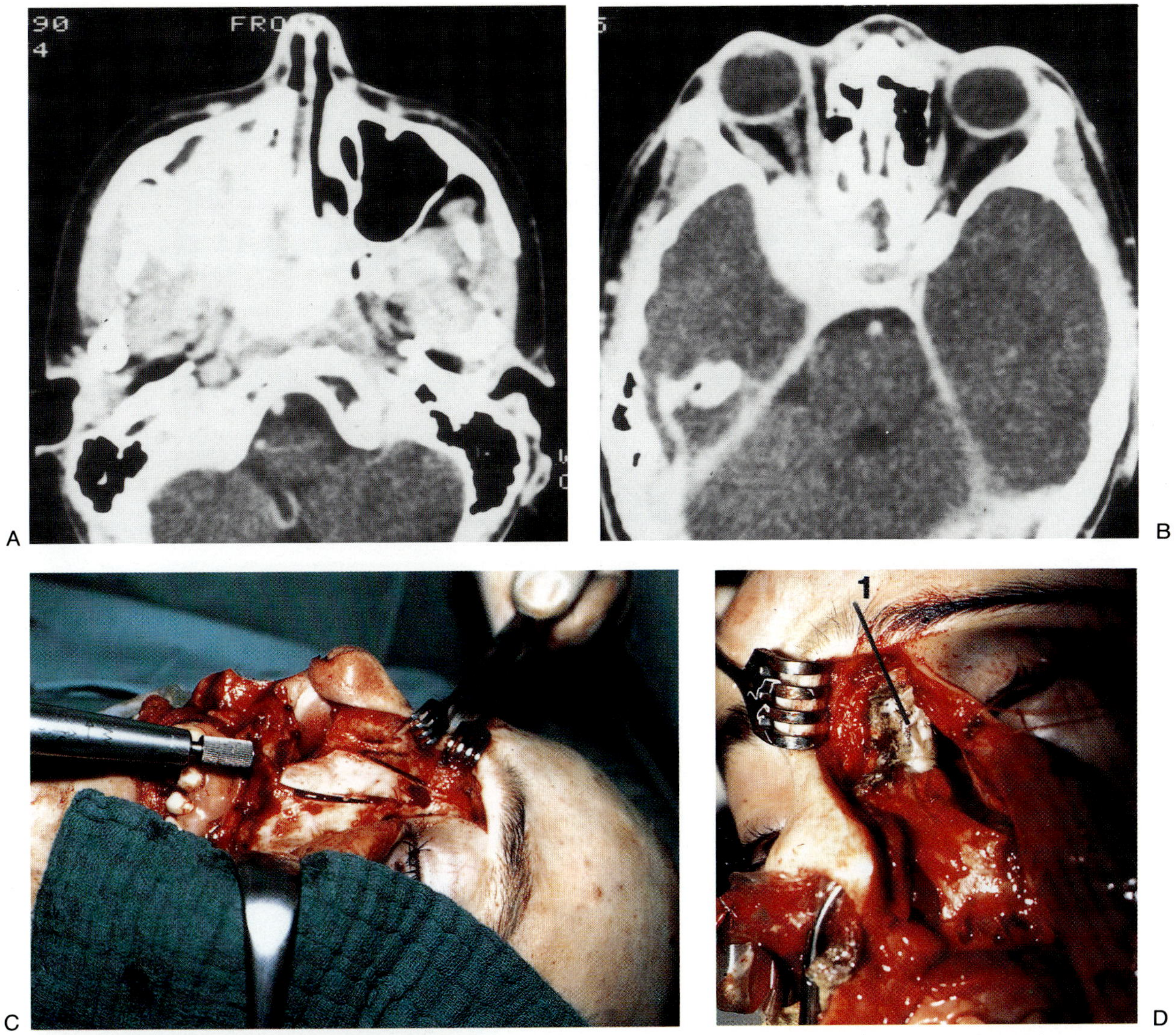

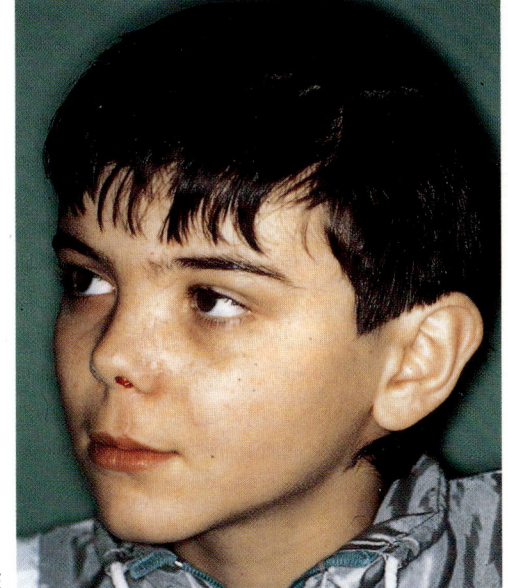

FIG. 5. Extremely extensive juvenile angiofibroma in a 12-year-old boy with compression of the cavernous sinus. Transfacial osteoplastic technique was employed. Reconstruction of facial skeleton was done with new glass-ionomer bone cement. **A:** Axial CT scan showing a large tumor. **B:** Intracranial part of the tumor, compressing the cavernous sinus. **C:** Outline of the bone grafts with a saw. **D:** Reconstruction of facial skeleton with bone cement (1). **E:** The boy, 6 months after surgery.

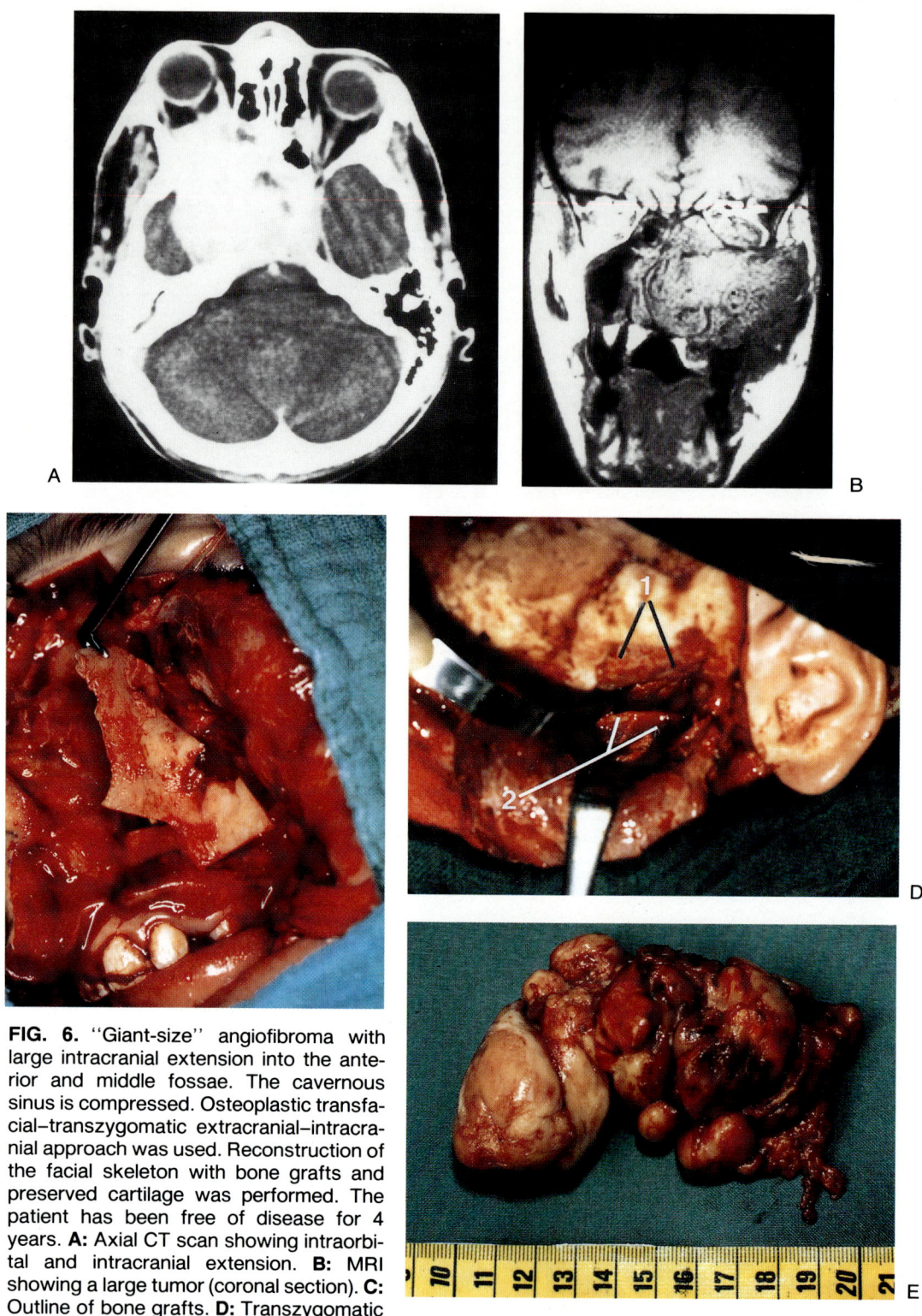

FIG. 6. "Giant-size" angiofibroma with large intracranial extension into the anterior and middle fossae. The cavernous sinus is compressed. Osteoplastic transfacial–transzygomatic extracranial–intracranial approach was used. Reconstruction of the facial skeleton with bone grafts and preserved cartilage was performed. The patient has been free of disease for 4 years. **A:** Axial CT scan showing intraorbital and intracranial extension. **B:** MRI showing a large tumor (coronal section). **C:** Outline of bone grafts. **D:** Transzygomatic approach with partial removal of squama temporalis. 1, Temporal lobe; 2, lateral part of intracranial tumor. **E:** Tumor specimen —left nasal, right lateral part.

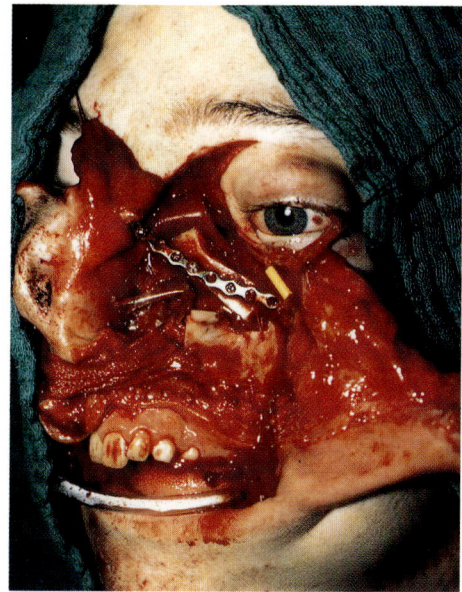
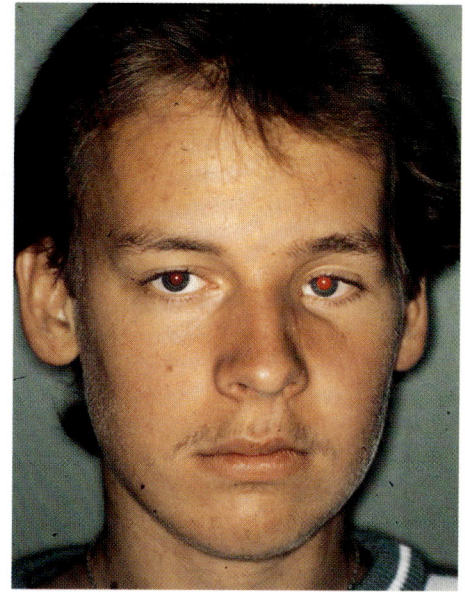

FIG. 6. *Continued.* **F:** Facial reconstruction. Infraorbital nerve was preserved. Miniplate with preserved cartilage was used for reconstruction of the infraorbital rim. **G:** The boy 1 year after surgery.

right vertebral artery. The tumor was approached by a combined transfacial transzygomatic macrosurgical–microsurgical extracranial–intracranial approach. The cell-saver was used. This proved to be of the utmost importance in saving the patient's life. The combined approach allowed complete tumor removal without excessive bone resection.

AUTHOR'S EXPERIENCE

Since 1980, we have treated 11 cases in our department, all males between 6 and 24 years of age. All but one had the tumor on the left side. We could not find any explanation for that. The majority of the patients had very large tumors involving the paranasal sinuses, pterygopalatine, pterygoid, and infratemporal fossae, and the orbit. Three cases had tumor extension into the parasellar region and the cavernous sinus.

In three cases, vision had deteriorated preoperatively. After decompression of the orbit and optic nerve, the visual field improved. No further deterioration of vision occurred postoperatively.

All cases but one (early angiofibroma) have been embolized preoperatively. In one patient, a transient hemiparesis occurred as a complication after embolization in another hospital. There were no major permanent neurological deficits. The patient is free of tumor 8 years after surgery.

One 6-year-old boy was operated by our endonasal micro-endoscopic technique because the tumor was restricted to the sphenoid sinus floor on one side. Two different pathologists made the diagnosis of JNA.

Except for two cases, all the other patients have been operated transfacially via a lateral rhinotomy approach, the first half of the patients without reconstruction of the facial skeleton, the second half with reconstructive techniques.

In two cases, a combined approach was necessary. In one patient, because of tumor recurrence, the transfacial-transpalatal approach was used; in the second a transfacial-transzygomatic approach was applied. None of the patients had lacrimal problems postoperatively. The infraorbital nerve was preserved in the latter two-thirds of our patients.

In this series, there was one recurrence in the first case in 1980. We believe that the real tumor extension was not clearly defined by CT of the first generation. Therefore a smaller part in the lateral pterygopalatine fissure was missed during surgery. The recurrence became obvious 2 years later. At that time, we combined the transpalatal and transfacial approach to resect the tumor. In addition, radiotherapy was performed postoperatively. This young man is now free of disease for 8 years. The other cases do not show any evidence of recurrence within a postoperative follow-up between 1 and 11 years.

At present, we believe that the transfacial osteoplastic macroscopic–microscopic approach is suitable in most cases. It allows preservation of facial contour, nasolacrimal drainage, and the infraorbital nerve as well as vision. In some cases, the visual field can be improved by decompression of the orbit and the optic nerve. For small early stage tumors, the endonasal micro-endoscopical route is an ideal one. In larger, but not too extensive, tumors, the midfacial degloving procedure may be used. Only "giant-sized" angiofibromas require the combined extracranial–intracranial approach. Embolization and the cell-saver machine are indispensable to reduce blood loss.

ACKNOWLEDGMENTS

We would like to acknowledge the cooperation of and to express our profound thanks to Professor Dr. R. Bässler, Director of the Institute of Pathology, Fulda Hospital; Professor Dr. J. P. Haas, Director of Radiologic Institute, Fulda Hospital; Dr. G. Kahle, Senior Assistant in our Radiologic Institute; Professor Dr. H. P. Richter, former Director of the Department of Neurosurgery, Fulda Hospital, now head of the Department of Neurosurgery, University of Ulm-Günzburg; and Professor Dr. M. Samii, Director of the Department of Neurosurgery, Nordstadt Hospital Hannover, Medizinische Hochschule Hannover.

REFERENCES

1. Berghaus A. The midfacial degloving. *HNO* 1990;38:7–11.
2. Bryant TDR, Fitzpatrick PJ, Book H. The radiological treatment of juvenile nasopharyngeal angiofibromas. *ORL* 1970;79:1108.
3. Casson PR, Bonnano PC, Converse JM. The midfacial degloving procedure. *Plast Reconstr Surg* 1974;53:102–113.
4. Conley JJ, Price. Sublabial approach to the nasal and nasopharyngeal cavities. *Am J Surg* 1979;138:615–618.
5. Cummings BJ. Relative risk factors in the treatment of juvenile nasopharyngeal angiofibroma. *Otolaryngol Head Neck Surg* 1980;3:21.
6. Draf W. Surgery of the anterior skull base (course). Hannover, 1980.
7. Goepfert H, Cangir A, Lee Y. Chemotherapy for aggressive juvenile nasopharyngeal angiofibroma. *Arch Otolaryngol* 1985;111:285–289.
8. Krause ChJ, Baker SR. Extended transantral approach to pterygomaxillary tumors. *Ann Otolaryngol* 1982;91:391–398.
9. Lasjaunias P, Berenstein A. *Surgical neuroangiography*. Berlin: Springer, 1987.
10. Luhr HG. Indications for use of a microsystem for internal fixation in craniofacial surgery. *J Craniofac Surg* 1988;1:35–51.
11. Martin H, Ehrlich HE, Abels JC. Juvenile nasopharyngeal fibroma. *Ann Surg* 1948;127:513–536.
12. McCombe A, Lund VJ, Howard DJ. Recurrence in juvenile angiofibromas. *Rhinology* 1990;28:97–102.
13. Moure P. Extracranial approach to the anterior skull base with preservation of the orbital content and lacrimal drainage system. (1902, quoted by Zange.) In: Thiel R, ed. *Ophthalmologische Operationlehre*. Leipzig: Thieme, 1959.
14. Neel III HB, Whicker JH, Devine DK, Weiland LH. Juvenile angiofibroma: review of 120 cases. *Am J Surg* 1973;126:547–556.
15. Panje WR, Gross CE. In: Thawley StE, Panje WR, eds. *Comprehensive management of head and neck tumors*. Philadelphia: Saunders, 1987; 678ff.
16. Samii M, Draf W. *Surgery of the skull base. An interdisciplinary approach*. Berlin: Springer, 1989;160,200.
17. Waldmann STR, Levine HL, Astor F, Wood BG, Weinstein M, Tucker HM. Surgical experience with nasopharyngeal angiofibroma. *Arch Otolaryngol* 1981;107:677–682.
18. Ward PH, Thompson R, Calcaterra Th, Kadin MR. Juvenile angiofibroma: a more rational therapeutic approach based upon clinical and experimental evidence. *Laryngoscope* 1974;84:2181–2194.
19. Zehm S. Geschwülste des Nasenrachens. In: Berendes J, Link R, Zöllner F, eds. *Hals-Nasen-Ohren-Heilkunde in Praxis und Klinik, vol 2. Obere und untere Luftwege*. Stuttgart: Thieme, 1977.

CHAPTER 35

Nasal/Paranasal Sinus Carcinoma

Ivo P. Janecka, Laligam N. Sekhar, and Eugene N. Myers

Neoplasms of paranasal sinuses are rare with annual incidence, in the general population, of approximately 0.07/100,000. In this group of neoplasms, malignant tumors are more frequent than benign ones (6.7:1) and the majority of them originate in the maxillary sinus. Histologically, squamous cell carcinoma is most prevalent (1).

The topographic proximity of all paranasal sinuses to key anatomic structures (brain, eye, internal carotid artery) makes malignant neoplasms involving these sinuses difficult to treat. The frequently encountered delays in establishing a diagnosis contribute to the development of the advanced stage of most malignant paranasal sinus tumors prior to treatment.

Patients with paranasal sinus carcinoma demonstrate only 25–30% five-year survival despite combined treatment with surgery and radiotherapy (2,3). Several factors contribute to the limited benefit of traditional surgical therapy: (a) large tumor volume and (b) frequently positive surgical margins. Both of these factors have great negative influence on patients' overall oncological prognosis.

New techniques of cranial base surgery can extend the available anatomic margin for oncological surgery of paranasal sinus cancer. This is reflected in a greater number of tumor-free margins of surgical specimens, which should ultimately be expressed in greater oncologic control of paranasal sinus malignancies.

I. P. Janecka: Center for Cranial Base Surgery, University of Pittsburgh School of Medicine, Presbyterian University Hospital, and Department of Otolaryngology, Eye and Ear Institute, Pittsburgh, Pennsylvania 15213.
L. N. Sekhar: Department of Neurosurgery, Center for Cranial Base Surgery, University of Pittsburgh School of Medicine, Presbyterian University Hospital, Pittsburgh, Pennsylvania 15213.
E. N. Myers: Department of Otolaryngology, University of Pittsburgh School of Medicine, and Eye and Ear Institute, Pittsburgh, Pennsylvania 15213.

DIAGNOSIS

The first symptoms of paranasal sinus neoplasia are usually related to sinus obstruction/inflammation or cranial nerve involvement (cranial nerves I–VI). Nasal bleeding and eustachian tube obstruction are more related to specific tumors (angiofibroma, olfactory neuroblastoma) or a particular site (lateral nasopharynx or infratemporal fossa).

Diagnostic evaluation of suspected paranasal sinus malignancy is directed toward several goals:

1. The determination of tumor extent—its size as well as the tumor's extracranial and/or intracranial relationship to key anatomic structures.
2. The classification of tumor biology (benign versus malignant, histologic type, tumor vascularity, and status of pertinent major vessels and their contribution to cerebral circulation).
3. The exploration of therapeutic options (single or multiple modality) and their time sequence.
4. Systemic evaluation in order to rule out metastatic disease and also to determine the extent of patient's tolerance to potential therapeutic options.
5. Procurement of patient's participation (understanding of diagnosis and therapeutic options).

The determination of *tumor extent* is currently performed with CT or MRI scans. CT utilizes the advantages of bone visibility or evidence of its destruction, especially using bony algorithms. Contrast enhanced images suggest tumor perimeter. MRI complements the CT evaluation in terms of tumor extent and its relationship to the CNS, eye, and ICA. It also helps in distinguishing the presence of blood/mucus from the tumor in the paranasal sinus. In addition, it further highlights the neoplastic components of the main tumor mass (e.g., vessels, necrotic areas). As in other cranial base regions, CT is the preferred imaging modality for osseous, fibro-osseous, or chondroid lesions. MRI is the primary modality for soft tissue tumors.

The possible pitfalls of imaging include the following:

1. Recent bleeding, mucus obstruction, biopsy-induced swelling—all may erroneously suggest a more extensive tumor.
2. Signal voids on MRI that are frequently a reflection of tumor vasculature may represent signal voids from spicules of bone within the tumor.

The diagnostic evaluation of *tumor biology* is best determined preoperatively by a biopsy. CT and MRI may give a strong clue as to the tumor type, but there is no substitution for knowing the histology. Current endoscopic armamentarium permits access for biopsy to most tumors of the paranasal sinuses. Occasionally, deep-seated tumors may not lend themselves to direct preoperative biopsy even with a CT guided needle. In such instances, intraoperative frozen section may have to be used.

Preoperative assessment of *tumor vascularity,* its origin and relationship to major vessels, as well as the status of cerebral collaterals is best achieved by angiography, temporary balloon occlusion test, and a xenon blood flow study (4). In paranasal sinus tumors, it is the relationship of the internal carotid artery to the neoplasm seen on CT or MRI that determines the indication for invasive vascular studies.

Therapeutic options for paranasal sinus carcinoma become evident from the diagnostic workup. In most cases, surgery and radiation used in sequence are employed as a combined treatment modality.

Systemic evaluation of the patient seldom reveals a distant metastatic disease in primary paranasal sinus carcinomas. Local and/or regional recurrences are seen more frequently than distant metastatic disease even following treatment failure at the primary site. Medical evaluation assesses the patient's overall tolerance to anticipated craniofacial or maxillofacial surgery.

The *patient's participation* in a diagnostic workup and therapeutic program is essential. Craniofacial resection of a paranasal sinus tumor does have a potential for esthetic deformity as well as functional impairment, for example, loss of smell and loss of vision or eye mobility.

PLANNING

Surgical strategy for treatment of paranasal sinus carcinoma develops from accurate histologic diagnosis and estimation of tumor extent, as well as knowledge of specific applications of craniofacial, oncologic, and reconstructive procedures. The strong possibility of achieving tumor-free surgical margins with maximum safety should be an integral part of a surgical therapeutic program.

Important considerations of regional anatomy include the following:

1. *Cribriform plate.* Jointly with the ethmoid labyrinth, the cribriform plate forms the roof of the nasal cavity. The cribriform plate is included in the craniofacial resection of an olfactory neuroblastoma and is often incorporated with resection of an ethmoid carcinoma. Even if direct erosion cannot be demonstrated on CT, the presence of numerous preformed anatomic spaces in the plate (for olfactory nerve terminal branches) should warrant consideration for its incorporation into the surgical specimen.

2. *Dura.* The intimate relationship of the dura and the cribriform plate is attributable to dural sleeves along the course of the olfactory nerve branches. Elevation of the dura from this region often results in multiple perforations, which must subsequently be repaired. If cribriform plate/ethmoid tumor is in contact with dura, an appropriate segment of the dura is resected. Removal of both olfactory nerves (done in most anterior craniofacial resections) results in total anosmia. This affects patients' perception of flavor, which they often interpret as a loss of taste.

3. *Cavernous sinus.* This dural duplication containing ICA and multiple cranial nerves (III, IV, V_1, VI) abuts the lateral wall of the sphenoid sinus. The ICA bulges into the sphenoid sinus to a variable extent, and, in most cases, it is covered by bone. The potential for anatomic bony dehiscence over the ICA within the sphenoid sinus may be present in up to 20% of the cases.

4. *Trigeminal nerve, second division.* This is the most commonly involved cranial nerve in paranasal sinus malignancies. Its long course from the foramen rotundum via the infraorbital canal to the skin of the cheek is vulnerable to tumor involvement. Clinical hypoesthesia or anesthesia of the cheek skin is an ominous oncologic sign. In tumors with great nerve affinity (e.g., adenoid cystic carcinoma) CT may show an abnormality at the foramen rotundum. MRI may further elucidate the more proximal nerve course and its possible involvement including the gasserian ganglion.

5. *Orbital content.* The CT evidence of bony orbital deficiency in paranasal sinus malignancies is not a *sine qua non* as an indication for orbital exenteration. The direct neoplastic involvement of orbital soft tissues is best verified by direct intraoperative exploration and frozen section. Especially in tumor recurrences following primary radiotherapy, obstructive sinus disease may present a deceiving picture on the CT of an extensive tumor. If orbital content is preserved, the bony orbit must be reconstructed to maintain eye position in all three planes and permit eye movement.

6. *Hard palate.* The hard palate, with dental arch, provides the roof of the oral cavity. Posteriorly it suspends the soft palate and assists in its function. Prior to

the removal of the hard palate, several reconstructive options may be considered. The defect may eventually be covered with a maxillary prosthesis (in most cases) or by muscle transfer (regional temporalis or distant microvascular muscle transfer), which can obliterate the skull base as well as the palatal defect.

PREOPERATIVE PREPARATION

1. *Airway.* Most patients with paranasal sinus tumors undergoing cranial base surgery are managed with an oral endotracheal tube. It is usually wired to the opposite mandible (via stable dentition or by circum-mandibular fixation). This allows safer movement of the patient's head intraoperatively.
2. *Eye protection.* In cases of planned eye preservation, the cornea is protected intraoperatively with either a large contact lens or a modified tarsorrhaphy.
3. *Position.* Patient is supine with head resting on a Mayfield headrest. The lower extremities are covered with automatic air compression stockings. The overall surgical access to the craniofacial region should allow for unhindered craniotomy as well as facial exposures.
4. *Neuroanesthesia.* Specifics as well as timing and duration of muscle relaxant usage are discussed with the anesthesiologist. The need for specific monitoring (e.g., cranial nerves or somatosensory evoked responses) is considered.
5. *Antibiotics.* Currently, a single agent (Cefuroxime) is used perioperatively. It is discontinued when external drains are removed (48–72 hr).
6. *Instrumentation.* The most useful special instrument for paranasal sinus resection has been the reciprocating and oscillating saws (electrically powered). The availability of multiple hand-held drives permits a quick switch during surgery while performing various osteotomies. During reconstruction, the same tools may be used for microplating of the craniofacial skeleton.

PROCEDURE

Goals

The goals of the procedure are as follows:

1. Safety.
2. Excision of tumor with microscopic free margins.
3. Adequate functional and esthetic reconstruction.
4. Tolerance of adjuvant therapy.

Safety of the Procedure

Protection of the CNS (structural and vascular) is the primary concern. Adequate craniotomy for visualization, protection, and possible repair of key structures is essential. This is assisted by the use of a spinal drain, which lessens the impact of retraction on the cerebral cortex. Control of the ICA requires cervical or petrous carotid access (proximal) as well as exposure of the supraclinoid segment (distal control) when the lateral sphenoid/cavernous sinus region is approached.

Wound contamination by nasopharyngeal and sinus microbial flora is unavoidable. Therefore special emphasis must be placed on CSF containment (dural repair) and elimination of surgical dead space with vascularized tissue (e.g., muscle flaps). The stability of the replaced craniofacial skeleton and its soft tissue coverage is a prerequisite for adequate bone healing. Small segments of the membranous facial skeleton may be "internally" exposed, providing they are stable and have satisfactory external vascularized coverage. The duration of the procedure has a rather profound impact on the patient's homeostasis. Longer procedures usually result in greater blood loss and an increase in overall contamination, as well as coagulation abnormalities. In general, cranial base procedures for paranasal sinus cancer range from 6 to 12 hr with extensions when a free flap is needed (additional 4–5 hr).

Containment of Tumor

Adequate visualization at the "oncologic" plane of resection is the key to providing a margin of normal tissue to the tumor specimen. Extensive paranasal sinus tumors often preclude safe visualization and protection of key structures. In such cases, it is possible to remove the tumor in segments. The segments must be precisely oriented to assist the pathologist in the evaluation of the entire surgical specimen.

Functional and Esthetic Results

The central location of paranasal sinuses within the craniofacial skeleton demands great emphasis on functional and esthetic reconstruction following oncologic surgery. Specifically, support of the eye and the contribution of the maxillary sinuses to facial contour must be considered. The preservation of the ipsilateral nasal airway is important for maintaining the continuity of nasal air and mucus flow into the nasopharynx. The medial and inferior orbital walls, most frequently resected in maxilloethmoidal tumors, should be reconstructed to achieve adequate eye support. Transferred temporalis muscle often used for dural coverage following cranial base surgery is, however, seldom enough to maintain the precise vertical, sagittal, and anteroposterior eye support. Enophthalmos with some inferior globe displacement is a frequent sequela of such reconstruction. The new mini/microplates (titanium or vitallium) used for stabilization of cranial bone grafts offer greater precision in three-dimensional support of the globe.

The placement of facial incisions may affect not only the eventual facial appearance but also the lid and lacrimal function through unfavorable scar formation. A lateral rhinotomy incision is placed at the junction of nasal and cheek skin with possible addition of an upper lip split. The horizontal cheek incision (e.g., traditional subciliary Weber–Ferguson) may be modified (see Janecka et al., Facial Translocation Approach to Nasopharynx, Clivus, and Infratemporal Fossa) by preserving the lower lid as a neuromuscular functioning unit. The nasolacrimal duct can usually be preserved in its proximal course. An oblique transection of the duct lessens the chances for its postoperative obstruction by scar. If a higher transection of the lacrimal system (saccus canaliculi) is necessary, postoperative stenting (for over 6 weeks) is warranted. Temporary tarsorrhaphy (sutures only) may be used to assist in proper lower lid healing by diminishing the chances of an ectropion as well as affording corneal protection in the immediate postoperative period.

Tolerance to Adjuvant Therapy

The large extent of most paranasal sinus malignancies warrants inclusion of radiotherapy in the postoperative management. The rapid healing of soft and bony tissues postoperatively is important in permitting timely application of the adjuvant therapy. The area of facial soft tissue most frequently demonstrating secondary healing problems after radiotherapy is the region of the medial canthus. This area contains the thinnest skin and is the most distal end of the cheek flap raised during surgery. Avoidance of tension at surgical closure or adding a support to this area by transferred temporalis muscle can lessen the frequency of this problem. The stability of the remaining craniofacial skeleton, especially the lateral orbital, malar eminence, and zygomatic arch segments, is assisted by three-plane fixation.

CASE PRESENTATIONS

Anterior Craniofacial Resection for Ethmoid Sinus Carcinoma

J.V. was a 57-year-old patient with a long history of inverted papilloma in the nasal cavity who was found to have squamous cell carcinoma of the ethmoid sinuses. His CT scan showed involvement of the ethmoid sinuses as well as the nasal cavity up to the cribriform plate (Fig. 1A). He was treated with anterior craniofacial resection using bifrontal craniotomy and facial incisions (horizontal transnasal and bilateral periorbital). The specimen (Fig. 1B) included the entire ethmoid labyrinth in conjunction with both medial walls of the orbits, the anterior aspect of the frontal bone, and the anterior face of the sphenoid sinus. Reconstruction (Fig. 1C) included cranial bone graft for the nasofrontal region as well as a pericranial flap (Fig. 1D) for reconstruction of the floor of the anterior cranial fossa. For tumor resection (Fig. 1E) the reciprocating saw was used. One year postoperatively (Fig. 1F), the patient demonstrated symmetrical position of his eyes as well as healed transverse nasal and periorbital scars.

Anterior Craniofacial Resection Including Brain Tissue

R.C. was a 52-year-old patient with an extensive transcranial olfactory neuroblastoma (Fig. 2A). The surgical approach used a midfacial split (Fig. 2B), which allowed resection of the transcranial tumor (Fig. 2C) in addition to the intracerebral tumor, which was done through a bifrontal craniotomy. The interorbital space reconstruction was done with split cranial bone grafts (Fig. 2D), rebuilding the medial walls of both orbits (Fig. 2E). One month after surgery (Fig. 2F), the patient demonstrated symmetrical eye position as well as healing nasal and periorbital scars.

Anterior Cranio-orbital Resection

M.K. was a 45-year-old patient with an orbital and paranasal sinus rhabdomyosarcoma (Fig. 3A). His tumor was resected via bifrontal craniotomy, periorbital/facial incisions, and craniofacial osteotomies (Fig. 3B). For reconstruction, a titanium miniplating was used (Fig. 3C) to stabilize the supraorbital and frontal skeleton. For soft tissue reconstruction, pericranial and temporalis muscle flaps (Fig. 3D) were used.

Anterior Cranio-orbital Resection with Free-Flap Reconstruction

T.G. was a 47-year-old patient with an extensive adenoid cystic carcinoma (Fig. 4A) extending from the soft palate to the cavernous sinus. The tumor was resected through a bifrontal and facial approach (Fig. 4B). Surgical specimen included maxillary and ethmoid sinuses, orbit, and cavernous sinus, as well as soft and hard palate. Reconstruction was carried out with replacement of the craniofacial skeleton (Fig. 4C) as well as a microvascular free-flap for soft tissue reconstruction. Postoperatively, a right external orbital prosthesis was fashioned (Fig. 4D).

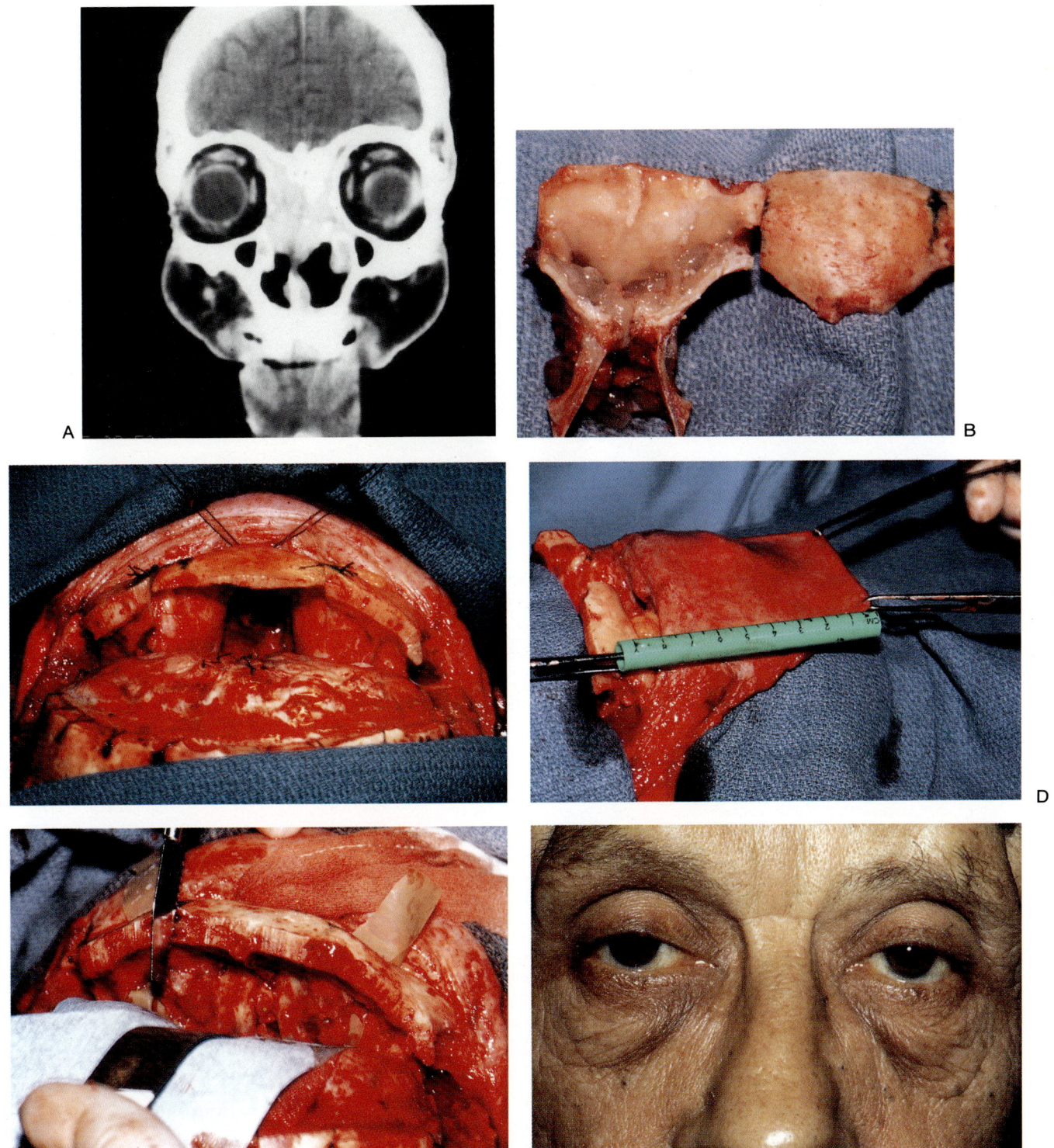

FIG. 1. A: Coronal CT scan with contrast demonstrating ethmoid mass. **B:** Specimen of anterior skull base. **C:** Superior view of defect in the anterior cranial base and bone graft in the low frontal region. **D:** Lateral view of raised pericranial flap. **E:** Reciprocating blade used for anterior cranial base resection; superior view; frontal lobes are retracted. **F:** Postoperative view one year later.

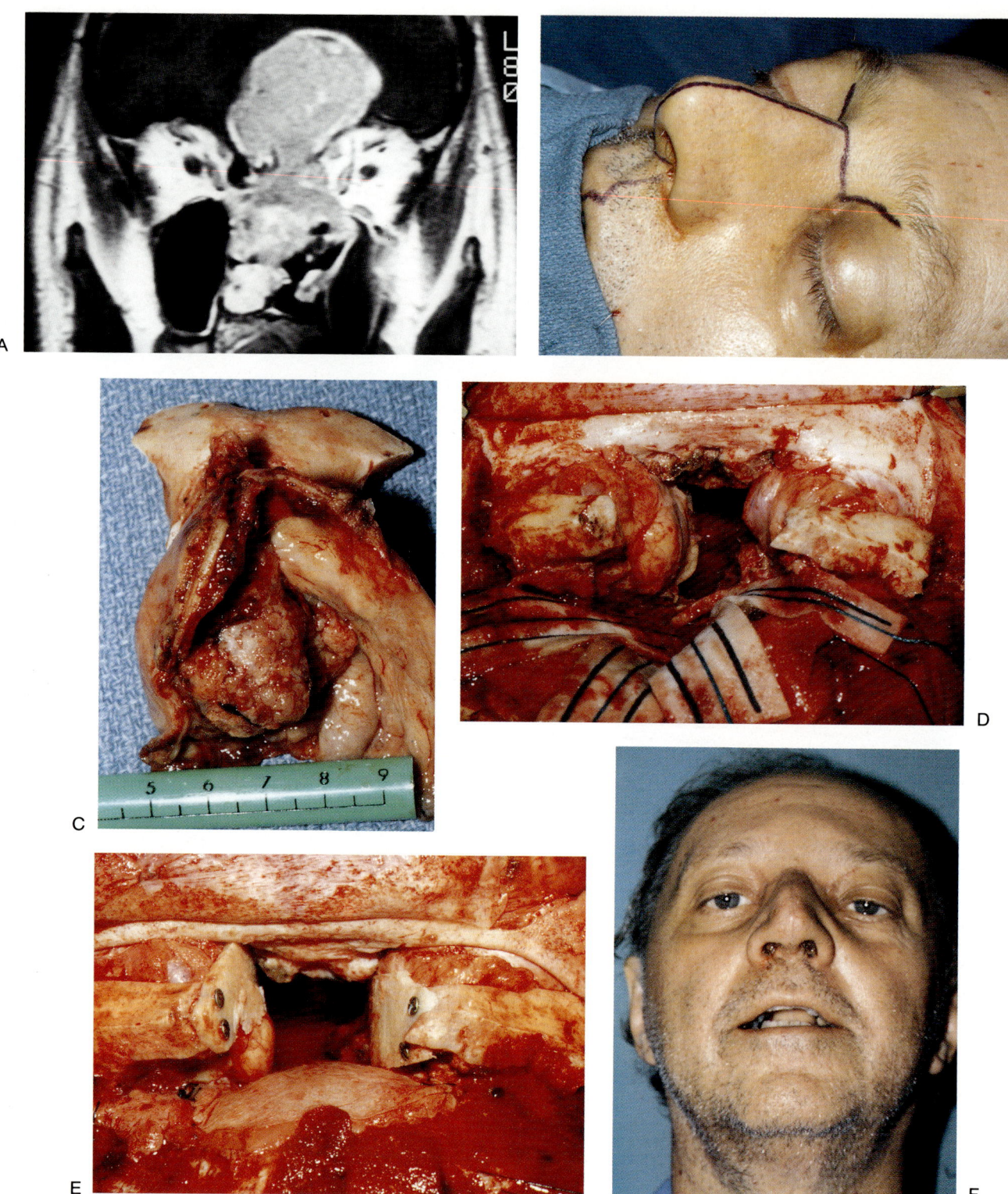

FIG. 2. A: Coronal CT scan with contrast demonstrating a transcranial extent of an olfactory neuroblastoma. **B:** Outline of incisions for midfacial split. **C:** Specimen of olfactory neuroblastoma following craniofacial resection; central frontal bone is seen superiorly; mass is enclosed by nasal septum on the right and lateral nasal wall on the left. **D:** Surgical defect (seen from above) of interorbital space. **E:** Both medial walls of orbits were reconstructed with split cranial bone graft affixed with titanium screws to supraorbital bar. **F:** Symmetrical facial appearance one month postoperatively.

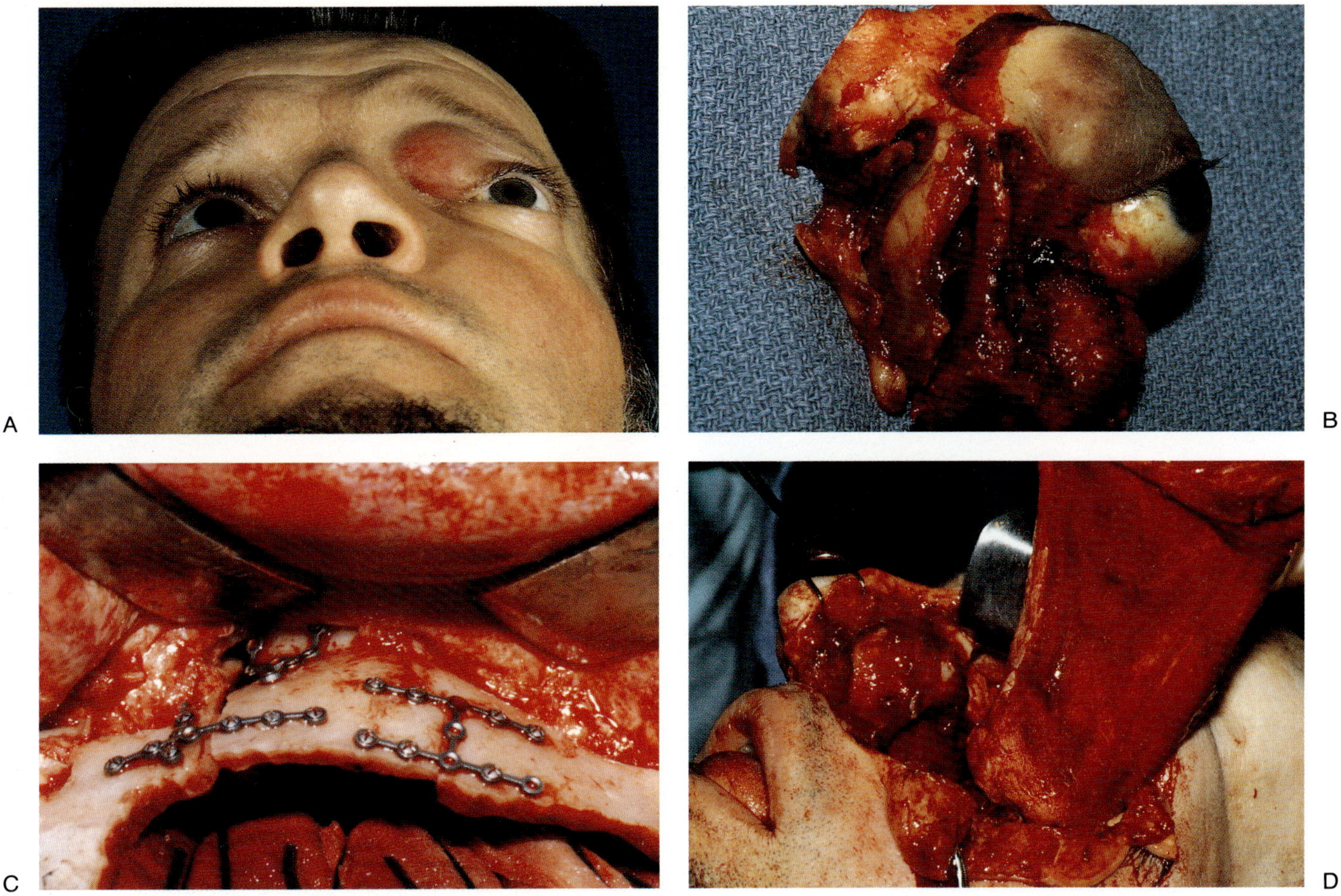

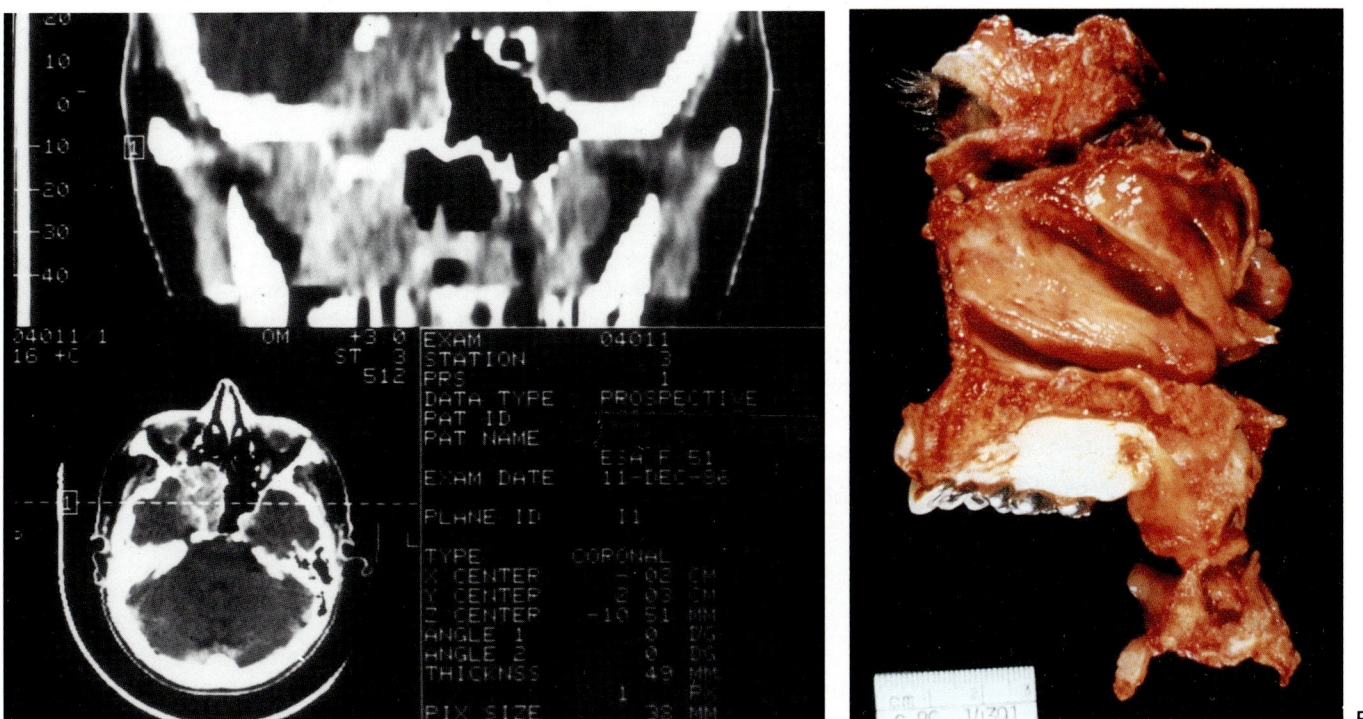

FIG. 3. A: Clinical photograph of left orbital rhabdomyosarcoma. **B:** Resected tumor following craniofacial surgery. **C:** Rigid fixation of supraorbital bone with titanium miniplate. **D:** Left temporalis muscle was rotated into the surgical defect for reconstruction.

FIG. 4. A: Coronal CT reconstruction demonstrating an extensive tumor in right sphenoid and cavernous sinuses as well as the infratemporal fossa. **B:** Resected specimen extends from right cavernous sinus to the soft palate. **C:** Temporarily removed craniofacial skeleton. **D:** Patient's appearance postoperatively with right orbital prosthesis.

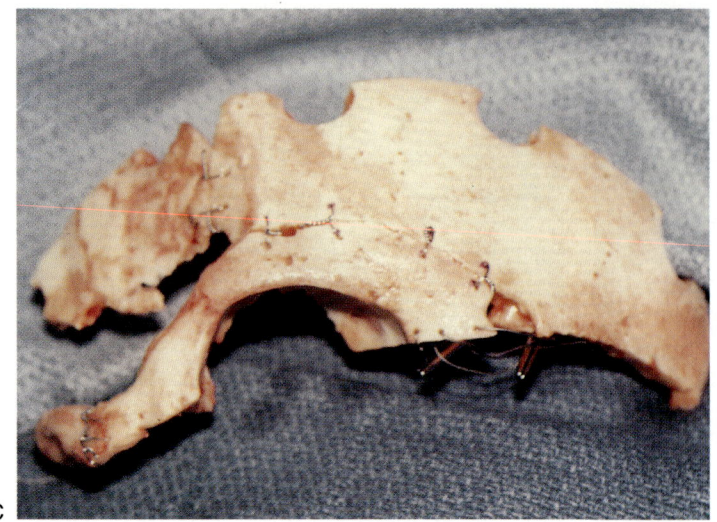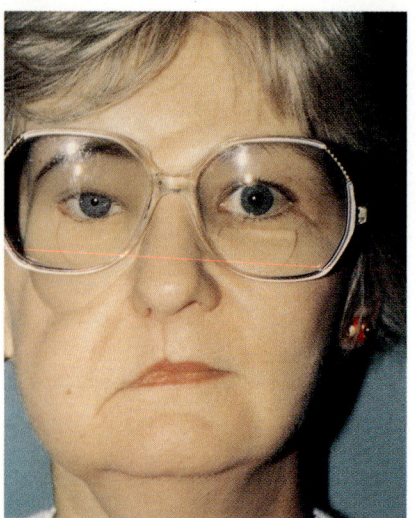

FIG. 4. *Continued.*

COMPLICATIONS

Craniofacial resection of paranasal sinus tumors creates a transcranial defect with potential for numerous complications. Minimal brain retraction, microsurgical techniques, and primary reconstruction using autogenous tissues are some of the best ways to prevent detrimental complications.

Prevention of Complications: Goals

1. Containment of CSF with dural reconstruction.
2. Reenforcement of dural reconstruction and support of anterior cranial floor. This is most frequently accomplished with a pericranial flap. In addition, a split cranial bone graft may be used in larger defects.
3. Stability of craniofacial skeleton, especially the nasal and orbital skeletal support. This is best done with a split cranial bone graft affixed by titanium screws and miniplates.
4. Acceptable facial scarring and function of the nasolacrimal duct. Placement of incisions in esthetic lines gives foundation for satisfactory healing. Protection of preservable segments of the nasolacrimal duct permits adequate drainage postoperatively in most cases.

Treatment of Complications

Pneumocephalus

A certain amount of postoperative air in the epidural space is frequently encountered and does not constitute a complication. However, development of an increasing amount of intracranial air is a reflection of an ongoing escape of nasal air into the cranial cavity and must be vigorously treated. It is often accompanied by a change in the patient's mental status due to frontal lobe compression. On an emergency basis, aspiration of air through the frontal skin and an underlying burr hole may dramatically reverse a patient's deteriorated mental status. Any partial upper airway obstruction should be corrected at this point. Such simple maneuvers as placement of nasopharyngeal airways may prove very valuable. Sometimes even tracheostomy or reexploration of the floor of the anterior cranial fossa may be necessary. Close CT follow-up is essential to ascertain the progressive diminution in intracranial air.

CSF Leakage

CSF leakage, in small amounts, may be present in many patients postoperatively for the first several days but frequently ceases spontaneously. A large amount of CSF leak (demonstrated clearly by dependent position of the head), however, must be treated. The first step in treating CSF leak may be spinal drainage and placement of the patient in a supine position. The CSF leak often stops with this treatment within several days. Large or persistent leaks should be reexplored and the site of the leak should be repaired.

Vision Loss

If optic nerve decompression is done as part of the tumor resection, intraoperative steroids are administered to limit intraneural swelling. However, the risk of permanent optic nerve injury always exists in such cases. Sudden loss of vision postoperatively should be evaluated with CT scan, looking for optic nerve/globe compression. Bone fragments or hematoma suspected of compressing the optic nerve should be surgically removed. Otherwise, intravenous steroids are used in an attempt to salvage the vision.

In cavernous sinus dissections, there frequently is a loss of function of several cranial nerves (III, IV, V_1, VI). If the continuity of nerves was preserved, an improvement in eye muscle function should occur within several months. If it does not recover, eye muscle surgery may be considered.

Ocular Dystopia

Resection of the medial walls of both orbits, especially in conjunction with resection of some portion of the orbital floor, may result in significant ocular displacement (posterior and/or inferior). Reestablishment of the normal orbital anatomy can be achieved with cranial bone grafts and transferred temporalis muscle. A persistent ocular dystopia requires secondary surgery.

Infection

An infection developing in the interorbital and nasal space is frequently related to the secondary healing of this area. To facilitate secondary healing of intranasal surfaces postoperatively, close attention to nasal hygiene is required. Once infection develops, it is treated with appropriate antibiotics and more intense nasal hygiene, including removal of nasal debris.

Intracranial infection (epidural or subdural) is usually a manifestation of direct intracranial communication with the nasal cavity, with or without CSF leak. Obliteration of epidural dead space, closure of CSF leak, and antibiotic coverage are important steps in treating intracranial infection.

STATISTICS

Paranasal sinus malignancies have a poor prognosis and local tumor control is a major therapeutic problem. Most of the malignancies (75%) are found to extend beyond the sinus cavity at the time of diagnosis and 45% are found to invade the orbit (5). The maxillary sinus is the overwhelming primary site (80%).

The literature points to the tumor stage as a statistically significant determinant of 5-year survival: T_1, 100%; T_2, 86%; T_3, 32%; T_4, 7%. The overall 5-year survival rate for paranasal sinus carcinoma is 38% (6).

RECOMMENDATIONS

1. Immunohistochemistry on all biopsies of paranasal sinus malignancy demonstrating "small cell" or "undifferentiated" tumors to better isolate cell of origin.
2. Resection of paranasal sinus malignant tumors with clear surgical margins.
3. Orbital exenteration when orbital soft tissue involvement is verified by histology.
4. Combined therapy (surgery and radiotherapy).
5. Surgical treatment of neck metastases when they develop.

REFERENCES

1. Freedmann I, Osbornda DA. Tumors of the nose and sinuses—material and classification. In: *Pathology of granulomas and neoplasms of the nose and paranasal sinuses.* Edinburgh: Churchill Livingstone, 1982;100–102.
2. Sisson GA. Symposium—paranasal sinuses. Discussion and summary. *Laryngoscope* 1970;80:945–953.
3. Carrau RL, Myers EN, Johnson JT. Cancer involving the nose and the paranasal sinuses. *Oncology* 1992;6:43–50.
4. deVries EJ, Sekhar LN, Horton JA, Yonas H, Eibling DE, Janecka IP, Schramm VL. A new method to predict safe resection of the internal carotid artery. *Laryngoscope* 1989;100:85–88.
5. Zamora RL, Harvey JE, Sessions DG, Spector JG, Spitznagel EL. Clinical classification and staging for primary malignancies of the maxillary antrum. *Laryngoscope* 1990;100:1106–1112.
6. Lavertu P, et al. Squamous cell carcinoma of the paranasal sinuses: the Cleveland Clinic experience 1977–1986. *Laryngoscope* 1989;99:1130–1136.

CHAPTER 36

Tuberculum Sella and Olfactory Groove Meningiomas

Ossama Al-Mefty

Separated in origin by approximately 2 cm, olfactory groove meningiomas and tuberculum sella meningiomas are quite dissimilar in symptoms, radiological findings, and surgical considerations. Clearly distinguishing them, Cushing and Eisenhardt devoted a separate chapter to each of these two locations in their classic book on meningiomas (5). Surgical removal of olfactory groove meningiomas is usually straightforward and less challenging than that of other basal meningiomas. The operation becomes more complex, however, when the tumor reaches a giant size, involving suprasellar vital structures, or when it extends into the ethmoidal sinuses or involves extensively the bony floor of the frontal fossa. Tuberculum sella meningiomas are noteworthy in their encroachment against and around the carotid arteries and the optic nerves laterally as well as against the hypothalamus with extension into the interpeduncular cistern and frontal fossa.

The overwhelming number of meningiomas are benign and potentially curable by surgery. The objective of operation is total removal of the meningioma including the involved dura and bone. Evidence indicates that the completeness of surgical removal is the single most important factor in the likelihood of recurrence and long-term prognosis (12). A considerable increase in mortality, morbidity, and failure of visual improvement occurs in cases in which the tumor size exceeds 3 cm (7,13). Likewise, the ability to achieve total removal is related to tumor size. A giant size, however, should not temper the surgeon's zeal for total removal of these benign neoplasms (1,2). The arachnoid membrane, providing a plane of dissection even when tumor totally engulfs the cerebral vessels and the optic apparatus, is the best ally of the surgeon. Thus, the best chance to achieve total removal is at the first operation when the arachnoid membrane has not been violated. Having stressed a zealous and aggressive attitude toward total removal of this tumor at the first operation, I should equally stress that "one should always remember that it is not the tumor that is the trophy but a viable patient." Technical ability should not blind the surgeon's judgment of the goal to preserve or improve neurological function (8).

DIAGNOSTIC CONSIDERATIONS

Modern imaging procedures, such as high resolution CT scanning, magnetic resonance imaging (MRI), and selective angiography are indispensable in the workup of these patients. These studies are important not only for identification of the lesion but also for visualization of extension and encroachment on surrounding neurovascular structures. Despite the remarkable advances in nonangiographic imaging techniques, cerebral angiography, both carotid and vertebral, is still a necessary preoperative investigation (1). Angiography delineates cerebral vasculature anatomy, identifies arterial encasement and displacement, demonstrates feeding vessels, and reveals associated vascular lesions. MRI angiography, however, might prove to be quite adequate and soon will replace conventional angiography in this role. As with other juxtasellar lesions, a documented visual field and acuity and complete endocrinological studies are an integral part of the preoperative evaluation of these patients.

PATIENT SELECTION

Tuberculum sella meningiomas are notorious in their production of visual loss. The visual prognosis and the

---

O. Al-Mefty: Division of Neurological Surgery, Loyola University Medical Center, Maywood, Illinois 60153.

overall mortality and morbidity depend on the size of the tumor. It has been frequently stated, and it cannot be overemphasized, that they should be diagnosed as early as possible and removed totally. Cavernous sinus involvement is no longer a deterrent to total removal (3,10). Unless serious systemic disease contraindicates major surgery, these tumors are recommended for surgical treatment. Olfactory groove meningiomas might have insidious growth and they frequently reach large size before they come to diagnosis (4). However, clinical and radiological observations are quite justified in an elderly patient with a small asymptomatic meningioma of the olfactory groove.

OPERATIVE TECHNIQUE

Anesthetic Considerations

As with other cranial base tumors, the successful removal of an anterior fossa meningioma is inextricably intertwined with the flawless administration of anesthesia. Premedication is usually withheld from a patient undergoing meningioma surgery. Induction should be smooth and rapid and should be accomplished with agents that reduce intracranial pressure (ICP). Lidocaine given intravenously after theopental induction decreases the intubation-induced hypertensive response. Although the choice of anesthetic agent should be flexible and tailored to suit the circumstances of each case, avoiding intracranial hypertension and maintaining adequate cerebral perfusion are mandates of anesthesia. It should be noted, however, that in patients with severely decreased brain function the response of cerebral blood flow to hyperventilation may be attenuated, and the technique may not prevent an increase in ICP when a volatile anesthetic is given (11). Normotension is the goal, and in my procedures I avoid any hypotension. Should temporary vascular occlusion be necessary during the surgical resection of the tumor, a barbiturate is given for its known cerebral protective effect. To avoid consumption coagulopathy with intraoperative diathesis, adequate blood replacement, platelet transfusion, and coagulation factor replacement through fresh frozen plasma transfusion should be given in appropriate amounts and in a timely manner.

Despite the pressing need for intraoperative monitoring of visual pathways during surgery of olfactory groove and tuberculum sella meningiomas, visual evoked potential monitoring has failed to gain wide intraoperative use. Intraoperative use of visual evoked potential monitoring is hindered by many factors related to its nature, stimulation and recording techniques, influence of other agents and condition, and finally the reliability of interpretation and significance.

Positioning

The patient is placed supine with the head at the foot-end of the table. In small and moderate sized tumors, a spinal needle is inserted through a split mattress and connected to a sterile collection bag. A flow control clamp is applied to the draining tube to avoid rapid CSF loss. The table is adjusted so the trunk and head are elevated 20°. The head is then carefully and moderately hyperextended and fixed in the Mayfield headrest to allow the frontal lobe to fall backward. To avoid compromising the bicoronal incision, the surgeon must not place the pins too far anteriorly. The head is kept straight to facilitate anatomical orientation (Fig. 1).

Operative Technique for Tuberculum Sella Meningioma

Supraorbital Approach

Both McArthur, in 1912, and Frazier, in 1913, removed the supraorbital arch to approach the hypophysis. Recently, Jane et al. (6) modified and revived this approach and consider it the approach of choice for orbital tumors. I have used this technique for all procedures requiring a subfrontal approach.

The scalp incision of the supraorbital approach is begun 1 cm anterior to the tragus and proceeds in a curvi-

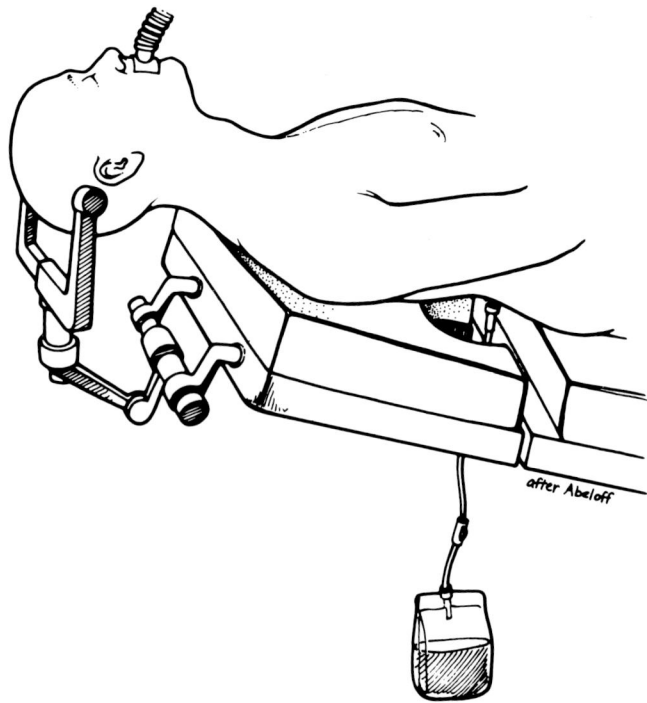

FIG. 1. Artist's illustration of patient's position. The head is elevated about 20°; the lumbar spinal needle is in place. The neck is extended to allow the frontal lobes to fall backward. The head is kept straight to facilitate orientation in the suprasellar area.

linear fashion behind the hairline to the level of the superior temporal line on the opposite side. In this manner, the superficial temporal artery courses posterior to the incision while the facial nerve branches are located anteriorly. As the scalp is turned anteriorly, the temporal muscle gives way to a temporal fat pad projecting anteriorly between the muscle and the frontozygomatic surface. The temporalis fascia actually splits into two layers, which contain the fat pad and the facial nerve branches. The temporalis fascia is incised and reflected anteriorly with the fat layer and nerves along with the scalp flap. The temporalis muscle is detached from its insertion anteriorly as far as the zygomatic arch; the muscle is then retracted posteriorly, exposing the junction of the zygomatic, sphenoidal, and frontal bones.

The periosteum of the frontal bone is incised as far posteriorly as possible, dissected forward, and reflected over the anteriorly-turned scalp flap. The intact base of this periosteum is then dissected free from the roof and lateral wall of the orbit. It may be necessary to use a high-speed air drill around the supraorbital notch to free the supraorbital nerve.

To begin the supraorbital approach, two burr holes are drilled. The first, MacCarty's keyhole, is made in the temporal fossa at the frontosphenoidal junction, just behind the zygomatic process of the frontal bone. When the hole is drilled, the surgeon will see that its upper half exposes the dura mater and its lower half exposes the periorbita, the two membranes being separated by the roof of the orbit. The second hole is made in the frontal bone above the nasion. To keep it as small as possible, this hole is made with a high-speed drill such as the Midas Rex (Fort Worth, Texas). In adults, this hole will invariably pass through the anterior and posterior walls of the frontal sinus. The mucosa is removed, and the sinus is packed with a small piece of temporalis muscle.

The two holes are joined by two bony cuts. The first cut is made with the foot attachment of the Midas Rex drill, which passes through the frontal bone about 4 cm above the superior orbital rim, as shown in Fig. 2. The second cut interconnects the two holes, crossing the roof of the orbit. This bony cut may be performed with the B1 attachment of the Midas Rex drill or by the use of a Gigli saw. Using a fine bit high-speed air drill, a groove is made from the burr hole through the medial part of the superior orbital rim. This groove helps direct the cut of a Gigli saw through the orbital roof. A Gigli saw guide is then passed between the two burr holes over the roof of the orbit in the epidural space (Fig. 3). The orbital roof is cut as shown in Fig. 4. This bony incision is carried laterally and inferiorly and is continued through the lateral orbital rim. During this process, the contents of the orbit are protected with a brain spatula. The surgeon should pay particular attention to keeping the periorbita intact. Injury to the supraorbital nerve and the trochlear attachment of the superior oblique muscle should be avoided.

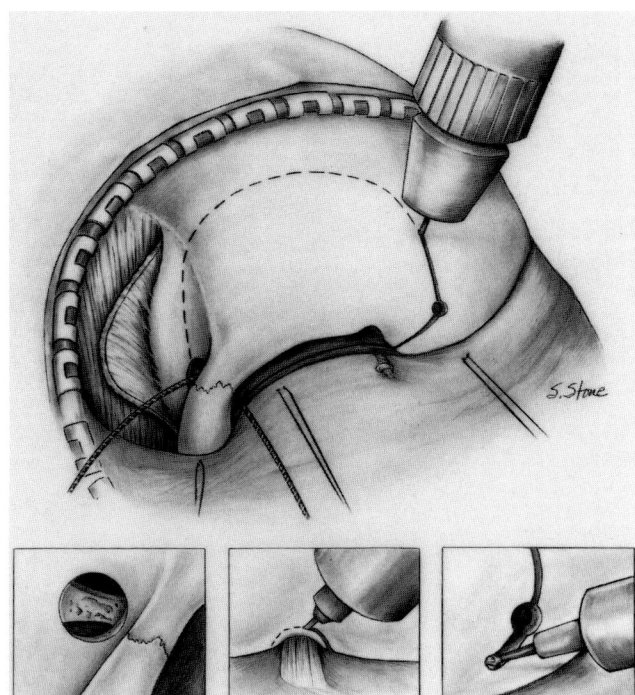

FIG. 2. Artist's illustration demonstrating the removal of the supraorbital bone flap. The midline hole and the keyhole are connected by a cut through the frontal bone using the craniotome and through the orbital roof using a Gigli saw. **Insert:** (*left*) the position of the keyhole; (*center*) freeing the supraorbital nerve from its canal; (*right*) grooving the medial supraorbital rim.

The removed and preserved craniotomy flap thus includes the superior and the upper half of the lateral orbital rim, the anterior portion of the orbital roof, and the adjacent frontal bone. The low frontal exposure is illustrated in Fig. 5.

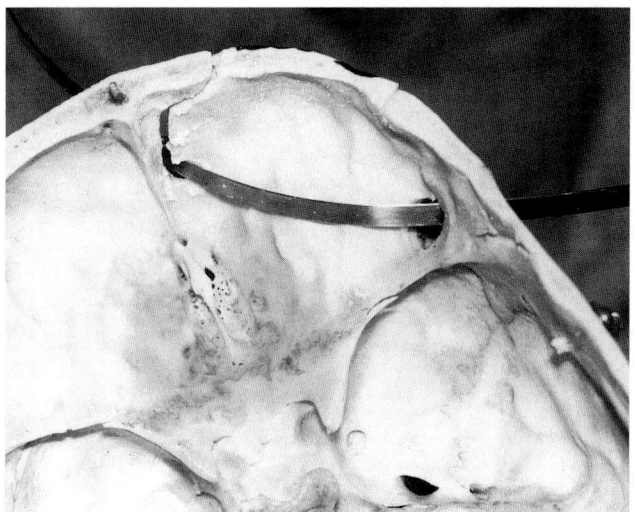

FIG. 3. Intracranial view of Gigli saw guide in skull model.

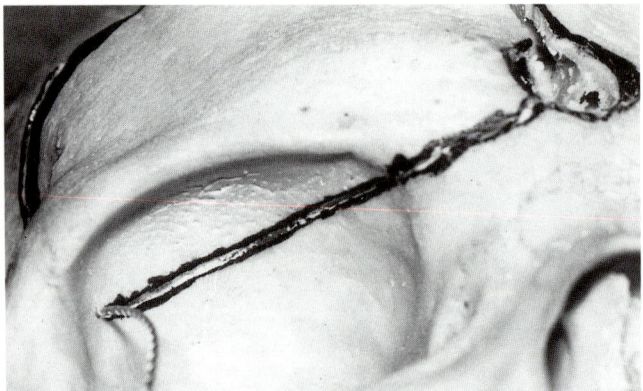

FIG. 4. Skull model with orbital roof view of Gigli saw incision.

Tissue Dissection and Tumor Resection

Upon removal of the bone flap, the dura is tacked up. The operating microscope (mounted on a Contraves stand) is brought into the field to open the dura. Opening the dura under the microscope provides a transitional adjustment of the surgeon's dexterity from bony work to fine microsurgical dissection.

With the aid of hyperventilation, partial release of CSF from the previously inserted spinal drainage, and the optional use of mannitol, the relaxed frontal lobe is held by a self-retaining retractor. Elevation of the frontal lobe should be minimal; a distance of 1.5 cm is adequate for tumor resection. The olfactory nerve is located and preserved by dissecting it for some distance from the base of the frontal lobe (Fig. 6). Preservation of the olfac-

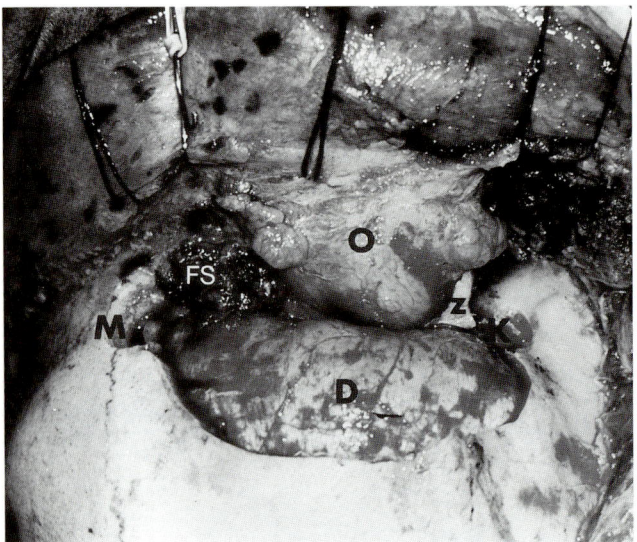

FIG. 5. Operative photograph: surgeon's view after bone flap removal. O, orbit; D, frontal lobe dura; K, keyhole; M, midline hole; FS, frontal sinus packed with muscle; Z, frontal process of the zygomatic bone.

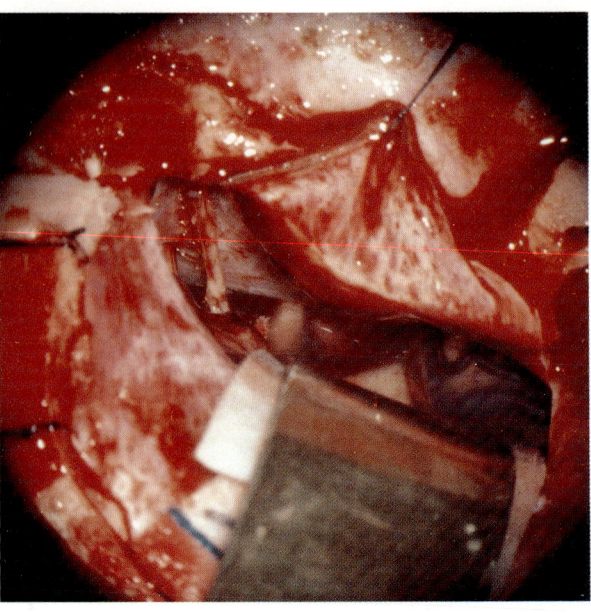

FIG. 6. Color operative photograph: surgeon's view through the supraorbital approach. The dura is incised transversely and reflected over the orbit. Elevation of the frontal lobe does not exceed 1.5 cm. The olfactory tract is dissected and preserved. The optic nerve and carotid cistern are well visualized. Retractors hold the frontal lobe, which is covered by the dura.

tory nerve deters excessive frontal lobe retraction, which results in its avulsion, and leaves the olfactory sense intact. Early interception of the arterial feeders is a crucial step. These feeders usually come from the posterior ethmoidal artery or travel along the lesser wing of the sphenoid bone. The tumor may be retracted gently backward until these feeders are exposed, coagulated, and severed. An alternative approach is to use the CO_2 laser to remove a slice from the tumor base to reach the blood supply without elevating the tumor mass against the frontal lobes (Fig. 7). The tumor is then debulked using the laser or the ultrasonic aspirator. The traditional method of debulking the meningioma using an electrocautery loop is discouraged since it creates a tremendous amount of heat. Once dissection approaches the neurovascular structures, only bipolar cautery should be used.

Optic Nerves

Tuberculum sella meningiomas typically displace both nerves outward and backward, often to the extent that the optic nerve lies above and lateral to the internal carotid artery, with the chiasm stretched far back from the tuberculum sella (2). At times, optic nerve identification is quite difficult when the nerve is completely engulfed by the tumor or when the nerve has been distorted to an almost unrecognizable thin band in the tumor capsule. Extreme caution and piecemeal removal of the tu-

optic nerves and chiasm should be preserved by the same method of tumor dissection (Fig. 9). In my opinion, the surgeon should not sacrifice the optic nerve to obtain better exposure of the tumor, even in a totally blind eye. This opinion is supported by occasional observations of visual recovery after total blindness (9).

Arterial Dissection

As in tumor dissection from the optic nerves, the carotid artery is dissected free from tumor using an array of microinstruments including bipolar forceps, microdissectors, and scissors. Adherence and encasement of the cerebral vessel should not deter the surgeon from attempting to dissect the tumor free from the involved arteries. Dissection of a tumor from the carotid artery employs the same techniques as dissection of the optic nerves. Carotid dissection continues to free the ophthalmic artery, the posterior communicating artery, the anterior thalamic perforators, and the choroidal artery. Further carotid dissection of the tumor progresses to the bifurcation of the internal carotid artery, and into the Sylvian fissure. Dissection continues to free the middle and anterior cerebral arteries. Tumor tissue has either simply displaced these vessels and their perforators or actually engulfed them. The A-1 segments in particular are usually severely stretched or adherent and tend to tear. Should this occur, the surgeon should remain calm, apply a temporary vascular clip (30 cm/mm^2) distal and proximal to the bleeding point, and suture the arterial wall with fine 10-0 sutures. A graft clip of appropriate size may also be used (Fig. 10).

While the tumor may be supplied by arterial twigs of the anterior cerebral arteries, the surgeon must first be

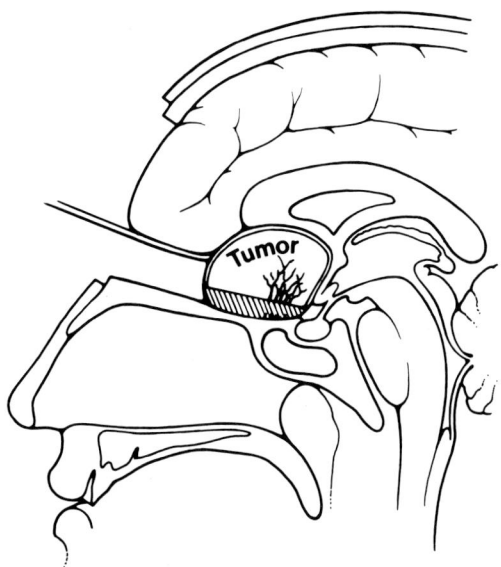

FIG. 7. Artist's illustration: the arterial blood supply at the base of a meningioma is interrupted early in the procedure. *Shaded area* of the tumor presents a slice of the tumor vaporized by laser to reach the arterial feeder.

mor, using fine-tipped bipolar forceps and microdissectors, are necessary. The tumor is slowly stripped from the flattened and engulfed nerve. Despite apparent encasement or severe adherence, a plane of dissection can be obtained under high magnification (Fig. 8).

In some instances, the easily identifiable and dissectable optic nerve belongs to the eye with total visual loss, while the optic nerve with residual function is encased in the tumor. To preserve the remaining vision, dissection of the nerve and its blood supply must be cautious and meticulous. At times it may be necessary to start the dissection at the chiasm to locate and dissect an obscure optic nerve on the other side. The arterial supply to the

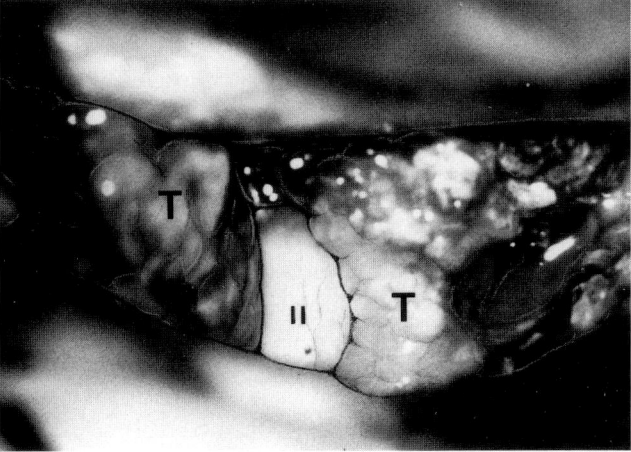

FIG. 8. Enhanced operative photograph: optic nerve (II) on the right is totally engulfed in the tumor (T). A small portion of it has been identified and a plane of dissection has been established.

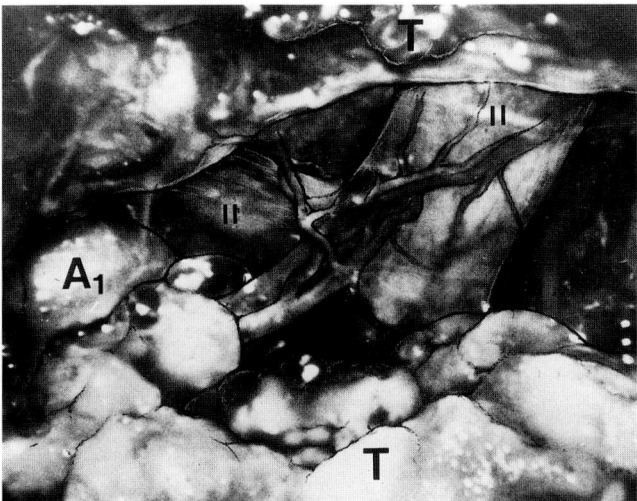

FIG. 9. Enhanced operative photograph: surgeon's view during dissection of a meningioma. The blood supply to the optic nerve (II) and chiasm was preserved after tedious dissection. T, tumor; A1, anterior cerebral artery.

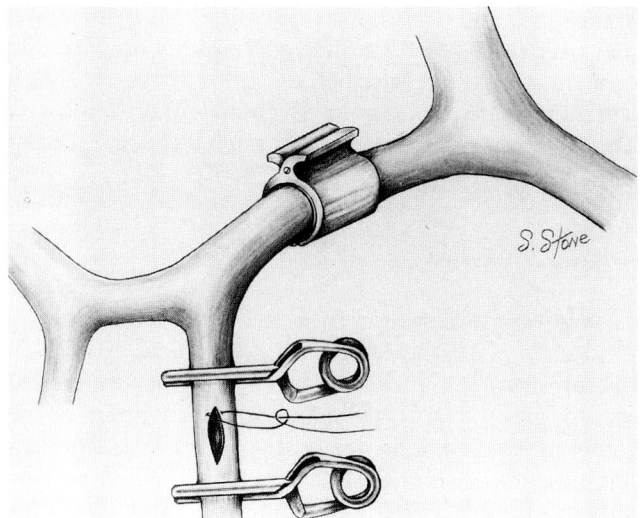

FIG. 10. Artist's illustration depicting arterial repair. Two temporary clips are applied distally and proximally to the arterial hole and a 10-0 suture is used to repair the artery, or a graft clip is applied to the injured segment.

certain that they are tumor feeders and not hypothalamic perforators or optic blood supply. Thus, each arterial branch should be dissected and followed to ascertain its eventual course (Fig. 11). Particular precision is needed to spare the artery of Heubner and the vital branches to the striatum. As dissection continues, both A-1 and anterior communicating arteries are freed from the tumor. The Liliequist membrane is intact in most cases; consequently, tumor removal from the posteriorly displaced basilar artery is usually easy (Fig. 12).

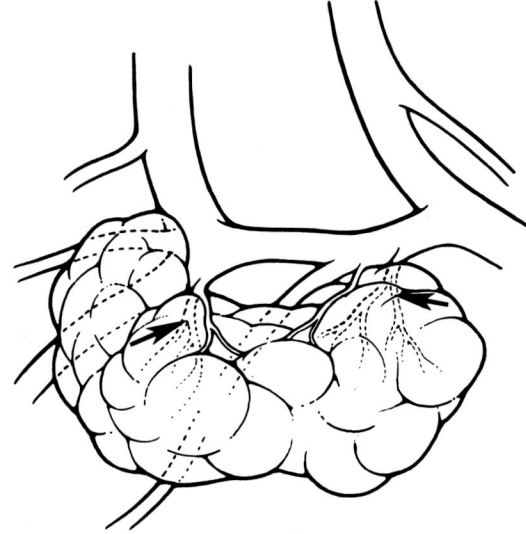

FIG. 11. Artist's illustration demonstrating the dissection of arterial branches from the A-1 segment. Only the arterial twigs terminating in the tumor (*arrows*) are coagulated while the perforators are preserved.

Dissection of the Pituitary Stalk and Hypothalamus

The pituitary stalk can be recognized by its distinctive color and vascular network. A tumor extending backward under the hypothalamus usually displaces the pituitary stalk backward and to one side (Fig. 13). Requiring meticulous and tedious dissection, some tumors totally engulf the pituitary stalk. A tumor impinging on the hypothalamus can be gently removed by maintaining a plane of cleavage. However, excessive downward retraction on the tumor should be avoided. The arachnoid membrane of Liliequist provides an excellent dissection plane for tumor removal. Often this membrane comes away with the tumor, leaving the rostral pons, midbrain, oculomotor nerves, and basilar artery and its branches in full view (Fig. 14).

Cavernous Sinus and Optic Canal

When the tumor extends into the cavernous sinus and/or the optic canal, the anterior clinoid process, the optic canal, and the roof of the superior orbital fissure are drilled away with a diamond bit on a high-speed air drill. The dura propria is opened. Tumor tissue around the optic nerve is removed with bipolar coagulation and microdissectors, paying particular attention to preserve the ophthalmic artery and the central retinal artery (Fig. 15).

The above bony drilling exposes the superior aspect of the cavernous sinus. The internal carotid artery emerges through the superior wall surrounded and firmly anchored by the dural ring. Starting at this emergence, an incision is made in the exposed dura and extended posteriorly toward the posterior clinoid process. The internal carotid artery is then followed in retrograde fashion into the cavernous sinus, where it is dissected. In the cavernous sinus space, the tumor is dissected using the bipolar coagulation technique along with microdissectors (Fig. 16). Venous hemorrhage is not encountered until near the completion of tumor removal because of the compressed venous plexus (3,10). The abducens nerve is the only one that courses through the middle of the space lateral to the carotid artery. Its identification, dissection, and preservation demand particular attention.

If a tear occurs in the arterial wall, the surgeon should be prepared to apply temporary vascular clips of 30–40 g/mm^2 pressure and repair the arterial injury with fine microsutures. If sacrifice of the artery is necessary, the artery can be reconstructed using a venous graft or an EC-IC anastomosis can be performed (10). Details of surgery of the cavernous sinus tumor are described by Sekhar et al. (Cavernous Sinus and Sphenocavernous Neoplasms).

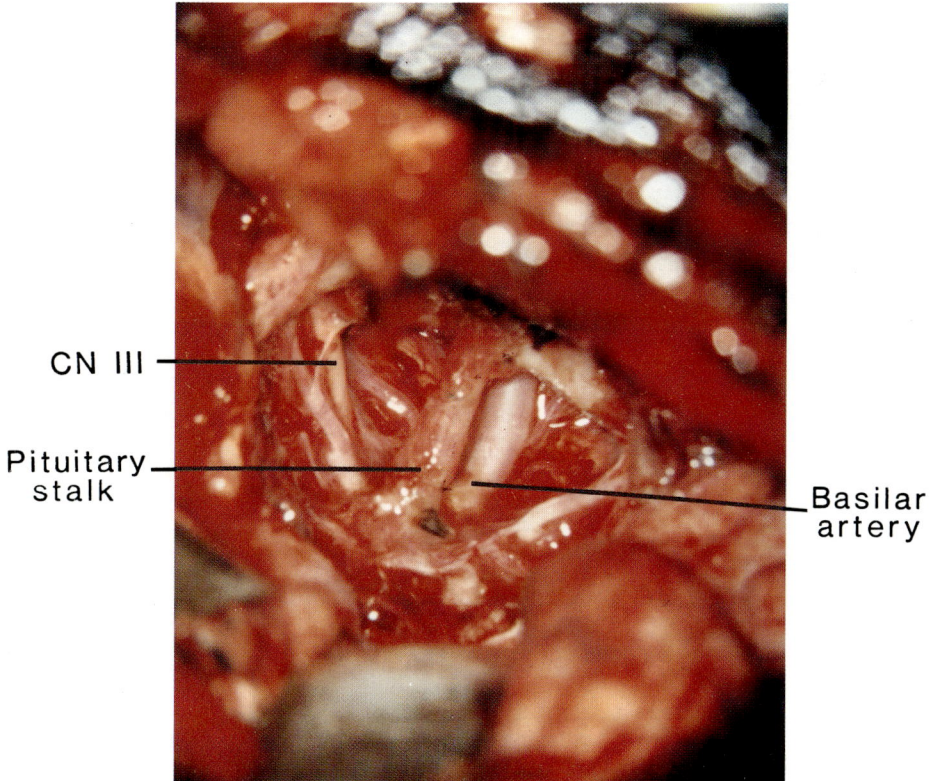

FIG. 12. Color operative photograph: surgeon's view of the tumor site after removal of its posterior extension. In the center is the pituitary stalk entering the diaphragma sella, arising behind the optic chiasm. The optic nerves are displaced laterally beyond the internal carotid artery. The basilar artery and the superior cerebellar artery are seen posterior to the dorsum sellae, and the oculomotor nerve and the posterior thalamic perforators are seen at the left.

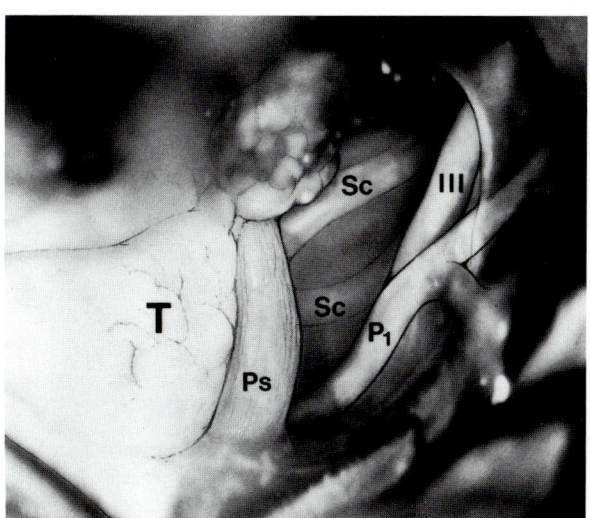

FIG. 13. Enhanced operative photograph: surgeon's view during removal of a meningioma from the interpeduncular cistern. The remaining tumor (T) displaces the pituitary stalk (Ps) to the right. The oculomotor nerve (III) and posterior cerebral artery (P-1) on the right are dissected free. Anatomical variant of a duplicate superior cerebellar artery (Sc) is seen.

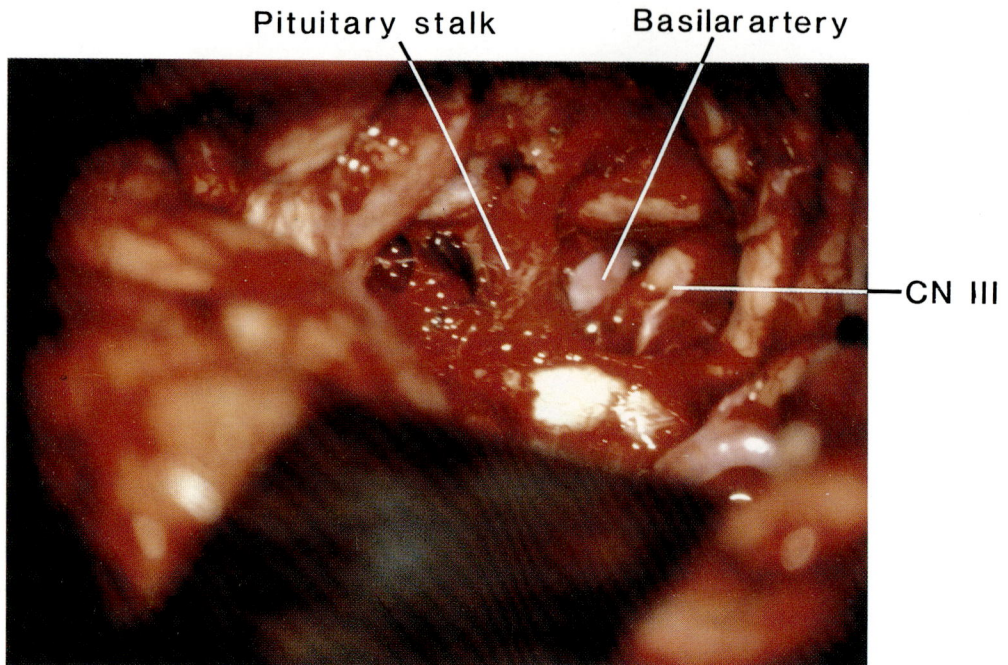

FIG. 14. Color operative photograph: surgeon's view of the interpeduncular cistern at the completion of tumor excision. The pituitary stalk and pituitary gland are seen in the center. The basilar artery, its branches, and cranial nerve III are seen behind the dorsum sellae.

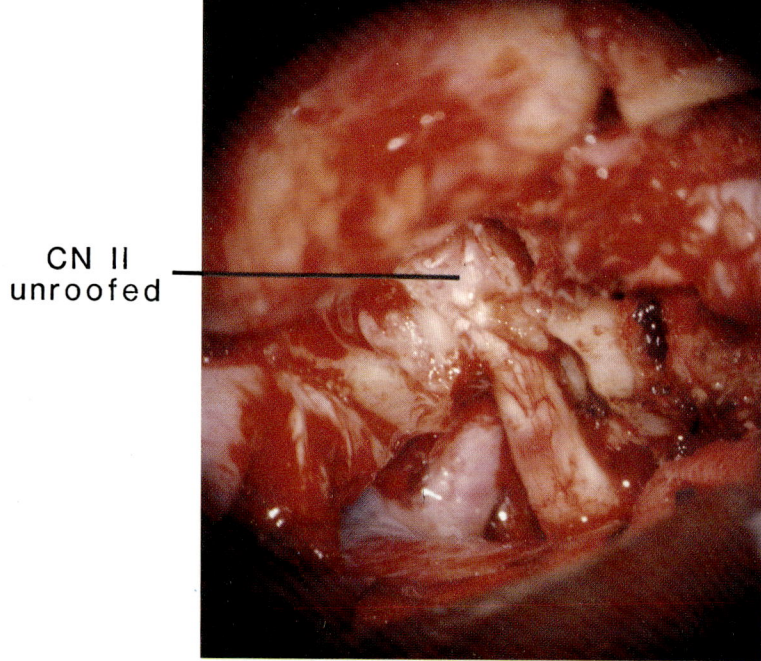

FIG. 15. Color operative photograph: surgeon's view of the unroofed left optic canal during removal of a tuberculum sella meningioma extending along the optic nerve.

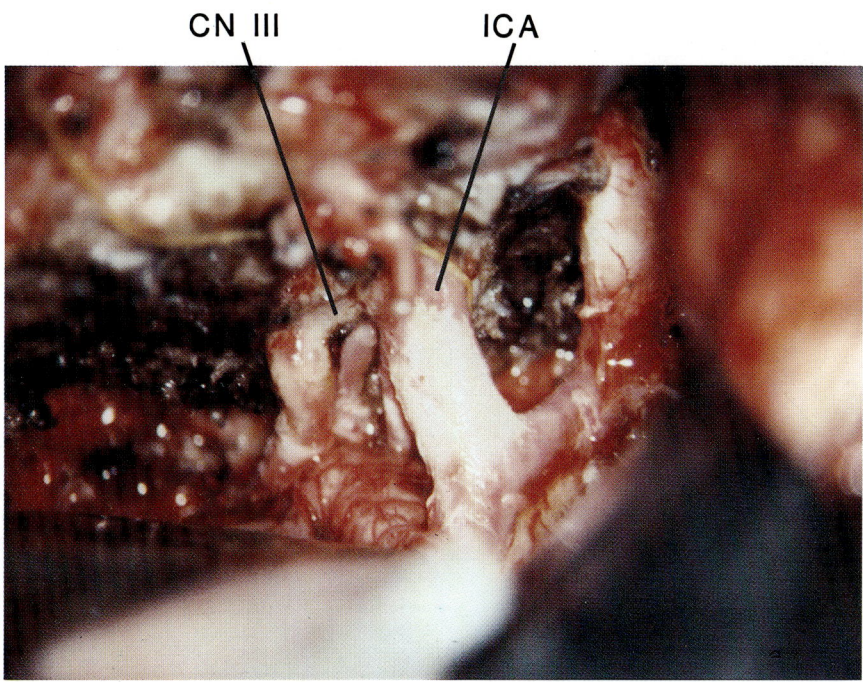

FIG. 16. Color operative photograph: surgeon's view during removal of a meningioma extending into the cavernous sinus; the superior and lateral cavernous sinus walls are opened. The internal carotid artery (ICA) and cranial nerve III are in view and being dissected from the surrounding tumor.

Tumor Attachment

When tumor removal is complete, the dura attachment should be resected. If dura resection is not possible, coagulation using the CO_2 laser is an alternative. If a laser is used, all neurovascular structures must be covered with wet surgical patties for protection. Involved bone can be removed using a diamond bit on a high-speed air drill, drilling the tuberculum sella, the anterior clinoid process, or ethmoid bone. The opening into the nasal sinus requires thorough repair of the dural defect. This is best done with a large piece of fascia lata. The fascia graft, which is laid intradurally, is secured with a few sutures along the lesser sphenoid wing. It is then spread to cover the frontal fossa and then is sutured to the frontal dura. Extradural coverage with a pericranial flap is described later.

Closure

At the conclusion of the procedure, the dura is made watertight. To avoid rhinorrhea, the preserved pericranium in the frontal region is turned over the frontal sinus and sutured to the dura mater. A heavy suture is used to reattach the bone flap to the cranial vault (Fig. 17). The temporalis muscle is sutured back to the fascia at the lateral orbital rim, and the skin is closed in two layers.

Operative Technique for Olfactory Groove Meningiomas

Olfactory groove meningiomas are approached through a bifrontal craniotomy. We prefer the inclusion of the supraorbital approach on the right side of the flap (Fig. 18). The base of the pericranial flap remains intact.

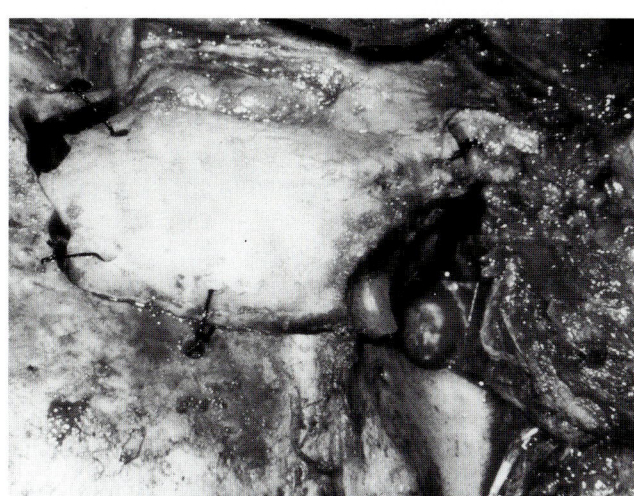

FIG. 17. Operative photograph: surgeon's view of the supraorbital flap secured with heavy sutures. The pericranial flap is turned over the frontal sinus under the bone flap.

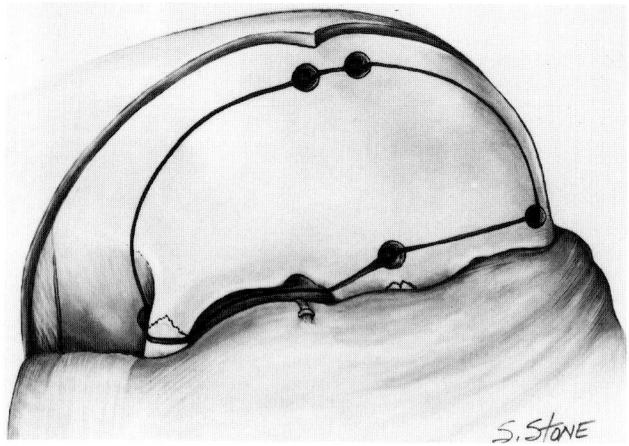

FIG. 18. Artist's illustration demonstrating the supraorbital bifrontal bone flap. Note the position of the holes and bony cuts.

The dura incision is made transversely over the medial inferior frontal lobes. The sagittal sinus is divided between two silk sutures and the falx is cut. The frontal lobes are carefully elevated and held by a brain spatula. The tumor comes into view in the midline and is readily exposed. The anterior aspect of the tumor's capsule is readily dissected free from the frontal lobes. The base of the tumor in the midline is gradually separated from the underlying bone, intercepting the tumor blood supply. Internal debulking is performed with the CUSA, or a CO_2 laser is used to remove a basal slice of the tumor. After the tumor is debulked, the capsule can be reflected into the hollowed area and gently dissected from the frontal lobes. Particular attention is paid to the dissection of the posterior pole of the tumor to free it from the pericallosal arteries and then the A-2 segment of the anterior cerebral arteries. A large tumor extending suprasellarly usually displaces the optic nerve and chiasm inferiorly. Maintaining an arachnoid cleavage assists in dissecting these structures free from the tumor. After the tumor is removed, the involved dura is excised and the involved bone is removed with a drill. If an extension into the ethmoid is present, this extension is followed and removed. The defect is closed by a sacral graft tied intradurally and then reflecting the vascularized pericranial flap extradurally over the defect. When the bony defect in the floor of the frontal fossa is large, a split thickness bone from the cranium is used to bridge the defect.

POSTOPERATIVE MANAGEMENT

We prefer prompt emergence from anesthesia and neurological evaluation of the patient. Fluid and electrolyte balance is monitored closely for possible diabetes insipidus. Steroids are tapered gradually in the postoperative period. In seizure-free patients, anticonvulsants are discontinued after 6 months.

COMPLICATIONS AND THEIR MANAGEMENT

A myriad of potential and reported complications are associated with removal of olfactory groove and tuberculum sella meningiomas and are detailed elsewhere (1). Although not necessarily a result of surgery, tumor recurrence testifies to surgical failure. Although true recurrence does occur, the tumor frequently recurs from subtotal removal or from conservative handling of tumor attachments or from missing a piece of tumor during intraoperative inspection.

Maintaining an adequate base and blood supply to the skin flap is a basic neurosurgical technique. Injury to the superior branches of the facial nerves can be avoided by following intrafascial dissection. Orbital swelling occurs more often, but it does not add significant morbidity during approaches that excise the orbital rim and roof. Entering the frontal sinus presents a potential source of septic complication and CSF leak. Important precautions to avoid this complication include exenteration of the mucosa, drilling the wall of the frontal sinus, packing the sinus with muscle, and covering it with a pericranial flap. The instruments used while handling the frontal sinus are disposed of and the surgical team redresses.

Injury to cerebral vessels is the most serious intraoperative complication. The anterior cerebral artery complex is the most likely to be injured; the fear of disastrous or fatal injury to cerebral vessels has kept many surgeons content with subtotal removal. With the microsurgical technique, however, the cerebral vessels can be dissected freely and safely. Although the small perforators supplying the hypothalamus and brain stem may not produce catastrophic hemorrhage, injury to these vessels produces a devastating neurological deficit. The importance of their preservation cannot be overemphasized, particularly since these vessels are apt to be mistaken for feeding vessels. Intraoperative hemorrhagic diathesis is most likely produced by consumption coagulopathy. This occurs when a massive blood transfusion has been given without concomitant replacement of the coagulation factors, a condition that can easily be avoided by giving proper transfusions of fresh frozen plasma and platelets along with intraoperative monitoring of the coagulation profile. Two less frequent vascular complications are iatrogenic aneurysm and postoperative delayed vasospasm with cerebral ischemic sequelae similar to the condition of subarachnoid hemorrhage from a ruptured aneurysm.

When brain swelling occurs intraoperatively, intracerebral or extracranial hematoma should be considered and inspected as a possible cause of swelling. Likewise, hydrocephalus, correctible through ventricular drainage, should be considered a possible cause. Preserving cerebral veins and facilitating venous drainage by accurate positioning of the head are important preventive maneuvers that avoid cerebral edema. The progressive excision of a large meningioma is an effective means of controlling an increasing ICP. Intraoperative brain swelling is rarely encountered nowadays, mainly because of the use of microsurgery and basal approaches. The role of intraoperative adjuvants, however, should not be downplayed. These adjuvants include steroids, hyperventilation, CSF drainage, and administration of mannitol or lasix.

Immediate postoperative worsening of the patient's condition is most likely due to hematoma or brain swelling. A CT scan is particularly helpful in the diagnosis. Rapid deterioration of the patient, however, may justify prompt surgical reexploration.

Because of the intimate relationship between the optic apparatus and the tumor, visual impairment may occur as a result of a variety of causes: development of a suprasellar hematoma, direct damage from surgical instruments or manipulation, interruption of vascular supply to the optic nerve and chiasm, migration of the optic chiasm, compression by surgically induced material, or arachnoiditis. The most important related cause of visual loss is ischemia, which results from interruption of the blood supply to the optic apparatus. The decussating fibers in the central chiasm are supplied solely by the inferior group of arteries arising from the circle of Willis. Failure to improve vision due to inadequate tumor removal and optic apparatus decompression should be considered a surgical disappointment at least. A suprasellar hematoma causing visual loss should be removed promptly, even though the prognosis for visual recovery is guarded.

Diabetes insipidus, usually transient in meningioma cases, is a frequent complication of surgery in the parasellar area and requires adequate monitoring of electrolyte and serum osmolarity. Partial or complete pituitary deficiency may occur after surgery for a tuberculum sella meningioma. A full endocrinological workup before and after surgery is routine in all cases. Hormonal replacement therapy is administered as indicated. Anosmia, which might be present preoperatively in olfactory groove meningiomas, frequently occurs after a subfrontal approach. Cranial nerves III, IV, and VI may suffer temporary or permanent palsy when the tumor is followed in the cavernous sinus. Frontal lobe syndrome might be present preoperatively or might result postoperatively. Minimal retraction and preservation of the frontal veins should decrease its occurrence.

Pulmonary embolism is still a heartbreaking cause of mortality, especially in patients who recover without neurological deficit. There is compelling evidence indicating that meningiomas may have a higher incidence of pulmonary embolism. The high incidence of pulmonary embolism may be related to the suprasellar location or hypercoagulation state in patients who harbor tumor or due to the lengthy procedure.

ILLUSTRATIVE CASES

Case 1. A 30-year-old white male presented with a 6-week history of right periorbital pain and total visual loss in the right eye and stuffiness in his nose. MRI demonstrated a large olfactory groove meningioma with extension through the ethmoid into the right nostril (Fig. 19). He underwent a total removal of his tumor through a bifrontal craniotomy. The floor of the frontal fossa was repaired with a pericranial flap and split thickness skull bone reconstruction. His vision promptly recovered postoperatively to the point of being able to count fingers with the right eye on the second postoperative day.

Case 2. A 60-year-old male presented with a yearlong history of bilateral gradual visual loss, headache, loss of libido, and weight loss. His visual examination showed vision present only in the left lower nasal quadrant with acuity of counting fingers at a distance of 2 feet. The right eye was totally blind with no light perception. A CT scan depicted a tuberculum sella meningioma with extension in both optic canals (Fig. 20A). During surgery, profuse bleeding ensued from an avulsed branch of the right anterior cerebral artery. This was controlled and the arterial wall was repaired with 10-0 sutures. Postoperatively, the patient was awake and alert and moving all extremities. Five days later the patient became obtunded and hemiparetic. His course continued to deteriorate. An arteriogram on the ninth postoperative day confirmed postoperative vasospasm (Fig. 20B). The patient declined into a vegetative a state and eventually expired 5 months later.

CASE MATERIAL

My series includes 35 tuberculum sella meningiomas and 14 olfactory groove meningiomas operated on during the past 8 years. Some of these patients were included in previous publications (2,3). All the tumors but one exceeded 4 cm in diameter. Visual loss was the main presenting syndrome in the tuberculum sella meningiomas, while frontal lobe syndrome, seizures, and anosmia were the findings in olfactory groove meningiomas. Four patients had evidence of multiple meningiomas. Total tumor removal, as confirmed by postoperative enhanced CT or MRI, was achieved in all but three patients. There were three deaths, two due to pulmonary embolism and one patient with a progressive neurological deficit and postoperative delayed vasospasm. There was only one patient with postoperative visual worsening. Improvement of vision was encountered in 25% of the patients, including visual recovery of a totally blind eye in two

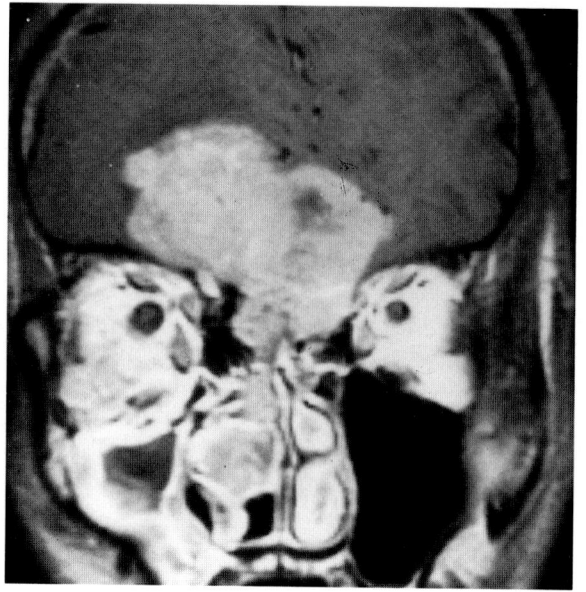 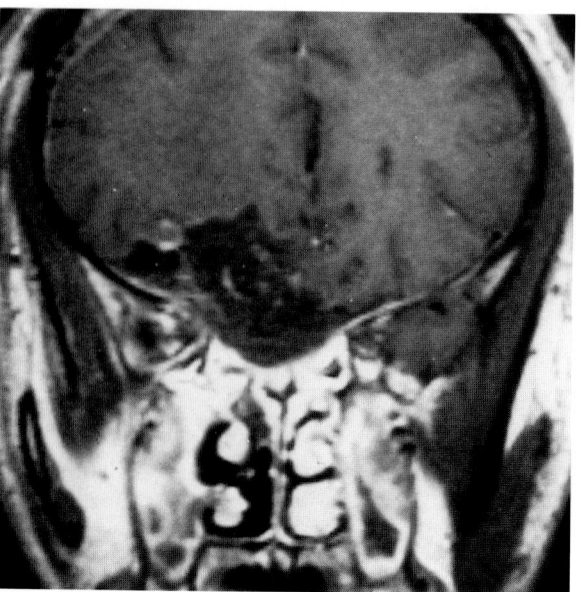

FIG. 19. Contrast enhanced coronal MRI scan demonstrating olfactory groove meningioma with nasal extension. **A:** Preoperative. **B:** Postoperative.

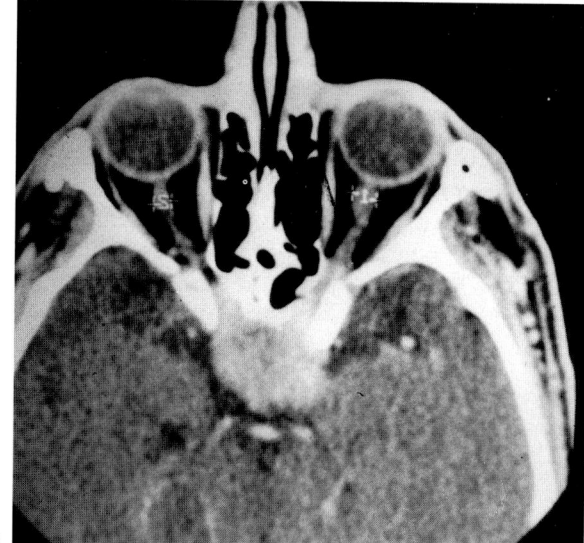 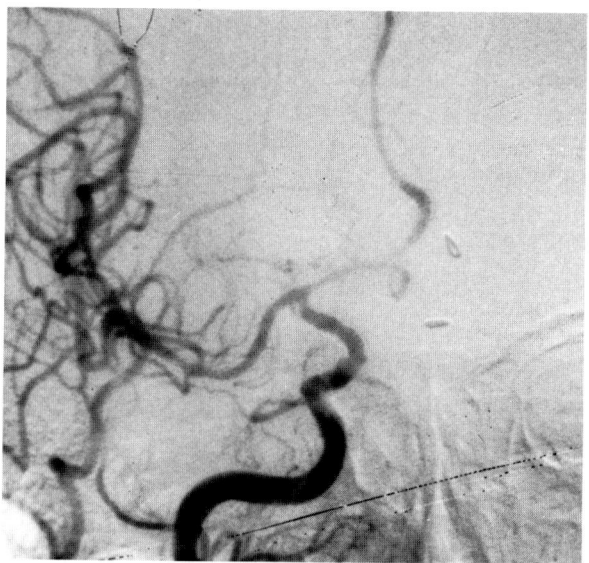

FIG. 20. A: A low cut of contrast enhanced CT scan of tuberculum sella meningioma with extension into both optic canal and right cavernous sinus. **B:** Nine days postoperative arteriogram depicting vasospasm.

patients where recovery was transient in one patient and sight remained functional in the other patient (Case 1). There was one delayed but transient hemiparesis. Two patients required a CSF shunting procedure for hydrocephalus. One epidural hematoma, remote from the surgical flap, was treated successfully. Two patients had transient hepatitis. One-third of the patients were treated for transient diabetes insipidus. The survivors left the hospital otherwise neurologically unchanged or improved, compared to their preoperative status.

REFERENCES

1. Al-Mefty O. *Surgery of the cranial base.* Boston: Kluwer Academic Publishers, 1989;31–126.
2. Al-Mefty O, Holoubi A, Rifai A, Fox JL. Microsurgical removal of suprasellar meningiomas. *Neurosurgery* 1985;16:364–372.
3. Al-Mefty O, Smith RR. Surgery of tumors invading the cavernous sinus. *Surg Neurol* 1988;30:370–381.
4. Bakay L. Olfactory meningiomas: the missed diagnosis. *JAMA* 1984;251:53–55.
5. Cushing H, Eisenhardt L. *Meningiomas: their classification, regional behaviour, life history, and surgical end results.* Baltimore: Charles C. Thomas, 1938.
6. Jane JA, Park TS, Pobereskin LH, Winn HR, Butler AB. The supraorbital approach: technical note. *Neurosurgery* 1982;11:537–542.
7. Kadis GN, Mount LA, Ganti SR. The importance of early diagnosis and treatment of the meningiomas of the planum sphenoidale and tuberculum sellae: a retrospective study of 105 cases. *Surg Neurol* 1979;12:367–371.
8. Ojemann RG, Swann KW. Meningiomas of the anterior cranial base. In: Sekhar LN, Schramm VL, eds. *Tumors of the cranial base: diagnosis and treatment.* Mount Kisco, NY: Futura Publishing Company, 1987;279–294.
9. Parent AD, Al-Mefty O. Visual recovery after blindness from compressive neuropathy (poster). AANS Annual Meeting, April 1988, Toronto, Canada.
10. Sekhar LN, Sen CN, Jho HD, Janecka IP. Surgical treatment of intracavernous neoplasms: a four-year experience. *Neurosurgery* 1989;24:18–30.
11. Shapiro HM. Neurosurgical anesthesia and intracranial hypertension. In: Miller RD, ed. *Anesthesia,* vol 3, 2nd ed. New York: Churchill Livingstone, 1986;1249–1620.
12. Simpson D. The recurrence of intracranial meningiomas after surgical treatment. *J Neurol Neurosurg Psychiatry* 1957;20:22–39.
13. Symon L, Rosenstein J. Surgical management of suprasellar meningioma. Part 1: The influence of tumor size, duration of symptoms, and microsurgery on surgical outcome in 101 consecutive cases. *J Neurosurg* 1984;61:633–641.

CHAPTER 37

Cavernous Sinus and Sphenocavernous Neoplasms

Anatomy and Surgery

Laligam N. Sekhar, Donald A. Ross, and Chandranath Sen

With improved neuroanatomical knowledge, imaging, and surgical techniques, direct surgery within the cavernous sinus (CS) is gaining wider acceptance (1,4,11,12,23,26). The practice of cavernous sinus surgery requires a detailed and practical knowledge of the relevant anatomy, and the reader is referred to the many excellent reviews in this area for detailed information (14,18,19,24,31,32,34). The surgeon who wants to learn surgery of CS lesions must be expert in general microsurgery and must learn the anatomy and approaches to CS lesions through cadaveric dissections and by observation of experienced surgeons who work in this area.

The cavernous sinus itself contains the internal carotid artery (ICA), the sixth cranial nerve (CN), and the sympathetic nerve. The third nerve, fourth nerve, first division of the fifth nerve (V_1), and the second division of the fifth (V_2) nerve are contained between the two dural leaves comprising the lateral wall of the cavernous sinus.

The inner dural layer is thinner and is continuous with the periosteal covering of the temporal, clival, and sphenoid bones. The thicker outer layer is continuous with the dura of the middle fossa, the anterior clinoid space, the sella, the clivus, and the tentorium.

The cavernous ICA has two constant branches, the meningohypophyseal trunk and the inferolateral trunk (or artery of the inferior cavernous sinus). The capsular artery of McConnell, the ophthalmic artery, and other unnamed vessels may arise from it also. The cavernous ICA is surrounded by three fibrous rings. The first is a periosteal ring found at the entrance of the petrous ICA into the CS. At the distal cavernous ICA, two dural rings are found that fuse medially and are separated by the anterior clinoid process laterally. The second ring lies just medial to CN III. The third ring or the dural ring surrounds the exit of the ICA from the CS. Although some authors feel that the space exposed by the removal of the anterior clinoid process ("the clinoid space") is not actually within the CS, we believe that this clinoid space is part of the cavernous plexus of veins. During anatomical dissections and at operation, a fine periosteal layer is seen to surround the clinoidal segment of the cavernous ICA. When this layer is opened, a venous plexus is found in the clinoid space, which is continuous with the remainder of the cavernous plexus. The surgical anatomy of the CS appears in Figs. 1–21.

L. N. Sekhar: Department of Neurosurgery, Center for Cranial Base Surgery, University of Pittsburgh School of Medicine, and Presbyterian University Hospital, Pittsburgh, Pennsylvania 15213.
D. A. Ross: Section of Neurological Surgery, University of Michigan, Ann Arbor, Michigan 48109.
C. Sen: Department of Neurosurgery, Mount Sinai Medical Center, New York, New York 10029.

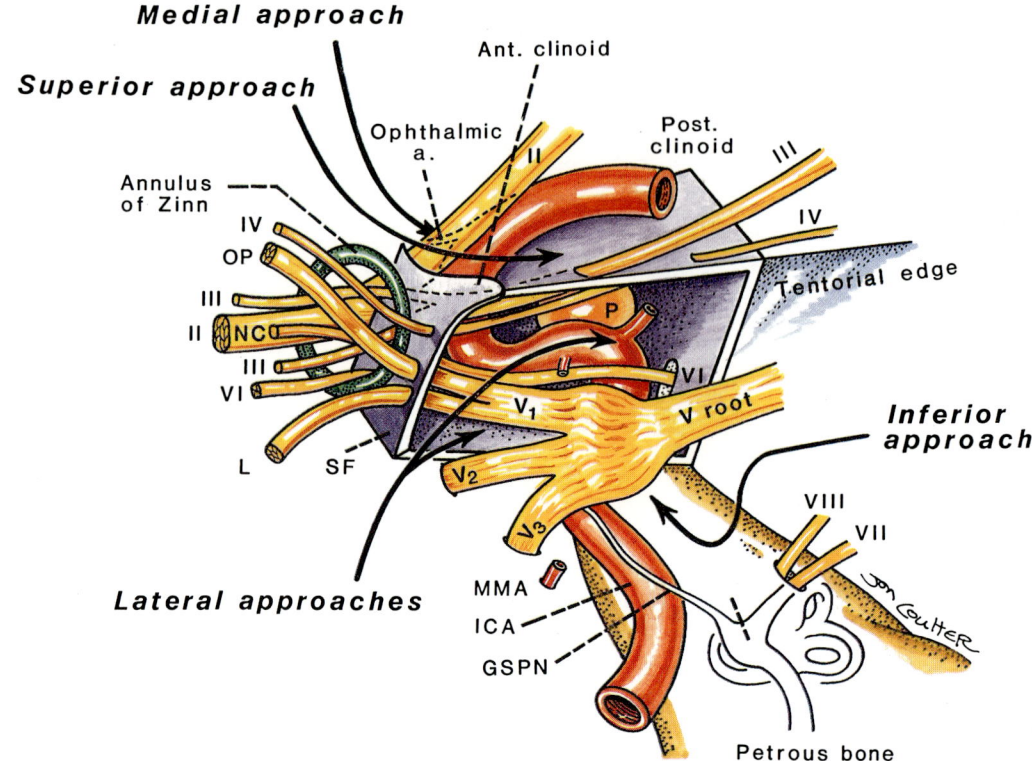

FIG. 1. This schematic diagram illustrates the anatomy of the cavernous sinus, and the related cranial nerves and vessels. The inferior, lateral, superior, and medial approaches to the cavernous sinus are shown with *arrows*. II–VIII, cranial nerves; ICA, internal carotid artery; MM, middle meningeal artery; MA, meningohypophyseal artery; P, pituitary gland; DC, Dorello's canal; GSPN, greater superficial petrosal nerve; GG, geniculate ganglion; SF, superior orbital fissure; NC, nasociliary nerve; L, lacrimal nerve. (From ref. 24, with permission.)

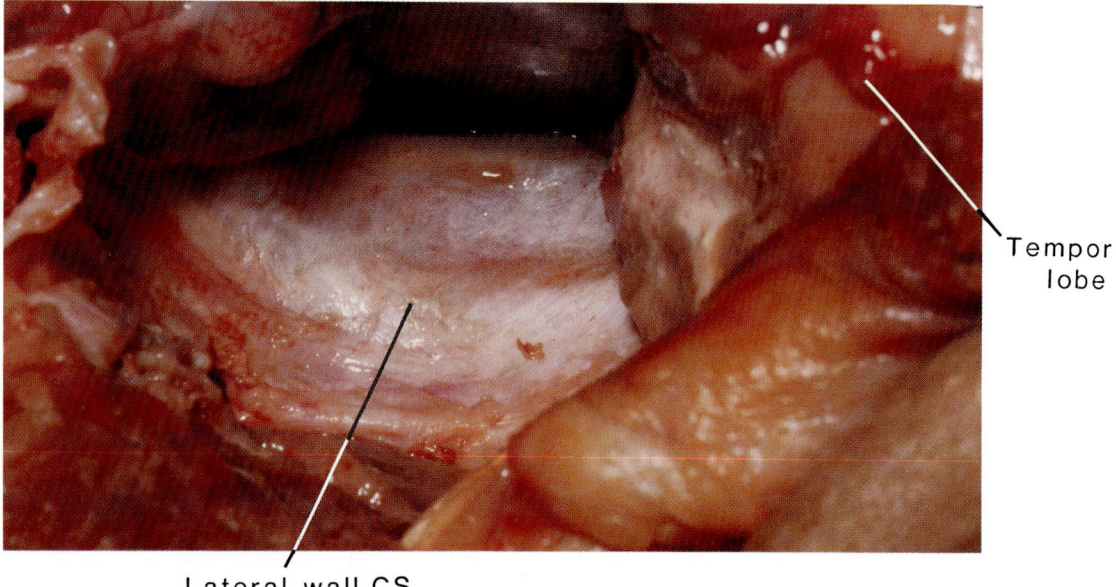

FIG. 2. Illustration of the anatomy of the cavernous sinus area in cadaveric dissections on the left side (see Figs. 3–9). The temporal lobe has been partially excised and retracted in this fresh cadaver specimen. The lateral dural wall of the CS is seen.

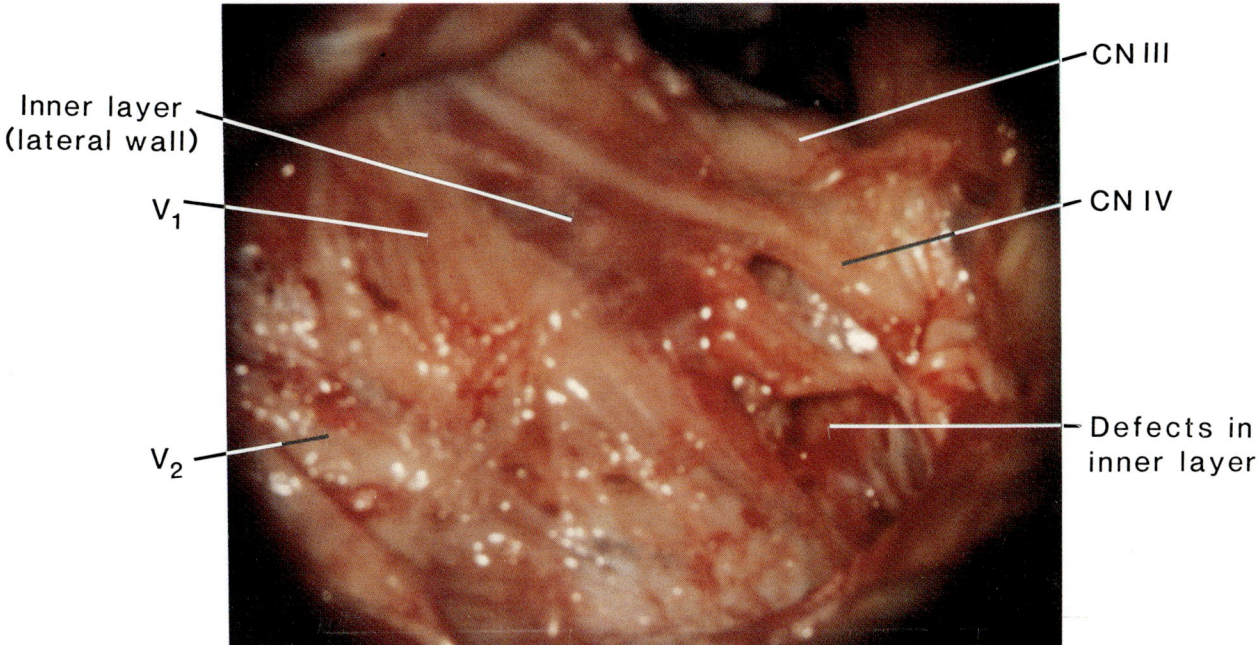

FIG. 3. The outer layer of the lateral wall has been peeled away. It can be seen that the inner layer is thin and envelops cranial nerves III, IV, and V. It is also incomplete in places. The lateral wall of the CS may be thinned in patients with intracavernous neurilemomas, chordomas, or chondrosarcomas. Meningiomas involving the lateral wall and prior surgery make the lateral wall much thicker.

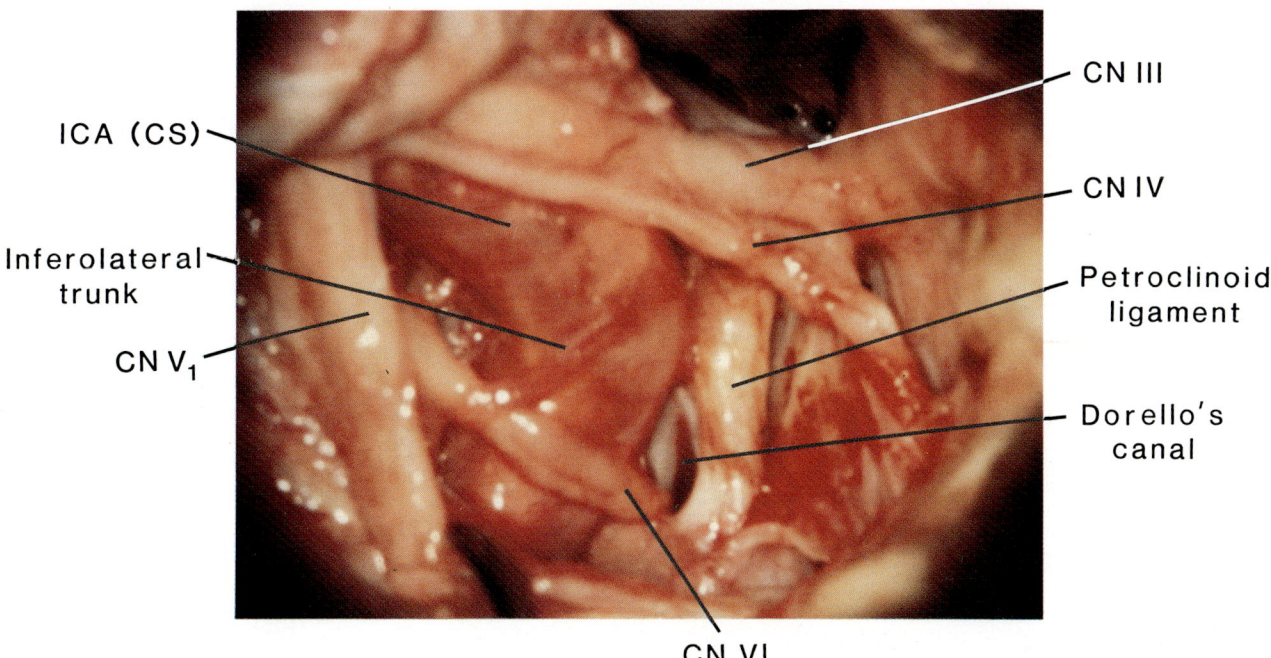

FIG. 4. The inner layer has been peeled away to expose the cranial nerves and the intracavernous ICA. The ophthalmic nerve (V_1) is being depressed to expose the abducens nerve. CN VI is entering the CS through Dorello's canal and is being crossed by the inferolateral trunk. V_1 crosses it at an angle such that, at the anterior end of the CS, CN VI lies slightly inferior to V_2. In this specimen, one sees the "open Parkinson's triangle" because CN IV closely follows the course of CN III. However, in other cases, the trochlear nerve may have a sharp inferior dip to become parallel to V_1 such that Parkinson's triangle becomes a "closed" one.

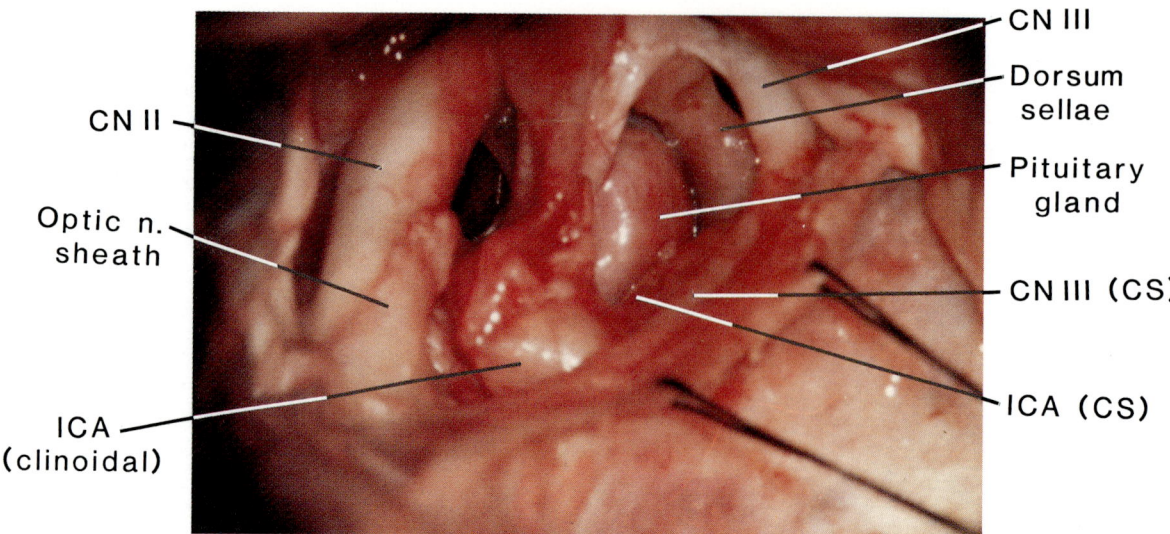

FIG. 5. The superior approach is shown here. The supraclinoid ICA is collapsed in this uninjected specimen. The tentorial edge containing the oculomotor nerve has been retracted laterally with sutures. The horizontal segment of the intracavernous ICA, the pituitary gland, and the dorsum sellae are exposed by this approach. When there is no intracavernous mass (the intracavernous ICA can be exposed back to the posterior bend by this approach), this approach is adequate for most paraclinoidal aneurysms.

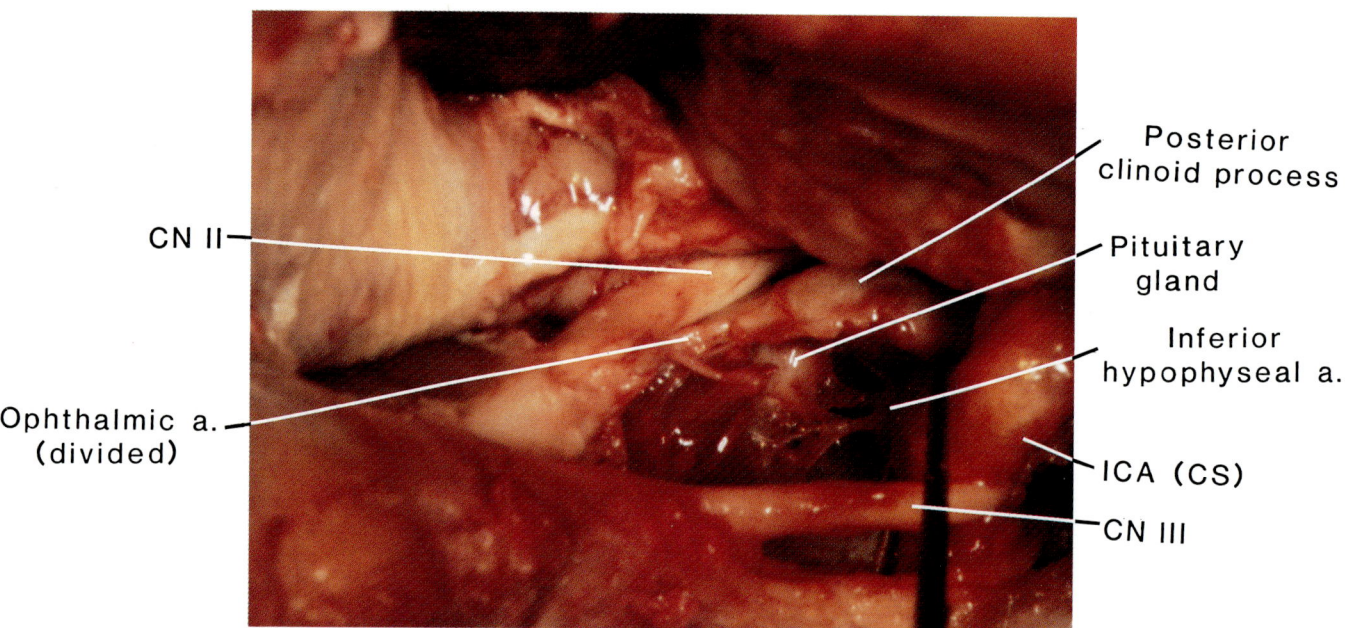

FIG. 6. Superior approach. The trochlear nerve and the ophthalmic artery have been divided. The intracavernous ICA has been elevated out of the CS to reveal the medial course of the inferior hypophyseal artery.

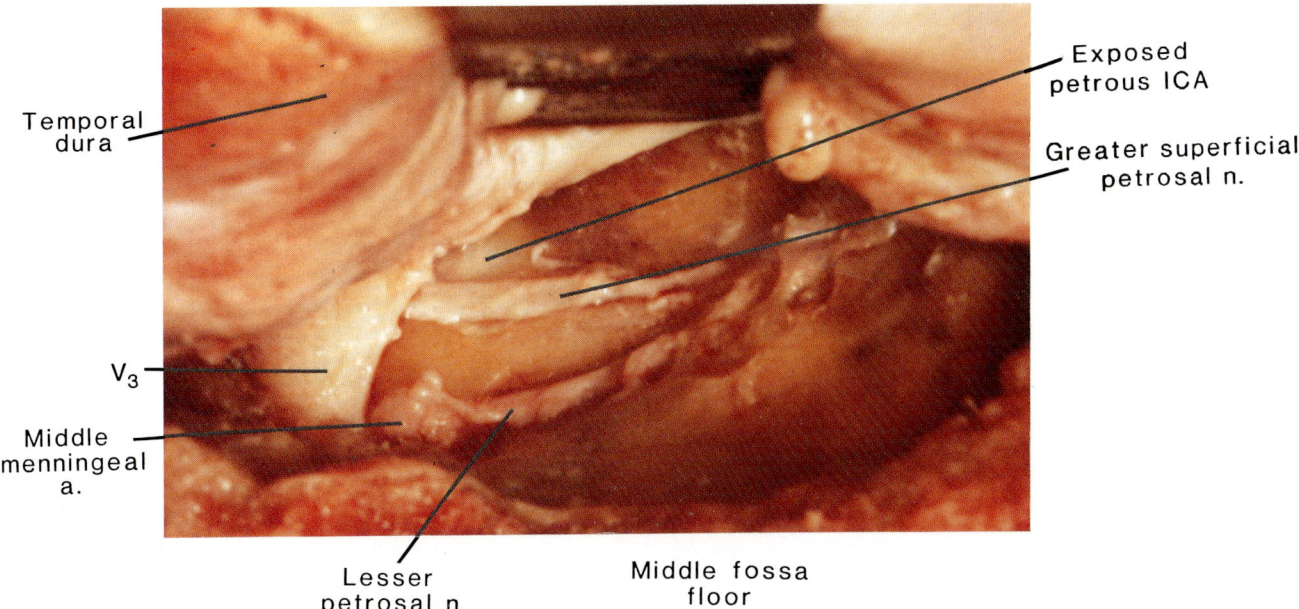

FIG. 7. Extradural middle fossa dissection and inferior approach. The arcuate eminence and the tegmen tympani are not shown. The remaining landmarks, including petrous ICA partially uncovered by bone, are visible.

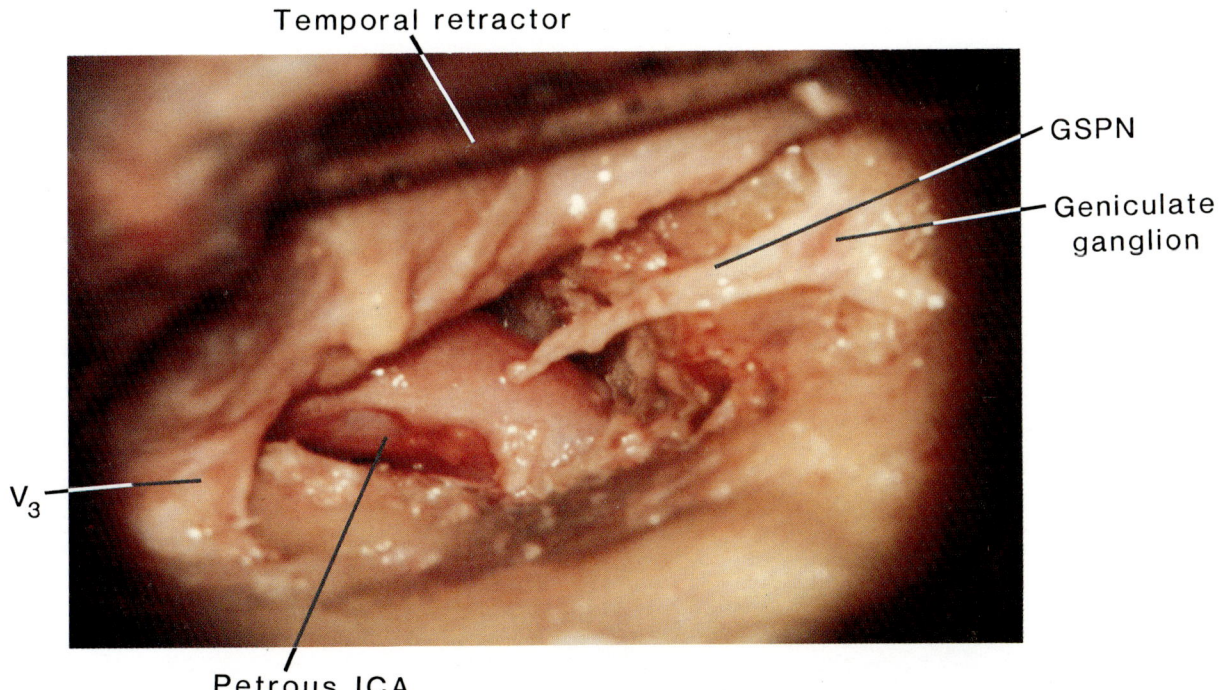

FIG. 8. Inferior approach. The horizontal segment of the petrous ICA has been exposed by drilling away bone. The facial nerve has been exposed to illustrate the relationship.

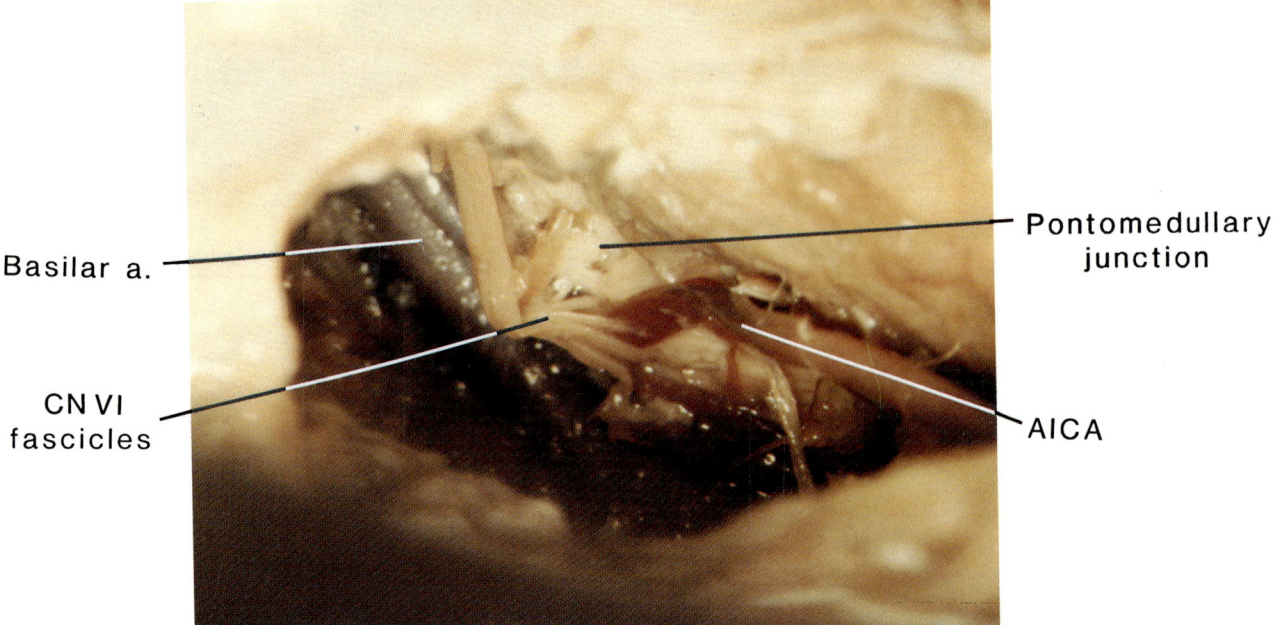

FIG. 9. Inferior approach. The petrous apex has been drilled away lateral to the trigeminal root and posteromedial to the horizontal petrous ICA, and the dura has been opened. One can see the basilar artery, pontomedullary junction area, the fascicles of origin of the abducens nerve, and the anterior-inferior cerebellar artery coursing between the fascicles. The abducens nerve is seen to be ascending toward Dorello's canal. This technique is useful to expose small extensions of cavernous sinus tumors and also to expose the abducens nerve before it enters the CS. The petrous apex and the clival bone medial to the trigeminal nerve cannot be removed extradurally. It is easier to remove it by working through the CS after the excision of intracavernous tumor.

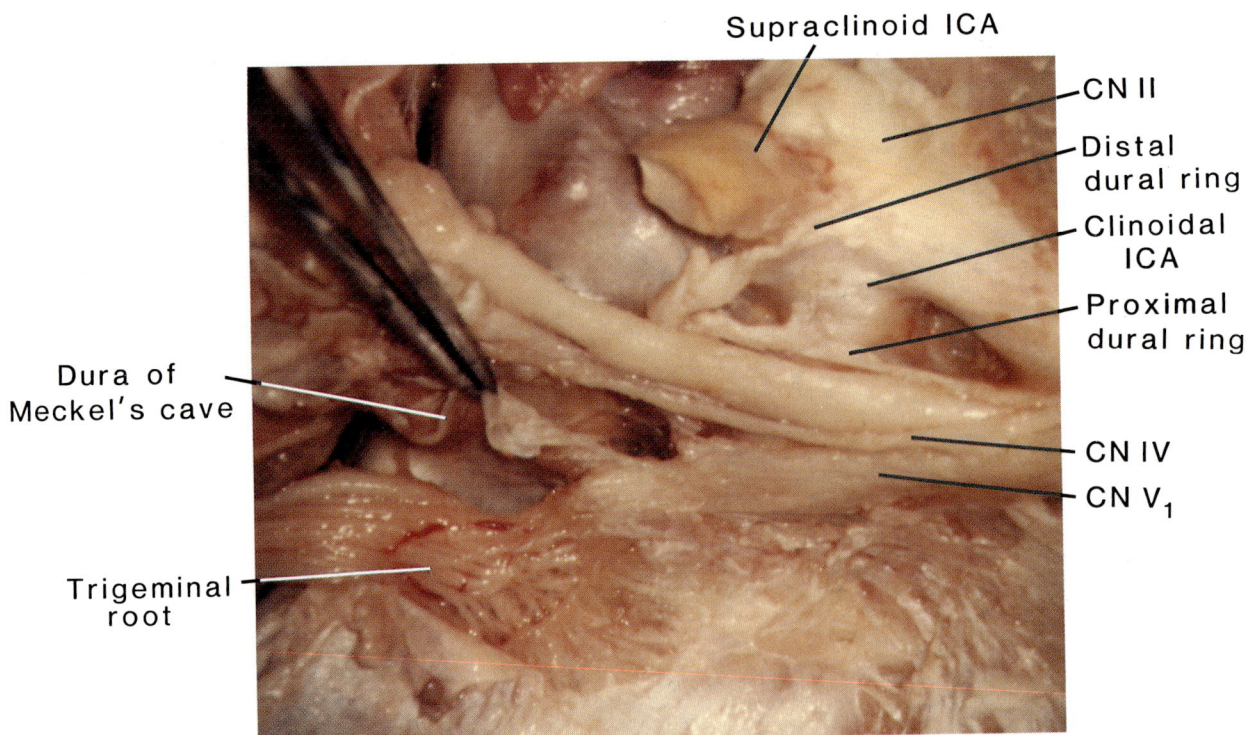

FIG. 10. The series of dissections shown in this figure through Fig. 19 illustrate the cavernous sinus anatomy on the right side. In this dissection, the clinoid process has been removed and the optic nerve canal unroofed. The clinoid space is clearly visible, with the distal two "rings" around the clinoidal ICA. The sheath of the third cranial nerve has been opened and Meckel's cave unroofed to show the trigeminal roof, ganglion, and V_1.

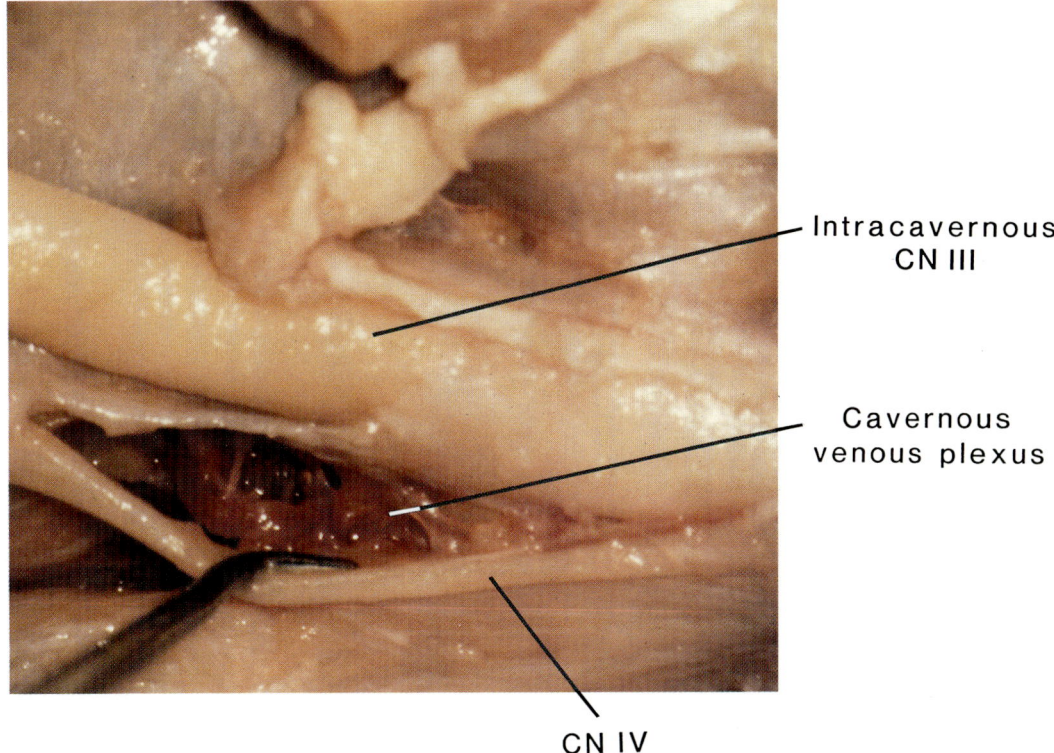

FIG. 11. Close-up view of the entrance area of CN III into the CS. Its dural sheath has been opened to reveal a still persistent arachnoidal covering. CN IV has been depressed. The venous plexus within the CS is clearly visible in this specimen.

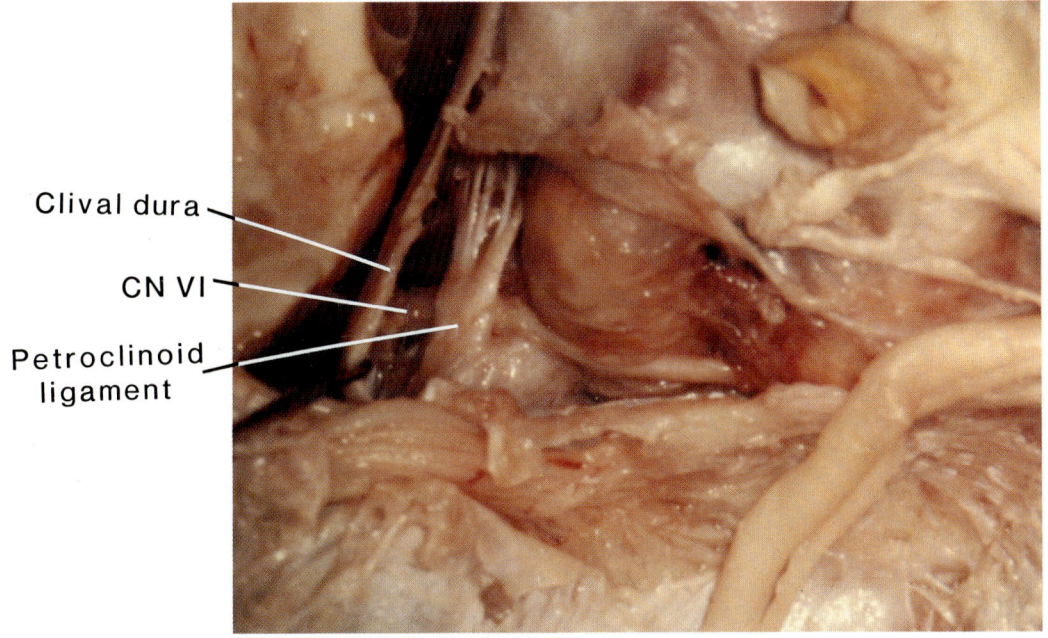

FIG. 12. Cranial nerves III and IV have been moved away, and some of the medial wall of Meckel's cave has been removed to show the abducens nerve. It can be seen that CN VI enters the clival dura first, and then Dorello's canal, with a segment interposed.

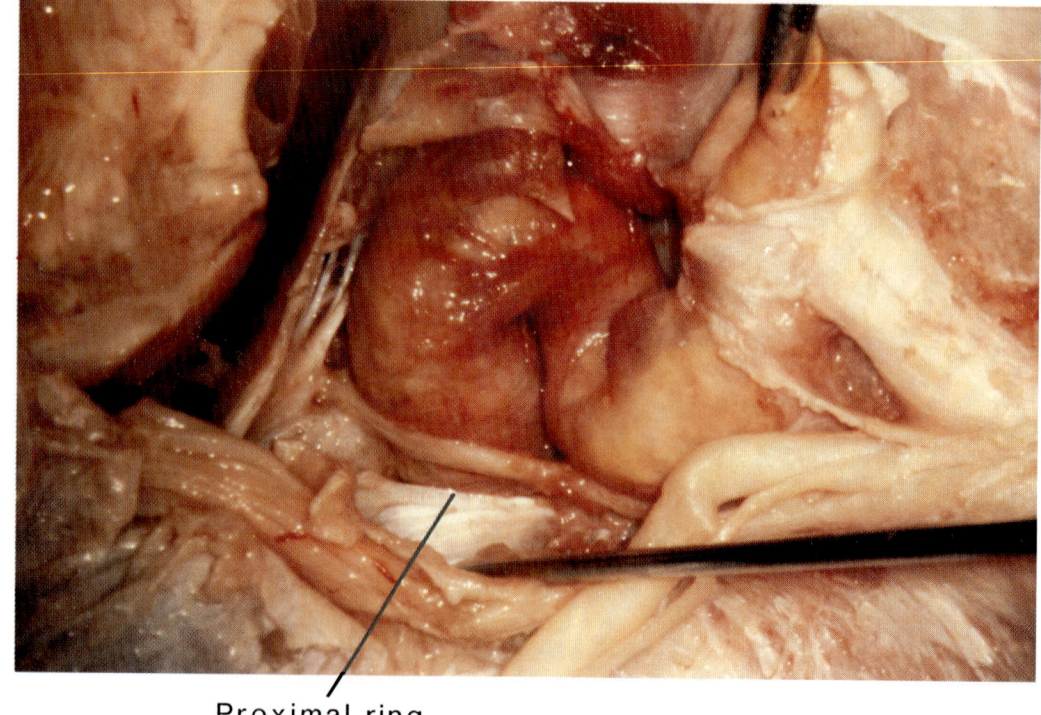

FIG. 13. In this dissection, the entire intracavernous ICA and all three rings around it are exposed. This intracavernous carotid artery is S-shaped.

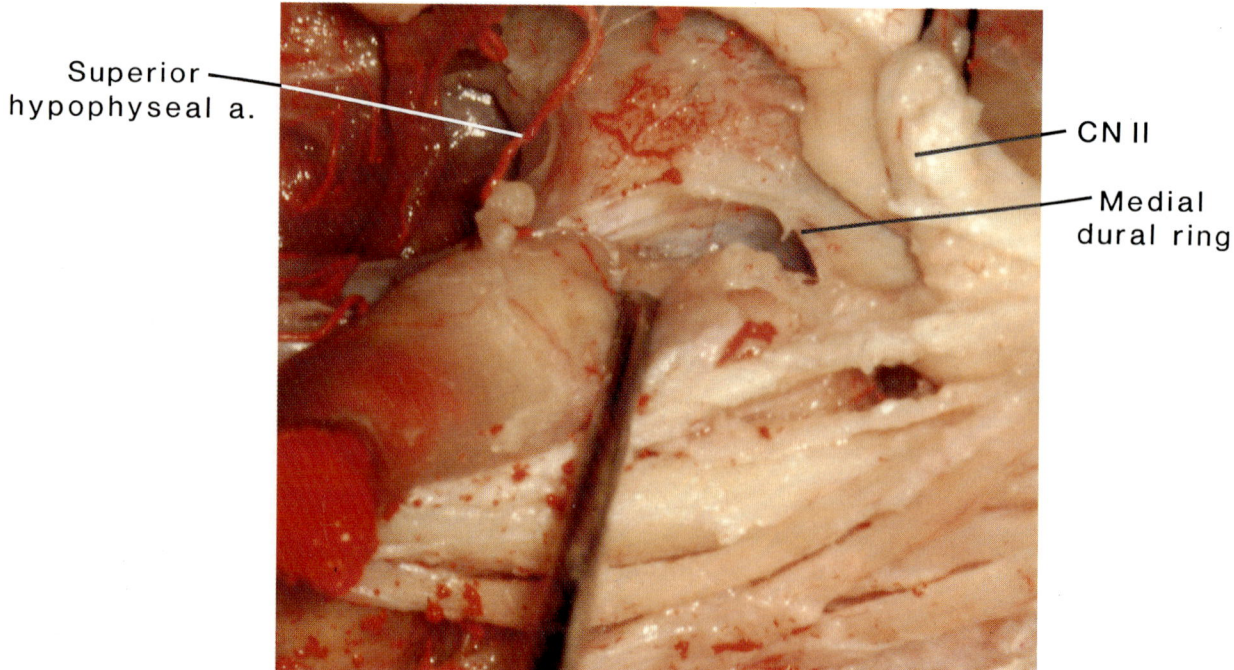

FIG. 14. The medial aspect of the dural ring is exposed by a section of the ophthalmic artery and the elevation of the optic nerve. The distal and middle dural rings fuse medially to form a single ring. The superior hypophyseal artery is also exposed.

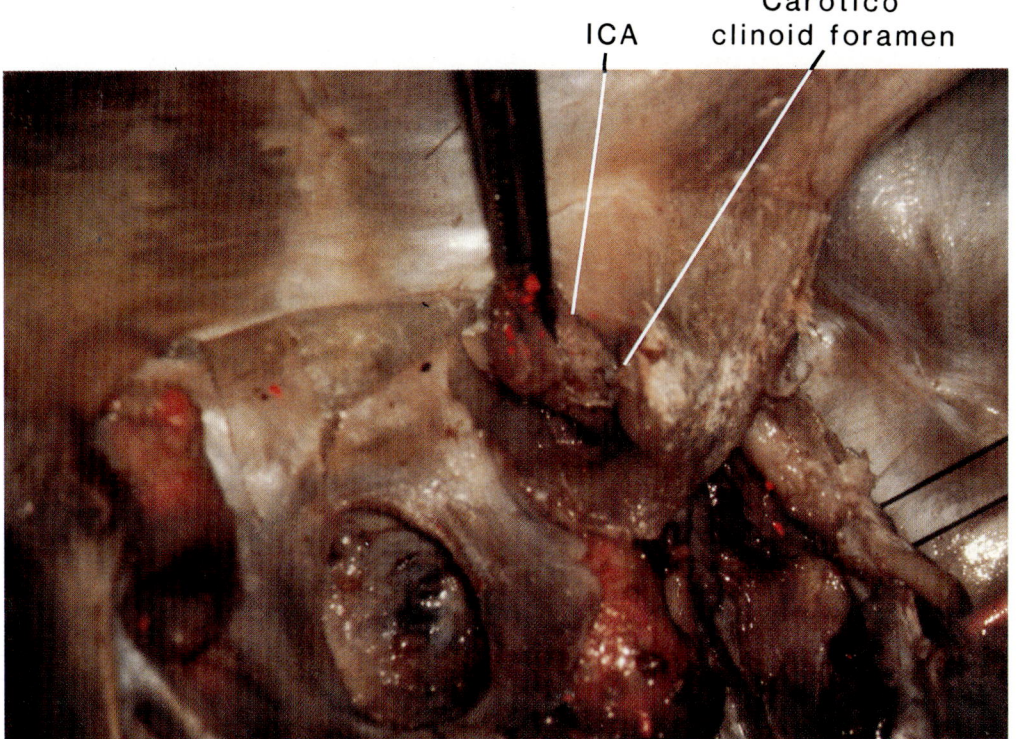

FIG. 15. The formation of a bony ring around the exit of the intracavernous ICA is seen. This would obviously present a problem for extradural resection of the clinoid process.

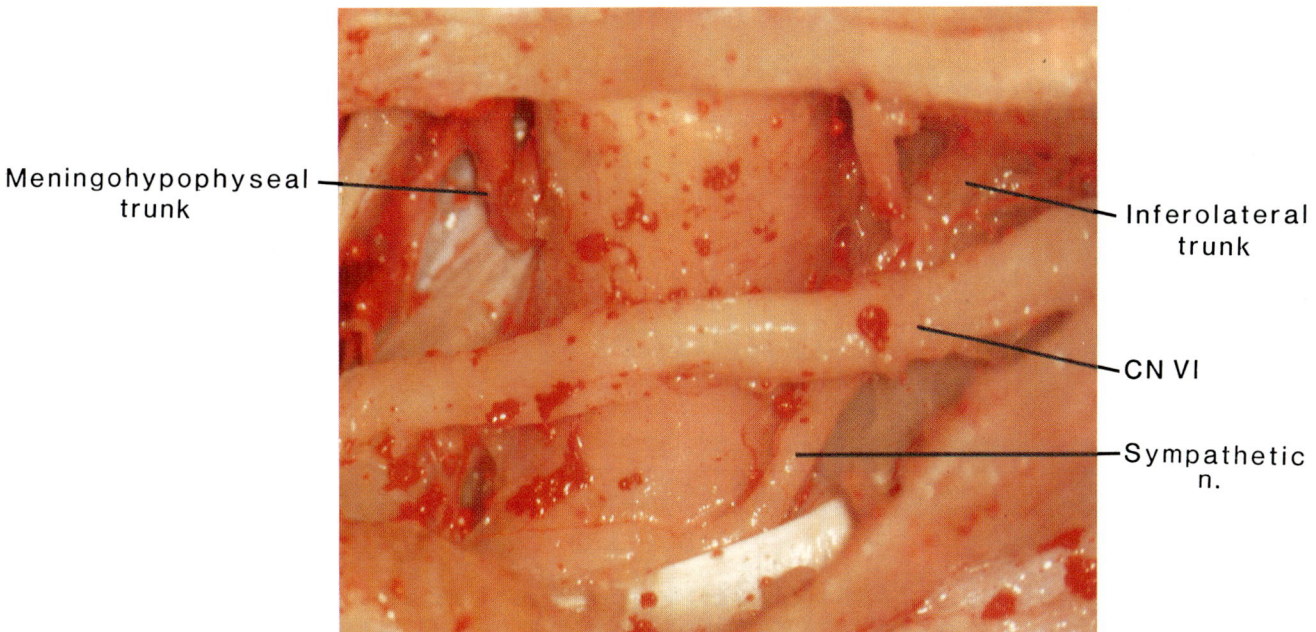

FIG. 16. Magnified view through Parkinson's triangle showing the sympathetic nerve joining the abducens nerve. The meningohypophyseal and inferolateral trunks are also seen.

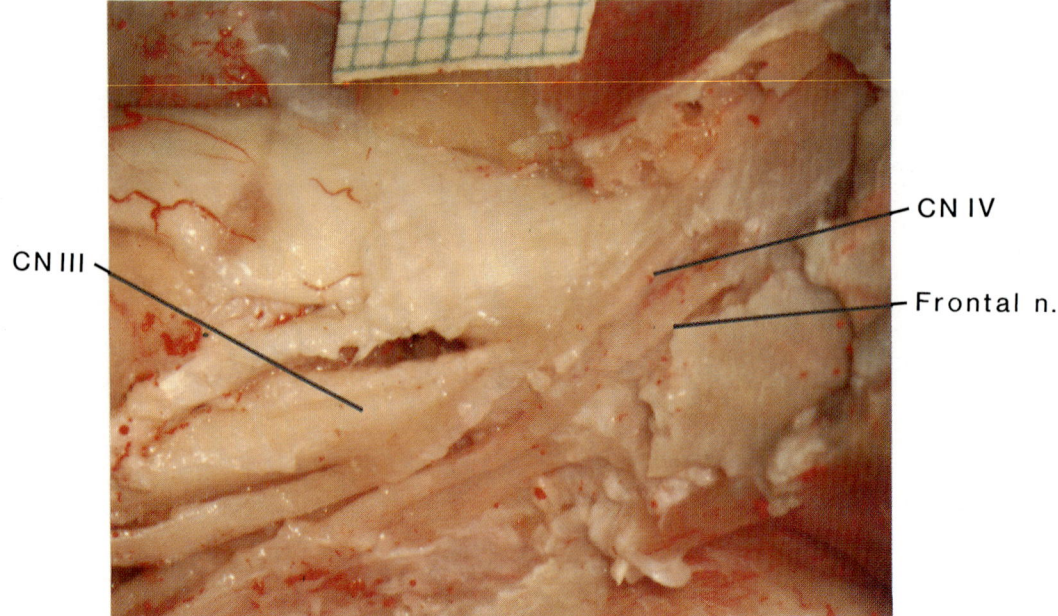

FIG. 17. At the apex of the cavernous sinus, the fourth cranial nerve and the frontal branch of the ophthalmic nerve cross lateral to the oculomotor nerve to enter the orbital apex area, outside the muscle cone.

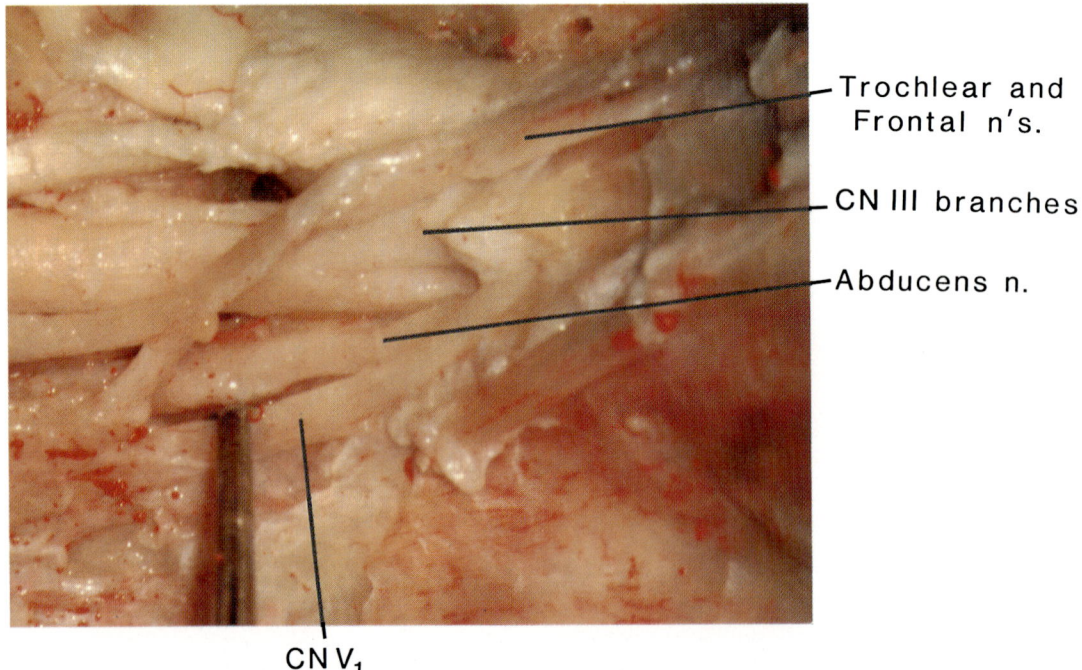

FIG. 18. At the apex of the cavernous sinus, the trochlear nerve and the frontal nerve have been elevated. Note the division of the oculomotor nerve into two branches, and the abducens nerve between the frontal nerve, and the remainder of the ophthalmic nerve. The ophthalmic nerve further divides into nasociliary and lacrimal branches.

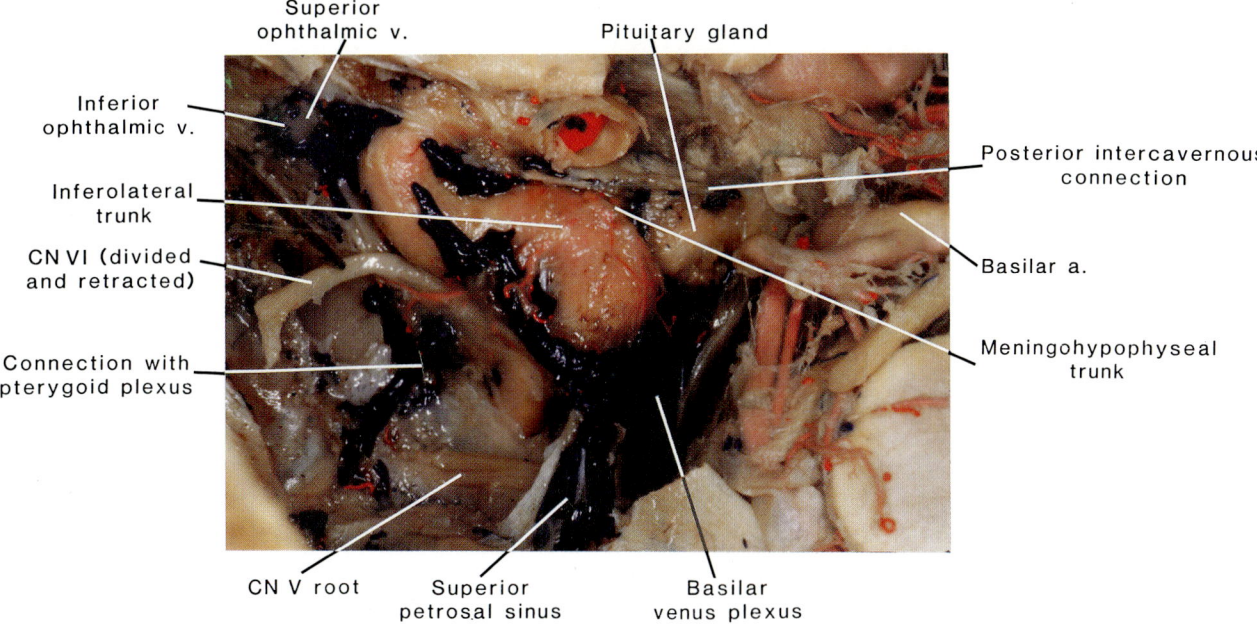

FIG. 19. In this specimen, the veins have been injected to illustrate the connections of the cavernous venous plexus.

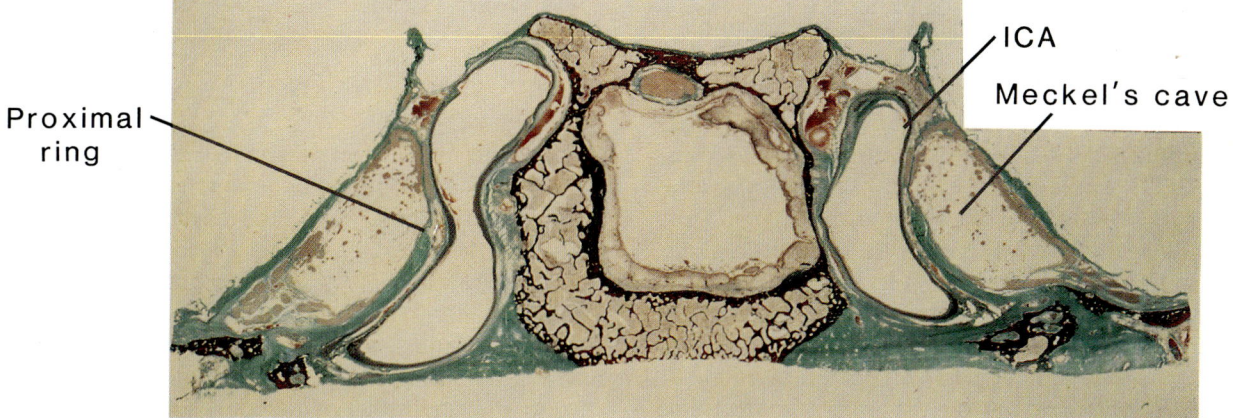

FIG. 20. Coronal section through a decalcified specimen stained with Masson trichrome (courtesy of Dr. Gutti R. Rao). Note that the outer dural layer is continuous with the diaphragma sellae. The inner layer of the lateral wall may be formed by the epineurium around CNs III, IV, and V. Smaller and larger venous spaces within the CS are visible. The medial periosteal layer continues across to the other side. The dural envelope of the pituitary gland, which forms the medial wall of the CS, is separated from the periosteal layer by various spaces. This provides one route for spread of tumor from one CS to the other, and also a way to reach the other CS from the ipsilateral side, when the intracavernous ICA has been excised or reconstructed with a graft.

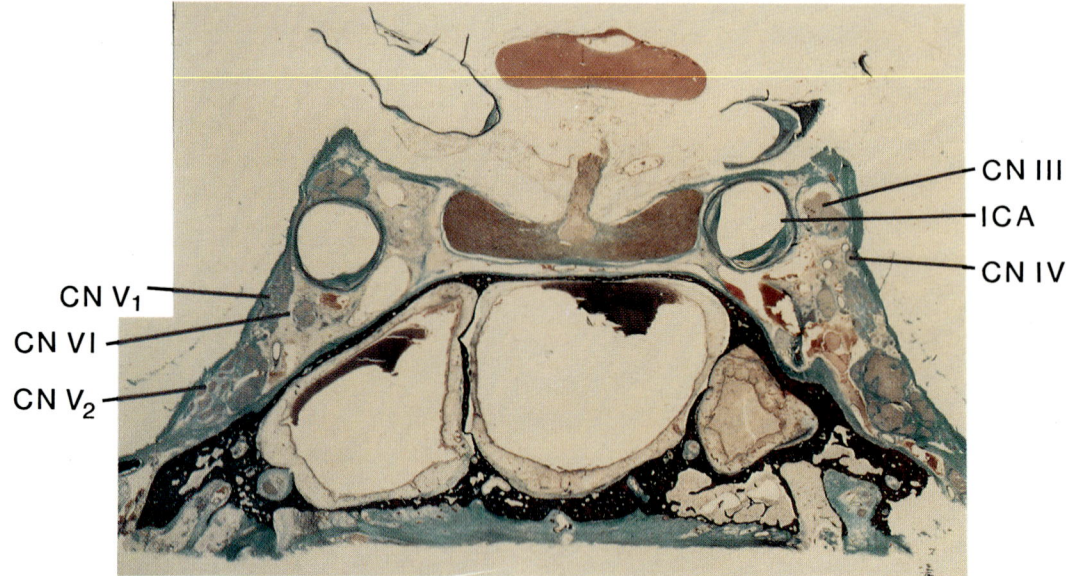

FIG. 21. Coronal section more posteriorly through the Meckel's cave area. Note the portion of the intracavernous ICA that lies medial to Meckel's cave. Note the proximal ring at the entrance of the ICA into the CS.

CLASSIFICATION OF CAVERNOUS SINUS TUMORS

A rational classification of cavernous sinus tumors is necessary to assess the technical difficulty of resection and for comparison of the results of surgery. The following classification system (Table 1) is based on magnetic resonance imaging (MRI) and is particularly suited to intracavernous meningiomas, although also applicable to other benign lesions. Grade I tumors are those that occupy only a single area of the cavernous sinus and do not encase the carotid artery. Grade II lesions occupy multiple areas of the cavernous sinus and displace but do not surround the carotid artery. Grade III lesions have encased the artery without narrowing, while Grade IV tumors both encase and narrow the artery. Grade V tumors are those involving both cavernous sinuses and with carotid encasement. Grade I and II tumors are much easier to resect since they can be peeled from intracavernous ICA, whereas tumors in grades III–V often require graft reconstruction and excision of the intracavernous ICA. The dural involvement is much more extensive in meningiomas of grades III–V.

IMAGING OF CAVERNOUS SINUS TUMORS

Although MRI, computerized tomography (CT), and angiography are complementary in the evaluation of cavernous sinus lesions, MRI in the axial and coronal planes is the best screening procedure for suspected cavernous sinus involvement (13). MRI has greater sensitivity in this region than CT, can better distinguish vascular from neoplastic lesions, can often reveal intradural extension, and clearly shows the relationship of the lesion to the carotid artery. Because of its superiority in defining bony anatomy, thin section axial and coronal CT with bone windows should be done when a lesion has been detected by MRI. With both CT and MRI, careful assessment should be made of structures adjacent to the cavernous

TABLE 1. Classification of intracavernous neoplasms

Grade	Cavernous sinus involvement	Intracavernous ICA
I	One area only (A, P, L, or M)	Not involved
II	More than one area	Displaced, not totally encased
III	Entire CS	Totally encased, at least a short length
IV	Entire CS	Encased, with narrowing, pseudoaneurysm or occlusion
V	Bilateral CS	Encased

From ref. 29, with permission.
Abbreviations: ICA, internal carotid artery; A, anterior; P, posterior; L, lateral; M, medial; CS, cavernous sinus.

sinus including the sella turcica, sphenoid bone and sinus, petroclival bone and dura, tentorial notch, orbit, middle cranial fossa, and neighboring cisterns. In the postoperative period, MRI cannot readily distinguish between surgical changes and residual tumor, and protracted follow-up will sometimes be needed to make this distinction.

Angiography remains a critical part of the preoperative evaluation in patients with cavernous sinus lesions. In addition to defining the exact nature and origin of vascular lesions within the cavernous sinus (26), angiography defines the degree of involvement of the carotid artery by neoplastic processes, reveals the degree and sources of vascularity of neoplasms, allows for embolization of tumor blood supply when feasible, reveals coexisting vascular pathology (such as contralateral carotid artery disease), which may affect surgical decision-making, and allows for the performance of a balloon test occlusion (BTO) of the ipsilateral internal carotid artery (ICA).

Surgery within the cavernous sinus may require temporary or permanent occlusion of the ICA. While approximately 80% of patients will tolerate occlusion of one ICA without neurological deficit, one cannot determine from clinical or radiographic data which patients are among the 20% at risk for massive infarction. BTO of the ICA with clinical examination alone will reveal patients at risk for immediate ischemia but may miss a group of patients who tolerate temporary occlusion but have greatly reduced cerebrovascular reserve and are thus at risk for delayed cerebral ischemia (15,21,33). BTO of the ICA including neurologic examination and stable xenon CT blood flow determination allows the risk of stroke with carotid occlusion to be more precisely quantified (6). Patients with no change in clinical exam or cerebral blood flow (CBF) during occlusion (CBF above 35 cc/100 g/min) are considered to be at low risk (approximately 75% of patients tested), patients with no change in exam but diminished blood flow (CBF 10–35 ml/100 g/min) may be considered at intermediate risk (approximately 15%), and patients with neurologic deficits during test occlusion are considered to be at high risk (approximately 10%). With this information, the need for graft reconstruction of the ICA and cerebral protective agents during temporary ICA occlusion can be assessed. All patients who require cavernous sinus surgery should undergo BTO of the ICA (see Horton et al.). This is especially important for patients with tumor grades III–V.

In addition to the immediate risk of stroke from carotid occlusion, there are other reasons for preferring carotid reconstruction to sacrifice. Some data suggest that the loss of cerebrovascular reserve secondary to carotid sacrifice may put patients at risk for delayed ipsilateral cerebral ischemia (2,8,9,17,35). The risk of contralateral *de novo* aneurysm formation (5) or the growth or rupture of existing contralateral aneurysms (3,7,21) appears to be increased by ligation of one ICA. In addition, many lesions that involve the cavernous sinus (especially meningiomas or aneurysms) have a tendency to involve the contralateral side. If the ipsilateral ICA is occluded, treatment of the contralateral ICA lesion becomes very risky. Therefore reconstruction of the ICA is preferred, especially in younger patients, with benign or low-grade malignant tumors.

TECHNIQUES OF CAVERNOUS SINUS SURGERY

Indications for Surgery

Meningiomas

Our current indications for operating on cavernous sinus meningiomas include progressive tumor growth on serial imaging studies and/or progression of cranial nerve deficits. In addition, there must be the possibility of total resection or of subtotal removal and stereotactic radiosurgery of a small remnant. Meningiomas originating outside the cavernous sinus and involving it secondarily are easier to remove completely than meningiomas originating within the cavernous sinus. Many meningiomas involving the CS with minimal symptoms and no growth on serial imaging studies are being followed, without operation. We are also more cautious in patients with tumors in grades III–V.

Other Benign Tumors

Neurilemomas, cavernous hemangiomas, juvenile angiofibromas, craniopharyngiomas, pituitary adenomas, and other benign tumors involving the CS are relatively easy to remove. Removal of the portion of tumor from the CS should be performed whenever it is elected to treat such patients with operation, with intent to perform complete excision.

Chordoma and Chondrosarcoma

Chordomas and chondrosarcomas are usually easy to remove completely from the cavernous sinus, and cavernous sinus involvement should not be an impediment to total excision, even if both cavernous sinuses are involved.

Malignant Lesions

The indications for operative excision of high-grade malignant lesions (e.g., squamous cell carcinoma) involving the cavernous sinus are controversial. With such cases, the cavernous sinus is not entered during the operation; rather, an en bloc resection is performed. The tumor should be removable from all areas outside the cavernous sinus to justify radical surgery. Bilateral cavernous sinus involvement precludes operation.

Anesthesia

Adequate autologous or homologous blood reserves should be available. The availability of autologous or homologous fibrinogen for the making of fibrin glue is useful (26). Thigh-high elastic stockings and intermittent pneumatic compression stockings should be placed on the patient prior to the induction of anesthesia (16). Large bore intravenous access and catheter drainage of the bladder should be established. All pressure points should be adequately padded for a lengthy procedure. Prophylactic antibiotics and high-dose steroids are administered. Precordial Doppler monitoring for detection of venous air embolism is mandatory.

Anesthetic agents are chosen to allow neurophysiologic monitoring of the intracavernous cranial nerves and the function of the cerebral hemispheres. Long-acting neuromuscular blockers are avoided. A constant low-dose barbiturate infusion, usually thiopental 2 mg/kg/hr, minimizes the need for inhalational agents and assists in brain relaxation. If temporary carotid occlusion is necessary, cerebral protection is achieved with moderate hypothermia to 32°C, by inducing barbiturate or etomidate coma to the level of burst suppression on EEG, and by inducing hypertension of 20–30 torr above the preoperative mean pressure. Cholinergic blocking agents should be available in the event that cranial nerve manipulation induces bradycardia. When the resection is finished and closure underway, the patient may be pharmacologically paralyzed and the barbiturate infusion stopped to allow for a rapid, smooth emergence from anesthesia.

Monitoring

Monitoring of the electroencephalogram (EEG), somatosensory evoked potentials (SSEPs), and brain stem evoked responses (BSERs) by stimulation of the contralateral ear allow continuous assessment of the function of the ipsilateral brain stem and cerebral hemisphere caused by retraction or by alterations in blood flow. Electromyographic (EMG) monitoring of cranial nerves III, VI, and VII with electrodes placed prior to draping is helpful for detection of injury to cranial nerves and for the identification of cranial nerves by the use of an intraoperative stimulating electrode (23).

Incisions

Operative approaches must allow the eventual achievement of a number of goals, including a low basal approach that minimizes brain retraction, adequate exposure of the lesion, proximal and distal control of the carotid artery, reconstruction of related arteries and nerves, and reconstruction of the cranial base to prevent cerebrospinal fluid leakage and for cosmetic reasons.

Meningioma

With ICA Grafting

Patients with poor tolerance for BTO are at high risk for ischemic complications of surgery. If operation is strongly indicated, then revascularization with appropriate pharmacological cerebral protection is necessary and appropriate preparation must be made. The proximal thigh should be prepared and draped out and the most proximal 8–10 cm of the saphenous vein exposed early in the operation. The incision should begin over the femoral ring just medial to the femoral artery pulse and extend for about 10 cm inferomedially along the course of the proximal saphenous vein. Careful dissection through the subcutaneous fat will expose the vein itself or a branch may have to be followed to the main vein. Approximately 8 cm of the vein should be exposed below the femoral ring. The vein should be at least 4 mm in diameter to provide adequate flow. Branches should be ligated and the vein fully mobilized, but the vein should not be removed until just before graft reconstruction of the ICA, to avoid endothelial injury during storage of the graft. Manipulation of the vein will result in spasm, so the adventitia should be injected with dilute (1:10) papaverine using a fine gauge needle. Care must be taken that the vein is not reversed after harvesting (30). Fat may also be obtained from this area for reconstruction. However, if fascia lata is required, a separate incision placed more laterally is preferred.

Generally, exposure of the internal carotid artery in the neck is not necessary for proximal control, except in patients in whom the horizontal segment of the petrous ICA is very short or is obscured by severe bony hyperostosis or tumor. Exposure of the petrous ICA is preferred in every patient since it is a good landmark during the tumor operation, allows an ICA–ICA vein graft reconstruction if necessary, and is also easier to locate and temporarily occlude during the operation in the event of ICA injury.

The scalp incision must allow for a generous frontotemporal craniotomy and for the removal of the zygomatic arch and orbital rim; therefore a bicoronal or curvilinear incision is made extending below the zygomatic arch. The inferior part of the incision should be placed about 1–2 mm anterior to the tragus so as to preserve the frontal branches of the facial nerve and the superficial temporal artery (Fig. 22). Electrical stimulation of the facial nerve aids in locating and preserving frontal

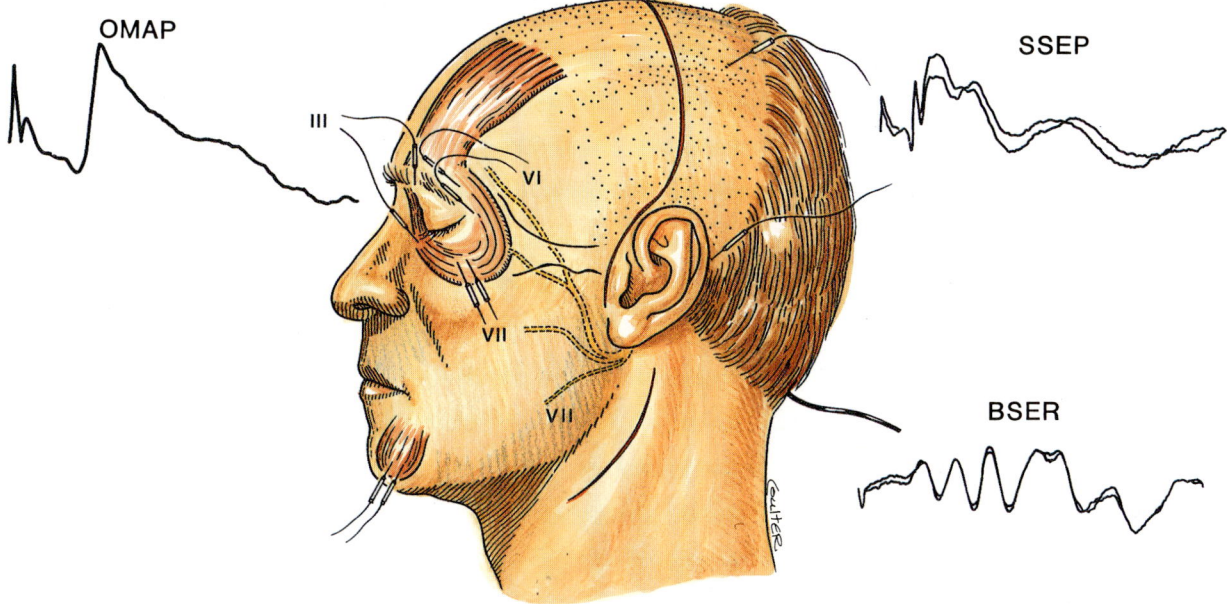

FIG. 22. The cervical and cranial incisions used for cavernous sinus exposure and monitoring modalities are shown. These include somatosensory evoked potentials (SSEP), auditory brain stem evoked responses (BSER), and the electromyographic potentials in muscles supplied by CNs III, VI, and VII.

branches. The scalp flap is elevated in the subperiosteal plane with care to take the frontal branches of the facial nerve with the scalp (36) and should be brought forward to expose the orbital rim and the entire zygoma. The scalp flap is mobilized from a superior to inferior direction. The superficial layer of temporal fascia blends with the pericranium, then with the periosteum of the orbit and zygoma. The surgeon works between the superficial and deep layers of the temporal fascia and then deep to the parotid gland, between it and the masseteric fascia. This will avoid injury to the facial nerve. The temporalis muscle should be completely mobilized and the periorbita carefully dissected from the orbital roof to just anterior to the superior orbital fissure, and from the lateral wall to the inferior orbital fissure.

Without ICA Grafting

When graft reconstruction of the carotid artery is not anticipated, then it is adequate to obtain proximal control by exposure of the horizontal segment of the petrous carotid. The thigh should be prepared in a sterile fashion in case a vein graft becomes necessary, and for the harvesting of fat or fascia if needed. The incision is as described previously. In patients with neurilemomas or other grade II lesions where ICA injury is exceptional, the experienced surgeon may work without proximal ICA control, but this is not generally recommended.

Chordoma or Chondrosarcoma

When a chordoma or a chondrosarcoma involves the petroclival or sphenoid bone as well as the cavernous sinus, the tumor is usually removed by a subtemporal and infratemporal approach with or without combination with an extended frontal approach (25). A bicoronal incision is therefore necessary to permit a bifrontal craniotomy and a long galeopericranial flap. The coronal incision should be placed at least 15 cm superior to the nasion so as to allow the elevation of a galeopericranial flap of sufficient size to reach the sphenoid sinus should this cavity be entered (Fig. 22). The pericranium should be elevated with the scalp and meticulously preserved. In many patients with chordoma or chondrosarcoma, the entire petrous ICA may need to be exposed to permit resection of the petroclival tumor (see Sekhar et al., Anterior, Anterolateral, and Lateral Approaches to Extradural Petroclival Tumors).

Craniotomy

A frontotemporal craniotomy is performed, bringing the bone cuts as low as possible along the orbital rim and in the temporal fossa. The medial extent is usually the supraorbital notch. The lateral extent depends on the posterior extension of the tumor (Fig. 23A). If only the middle fossa is involved, the craniotomy stops at the root of the zygoma. If the posterior fossa is involved as well, the craniotomy is continued 2 or 3 cm posterior to the root of the zygoma. All bone uninvolved by tumor is saved for use in the reconstruction. The subfrontal dura is separated from the orbital roof back to the superior orbital fissure. Some of the bone of the pterional area and the squamous temporal bone are rongeured away. The subtemporal dura is elevated extradurally to expose

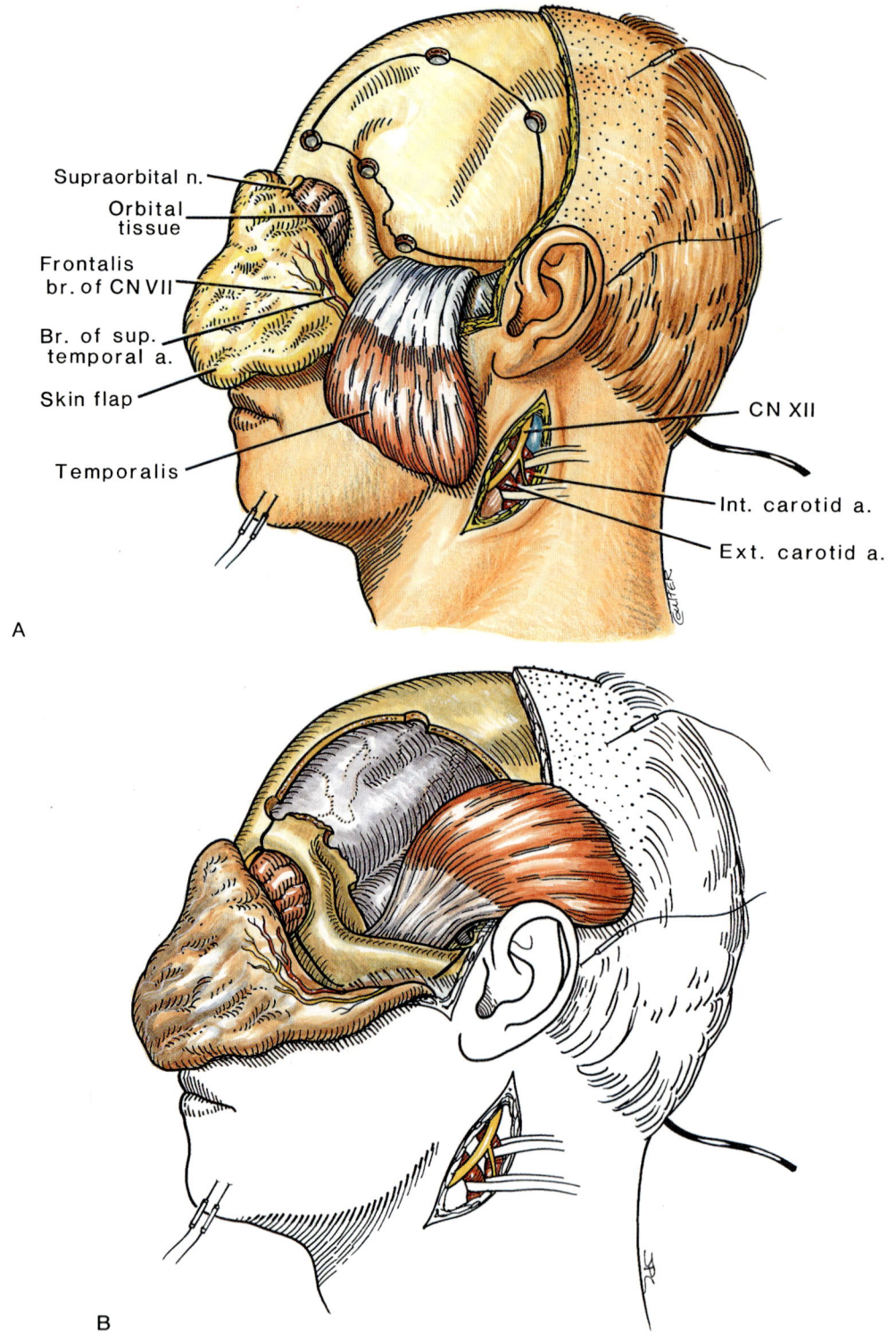

FIG. 23. Cervical exposure of the ICA has been performed here, which is usually not necessary. **A:** A frontotemporal craniotomy has been performed. **B:** The next step of orbitozygomatic osteotomy.

the roof of the condylar fossa and other landmarks (see Sekhar et al., Anterior, Anterolateral, and Lateral Approaches to Extradural Petroclival Tumors). From the orbital side, the periorbita is separated from the roof of the orbit for about 3 cm posteriorly. The periorbita is also separated from the lateral wall of the orbit to reach the inferior orbital fissure. Some brain relaxation is necessary for this procedure, achieved either with diuretics or with cisternal CSF drainage.

Extradural Approach

Orbitozygomatic Osteotomy

Using malleable brain retractors to protect the brain and orbital contents, a reciprocating saw is used to remove the rim and roof and lateral wall of the orbit and the zygomatic arch as a single piece. This procedure reduces the extent of brain retraction. A cut is first made in the sagittal plane at the medial aspect of the orbit across the superior rim and wall of the orbit at or near the supraorbital notch and extending about 2.5 cm posteriorly. A second cut is made in the coronal plane across the orbital roof and then across the lateral wall of the orbit to the inferior orbital fissure. This cut is usually about 1 cm anterior to the superior orbital fissure. The anterior zygomatic osteotomy is made at or lateral to the zygomaticomaxillary suture (Figs. 23B and 24). Beginning this cut from the inferior orbital fissure and working laterally will avoid entry into the maxillary sinus. The temporomandibular joint capsule is opened and the meniscus separated from the condylar fossa. The posterior zygomatic osteotomy is then made through the condylar fossa, but staying within its confines to avoid entry into the middle ear or the petrous ICA canal. The entire orbital rim, zygomatic arch, and condylar fossa may then be removed

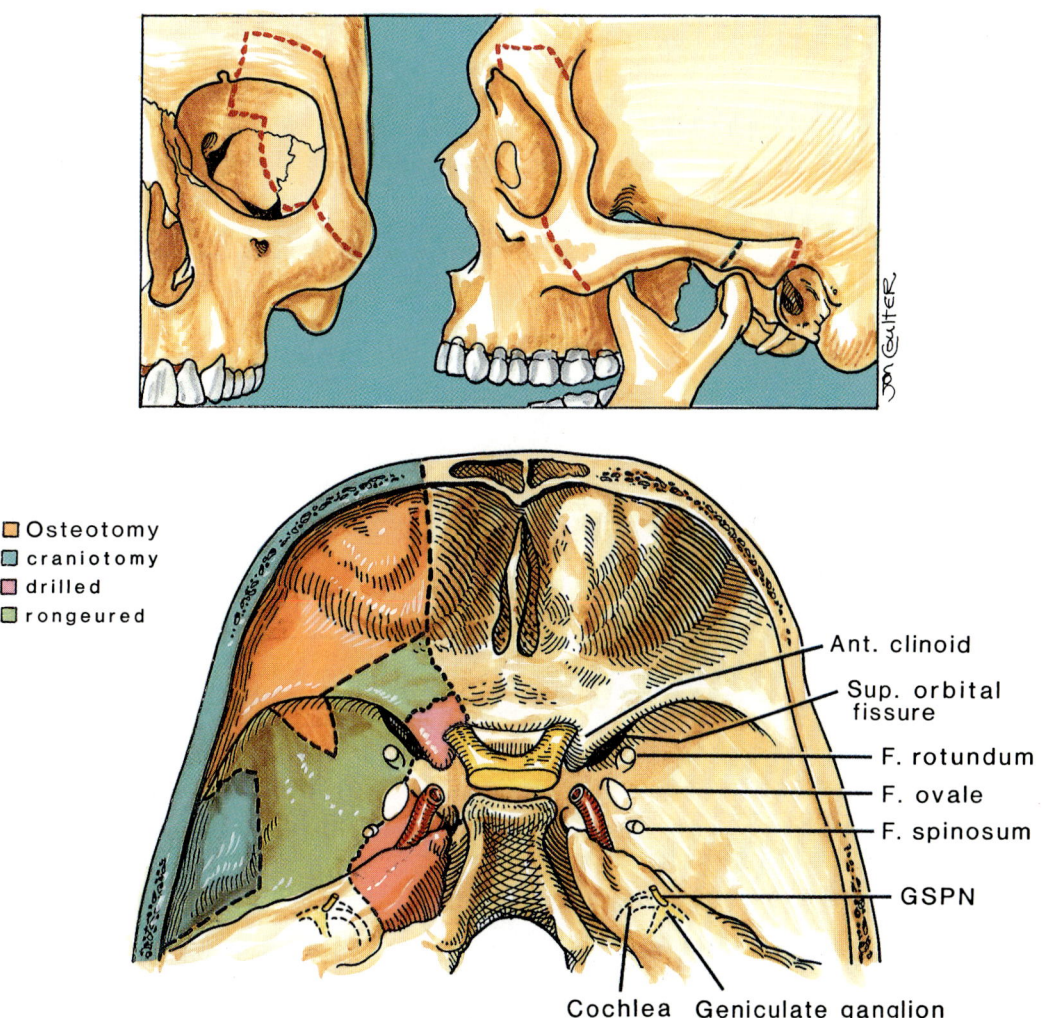

FIG. 24. The orbitozygomatic osteotomy is performed after the frontotemporal craniotomy. It may or may not include the condylar fossa. The areas of bone shown in *green* are rongeured away. The petrous ICA is exposed with drills and rongeurs. Optic canal unroofing and the resection of the anterior clinoid process are performed *intradurally* with drill and rongeurs.

as a single piece. Removal of the condylar fossa in this manner allows more freedom of movement in working with the horizontal segment of the petrous carotid and allows restoration of the temporomandibular joint. However, when the vein graft reconstruction of the ICA is unlikely, as in patients with grade I or II tumors, the zygomatic osteotomy is usually made anterior to the condylar fossa (Fig. 25).

Condylar Resection

When exposure of the vertical segment of the petrous carotid is necessary, then the mandibular condyle must be resected. The disability caused by unilateral condylar resection is surprisingly minimal and is less than that due to dislocation of the mandibular condyle. After freeing all soft tissue attachments to the condyle and superior aspect of the ascending ramus of the mandible by cutting the pterygoid muscles and the sphenomandibular ligament, the condyle is cut at its neck with a reciprocating saw, taking care to avoid injury to the internal maxillary artery, which courses medial to the condyle, and the superficial temporal artery and facial nerve, which lie in the substance of the parotid gland.

Exposure of the Petrous Carotid Artery

A clear understanding of the relevant anatomy is mandatory before attempting surgical exposure of the petrous carotid artery. The bony anatomy of the floor of the middle fossa, the location of the cochlea, and the course of the facial nerve, eustachian tube, middle meningeal artery, and the trigeminal nerve should be well known to the surgeon (24). Bone window CT scans of the area should be studied preoperatively to reveal anatomical variations.

Horizontal Portion

The exposure of the horizontal portion (Fig. 25) of the petrous carotid artery is begun by gently elevating the dura from the floor of the middle fossa in a posterior to anterior direction. The tegmen tympani, arcuate eminence, middle meningeal artery, the third division of the trigeminal nerve, and the lesser and greater superficial petrosal nerves (LSPN and GSPN) should be clearly identified. The location of the foramen ovale can be confirmed by infratemporal dissection as well. The GSPN can be positively identified by stimulation of its exit foramen with facial nerve monitoring. The horizontal petrous ICA is usually visible without a bony covering just inferior to the GSPN. The GSPN should be divided to prevent traction on the facial nerve. The petrous apex area posteromedial to the ICA is first drilled away while the ICA remains protected by bone. Then the bone over the ICA is removed with a drill and fine rongeurs. The periosteum is then separated from the bone. Bone re-

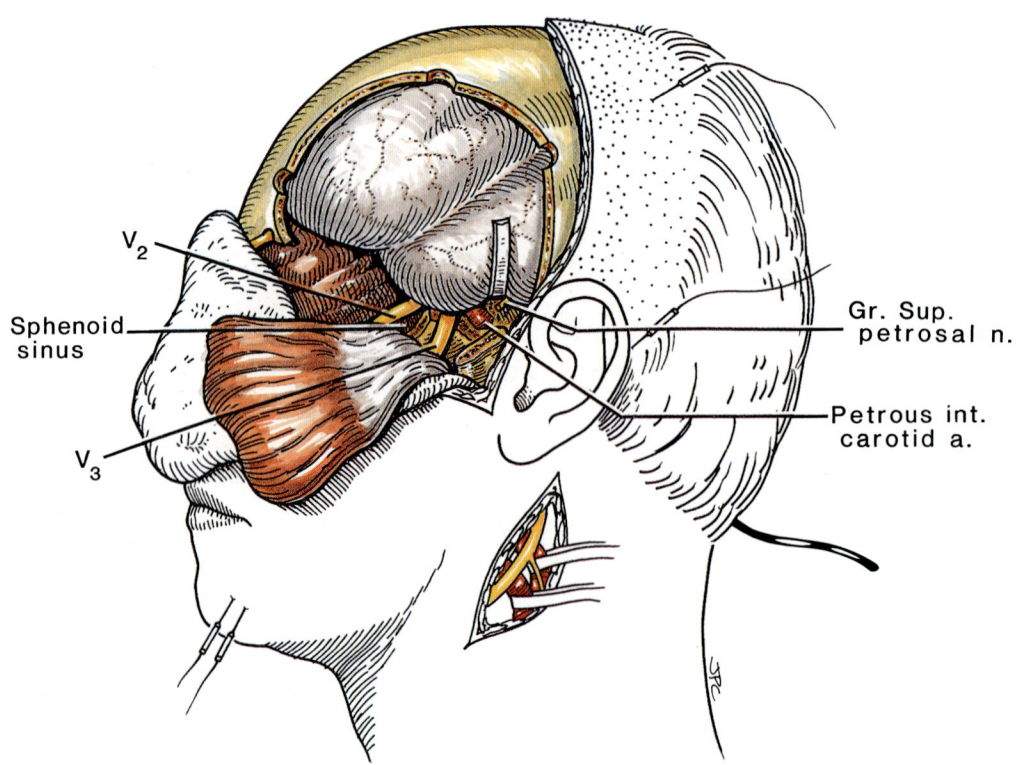

FIG. 25. The final appearance obtained after extradural work is completed, for a meningioma. The petrous ICA has been exposed in the horizontal segment.

moval should not be carried too far inferolaterally or the eustachian tube will be opened. The tensor tympani muscle serves to warn the surgeon of the proximity of the eustachian tube. If the tube is opened, the opening must be closed with autologous fat to prevent a CSF leak, and the patient may require an elective tympanostomy postoperatively. The location of the cochlea is variable, and the bone windowed CT should be carefully studied to avoid entering this structure. The location of the GSPN is the best intraoperative guide to the location of the cochlea. Exposure of the ICA is carried out from the genu proximally to the cavernous sinus distally. If ICA reconstruction is anticipated, then the periosteum of the carotid canal should be opened. The sheath contains a venous plexus and the sympathetic nerve in addition to the artery.

Entire Petrous Carotid Artery

When exposure of the entire petrous carotid artery (Fig. 26) is planned, the mandibular condyle should be resected during the exposure. Bone of the lateral floor of the middle fossa should be rongeured away, unroofing the bony canal of V_3 (foramen ovale). Bone removal at the junction of the middle fossa floor and the condylar fossa will expose first the eustachian tube and then the carotid artery. The eustachian tube is excised at the junction between the bony and cartilaginous segments. The cartilaginous end of the tube is occluded with autologous fat and sutured shut, medial to V_3. After exposure of the horizontal segment as described previously, the carotid exposure is carried inferiorly until the fibrous ring at the entrance to the carotid canal is opened. If transposition of the petrous ICA is needed, the upper cervical segment of the internal carotid artery (superior to the styloid process) must also be freed up from soft tissues and all attachments of the ICA to the fibrous ring have to be divided.

Inferior Approach

As only about 8 mm of the horizontal segment of the petrous carotid may be exposed lateral to the trigeminal root (24), the inferior approach is possible only when the third division of the trigeminal nerve is divided due to tumor invasion, or when the third division of the trigeminal nerve and the petrous internal carotid artery are completely mobilized from their bony canals by the subtemporal–infratemporal approach. The carotid artery is followed from its horizontal petrous segment into the cavernous sinus. The sixth nerve should be identified early on as it crosses the carotid artery medial to the trigeminal root. When the involvement of the CS by tumor is extensive, this approach alone is inadequate.

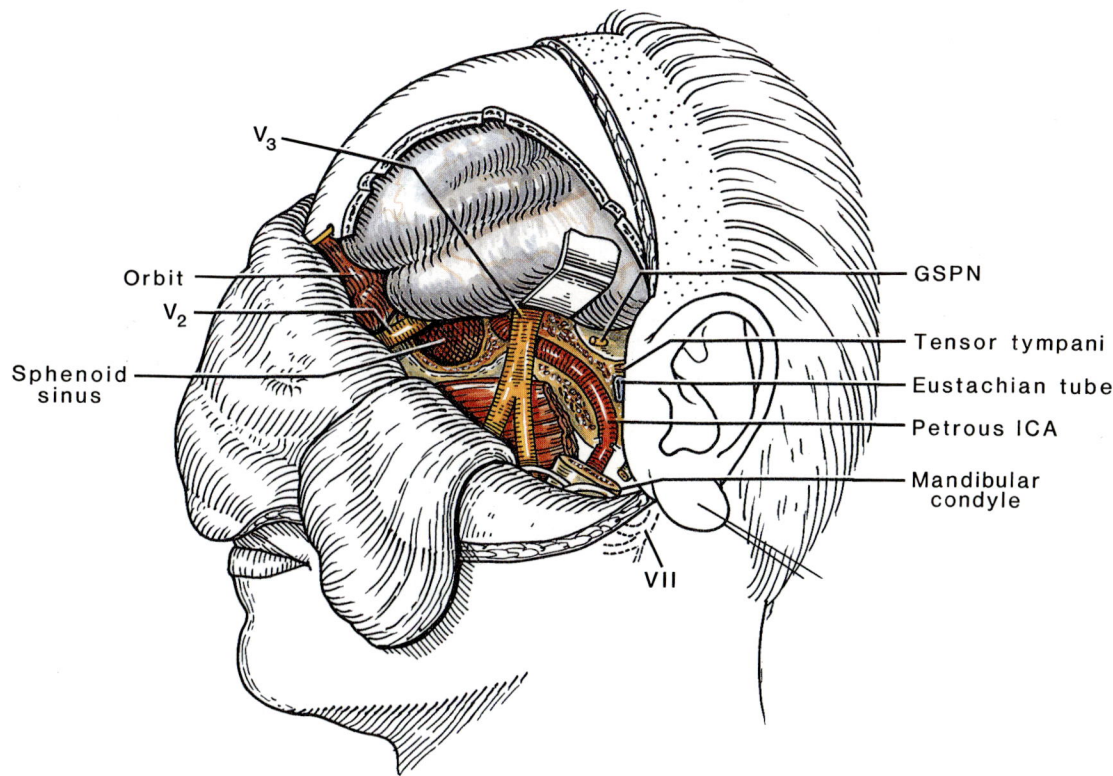

FIG. 26. For lesions arising from the petroclival bone, such as chordoma or chondrosarcoma, a more extensive exposure of the petrous ICA is performed with the resection of the condyle if necessary.

Anterolateral Approach

This approach (Fig. 27) may be indicated for juvenile angiofibromas, for palliative resection of some adenoid cystic carcinomas, and for some trigeminal neurilemomas that are intracavernous and extracavernous. It is an extradural approach between the second and third divisions or between the first and second divisions of the trigeminal nerve.

Medial Approach

This approach (Fig. 28) is useful for some chordomas, craniopharyngiomas, and pituitary adenomas that lie medial to the cavernous ICA. Limited involvement of the contralateral CS by meningiomas can also be resected by this approach. The ipsilateral optic nerve is unroofed and the sphenoid sinus is entered by opening the planum sphenoidale. The lateral bony wall of the sphenoid sinus is then removed from an anterior to posterior direction to expose the cavernous sinus. The medial aspect of the intracavernous ICA and CS can be exposed by this approach. This approach can be combined well with the superior approach to the cavernous sinus intradurally. Proximal control of the ICA must still be obtained in the petrous bone or the neck. The exposure of the cavernous sinus is better on the contralateral side, and this approach usually requires sacrifice of the ipsilateral olfactory bulb. Before opening the contralateral CS, the ICA can be exposed through the sphenoid sinus as it enters the CS to obtain proximal control. When the sphenoid sinus has been opened, adequate reconstruction with a galeopericranial flap, fat, and fascia lata must be performed.

Intradural Approach

Meningioma

Meningiomas always require an intradural approach, as do all large intracavernous tumors.

Sylvian Dissection

After the dura is opened, the brain is protected from surface contusions with rubber dams and cottonoids and/or sponges. The sylvian fissure is opened widely from a lateral to a medial direction, under magnification. Temporal tip bridging veins usually will need to be divided. Wide opening of the sylvian fissure allows manipulation of the frontal and temporal lobes independently and improves exposure. Additionally, when the tumor involves the supraclinoid ICA, this technique allows the surgeon to dissect the arteries from a normal (MCA) to an abnormal (ICA) area. Using a fine suction with variable vacuum and bipolar forceps, arachnoid and veins bridging the fissure are dissected and sharply sectioned until the entire MCA and supraclinoid ICA are fully exposed.

Temporal Lobe Resection

In cases requiring prolonged or forceful temporal lobe retraction, as for tumors extending into the tentorial incisura or onto the clivus, it is better to resect about 4 cm of the inferior temporal gyrus including the temporal tip rather than injure the brain by excessive retraction with resulting postoperative swelling. This type of resection has not been found to cause any permanent problems of cognition, and the appearance on late postoperative CT or MRI scans is similar to patients who have not had the brain resection.

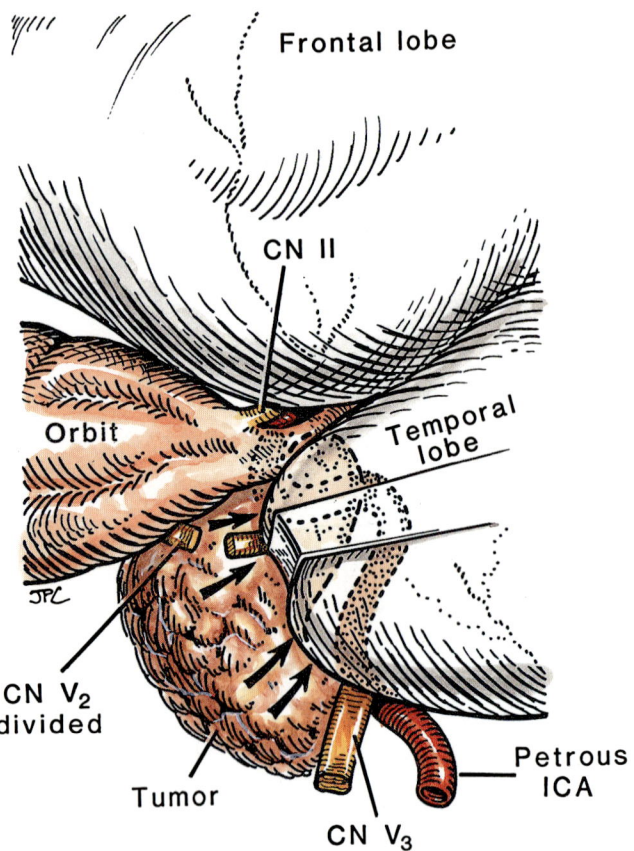

FIG. 27. For predominantly extradural lesions such as a juvenile angiofibroma with a small extension into the cavernous sinus, an entirely extradural approach into the CS is possible, as shown in this figure. It is not usually necessary to divide V_2 as shown in the figure. The surgeon follows the path taken by the tumor.

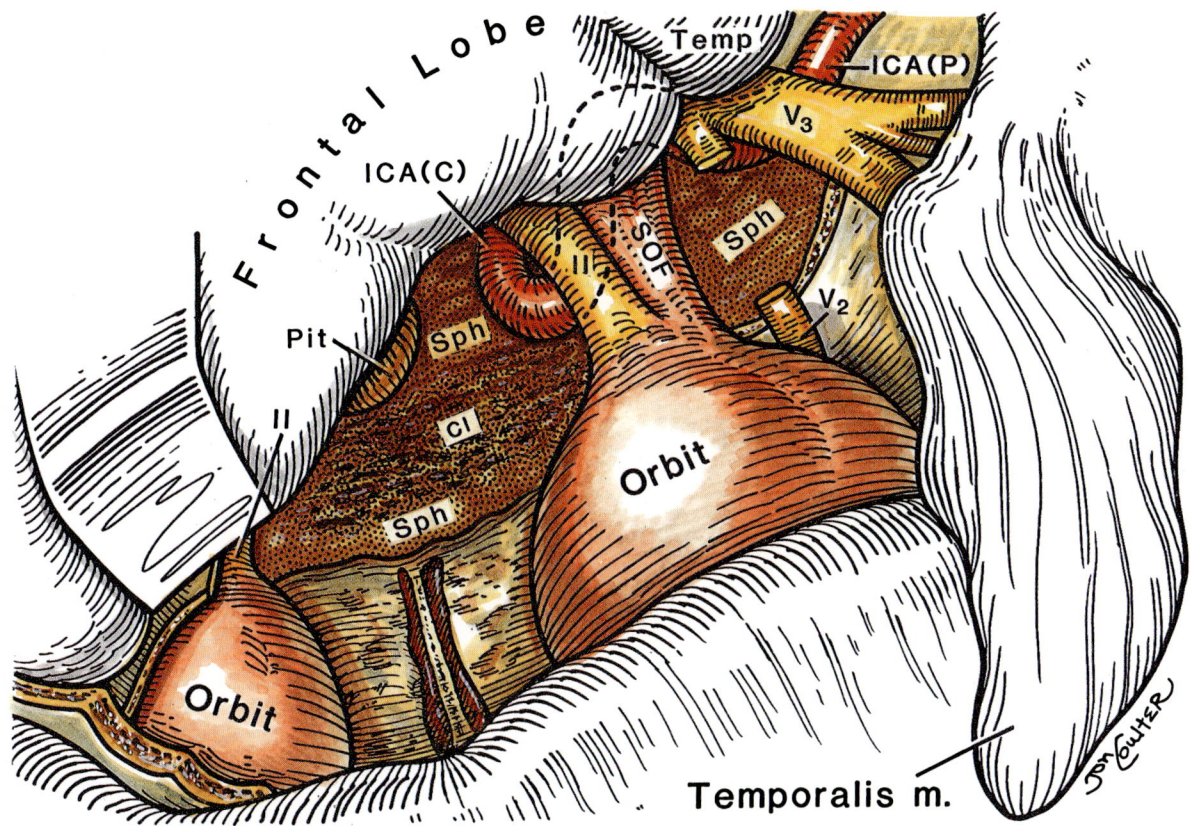

FIG. 28. For chordomas or chondrosarcomas extending medially into the sphenoid sinus and into the clivus across the midline, a basal frontal approach is performed. The sphenoid sinus is opened widely with the ipsilateral optic nerve being unroofed. This, combined with the infratemporal exposure and the transcavernous exposure, permits an excellent tumor resection. Reconstruction is similar to Fig. 38, but a portion of the temporalis muscle may also be split and rotated into the operative cavity laterally.

Subdural Tumor Resection

When there is considerable tumor in the subdural compartment, it is resected at this time, including tumor in the anterior and middle fossae and in the tentorial notch area. We generally use the suction or suction irrigation, the bipolar cautery, and pituitary forceps to remove this portion of the tumor. The CO_2 laser or the ultrasonic aspirator is rarely used.

Anterior Clinoid Process and Optic Nerve

When tumor enters the orbital apex or the superior approach to the cavernous sinus is to be used, then the anterior clinoid process, roof of the optic canal, and optic strut must be removed. The dura over the anterior clinoid process and optic canal is then coagulated and opened sharply (Fig. 29). A Cottle elevator is used to strip the dura back sufficiently to expose the anterior clinoid process and the roof of the optic canal. Small strips of Gelfoam should be placed in the cisterns to prevent the dissemination of bone dust in the subarachnoid space. Using copious irrigation to prevent heating and obscuration of the field by bone dust, a diamond burr is used to remove the anterior clinoid process and expose the dura propria of the optic canal. The ethmoid or sphenoid sinus may be encountered medial to the optic nerve or in the optic strut. If air cells are encountered in the clinoid or optic strut, these must be closed at the end of the case with autologous fat and fibrin glue to prevent a CSF leak. The best way to remove the anterior clinoid process is to hollow it out into a thin shell and then remove it with fine rongeurs (Fig. 30). The intracavernous CN III lies inferolateral to it, the clinoidal segment of the ICA is inferior to it, and the optic nerve is medial to it. The optic strut is also removed and the optic nerve is unroofed superiorly, laterally, and inferiorly. Occasionally, anatomical variations such as a middle clinoid process or a bony ring around the ICA may be encountered (14) (Fig. 14). For these reasons, and for reasons of safety, we always remove the clinoid process intradurally, rather than extradurally.

The ophthalmic artery should be clearly identified. The dura propria of the optic nerve is opened to allow mobilization of the nerve and identification of the ophthalmic artery.

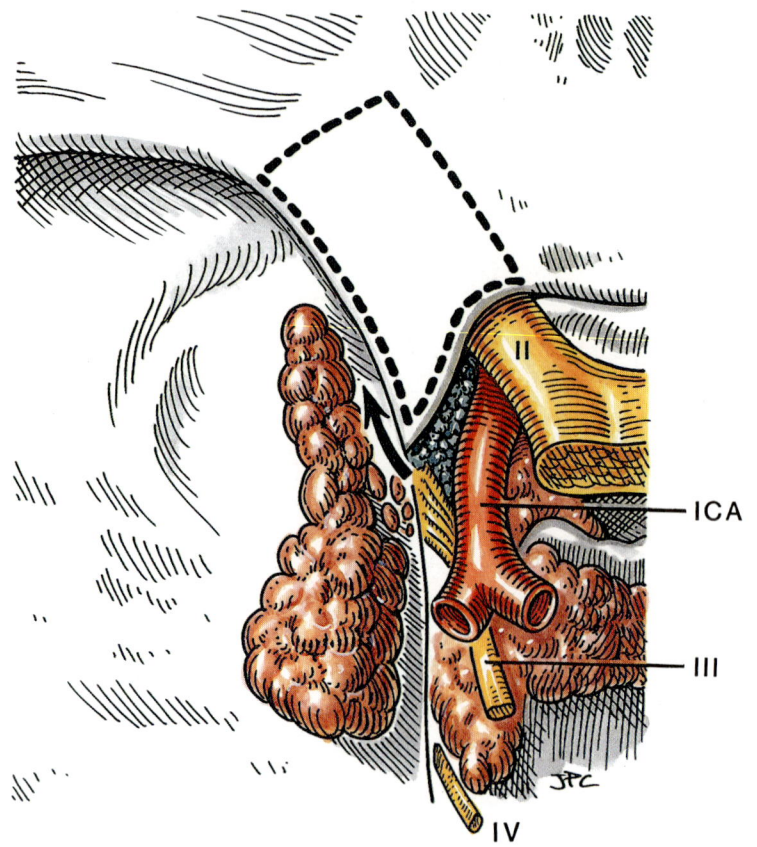

FIG. 29. After the dura is opened, the sylvian fissure is split and the frontal and temporal lobes are separated. The subdural tumor is removed first. The next step shown in this figure is to excise the dura over the anterior clinoid process and optic canal and proceed to unroof the extradural optic nerve and the clinoid space.

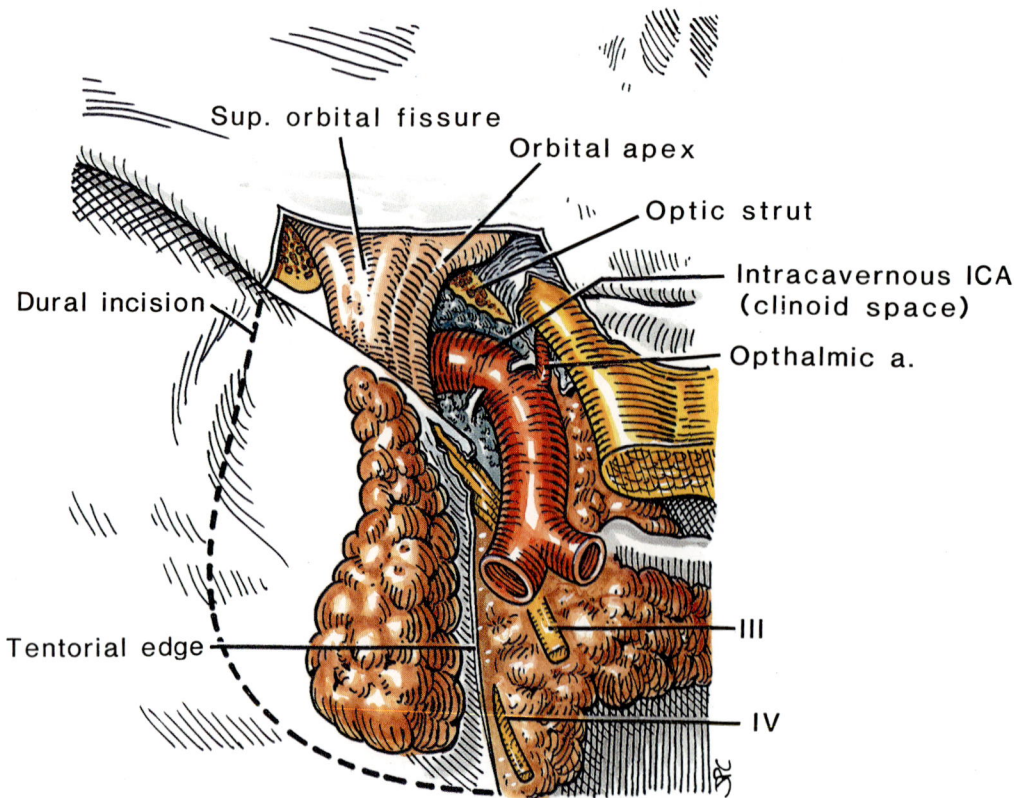

FIG. 30. The distal dural ring has been excised, and the superior wall of the cavernous sinus has been opened, providing the superior approach. The dural incision for the lateral approach is shown. Also seen is a 2–3-mm incision along the course of CN III.

Superior Approach

The superior approach (Fig. 31) to the cavernous sinus provides good exposure of the region superior and medial to the horizontal portion of the cavernous carotid, of the anterior genu and vertical segments of the intracavernous carotid, and of the sella turcica. In some patients, the horizontal segment of the intracavernous ICA may be exposed back to the posterior bend. This exposure requires removal of the anterior clinoid process, unroofing of the optic canal, and opening of the dura propria of the optic nerve (24). The removal of the clinoid process and unroofing of the optic nerve expose the clinoid segment of the internal carotid artery. It is surrounded by a thin periosteal membrane, the opening of which will produce bleeding from the cavernous sinus. The clinoid segment of the carotid artery is then followed distally until the third or dural ring is encountered. The ring is opened and excised to allow mobilization of the distal intracavernous carotid.

The incision in the superior wall begins in the clinoid space and extends toward the posterior clinoid. The tentorial edge may be retracted laterally with a suture to improve the exposure. Even when tumor or aneurysm is readily visible from this approach, caution is warranted. The intracavernous ICA may be adherent to the superior wall and consequently may be torn on opening the dura. The MRI scan will show the course of the carotid and allow this problem to be anticipated. The ICA must be followed from the dural ring to the posterior bend to avoid injury to the vessel. The oculomotor nerve lies just lateral of the clinoid space and may also be injured during the opening. Adhesions between the ICA and the pituitary gland and the lateral wall of the sinus are lysed. The posterior vertical segment and bend of the ICA are not well seen by this approach. Although the sixth nerve may sometimes be seen by this approach, and CN III can be exposed in its short intracavernous course, the remaining cranial nerves are not well seen. When combined with the lateral approach, all the cranial nerves, most of the intracavernous ICA, and all of the spaces of the cavernous sinus are well exposed (24).

Lateral Wall Dissection

The lateral approach is useful for neurilemomas, cartilaginous tumors, and meningiomas of the cavernous sinus. For neurilemomas or chordomas, a horizontal incision may be made parallel to and below the fourth nerve to enter the sinus (24). An intersecting vertical incision (T-shaped) may be made over the bulge of the tumor to enlarge the opening. Extensive dissection of CNs IV and III is unnecessary for these tumors (Figs. 32 and 33).

For meningiomas, a complete dissection of the lateral wall is necessary (Fig. 34). Since CN III is often splayed

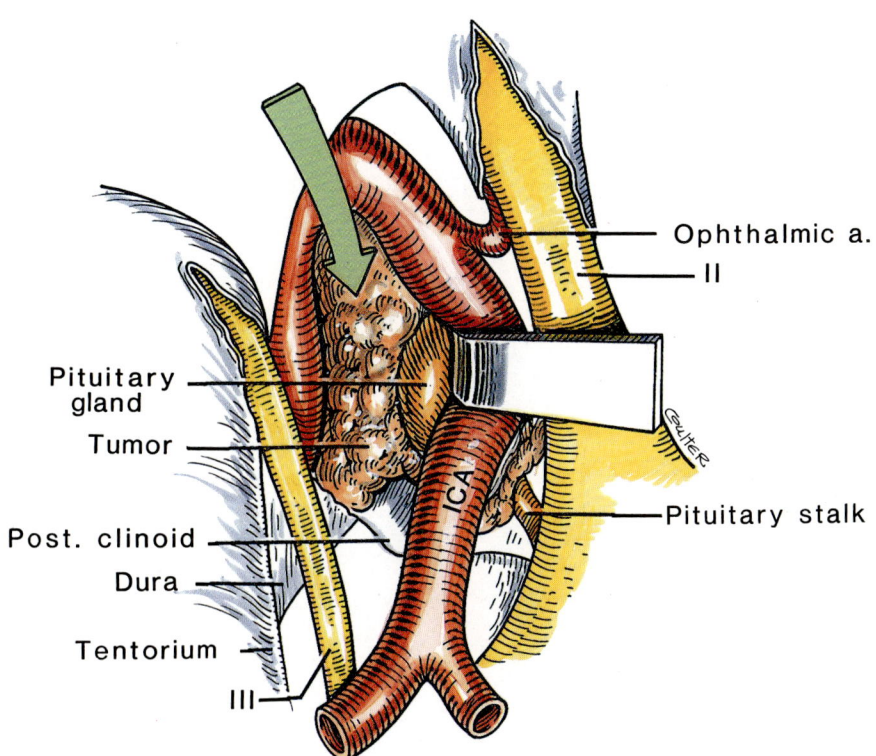

FIG. 31. The superior approach to the cavernous sinus is shown here. This approach is adequate for most anterior segment aneurysms of the intracavernous ICA as well.

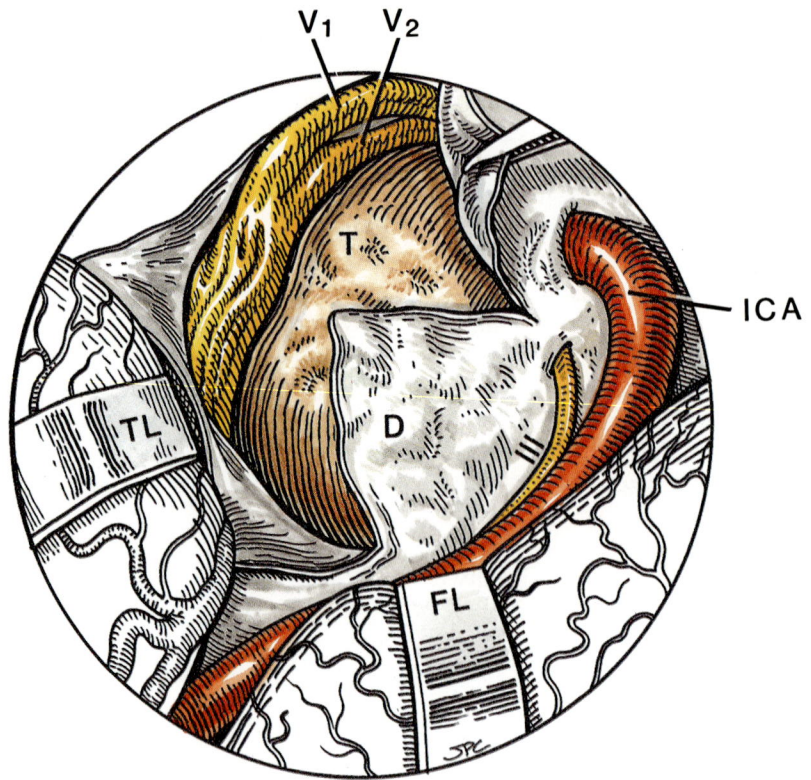

FIG. 32. The removal of intracavernous chordoma or chondrosarcoma and neurilemomas is technically easier than meningiomas. It is adequate to make a cruciate dural incision over the Parkinson's triangle and V_1 area (or the most prominent portion of the tumor) and peel away the dural layer. Cranial nerves V and IV may be exposed, but extensive dissection of CN III is avoided.

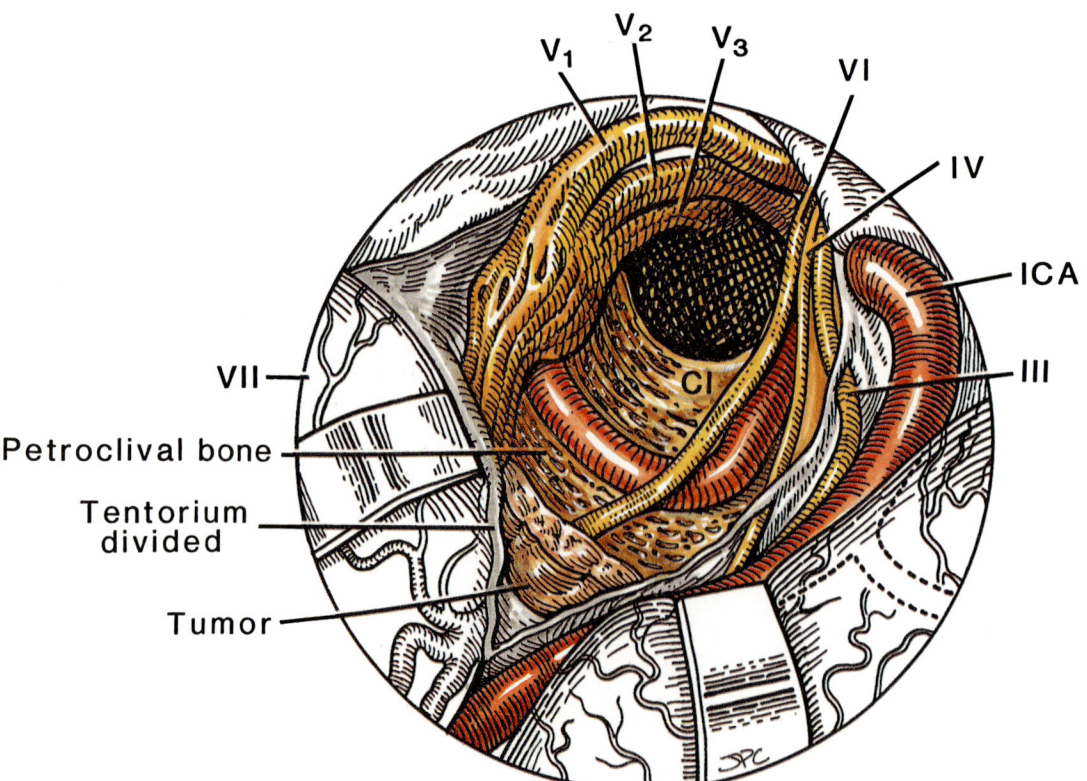

FIG. 33. Tumor removal then proceeds inside the cavernous sinus, with debulking and then dissection from surrounding structures. The clival and sphenoidal bone may even be drilled away, working through the cavernous sinus after tumor resection. For posterior fossa extensions of lesions, such as trigeminal neurilemoma, the tentorium overlying Meckel's cave can be opened, exposing the prepontine and interpeduncular area, and completing the tumor resection.

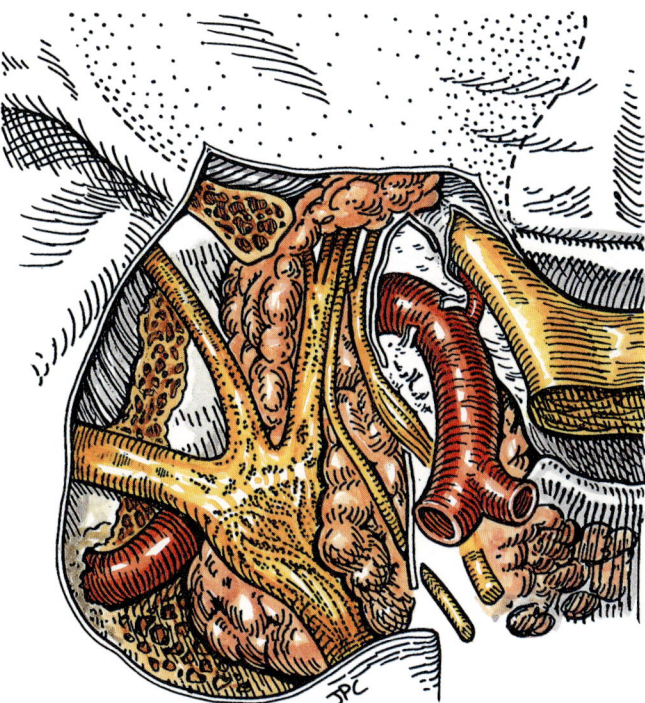

FIG. 34. For intracavernous meningiomas, a more extensive lateral wall dissection is needed. The dura of the lateral wall of the CS has been peeled away, exposing cranial nerves III, IV, and V. Note the course of the trochlear nerve, which results in a "closed Parkinson's triangle."

and deformed by tumor at its entry into the CS, it is useful to open the dura at its entry point for about 2–3 mm to decompress it. Further opening from a posterior to anterior direction may result in injury to CN IV and the frontal branch of V_1, which cross CN III laterally. The outer dural layer of the lateral wall of the cavernous sinus is then peeled entirely away, working from the sphenoparietal sinus anteriorly, the second and third divisions of the trigeminal nerve inferiorly, the tentorial edge superiorly, and the region of the superior petrosal sinus posteriorly. A Rosen dissector or a Cottle elevator may be used for this dissection. Alternatively, the assistant provides suction while the surgeon grasps the outer dural wall with an instrument and pulls on it, while sharply dissecting it from cranial nerves III, IV, and V with microscissors held in the other hand. If the third and fourth cranial nerves are not immediately identified in the lateral wall, then they should be traced from their subarachnoid segments into the cavernous sinus for positive identification. The first division of the trigeminal nerve may also be followed anteriorly from the trigeminal ganglion in Meckel's cave. As the fourth nerve may be quite attenuated, it is often wise to leave a small cuff of dura on the nerve until later in the operation. Intraoperative stimulation is very helpful in the identification of the cranial nerves and in avoidance of injury to them, but the surgeon should not rely on it entirely. The inner layer of dura may be quite thin or incomplete in nonmeningomatous tumors. With meningiomas, however, this layer is often thickened and quite fibrous.

Intracavernous Dissection

Cranial Nerves. Once cranial nerves III–V have been identified, the cavernous sinus itself is entered through Parkinson's triangle between the trochlear nerve and the first division of the trigeminal nerve, between cranial nerves III and IV, between the first and second divisions of the trigeminal nerve, and posterior to the third division of the trigeminal nerve. The trochlear nerve has a variable course and is therefore most susceptible to injury. The fourth nerve crosses lateral to the third nerve near the orbital apex.

It is critical to locate the intracavernous carotid artery and the sixth nerve. The sixth nerve is most likely to be injured during the tumor resection and may be found at the anterior end of the cavernous sinus between the first and second divisions of the trigeminal nerve, or at the posterior end of the cavernous sinus medial to the trigeminal root. If the nerve is not found in either of these places, then it is best to remove the petrous apex subtemporally to expose the clivus dura, open the dura into the posterior fossa, and expose the subarachnoid segment of the nerve posterior to Dorello's canal. The sixth nerve may temporarily divide into several fascicles within the cavernous sinus (24). If possible, the sympathetic nerve should also be identified and preserved. Since the sympathetic nerve may travel with the sixth nerve before joining the first division of the trigeminal nerve (24), the sixth nerve should only be retracted inferiorly toward the first division of the trigeminal nerve (19) (Fig. 35).

There is a blind area medial to the gasserian ganglion and the trigeminal root (medial to Meckel's cave) where tumor may be left if this area is not explored. The trigeminal root and ganglion may be split along the junction of V_2 and V_3 or occasionally between V_1 and V_2 to gain exposure to this area. This "transtrigeminal approach" has not resulted in any additional sensory deficit in six patients in whom this technique was used (Fig. 36).

Carotid Artery. Usually a plane can be developed between the tumor and the carotid artery with the Rosen dissector and bipolar forceps, or with a gentle spreading action of the microscissors. The surgeon should be prepared at all times to place temporary clips on the artery should the ICA be injured. Lacerations of the carotid artery may be repaired directly while temporary clips are used to control bleeding (4,11,23). Simple packing of arterial hemorrhage is not acceptable as the definitive means of controlling bleeding and may lead to postoperative hemorrhage, pseudoaneurysm formation, or ICA occlusion. Arterial hemorrhage may also ensue when in-

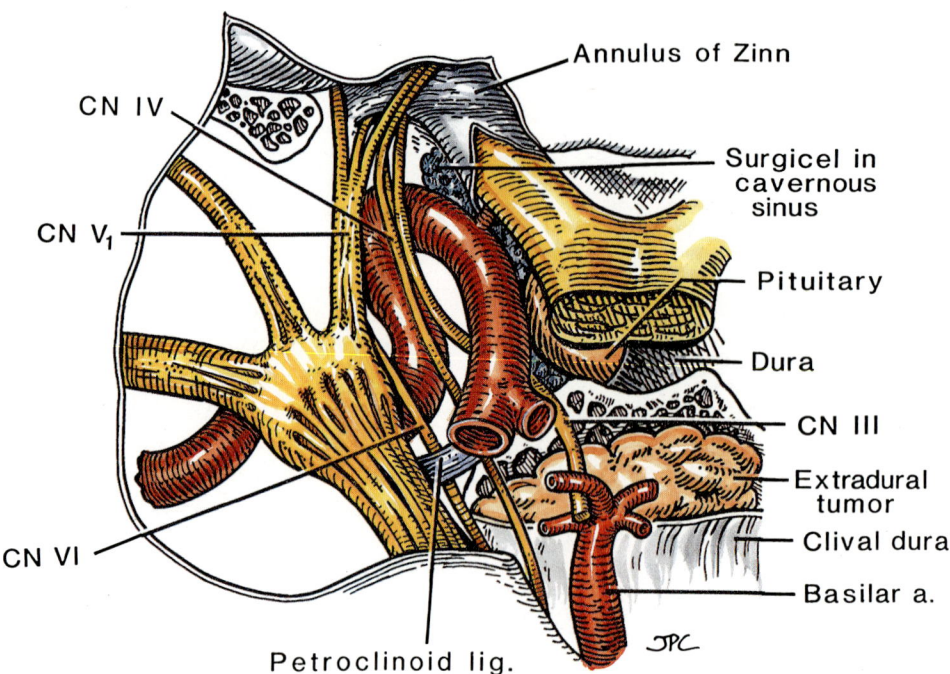

FIG. 35. The tumor has been removed from the cavernous sinus, with the preservation of the cranial nerves and the carotid artery. After removal of the intracavernous tumor, remaining tumor in the upper clival region can readily be removed.

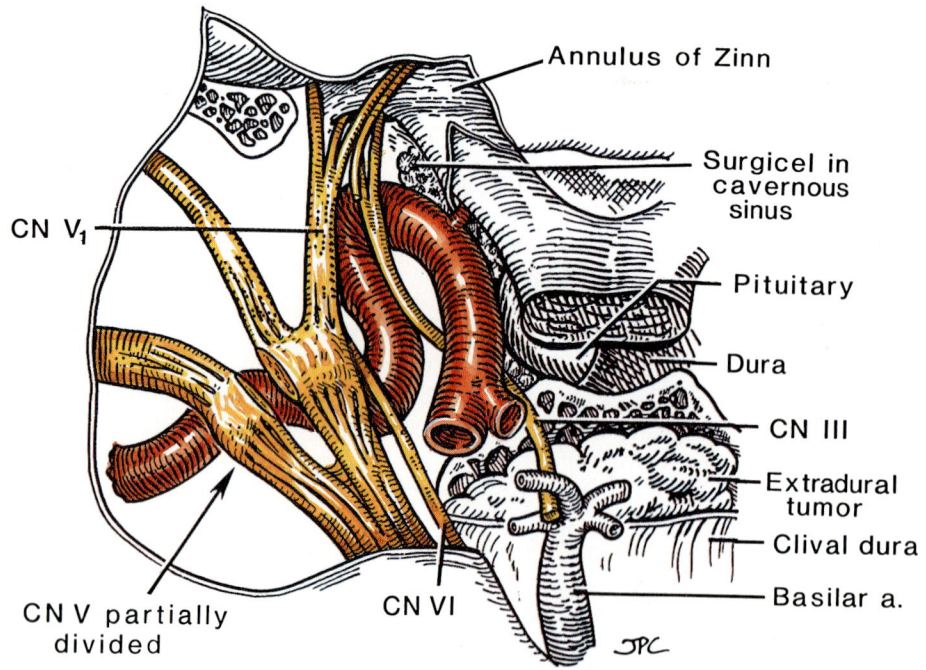

FIG. 36. This figure illustrates a transtrigeminal approach to the posteroinferior aspect of the cavernous sinus.

tracavernous branches of the carotid artery are encountered. The meningohypophyseal trunk is the most frequently encountered branch, usually arising from the posterior bend of the carotid (24). When an intracavernous tumor is present, other branches such as the inferolateral trunk are often enlarged. Bipolar coagulation is sufficient to control this type of bleeding once it is certain that the source is not the carotid itself. With grade III and IV meningiomas, it is usually not possible to strip the tumor from the carotid artery, which should then be excised and grafted.

Veins. Venous bleeding is controlled with gentle packing with Surgicel (Johnson & Johnson, New Brunswick, NJ). The bleeding may be profuse, and when arterial oxygen tension is high, it may be difficult to distinguish arterial from venous bleeding. It may be necessary to ask the anesthesiologist to lower the inspired oxygen concentration to normal levels to aid in this determination. Slight elevation of the head is also useful in controlling venous bleeding, but it increases the risk of air embolism. Venous bleeding is usually encountered when the margins of the tumor are reached. Once the resection is complete, the packing should be sequentially removed and replaced to be certain no tumor has been left behind, and also to reduce the amount of packing used.

Vascular Reconstruction

If ICA reconstruction (Fig. 37) is necessary, the most proximal 8–10 cm of the saphenous vein should be exposed at the beginning of the procedure as described previously. When the vein is harvested, care must be taken to maintain the proper orientation of the vessel. In patients with a compromised collateral circulation, brain protection with moderate hypothermia, induced hypertension, and etomidate or barbiturate coma is utilized. Temporary clips are placed on the petrous ICA and on the supraclinoid ICA proximal to the posterior communicating artery to allow continued perfusion of the hemisphere through that anastomotic channel. A fine temporary clip will also have to be placed on the ophthalmic artery. The ICA is transected and any bleeding from the intracavernous segment (due to collateral intracavernous channels) is controlled by packing the lumen. A

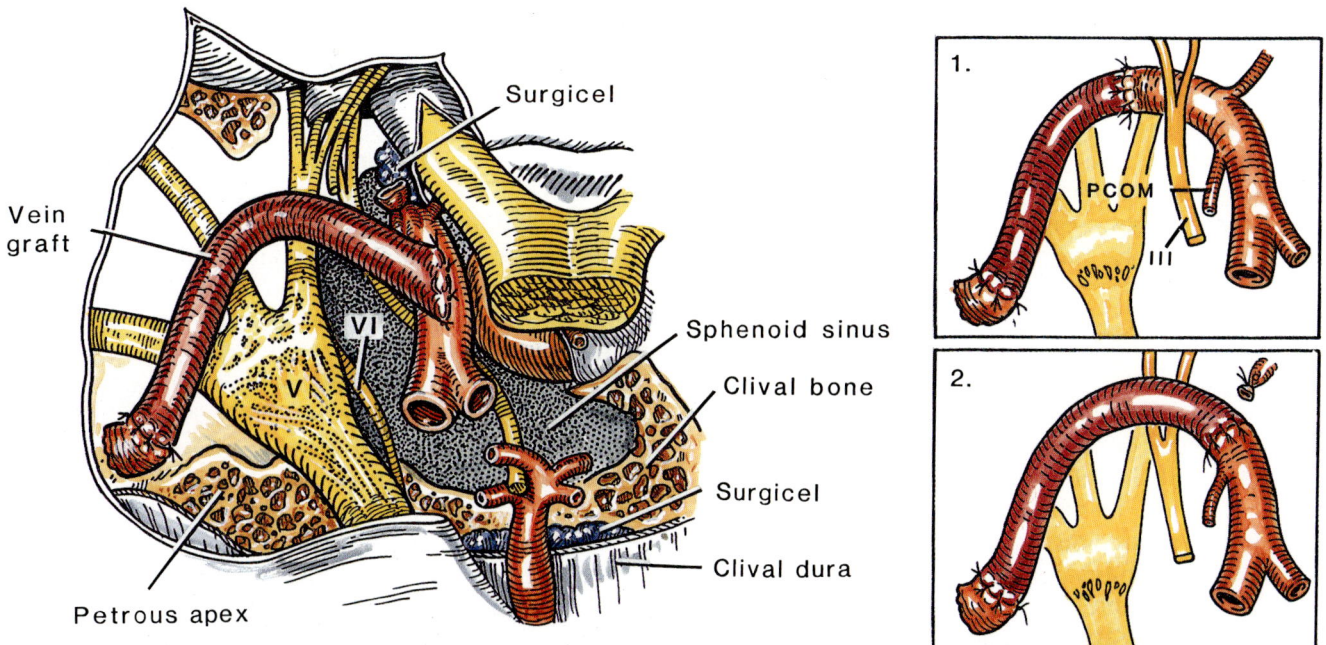

FIG. 37. In patients with grade III–V tumors, a saphenous vein graft is performed from the petrous to the supraclinoid ICA, and then the intracavernous tumor is completely excised. The distal anastomosis is end-to-side, while the proximal anastomosis is end-to-end. After tumor resection, it is easy to remove the petroclival and sphenoidal bone, extradural tumor in the clival area, and tumor involving the sphenoid sinus. Two variations of saphenous vein graft technique are shown. One involves a distal end-to-end anastomosis when the ophthalmic artery can be sacrificed. The second involves a distal clinoidal or infraclinoidal anastomosis, when a healthy clinoidal or infraclinoidal segment is available. This technique will not interrupt collateral flow through the ophthalmic artery during the operation, since the temporary clip can be placed proximal to it.

large dose of intravenous steroid is then given to prevent loss of the endothelium from the graft (20).

The distal anastomosis is performed first, in either an end-to-end or end-to-side fashion, depending on the status of the ophthalmic artery. If the ophthalmic artery is to be preserved and the usable infraclinoid segment is short, then an end-to-side anastomosis just distal to the ophthalmic artery is indicated. If the infraclinoid segment is sufficiently long, then an end-to-end anastomosis can be performed sparing the ophthalmic artery as well. If the ophthalmic artery is to be sacrificed, then an end-to-end supraclinoid anastomosis may be performed. The 7-0 or 8-0 monofilament suture is used in interrupted fashion. The graft is trimmed to the proper length so as to be under no tension but to avoid redundancy. Sufficient length should remain to allow the graft to be retracted out of the way of subsequent tumor removal. The proximal anastomosis is then performed but not completed until the graft has again been flushed with heparinized saline and back-bleeding from both temporary clips has flushed any air or clot from the graft (27).

Intraoperative anticoagulation is not usually necessary for grafting but was used in two patients following thrombosis at the proximal anastomotic site, and in one patient with ICA dissection caused by the balloon test occlusion. In such patients, a low dose of heparin, about 400–600 units/hr, was used to raise the partial thromboplastin time (PTT) to the upper limits of the normal range. All patients are maintained on subcutaneous heparin, 5000 units three times daily, for 1 month postoperatively. In addition, 325 mg of aspirin by mouth daily is begun several days postoperatively and continued indefinitely. All patients who have extensive manipulation of the ICA or have had graft reconstruction undergo a carotid angiogram postoperatively. In addition, all patients with ICA vein grafts undergo a yearly MRI angiogram.

Pituitary Gland

During resection of grade III–V meningiomas, the lateral and inferior dural wall of the sella turcica (medial wall of the CS) should be removed because the tumor invades this dura. This allows the surgeon to inspect the opposite cavernous sinus as well. Because resection of intracavernous tumors may deprive the pituitary gland of its vascular supply, careful postoperative endocrine evaluation is necessary before steroid coverage is discontinued. Diabetes insipidus or SIADH may occur postoperatively, but they are usually transient.

Petroclival Bone and Apex Region

When resecting intracavernous meningiomas, the petrous apex and dorsum sellae should be removed intradurally through the cavernous sinus with a drill and fine rongeurs. For higher grade tumors, all the dura of the medial wall of the cavernous sinus, the lateral wall of the sella, and the upper clivus should also be removed. Small tumor extensions into the opposite cavernous sinus may be removed through this approach as well. Removal of the lateral wall of the sphenoid sinus and tumor in the sphenoid sinus is much easier when the carotid has been grafted.

Grade III and IV tumors often involve the petroclival and sphenoid bone, which will have to be removed to effect complete tumor resection. When tumor extends into the apex of the cavernous sinus, then a combination of the superior and lateral approaches is usually adequate to complete the resection. This is the most difficult area of the CS from which to remove tumor. When tumor extends into the orbital apex, then the periorbita must be opened and the operation extended into the orbit itself as necessary. Opening of the annulus of Zinn may also be necessary.

Reconstruction

Cranial Nerves. Even when ophthalmoplegia follows a cavernous sinus operation, it is usually temporary, and a good recovery of function can be expected if the nerves were preserved in continuity and appear healthy at the end of the operation (23). When only ophthalmoparesis is observed, recovery is generally rapid and complete. Grafting should be undertaken for injured nerves, as good results of cranial nerve reconstruction have been reported (10,22) and have been obtained by us (see Table 9). If cranial nerve grafting is necessary, the greater auricular nerve or sural nerve should be harvested. Exposure of the proximal end of CN VI may require drilling of the petrous apex (24). Division of the inferior petrosal sinus will further increase the posterior fossa exposure. Distal nerve stump exposure may require the exploration of the orbital apex tissues. The periorbita is opened and orbital fat carefully removed to expose the orbital contents. The sixth nerve is the most lateral nerve within the muscle cone, running on the medial surface of the lateral rectus muscle. The anatomy of the anterior end of the cavernous sinus and orbital apex is complex and requires careful study (24). For nerve suturing, 10-0 nylon suture is most often used. Reconstruction of CN VI by graft or suture was performed in nine patients, with five showing recovery (see Table 9 and Fig. 90).

The third nerve may be grafted, but this has only been done in one patient who had poor preoperative function with no binocular vision (see Fig. 81). Another patient with poor preoperative function underwent resuture of CN III with some recovery. CN IV is usually not reconstructed since the disability is minimal or easily corrected by oculoplastic surgeons. It is done if the reconstruction will not excessively increase the operative time. The trigeminal nerve and root must be reconstructed whenever possible, because ocular and facial sensation is extremely important. In our patient population, reconstruction of V_1 was performed in three patients with partial recovery in two, and the trigeminal root was reconstructed in one patient, also with some recovery of sensation (see Figs. 56 and 71).

Cranial Base. If the sphenoid sinus has been entered during the tumor resection, then careful reconstruction is required to prevent a cerebrospinal fluid leak. Autologous fat is used to pack the sinus, and the dura is reconstructed as well as possible with a fascia lata or pericranial graft. This free graft is sutured circumferentially, and autologous fibrin glue may be used to reinforce the suture line. For larger openings into the sphenoid sinus, a pedicled pericranial or galeopericranial flap is used to line the surface of the sphenoid sinus. This is held in apposition to the bone with autologous fat packing (Fig. 38).

In patients with extensive tumors who have a large defect of the infratemporal fossa and the sphenoid sinus, a vascularized flap repair is necessary. However, it is difficult to fill the sphenoid sinus completely with such flaps, and reoperation to fill the sphenoid sinus with fat or to close the dura may become necessary.

If it was opened, the eustachian tube should be checked again to ensure that it has been occluded, and its proximal end and any other openings into the middle ear are occluded with fat. Large infratemporal defects may be repaired by rotation of the temporalis muscle into the infratemporal fossa.

The dura is closed completely, and where primary closure is not possible, pieces of fat are secured to the dura to fill the gaps. Pericranial or fascia lata grafts may be necessary for dural repair.

The orbitozygomatic osteotomy is replaced with the temporalis muscle beneath it and secured with 2-0 Neurolon sutures. After the dura is tacked up, the craniotomy bone flap is replaced. Burr holes are filled with bone chips and the temporalis muscle closed carefully, especially inferiorly, to prevent CSF leakage. A subgaleal drain is placed prior to scalp closure and hooked to gravity drainage only for 24–48 hr. Suction drainage is not used, for fear of provoking a CSF leak.

Chordoma and Chondrosarcoma

Chordomas and chondrosarcomas are less adherent to intracavernous structures than meningiomas and are therefore easier to remove. While a combination of multiple approaches to the cavernous sinus is usually neces-

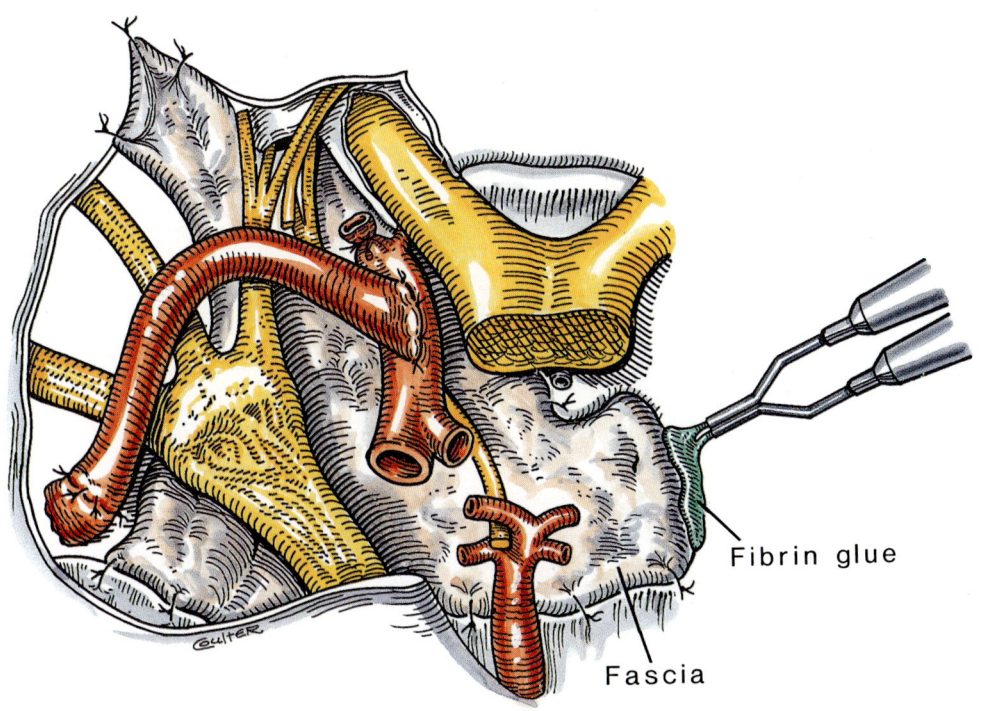

FIG. 38. Reconstruction technique after extensive sphenoidal sinus opening is shown. A galeopericranial flap is used to line the inner surface of the sphenoid sinus, not shown in the figure. The sphenoid sinus is then packed with autologous fat, and the dural opening is closed with a free fascia lata graft. It is impossible to achieve a watertight closure of the fascia lata, but circumferential sutures and autologous fibrin glue are adequate.

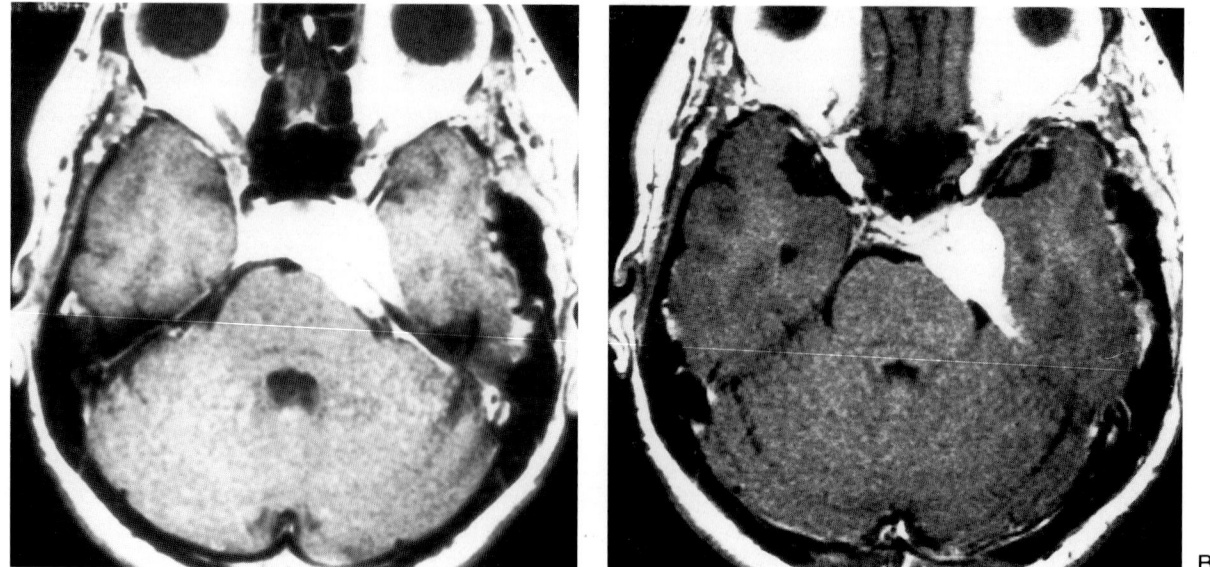

FIG. 39. A,B: Preoperative axial MRI images reveal a tumor involving the cavernous sinus and the tentorial notch area.

sary for meningioma resection, these tumors can often be removed through a single approach.

Highly Malignant Tumors

Highly malignant tumors such as squamous cell carcinoma are resected *en bloc* without actually entering the CS. Excision of the cranial nerves and ICA is necessary. Vascular and cranial base reconstruction is performed as needed.

CASE EXAMPLES

K.R.: Grade II Meningioma

This 38-year-old woman presented with a long history of migraine headaches, and the recent onset of deficits of CNs V_1 and VI. Biopsy at another institution had revealed a meningioma. Preoperative axial MRI images (Fig. 39A,B) revealed a tumor involving the cavernous sinus and the tentorial notch area. Coronal MRI images (Fig. 40A) showed that the tumor has mostly displaced

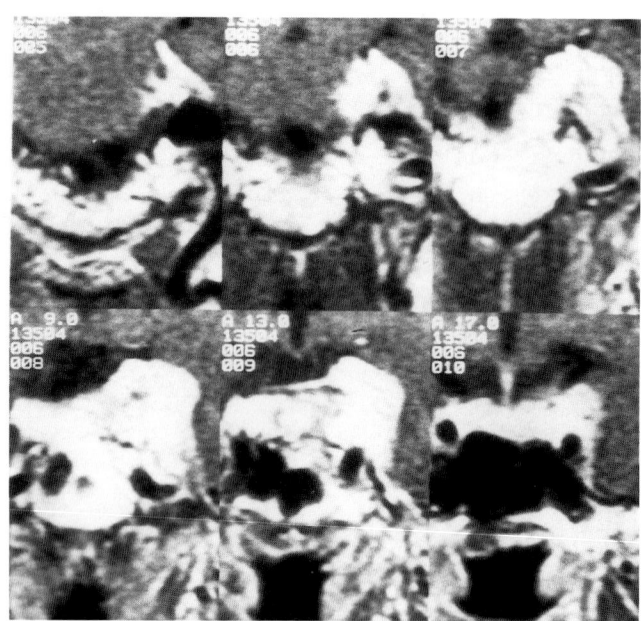
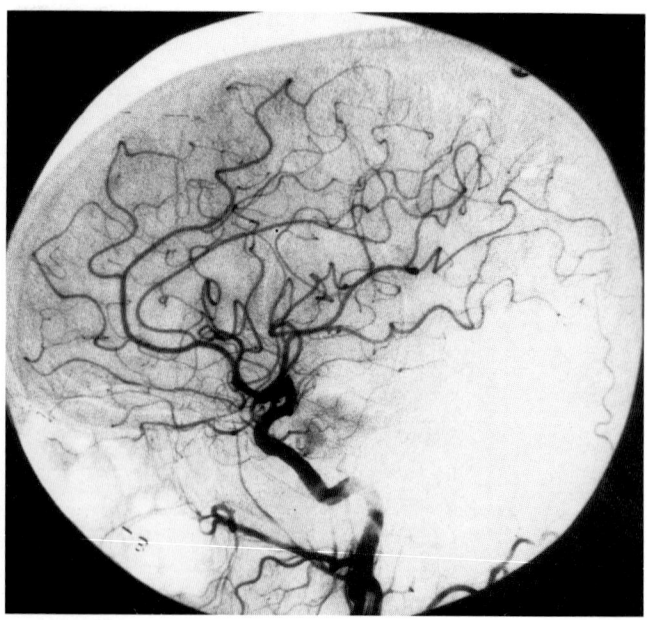

FIG. 40. A: Coronal MRI images show that the tumor has mostly displaced the intracavernous ICA interoinferiorly, with partial but not total encasement. **B:** Angiography shows the blood supply to the tumor.

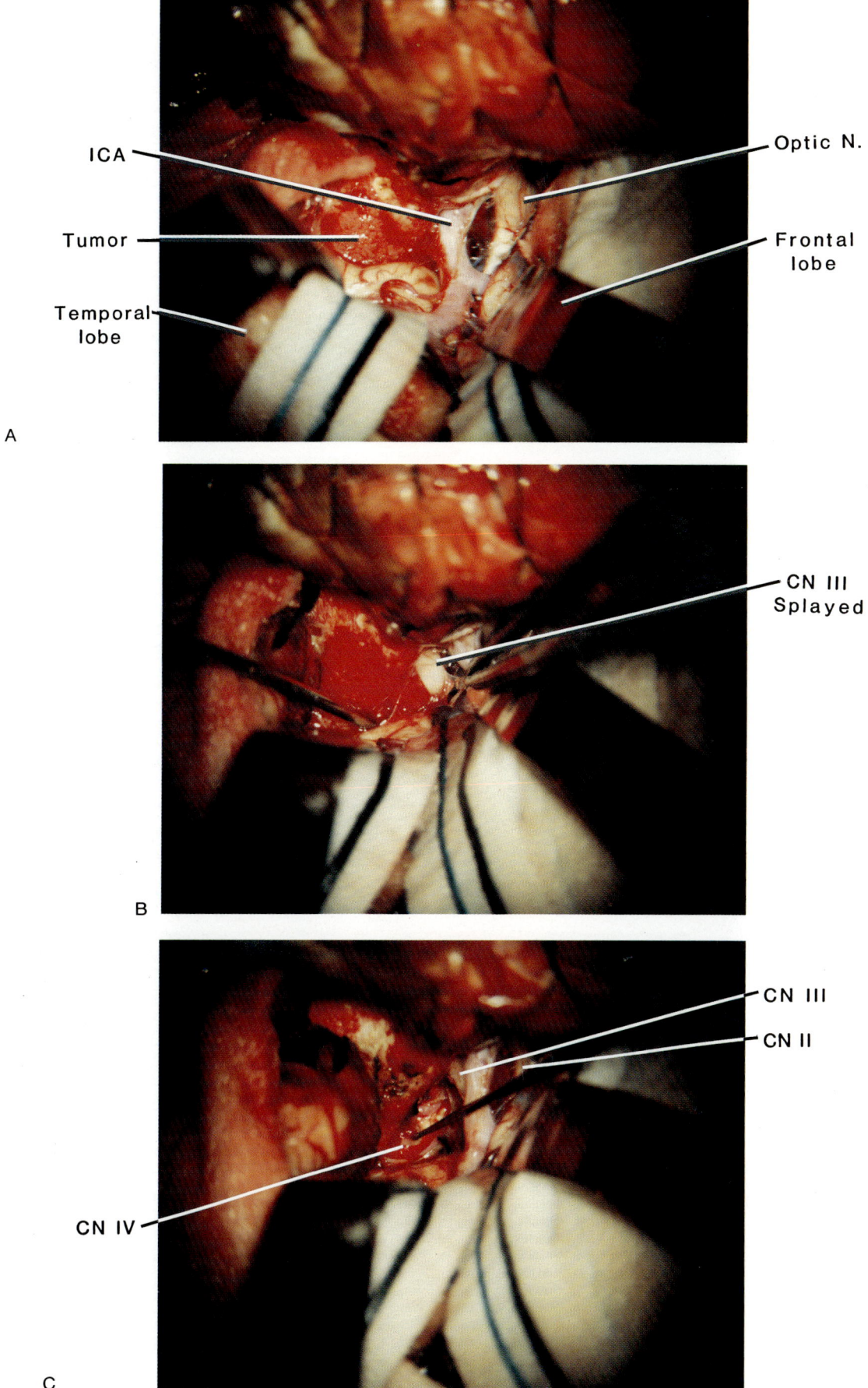

FIG. 41. A: The frontal and temporal lobes after splitting the sylvian fissure, and the subdural tumor. **B:** CN III was splayed by tumor at its entrance into the cavernous sinus and is seen during tumor removal. **C:** After removal of all subdural tumor, CN IV and the tentorial notch structures are clearly seen.

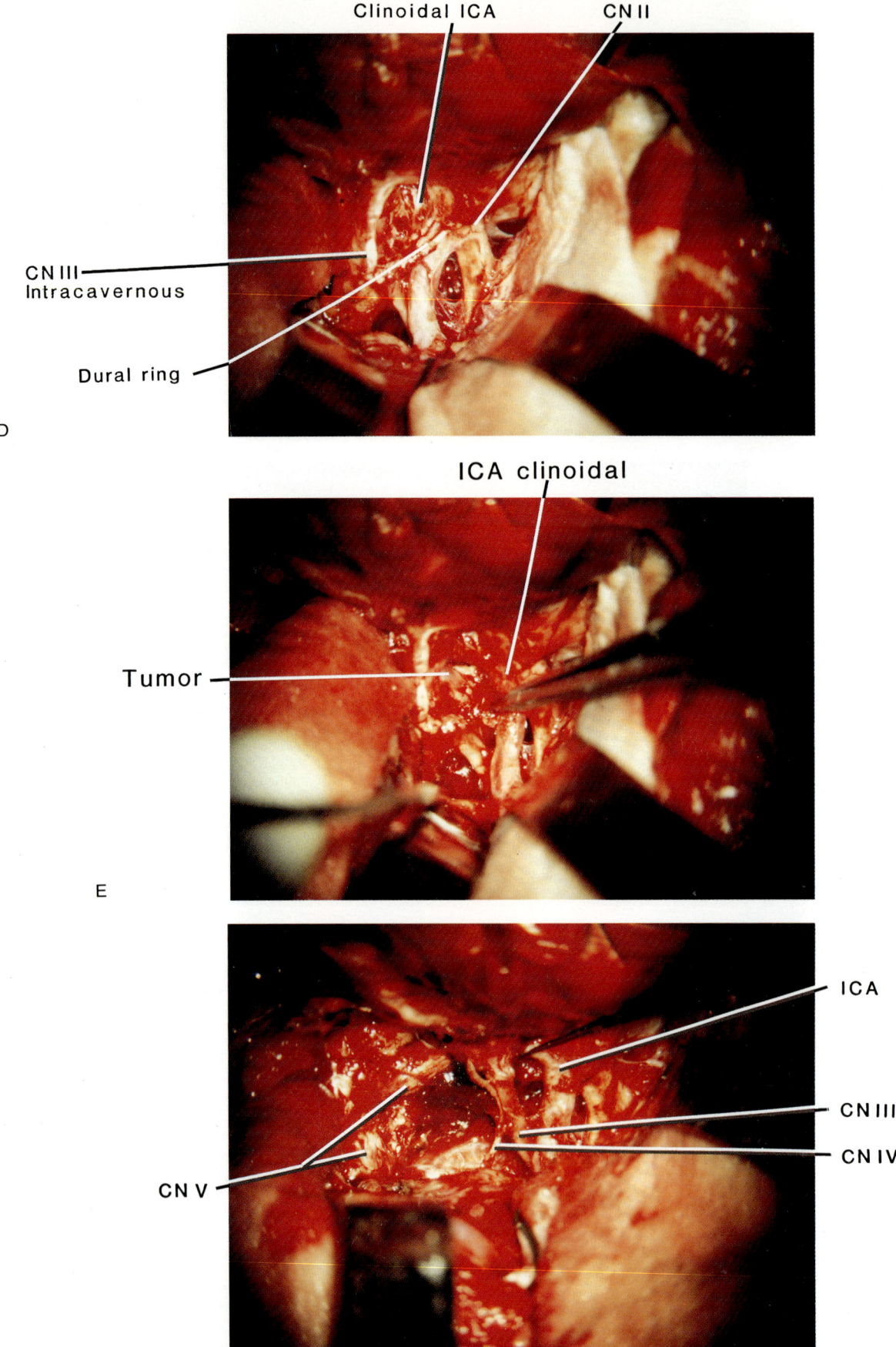

FIG. 41. *Continued.* **D:** The optic nerve has been unroofed and the anterior clinoid process removed. The clinoid space is clearly visible. **E:** The dural ring has been excised, and the superior wall of the cavernous sinus opened with tumor visualized within. **F:** The appearance after tumor resection.

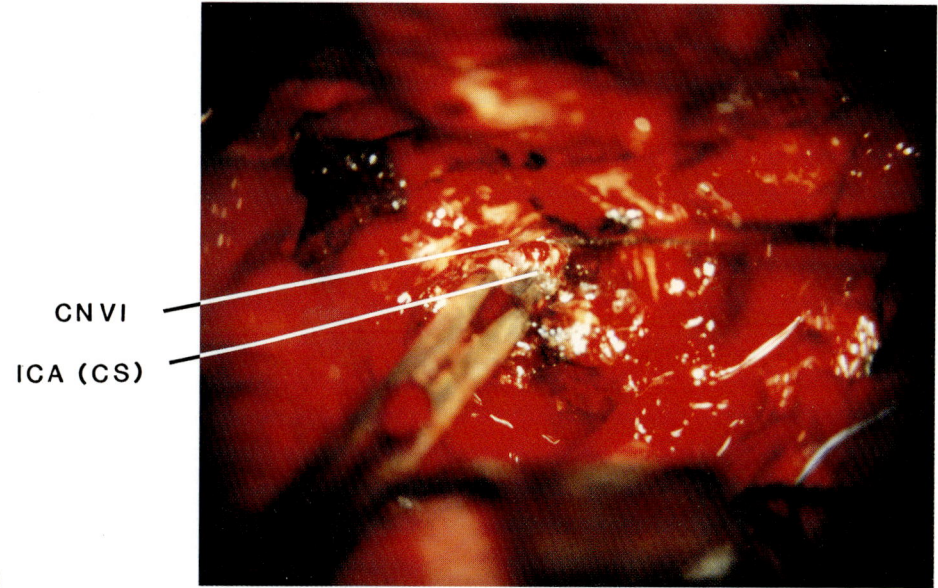

FIG. 41. *Continued.* **G:** The intracavernous CN VI and ICA are seen to be displaced anteroinferiorly.

the intracavernous ICA anteroinferiorly, with partial but not total encasement. This was confirmed by angiography (Fig. 40B), which also showed the blood supply to the tumor.

At operation, the tumor was found to be subdural and intracavernous. Figure 41A shows the frontal and temporal lobes, after splitting the sylvian fissure, and the subdural tumor. CN III was splayed by tumor at its entrance into the cavernous sinus and is seen during tumor removal in Fig. 41B. After removal of all subdural tumor (Fig. 41C), CN IV and the tentorial notch structures are clearly seen. In Fig. 41D, the optic nerve has been unroofed, and the anterior clinoid process removed, with the clinoid space clearly visible. In Fig. 41E, the dural ring has been excised, and the superior wall of the cavernous sinus opened, with tumor visualized within. The clinoidal segment of the ICA is clearly visible. Figure 41F shows the appearance after tumor resection. CN III has been dissected entirely and is seen to be branching anteriorly. CN IV has been dissected and displaced superiorly, to open up Parkinson's triangle. The trigeminal root, ganglion, and V_1 are clearly visible. The cavernous sinus has been packed with Surgicel. In Fig. 41G, the intracavernous CN VI and ICA are seen to be displaced anteroinferiorly.

Postoperative enhanced axial CT images (Fig. 42A,B)

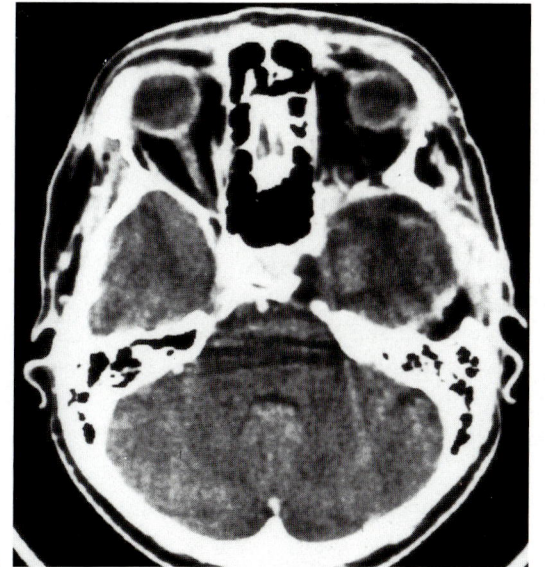
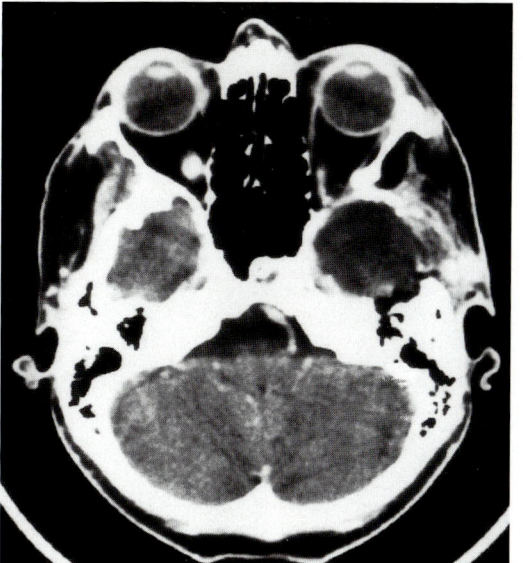

FIG. 42. A,B: Postoperative enhanced axial CT images reveal the absence of tumor two years later.

reveal the absence of tumor, 2 years later. The patient recovered considerable extraocular muscle function. She was left with a paresis of CN VI and normal pituitary function. She was able to achieve binocular vision with prism glasses (Fig. 43) (photograph reproduced with patient's permission).

A.G.: Grade II Intracavernous Meningioma

This 64-year-old woman presented with a severe facial pain syndrome and complete ophthalmoplegia of 3 months' duration (Fig. 44). MRI revealed an intracavernous tumor displacing the ICA but not encasing it, thought to be a neurilemoma (Fig. 45A,B). At operation, a meningioma was found and removed totally. She made a surprisingly good recovery of extraocular muscle function (Fig. 46). The facial pain syndrome was im-

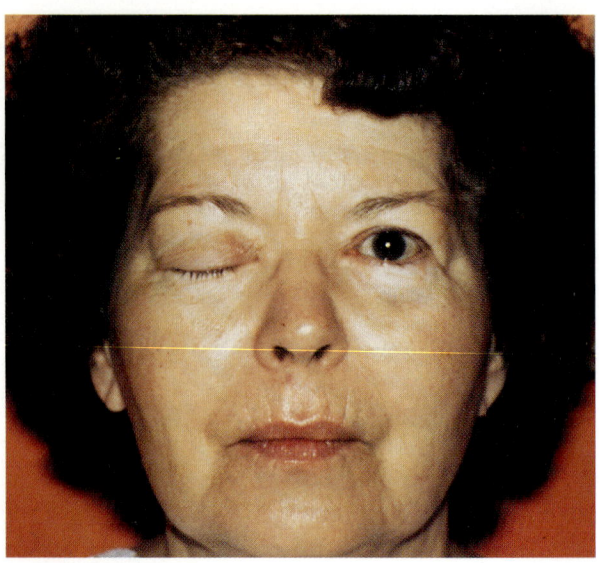

FIG. 44. A 64-year-old woman presented with a severe facial pain syndrome and complete ophthalmoplegia of 3 months' duration.

proved but not completely abated (photographs reproduced with the patient's permission).

V.O.: Grade III Sphenocavernous Meningioma

This 24-year-old woman had undergone a partial resection of a sphenoid wing meningioma previously. She presented with progressive tumor regrowth, a seizure, and visual loss during pregnancy. Because of the absence of significant brain compression, she was managed without operation until the delivery of a baby by cesarean section at 35 weeks gestation. Gadolinium enhanced MRI scans (Fig. 47A–D) revealed a tumor involving the cavernous sinus, orbit, middle fossa, infratemporal fossa, and the sphenoid bone. At operation, the intracavernous tumor could be peeled off the ICA. An extensive bone resection was necessary to remove all the tumor. The abducens nerve was partially injured and was reconstructed with a graft. Cranial base reconstruction was performed with autologous fat and temporalis muscle. Postoperatively, her extraocular muscle movements were almost normal, with mild ptosis (Fig. 48). Numbness in the V_1 distribution persisted, and vision improved to 20/70. No tumor recurrence was seen 2 years later, and the axial and coronal enhanced CT scan reveals the absence of tumor and the fat packing, and bone window CT scan reveals the extent of the bone removal (Fig. 49A–D).

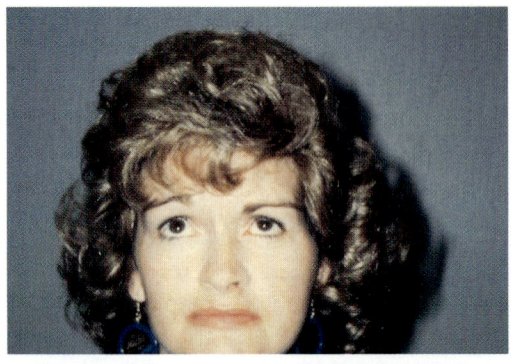
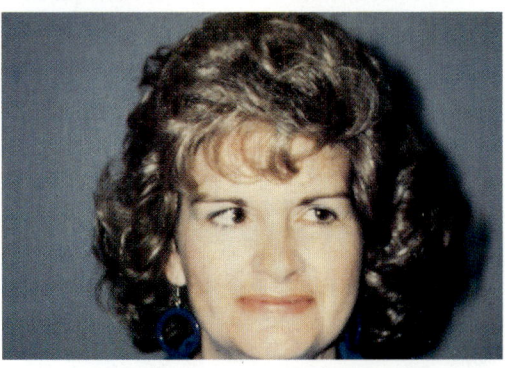
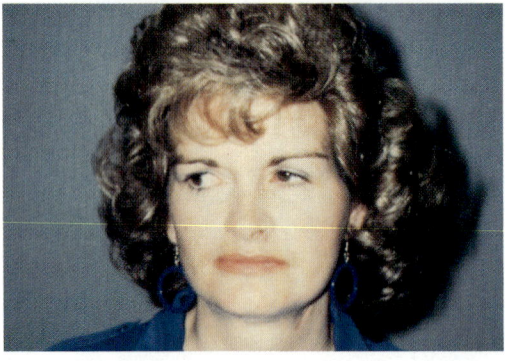

FIG. 43. The patient was able to achieve binocular vision with prism glasses.

G.G.: Intracavernous Hemangioma Grade III

This 62-year-old woman presented with long-standing visual loss and ophthalmoplegia in the right eye and re-

CAVERNOUS SINUS AND SPHENOCAVERNOUS NEOPLASMS / 555

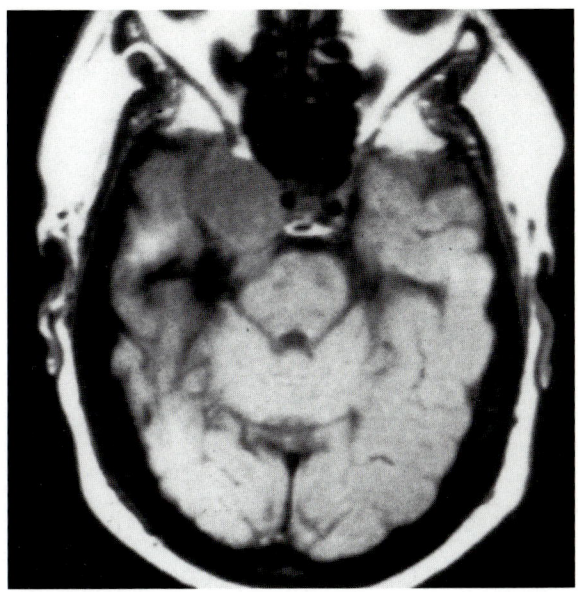
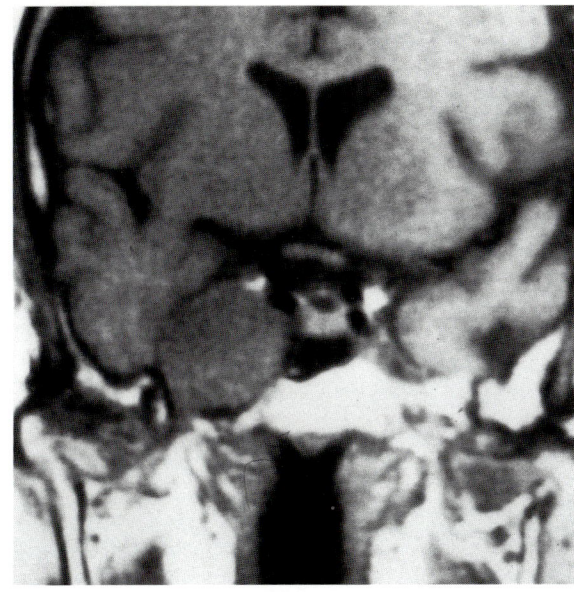

FIG. 45. A,B: MRI revealed an intracavernous tumor displacing the ICA but not encasing it, thought to be a neurilemoma.

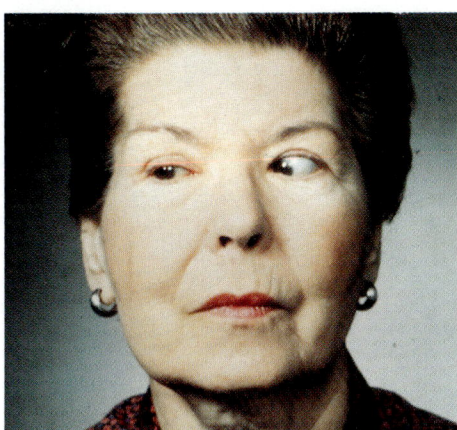
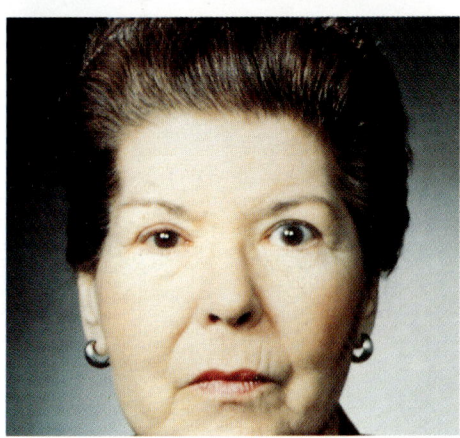

FIG. 46. The patient made good recovery of extraocular muscle function.

cently worsening vision in the left eye. The tumor had been explored twice previously with the presumption of a meningioma, and the operation had been stopped because of excessive bleeding. Preoperative nonenhanced, T1-weighted coronal (Fig. 50A) and sagittal (Fig. 50B) MRI scans, and enhanced coronal MRI scans (Fig. 50C,D) reveal a large tumor that occupied the middle and posterior cranial fossae. The tumor is isodense on T1-weighted images, hyperdense on T2-weighted images (not shown here), and enhances brightly after gadolinium. Cerebral angiogram reveals a blush after both selective external (Fig. 51A) and internal (Fig. 51B) injection.

At operation, the lesion was very vascular and spongy, typical for hemangioma. The lesion was encasing the ICA but could be dissected free. Removal was done very quickly (60 min) because of the bleeding from feeding vessels, and the technique was similar to the excision of an arteriovenous malformation. Figure 52A shows the lesion isolated from all the feeding vessels. Figure 52B shows the cavernous sinus packed with Surgicel, the supraclinoid ICA, optic nerve, basilar artery, and pituitary stalk. The ipsilateral CNs III, IV, and VI were excised with the lesion. Figure 52C shows the reconstruction of the cranial base with autologous fat and fascia lata graft. The patient needed reexploration and closure of an opening into the sphenoid sinus medial to the optic nerve.

The pathological examination revealed a cavernous angioma (Fig. 53) (photograph courtesy of J. Martinez). Postoperative enhanced CT scan (Fig. 54A,B) and en-

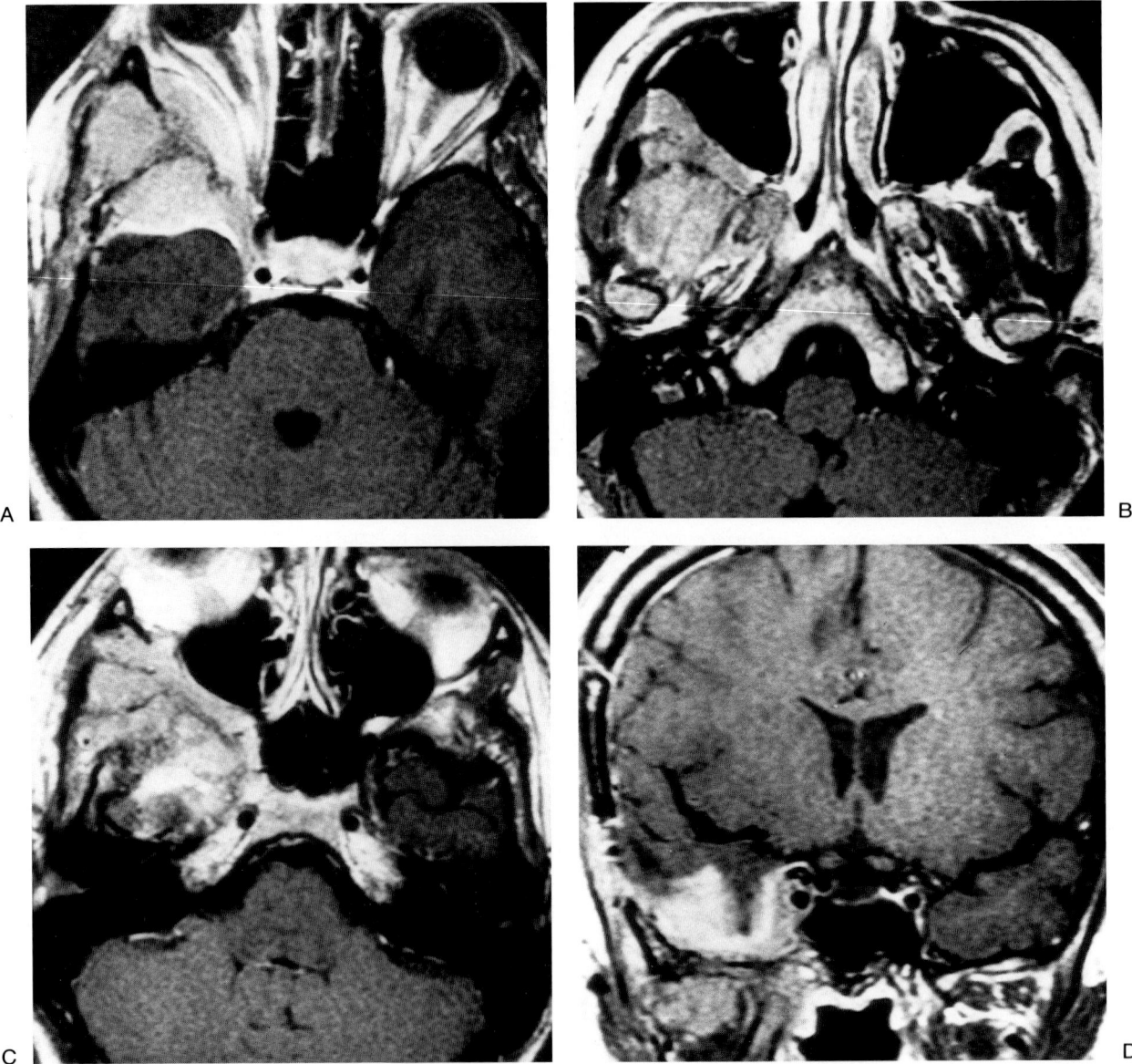

FIG. 47. Patient V.O. **A–D:** Gadolinium enhanced MRI scans reveal a tumor involving the cavernous sinus, orbit, middle fossa, infratemporal fossa, and the sphenoid bone.

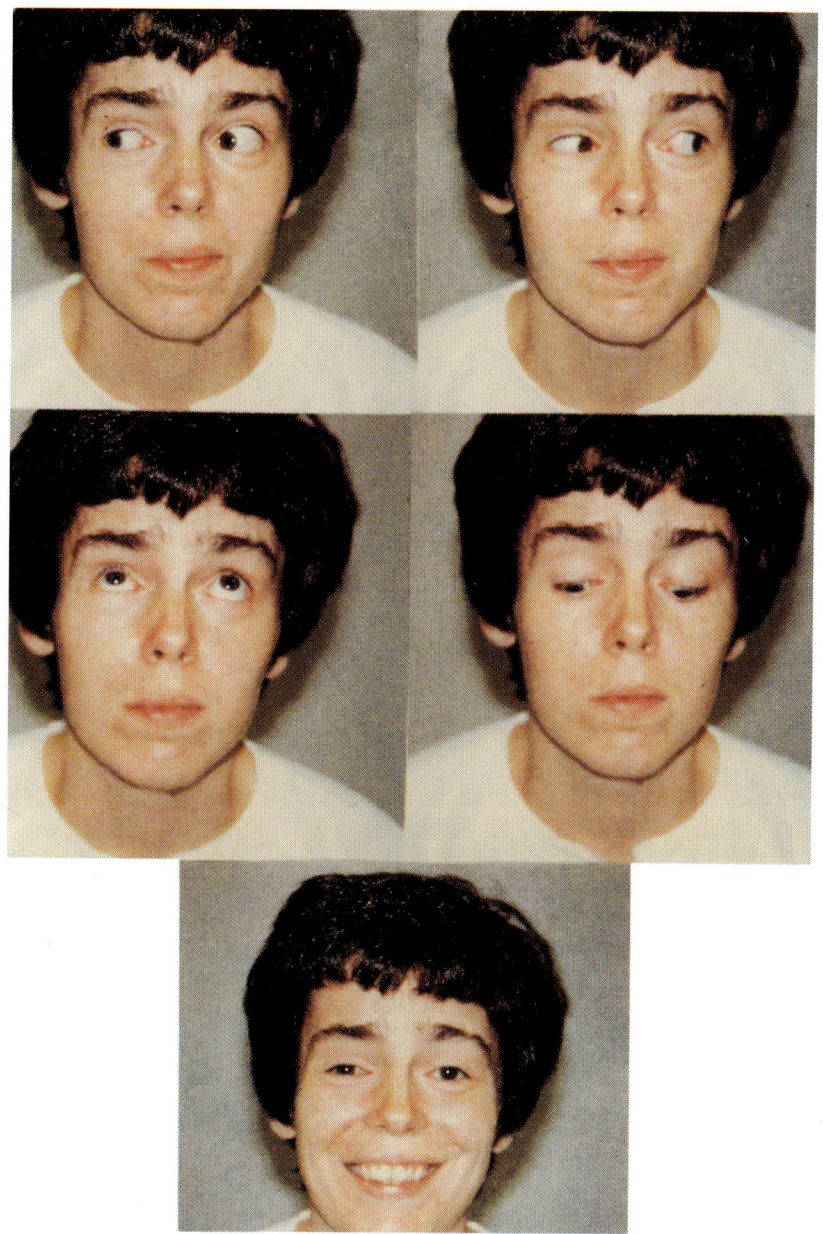

FIG. 48. Patient V.O. Postoperatively, the patient's extraocular movements were almost normal, with mild ptosis.

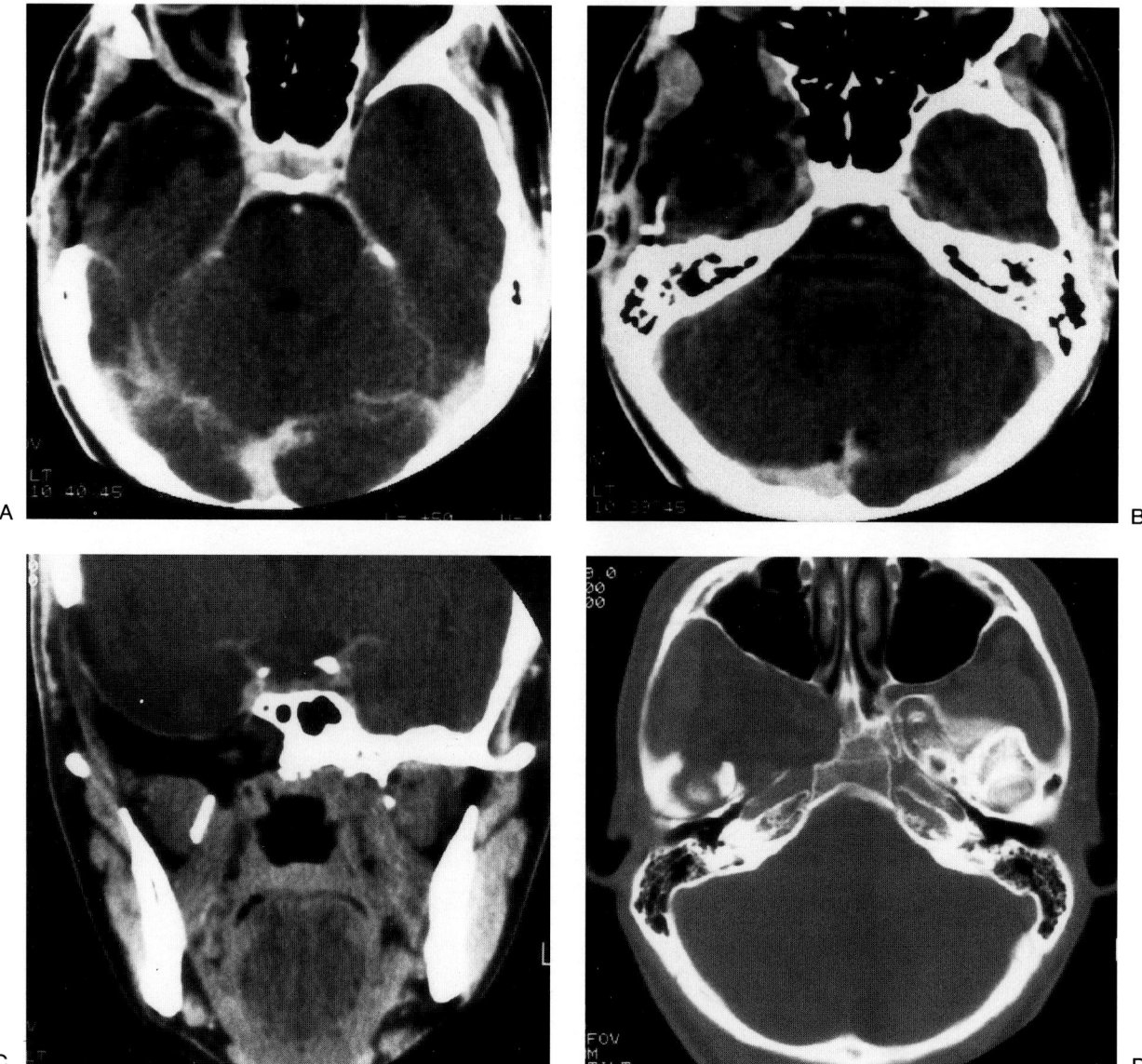

FIG. 49. Patient V.O. **A–D:** Axial and coronal enhanced CT scan reveals the absence of tumor; the fat packing and bone window CT scan reveals the extent of the bone removal.

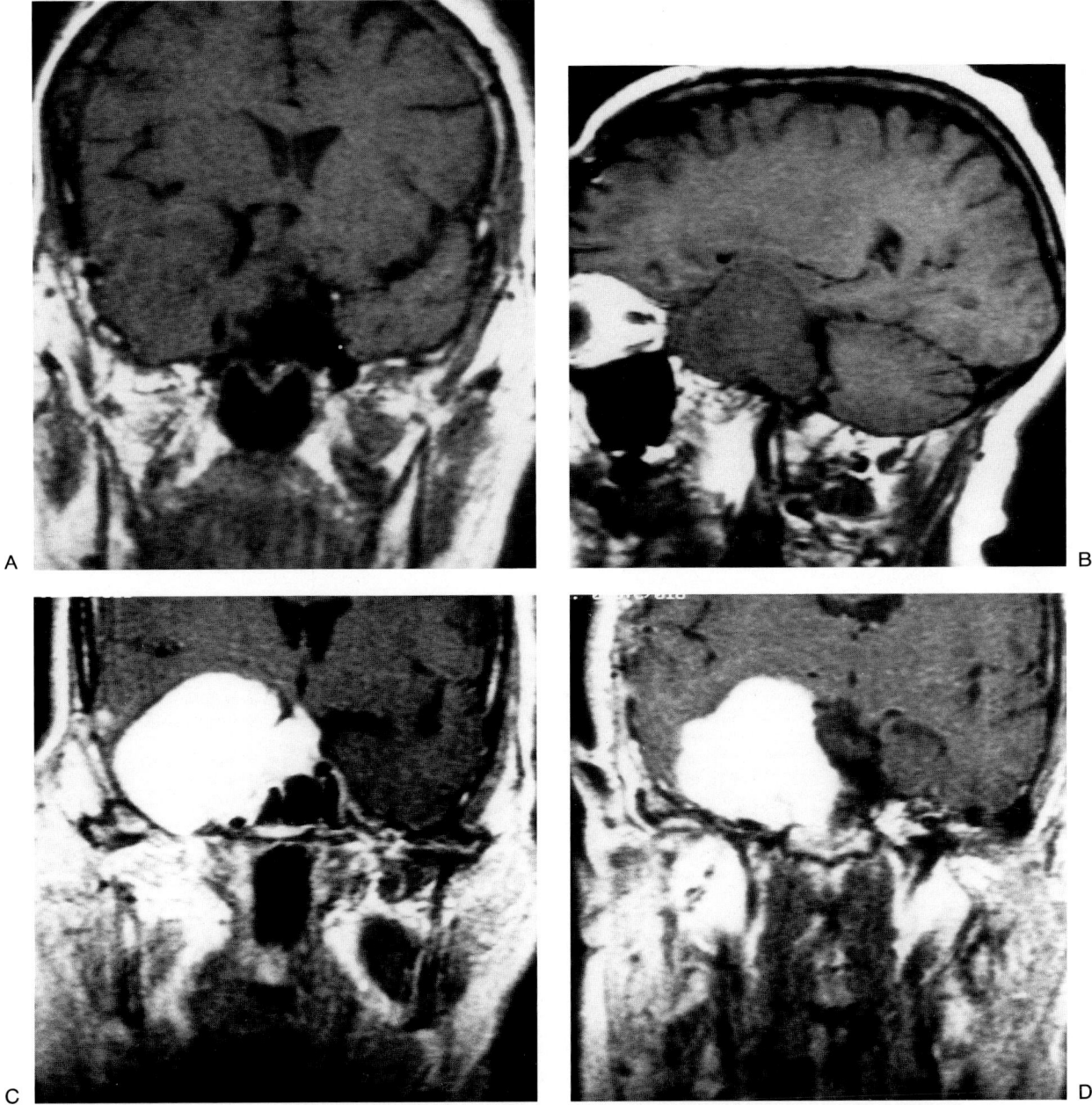

FIG. 50. Patient G.G. **A–D:** Preoperative nonenhanced T1-weighted coronal (**A**) and sagittal (**B**) MRI scans and enhanced coronal MRI scans (**C, D**) reveal a large tumor that occupied the middle and posterior cranial fossae.

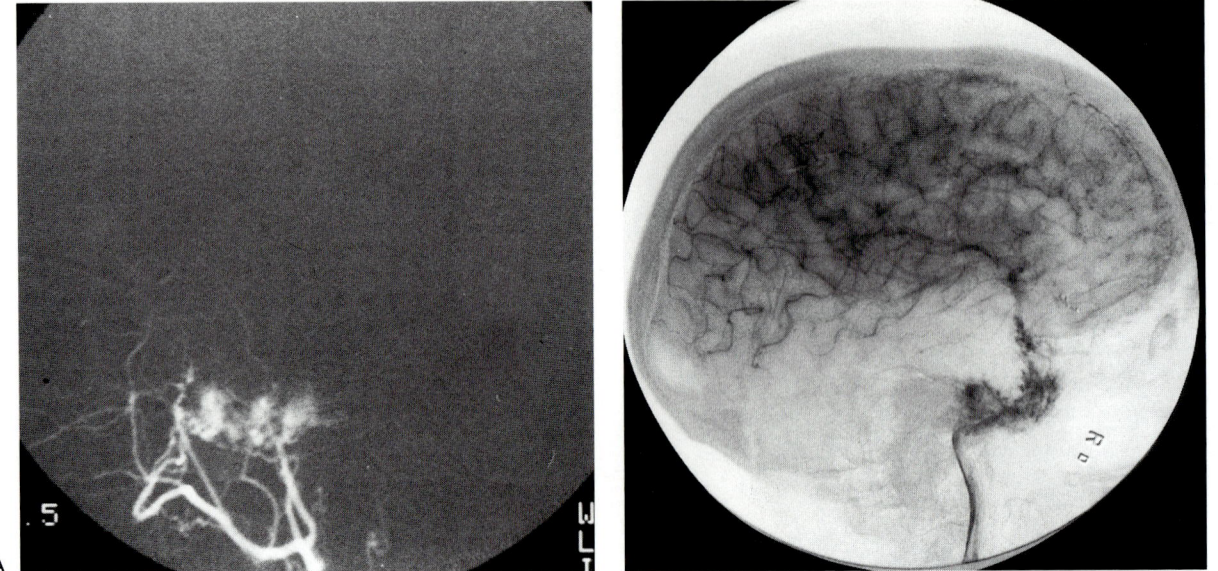

FIG. 51. Patient G.G. Cerebral angiogram reveals a blush after (**A**) selective external and (**B**) selective internal injection.

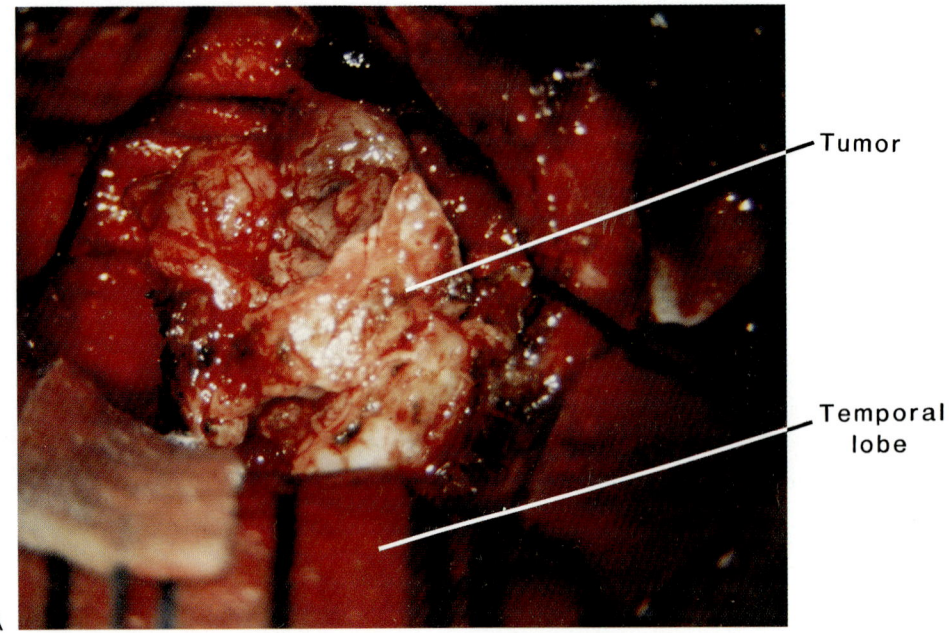

FIG. 52. Patient G.G. **A:** The tumor isolated from all the feeding vessels. **B:** The cavernous sinus is packed with Surgicel. The supraclinoid ICA, optic nerve, basilar artery, and the pituitary stalk are also seen. **C:** The reconstruction of the cranial base with autologous fat and fascia lata graft is seen.

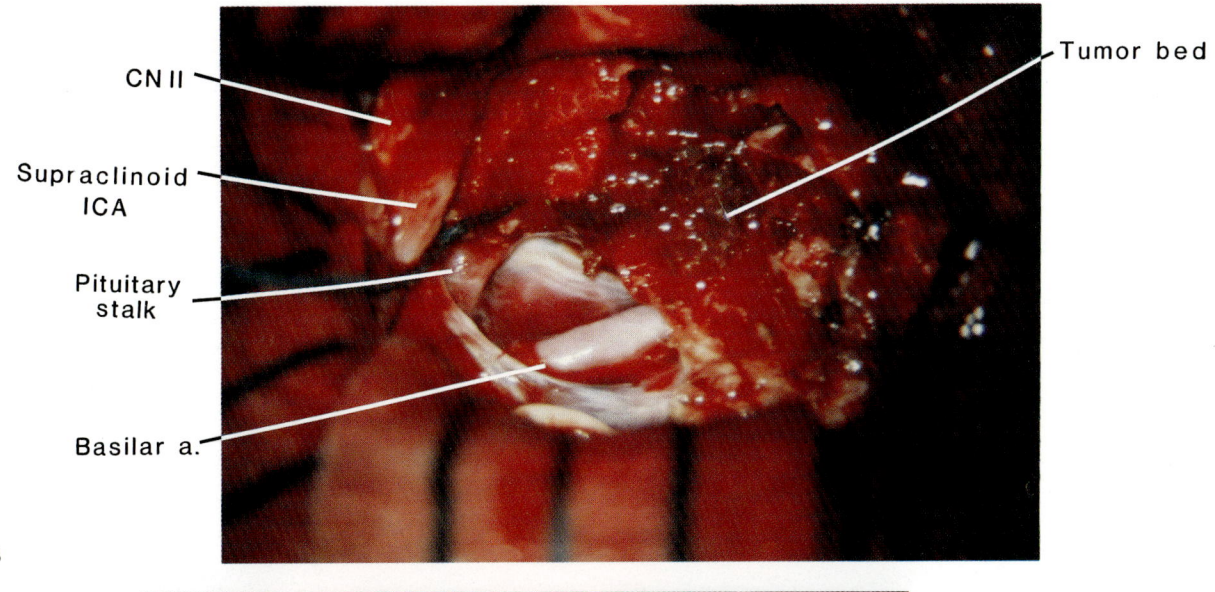

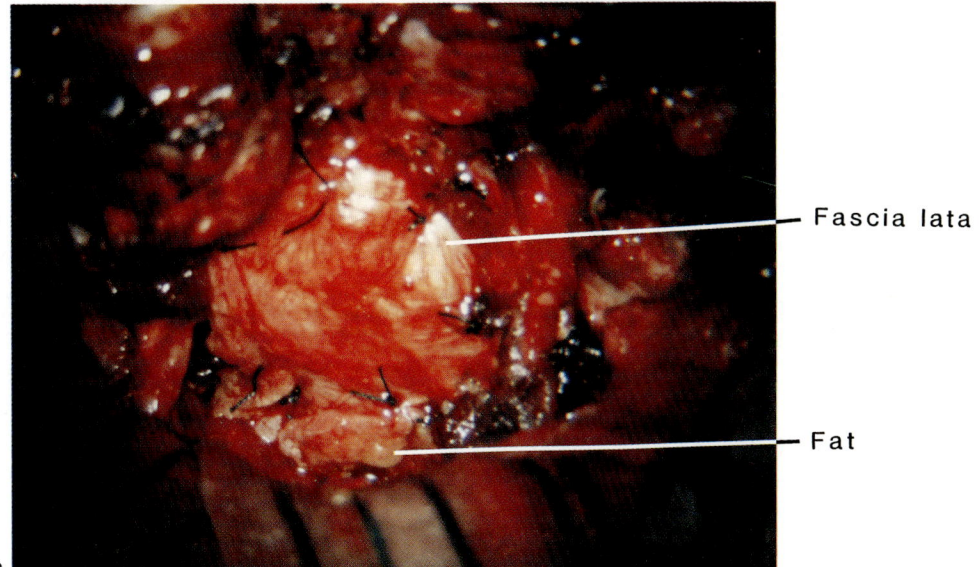

FIG. 52. Continued.

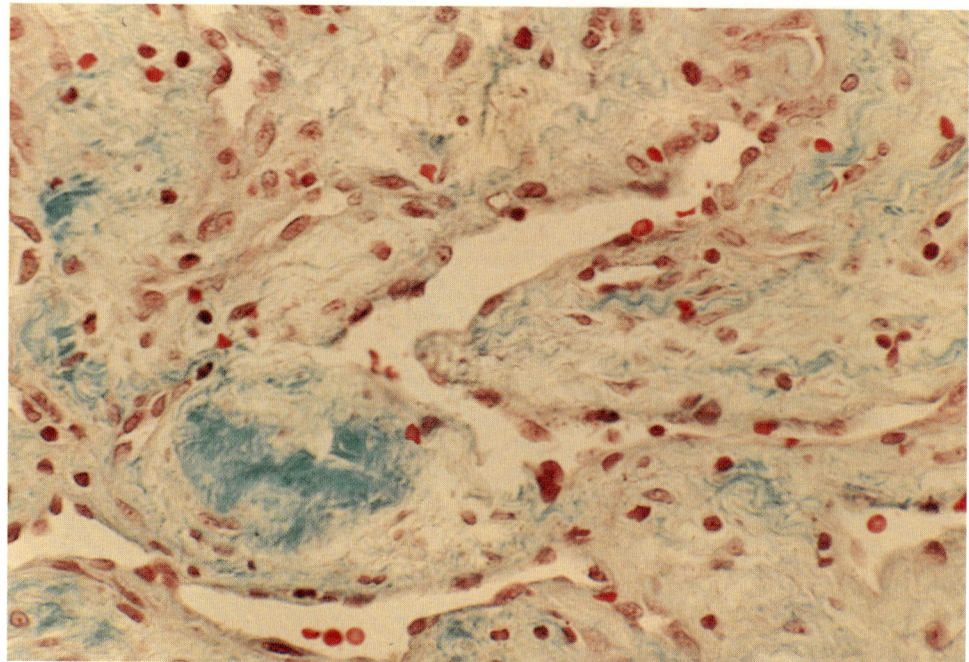

FIG. 53. Patient G.G. Pathological examination shows a cavernous angioma.

hanced MRI scans (Fig. 54C,D) revealed the absence of lesion, and the fat and fascia used for reconstruction, especially in the sphenoid sinus.

K.H.: Sphenocavernous–Orbital Meningioma Grade II

This 30-year-old woman presented with exophthalmos, loss of vision, and partial oculomotor palsy during pregnancy due to the tumor shown in the figures. After delivery of her child, the tumor was removed by us. The preoperative coronal and axial CT scans revealed a tumor involving the sphenocavernous and the orbital area (Fig. 55A,B). T1- and T2-weighted MRI scans (Fig. 55C) revealed tumor involvement of the cavernous sinus. Even though the intracavernous ICA is narrowed, it is predominantly displaced with partial encasement only. The ICA angiogram (Fig. 55D) shows the tumor blush and the elevation of the middle cerebral artery by the tumor.

During operation to remove the tumor, the most important first intradural step is to split the sylvian fissure from a lateral to a medial direction and find the distal branches of the middle cerebral artery (Fig. 56A). The tumor is then progressively dissected away from the branches (Fig. 56B), then the MCA and the ICA. At the conclusion of tumor resection (several other steps not shown), the intracavernous ICA and the maxillary nerve are seen (Fig. 56C), the ophthalmic nerve being resected due to tumor invasion. It was reconstructed with sural nerve graft (Fig. 56D). Postoperative CT scan (Fig. 57) suggests residual tumor in the orbital apex area, unchanged upon follow-up for 3 years. Her oculomotor palsy was slightly worsened, vision was unchanged, and sensation in V_1 distribution partially recovered upon follow-up.

R.P.: Craniopharyngioma

This 50-year-old man had previously undergone the transsphenoidal resection of a craniopharyngioma and radiation therapy for recurrence. He presented with a sizable tumor recurrence. He was blind in the left eye with a left abducens palsy, had a partial CN III palsy, and had complete loss of anterior pituitary function on the right. MRI scans with gadolinium enhancement in the coronal plane (Fig. 58A,B), axial plane (Fig. 58C), and nonenhanced T1-weighted images (Fig. 58D) are shown. A tumor involving the sella, suprasellar region, upper clivus, and the predominantly right cavernous sinus is seen.

The operation was performed through a right subfrontal, subfrontal and transsylvian approach, both cavernous sinuses being entered by a medial route, and the right CS also through a superior route. Figure 59A shows the right transsylvian and subfrontal exposure. The optic chiasm is prefixed. The tumor is seen. In Fig. 59B, the

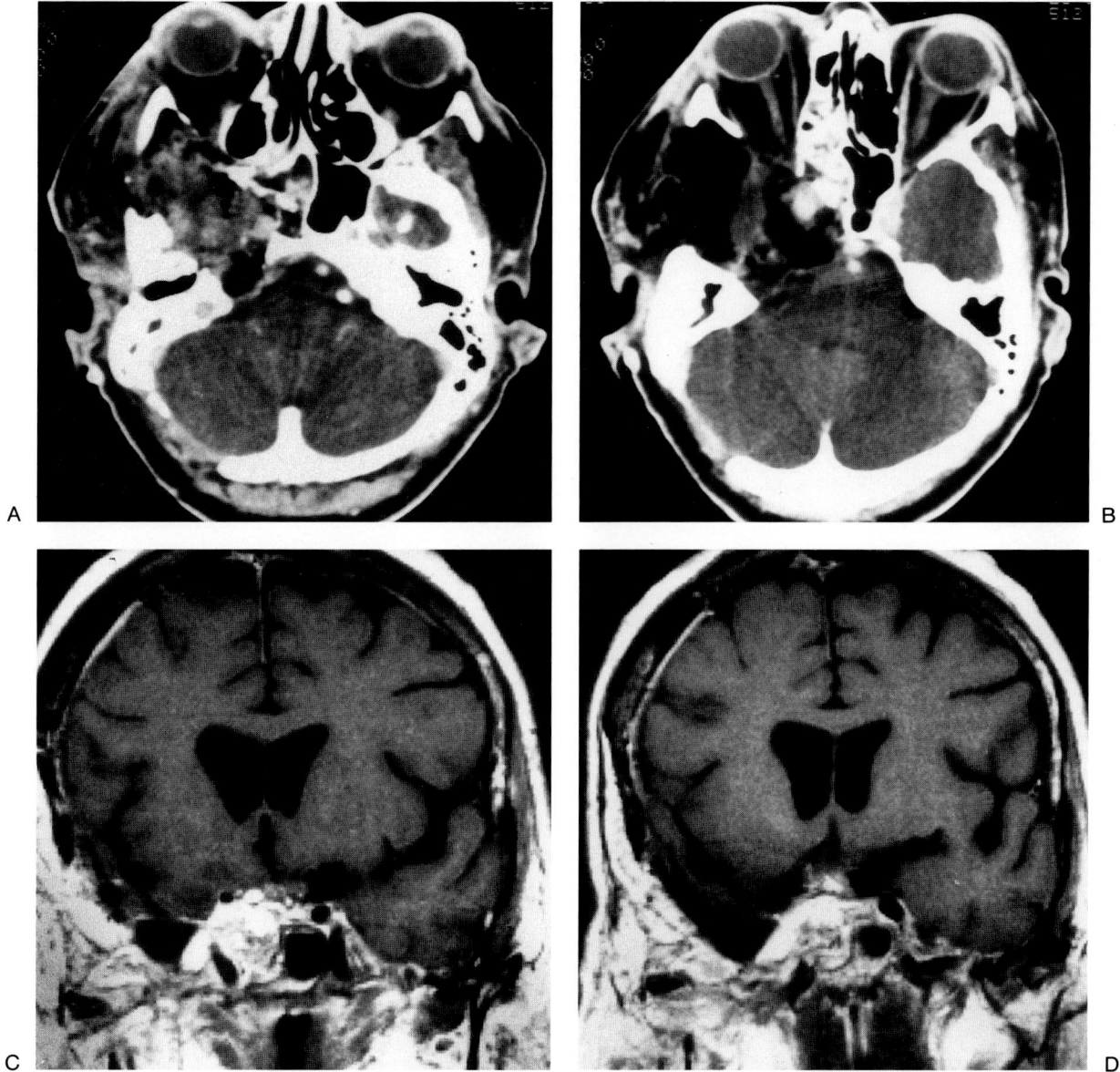

FIG. 54. Patient G.G. **A–D:** Postoperative enhanced CT scan (**A, B**) reveals absence of lesion; postoperative enhanced MRI scans (**C, D**) reveal absence of lesion and the scar tissue from reconstruction.

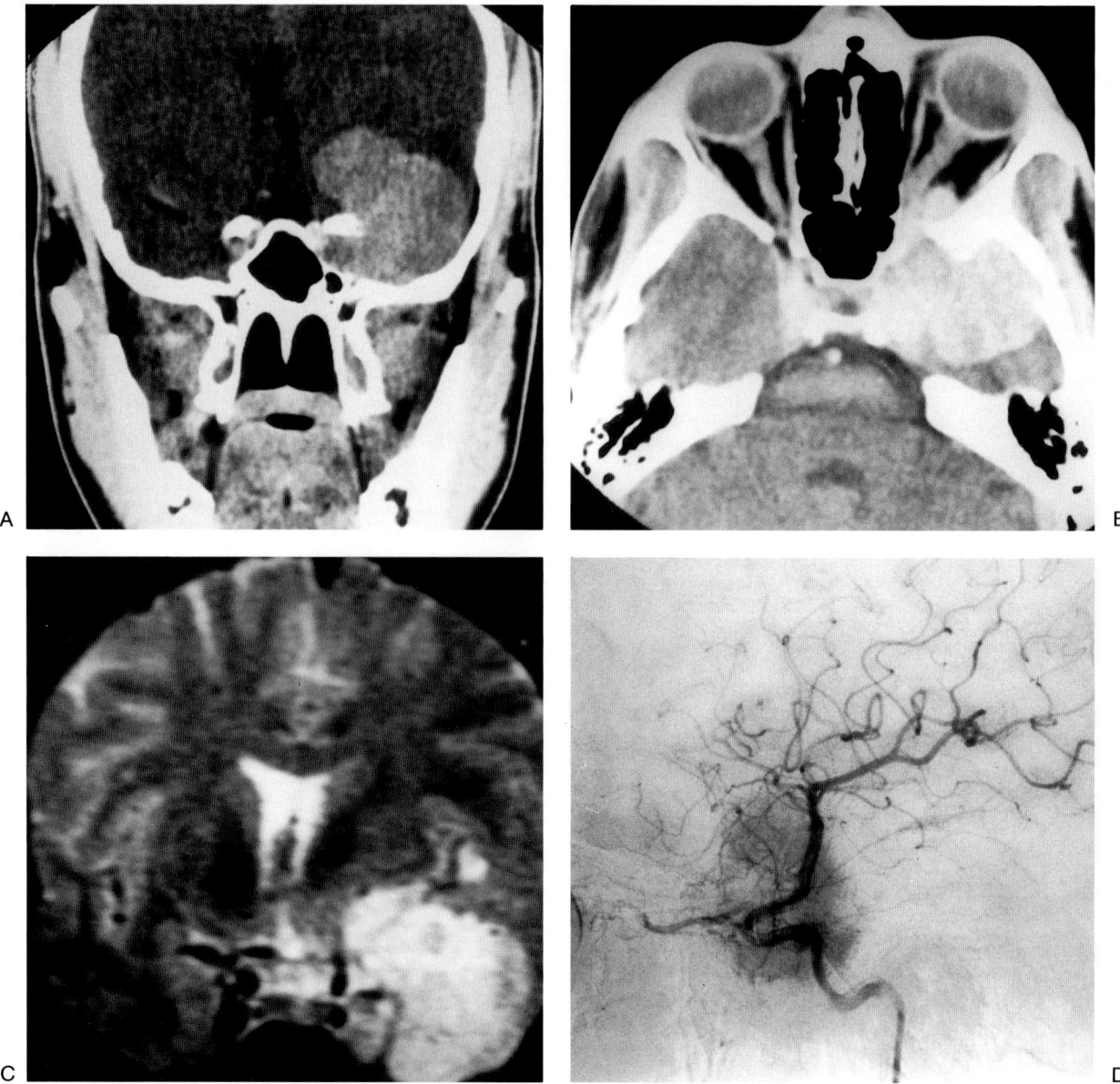

FIG. 55. Patient K.H. **A,B:** Preoperative coronal and axial CT scans reveal a tumor involving the sphenocavernous and the orbital area. **C:** T2-weighted MRI scan reveals tumor involvement of the cavernous sinus and the middle fossa. **D:** The ICA angiogram shows the tumor blush and the elevation of the middle cerebral artery by the tumor.

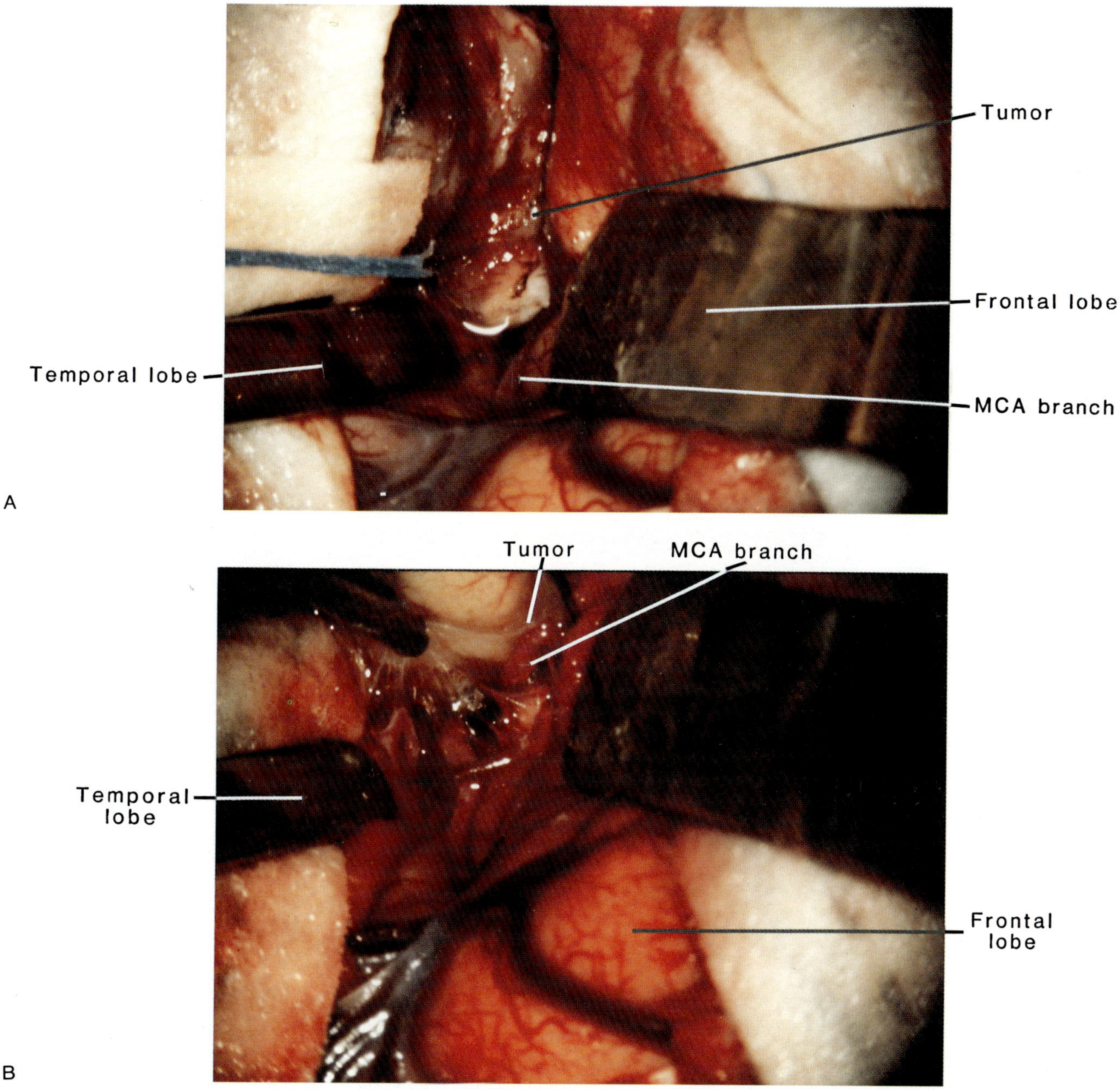

FIG. 56. Patient K.H. **A:** During the operation to remove the tumor, the sylvian fissure is split from a lateral to a medial direction and the distal branches of the middle cerebral artery are seen. **B:** The tumor is progressively dissected away from the branches of the MCA, then the MCA and the ICA.

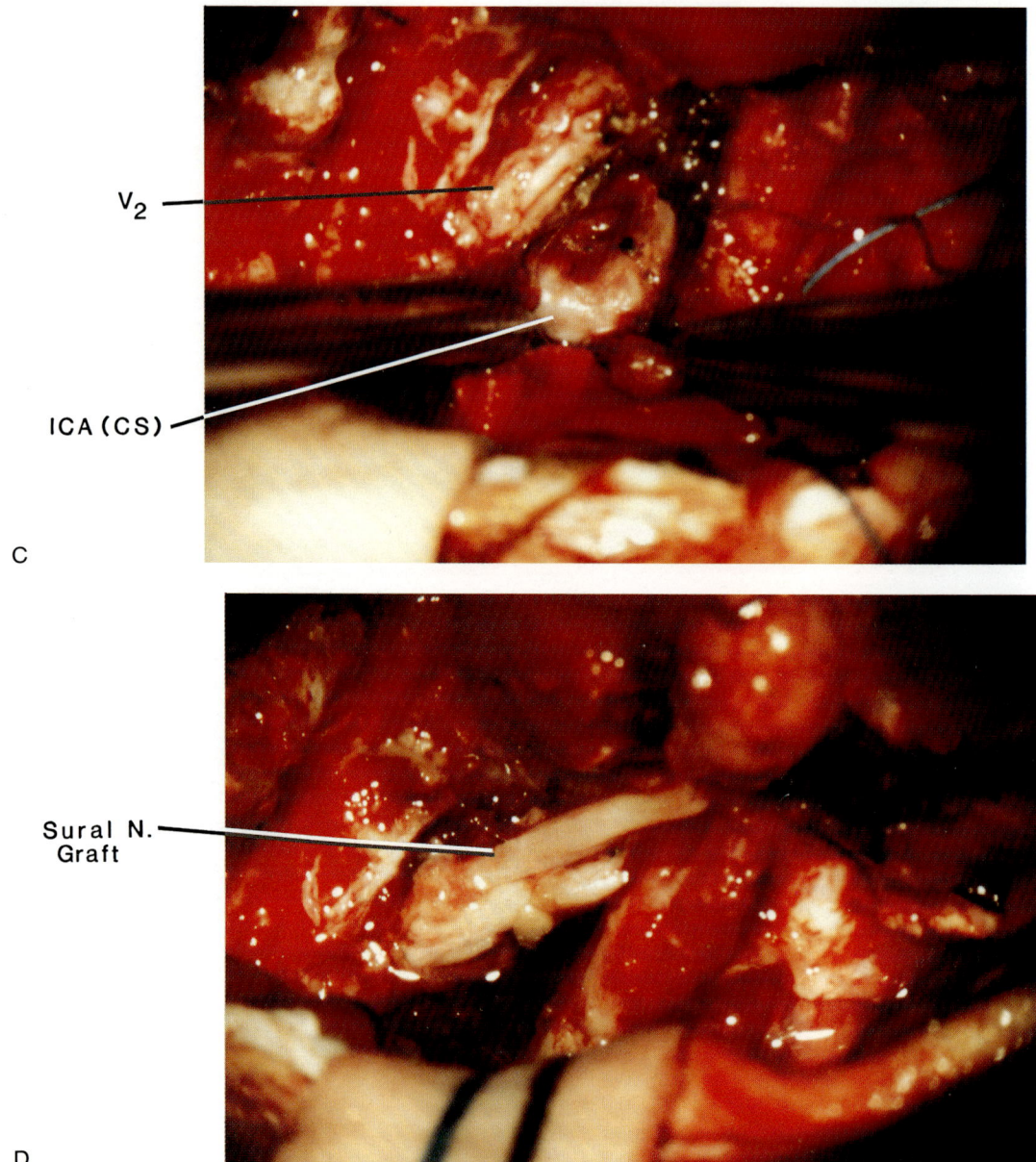

FIG. 56. *Continued.* **C:** At the conclusion of tumor resection, the intracavernous ICA and the maxillary nerve are seen. **D:** The ophthalmic nerve has been reconstructed with sural nerve graft.

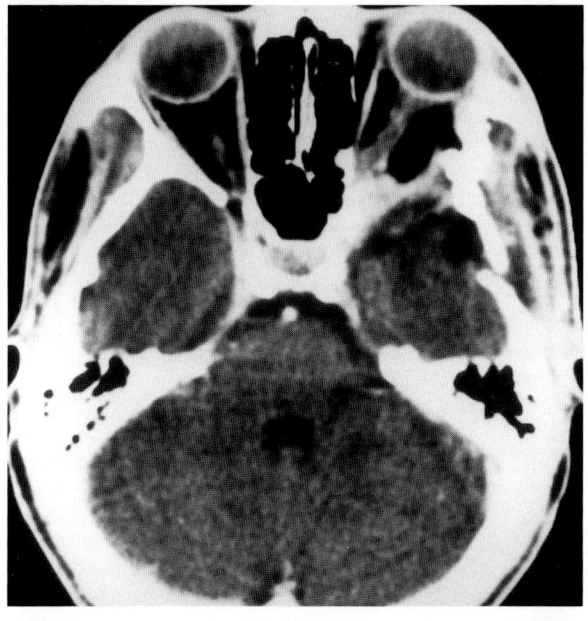

FIG. 57. Patient K.H. Postoperative CT scan suggests residual tumor in the orbital apex area, unchanged upon follow-up for 3 years.

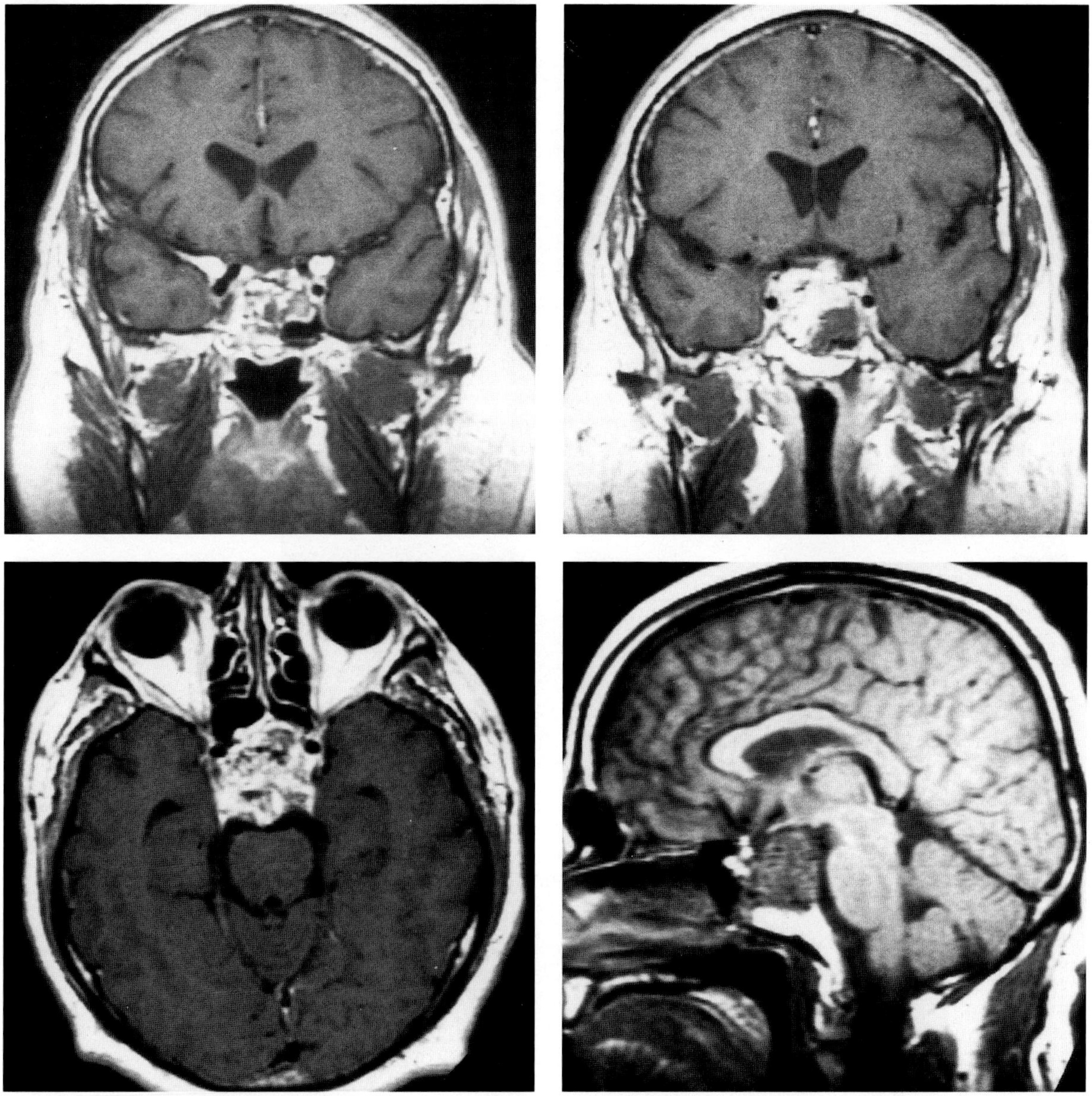

FIG. 58. Patient R.P. **A–D:** MRI scans with gadolinium enhancement in the coronal plane (**A,B**) and the axial plane (**C**) and nonenhanced T1-weighted sagittal images (**D**) reveal a tumor involving the sella, suprasellar region, upper clivus, and the predominantly right cavernous sinus.

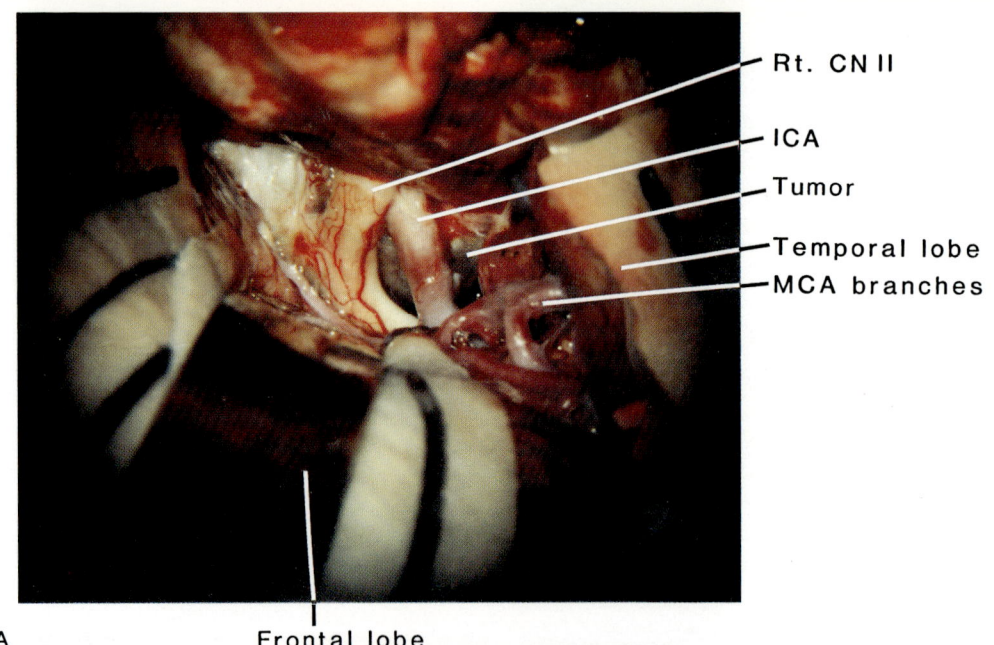

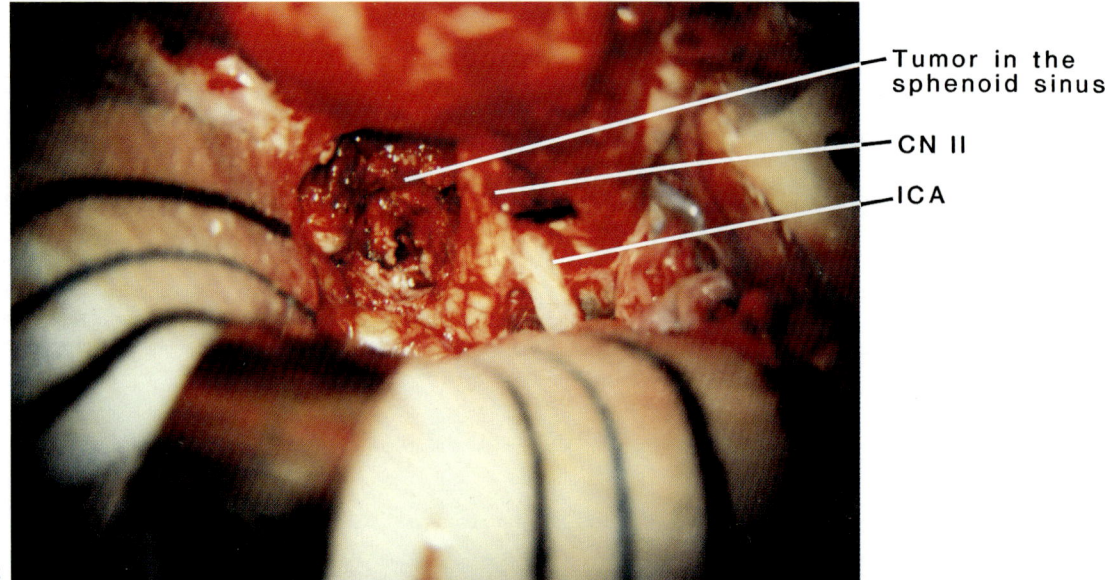
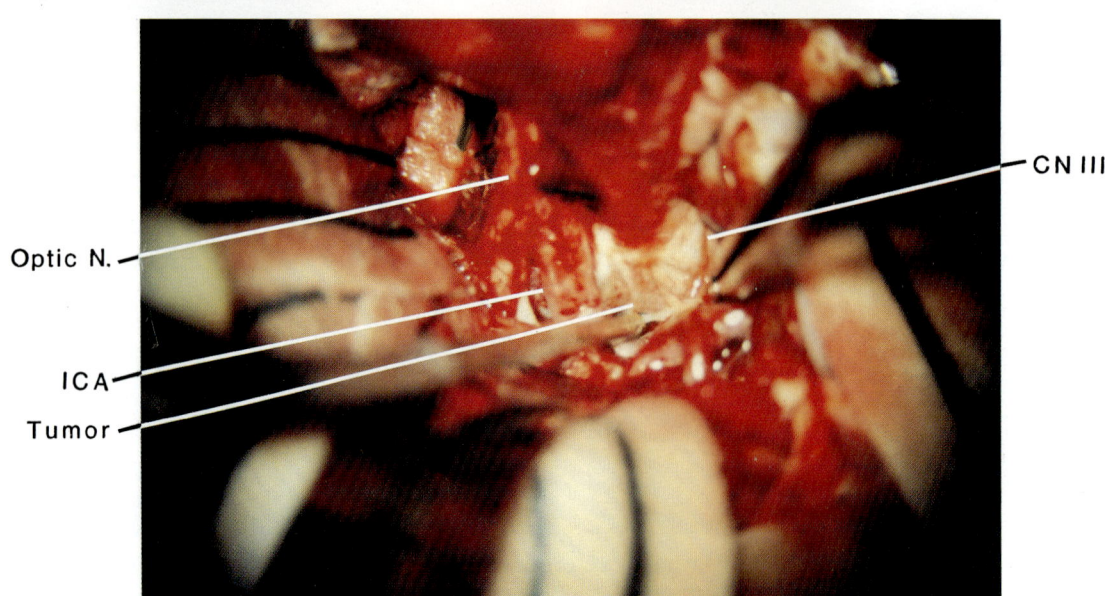

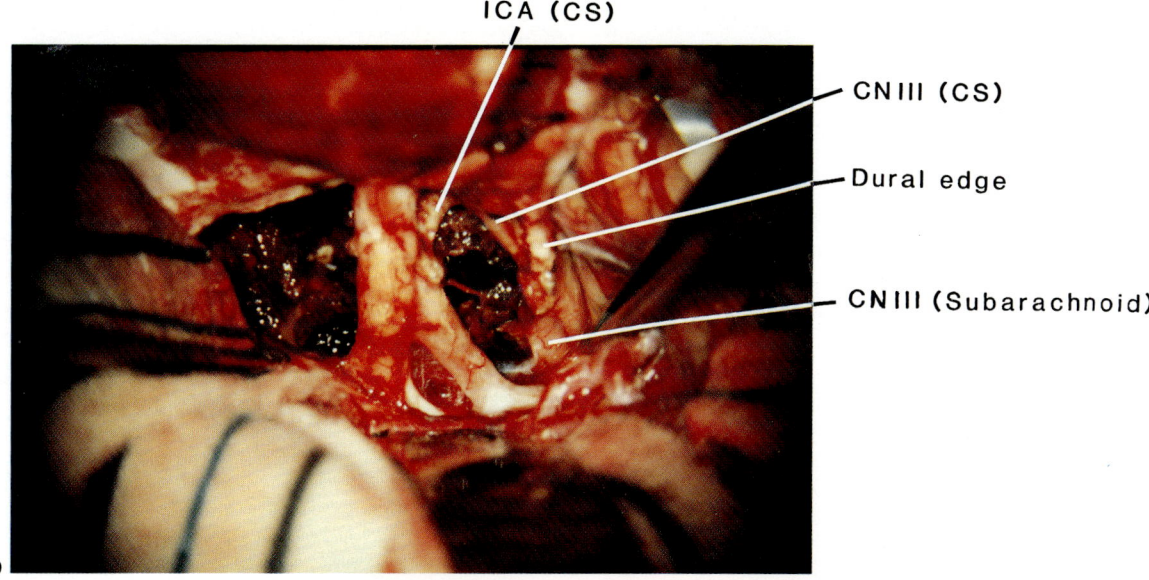

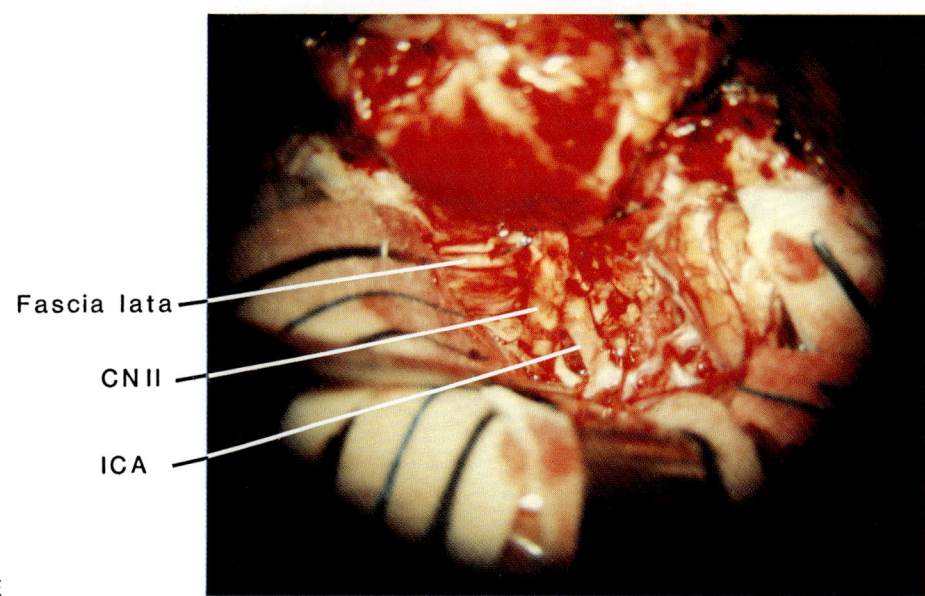

FIG. 59. Patient R.P. A: Right transSylvian and subfrontal exposure. B: The sphenoid sinus has been entered through the planum sphenoidale and tumor is being removed from the subchiasmatic and sphenoidal areas. C: The markedly stretched CN III is seen as it enters the cavernous sinus. D: The cavernous sinus has been opened widely by the superior and medial approaches, enabling total resection of the tumor. E: Reconstruction of the cranial base with fascia lata and autologous fat packing (not seen) of the sphenoid sinus is shown.

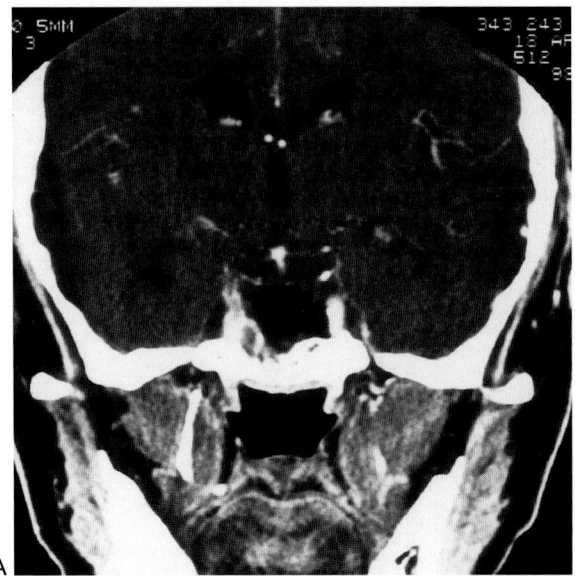
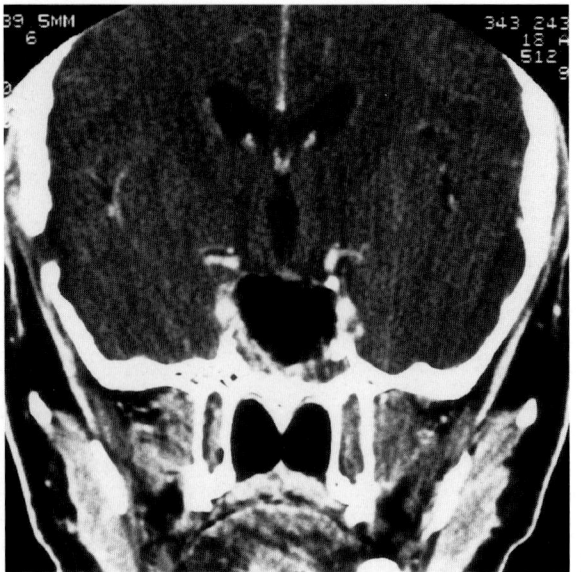

FIG. 60. Patient R.P. **A,B:** Enhanced coronal CT scans, obtained 6 months postoperatively, reveal the absence of tumor.

sphenoid sinus has been entered through the planum sphenoidale and tumor is being removed from the subchiasmatic and sphenoidal areas. In Fig. 59C, the markedly stretched CN III is seen as it enters the cavernous sinus. In Fig. 59D, the cavernous sinus has been opened widely by the superior and medial approaches, enabling the total resection of the tumor. In Fig. 59E, reconstruction of the cranial base with fascia lata and autologous fat packing (not seen) of the sphenoid sinus is shown.

Enhanced coronal CT scans (Fig. 60A,B), obtained 6 months postoperatively, reveal the absence of tumor. The patient made a good recovery of CN III function, without any impairment of vision in the right eye. However, 7 months postoperatively, a rapid regrowth of the same tumor occurred, involving the lower and midclival area. The pathology of the tumor was the same, but the biology was malignant.

D.M.: Grade IV Meningioma

This 36-year-old woman presented with rapidly progressive sixth nerve palsy secondary to a predominantly intracavernous tumor, with extension onto the petrous ridge, as seen in gadolinium enhanced coronal (Fig. 61A,B), axial (Fig. 61C), and sagittal (Fig. 61D) images.

This patient's tumor was removed in two operations. The first operation consisted of a subdural tumor resection and a petrous to supraclinoid ICA vein graft. Figure 62A shows the proximal end-to-end anastomosis between the petrous ICA and the graft. Figure 62B shows the distal end-to-side anastomosis between the graft and the artery. At a second operation 1 week later, the remaining tumor was resected. Figure 62C shows the dissection of CN VI from the tumor and the use of monopolar stimulation to identify it. CN IV could not be preserved. In Figs. 62D and 62E, the appearance after tumor resection is seen.

The patients' preoperative (Fig. 63A) and postoperative (Fig. 63B) angiograms are seen. Further follow-up has been performed with MRI angiography (Fig. 64A,B). One year after the operation, the patient had achieved binocular vision, with persisting mild paresis of CN VI, and hypoesthesia of the cornea (Fig. 65). There was no evidence of tumor residue on follow-up nonenhanced and enhanced MRI exam (Fig. 66A,B).

L.W.: Grade V Meningioma

This 25-year-old woman presented with a 2-year history of blindness and paralysis of CNs III–VI. She was starting to have a decrease of vision in the contralateral eye. Preoperative CT scan (Fig. 67A) reveals an extensive tumor involving the orbit, cavernous sinus, middle fossa, sella, sphenoid sinus, and infratemporal fossa, with some extension into the posterior fossa. Coronal enhanced MRI (Fig. 67B) and the preoperative internal carotid and external carotid angiograms (Fig. 67C,D) reveal the encased and narrowed intracavernous ICA. This tumor was resected in two operations, with saphenous vein graft reconstruction of the ICA. No attempt was made to preserve ipsilateral CNs III–VI. The tumor extended partly into the contralateral cavernous sinus. Re-

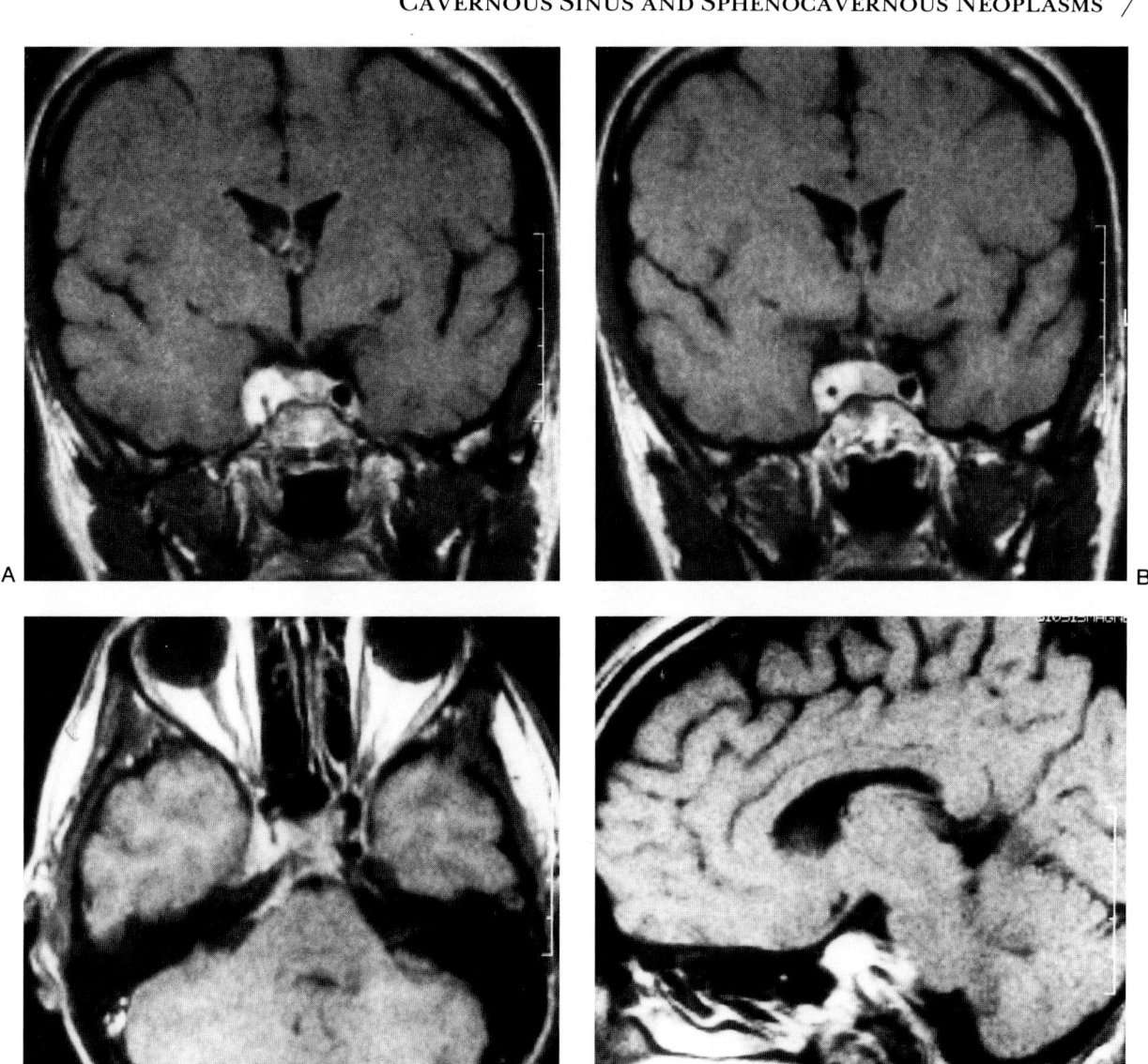

FIG. 61. Patient D.M. **A–D:** Intracavernous tumor with extension onto the petrous ridge, as seen in gadolinium enhanced coronal (**A,B**), axial (**C**), and sagittal (**D**) images.

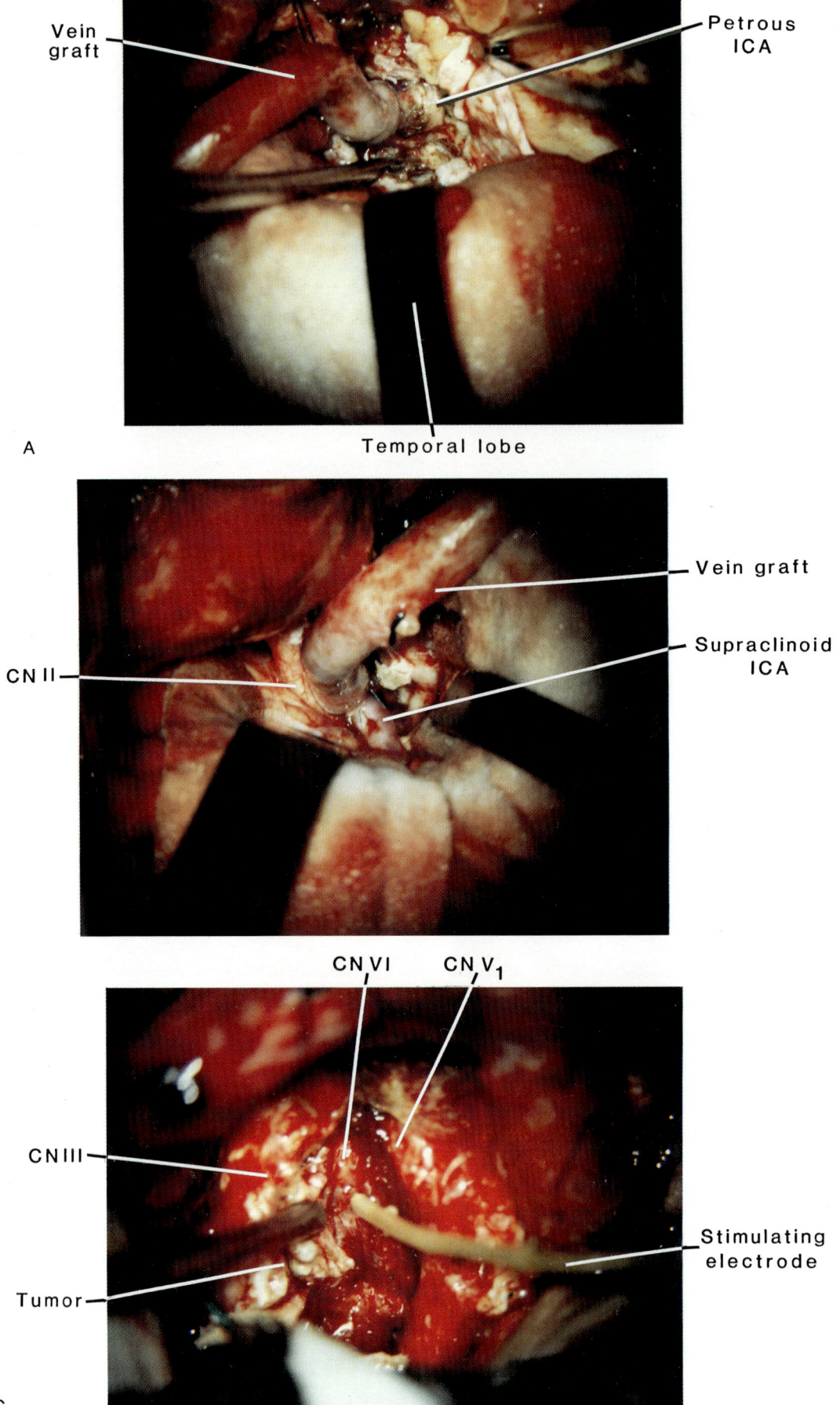

FIG. 62. Patient D.M. **A:** The proximal end-to-end anastomosis between the petrous ICA and the graft. **B:** The distal end-to-side anastomosis between the graft and the artery. **C:** The dissection of CN VI from the tumor and the use of monopolar stimulation to identify it.

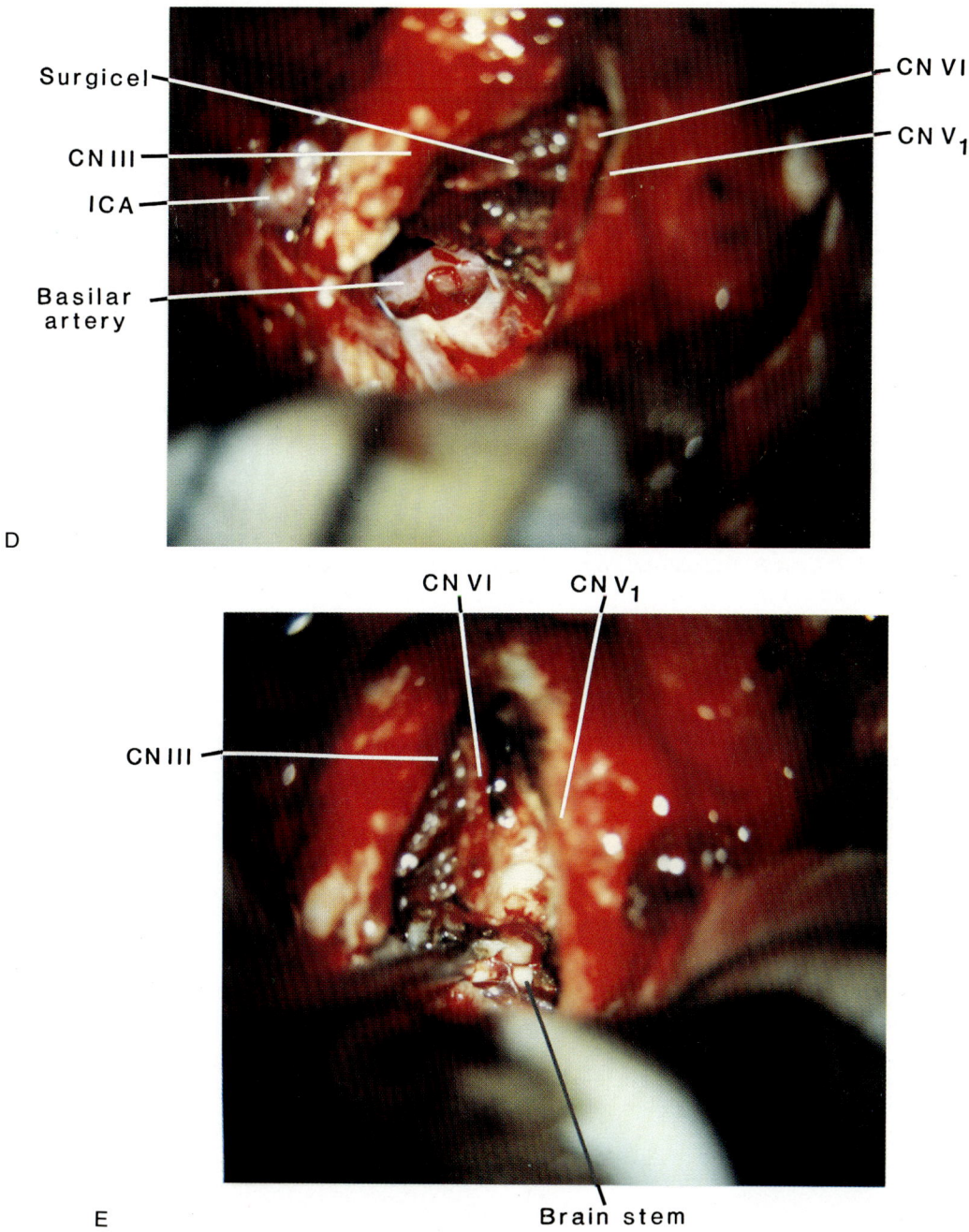

FIG. 62. *Continued.* **D,E:** The appearance after tumor resection.

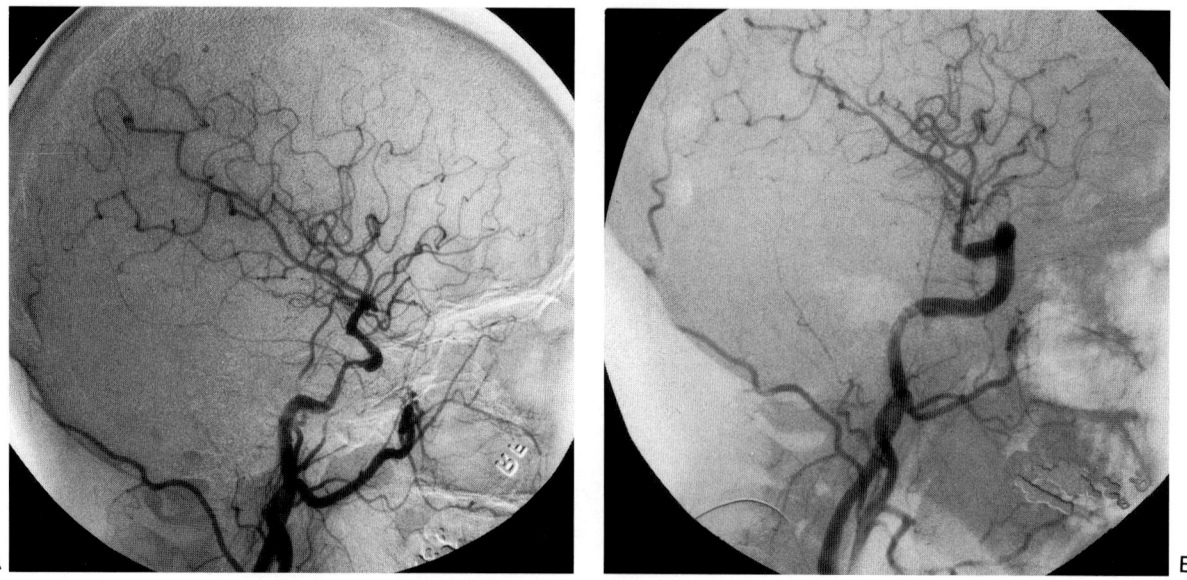

FIG. 63. Patient D.M. **A,B:** The patient's preoperative (**A**) and postoperative (**B**) angiograms are shown. (Note the vein graft in **B**.)

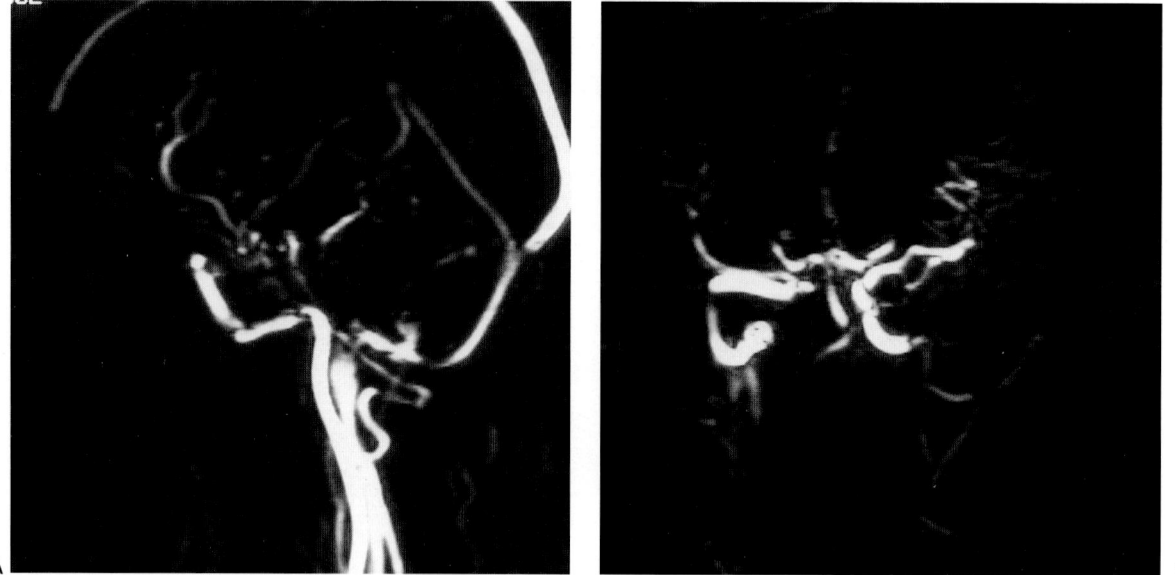

FIG. 64. Patient D.M. **A,B:** Further follow-up has been performed with MRI angiography, which shows the vein graft clearly.

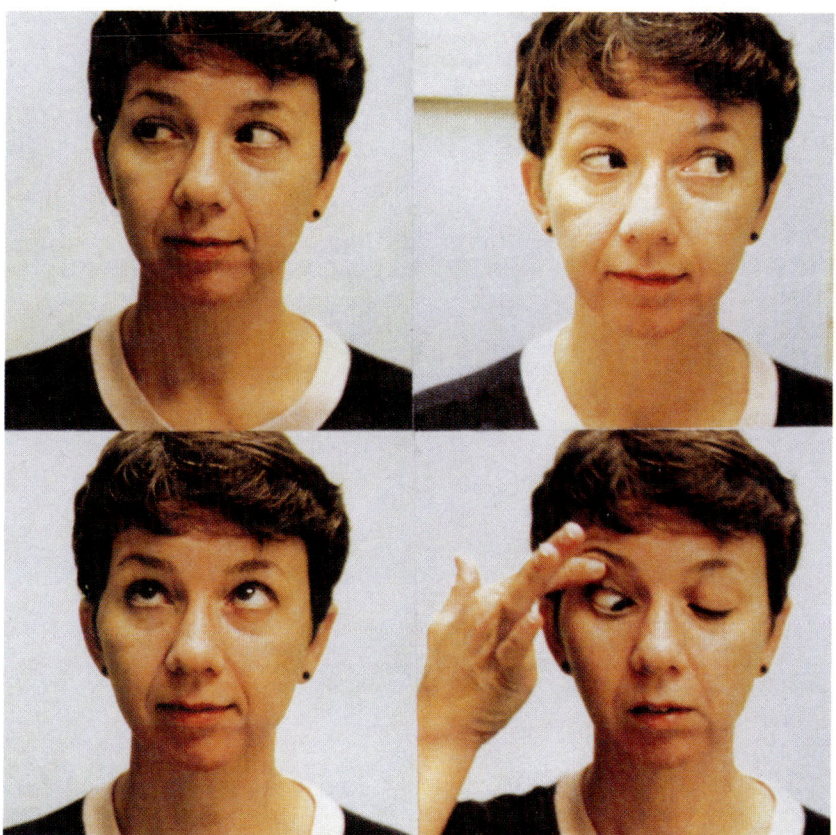

FIG. 65. One year after the operation, the patient D.M. had achieved binocular vision with persisting mild paresis of CN VI and hypesthesia of the cornea.

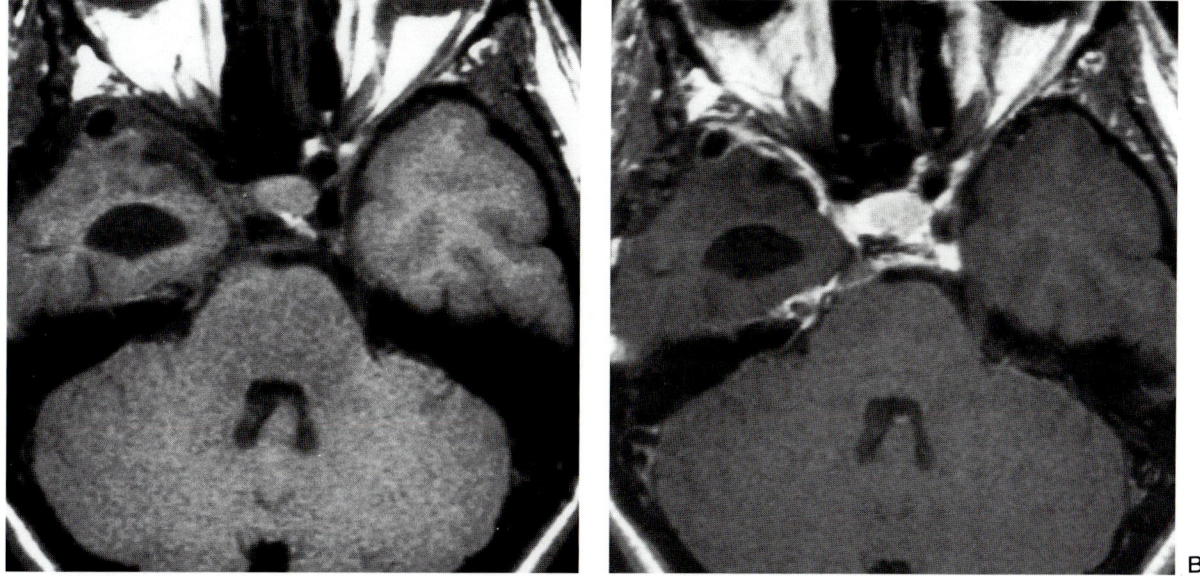

FIG. 66. Patient D.M. **A,B:** There was no evidence of tumor residue on follow-up nonenhanced and enhanced MRI exam. Enhancing scar tissue is seen.

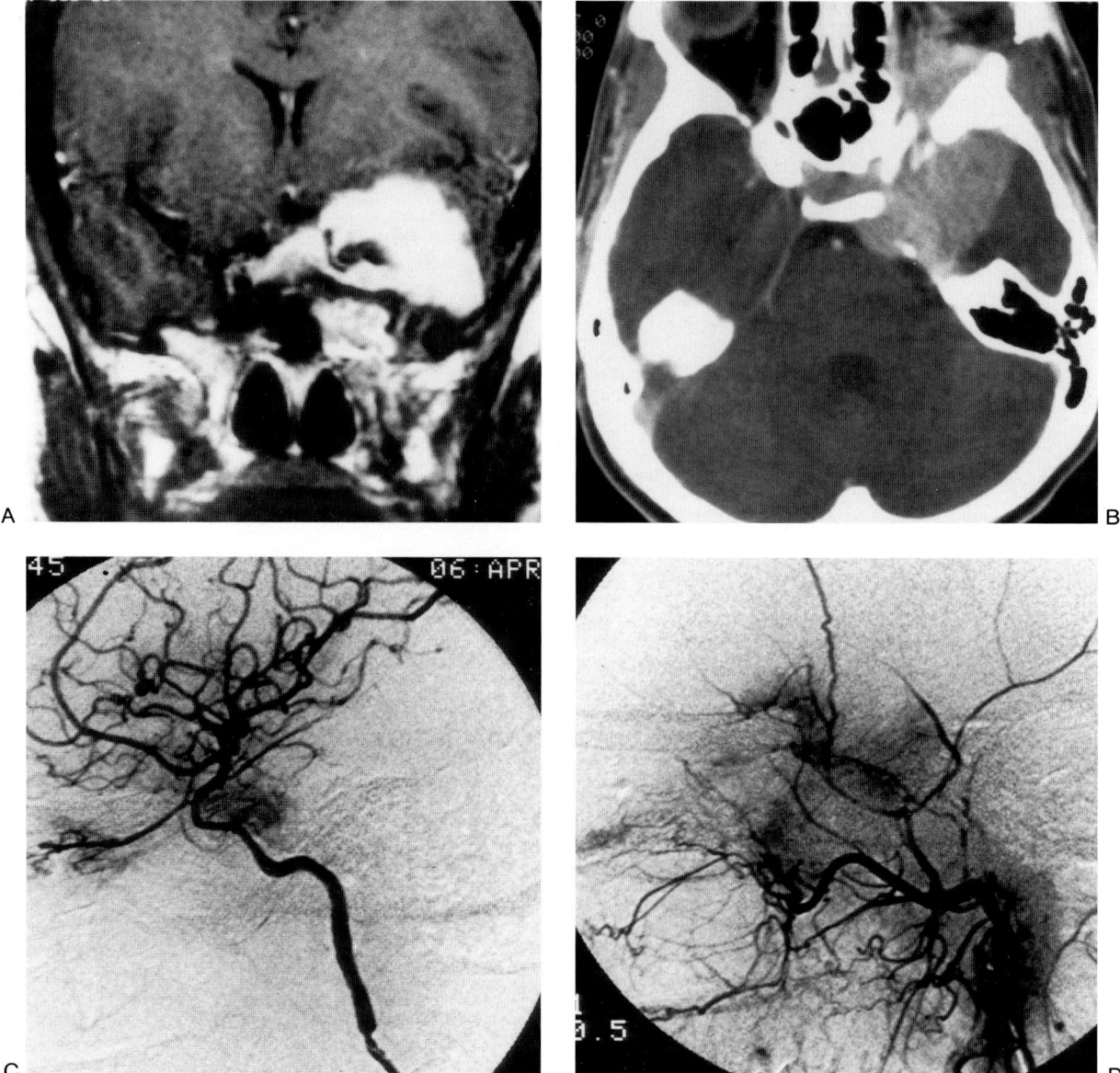

FIG. 67. Patient L.W. **A–D:** Preoperative CT scan (**A**) reveals an extensive tumor involving the orbit, cavernous sinus, middle fossa, sella, sphenoid sinus, and infratemporal fossa, with some extension into the posterior fossa. Coronal enhanced MRI (**B**) and the preoperative internal carotid arteriogram (**C**) reveal encased and narrowed intracavernous ICA. The vascular supply of the tumor is also derived from the external carotid artery (**D**).

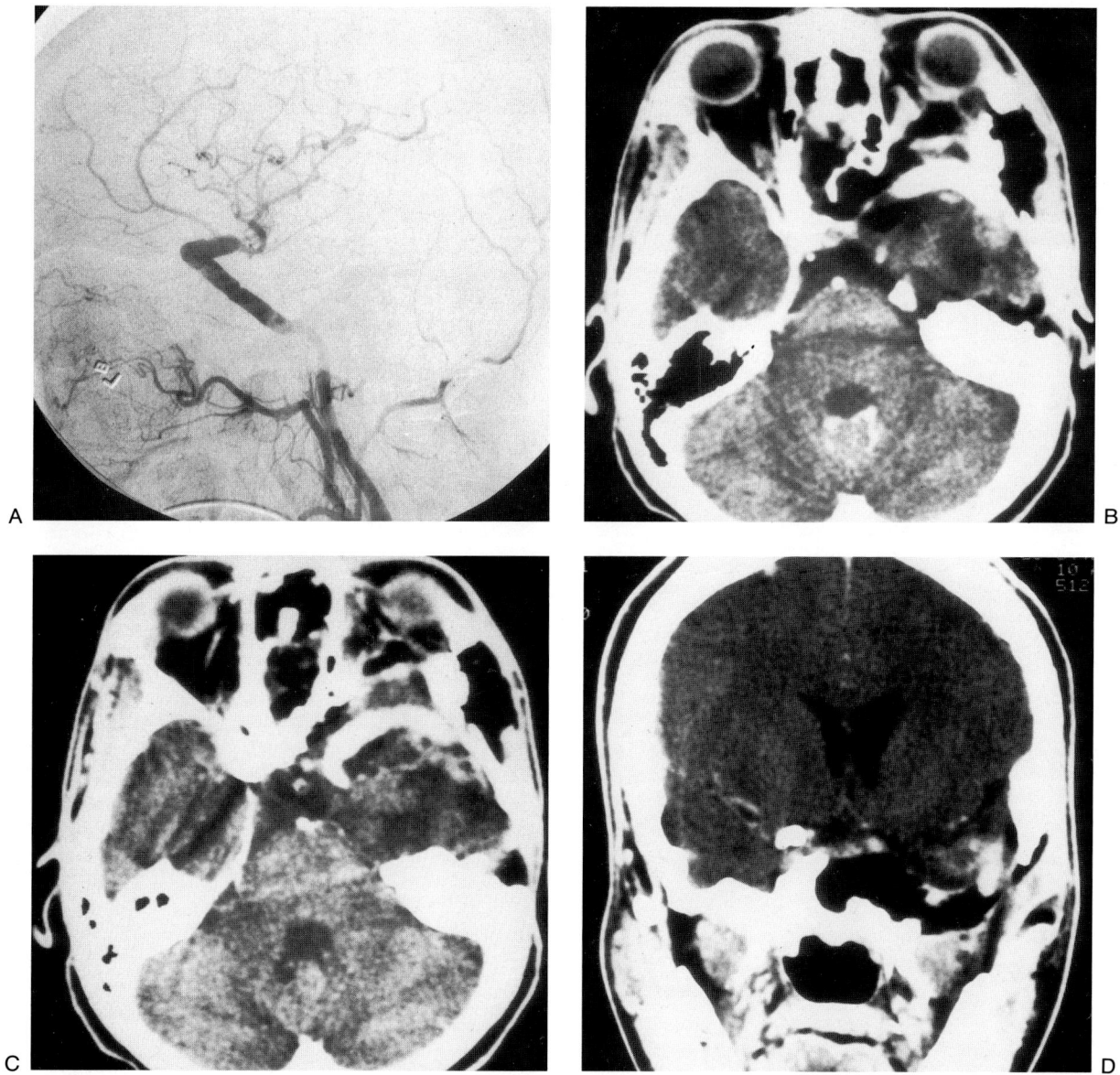

FIG. 68. Patient L.W. **A:** Postoperative angiogram reveals the vein graft. **B,C:** Postoperative, enhanced axial CT scans reveal the absence of tumor and the enhancing vein graft. **D:** The coronal CT scan shows the fat used for reconstruction.

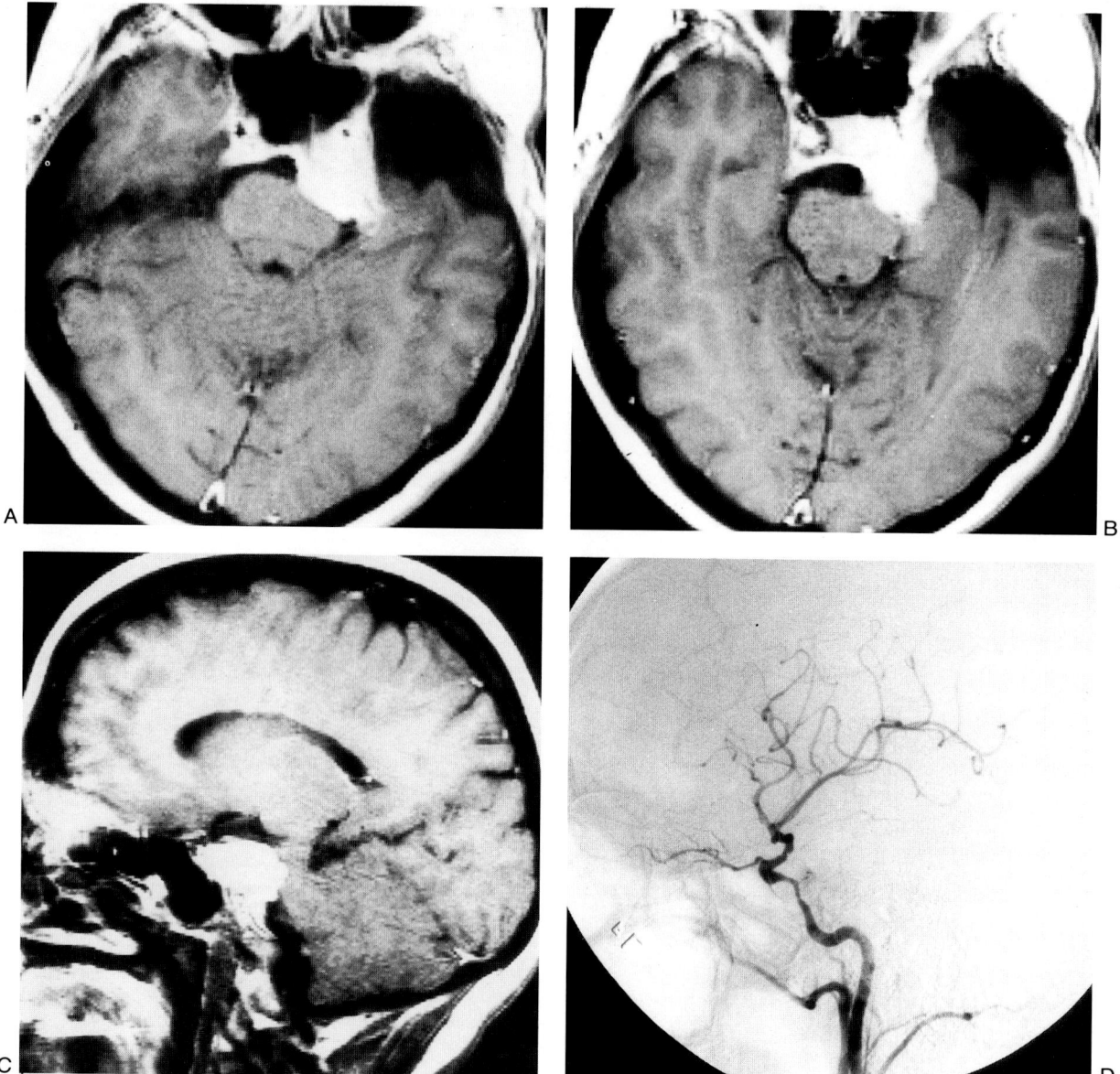

FIG. 69. Patient G.M. **A–C:** Preoperative enhanced MRI scans reveal tumor involvement of the cavernous sinus and petroclival area with encasement and narrowing of the cavernous ICA. **D:** Preoperative angiogram reveals mainly the posterior vertical segment and the horizontal segment of the ICA to be involved by tumor.

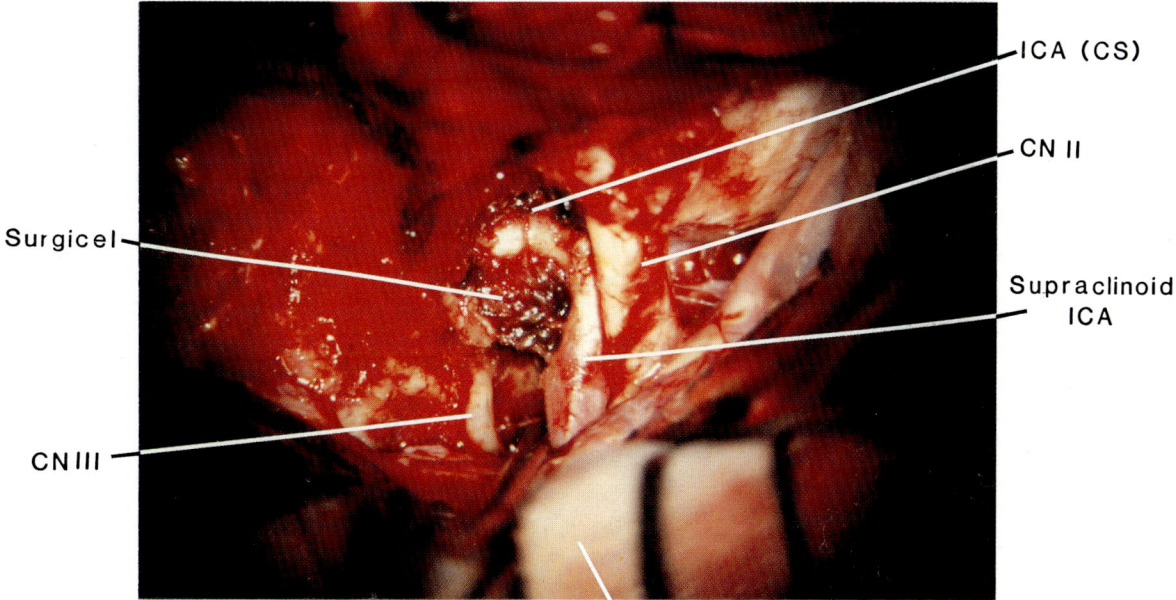

FIG. 70. Patient G.M. **A:** The superior approach to the cavernous sinus. **B:** A saphenous vein graft has been placed from the petrous ICA to the anterior genu of the intracavernous ICA.

construction was performed with fascia lata, autologous fat, and pericranial flap. The postoperative angiogram reveals the vein graft (Fig. 68A). Postoperative, enhanced axial CT scans (Fig. 68B,C) reveal the absence of tumor. The coronal CT scan shows the fat used for reconstruction (Fig. 68D).

G.M.: Grade VI Petroclival and Cavernous Sinus Meningioma

This 45-year-old woman had undergone the resection of a basal meningioma several years previously and now presented with progressive tumor regrowth. Her neurological deficits included a memory disorder, complete palsy of CNs IV and VI, and paresis of CNs VI and V. The preoperative enhanced MRI scans reveal tumor involvement of the cavernous sinus and petroclival area (Fig. 69A–C) with encasement and narrowing of the cavernous ICA. Preoperative angiogram reveals mainly the posterior vertical segment and horizontal segment of the ICA to be involved by tumor (Fig. 69D).

At operation, the tumor was totally removed. Figure 70A shows the superior approach to the cavernous sinus. The clinoidal segment and the anterior bend of the ICA have been dissected free of tumor. In Fig. 70B, a saphenous vein graft has been placed from the petrous ICA to the anterior genu of the intracavernous ICA. CN III has been dissected and preserved. The trigeminal root was atrophic and partially injured by tumor dissection. It was reconstructed with a greater auricular nerve graft. CNs VI and IV were absent because of the prior operation.

At $1\frac{1}{2}$ years postoperatively, the patient has achieved a cosmetically acceptable level of eye function but achieves biocular vision only by turning her head to a certain position (Fig. 71). This is unchanged from her preoperative condition. The patient has returned to prior employment. Postoperative MRI scans (Fig. 72A–C) after contrast reveal no evidence of residual tumor. The angiogram shows the patent vein graft (Fig. 72D).

R.P.: Grade V Cavernous Sinus and Clival Meningioma

This 49-year-old man presented with facial pain, numbness, and mild hemiparesis and hemihypoesthesia.

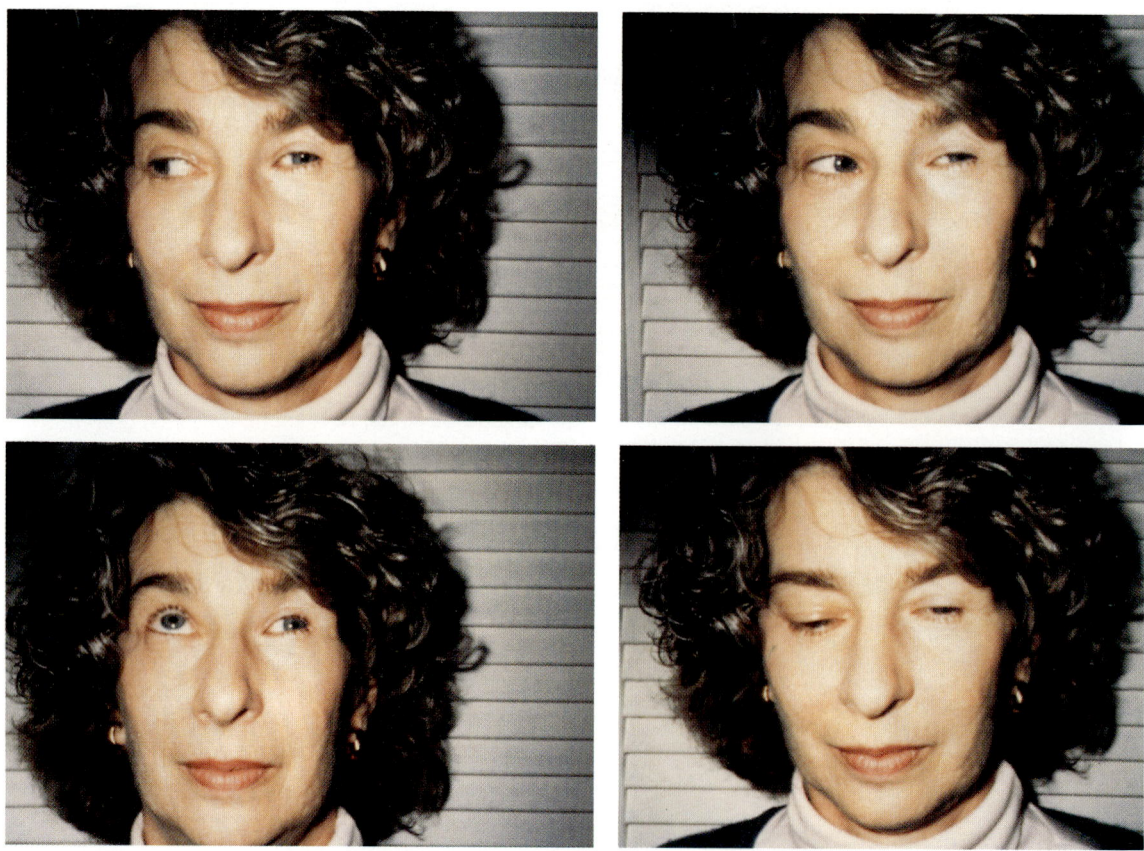

FIG. 71. At $1\frac{1}{2}$ years postoperatively, the patient G.M. has achieved a cosmetically acceptable level of eye function but achieves binocular vision only by turning her head to a certain position.

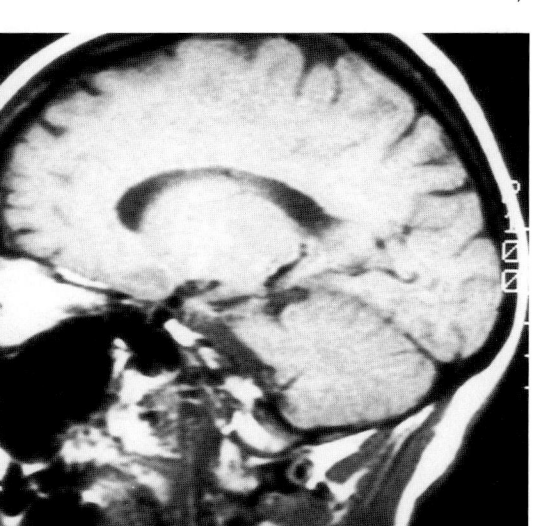
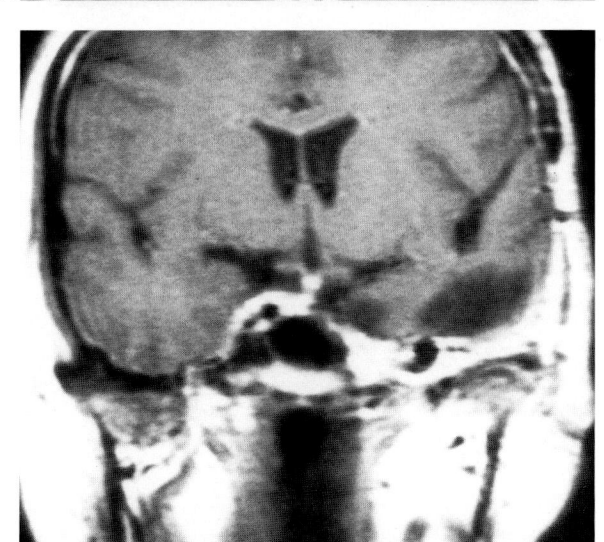
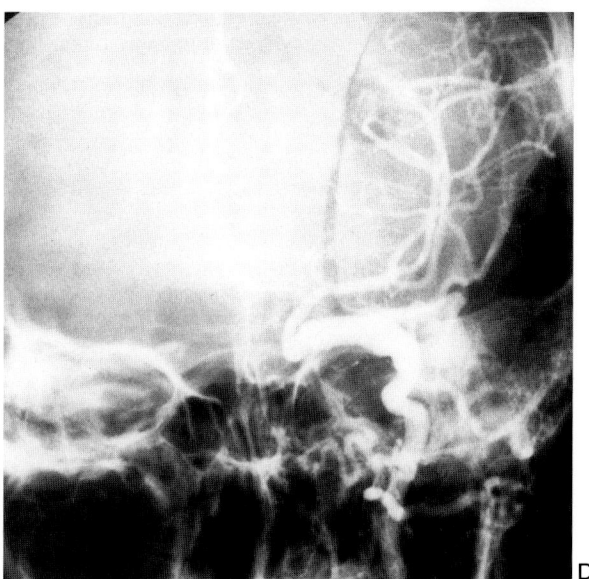

FIG. 72. Patient G.M. **A–C:** Postoperative MRI scans after contrast reveal no evidence of residual tumor. **D:** Postoperative angiogram shows a patent vein graft.

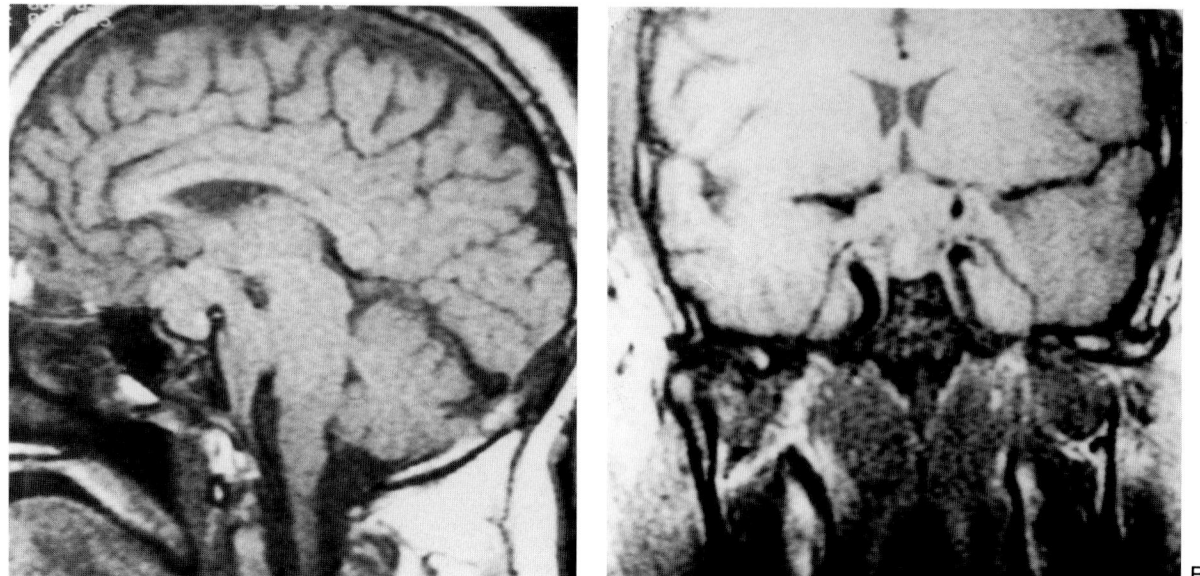

FIG. 73. Patient R.P. **A,B:** Preoperative MRI scans revealed a clival meningioma involving both cavernous sinuses extensively with extension into the suprasellar region.

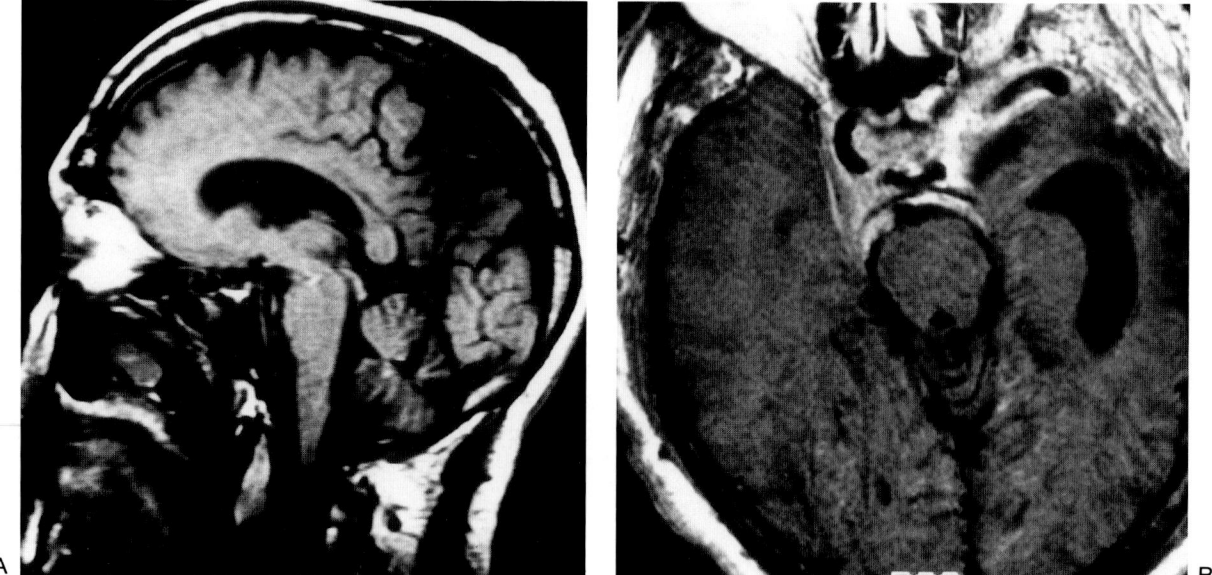

FIG. 74. Patient R.P. **A,B:** Postoperative enhanced MRI scans reveal the vein graft and scar on the left and residual tumor in the right CS.

Preoperative MRI scans revealed a clival meningioma involving both cavernous sinuses extensively with extension into the suprasellar region (Fig. 73A,B). His clival tumor was removed initially by a posterior subtemporal and presigmoid–transpetrous approach. The patient suffered significant temporal lobe and cerebellar swelling postoperatively, requiring a partial temporal lobectomy and cerebellectomy, and a very protracted recovery period. Subsequently, the left cavernous sinus and sellar–suprasellar lesion was removed after vein graft replacement of the ICA. The right cavernous sinus lesion is asymptomatic and is being watched. The postoperative enhanced MRI scans reveal the vein graft on the right, and scar residual tumor in the left CS (Fig. 74A,B).

The patient is living independently but is unable to return to prior employment because of memory difficulties (Karnofsky 70).

F.M.: Grade V Meningioma

This 47-year-old woman presented with a history of prior operation. At presentation, she was blind in the left eye with subtotal palsies of CNs III–VI. Preoperative enhanced CT scan revealed a tumor involving the orbit, cavernous sinus, middle fossa, and the petroclival area (Fig. 75A,B). Bone windowed CT scan revealed extensive hyperostosis of the sphenoid and petroclival bone (Fig. 76). The patient tolerated the balloon test occlusion of the ICA well. The soft tissue tumor and the bone tumor were resected totally from the above-mentioned areas, with the excision of the intracavernous ICA. Two years later, the tumor recurred at the margins of prior resection, namely, in the opposite cavernous sinus and in the petrous ridge area (Fig. 77A,B). Since the patient was asymptomatic and the ipsilateral ICA was absent, these lesions were treated by gamma knife radiosurgery and have remained stable for 1 year. This case illustrates the paths of spread of intracavernous meningiomas, where lesions might recur on long-term follow-up, and the importance of ICA reconstruction with graft, especially in younger patients. This patient is functioning independently at her preoperative level (Karnofsky 80).

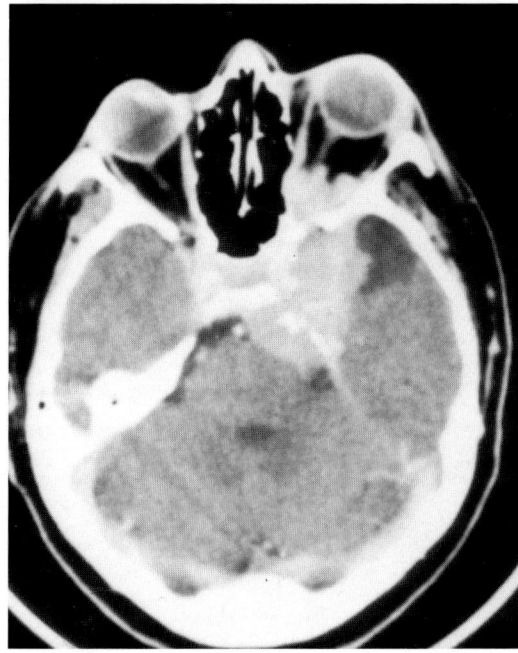

FIG. 75. A,B: Patient F.M. Preoperative enhanced CT scan reveals a tumor involving the orbit, cavernous sinus, middle fossa, and the petroclival area.

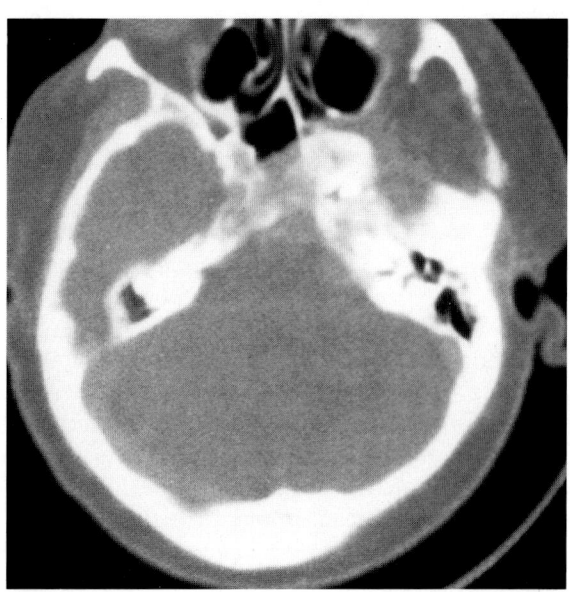

FIG. 76. Patient F.M. Bone windowed CT scan reveals extensive hyperostosis of the sphenoid and petroclival bone.

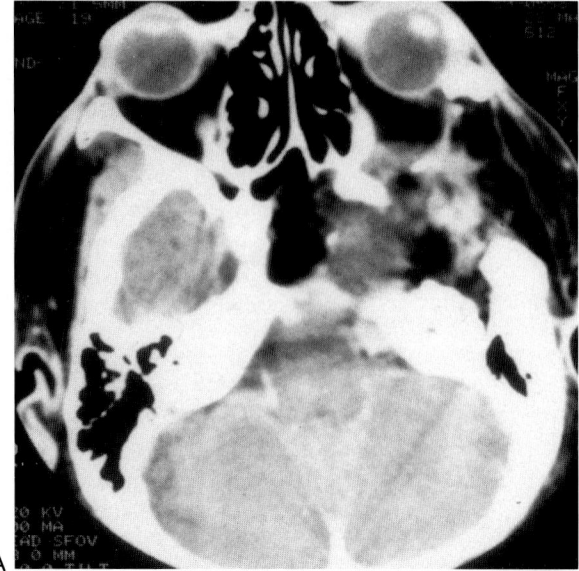

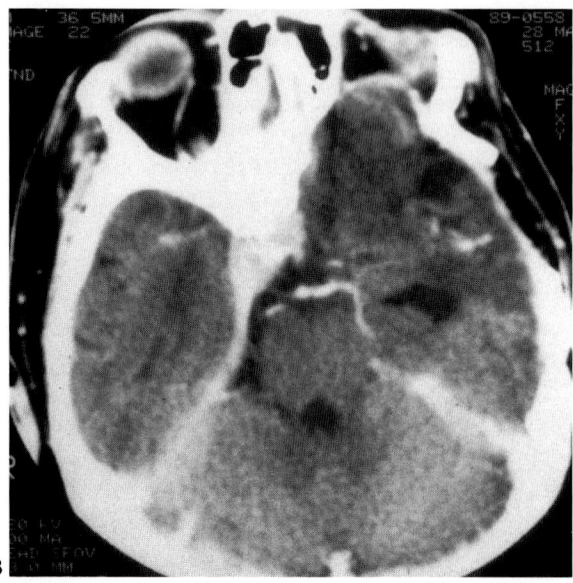

FIG. 77. Patient F.M. **A,B:** Two years later, the tumor recurred at the margins of prior resection, namely, in the opposite cavernous sinus and in the petrous ridge area.

J.H.: Invasive ACTH Secreting Pituitary Adenoma

This 51-year-old woman had previously undergone a bilateral adrenalectomy and cranial radiation therapy for Cushing's syndrome. She presented to us with progressive growth of an ACTH secreting adenoma, but with normal extraocular muscle function. She was markedly hyperpigmented (Nelson's syndrome). The preoperative enhanced MRI scans in the coronal (Fig. 78A) and sagittal (Fig. 78B) planes revealed a sellar tumor invading the cavernous sinus and clivus. The intracavernous ICA is occluded because of the tumor or because of the radiation therapy. Operation was elected because of the progressive tumor growth despite radiotherapy.

At operation (Fig. 79A), the supraclinoid ICA was atrophic and tumor was growing superiorly out of the cavernous sinus, markedly splaying CN III. CN IV was injured during tumor resection but was resutured at the end of the operation (Fig. 79B). The abducens nerve was totally tumor-invaded in the proximal intracavernous segment. The invaded segment was resected, and a sural nerve graft was placed from the subarachnoid segment to the distal intracavernous segment. Skull base reconstruction was with autologous fat, fascia lata, and a pericranial flap. In Fig. 79B, the arrows show the sites of nerve anastomoses.

J.P.: Cavernous Sinus and Supracavernous Epidermoid

This 40-year-old woman presented with a history of progressively increasing intermittent headaches and marked paresis of CN III. She did not have binocular vision. Preoperative MRI scans (Fig. 80A–D) reveal a low-density lesion involving the cavernous sinus, supracavernous area, and interpeduncular area.

At operation, a typical epidermoid cyst was found in the areas mentioned. The capsule was thin in the subarachnoid areas (Fig. 81A) but very thick in the cavernous sinus. CN III was splayed inferolaterally by the tumor and was invaded by the capsule. A conservative resection was considered, but the patient had a long-standing significant oculomotor paresis, and there was no prospect of her achieving binocular vision, even with conservative resection, and the risk of tumor recurrence in future was much greater if the capsule was left behind. The entire tumor capsule along with the invaded CN III was removed. Figure 81B shows the appearance at the conclusion of tumor resection, the CS being entered solely by a superior approach. Since good proximal and distal stumps of CN III were present, reconstruction was performed with a sural nerve graft (Fig. 81C), with the hope that the patient may achieve cosmetically acceptable recovery. After 8 months, the patient was showing progressive recovery of oculomotor function, recovery being more pronounced in the levator palpebrae superioris and medial rectus muscles. She was able to achieve binocular vision in primary position of gaze, but not in the reading position. Her headaches were relieved (Fig. 81D).

D.H.: Sphenoid Wing, Planum and Suprasellar Meningioma

This 52-year-old woman had previously undergone surgical resection of a basal meningioma, with resulting blindness of the left eye. She presented to us with head-

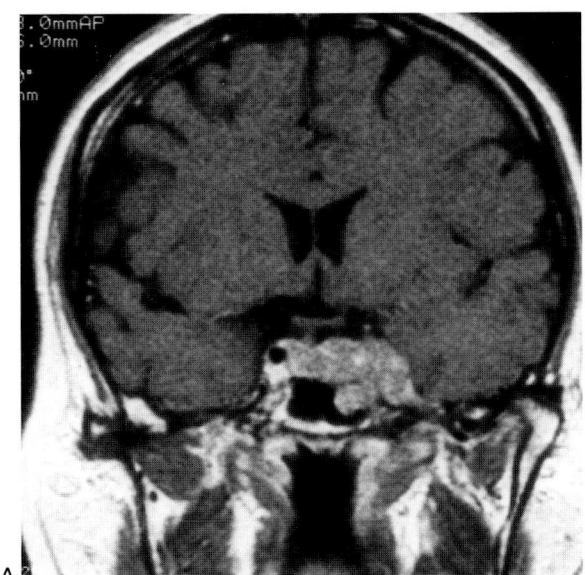 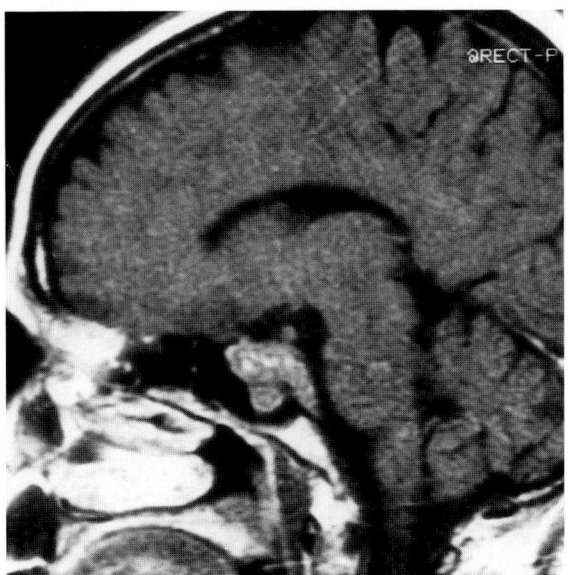

FIG. 78. Patient J.H. **A,B:** Preoperative enhanced MRI scans in the (**A**) coronal and (**B**) sagittal planes reveal a sellar tumor invading the cavernous sinus and clivus.

aches, right-sided visual loss, and a recurrent tumor. The enhanced CT scan (Fig. 82A) shows the tumor well but gives no idea about whether vascular encasement is present, which is seen well in an enhanced MRI scan in the same position (Fig. 82B). The enhanced coronal (Fig. 83A), axial (Fig. 83B,C), and sagittal (Fig. 83D) MRI scans show clearly that the left internal carotid artery and the entire anterior cerebral artery complex are encased by tumor. The cavernous sinuses are mostly free of tumor.

Operation was performed through a left frontotemporal craniotomy crossing the midline, orbital osteotomy, and a basal frontal approach (extradurally) into the sphenoid sinus. In Fig. 84A, the sylvian fissure has been split, and tumor is visible between the frontal and temporal lobes, as are the distal branches of the middle cerebral artery. In Fig. 84B, the tumor is being removed with bipolar cautery, and the MCA is being followed to the ICA. In Fig. 84C, the tumor-encased ICA is being dissected, and a medial lenticulostriate artery has been dissected free of tumor. Figures 84D and 84E reveal the encasement of the perforators and their dissection. Tumor can be seen behind the ICA and the anterior cerebral artery. In Fig. 84F, the tumor has been dissected from the medial lenticulostriate artery. In Fig. 84G, the entire ipsilateral and contralateral anterior cerebral complex has been dissected free. In Fig. 84H, the ipsilateral atrophic optic nerve has been removed with the tumor. A nice view of the basilar artery, pituitary stalk, contralateral ICA, and contralateral CN III is obtained. The hyperostotic planum sphenoidale was removed and reconstruction of the skull base performed.

Postoperatively, the patient sustained a visual loss in the right temporal field, which improved gradually. The postoperative enhanced axial and coronal MRI images show no evidence of tumor (Fig. 85A–D).

G.W.: Petroclival and Cavernous Sinus Meningioma

This 49-year-old woman presented with headaches and a partial third cranial nerve palsy. MRI scan revealed a grade IV tumor involving the cavernous sinus and the petroclival area, as seen on nonenhanced T1-weighted sagittal (Fig. 86A), enhanced axial (Fig. 86B,C), and enhanced coronal (Fig. 86D) views.

Operation to remove the tumor was performed in two stages. During the first operation (Fig. 87A), tumor has been exposed after splitting the sylvian fissure. The oculomotor nerve, which was tumor encased, was freed up. A saphenous vein graft was anastomosed end-to-end to the petrous ICA and the clinoidal segment of the ICA just inferior to the ophthalmic artery (Fig. 87B). The second operation was delayed because of left-sided brain swelling. Six weeks after the first operation, the vein graft is seen to be covered with fibrous tissue. Tumor was removed but the encased CN VI could not be preserved (Fig. 87C). It was reconstructed with a graft. In figure 87D, the proximal stump of CN VI is seen to be lying on the brain stem. A sural nerve graft was then anastomosed proximally to the subarachnoid segment in the posterior fossa, brought out through the dura of the middle fossa, and anastomosed to the abducens nerve in the orbit on the medial surface of the lateral rectus muscle. Figure 87E shows the proximal anastomosis. Figure 87F shows the graft being brought out through the middle fossa

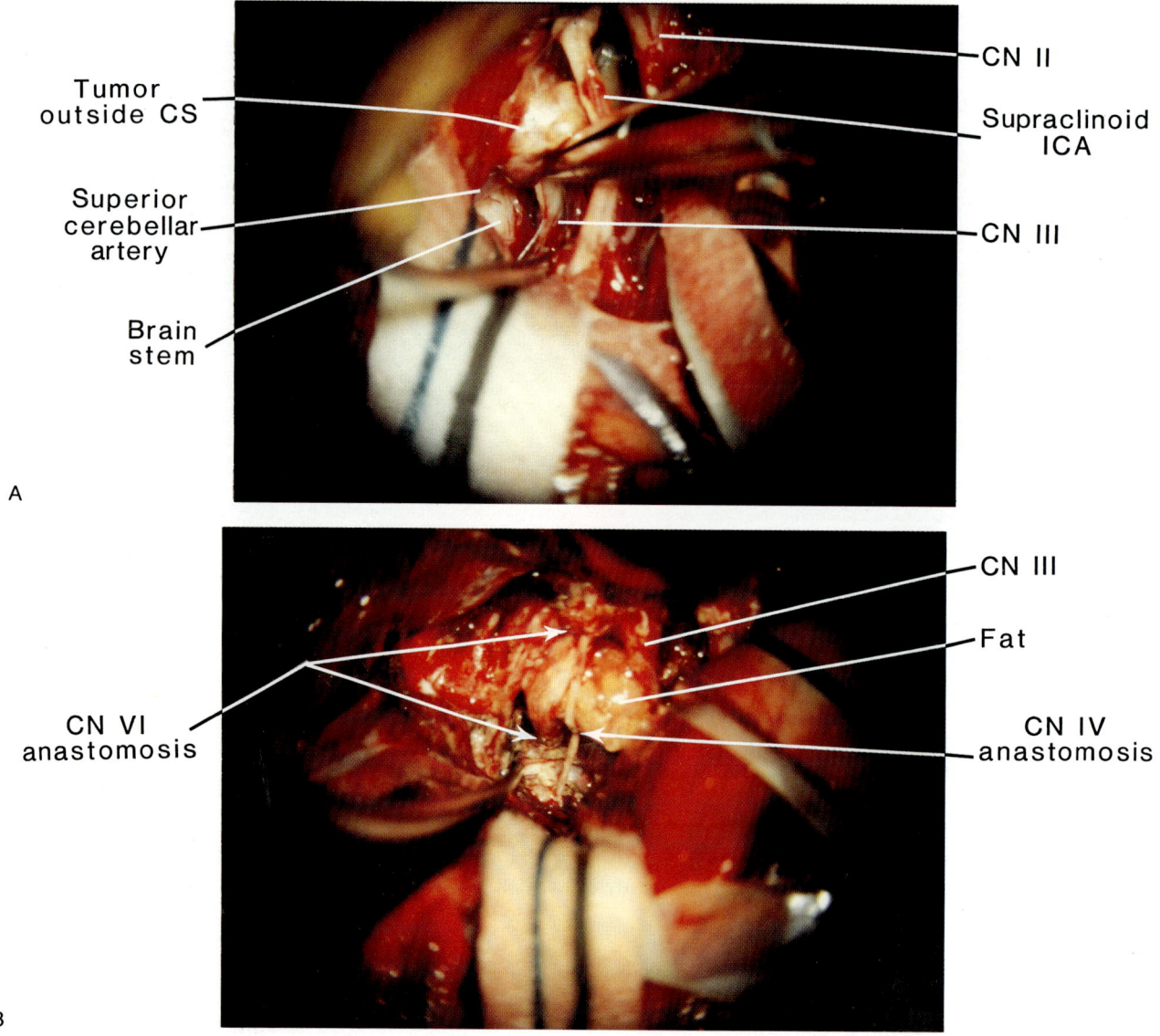

FIG. 79. Patient J.H. **A:** At operation, the supraclinoid ICA was atrophic and tumor was growing superiorly out of the cavernous sinus, markedly splaying CN III. **B:** CN IV was injured during tumor resection but was resutured at the end of the operation. The reconstruction of the abducens nerve with a graft is also seen.

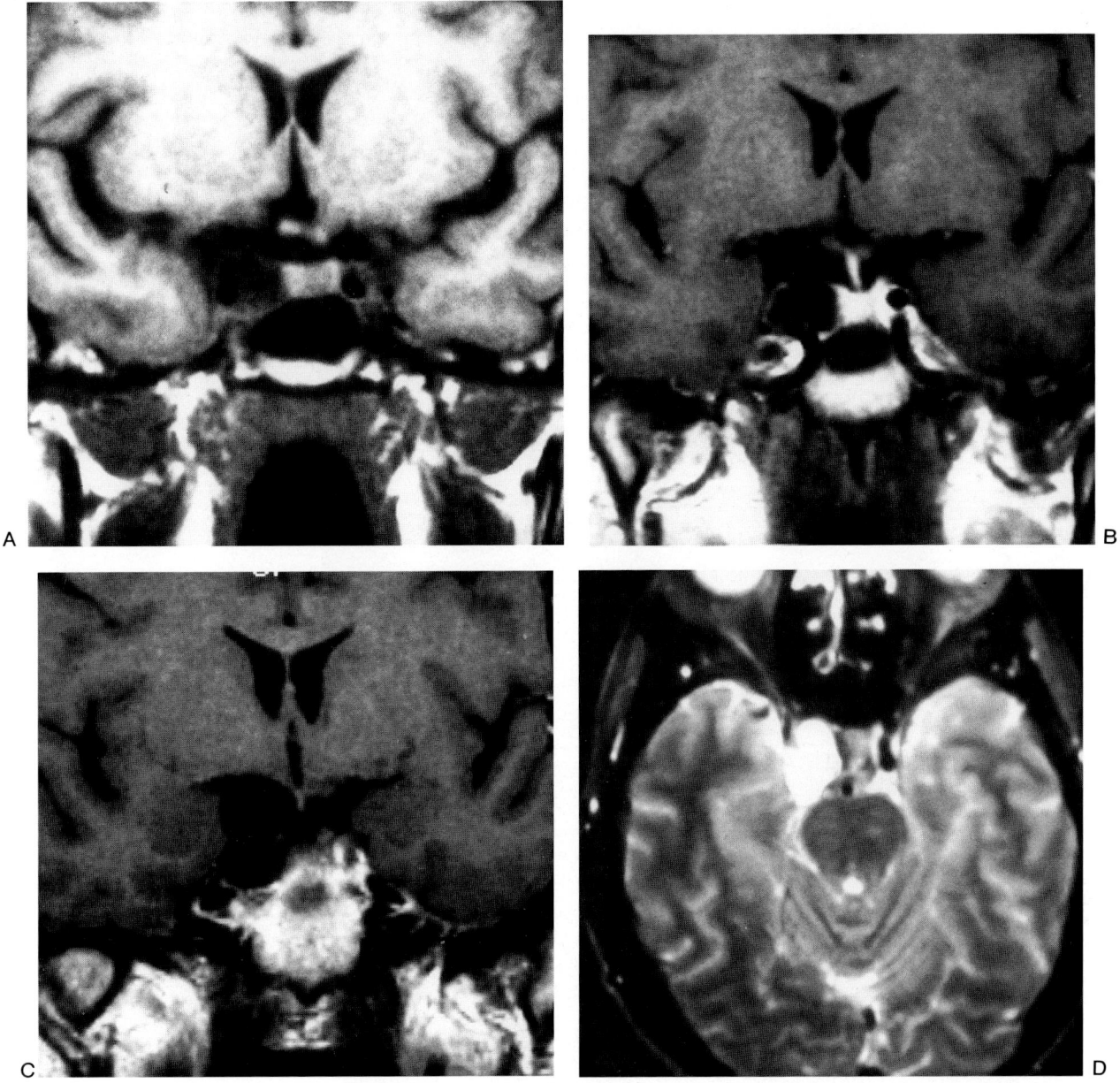

FIG. 80. Patient J.P. **A–D:** A low-density lesion involving the cavernous sinus, supracavernous, and the interpeduncular area is shown on preoperative MRI scans.

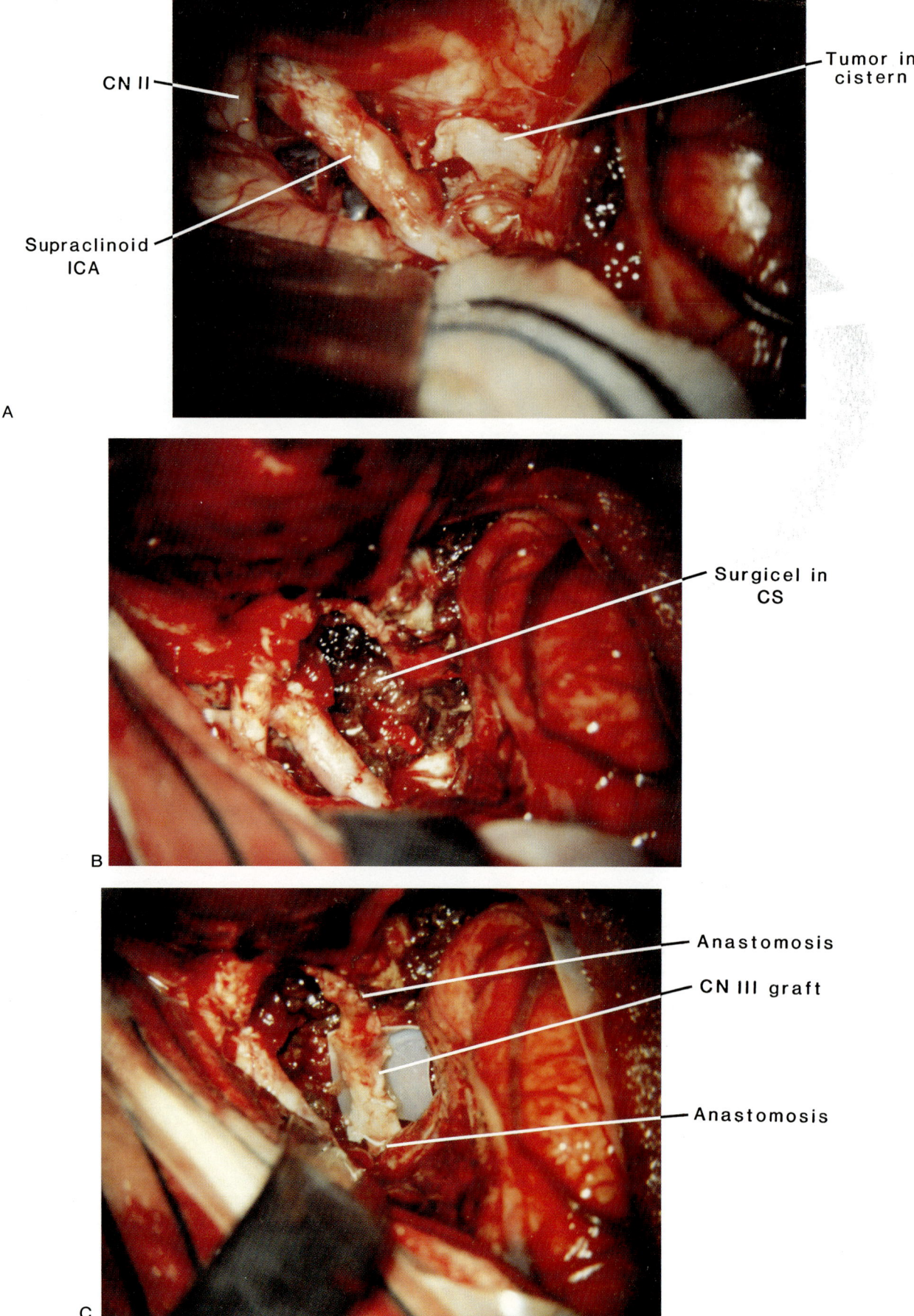

FIG. 81. Patient J.P. **A:** The tumor with its typical contents. **B:** The appearance at the conclusion of tumor resection, the CS being entered solely by a superior approach. **C:** Reconstruction of the oculomotor nerve was performed with a sural nerve graft.

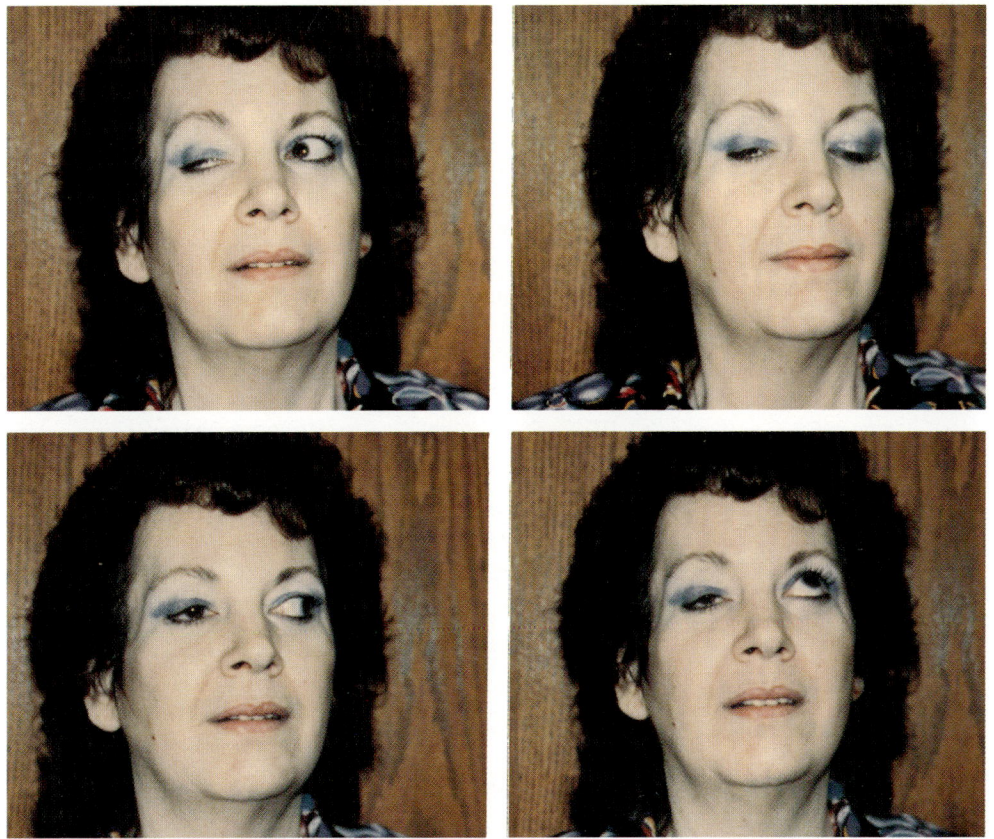

FIG. 81. *Continued.* **D:** Patient (J.P.) was able to achieve binocular vision in primary position of gaze, but not in the reading position.

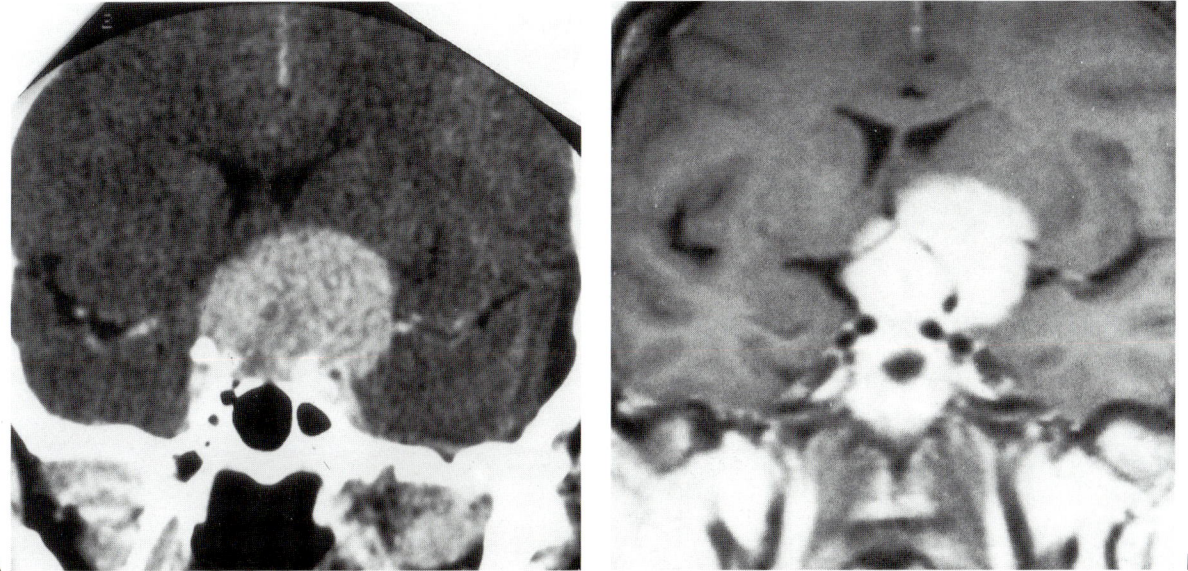

FIG. 82. Patient D.H. **A:** Enhanced CT scan shows the tumor well but gives no idea about whether vascular encasement is present. **B:** Vascular encasement is clearly visible in an enhanced MRI scan in the same position.

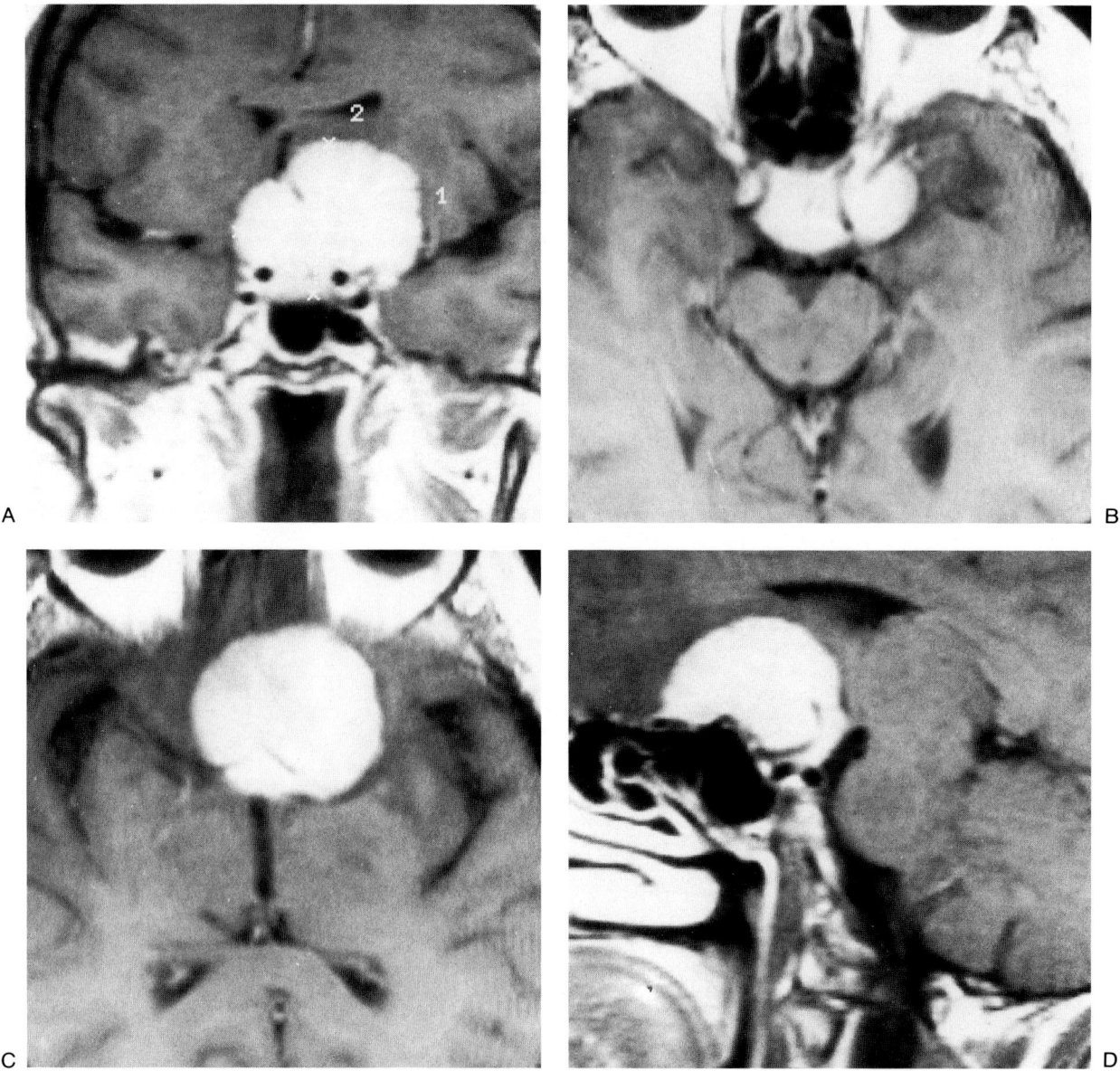

FIG. 83. Patient D.H. **A–D:** The enhanced coronal (**A**) axial (**B,C**), and sagittal (**D**) MRI scans show clearly that the left internal carotid artery and the entire anterior cerebral artery complex are encased by tumor.

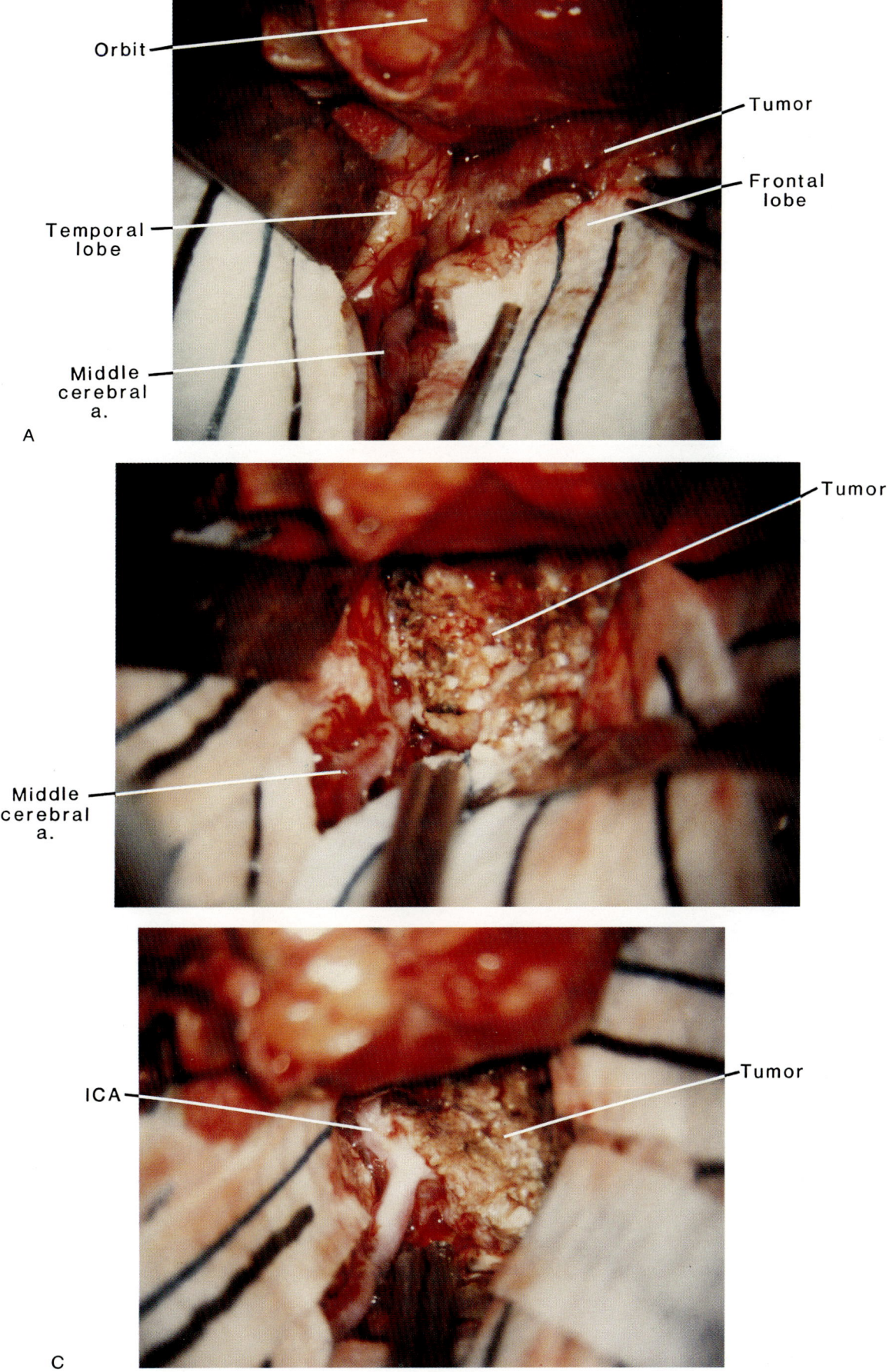

FIG. 84. Patient D.H. **A:** The sylvian fissure has been split, and tumor is visible between the frontal and temporal lobes, as are the distal branches of the middle cerebral artery. **B:** The tumor is being removed with bipolar cautery, and the MCA is being followed to the ICA. **C:** The tumor-encased ICA is being dissected, and a medial lenticulostriate artery has been dissected free of tumor.

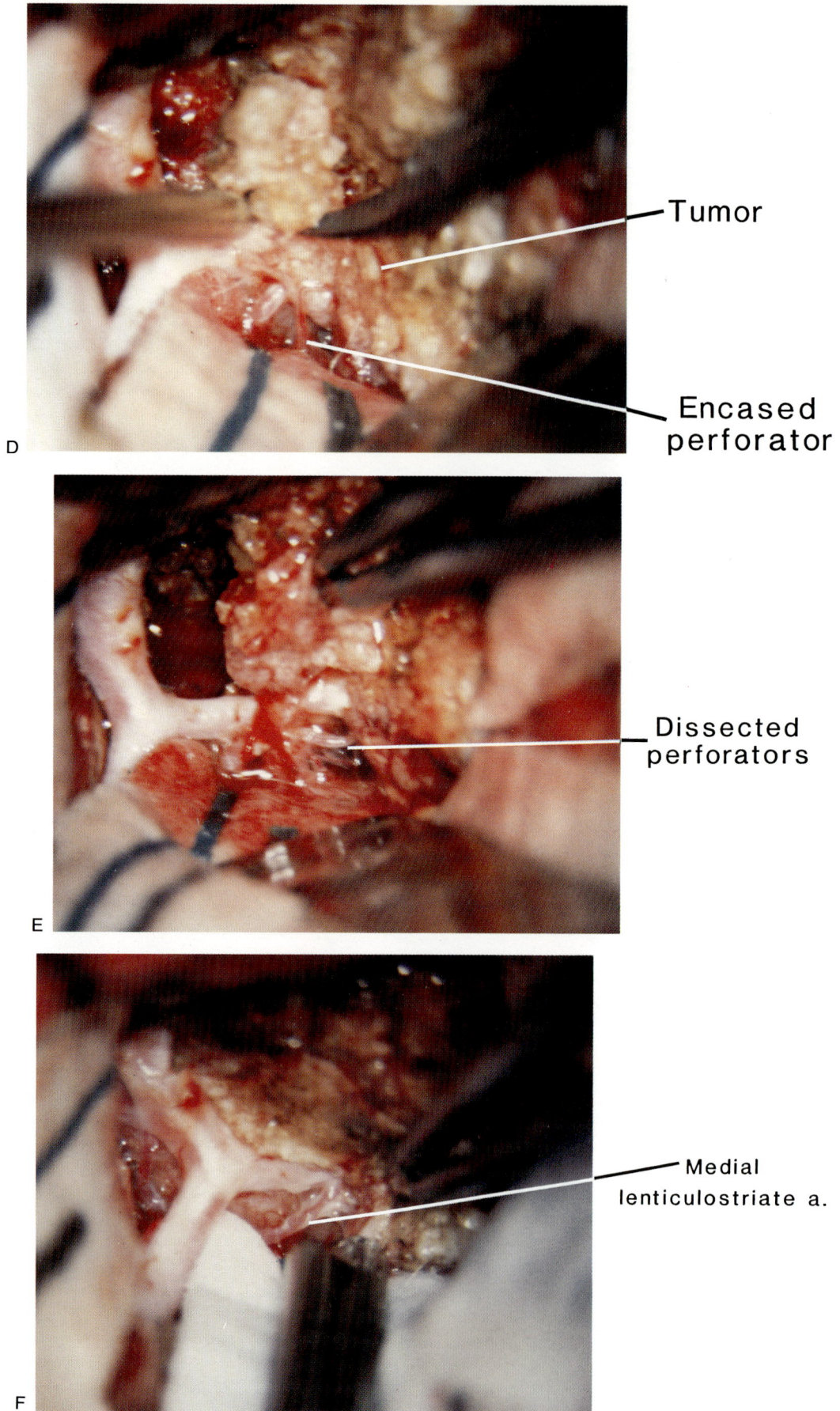

FIG. 84. *Continued.* **D,E:** The encasement of the perforators and their dissection is seen. **F:** The tumor has been dissected from the medial lenticulostriate artery.

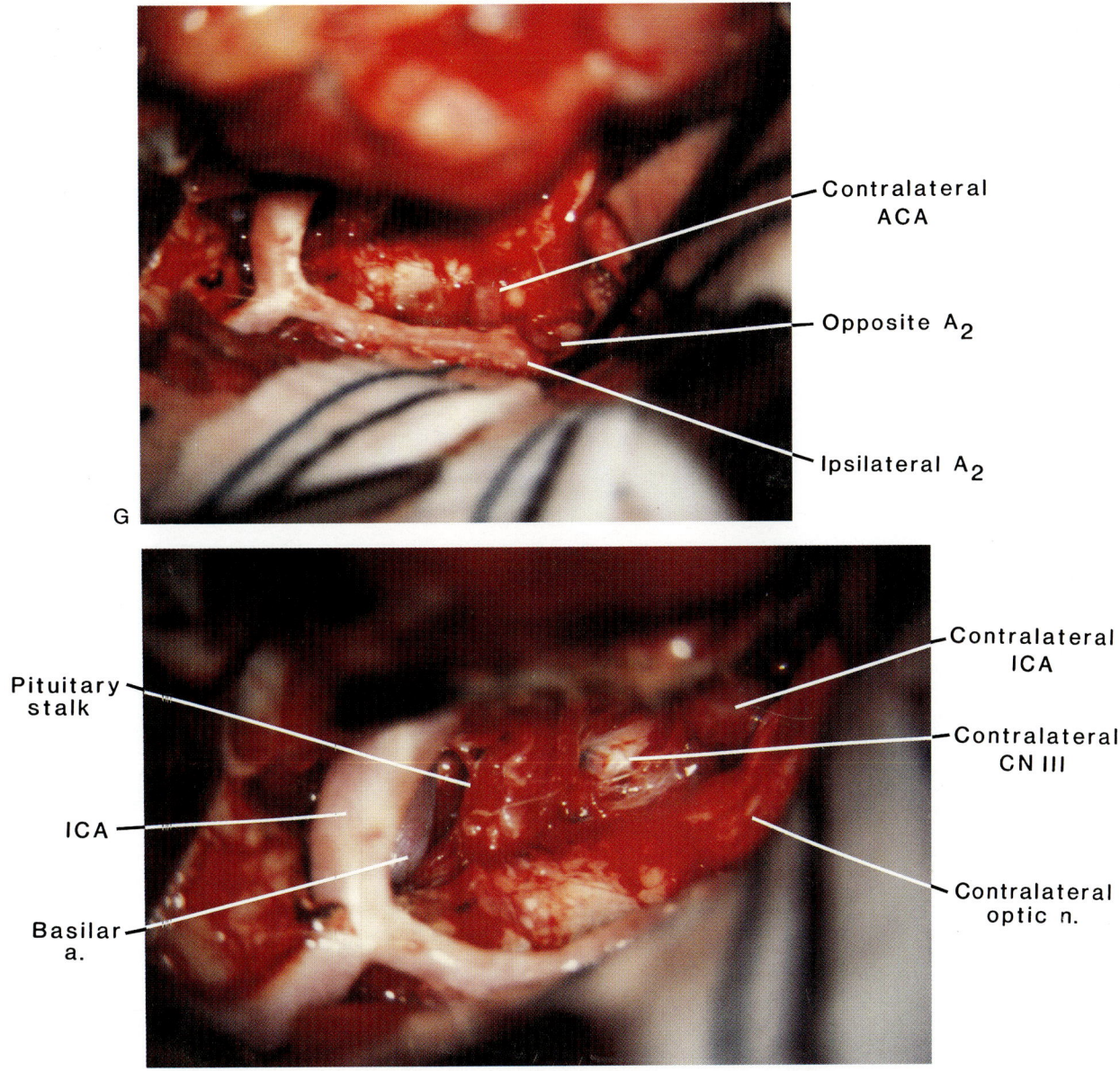

FIG. 84. *Continued.* **G:** The entire ipsilateral and contralateral anterior cerebral complex has been dissected free. **H:** The ipsilateral atrophic optic nerve has been removed with the tumor. An excellent view of the various important structures is obtained after tumor resection.

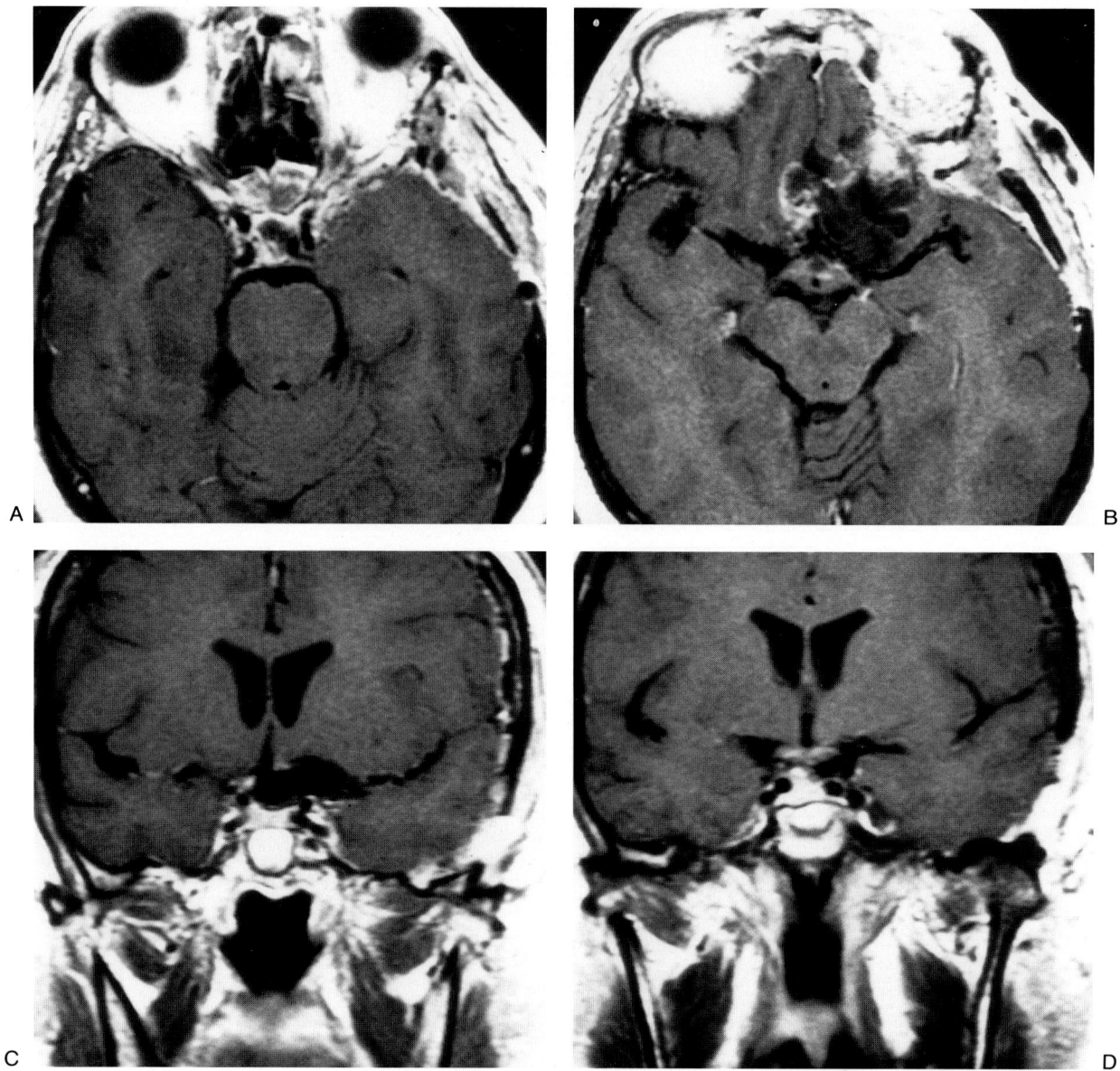

FIG. 85. Patient D.H. **A–D:** The postoperative enhanced axial and coronal MRI images show no evidence of tumor.

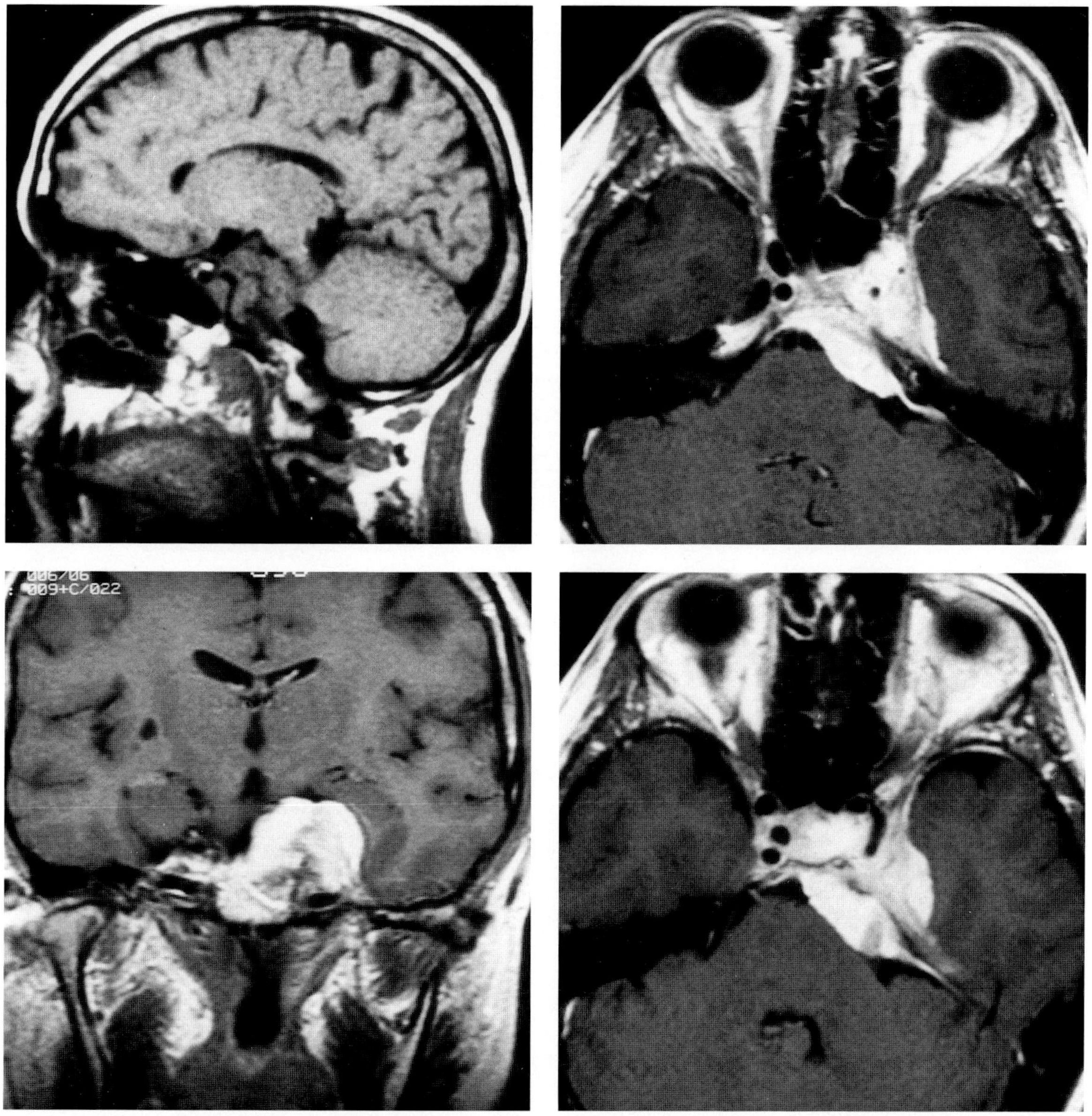

FIG. 86. Patient G.W. **A–D:** MRI scan revealed a grade IV tumor involving the cavernous sinus and the petroclival area, as seen on nonenhanced T1-weighted sagittal (**A**), enhanced axial (**B,C**), and enhanced coronal (**D**) views.

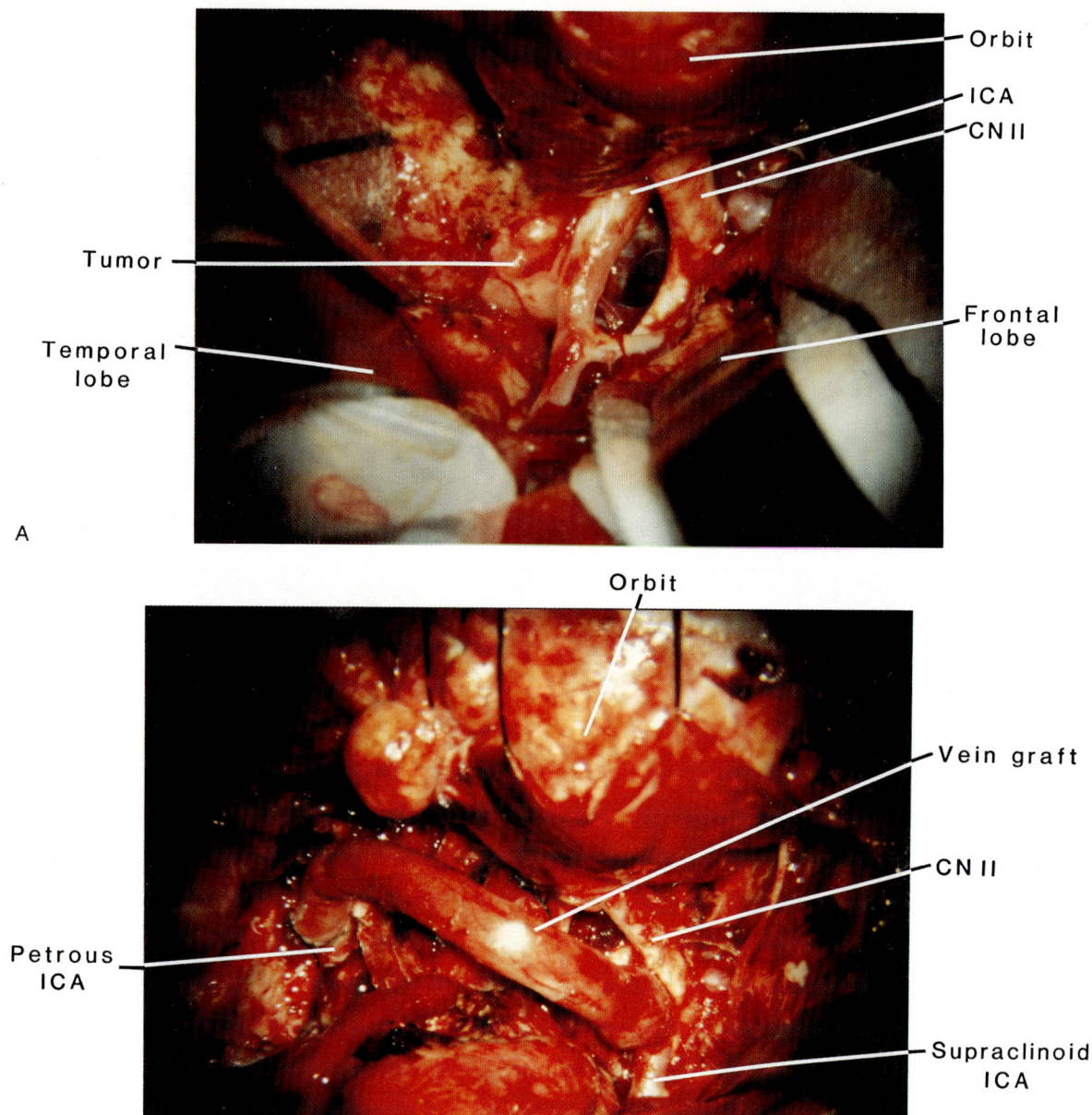

FIG. 87. Patient G.W. **A:** Operation to remove the tumor was performed in two stages. During the first operation, tumor has been exposed after splitting the sylvian fissure. **B:** A saphenous vein graft was anastomosed end-to-end to the petrous ICA and the clinoidal segment of the ICA just inferior to the ophthalmic artery.

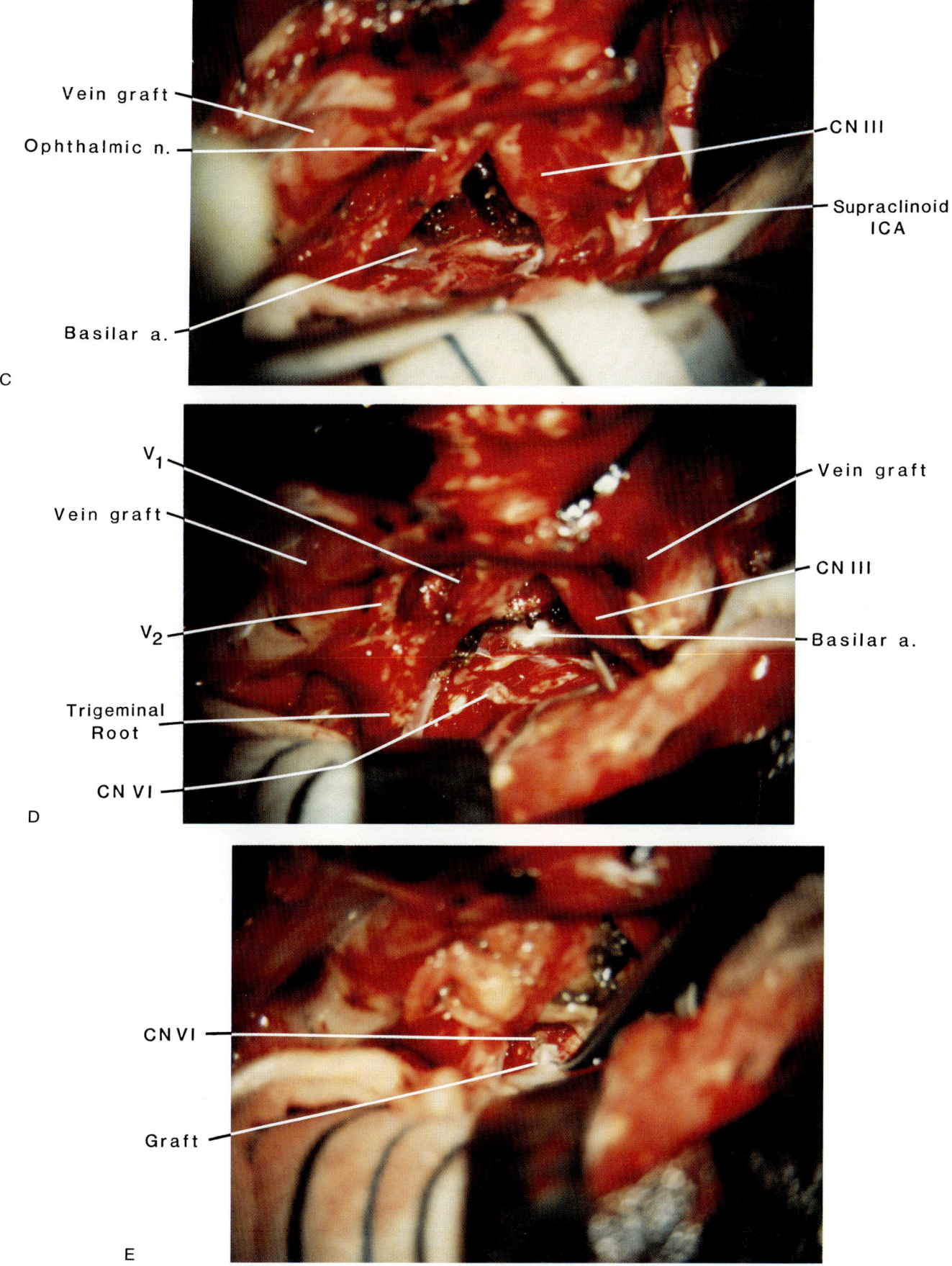

FIG. 87. *Continued.* **C:** Six weeks after the first operation, the second operation was performed. The vein graft is covered by scar tissue. The oculomotor and trigeminal nerves were preserved, but the abducens nerve was not. Tumor was totally removed. **D:** The proximal stump of the abducens nerve is seen near the brain stem. **E:** The proximal anastomosis between the abducens nerve stump and the sural nerve graft is seen.

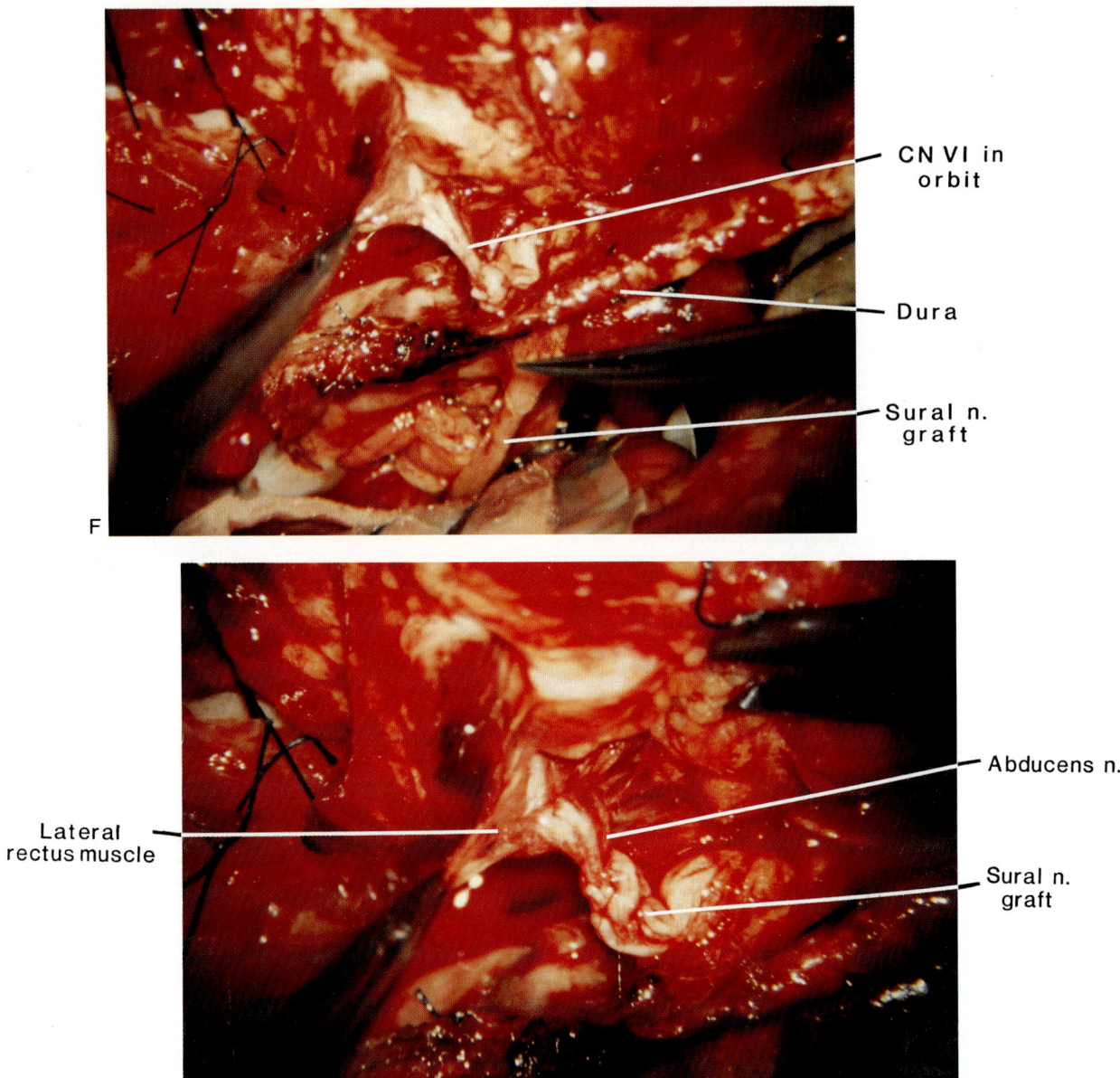

FIG. 87. *Continued.* **F:** The sural nerve graft has been brought out through the middle fossa dura to the abducens nerve in the orbit. **G:** The distal anastomosis of the nerve graft and the entry of the distal abducens nerve into the lateral rectus muscle are seen.

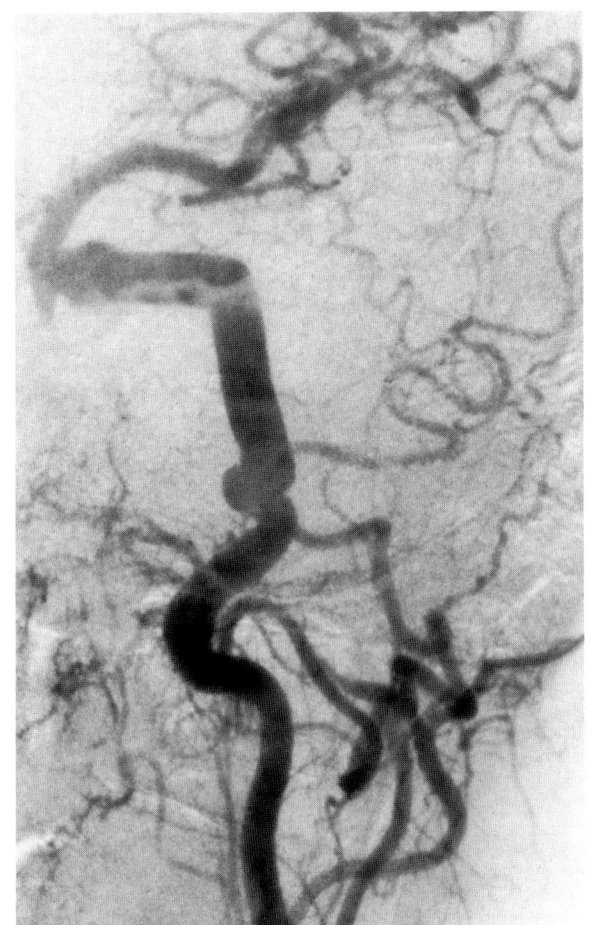
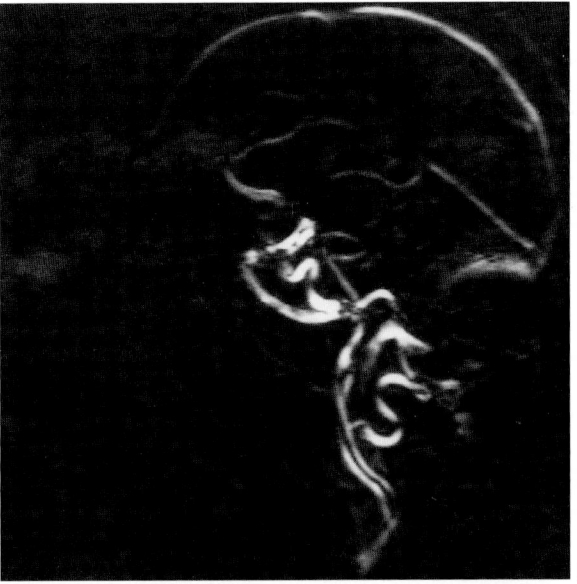

FIG. 88. Patient G.W. **A,B:** The postoperative contrast angiogram and an MRI angiogram one year later show the patency of the graft.

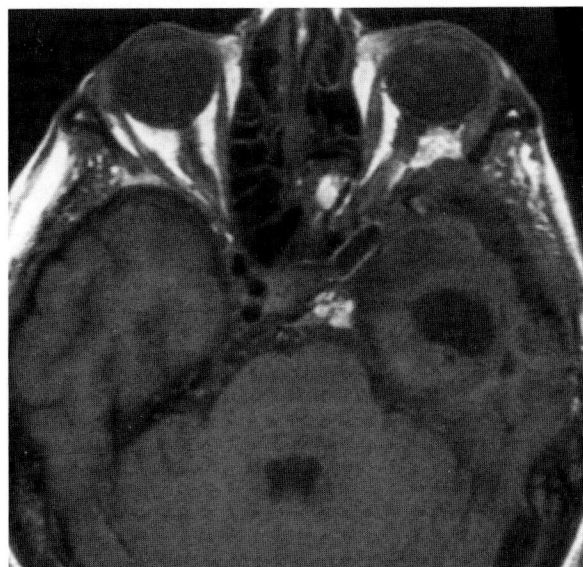
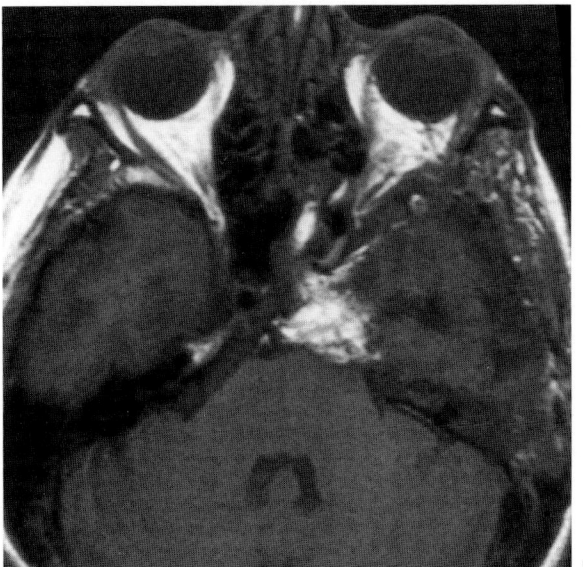

FIG. 89. Patient G.W. **A–D:** Six months after the operation, T1-weighted (**A,B**) and enhanced MRI scans (**C,D**) show no evidence of tumor, but do show scar and fat tissue in the area of tumor and sphenoid sinus.

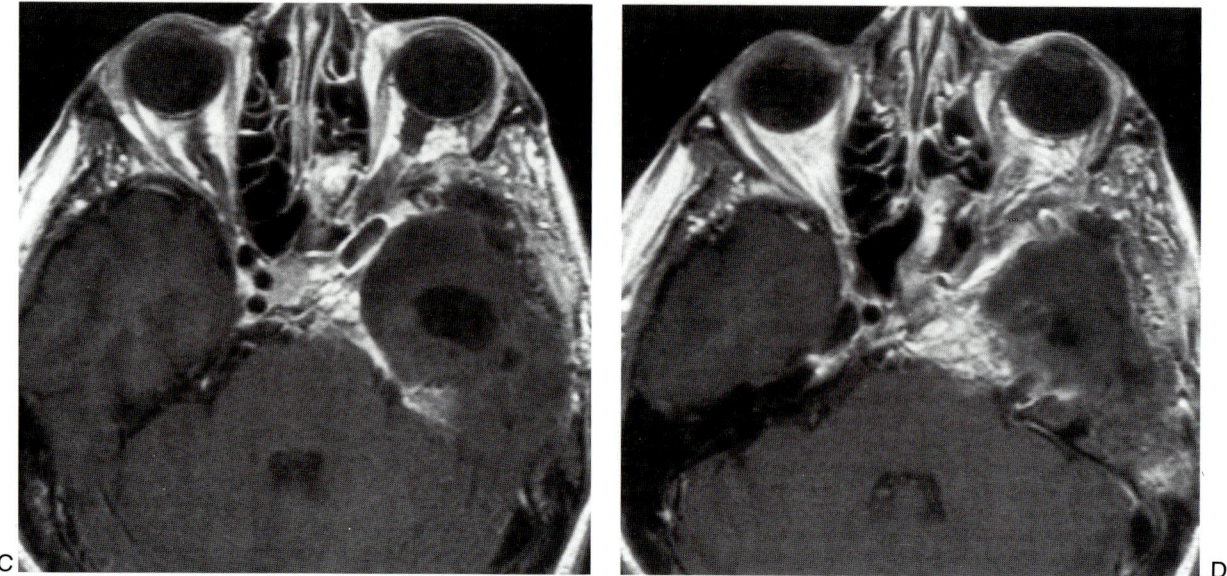

FIG. 89. *Continued.*

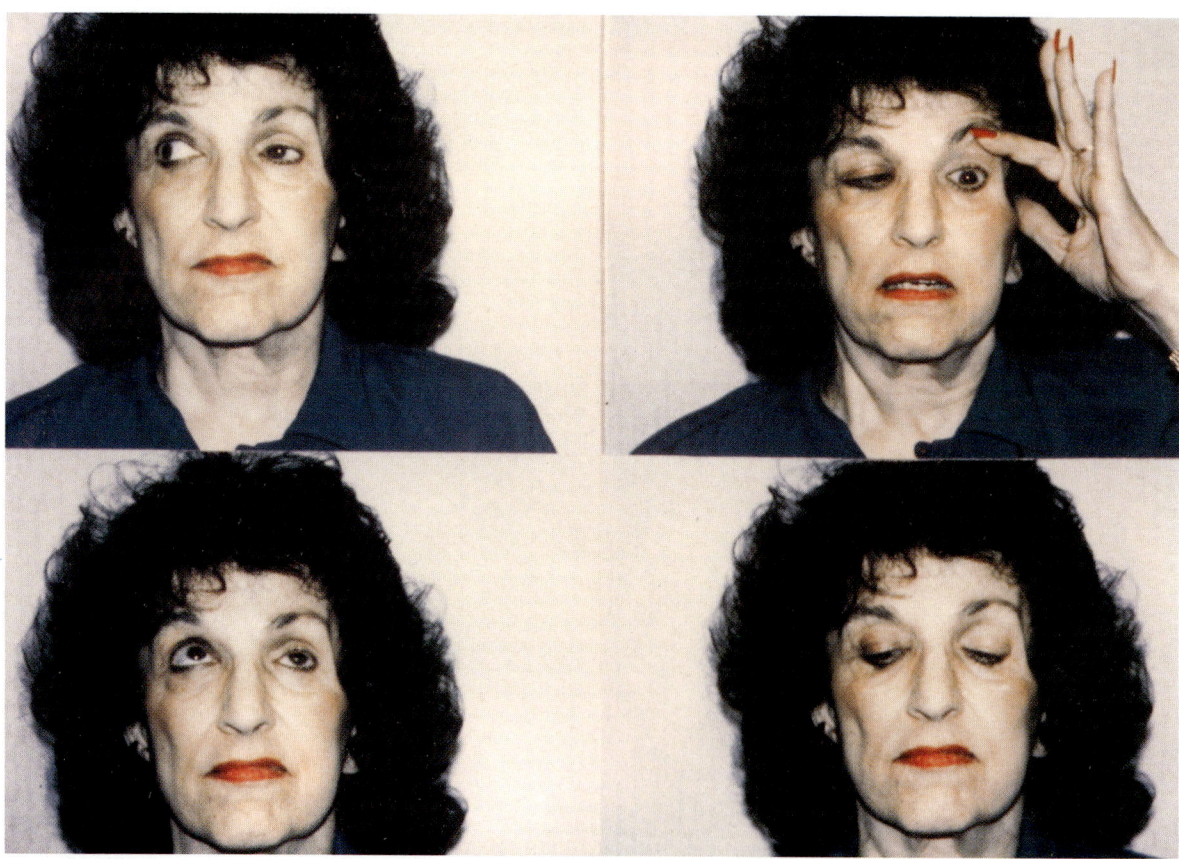

FIG. 90. The patient's third cranial function has recovered almost completely, and abducens function is recovering.

dura to the abducens nerve in the orbit. Figure 87G shows the distal anastomosis of the nerve graft and the entry of the distal abducens nerve into the lateral rectus muscle.

The postoperative contrast angiogram and a MRI angiogram 1 year later show the patency of the graft (Fig. 88A,B). Six months after the operation, T1-weighted (Fig. 89A,B) and enhanced MRI scans (Fig. 89C,D) show no evidence of tumor, but do show scar and fat tissue in the area of the tumor and sphenoid sinus. Her third cranial function has recovered almost completely, and abducens function is recovering (Fig. 90).

PATIENT SERIES

From 1983 to 1990, 148 patients with tumors involving the CS were operated on by either LNS or CSN or both. About two-thirds were benign tumors, while the remainder were malignant tumors (Table 2). During the same period, 25 intravenous and pericavernous vascular lesions were also operated on.

The complications relating to these 148 patients are shown in Table 3. Two deaths occurred in the postoperative period. One patient with a recurrent malignant meningioma underwent vein graft reconstruction of the ICA

TABLE 2. *Surgical management of 148 cavernous sinus neoplasms, 1983–1990*

Benign tumors		Malignant tumors	
Meningioma	68	Meningioma	2
Neurilemoma	12	Chordoma	14
Pituitary adenoma	8	Chondrosarcoma	10
Juvenile angiofibroma	6	Adenoid cystic carcinoma	6
Craniopharyngioma	2	Osteosarcoma	2
Epidermoid cyst	2	Squamous cell carcinoma	5
Chondroblastoma	1	Basal cell carcinoma	1
Teratoma	1	Malignant melanoma	1
Hemangioma	3	Plasmacytoma	1
Total	103	Malignant fibrous histiocytoma	1
		Malignant neurilemoma	1
		Hypernephroma	1
		Total	45

TABLE 3. *Operated cavernous sinus tumors, 1983–1990: surgical complications (137 cases)*

Death (ICA dissection; sepsis and pulmonary embolism)	2
Cerebral infarction	
Superior cerebellar artery occlusion, small infarct	1
Postoperative vasospasm, small caudate infarct	1
Cerebral ischemia	
Temporary hemiparesis/aphasia, <1 week, no infarct	6
Hematomas	
Frontal	1 (Evacuated)
Subdural	1 (Evacuated)
Brain edema	
Temporal lobe	2
Temporal lobe herniation 2° excessive CSF drainage	1 (Reoperation)
CSF leak	
Wound	2
Sphenoid sinus	10 (8 Reoperations)
Eustachian tube	2 (1 Repoperation)
External ear canal	1 (Reoperation)
Infections	
Meningitis—following CSF leak	3
Meningitis—without CSF leak	2
Wound infection with carotid pseudoaneurysm	1
Pneumonia	1
Seizures, postoperative	2
Diabetes insipidus, transient	6
Deep vein thrombophlebitis	2
Pulmonary embolism	4
Outcome of surgical complications	
Death	2
Disabled, requiring assistance in daily life	2

TABLE 4. *Operated cavernous sinus tumors, 1983–1990: permanent cranial nerve palsies/worsening[a]*

I	Olfactory	3 (Expected)
III	Oculomotor	6
IV	Trochlear	11 (3 Expected)
V₁	Ophthalmic	10 (Expected)
V₂	Maxillary	7 (Expected)
V₃	Mandibular	5 (4 Expected)
VI	Abducens	10 (3 Expected)

[a] First 101 cases—minimum follow-up 6 months.

TABLE 5. *Extraocular muscle function: all cavernous sinus tumors[a], 1983–1989*

	Excellent	Good	Fair	Poor
Preoperative	35	22	13	21
Postoperative				
Excellent	25	6	—	—
Good	7	11	2	2
Fair	—	2	7	1
Poor	—	—	2	15
Indeterminate[b]	3	3	2	3

[a] First 91 cases.
[b] Too early to evaluate, or orbital exenteration for malignant tumor.

because of a reduction of CBF after BTO of the ICA. The distal ICA was severely atherosclerotic. The vein graft remained patent, but the patient developed an ICA dissection and occlusion, despite an attempt to revascularize the brain with an occipital–middle cerebral artery branch anastomosis. The second was a patient with previously operated and radiated chordoma. After an initially good recovery from operation, she developed sepsis and a probable pulmonary embolism.

Cerebral infarctions occurred in two patients: in one with a recurrent meningioma, the superior cerebellar artery was transected while dissecting through scar tissue. Reconstruction was unsuccessful. The patient developed brain stem infarction, but with rehabilitation recovered to independent living. No further tumor recurrence was observed. The second patient developed diffuse vasospasm and a small caudate infarct, with prolonged abulia, but made a good recovery.

Temporary hemiparesis and/or aphasia lasting less than a week and without any cerebral infarction was seen in patients with impaired collateral circulation who had prolonged ICA occlusion.

Cerebrospinal fluid leakage is the most common problem, especially when the operation involves entry into the sphenoid sinus and in patients who have had prior operation or radiation therapy. Most of these patients require reoperation and packing of the sphenoid sinus with more autologous fat. In two patients, a free flap had to be used to occlude the sinus because of infections. As of now, this is a yet unsolved problem since most free flaps are too bulky to occlude the sinus.

Transient diabetes insipidus is common in patients in whom the tumor has been dissected from around the pituitary gland, and in patients in whom the ICA is replaced with a vein graft. This may be due to the occlusion of the inferior hypophyseal artery. Only one patient developed permanent diabetes insipidus, requiring hormonal replacement. Patients who have not undergone radiation therapy rarely develop permanent anterior pituitary deficiency. However, testing of pituitary function is important prior to the patient's discharge. Inappropriate secretion of antidiuretic hormone (SIADH) occurred transiently in many patients.

Cranial nerve recovery has, for the most part, been acceptable. Instances of permanent worsening are shown in Table 4. When preoperative (combined) extraocular muscle (EOM) function was graded as excellent, good, fair, or poor, we found that most of the patients tend to remain in the same class as their preoperative function, although some notable improvements and deteriorations occur (Table 5). Thus it appears that while in patients with poor eye function, the patients have little to lose, they also have little to gain. It would appear that the experienced surgeon should preferably operate on patients before EOM function becomes poor. Yet the surgeon must avoid operating on patients with benign tumors in whom the tumor size and EOM function remain unchanged upon follow-up.

Neurotrophic keratitis of the cornea occurs in some patients. Although the loss of corneal sensation is common, only some patients develop this problem. This may be because of reduced tearing or because of viral infection. Some patients are treated effectively with a soft contact lens or lubricants. However, a few patients require a tarsorrhaphy, which considerably impairs the patient's ability to see.

TABLE 6. *Direct ICA vein graft reconstruction[a] of cavernous ICA: 1987–1991*

Diagnosis	Total patients	Intraoperative or postoperative occlusion	Hemispheric neurologic deficit	BTO–ICA
Neoplasm	16	3 (small vein; inflamed vein; ICA dissection)	2 Asymptomatic	Passed
			1 Death	Passed; P-Com, ophthalmic artery, occlusion
Aneurysm	2	—	2 minor strokes	1 Failed clinical; 1 failed CBF

[a] Patency rate, 83%.

TABLE 7. Cavernous sinus surgery, 1983-1990: cranial nerve reconstruction

Cranial nerve	Type of reconstruction	Number of patients	Preoperative function	Postoperative function
III	Resuture	1	Poor	Poor
	Graft	1	Fair	Too early
IV	Resuture	1	Good	Fair
	Graft	1	Good	Too early
V_1	Graft	3	Good	2 Fair 1 Poor
V Root	Graft	1	Fair	Fair
VI	Resuture	4	3 Good 1 Fair	3 Good 1 Poor
	Graft	5	4 Good 1 Poor	2 Fair 1 Poor 2 Too early

At the present time, all our patients with cavernous sinus disease who undergo operation are evaluated preoperatively and postoperatively (at 6 months and 1 year) by an ophthalmologist experienced in ocular muscle surgery. Some correction of eye muscle function is helpful to restore or improve binocular function at 1-year postsurgery. When corneal sensation is not severely compromised, some correction of ptosis is also beneficial. Even in patients with permanent ophthalmoplegia, a permanent opening of the eyelid and the implantation of the scleral shell can improve the appearance significantly. This collaborative effort with ophthalmologists will help us to select patients for surgery better in future, as well as to rehabilitate them better. Tables 6 and 7 show the patients who have had a vascular or nerve graft reconstruction.

FOLLOW-UP EXAMINATION

Follow-up of patients is with annual clinical examination and MRI or CT scans, except during the first year, when a baseline postoperative MRI scan is done 3 months after operation, and the patient is seen every 3–6 months as necessary. In postoperative MRI scans, scar tissue and flaps are sometimes difficult to distinguish from residual tumor because all these structures enhance with gadolinium. Only when there is a change in the MRI appearance can recurrence or regrowth of tumor be diagnosed.

One late problem related to surgery is the development of delayed hydrocephalus in patients who have had prior surgery or radiation therapy. This manifested in two patients in this group with cerebrospinal fluid leakage. When the problem is diagnosed, ventriculoperitoneal shunting will be necessary.

Delayed radiation problems may be seen in patients with malignant lesions. In our series, these problems have consisted of temporal bone osteoradionecrosis (one patient), optic nerve neuropathy (one patient), and pituitary insufficiency (one patient).

Among the patients with benign tumors, recurrence (after complete tumor resection) in the area of tumor resection was seen in one patient with a meningioma (Table 8). In this patient, a radiation-induced tumor appeared benign histologically but was malignant in its biological behavior. Recurrences at the margin of tumor resection occurred in three patients with meningiomas. This was in the clivus and in the opposite cavernous sinus, as expected from the patterns of tumor spread. Regrowth of an incompletely removed tumor necessitated reoperation. The majority of incomplete resections were earlier in our experience, before the development of vein graft reconstruction to deal with grade III and IV lesions.

Incomplete resections were more common with malignant tumors (Table 9). Residual tumor remained more commonly in areas outside the cavernous sinus. All patients with malignant tumors received adjuvant radia-

TABLE 8. Operated benign cavernous sinus lesions, 1983-1990: recurrence or regrowth in all areas

Neoplasm	Total number	Total resection	Recurrence (in CS)[a]	Partial resection	Regrowth (in CS)[a]
Meningioma	68	60	4 (2)	8	1 (1)
Neurilemoma	12	11	—	1	1 (0)
Pituitary adenoma	8	4	—	4	—
Juvenile angiofibroma	6	5	1	1	—
Other lesions	9	9	—	—	—
Totals	103	89 (86%)	5 (2)	14 (14%)	2 (1)

[a] Numbers in parentheses indicate tumors that recurred inside the cavernous sinus.

TABLE 9. *Malignant cavernous sinus neoplasms, 1983–1990: recurrence or regrowth in all areas*

Neoplasm	Total number	Total excision	Recurrence (in CS)[a]	Partial excision	Regrowth (in CS)[a]
Chordoma	14	9	1	5	3
Chondrosaroma	10	5	—	5	—
Adenoid cystic carcinoma	4	4	1 (0)	2	1
Squamous cell carcinoma	5	2	2 (0)	3	1
Meningioma	2	1	—	1	—
Other lesions	7	3	2 (2)	4	1 (1)
Totals	44	24 (55%)	6	20 (45%)	6 (1)

[a] Numbers in parentheses indicate tumors that recurred inside the cavernous sinus.

tion or chemotherapy. In general, patients with highly malignant tumors such as squamous cell carcinoma, osteogenic sarcoma, and fibrous histiocytoma fared poorly, with tumor recurrences. Patients with low-grade tumors such as chordoma, chondrosarcoma, or adenoid optic carcinoma have fared well.

REFERENCES

1. Al-Mefty O, Smith R. Surgery of tumors invading the cavernous sinus. *Surg Neurol* 1988;30:370–381.
2. Barnett HJM. Delayed cerebral ischemic episodes distal to occlusion of major cerebral arteries. *Neurology* 1978;28:769–774.
3. DeMorais JY, Lana-Peixoto MA. Bilateral intracavernous carotid aneurysms: treatment by bilateral carotid ligation. *Surg Neurol* 1978;9:379–381.
4. Dolenc VV. Direct microsurgical repair of intracavernous vascular lesions. *J Neurosurg* 1983;58:824–831.
5. Dyste GN, Beck DW. De novo aneurysm formation following carotid ligation: case report and review of the literature. *Neurosurgery* 1989;14:88–92.
6. Erba SM, Horton JA, Latchaw RE, Yonas H, Sekhar LN, Schramm V, Pentheny S. Balloon test occlusion of the internal carotid artery with stable xenon/CT cerebral blood flow imaging. *AJNR* 1988;9:533–538.
7. Faria MA, Fleischer AS, Spector RH. Bilateral giant intracavernous carotid aneurysms treated by bilateral carotid ligation. *Surg Neurol* 1980;14:207–210.
8. German WJ, Black SPW. Cervical ligation for internal carotid aneurysms: an extended follow-up. *J Neurosurg* 1965;23:572–577.
9. Gomensoro JB, Maslenikov V, Azambuga N, Fields WS, Lemak NA. Joint study of extracranial arterial occlusion. *JAMA* 1973;224:985–991.
10. Grimson BS, Ross MJ, Tyson G. Return of function after intracranial suture of the trochlear nerve. *J Neurosurg* 1984;61:191–192.
11. Hakuba A, Nishimura S, Tsukanoto M. Surgical approaches to the cavernous sinus: report of 19 cases. *Neurol Med Chir (Tokyo)* 1982;22:295–308.
12. Hakuba A, Tanaka K, Suzuki T, Nishimura S. A combined orbitozygomatic infratemporal epidural and subdural approach for lesions involving the entire cavernous sinus. *J Neurosurg* 1989;71:699–704.
13. Hirsch WL Jr, Hryshko FG, Sekhar LN, Brunberg J. Comparison of MR imaging, CT, and angiography in the evaluation of the enlarged cavernous sinus. *AJR* 1988;151:1015–1023.
14. Inoue T, Rhoton AL Jr, Theele D, Barry ME. Surgical approaches to the cavernous sinus: a microsurgical study. *Neurosurgery* 1990;26:903–932.
15. Matas R. Testing the efficiency of the collateral circulation as a preliminary to the occlusion of the great surgical arteries. *Ann Surg* 1911;53:1–43.
16. Mohr DN, Ryu JH, Litin SC, Rosenow EC III. Recent advances in the management of venous thromboembolism. *Mayo Clin Proc* 1988;63:281–290.
17. Oldershaw JB, Voris HC. Internal carotid artery ligation, follow-up study. *Neurology* 1966;16:937–938.
18. Parkinson D. Anatomy of the cavernous sinus. In: Pia HW, Langmaid C, Zierski J, eds. *Cerebral aneurysms: advances in diagnosis and therapy.* New York: Springer-Verlag, 1979;62–66.
19. Parkinson D. Surgical anatomy of the lateral sellar compartment (cavernous sinus). *Clin Neurosurg* 1990;36:219–239.
20. Pearce JE, Dujovny M, Ho KL, et al. Acute inflammation and endothelial injury in vein grafts. *Neurosurgery* 1985;17:626–634.
21. Poppen JL. Specific treatment of intracranial aneurysms. Experiences with 143 surgically treated patients. *J Neurosurg* 1951;8:75–102.
22. Samii M. Reconstruction of the trigeminal nerve. In: Samii M, Jannetta PJ, eds. *The cranial nerves.* New York: Springer-Verlag, 1981;352–358.
23. Sekhar LN, Moller AR. Operative management of tumors involving the cavernous sinus. *J Neurosurg* 1986;64:879–889.
24. Sekhar LN, Burgess J, Atkin O. Anatomical study of the cavernous sinus emphasizing operative approaches and related vascular and neural reconstruction. *Neurosurgery* 1987;21:806–816.
25. Sekhar LN, Janecka IP, Jones NF. Subtemporal-infratemporal and basal subfrontal approach to extensive cranial base tumours. *Acta Neurochir (Wien)* 1988;92:83–92.
26. Sekhar LN, Linskey ME, Sen CN, Altschuler E. Surgical management of lesions within the cavernous sinus. In: Black P McL, ed. *Clinical neurosurgery,* vol 37. Baltimore: Williams & Wilkins, 1990;440–489.
27. Sekhar LN, Sen CN, Jho HD. Saphenous vein graft bypass of the cavernous internal carotid artery. *J Neurosurg* 1990;72:35–41.
28. Shaffrey CI, Spotnitz WD, Shaffrey ME, Jane JA. Neurosurgical applications of fibrin glue: dural closure in 134 patients. *Neurosurgery* 1990;26:207–210.
29. Spetzler RF, Fukushima T, Martin N, Zobramski JM. Petrous carotid to intradural carotid saphenous vein graft for intracavernous giant aneurysm, tumor, and occlusive cerebrovascular disease. *J Neurosurg* 1990;73:496–501.
30. Sundt TM III, Sundt TM Jr. Principles of preparation of vein bypass grafts to maximize patency. *J Neurosurg* 1987;66:172–180.
31. Taptas JN. The so-called cavernous sinus: a review of the controversy and its implications for neurosurgeons. *Neurosurgery* 1982;11:712–717.
32. Umansky F, Nathan H. The lateral wall of the cavernous sinus, with special reference to the nerves related to it. *J Neurosurg* 1982;56:228–234.
33. Voris HC. Complications of ligation of the internal carotid artery. *J Neurosurg* 1951;8:119–131.
34. Willinsky R, Lausjaunias P, Berenstein A. Intracavernous branches of the internal carotid artery: comprehensive review of their variations. *Surg Radiol Anat* 1987;9:201–215.
35. Winn HR, Richardson AE, Jane JA. Late morbidity and mortality of common carotid ligation for posterior communicating aneurysms. A comparison of conservative treatment. *J Neurosurg* 1977;47:727–736.
36. Yasargil MG, Reichman MV, Kubik S. Preservation of the frontotemporal branch of the facial nerve using the interfascial temporalis flap for pterional craniotomy. *J Neurosurg* 1987;67:463–466.

CHAPTER 38

Petroclival Meningiomas

Laligam N. Sekhar, Tariq Javed, and Peter J. Jannetta

Meningiomas of the clivus and apical petrous bone are rare tumors that present both diagnostic and technical challenges to the neurosurgeon. Their natural history is one of slow but progressive growth, which, if left untreated, eventually leads to a fatal outcome (3). This slow growth pattern enables these tumors to achieve an enormous size before manifesting neurological symptoms. By the time they become clinically apparent, it is not unusual to find evidence of brain stem distortion and encasement or displacement of cranial nerves III–XII. In up to 25% of these tumors, there is encasement of the basilar artery and its branches (9). These factors combined with the relative inaccessibility of the petroclival area make radical surgical tumor excision a formidable undertaking.

Up until a few decades ago, the results of surgical treatment of petroclival meningiomas were so dismal (2,3,5,13,24) that it is little wonder that these tumors were felt to be incurable. Major advances in imaging modalities over the last two decades have permitted a more precise delineation of the anatomical extension of these tumors. Advances in cranial base surgery have provided improved exposure of these tumors by using different approaches, better methods for tumor removal, and innovative techniques to minimize injury to neural and vascular structures during tumor removal. These factors have enabled the surgeon to treat these tumors more effectively, with acceptable morbidity and mortality.

L. N. Sekhar: Department of Neurosurgery, Center for Cranial Base Surgery, University of Pittsburgh School of Medicine, and Presbyterian University Hospital, Pittsburgh, Pennsylvania 15213.
T. Javed and P. J. Jannetta: Department of Neurosurgery, Presbyterian University Hospital, Pittsburgh, Pennsylvania 15213.

SURGICAL ANATOMY AND CLASSIFICATION

The clivus is the inclined surface that extends from the basiocciput to the sphenoid, where it ends as the dorsum sellae. It forms the anterior–inferior boundary of the posterior fossa. The upper portion of the clivus develops from the sphenoid bone, while the lower portion is derived from the occipital bone. In early life, there is an articulation between the basal portion of the sphenoid and occipital bone, and this synchondrosis fuses at 18 years of age.

The clivus varies in length from 37 to 52 mm (mean 45 mm) and in width from 11 mm at the anterior narrow portion to 14.3 mm (range 8–20 mm) at the posterior widest portion. The posterior surface of the clivus is lined by a thick, two-layered, basilar dura that incorporates the basilar venous plexus. Immediately posterior to the basilar dura lie the brain stem and vertebrobasilar arteries and their branches. Anteriorly, it is related to (in superior to inferior order) the pituitary fossa, the sphenoid sinus, and the retropharyngeal space of the nasopharynx/oropharynx, which contains the insertion of the anterior cervical and pharyngeal muscles to the clivus.

Classification of petroclival meningiomas is important for the purposes of communicating precise anatomical tumor location, planning operative approaches, assessing difficulty of surgical excision, and having some parameter for comparison of results between different institutions. Unfortunately, no ideal classification system presently exists which takes all these factors into account. We have devised our own classification system for petroclival meningiomas based on anatomical location with reference to the clivus and on the size and volume of the tumor. This has been found to be very useful for making rational decisions in selecting operative ap-

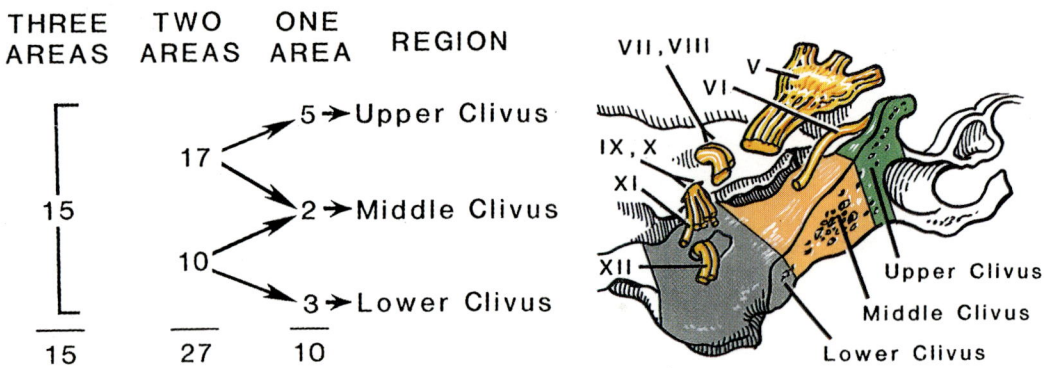

FIG. 1. Anatomical classification of clivus into upper, middle, and lower clival regions with areas of involvement by tumor.

proaches and in considering areas of potential tumor invasion.

Our anatomical classification divides the clivus into three separate anatomical regions: upper, middle, and lower clivus (Fig. 1). The *upper clivus* lying above the exit of the trigeminal nerve includes the dorsum sellae and the posterior clinoid processes. The *middle clivus* lies between the exits of the trigeminal nerve and the glossopharyngeal nerve. The *lower clivus* extends from the glossopharyngeal nerve to the foramen magnum. Areas that are in close proximity to the clival dura may often be involved by tumor. These include the cavernous sinus, sella turcica, Meckel's cave, and tentorial notch for tumors arising in the upper clivus; the internal auditory meatus for midclival tumors; and the jugular bulb, hypoglossal foramina, and the upper cervical dura for lower clival tumors. Additionally, the petroclival bone, the sphenoid sinus, and the infratemporal fossa may be involved by extensive lesions.

The second criterion of our classification system divides these tumors according to their size and volume into the following three categories: medium (up to 2.5 cm average diameter), large (2.5–4.4 cm average diameter), and giant (>4.5 cm). Measurement of size and volume are taken directly from the magnetic resonance imaging (MRI) or high resolution computerized tomography (CT) scans. The tumor volume can be calculated based on the assumption that the tumor is ellipsoid. The ellipsoid volume can be equated to a sphere of an equivalent volume and a tumor equivalent diameter can be computed as the diameter of the sphere.

Other factors related to both the tumor and the patient must also be taken into consideration when evaluating tumor resectability. Although not incorporated into the present classification, factors relating to the tumor such as arterial encasement, compromise of important venous structures, degree of brain stem compression, tumor vascularity, tumor consistency (soft as opposed to firm), and the presence (or absence) of a subarachnoid plane between the tumor and the brain stem are important variables that must be taken into account. Patient related factors such as functional status, rate of progression of clinical symptoms, and, most importantly, prior radiation therapy or surgery must be incorporated into any classification for comparison of results.

CLINICAL SIGNS AND SYMPTOMS

The clinical presentation of 52 patients operated on at the University of Pittsburgh between July 1983 and July 1990 are summarized in Table 1. Presenting symptoms by this group of patients were similar to those noted in previous reports (1,3,11,14,16,17,19). Cranial nerves (V, VI, VII, VIII, and IX–X complex) were most frequently involved because of close proximity to the tumor. Typically, the tumor distorted or encased these structures in its intradural course; less frequently, the tumor invaded the cavernous sinus or the extradural spaces. Other common neurological findings included dementia and gait ataxia, as well as motor and sensory deficits. Changes in mentation including dementia and visual acuity were frequently associated with hydrocephalus (secondary to aqueductal compression) and hence reflected increased intracranial pressure.

TABLE 1. *Clinical presentation in 52 patients with petroclival meningiomas*

Symptoms	Number of cases	Percentage
Headache	17	33
Seizures	3	6
Dementia	6	12
Motor weakness	7	13
Hemisensory loss	4	8
Gait ataxia	20	38
Limb ataxia	5	10
Cranial nerve problems		
II, decreased vision	3	10
V, pain	12	23
V, Sensory loss	13	25
VII, weakness	5	10
VIII, tinnitus	5	10
IX, X, paresis	10	19
XII, dysarthria	2	4

The decision concerning whether and when to operate is based on these key factors: location and extent of tumor invasion, patient's age and functional level, associated medical problems, progression of tumor growth as documented by MRI or CT scans, and progression of clinical symptoms and signs.

RADIOLOGICAL EVALUATION

Evaluation of the complex bony and soft tissue anatomy of the clivus and related areas has been revolutionized by the advent of high resolution CT scan and MRI. Thin section computerized tomography is performed in the axial and coronal planes with and without contrast agents using soft tissue and bone algorithms. The CT scan is presently the best imaging modality for defining the bony anatomy of the skull base. MRI in thin sections and in different planes is the best imaging modality for soft tissues. Three-millimeter sections are usually obtained using T1- and T2-weighted techniques with and without gadolinium contrast agent. Vascular encasement or displacement and location within tumor are best demonstrated by MRI. In the T2-weighted images, soft tumors appear white in contrast to firm tumors. The subarachnoid plane between the tumor and the brain stem is shown as a thin cerebrospinal fluid (CSF)-containing space. To date, we have used these two imaging modalities to complement each other in the evaluation of skull base meningiomas.

Cerebral angiography is performed on a routine basis and has three important functions: first, to define the relationship of the tumor to vascular structures; second, to evaluate the vascular supply of the tumor and subsequent embolization if this is deemed possible; and third, to evaluate tolerance to temporary vascular occlusion clinically and quantitatively using xenon/CT cerebral blood flow techniques. Petroclival meningiomas derive their blood supply predominantly from the meningohypophyseal branch of the internal carotid artery. When the tumor is supplied by the external carotid artery (ascending pharyngeal, middle meningeal branches, occipital artery), preoperative embolization of these external carotid artery feeders can be extremely helpful with tumor excision by reducing intraoperative bleeding. Embolization of the meningohypophyseal arteries is occasionally feasible.

A preoperative balloon test occlusion is performed in cases where the tumor is encasing petrous or cavernous carotid artery and radical tumor excision is planned. If the patient failed the occlusion test and vascular ligation becomes necessary intraoperatively, every effort must be made to reconstruct the vessel using saphenous vein grafts intracranially or using extracranial/intracranial (EC/IC) bypass (21,22).

OPERATIVE TECHNIQUES

Anesthesia and Monitoring

The role of the anesthesiologist is critical in maintaining hemodynamic stability, preventing increased intracranial pressure, enhancing surgical exposure, and allowing appropriate neurophysiological monitoring. Anesthesia is induced by using sodium thiopental and short-acting muscle relaxants. After intubation, anesthesia is maintained using a gaseous mixture of isoflurane, nitrous oxide, and oxygen. Muscle relaxants are avoided after induction to allow electromyographic (EMG) monitoring of cranial nerve function.

A continuous infusion of low-dose sodium thiopental (2–3 mg/kg/min) is useful to assist in the anesthesia and, when accompanied by standard hyperventilation techniques, provides adequate brain relaxation. Mannitol or furosemide is used sparingly to provide additional brain relaxation during the operation, if this is deemed necessary. Mild to moderate hypothermia (to 32°C) provides some brain protection, especially if vascular repair is necessary.

High-dose steroids are begun 24–48 hr preoperatively. To reduce the incidence of thromboembolic phenomena, intermittent pneumatic compression of the lower extremities is used intraoperatively.

Intraoperative monitoring of brain and cranial nerve functions has been an important cornerstone in the development of cranial base surgery, and nowhere is it as important as in the excision of petroclival meningiomas (12). It is important to obtain preoperative brain stem evoked response (BSER), somatosensory evoked potential (SSEP), or electroencephalogram (EEG) if such monitoring is contemplated intraoperatively. This provides a baseline for comparison intraoperatively. The BSERs are generally monitored by placing click electrodes in the opposite ear and using waves III–V as indicators of activity in the ipsilateral brain stem. SSEPs are monitored by median nerve stimulation at the opposite wrist. Cochlear nerve function can be monitored by BSER and by monitoring action potentials recorded by an electrode placed directly on the nerve. Facial nerve activity is monitored by EMG electrodes placed in the orbicularis oris, orbicularis oculi, and frontalis muscles. EMG of cranial nerves (CNs) III and VI is performed by electrodes placed in the appropriate muscles of the orbit percutaneously. Hypoglossal nerve function is recorded by placing electrodes on the tongue. Occasionally, electrodes are positioned under direct visualization on the vocal cords to monitor CN X.

It is important to have the capabilities to perform intraoperative direct nerve stimulation for anatomical localization of cranial nerves and to evaluate functional status of an anatomically intact nerve. This stimulation is performed with a hand-held monopolar electrode capable of delivering a 100–200-ms long rectangular pulse with a balanced charge.

SURGICAL APPROACHES

General Principles

In the last two decades, a number of surgical approaches to tumors of the petroclival area have been proposed (1,4,6,8,9,11,14,17,18,20,23) that reflect the considerable difficulty and morbidity associated with surgery by any approach, and the necessity to vary the approach, depending on the surgical anatomy. The surgeon should be familiar with all the skull base approaches and select the approach according to each individual tumor. The surgical goal should primarily be radical tumor excision, as this offers the only hope for cure.

Operative approaches can be divided into two types: *simple approaches,* which are adequate for small and medium size tumors, and *complex approaches,* which are more appropriate for large and giant tumors. Factors that are important when considering approach selection include tumor- and patient-related factors mentioned earlier and the goals of the surgery (radical versus subtotal removal).

In our experience, tumors requiring complex approaches include those encasing the basilar artery where good exposure is critical, large or giant tumors as previously mentioned, and tumors that are technically difficult to excise due to increased vascularity or the presence of scar tissue from previous surgery. Tumors that are *centrolateral,* thus providing a lateral window to the lesion, are easily managed with a simple approach. The lesions that are predominantly *central* in location require a complex approach since the lateral window is small. Tumors that are soft in consistency can generally be resected by a simple approach.

Simple Approaches

These approaches are most useful for smaller tumors and for tumors that are technically easier to resect. Table 2 summarizes various surgical approaches that have been used in our institution for exposure of tumors involving the three anatomical areas of the clivus. The object of the surgery is to select the approach that offers the best and widest exposure of the tumor with the least amount of brain retraction.

Frontotemporal-Transsylvian/Anterior Subtemporal Approach with Zygomatic Osteotomy

This approach provides excellent exposure for tumor resection in the upper clivus and tentorial notch. Using a frontotemporal scalp flap, an anterior and midtemporal craniotomy is performed in the standard fashion. A fron-

TABLE 2. *Approaches used for petroclival meningiomas*

Simple approaches
Upper clivus
   Frontotemporal transsylvian or anterior subtemporal approach with orbitozygomatic osteotomy
   Frontotemporal/orbitozygomatic transcavernous approach
Midclivus
   Retrosigmoid approach (small and medium sized tumors)
Lower clivus
   Extreme lateral transcondylar approach
Complex approaches
   Subtemporal–preauricular infratemporal fossa approach
   Posterior subtemporal, transzygomatic, and presigmoid transpetrous approach
   Total petrosectomy

totemporal craniotomy is performed if the tumor extends into the carotid and optic nerve cisterns. Exposure of the floor of the middle fossa is obtained by performing a zygomatic or orbitozygomatic osteotomy, including the condylar fossa, to enable the temporalis muscle to be reflected further inferiorly. The tumor can then be approached either by a subtemporal or a transsylvian approach. During the transsylvian approach, the sylvian fissure is opened widely from the lateral to medial direction by dividing some of the bridging veins of the medial temporal lobe. The medial temporal lobe is retracted laterally and the frontal lobe superiorly. This provides adequate exposure of the upper clivus on the ipsilateral side and anterior tentorial notch. The two major disadvantages of the approach are the limited working space available for tumor resection despite adequate exposure, and the risk of injury to vessels within the sylvian fissure (internal carotid artery [ICA] and middle cerebral artery [MCA]) during tumor resection.

For the anterior subtemporal approach, it is sometimes helpful to resect the anterior 4 cm of the inferior temporal gyrus, while sparing the medial temporal structures (uncus, hippocampus, amygdala). This provides a wide exposure of the tentorial notch, upper clivus, and cavernous sinus without the need for excessive temporal lobe retraction. Whenever possible, this anterior approach is preferred over the posterior subtemporal approach because of the higher morbidity associated with the latter and the greater risk of vascular injury to Labbé's vein due to potential temporal lobe retraction. This approach is particularly useful for tumors involving the upper clivus with extension into the cavernous sinus. This approach can be used in conjunction with the infratemporal fossa approach for tumors extending extradurally or involving the internal carotid artery.

Frontotemporal Transcavernous and Transpetrous Apex Approach

This approach is useful for tumors involving the cavernous sinus and the medial upper clival area, when re-

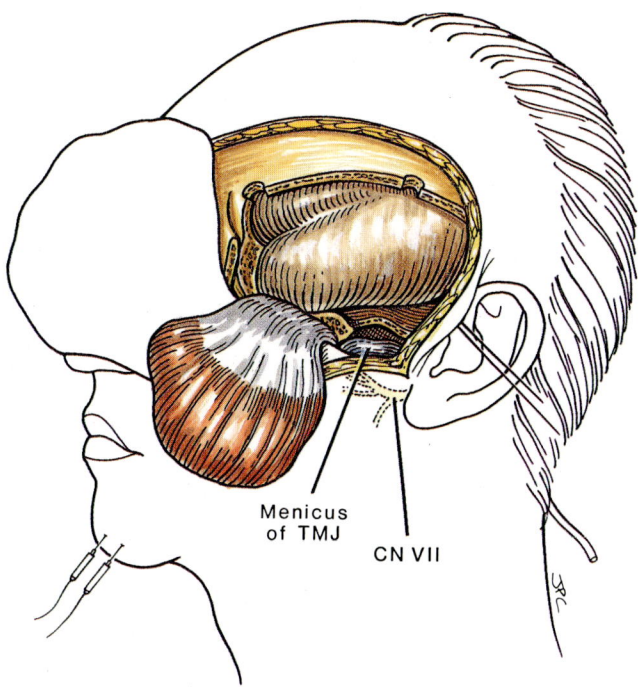

FIG. 2. Illustration of the skin flap and the extent of craniotomy necessary for the frontotemporal transcavernous approach to tumors of the upper clivus. A zygomatic osteotomy is an essential component of the osseous exposure.

moval of the intracavernous tumor is one of the goals of the operation. The use of this approach has been previously described in detail (21). A frontotemporal craniotomy is performed, followed by an orbitozygomatic osteotomy to minimize frontal and temporal lobe retraction (Fig. 2). Intracavernous tumor removal is performed as previously described (see Lang, Anatomy of the Posterior Cranial Fossa).

Access to the upper clival tumor is obtained by working between the supraclinoid ICA and CN III, between CNs III and IV, or between CNs IV and V_1. Prior intracavernous tumor removal usually provides adequate working space for removal of the dorsum sellae and ipsilateral posterior clinoid process, to facilitate exposure and resection of the tumor from the upper clival area. The petrous apex bone is removed intradurally, both lateral and medial to the trigeminal root. This improves the inferior exposure down to CN VI (Figs. 3 and 4). If the intracavernous carotid artery has to be excised as a part of the tumor resection (with or without ICA grafting), access to the sphenoid sinus can be obtained by removal of its lateral wall (Fig. 5). In this manner, further exposure of the clivus and tumor can be obtained by working through the sphenoid sinus. Adequate reconstruction is important to prevent postoperative CSF leakage. This is done by placing a pericranial flap to line the sphenoid

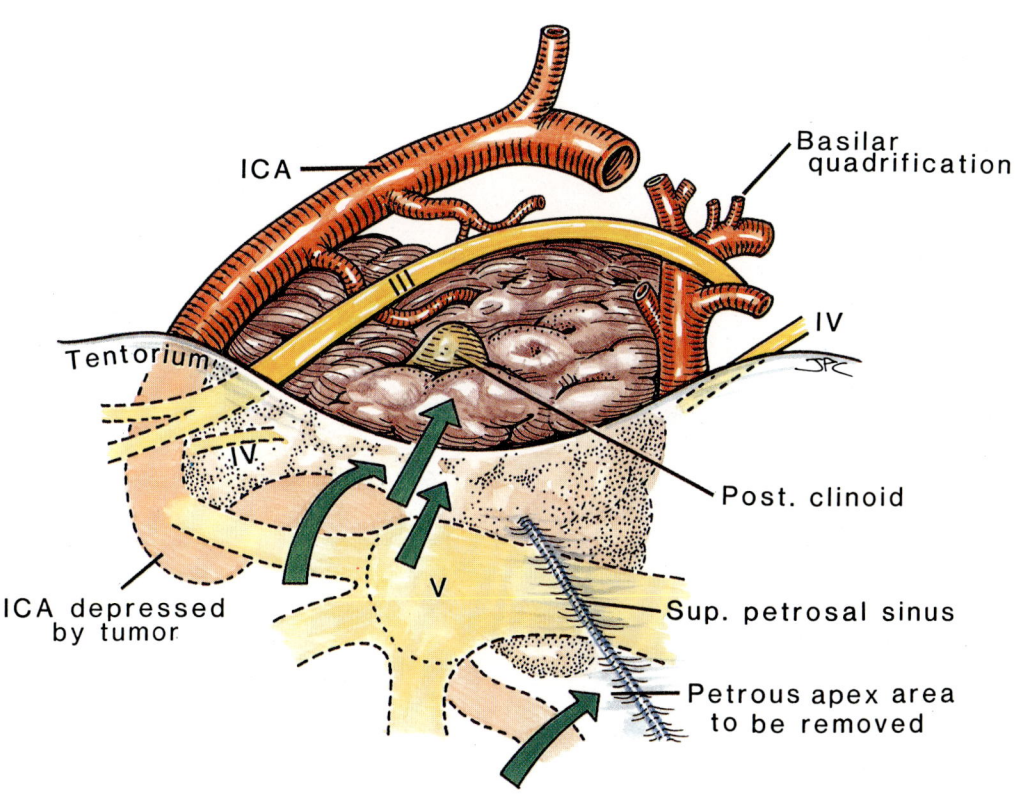

FIG. 3. Subtemporal transcavernous transpetrous approach. Note the cavernous sinus is entered through the medial wall of Meckel's cave (*arrows*) and between CNs III, IV, and V. The intracavernous tumor and dorsum sellae can be removed.

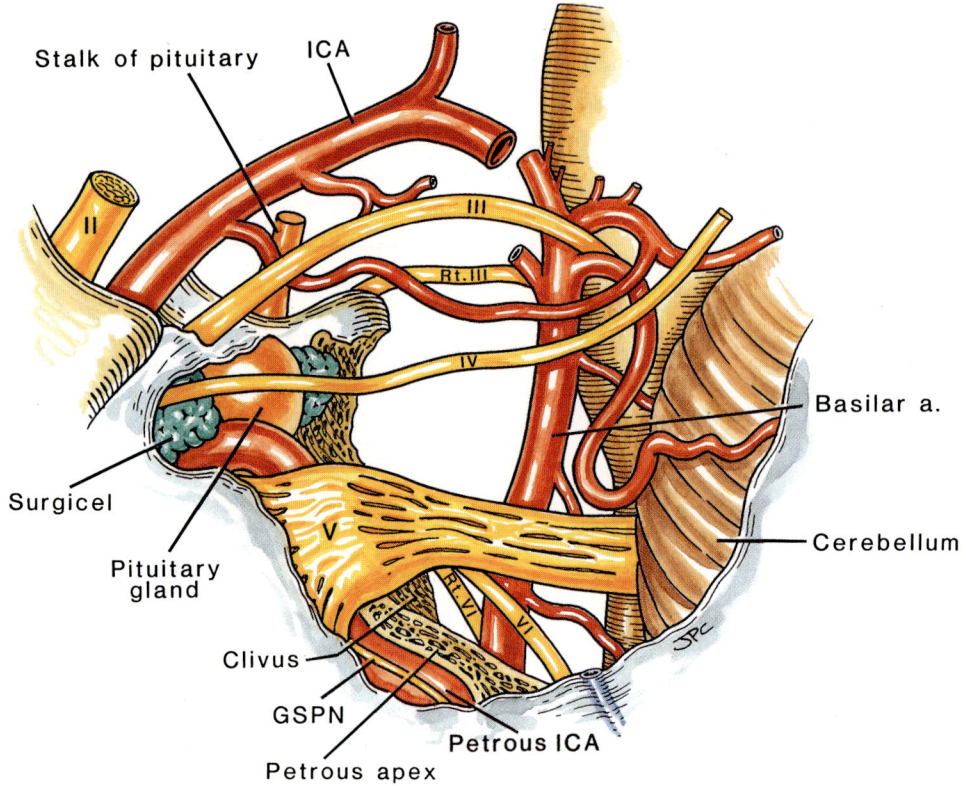

FIG. 4. Exposure obtained at the end of the procedure, when combined with petrous apex resection.

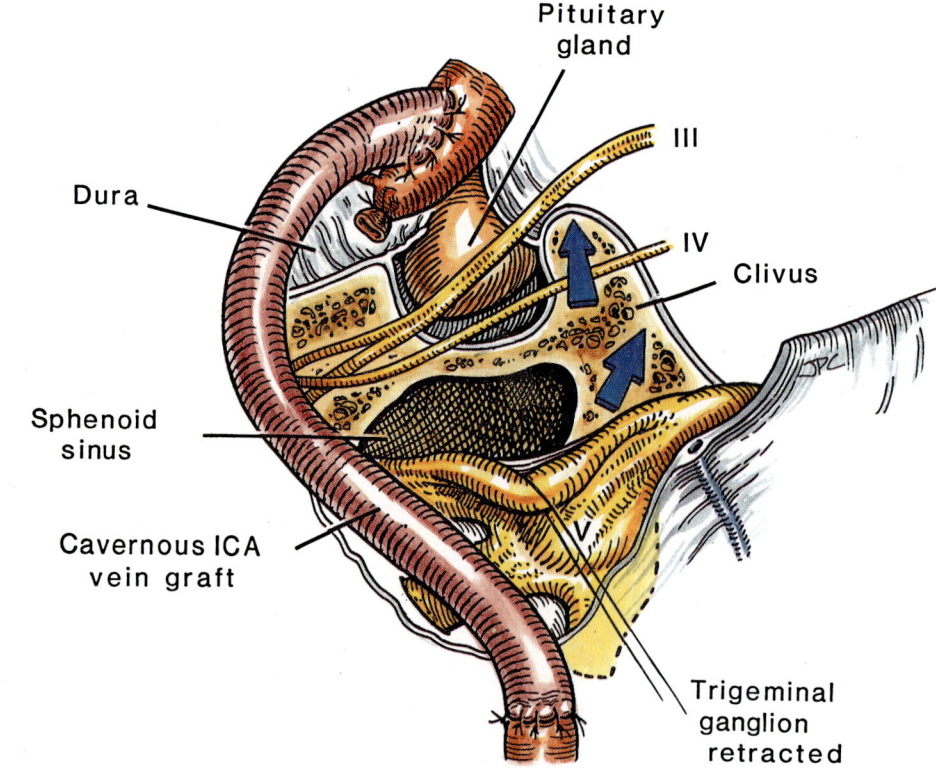

FIG. 5. Using the frontotemporal transcavernous approach, if the intracavernous carotid artery is excised as part of the tumor resection, access to the sphenoid sinus is obtained by removal of the lateral wall of the sphenoid sinus. A saphenous vein bypass graft has been performed to reconstruct the excised cavernous ICA in this case. The *arrows* indicate the areas that are accessible (after bone removal) by working through the cavernous sinus.

sinus, packing it with autologous fat, and then closing the dural defect with a fascia lata graft sutured to the edges of the dura circumferentially.

The major advantages of this approach are that the upper clivus can be approached through the middle cranial fossa without the need for posterior temporal lobe retraction, and that the tumor is devascularized at an early point in the operation. The disadvantage of the procedure lies in the increased morbidity associated with working within the cavernous sinus, and the restricted applicability of this approach to only those cases where the cavernous sinus is involved with tumor.

Retrosigmoid Approach

This approach provides rapid access to tumors that are centrolateral, medium to small in size, and involve the midclivus and the petrous apex region. The key to this approach is to ensure adequate bone removal over the sigmoid sinus laterally to allow the lateral rotation of the sigmoid sinus with the dura, and to minimize cerebellar retraction with adequate cisternal CSF drainage. The advantage of this approach is its ease, and that mild to moderate cerebellar retraction is generally well tolerated. The disadvantages of this approach are the need to work between the cranial nerves and blood vessels in the cerebellopontine angle and poor brain stem visualization, especially when there is severe distortion by the tumor. The approach also does not provide adequate exposure of more medial lesions and lesions extending contralaterally unless the tumor has provided a large lateral window. The anterior inferior cerebellar artery and CNs VIII, IX, and X are at greatest risk for injury during this operation.

Extreme Lateral Transcondylar Approach

This approach is useful for the management of lower clival and foramen magnum tumors with extension into the upper cervical spine, and where the vertebral artery or cranial nerves IX–XII may be encased by the tumor (23).

With the patient in the lateral position, an inverted U-shaped incision is made in the retroauricular area. The sternocleidomastoid and trapezius muscles are detached from their insertion to the mastoid and occiput and reflected inferiorly, and the internal jugular vein and spinal accessory nerve are identified. The splenius capitis, superior and inferior oblique, and the major and minor recti muscles are detached from the occipital bone, mastoid process, and transverse process of C1. The transverse process of C1 (the most prominent bony structure) is easily palpable and provides a reliable anatomical landmark for orientation and exposure of the extradural segment of the vertebral artery. The artery is surrounded by a venous plexus, which warns the surgeon about the location of the artery. The veins can be cauterized or packed. If necessary, the vertebral artery can also be exposed between the C1 and C2 transverse foramina and, after unroofing the C1 foramen, can be reflected inferomedially.

Following a small retrosigmoid craniectomy, a partial mastoidectomy extending up to the vertical segment of the facial canal is performed, and the sigmoid sinus is unroofed to the point where it turns to join the jugular bulb. The posterior half of the occipital condyle is removed with the aid of a high-speed drill, taking care not to injure the hypoglossal nerve and jugular bulb, which are in close proximity to the occipital condyle. The lateral third of the C1 lamina is removed to the foramen transversarium. The articular process of C1 is also removed in its posterior half, taking care not to injure the vertebral artery. The dural entry point of the vertebral artery is now the center of the exposure. The dura is opened vertically, just medial to the vertebral artery entrance point. There is a dural ring around the entrance of the vertebral artery, which is opened to release the artery. The dura is then opened transversely, just superior to the extradural vertebral artery, and tacked up. The C1 rootlets and the first dentate ligaments are divided, but C2 is carefully protected

Tumor is initially removed around the vertebral artery, which can then be mobilized laterally to avoid any risk of injury. The vertebral artery can be followed distally to its junction with the basilar artery. When a segment of the vertebral artery has to be resected due to tumor infiltration, it can be reconstructed using a saphenous vein graft. In patients in whom cranial nerves IX–XII are encased by the tumor, neurophysiological monitoring and nerve stimulation can aid with identification and preservation of these nerves. The main advantage of this approach is that it provides a very lateral exposure of the tumor and lower brain stem interface and allows tumor removal without brain or spinal cord retraction. Excellent exposure of the proximal and distal vertebral artery is obtained for vascular reconstruction if this becomes necessary. Removal of the posterior half of the occipital condyle has no effect on stability of the craniocervical junction. However, in cases where complete unilateral condylectomy is necessary for tumor involving the lower clivus and jugular bulb, an occiput to C1–C2 fusion is recommended. Watertight dural closure is usually not possible, and holes in the dura are plugged with autologous fat. Any opening into the middle ear cavity must be closed with bone wax and autologous fat. The muscles and more superficial tissues must be carefully reapproximated in layers to prevent postoperative CSF leak (See Sen and Sekhar, *Extreme Lateral Transcondyle Approach*).

Complex Approaches

Subtemporal–Preauricular Infratemporal Fossa Approach

This approach provides both intradural and extradural exposure, the details of which have been previously described (20). The intradural approach (frontotemporal craniotomy) as described previously provides adequate exposure of the upper clivus. The infratemporal approach allows the surgeon to extend the exposure further down the clivus and the details of the approach are presented by Sekhar et al. (Anterior, Anterolateral, and Lateral Approaches to Extradural Petroclival Tumors). The condyle of the mandible is resected to its neck. The horizontal and vertical segments of the petrous internal carotid artery are exposed and displaced anteriorly to enable removal of the petrous apex medial to the cochlea, and the middle and lower clival bone medial to the carotid canal. This exposes the petroclival dura from the level of the petrous apex to the foramen magnum (Fig. 6). Further exposure of the upper clival region is provided by entering the posterior cavernous sinus through the medial wall of Meckel's cave and working through the cavernous sinus.

The midsegment of the eustachian tube is excised during petrous ICA exposure. It is critical to close the cartilaginous eustachian tube with autologous fat and a suture at this stage to prevent postoperative CSF leaks. If the sphenoid sinus is entered, its mucosa is exenterated and it is closed with autologous fat, fascia, and fibrin glue. The dural defect is closed using fascial graft, and the extradural space is occluded with fat and a temporalis muscle rotation flap. The limitation of this approach is inadequate exposure of the ipsilateral cerebellopontine angle (CNs VII–VIII) and cerebellomedullary angle (CNs IX–XII). It also fails to provide control of the contralateral carotid artery should this be involved with tumor. Potential complications include CSF leaks from the sphenoid sinus or the eustachian tube and injury to the petrous ICA, the facial nerve, and the cochlea. The major advantage is the wide exposure of the middle and lower clivus, which is attained without retraction of the brain stem or the cerebellum, and an anterolateral view of the brain stem to allow tumor dissection.

Posterior Subtemporal/Transzygomatic and Presigmoid Transpetrous Approach

This approach has been popularized by Al-Mefty, Hakuba, Malis, and Samii (1,6,10,14) and is used by our

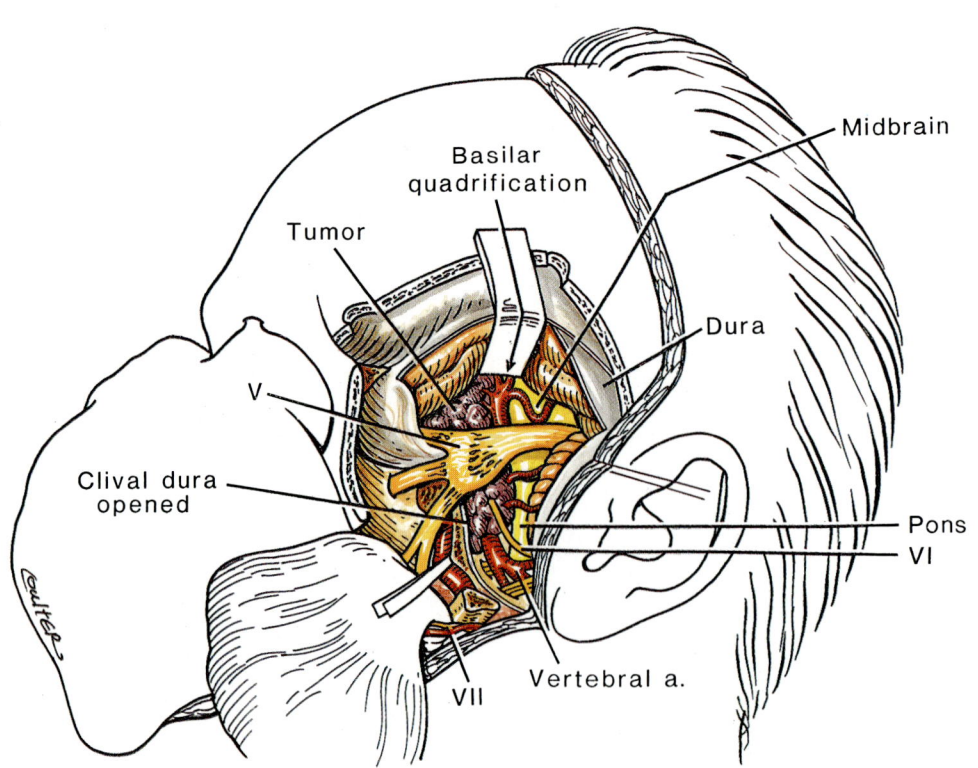

FIG. 6. The subtemporal–preauricular infratemporal fossa approach provides a lateral exposure of the lower aspect of the clivus and enables the neurosurgeon to work anteriorly to the brain stem and medially to CNs VII–XII.

group with modifications. It may also be combined with the preauricular infratemporal approach in the same or subsequent operation. In this approach, the dural opening is made in the presigmoid dura and the temporal dura, thus preserving the sigmoid sinus as described by Al-Mefty et al. (1). Malis (10) prefers to divide the transverse sinus with preservation of Labbé's vein blood flow via the opposite sinus for obtaining improved exposure of structures below the internal auditory canal. This can only be performed in patients with good communication between the transverse sinuses at the torcular Herophili and on the nondominant side. The advantage of this approach includes minimal cerebellar and temporal lobe retraction and shortening of the operative distance to the tumor by 3 cm when compared to the retrosigmoid approach. The surgeon has reasonable access to anterior and lateral aspects of the brain stem. However, the surgeon still has to work between CNs V and IX and is at a disadvantage when these nerves have not been stretched by the tumor. Posterior temporal lobe retraction, the possibility of injury to Labbé's vein, and the variable location and size of the temporal lobe draining veins are also disadvantages.

This approach is most suitable for centrolateral midclival and petrous apex lesions rather than tumors involving the central or contralateral clivus. Exposure of the upper clival region, although possible, may require considerable posterior temporal lobe retraction. Exposure of the lower clivus is limited by the jugular bulb, especially when it is high. It may only be obtained at the expense of division of the sinus or working posteriorly to it (Fig. 7). When CNs V–IX have not been chronically stretched by tumor, this approach puts the nerves at considerable risk for injury, and care must be taken. We combine this approach usually with a zygomatic osteotomy including the condylar fossa. *Petrous apex resection* is also performed, as needed. For such exposures, either two incisions can be used (as seen in Fig. 7) or a retroauricular incision can be made with the division of the pinna, which is resutured at the end of the operation. The labyrinth limits the exposure during the presigmoid approach. When the hearing in the ipsilateral ear is poor, and good in the contralateral ear, a *translabyrinthine* approach is combined with the subtemporal approach. This improves the exposure of the cerebellopontine angle considerably.

Total Petrosectomy Approach

A lateral extradural approach involving the posterior displacement of the infratemporal facial nerve and the removal of the cochlea was pioneered by House and Hitselberger under the name "transcochlear approach" (7,8). We have improved this approach with the anterior mobilization of the petrous ICA and the removal of the petroclival bone to call it the "total petrosectomy approach" (Figs. 8 and 9) (15). This approach has been used for the exposure of nine cases of giant and complex petroclival meningiomas and other tumors at Presbyterian University Hospital. In this approach, an incision in the form of a question mark is made starting in the temporal area and extending behind the ear and the mastoid region, and curving inferiorly in front of the sternomastoid area and behind the angle of the jaw. The skin flap is dissected in the subcutaneous plane from the underlying periosteum and reflected anteriorly. The external ear canal is divided at the junction of the cartilaginous and bony parts and sutured shut. The pericranium is reflected off the temporal and mastoid bone. The sternomastoid and the digastric muscles are divided at the point of attachment to the mastoid process and reflected downward. The splenius and semispinalis capitis muscles are detached from the suboccipital bone. The facial nerve trunk is dissected free near its exit from the stylomastoid foramen and followed distally into the parotid gland, exposing its major divisions.

The mandibular condyle and surrounding joint capsule are dissected from the glenoid fossa and the neck of the mandible is transected and the condyle removed. The zygomatic arch is divided with the glenoid fossa and the temporalis muscle reflected inferiorly. A temporal craniotomy is performed beginning near the pterion and extending posteriorly to the level of the sigmoid sinus. The petrous ICA and upper cervical ICA are then exposed entirely and translocated forward as described previously in this chapter. The greater superficial petrosal nerve will be divided during this phase of the operation. The petrosectomy part of the procedure begins with a mastoidectomy. After this, the remaining part of the external auditory canal, the tympanic membrane, and the middle ear contents are removed. The facial nerve is then unroofed using a diamond drill, beginning from the stylomastoid foramen up through the mastoid process and the middle ear to the geniculate ganglion. The bony labyrinth is drilled away to expose the facial nerve within the internal auditory canal. The chorda tympani is divided at its exit from the facial nerve, thus freeing up the facial nerve entirely. The infratemporal facial nerve is then mobilized and displaced posteriorly. The cochlear and vestibular nerves are divided within the internal auditory canal. After displacing the intrapetrous facial nerve posteroinferiorly, and the petrous ICA forward, the apex of the petrous temporal bone and much of the midclival bone can be removed in a piecemeal fashion. The jugular bulb is skeletonized and is the inferior limit to this approach. This approach provides a much wider exposure than the transcochlear approach (Figs. 8 and 9).

Tumor is removed with gentle cerebellar, temporal lobe, and petrous ICA retraction. The strategy is to first disconnect the tumor from the clival dura and the poste-

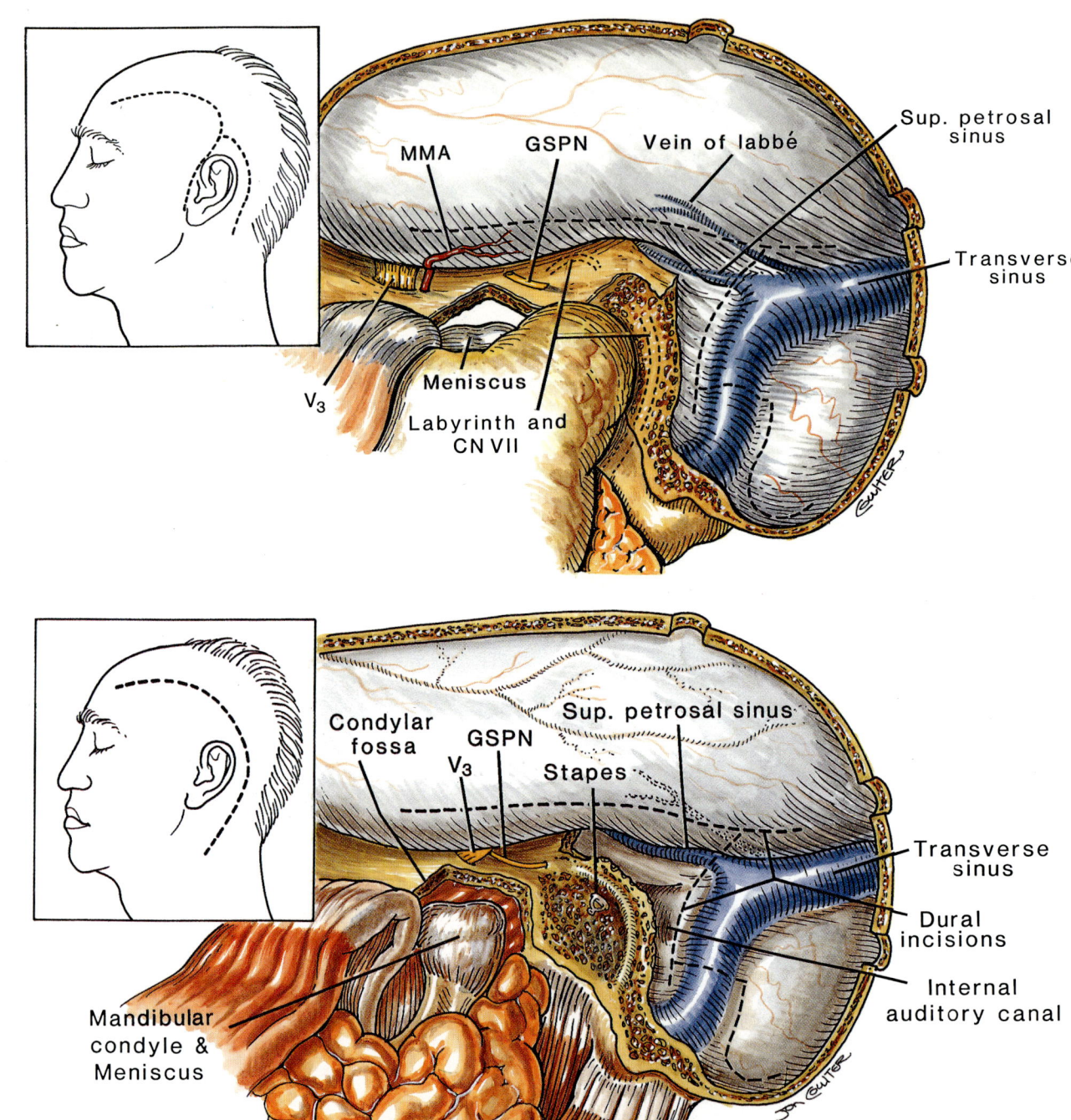

FIG. 7. Posterior subtemporal/presigmoid approach (petrosal approach) to midclival and petrous apex tumors. **A:** The approach with the preservation of the labrynth. The zygomatic arch has been removed, along with the condylar fossa. (The skin incision is shown in the *inset*.) The posterior flap should include the main trunk and posterior branch of the superficial temporal artery. **B:** The approach in **A** combined with a labrynthectomy. Since the external ear canal is divided and sutured shut, a retroauricular incision (*inset*) can be employed. The removal of the petrous apex (not shown) is an added help.

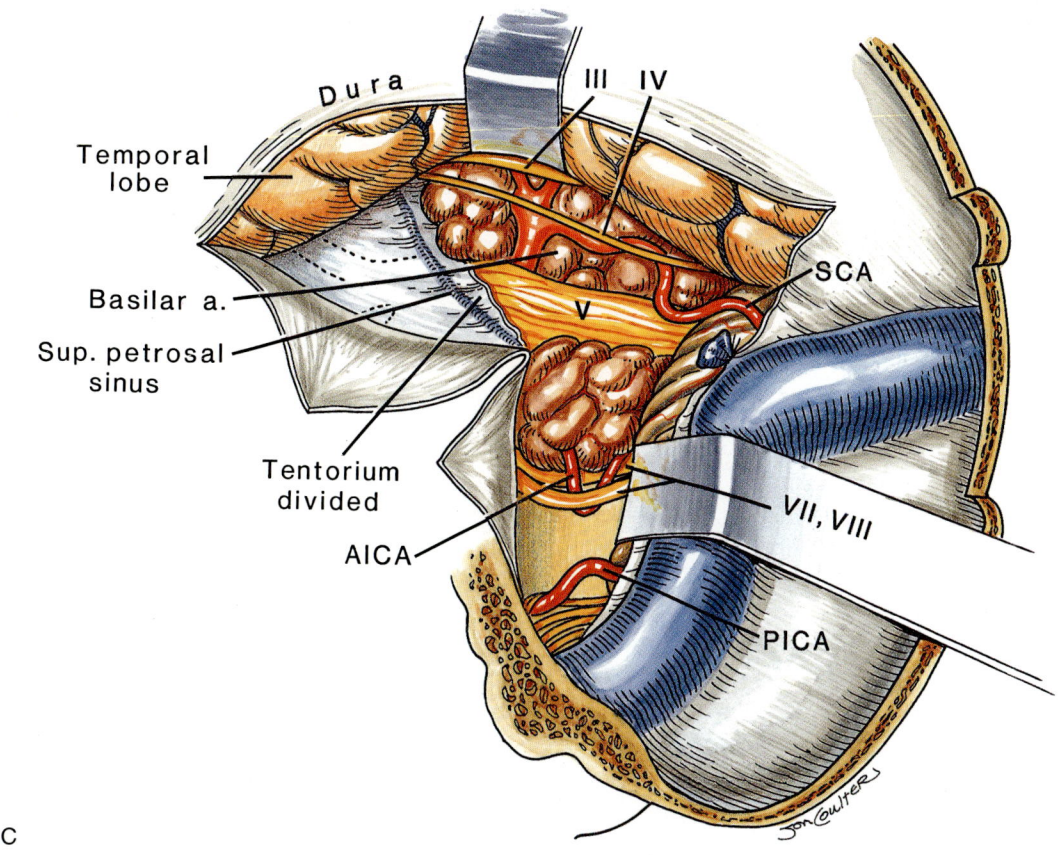

FIG. 7. *Continued.* **C:** The intradural exposure of the tumor. When the tumor extends well below the level of CNs VII and VIII, the surgeon will have to work retrosigmoid, or divide the sigmoid sinus (if it is nondominant and well collateralized).

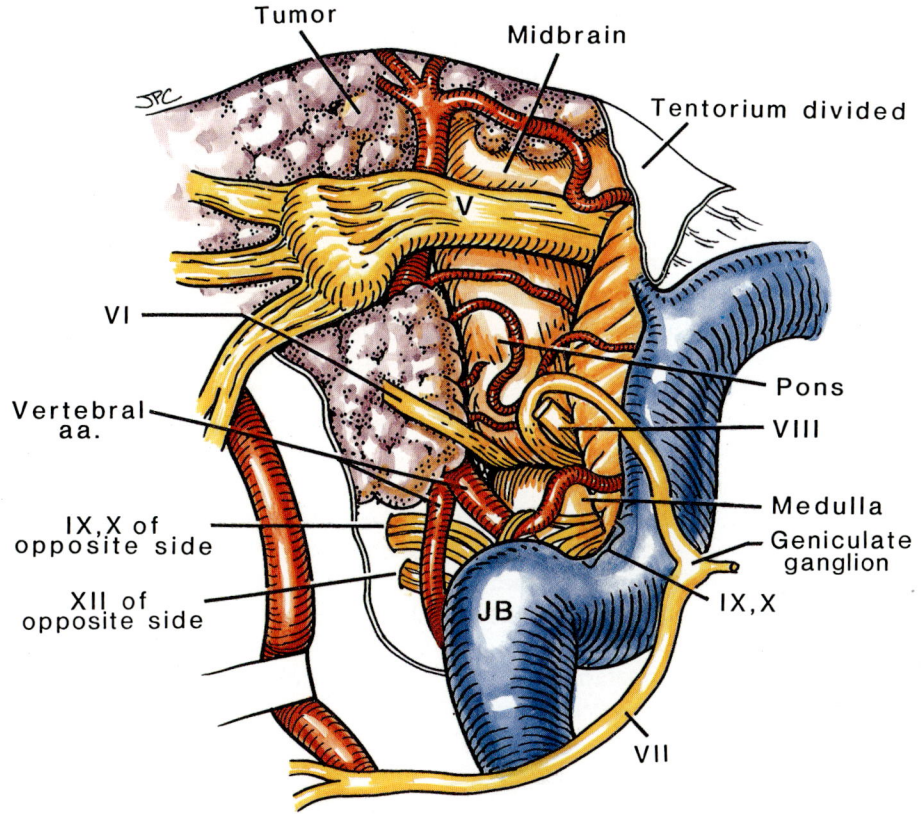

FIG. 8. Exposure obtained through total petrosectomy approach. The basilar artery and CN VI are encased by tumor. No graft was required for CN VII in this case.

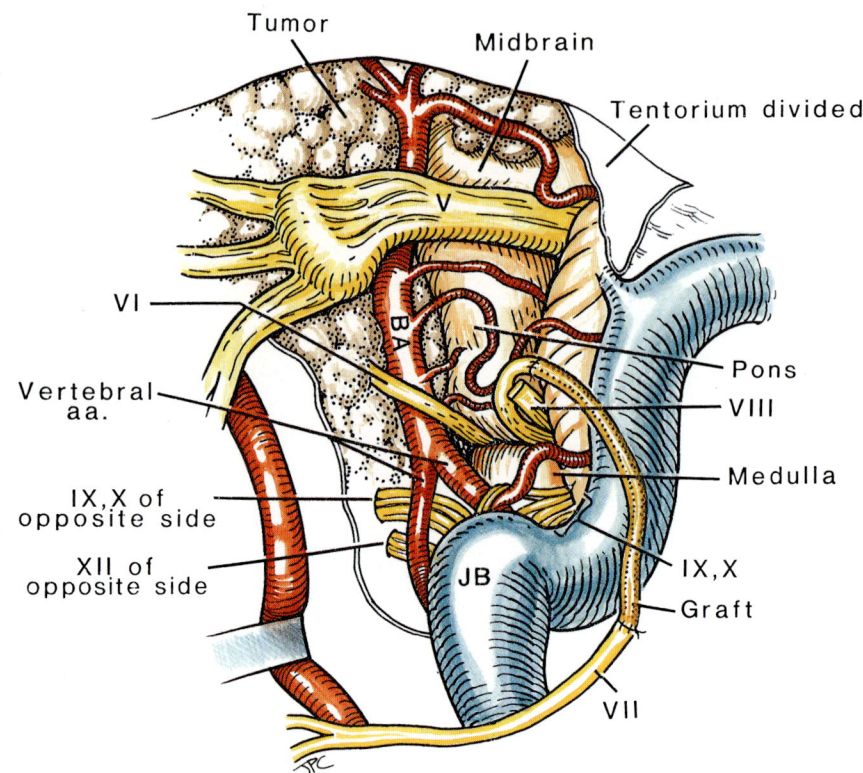

FIG. 9. Total petrosectomy approach for exposure of a giant petroclival meningioma. The petrous ICA has been displaced forward and the facial nerve displaced posteroinferiorly to improve exposure. The encased basilar artery is seen along with nerve grafting of the facial nerve. (From ref. 16, with permission.)

rior cavernous sinus, taking care to preserve CN VI. Reconstruction is performed by suturing a dural graft circumferentially to the defect (although a watertight closure is impossible). The dural closure is reinforced by reconstructing the extradural space using autologous fat and a temporalis muscle flap. The temporalis is rotated posteroinferiorly and sutured to the occipital and cervical muscles posteriorly, the temporal dura superiorly and parotid fascia inferiorly. Occasionally, when this does not suffice, a free rectus abdominis flap or another type of microvascular flap can be used to reconstruct this large defect (20). Although this approach provides the widest possible exposure of petroclival meningiomas, exposure of the ipsilateral lower clival area is limited inferiorly by the jugular bulb, and by CNs IX–XI, exiting the pars nervosa of the jugular foramen. This approach can be combined with the extreme lateral, transcondylar, transjugular approach to obtain lower exposure.

A prolonged postoperative facial paresis or palsy with some permanent loss of facial function always results from displacement of the facial nerve. Injury of the intrapetrous CN VII is common during this operation, and when it occurs, facial nerve reconstruction is performed by using an interposition graft. In our series, House grade III function has usually been achieved with grafting, equivalent to results obtained after facial nerve transposition. Complete loss of hearing is also an inevitable sequela of total petrosectomy. This limits its use to giant tumors where CN VIII is severely involved, or in patients with very difficult tumors such as those with scar from prior operation, or with basilar artery encasement.

Since the exposure itself may take from anywhere up to 6–7 hr, we usually postpone tumor resection until the second operation.

The extradural approaches to the clivus (transoral, transsphenoidal, transethmoidal, and bifrontal transbasal) are mentioned here for the sake of completeness. We do not usually use these approaches for intradural lesions. However, when used for midline intradural lesions by some surgeons (4), these approaches are fraught with complications related to CSF leakage. The only advantage they offer is that they require no brain retraction. These approaches can be used for resecting small midline tumors. However, their application is very limited because the exposure is restricted to the midline by the two ICAs, the surgeon is working at great depths in a very confined space, and dural repair is difficult at such depths, increasing the likelihood of CSF leak and subsequent meningitis. Since the neurovascular structures are not encountered until the completion of tumor resection, distortion of normal anatomy or the absence of a well-defined plane between tumor and brain stem poses a high risk of neurological damage. In contrast with the lateral approaches outlined here, the brain stem–tumor interface is well visualized allowing a good dissection.

TECHNICAL PRINCIPLES OF TUMOR RESECTION

It is important for the surgeon to formulate a well-defined plan for tumor excision preoperatively. This surgical strategy is based on the anatomical location of the tumor, the extent of neurovascular involvement, and the experience of the surgeon. The surgeon must decide whether the tumor can be removed by single approach, or multiple approaches, and if staged resection is necessary.

Staged resection of complicated skull base tumors depends to a large extent on the surgeon's personal preferences. We have routinely opted for staged resection of giant petroclival meningiomas and other skull base tumors for several important reasons. First, the operations are always long and tedious and prolonged anesthesia may result in a number of anesthesia-related complications postoperatively. Second, the surgical team may become fatigued during the most delicate part of the tumor resection. Furthermore, in our experience, there is a higher likelihood of obtaining a complete tumor resection when staging is used. Frequently, the exposure itself (e.g., total petrosectomy) can be such a lengthy procedure that it is better to close and begin the tumor resection at another time. The patient and immediate family members should be informed and psychologically prepared for the possibilities of requiring more than one operation for tumor removal.

It is important for the neurosurgeon to be physically and psychologically prepared for the possibility of intraoperative neurovascular injury and have the ability to repair injured blood vessels, including suture anastomosis and repair of cranial nerves with cable grafting.

Once tumor exposure has been obtained, it is important to spend a little time to become oriented to the distorted anatomy. Use of the monopolar nerve stimulator at this stage can be very helpful in the identification of cranial nerves, some of which may be very thin and splayed over the tumor capsule. The general principle of tumor resection includes early devascularization of the tumor if possible, and reducing tumor bulk by coring out the center of the tumor before attempting dissection from the brain stem. We initially work on the upper part of the tumor and thus obtain early control of its major vascular supply via the meningohypophyseal artery. Further control of the blood supply is obtained by disconnecting the tumor's attachment to the clival dura. The major drawback to initiating tumor resection with this approach is the high risk of injury to CN VI, since it runs through the central portion of the tumor, toward the cavernous sinus. In cases of basilar artery encasement, it is better to initially devascularize the tumor, as this makes subsequent vessel dissection somewhat easier.

Tumor resection is most effectively performed by a combination of bipolar cautery and suction irrigation. The ultrasonic aspirator has not been particularly helpful and is usually too large and cumbersome to use in these tumors, particularly when working close to the brain stem. The CO_2 laser can be very effective for coring out vascular or firm tumors or removing tumor from restricted spaces. When using the laser, one has to be extremely careful to prevent injury to exposed cranial nerves, artery, and brain stem from direct or reflected laser beam. Injury to the abducens and the facial nerves occurred in two cases in our series from reflected laser beam. The most crucial part of the tumor removal involves dissection of tumor from the brain stem, encased arteries, and nerves. This is best done using sharp dissection with the aid of an irrigating bipolar cautery.

For vascular and cranial nerve encasements, it is important to start working from areas of normal anatomy and to follow the neurovascular structures into the tumor. Frequently, a nice plane can be developed between tumor and blood vessel wall because of the arachnoidal membrane surrounding the blood vessel. Tumor bleeding during this part of surgery can make the dissection very difficult, pointing out the importance of early tumor devascularization. The most difficult aspect of resection of tumors with basilar artery encasement concerns the fate of the perforating vessels. Every effort must be made to carefully dissect and preserve all basilar artery perforators. A significant brain stem stroke can occur after injury to a single perforator. Reconstruction of these small arteries is still a problem that needs to be solved. Basilar artery laceration can be repaired by resuture, and injury to larger branches of the basilar artery can be repaired by reanastomosis. In cases where the basilar artery or nerves are encased by the tumor, it is best to start by disconnection of the tumor from the clival and tentorial dura before debulking the core of the tumor. Cranial nerve preservation in cases of complete encasement can be a difficult task. It is important to adhere to the same principles of dissection from normal to abnormal anatomy, carefully peeling away tumor from the nerve with the help of neurophysiological monitoring. The dissected nerve must be protected by a thin rubber sheet to prevent inadvertent injury during surgery. In cases where the nerve cannot be preserved, either end-to-end anastomosis or cable grafting can be performed using the greater auricular nerve or sural nerve as interposition graft.

Dissection of the tumor from the brain stem is best performed using sharp dissection, with the aid of a fine suction and the Malis irrigating bipolar cautery. Usually, there is a subarachnoid plane that can be developed between the tumor and pia of the brain stem. Sometimes, this plane is absent in those cases of giant-sized tumors and those that have been previously operated. The existence of this subarachnoid plane between the tumor and brain stem can frequently be predicted on the preoperative MRI scan. When a subarachnoid plane is absent, and dissection is difficult, occasionally it is necessary to leave a small piece of tumor on the brain stem.

RECONSTRUCTION

Reconstruction of the cranial base is just as important as the other aspects of skull base surgery. Inadequate reconstruction may result in postoperative CSF leakage, life-threatening intracranial infection, and prolonged hospital stay. The key points to preventing CSF leaks and central nervous system infections are to have as watertight a dural closure as possible, to ensure large cranial base defects are covered by well-vascularized tissues, and to manage elevated CSF pressure with adequate drainage. Common sources for CSF leaks include the eustachian tube and sphenoid sinus. The incidence of CSF leaks is higher with the complex approaches, and it is often necessary to use either a temporalis muscle rotation flap or free rectus/pectoralis muscle flap to cover the defect.

Some of these patients may develop a communicating hydrocephalus postoperatively, which may cause a secondary CSF leak. A spinal fluid drain, ventriculostomy, or a shunt may help control CSF pressure long enough to enable the area of the leak to seal. However, in most patients with preoperative obstructive hydrocephalus, a shunt is inserted preoperatively. In cases of progressive postoperative hydrocephalus, permanent shunt placement is recommended to prevent late recurrence of CSF leaks.

Postoperative Management and Rehabilitation

Patients are managed in the intensive care unit until neurological and vital signs have stabilized. It is important to check for the function of CNs IX–XI before initiating feeding. There should be no hesitation in performing a tracheostomy in patients with symptoms or signs of lower cranial nerve palsy. In cases presenting with paralysis of CNs IX, X, and XII, a tracheostomy may be performed as a part of the initial surgery. This will protect against aspiration and assist with pulmonary toilet in the immediate postoperative period. In these patients, a feeding gastrostomy or jejunostomy is also performed at the same time in order to initiate feeding at the earliest opportunity. Central hyperalimentation is rarely necessary. Patients with complete facial palsy or corneal anesthesia are at risk of exposure keratitis. They must be started on a regime of artificial tear drops and ointments, and usually either a lateral tarsorrhaphy or eyelid gold weight insertion is performed.

Postoperative pulmonary embolism is a frequent complication, occurring in 38% of the Al-Mefty series (1). This may be related to several factors including postsurgical hypercoaguable state, the length of the operation, and postsurgical immobilization. In most patients, deep venous thrombosis is prevented by the use of intermittent pneumatic compression of the lower extremities both intraoperatively and postoperatively, and low-dose subcutaneous heparin postoperatively. Rehabilitation therapy is begun as soon as the patient's medical condition has stabilized. The patient and family members should be well informed about the importance of an extended period of rehabilitation upon discharge from the hospital.

ILLUSTRATIVE CASE REPORTS

P.B.: Total Petrosectomy and Extreme Lateral Transcondylar Approach

This 45-year-old woman was referred with progressive tumor growth and hemiparesis. She had previously undergone partial tumor resection at another institution and two treatments with proton beam radiation. Upon admission, she had anacusis on the right, paresis of CNs VI, VII, IX, and X, and left hemiparesis. MRI scan showed a 3.5-cm petroclival meningioma, involving the

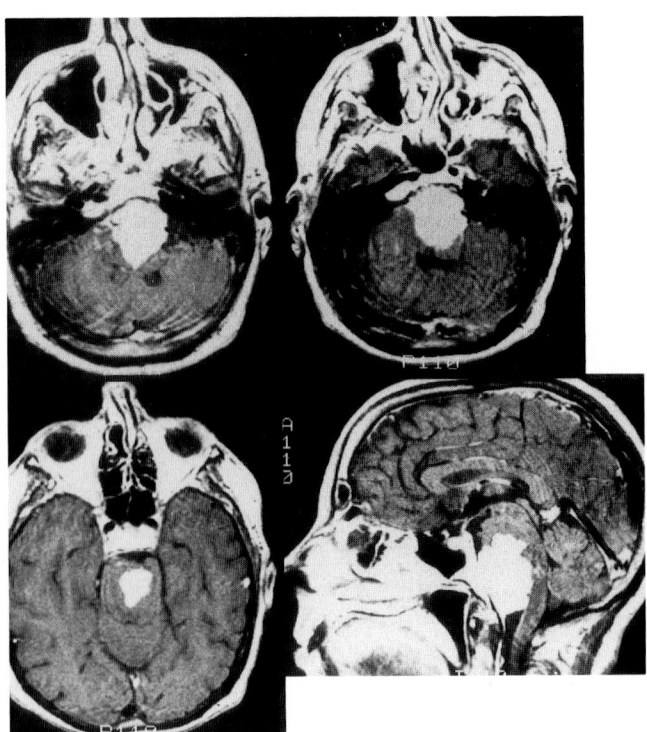

FIG. 10. (Figures 10–12 are of patient P.B.) Preoperative axial and sagittal MRI scans with intravenous contrast showing a large meningioma of the middle and lower clivus with extension to the foramen magnum (**bottom right**). Note a small island of tumor causing marked indentation of the brain stem at the superior aspect of the tumor (**bottom left**).

middle and lower clivus with invagination of tumor into the pons and encasement of the basilar artery (Fig. 10). The tumor was initially approached through a total petrosectomy. At surgery, the basilar artery and its branches were encased by a very fibrotic tumor, and all except one perforator vessel were successfully dissected free from the tumor. No subarachnoid plane was present between the tumor and the brain stem, but dissection was possible with difficulty. The upper 75% of the tumor was resected by the petrosectomy approach (Fig. 11). Residual tumor at the level of the foramen magnum was removed using the extreme lateral transcondylar approach. Postoperatively, she remained hemiparetic, with paralysis of CNs VI and VII (transected and reconstructed with nerve graft) and increased weakness of CNs IX and X, necessitating a tracheostomy. Postoperative MRI scan with intravenous contrast showed complete tumor resection (Fig. 12). Six months later, her hemiparesis was improving, and facial nerve recovery was in progress. This case highlights the difficulties associated with operating on patients who have undergone previous surgery and especially prior radiation therapy, and the benefits of optimal tumor exposure in such cases.

I.F.: Total Petrosectomy Plus a Subtemporal Transzygomatic Approach

This 61-year-old woman underwent a ventriculoperitoneal shunt 5 years previously for hydrocephalus associated with a petroclival meningioma, thought to be inoperable. Due to progressive tumor growth, she became quadriplegic, unable to speak or swallow, and suffered an episode of aspiration pneumonia. Shortly after admission to our institution, she had a respiratory arrest, which required a tracheostomy and ventilatory assistance. Upon examination, she was awake and yet could only communicate by blinking her eyes (Fig. 13). There was paralysis of lateral eye movement, paralysis of CNs IV–VII on the right, V_1 on the left, and IX and X bilaterally. She was quadriplegic except for slight movements of her left fingers. The tumor had almost doubled in size over the last 5 years and was now involving the whole clivus, petrous apex, tentorial notch, and cavernous sinus (Figs. 14 and 15). Angiography showed that the basilar artery was narrowed and displaced by the tumor (Fig. 16). The tumor was removed in three stages. Initially, the upper third was resected by a subtemporal transzygomatic approach. At surgery, the basilar artery was noted to be completely encased, and its upper third was dissected free from the heavily calcified and vascular tumor (Figs. 17 and 18). Because of the basilar artery encasement, a total petrosectomy approach was chosen. The remaining tumor was removed by a total petrosectomy approach in two stages (Figs. 19–21). The entire basilar artery and its branches that were encased by the tumor were successfully dissected free. One anterior–inferior cerebellar artery was injured in the process. The ipsilateral CNs V–VIII had been invaded and destroyed by the tumor beyond salvage and were therefore removed. Facial nerve graft reconstruction was not possible since the nerve was invaded by tumor up to its exit from the brain stem. Postoperative CT scans have not shown any tumor recurrence (Fig. 22). At 1 year postoperatively, she had recovered completely from her quadriparesis and had returned to independent living at home (Fig. 23).

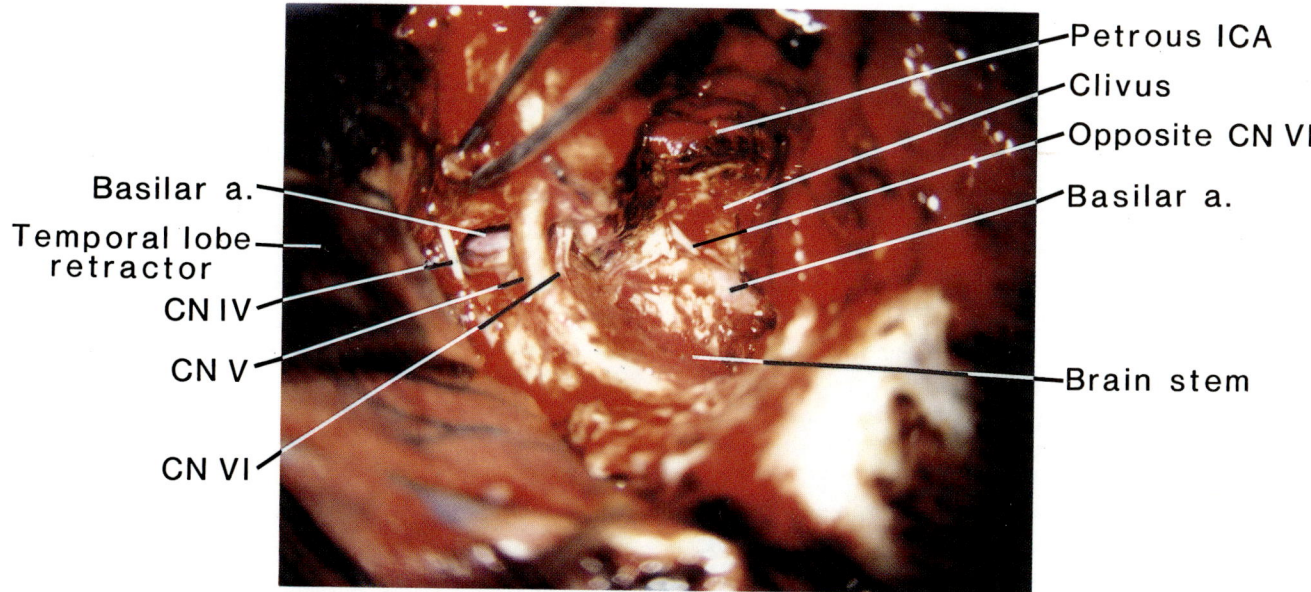

FIG. 11. Patient P.B. Tumor exposure obtained after total petrosectomy approach and resection of the upper three-quarters of tumor. Tumor dissection from the brain stem and vessels was very difficult due to prior surgeries and radiation therapy. An additional operation by the extreme lateral approach was necessary to remove the remaining lower one-quarter of the tumor.

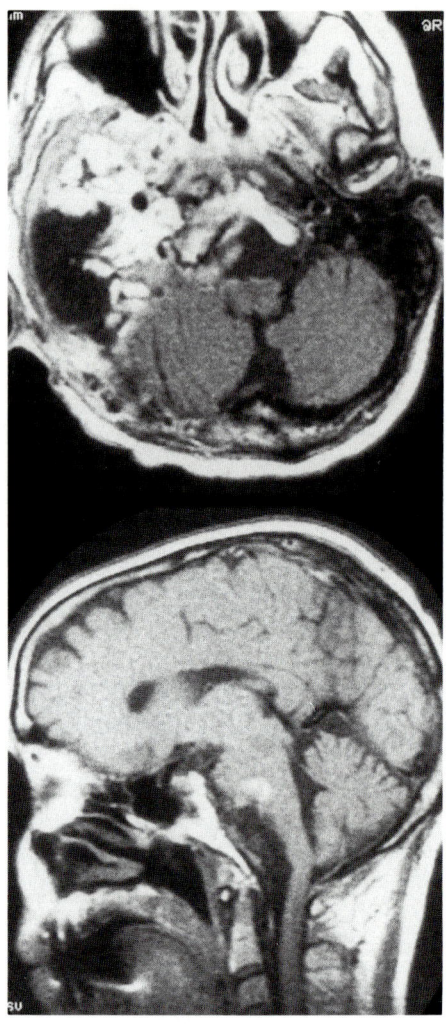

FIG. 12. Patient P.B. Postoperative axial and sagittal MRI scans showing complete tumor resection. A small blood clot is present where the superior aspect of the tumor was indenting the brain stem (**bottom**).

P.E.: Subtemporal/Preauricular Infratemporal Approach Plus a Retrosigmoid Approach

This 36-year-old woman was seen at another hospital with a history of diplopia. Discovery of a large petroclival meningioma led to two unsuccessful attempts at tumor resection followed by radiation therapy. Upon referral to us, she exhibited partial deficits of CNs III, V, and VII and absent hearing on the left. MRI scan showed a large petroclival meningioma involving the entire clivus and the left cavernous sinus, sella, Meckel's cave, and internal acoustic meatus with encasement of the ICA and basilar artery (Fig. 24). The tentorial branch of the meningohypophyseal artery was the major blood supply to the tumor (Fig. 25). Surgery was performed in two stages. During the first operation, the subtemporal preauricular infratemporal approach was employed (Fig.

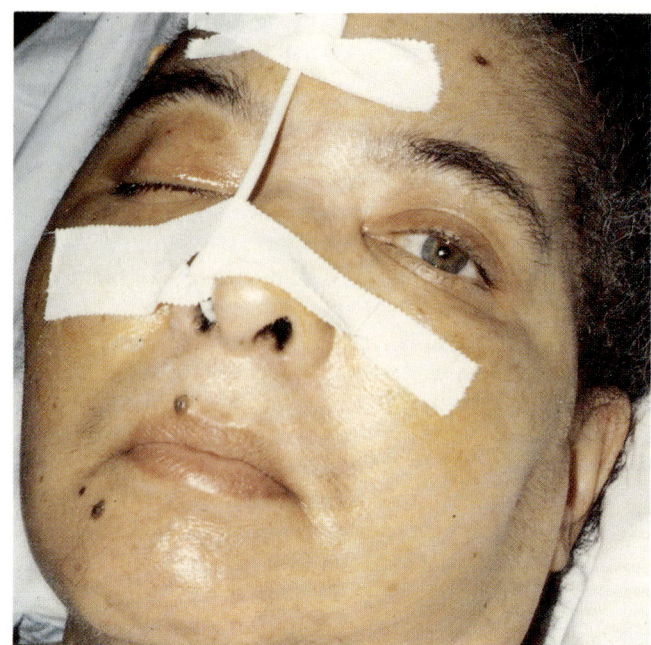

FIG. 13. (Figures 13–23 are of patient I.F.) Preoperative photograph of patient with tracheostomy and ventilator dependent. She is receiving alimentation through a nasogastric tube.

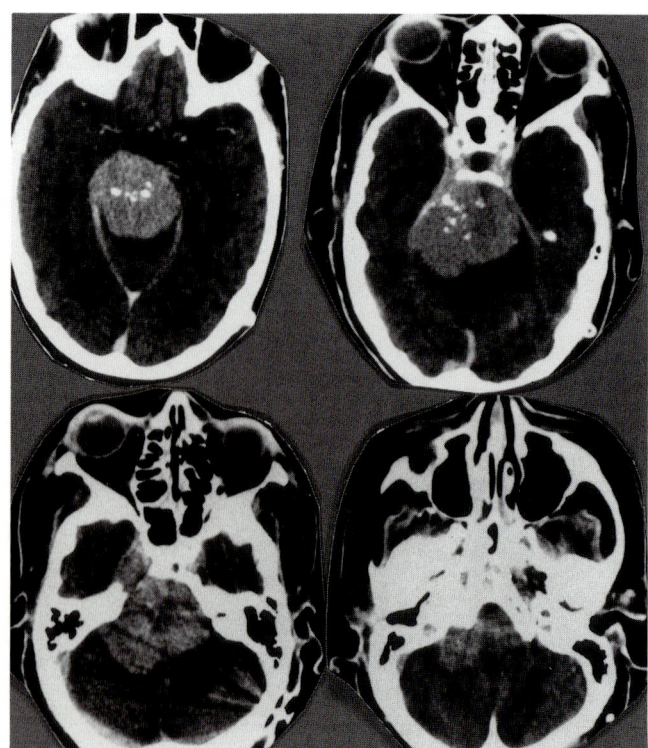

FIG. 14. Axial CT scans with intravenous contrast show a giant petroclival meningioma with extension into the cavernous sinus. Note that specks of calcification are present within the tumor.

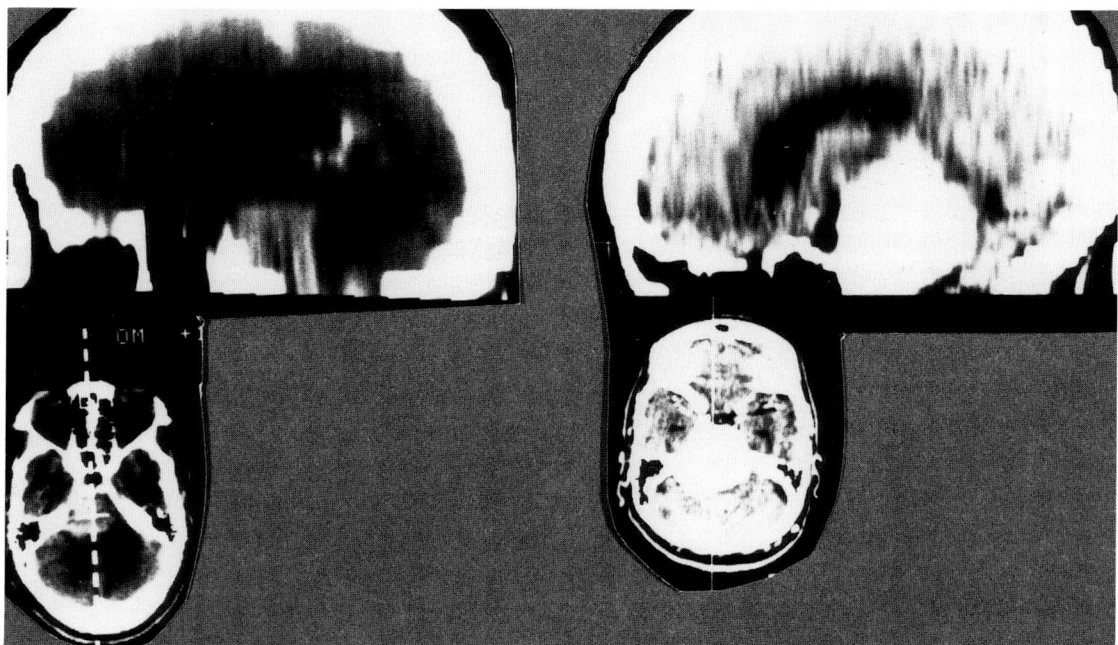

FIG. 15. Sagittal reconstruction of CT scans performed 4 years apart showing the increase in tumor size during this interval. Left, I.F. 1984, right, I.F. 1988.

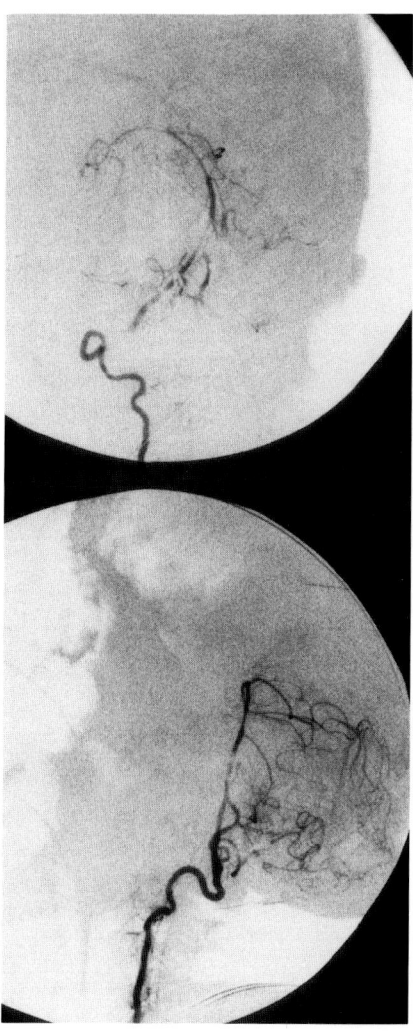

FIG. 16. AP and lateral cerebral angiograms following vertebral artery injection showing basilar artery displacement with stenosis of the distal basilar artery and its branches from tumor encasement.

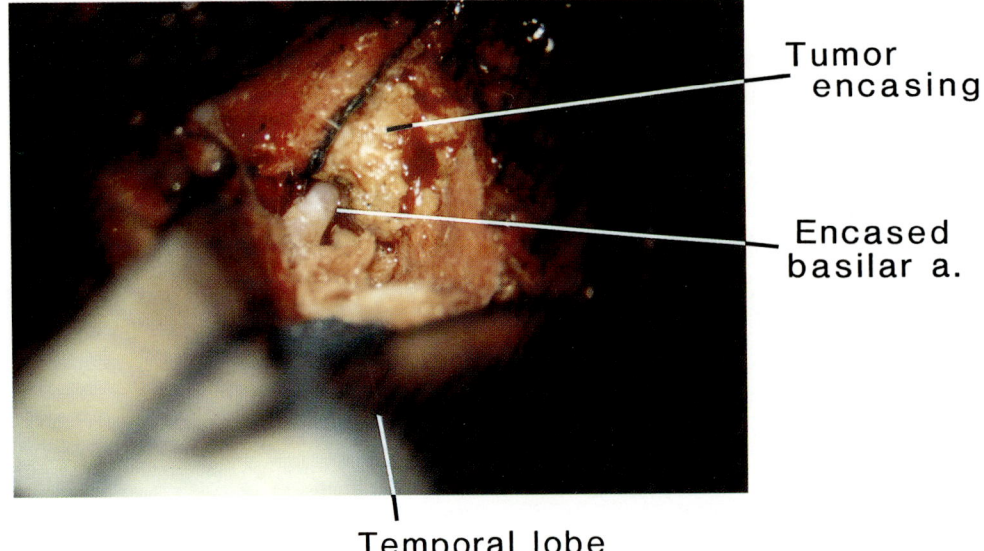

FIG. 17. During the first operation by a subtemporal transzygomatic approach, tumor encasement of the basilar artery is apparent.

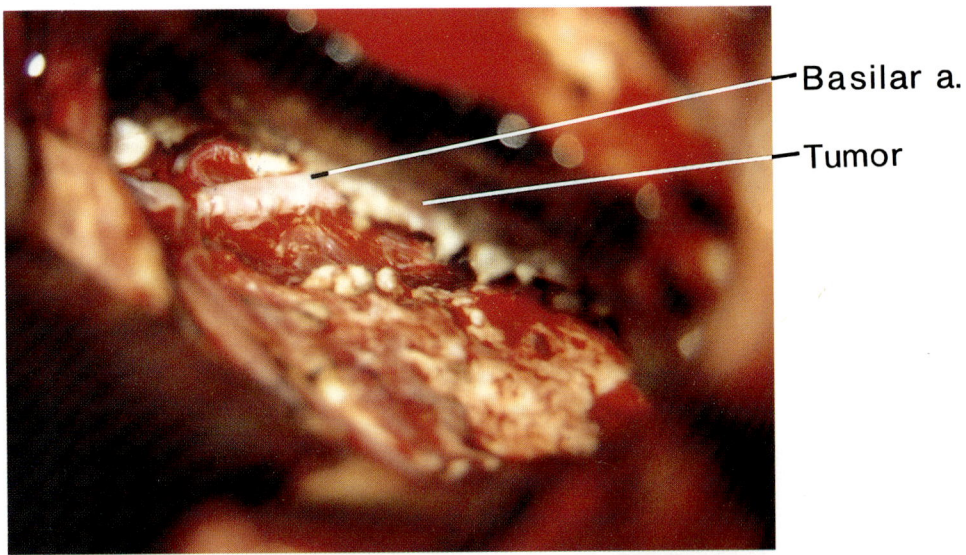

FIG. 18. At the end of the first operation, the upper portion of the basilar artery has been dissected free of tumor. The tumor was very firm in consistency with considerable calcification. It was apparent that adequate exposure may permit complete tumor removal. Because of this, a total petrosectomy was performed during a separate approach.

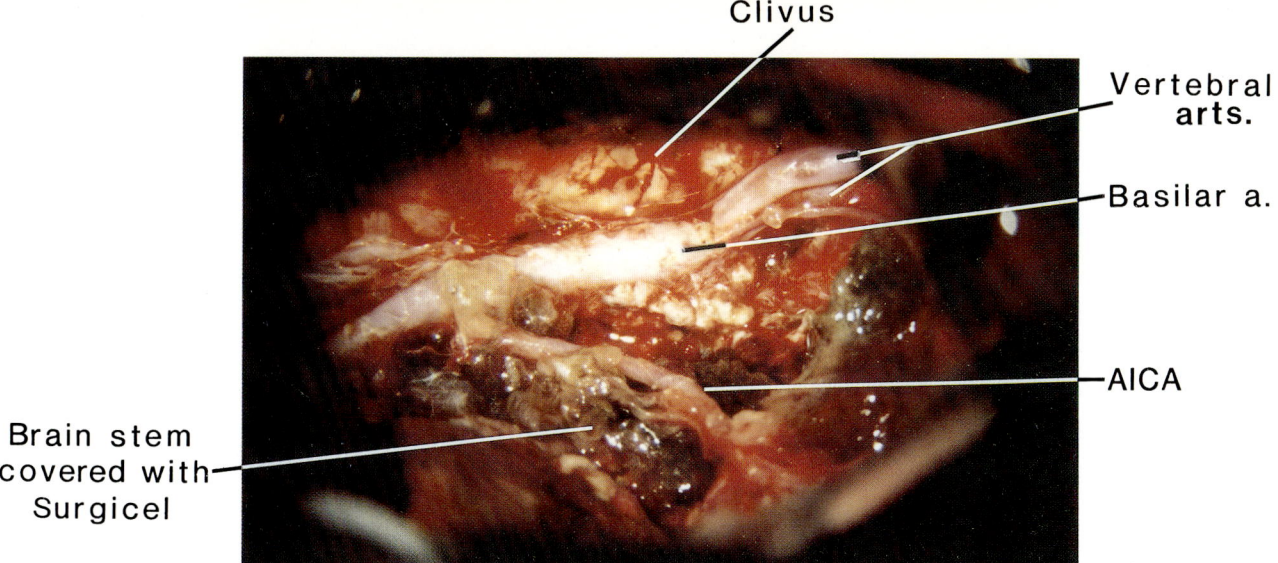

FIG. 19. At the end of the third operation, complete tumor resection has been accomplished in the clival area with successful dissection of basilar artery and its perforators from the surrounding tumor. Ipsilateral CNs V–VIII were invaded by tumor and had to be excised. This figure displays the vertebrobasilar junction, basilar artery, and clival dura. AICA, anterior inferior cerebellar artery.

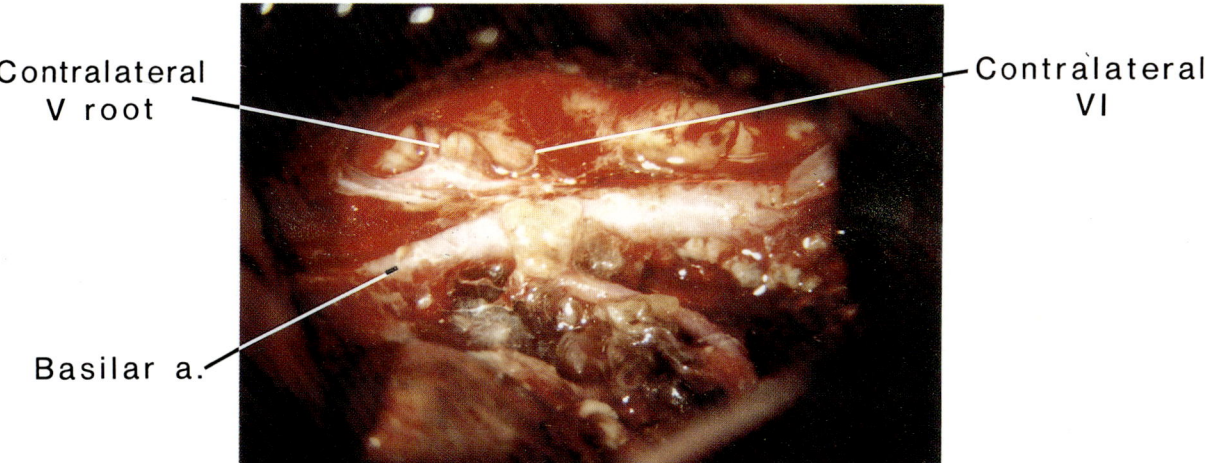

FIG. 20. Contralateral trigeminal nerve and abducens nerve.

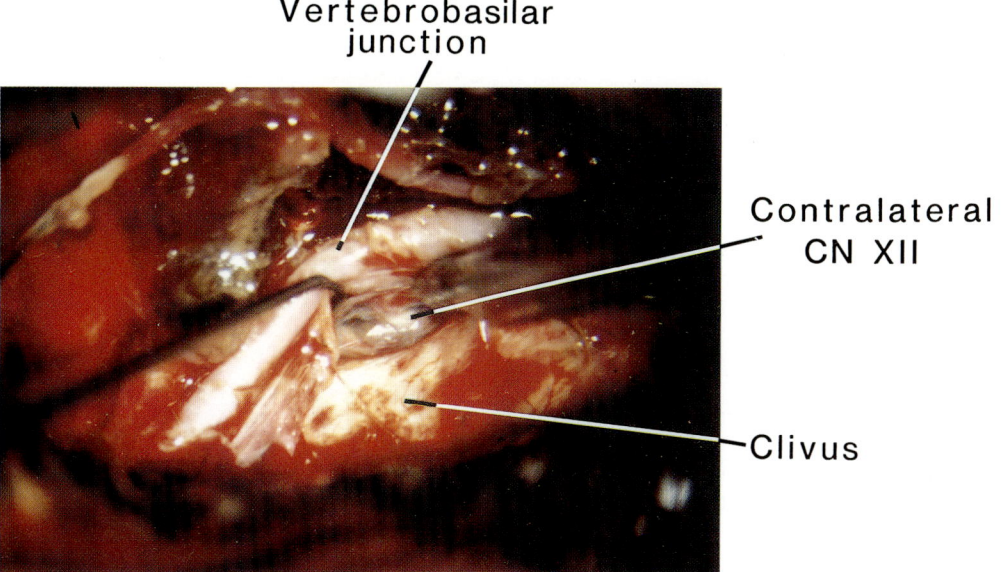

FIG. 21. Contralateral hypoglossal nerve under the arachnoid membrane after displacement of the vertebrobasilar junction.

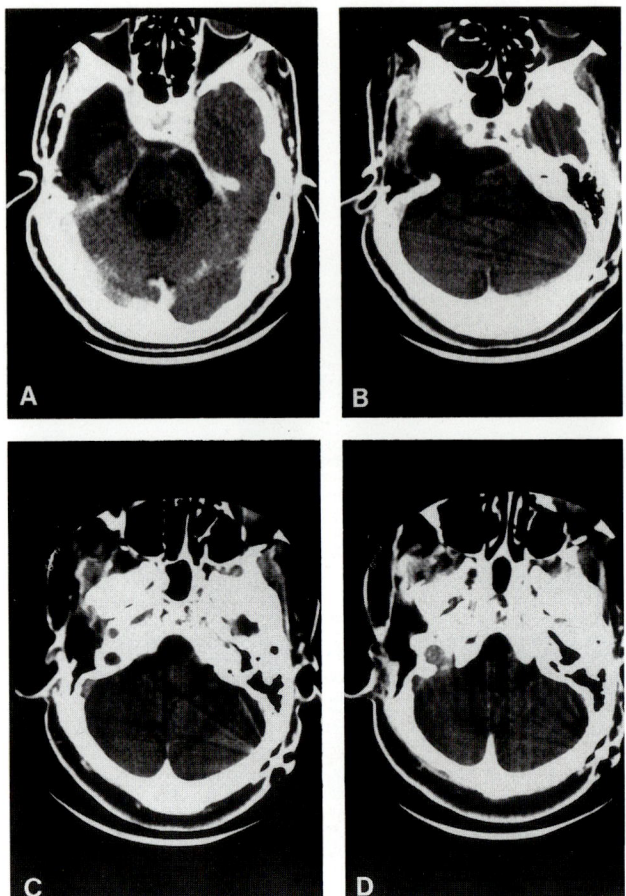

FIG. 22. Postoperative axial CT scans with contrast showing gross total tumor removal. Note the extent of petrous bone removal achieved by the total petrosectomy approach (**A–D**).

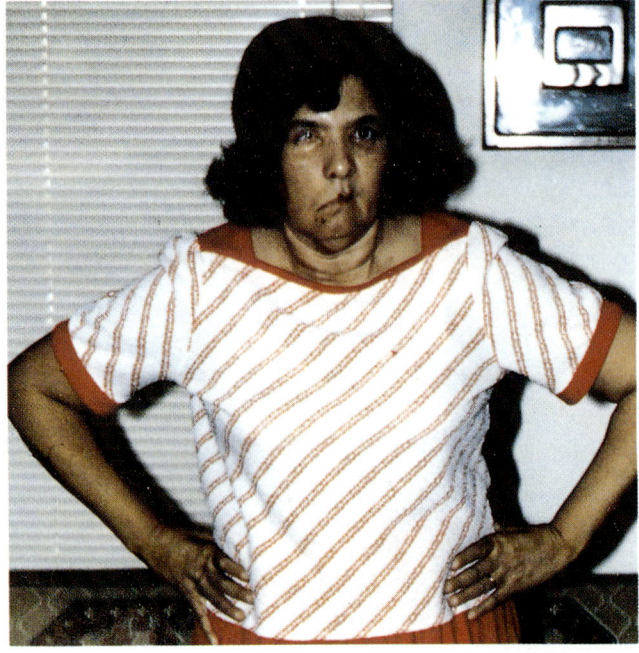

FIG. 23. Postoperative photograph shows persistent right facial palsy. The patient is functional at home.

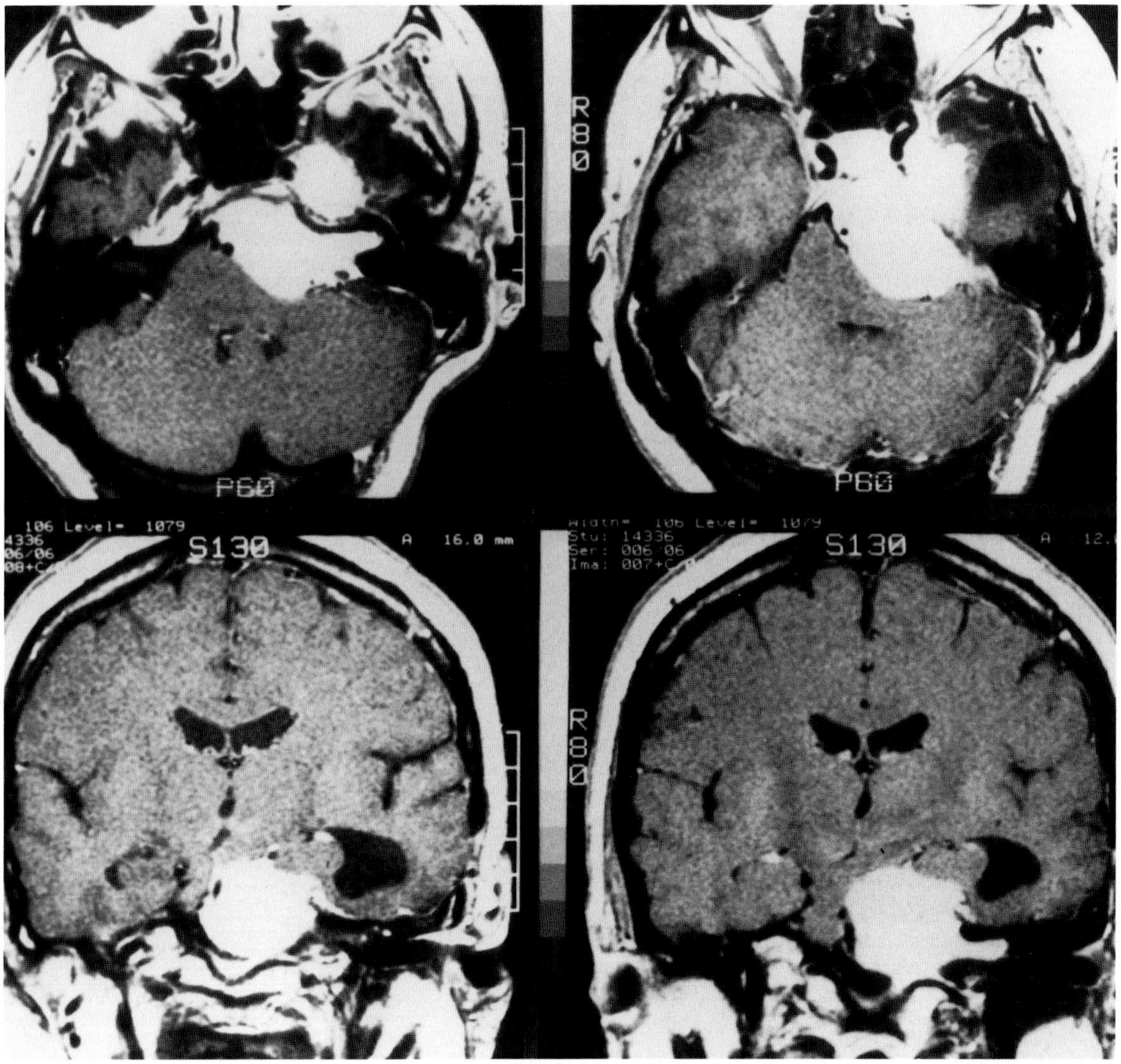

FIG. 24. (Figures 24–34 are of patient P.E.) Preoperative axial and coronal MRI scans with intravenous contrast show a giant petroclival meningioma with involvement of the left cavernous sinus, Meckel's cave, and a small tongue of tumor extending into the internal auditory canal. Note encasement and stenosis of the basilar artery and ICA by the tumor (**top right**).

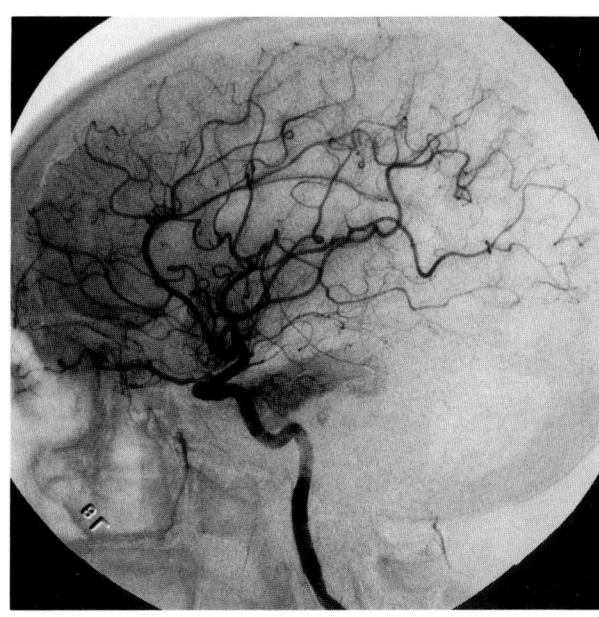

FIG. 25. Carotid angiogram showing tumor blood supply by the tentorial branch of the meningohypophyseal artery.

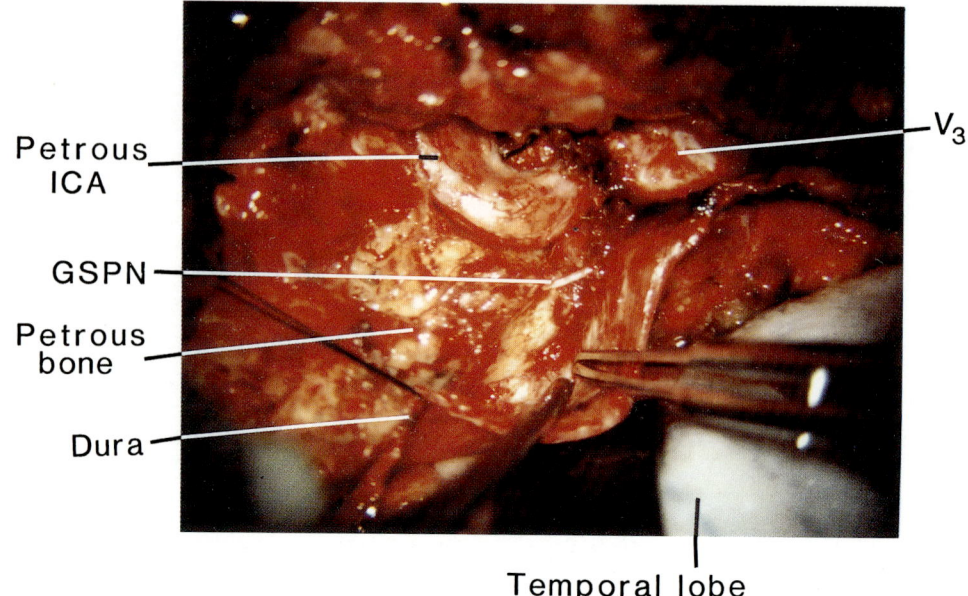

FIG. 26. Preauricular infratemporal and subtemporal approach showing the extradural exposure of the petrous ICA after removal of overlying bone. The ascending genu and horizontal segment of petrous ICA are seen, along with related anatomical landmarks.

26), and the tumor was removed from the cavernous sinus and clivus area. The intracavernous ICA was lacerated during tumor resection and required resuture. CN VI was injured (Fig. 27) but was reconstructed by end-to-end anastomosis. Scar tissue from prior operation and the basilar artery encasement made the procedure difficult (Figs. 28 and 29). After this operation, tumor remained in the internal auditory canal and the cerebellopontine angle (Fig. 30). This required a second operation by a retrosigmoid approach for complete removal (Figs. 31 and 32). At 1 year postoperatively, the patient had a mild paresis of CN III but had recovery of CN VI function (Fig. 33) and returned to her prior vocation (Karnofsky 80). CT scan and MRI scan did not show any evidence of tumor (Fig. 34).

F.B.: Extreme Lateral Transcondylar Approach

This 47-year-old woman presented with a 6-week history of headaches, unsteady gait, and urinary incontinence. MRI scan showed a meningioma growing from the lower clivus foramen magnum, extending down to C2 encasing the vertebral artery (Fig. 35). Following pre-

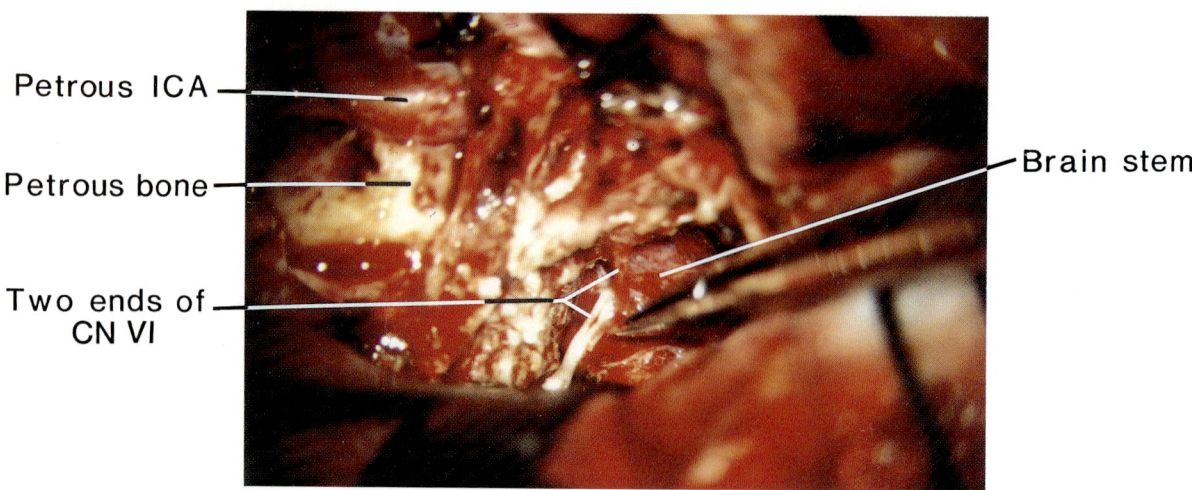

FIG. 27. Exposure of petrous ICA and intradural exposure of the two ends of the abducens nerve brought together (not sutured yet) after tumor resection.

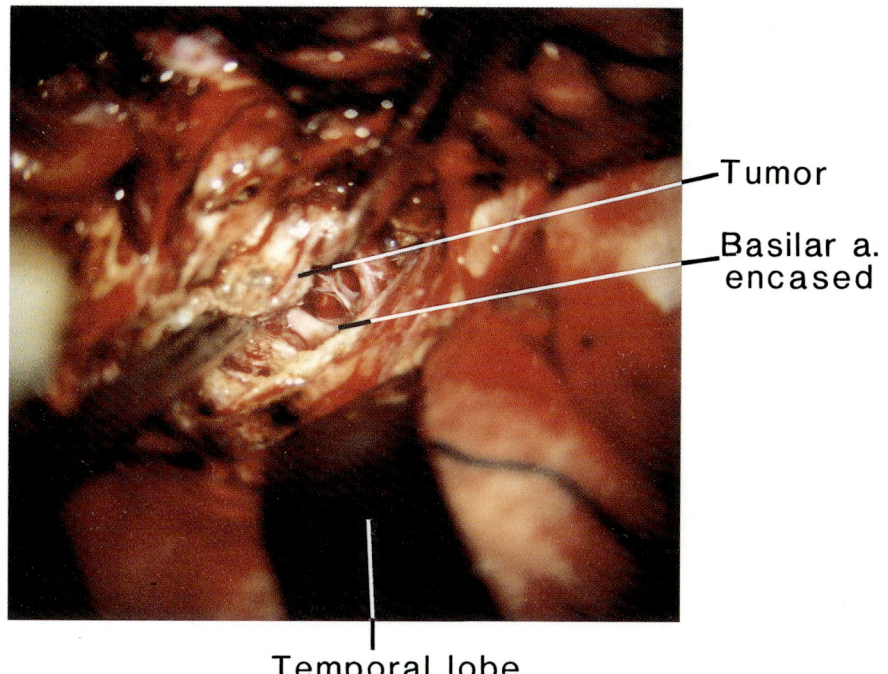

FIG. 28. Distal basilar artery encased by the tumor.

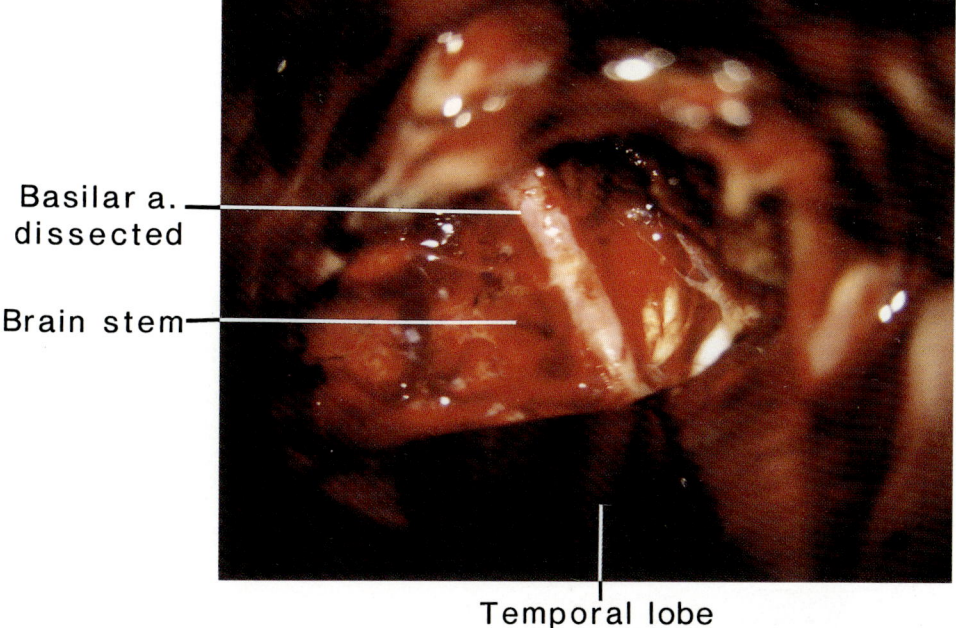

FIG. 29. Basilar artery dissected free of tumor and the brain stem.

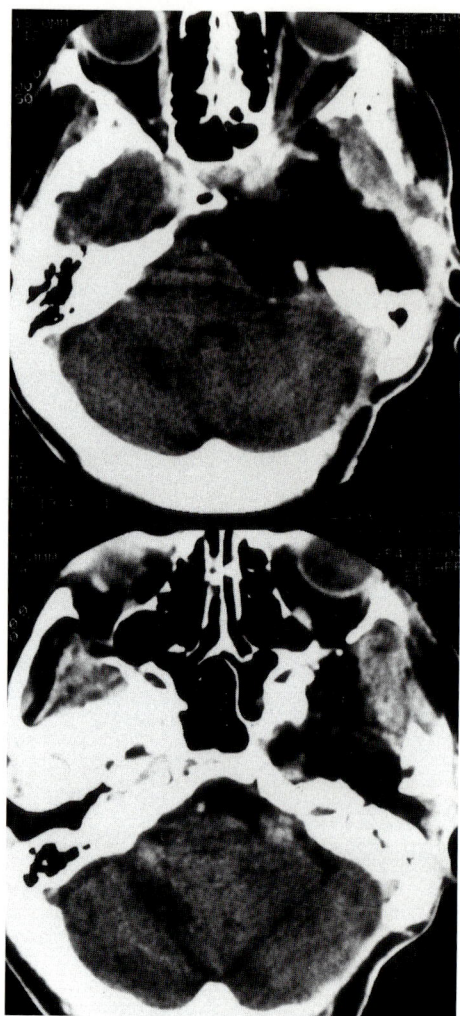

FIG. 30. Axial CT scan (**top**) shows the extent of bone removal during partial petrosectomy. The enhanced axial CT scan (**bottom**) shows the residual tumor in the internal auditory canal and cerebellopontine angle. This was removed at a second stage through a retrosigmoid approach.

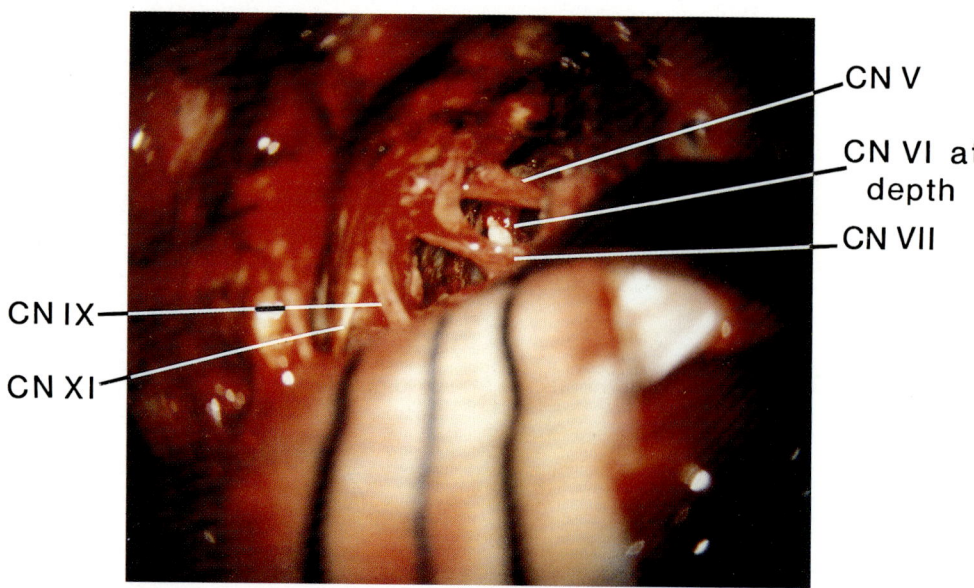

FIG. 31. During the second operation (retrosigmoid approach), residual tumor is seen around CNs V, VII, and VIII. The tumor is extending into the internal auditory canal. The sutured ends of CN VI are seen in the depth of the operative field.

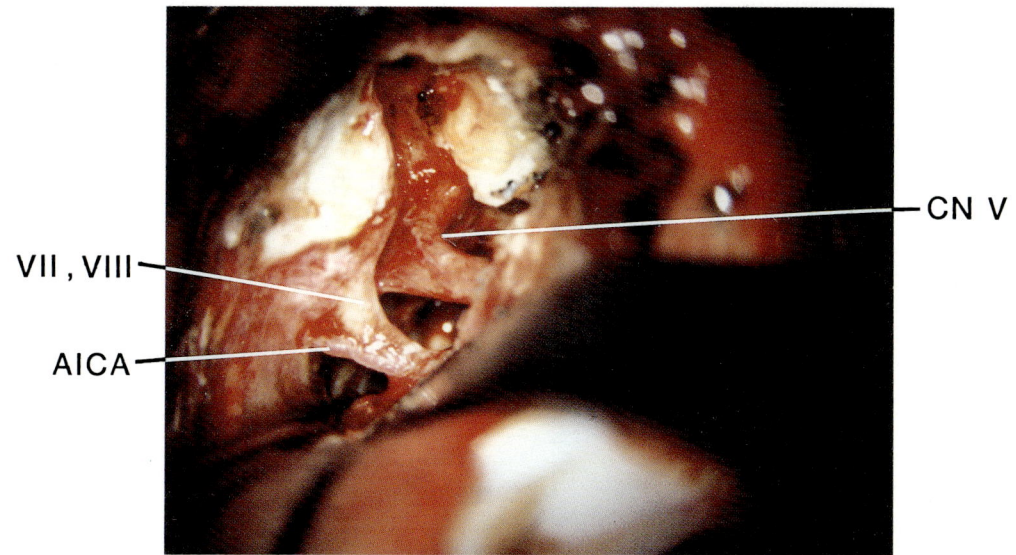

FIG. 32. The posterior aspect of the porus acusticus has been drilled away. The trigeminal nerve (CNV) is seen to be pushed downward toward the internal auditory canal and then courses upward. CNs VII and VIII and the anterior inferior cerebellar artery (AICA) are also seen.

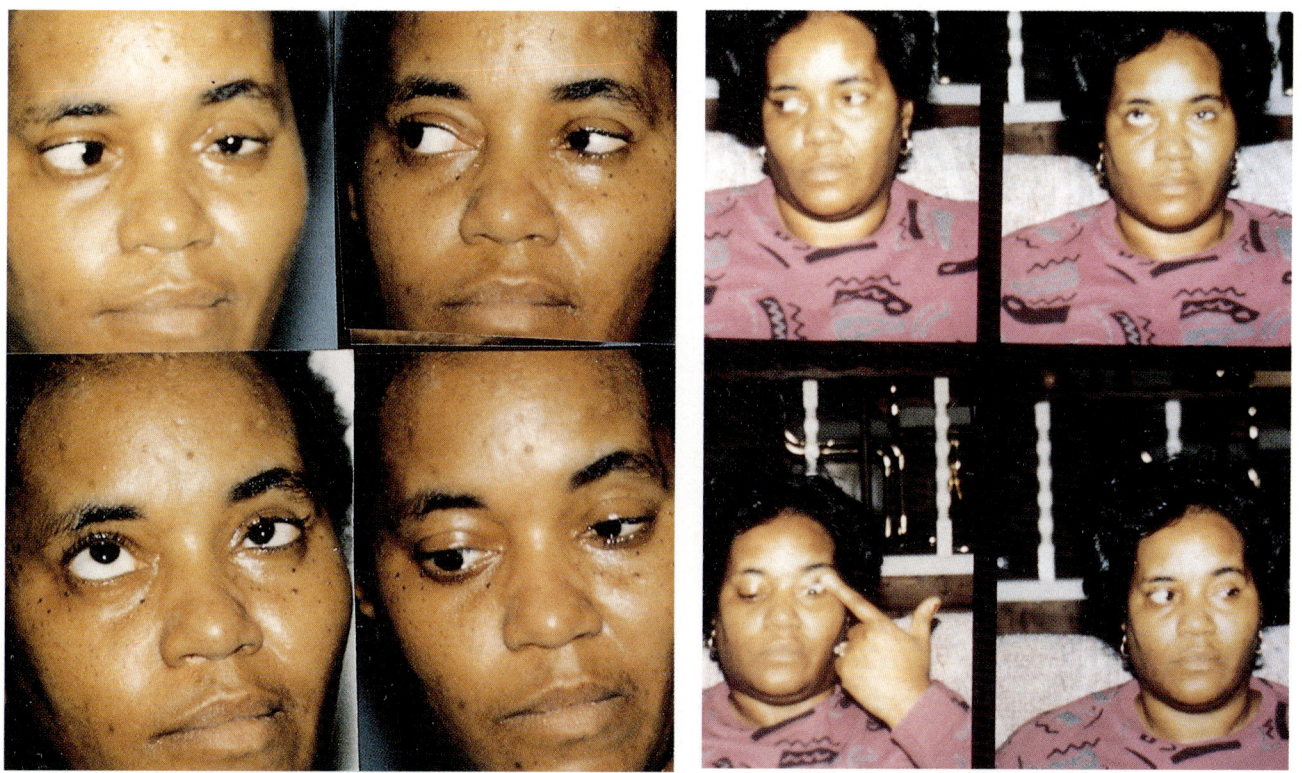

FIG. 33. Lateral rectus weakness immediately after surgery (**A**) and subsequent postoperative recovery of VIth nerve function (**B**).

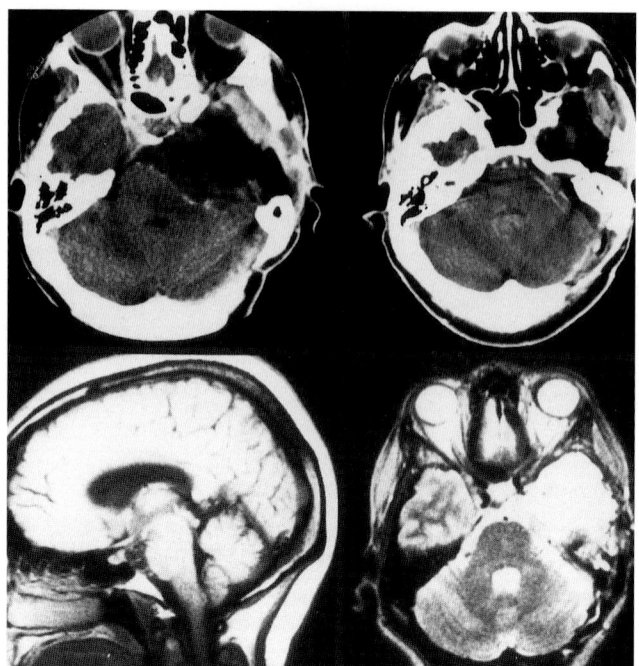

FIG. 34. Postoperative CT scans (**top**) and MRI scans (**bottom**) show total tumor excision.

operative embolization of tumor blood supply (via the ascending pharyngeal artery), the tumor was exposed by the extreme lateral transcondylar approach. At surgery, the tumor was dissected off the encased vertebral artery and CNs IX, X, and XII, with preservation of these neurovascular structures (Figs. 36–43). She had temporary postoperative left vocal cord paresis. Postoperative CT scans at 3 months showed complete tumor excision (Fig. 44). She has returned to her preoperative functional level (Karnofsky 90).

J.K.: Frontotemporal and Preauricular Infratemporal Approach with Clipping of an Anterior Communicating Artery Aneurysm and Vertebrobasilar Fenestration Aneurysm

This 54-year-old woman developed progressive diplopia and ptosis of the right eye for 2 years. Neurological examination was unremarkable, except for a subtotal right CN III palsy. Preoperative evaluation with MRI scans showed a right petroclival meningioma, involving the cavernous sinus, sella, and Meckel's cave (Fig. 45).

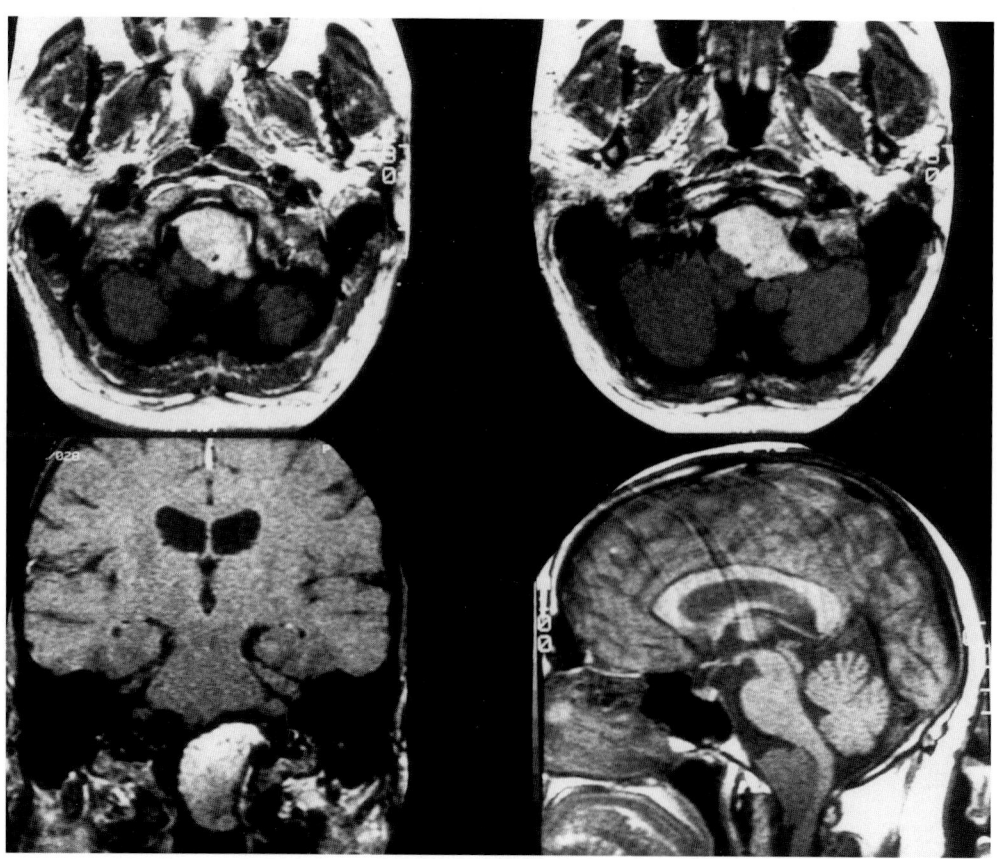

FIG. 35. (Figures 35–44 are of patient F.B.) Preoperative axial, coronal, and sagittal MRI scans showing a meningioma of the lower clivus and foramen magnum. Note encasement of the vertebral artery (**top left** and **bottom left**) The cervicomedullary junction is severely compressed (**bottom right**).

PETROCLIVAL MENINGIOMAS / 631

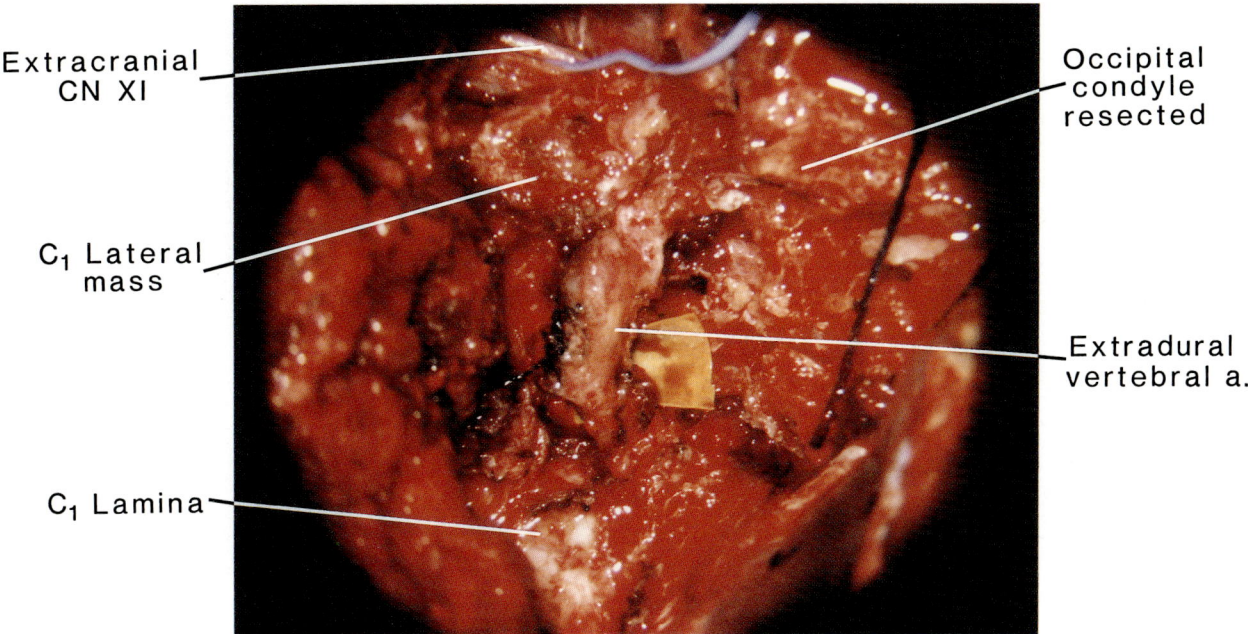

FIG. 36. Extradural exposure obtained through the extreme lateral transcondylar approach. The extradural vertebral artery and extracranial spinal accessory nerve are visible. The occipital condyle and lateral mass of C1 have been partially resected along with partial C1 laminectomy.

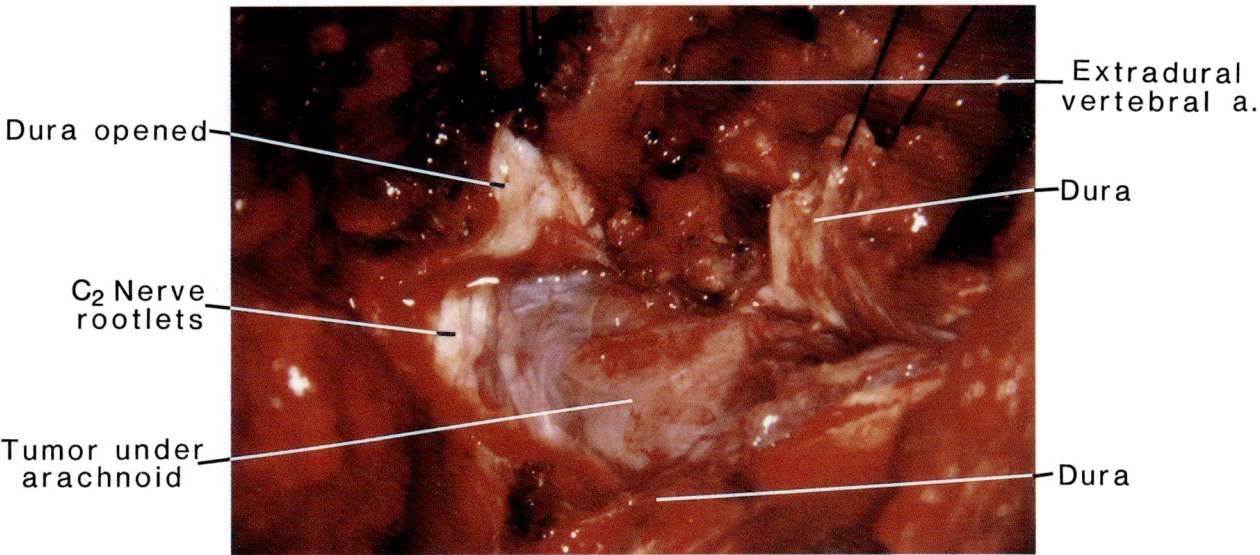

FIG. 37. The dura has been opened along with opening of the dural ring at the entrance of the vertebral artery into the posterior fossa. Tumor is visible in the subdural space. The rootlets of C2 are also seen. The first cervical rootlets and denticulate ligaments are divided. Note that the spinomedullary junction lies inferiorly and is not even seen at this stage; therefore no retraction is required.

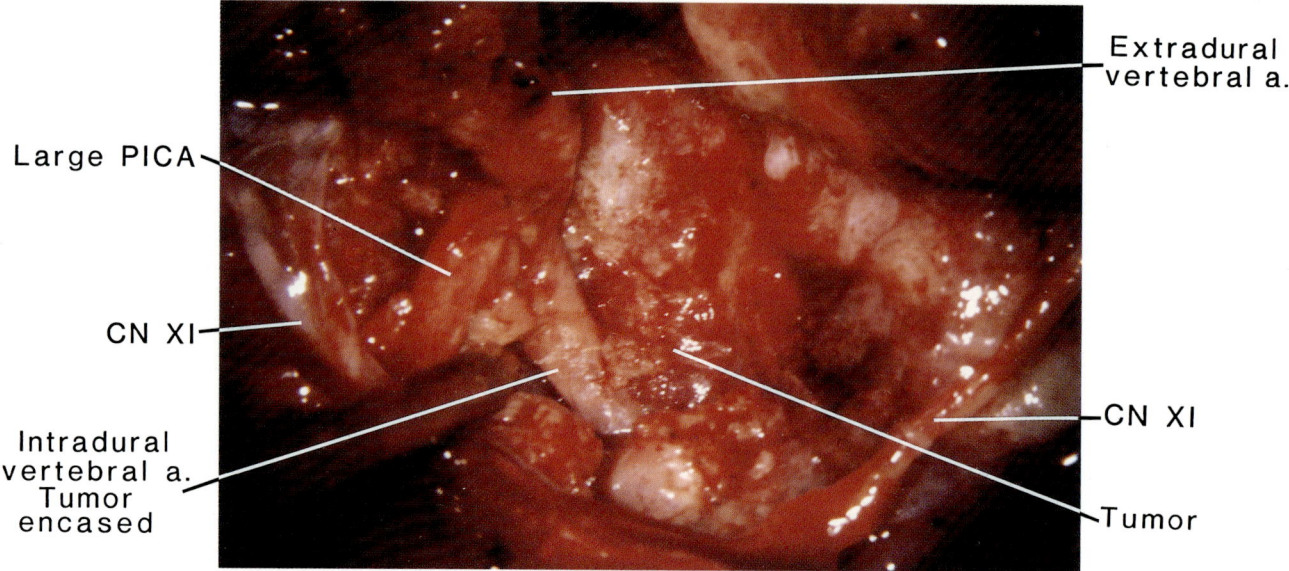

FIG. 38. The posterior inferior cerebellar artery (PICA), which was partially encased by tumor, has been dissected free. One can see complete encasement of the vertebral artery by tumor. It is being dissected free from normal to abnormal areas. The surgeon should be prepared for temporary arterial occlusion, primary repair, or saphenous vein bypass grafting in case of arterial injury.

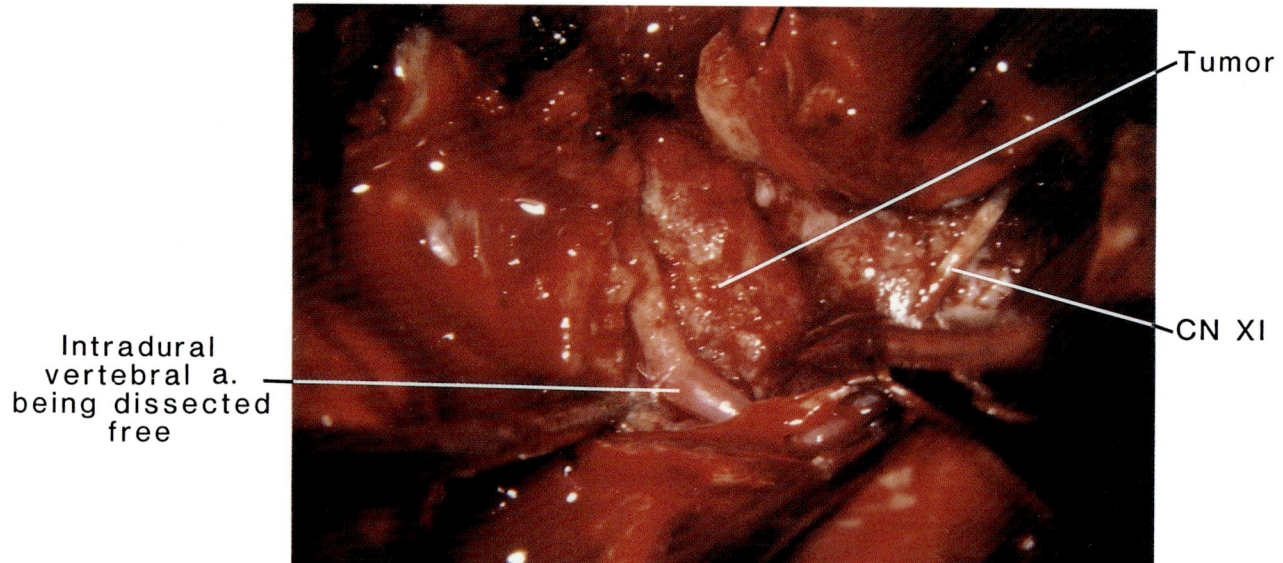

FIG. 39. Further dissection of vertebral artery from tumor.

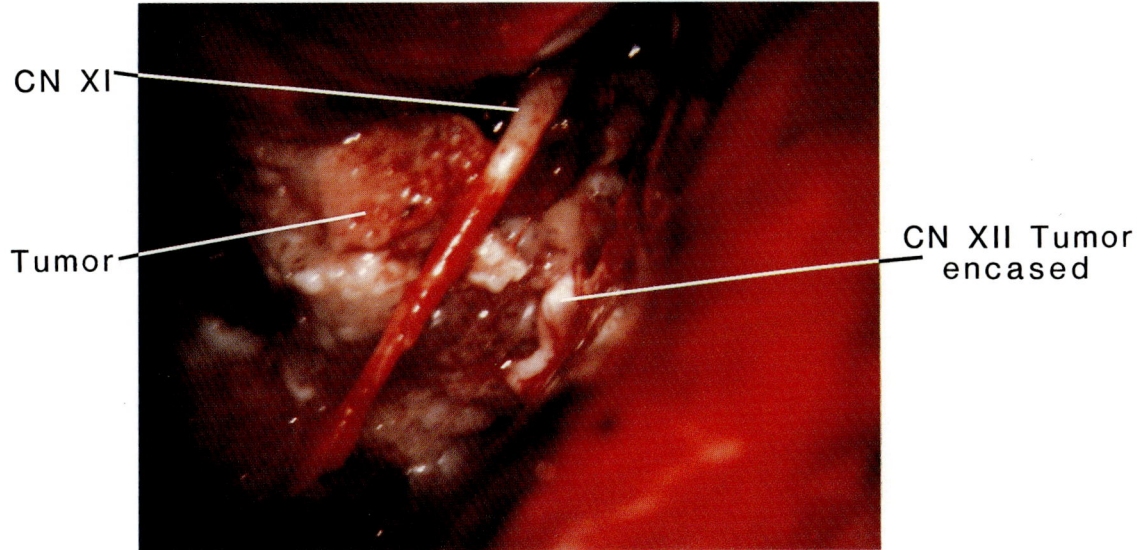

FIG. 40. CN XII rootlets are completely encased by tumor and are being dissected free. Neurophysiological monitoring of CN XII is useful during this phase of dissection. The tumor has been completely devascularized making dissection easier.

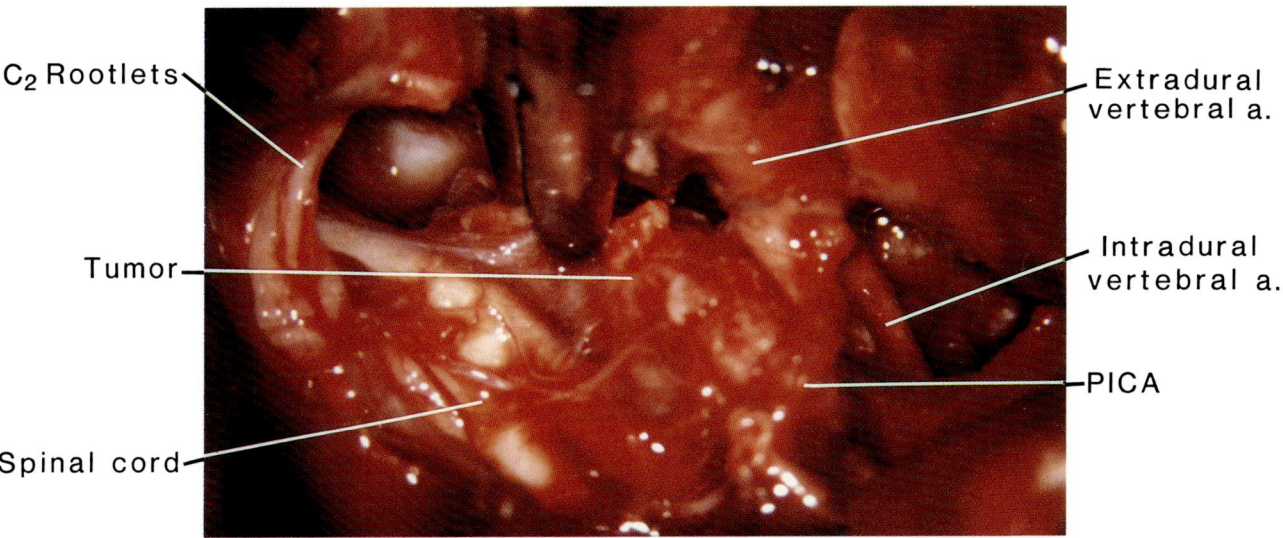

FIG. 41. The tumor is now being dissected from the spinomedullary junction. Note the very lateral view of tumor–brain interface.

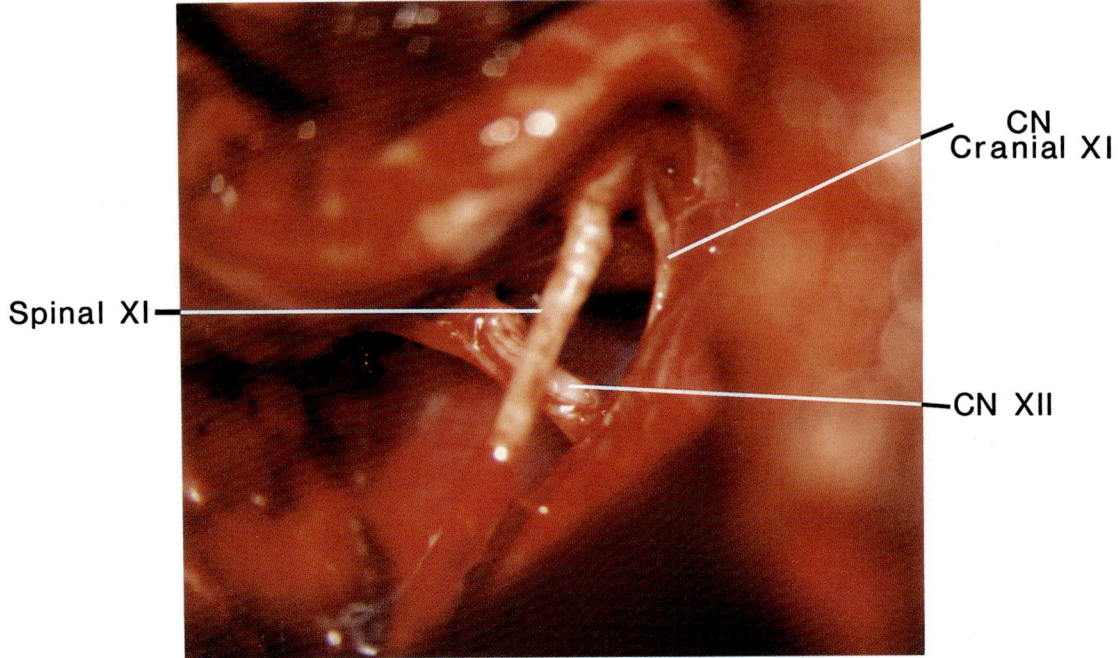

FIG. 42. After tumor removal, CN XI (spinal and cranial) and CN XII are seen.

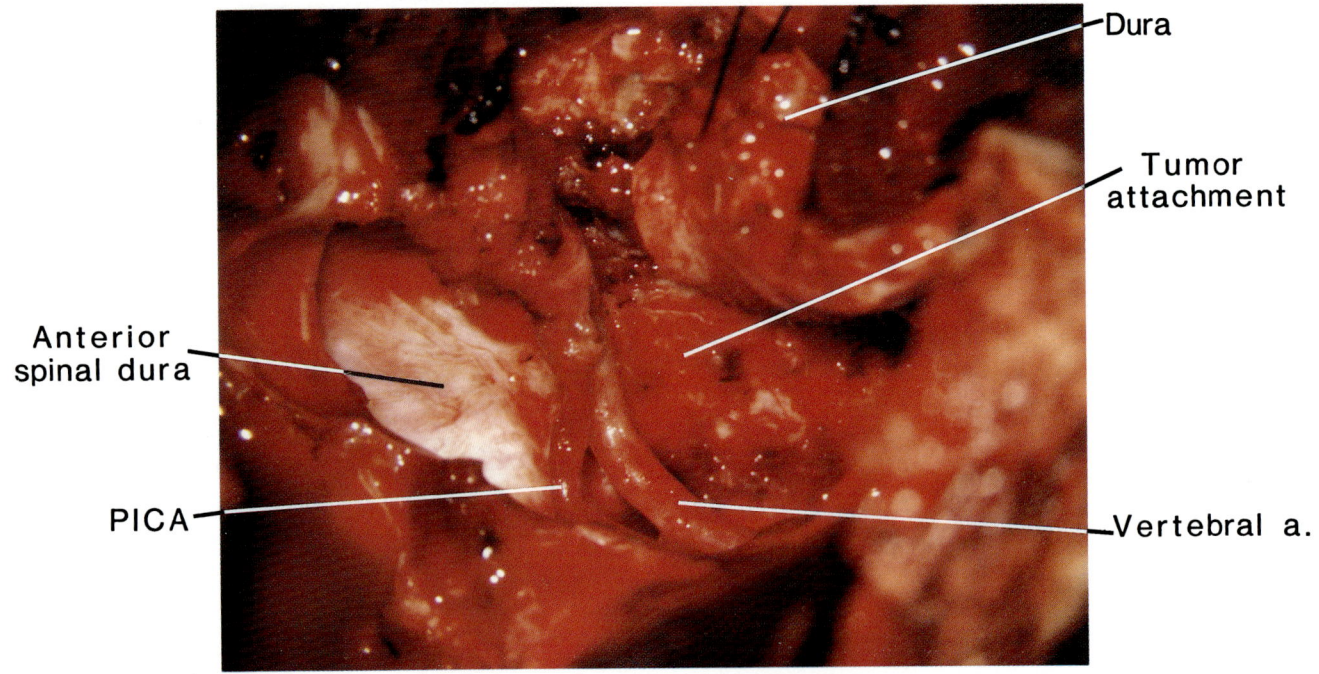

FIG. 43. Appearance after tumor resection. The dural base of the tumor was excised.

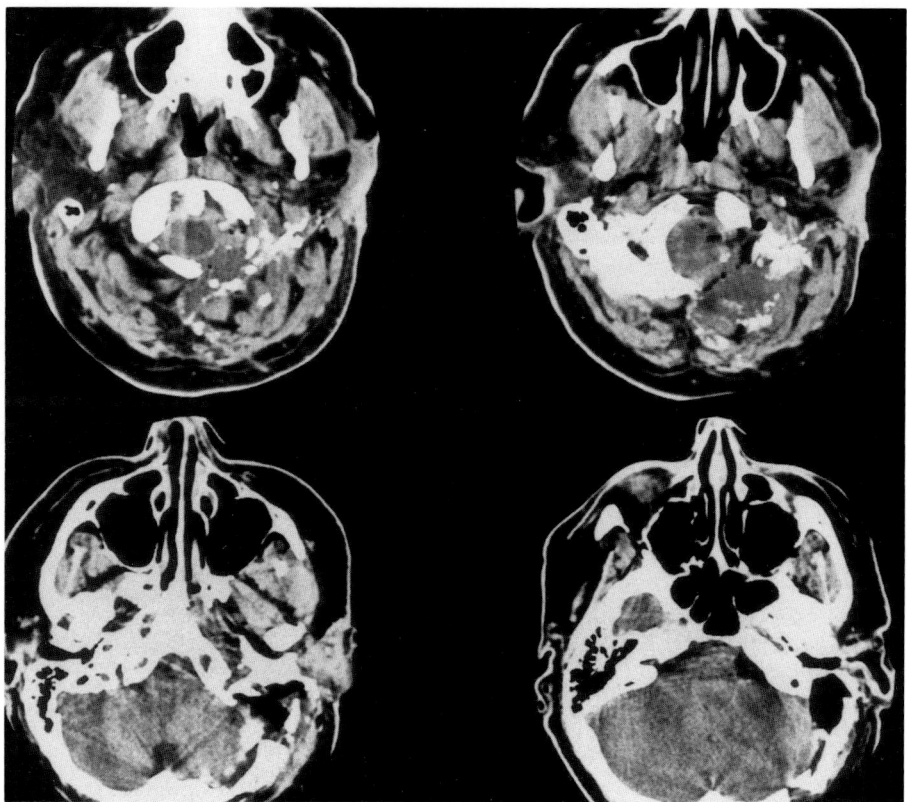

FIG. 44. CT scans with intravenous contrast show complete tumor resection. Note the extent of bone resection required with the extreme lateral transcondylar approach.

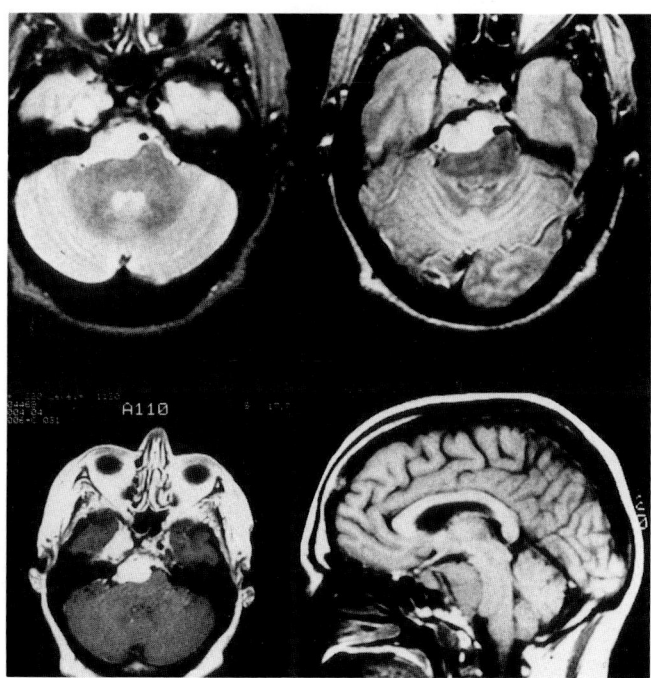

FIG. 45. (Figures 45–54 are of patient J.K.) Axial and sagittal MRI scans show a large petroclival meningioma with tumor involvement of the middle fossa, sella, cavernous sinus, and Meckel's cave.

Angiography showed right internal carotid artery occlusion, secondary to tumor encasement, and aneurysms at the anterior cerebral–anterior communicating artery junction and of the vertebrobasilar junctions (Figs. 46 and 47). Surgery was performed in two stages. Initially, the tumor was exposed by a frontotemporal and transzygomatic approach. Tumor was resected from the cavernous sinus, sella, and upper clival area, and the anterior communicating artery aneurysm was clipped (Figs. 48 and 49). Two weeks later, the remaining tumor and the vertebrobasilar fenestration aneurysm were exposed by further removal of clival bone by the infratemporal approach. The tumor was resected and the vertebrobasilar fenestration aneurysm was clipped (Figs. 50–53). At 1-year follow-up, her deficits of CNs III and VI persist on the right side, without significant improvement from the preoperative condition. There is no evidence of recurrent tumor on the follow-up CT scans (Fig. 54).

M.H.: Retrosigmoid Approach

This 68-year-old woman presented with a long history of trigeminal neuralgia and deteriorating gait, as well as a 1-month history of changes in mentation. Examination

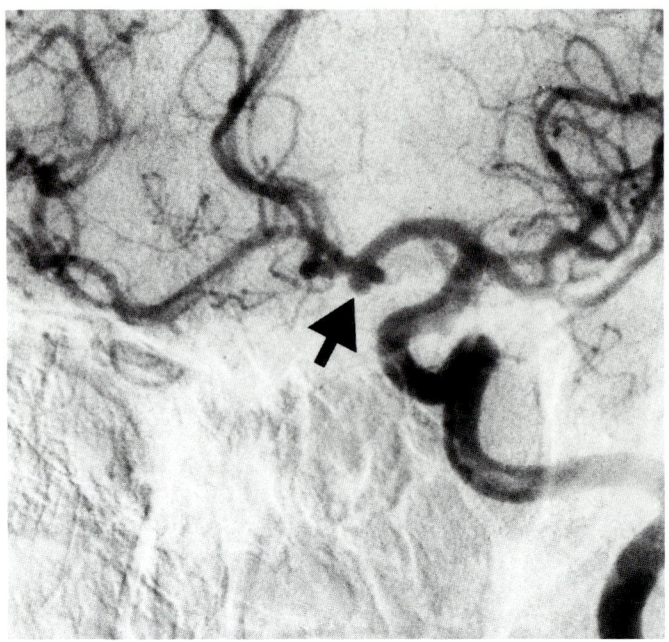

FIG. 46. Angiogram showing right ICA occlusion by tumor and aneurysm of anterior cerebral artery–anterior communicating artery junction (*arrow*).

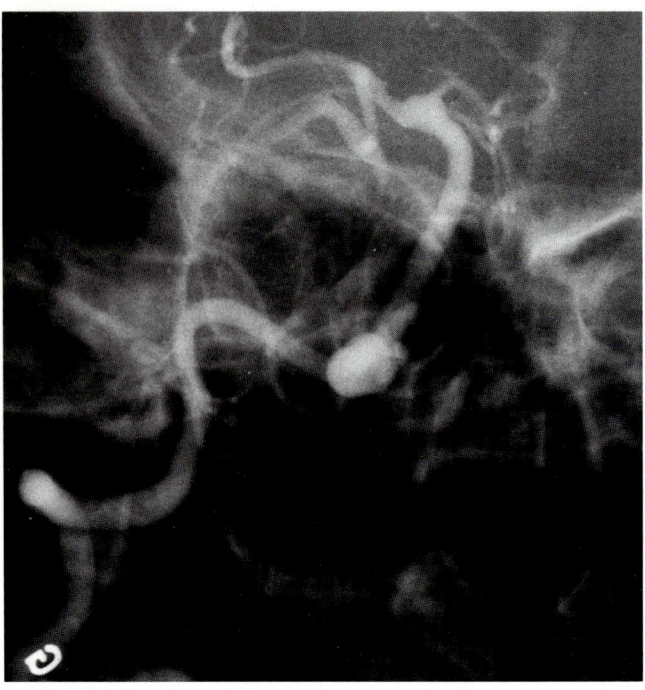

FIG. 47. Vertebral injection shows aneurysm of vertebrobasilar artery junction.

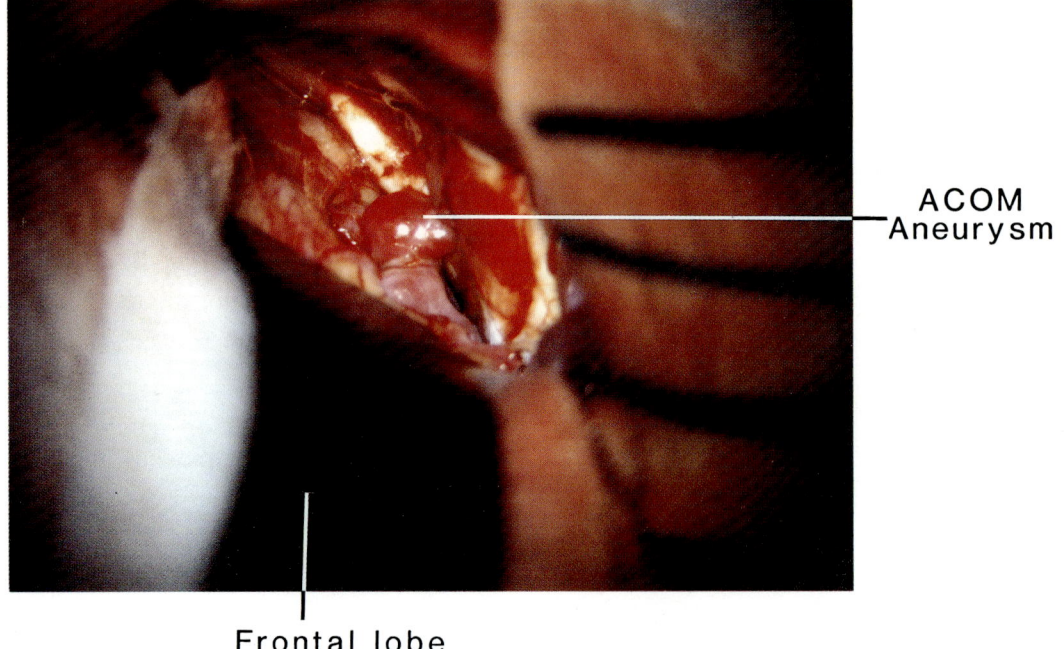

FIG. 48. During the first operation via a frontotemporal transzygomatic approach, the anterior communicating artery aneurysm has been exposed.

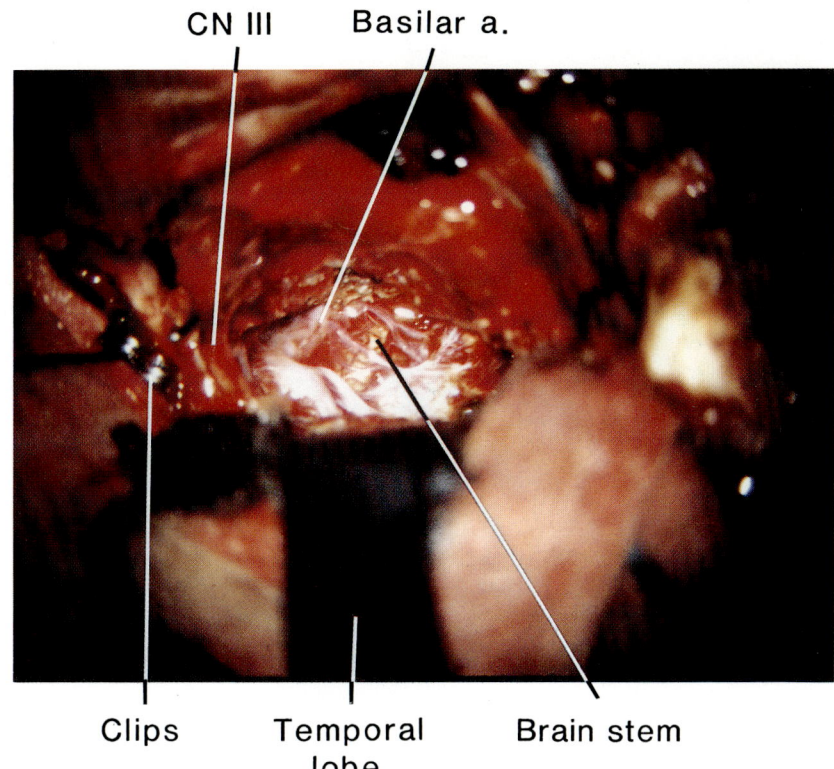

FIG. 49. During the first operation, the upper clival and cavernous sinus tumor has been removed, and the upper third of the basilar artery and brain stem are visible.

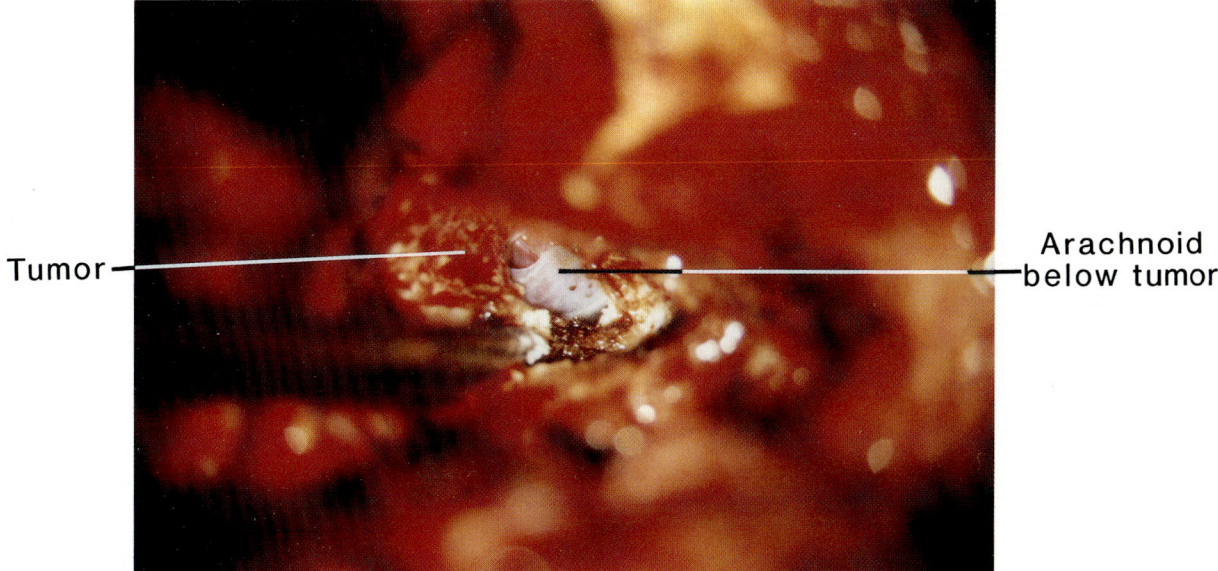

FIG. 50. During the second operation via a subtemporal and infratemporal approach, the dura and arachnoid have been opened below the level of the tumor.

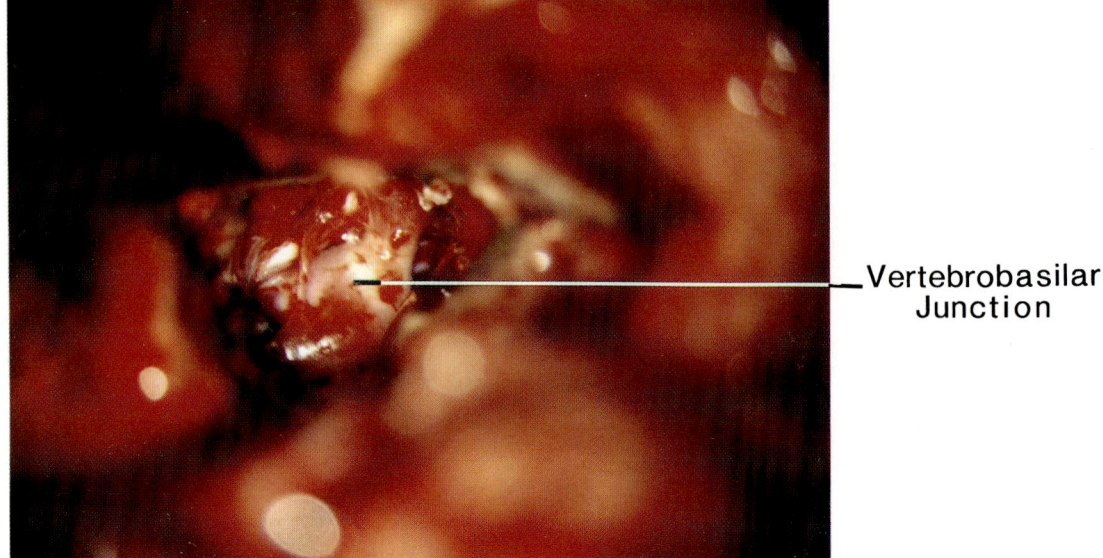

FIG. 51. The tumor has been removed and the bulbous vertebrobasilar junction has been exposed.

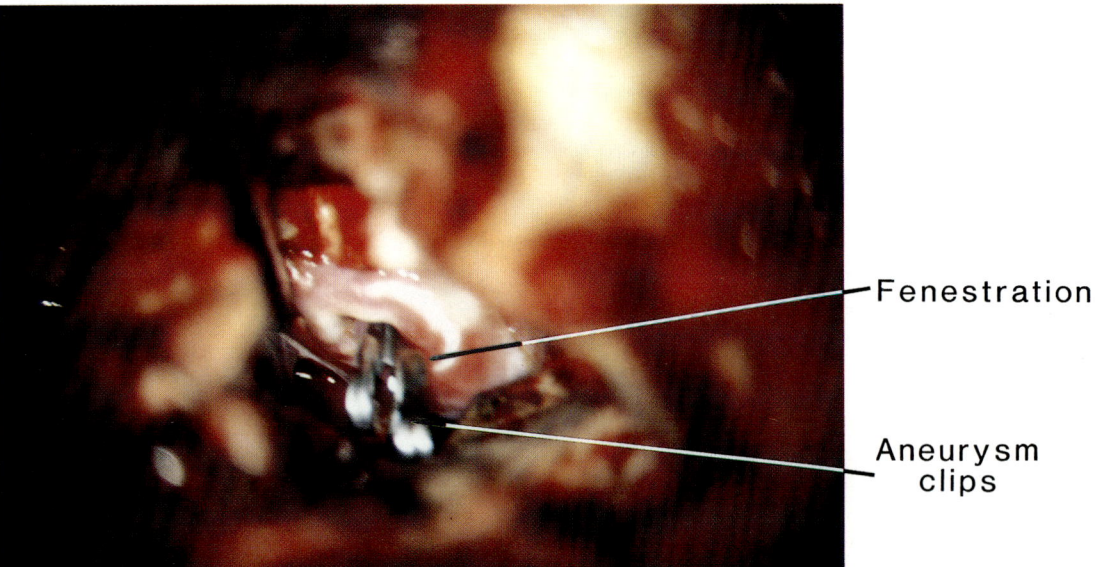

FIG. 52. The vertebrobasilar fenestration aneurysm has been clipped. The dissection was difficult because of its thin wall and tight adherence to the arterial wall.

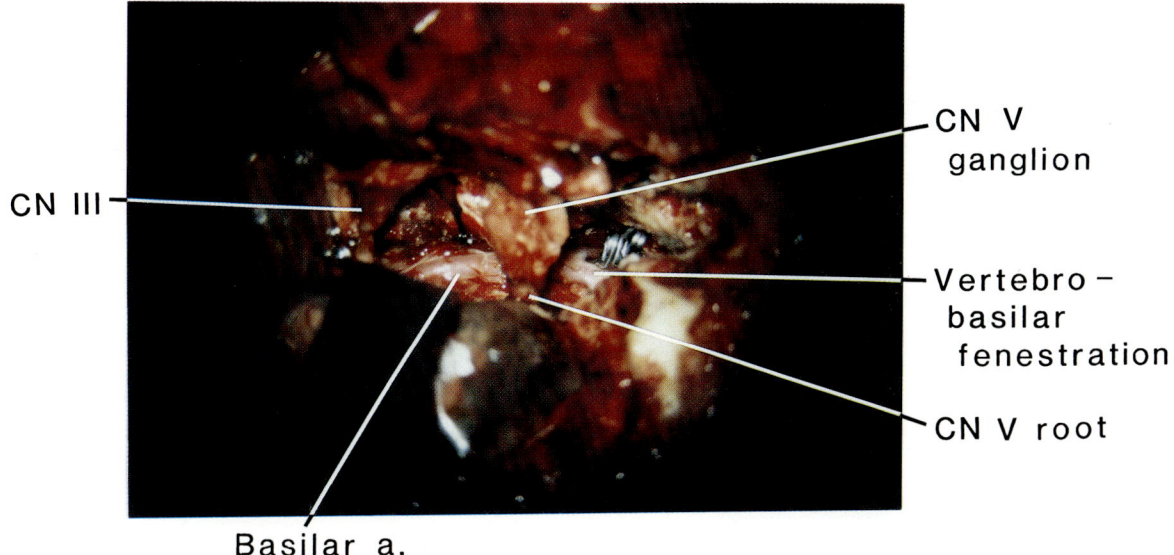

FIG. 53. Overview at the end of tumor resection reveals CN III, the brain stem, the ganglion and root of CN V, the lower two-thirds of the basilar artery, and the vertebrobasilar fenestration aneurysm, which has been clipped. The continuity of CN VI could not be preserved and reconstruction was not performed due to poor preoperative function of the extraocular muscles.

disclosed bilateral papilledema, decreased sensation in the right V_2–V_3 distributions, right palatal paresis, marked gait ataxia, and significant impairment of short-term memory. CT scan revealed a large petroclival meningioma extending to the foramen magnum inferiorly, with considerable brain stem distortion (Fig. 55). On cerebral angiogram, the basilar artery displacement was apparent (Fig. 56). After preoperative tumor embolization, the tumor was completely resected through a retromastoid craniectomy and C1 laminectomy (Figs. 57–62). The CO_2 laser was used to core the tumor and, working between the cranial nerves, it was completely resected. CN VI was injured by the laser. It was trimmed and resutured. CN VII was injured by reflected laser energy, but without an obvious anatomical lesion. Postoperatively, she had complete left CN VII deficit and partial deficits of CNs IX and X. Prophylactic tracheostomy was performed for airway protection and pulmonary toilet. Postoperative CT scans with contrast confirmed complete tumor resection (Fig. 63). She was making good progress and ambulating on the ward, when 10 days postoperatively she developed massive pneumonia and died suddenly, presumably secondary to a mucous plug. Consent for autopsy could not be obtained. This case illustrates how even large midclival tumors can be removed via a retrosigmoid approach if adequate cerebellar relaxation can be achieved. The value of postoperative intensive care is also apparent.

K.E.: Frontotemporal–Transcavernous and Presigmoid and Transsigmoid Transpetrous Approach

This 32-year-old woman was referred with a 2-year history of progressive supraorbital headaches and oculomotor paresis. Radiological studies showed a meningioma involving the right cavernous sinus, sellar and suprasellar region, extending into the tentorial notch and clivus down to the level of CNs IX and X (Fig. 64). The

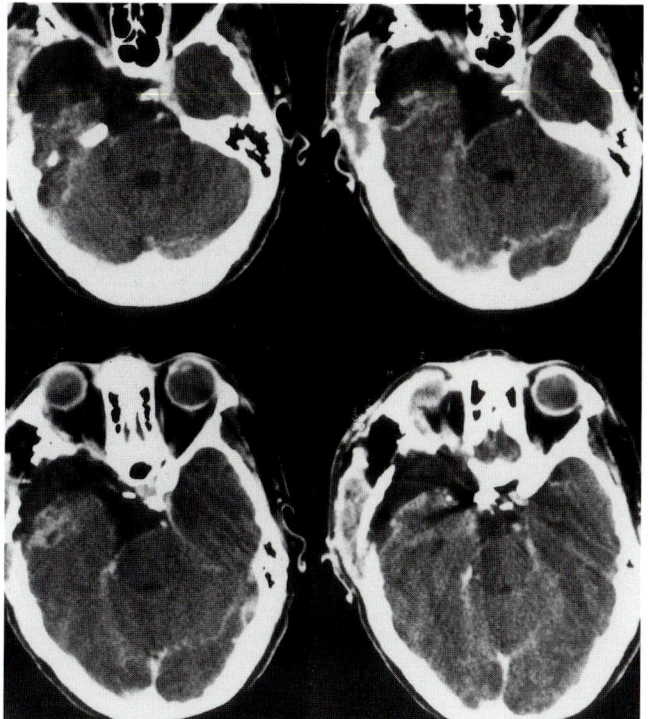

FIG. 54. Postoperative CT scan with intravenous contrast shows complete tumor resection.

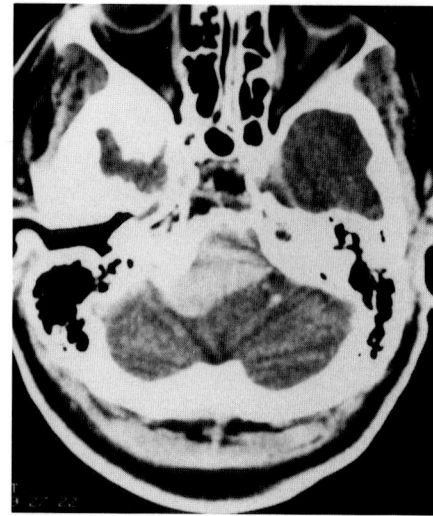

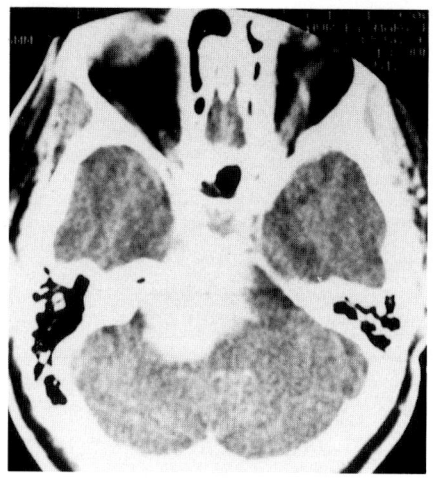

FIG. 55. (Figures 55–63 are of patient M.H.) Axial CT scan of head showing a large petroclival meningioma extending down to the foramen magnum.

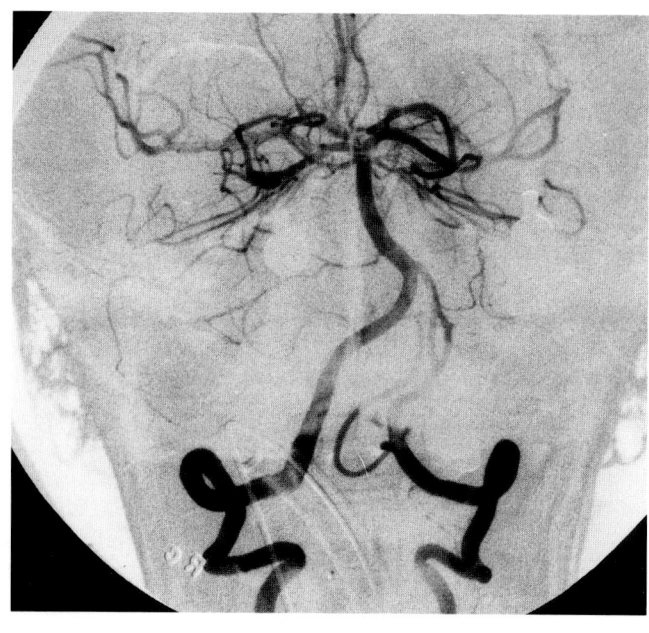

FIG. 56. Vertebral artery injection shows significant basilar artery displacement by tumor.

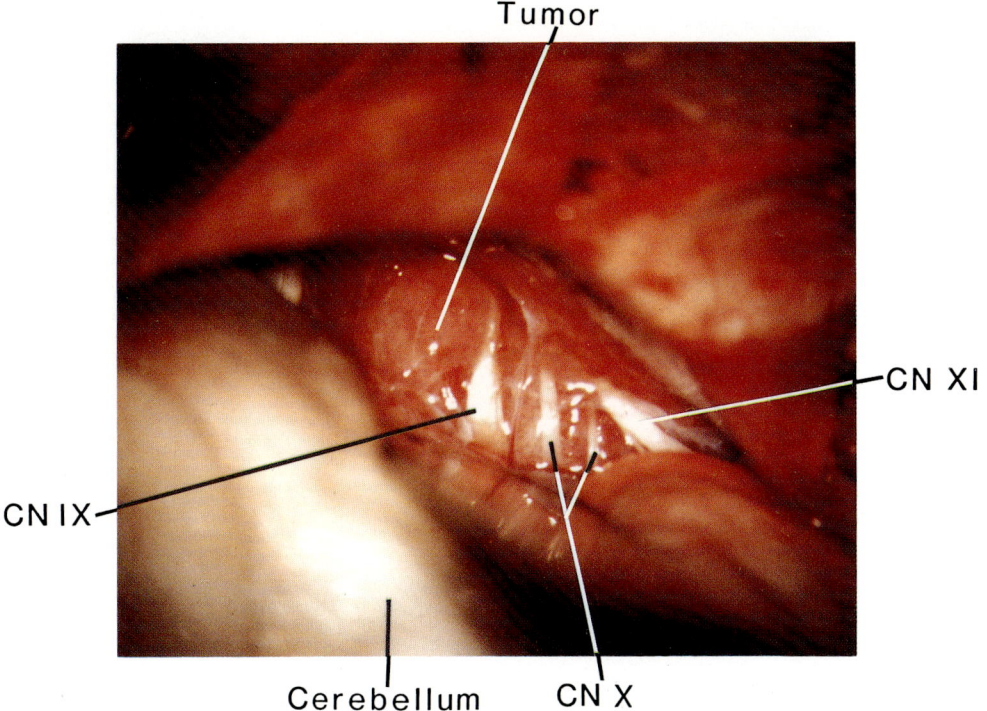

FIG. 57. This is a good example of exposure obtained through a retrosigmoid approach. CNs IX, X, and XI are extremely stretched over the tumor.

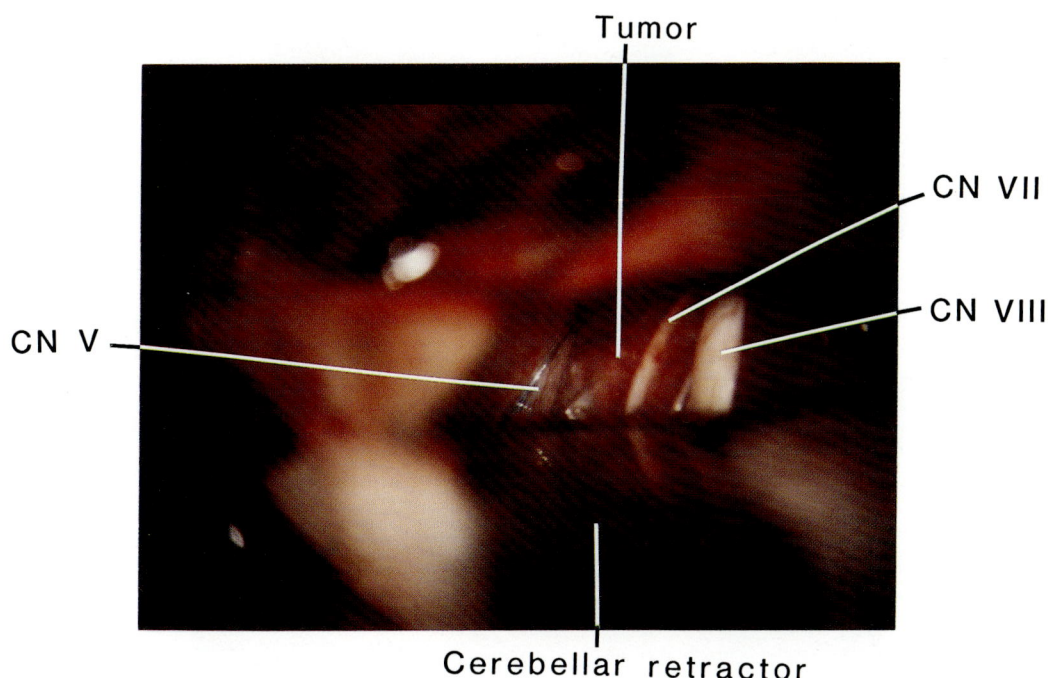

FIG. 58. Superior aspect of the tumor with CNs V, VII, and VIII draped over the tumor.

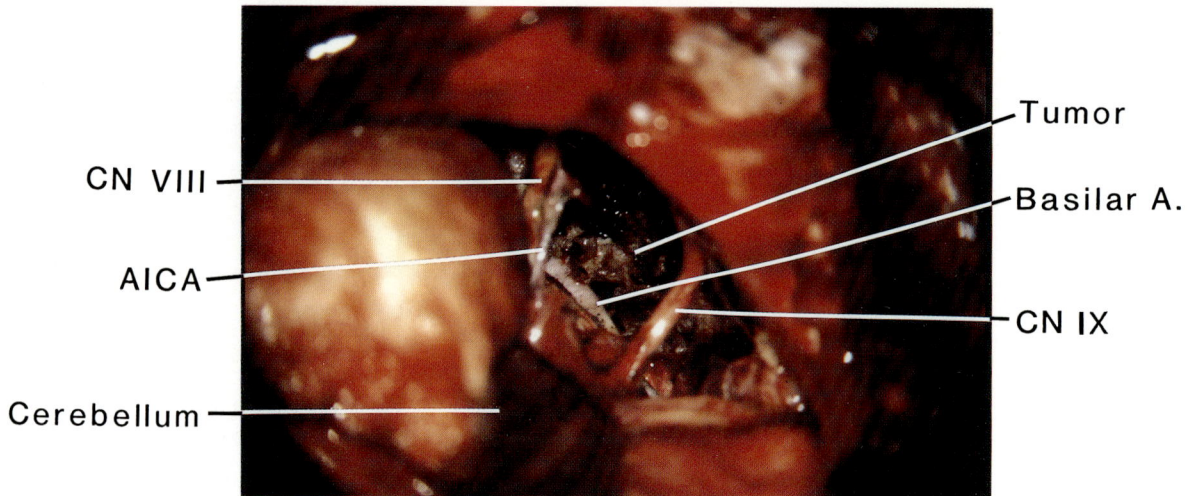

FIG. 59. Partial tumor debulking has been performed with the laser. CNs VIII and IX, the AICA, and the basilar artery are seen.

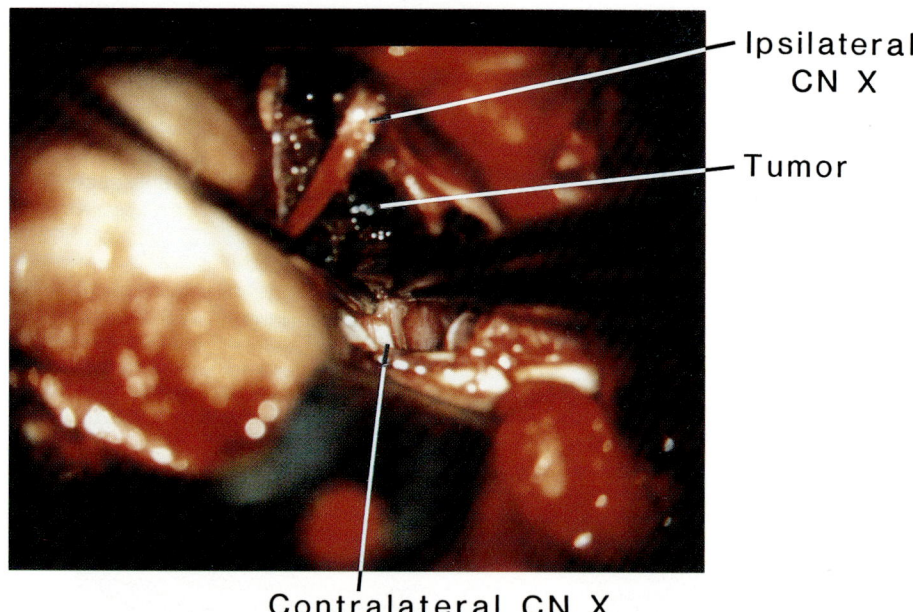

FIG. 60. Origin of contralateral CNs IX and X, tumor, and ipsilateral CN X are seen.

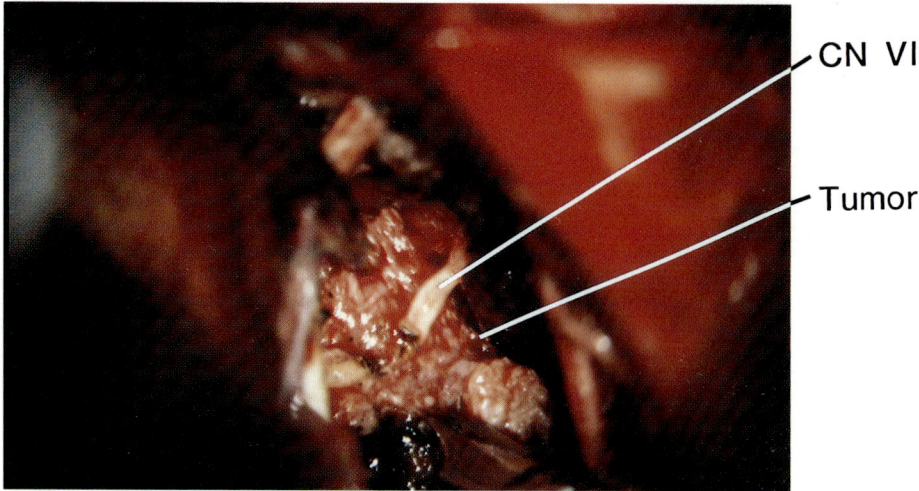

FIG. 61. Transection of the encased CN VI by laser beams. The two ends of the transected nerve are visible.

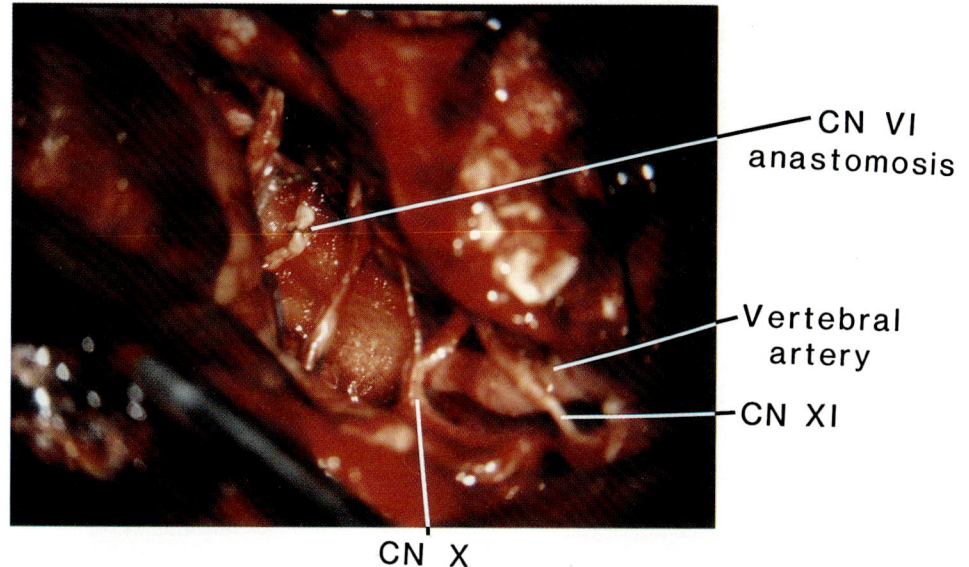

FIG. 62. Final appearance after tumor resection. The reconstructed CN VI, fascicles of CNs IX, X, and XI and the vertebral artery are seen.

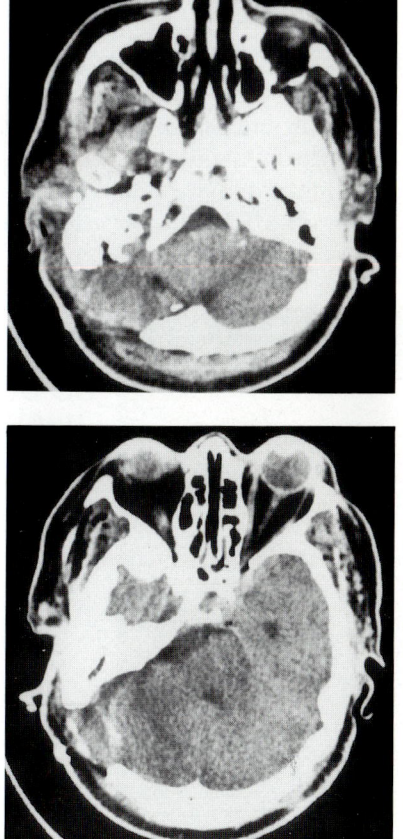

FIG. 63. Postoperative axial CT scans with intravenous contrast showing complete tumor resection.

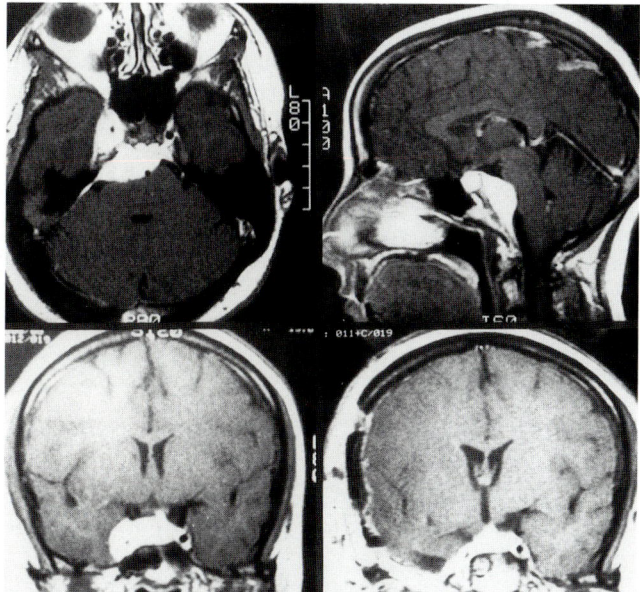

FIG. 64. (Figures 64–72 are of patient K.E.) Axial, sagittal, and coronal MRI scans with intravenous contrast show a petroclival meningioma involving the right cavernous sinus, sellar and suprasellar region, extending into the tentorial notch and clivus down to the level of CN X. Note the right ICA is completely encased by tumor and is severely stenosed. Xenon/cerebral blood flow studies were within normal range, after balloon test occlusion of the right ICA.

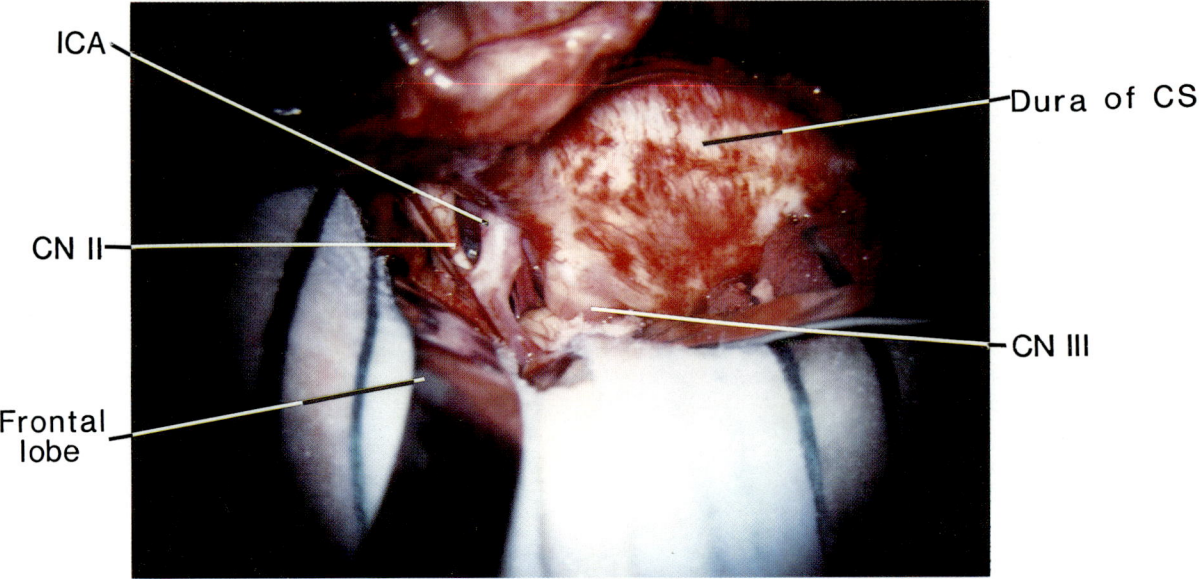

FIG. 65. During the first operation, via the frontotemporal orbitozygomatic approach, the tumor appears to be entirely within the cavernous sinus with marked bulging of the lateral wall of the cavernous sinus. The oculomotor nerve is splayed by the tumor.

right ICA was narrowed and completely encased by tumor. She tolerated a balloon test occlusion of the ICA with no changes in xenon blood flow studies. Through use of a frontotemporal approach with orbitozygomatic osteotomy, the tumor was completely removed from within the cavernous sinus, sellar region, and upper clival area (Figs. 65–68). All cranial nerves in the cavernous sinus were preserved anatomically. Although the ICA was encased and narrowed, the tumor was soft and could be dissected away from the artery. Postoperatively, she developed a complete CN VI palsy, a partial CN III palsy, and diminished sensation in the V_1 distribution. Six weeks later, she underwent a retromastoid, posterior subtemporal, and transpetrous approach with the division of the sigmoid sinus for resection of remaining clival tumor (Figs. 69 and 70). The sigmoid sinus was reconstructed at the end of surgery. Gross total tumor removal was achieved. Three years postoperatively, she has normal CN III function and paresis of CNs V and VI. Diplopia is present only on lateral gaze (Fig. 71). She has returned to full-time employment and has no evidence of recurrent tumor on MRI scan. Persistent enhancement

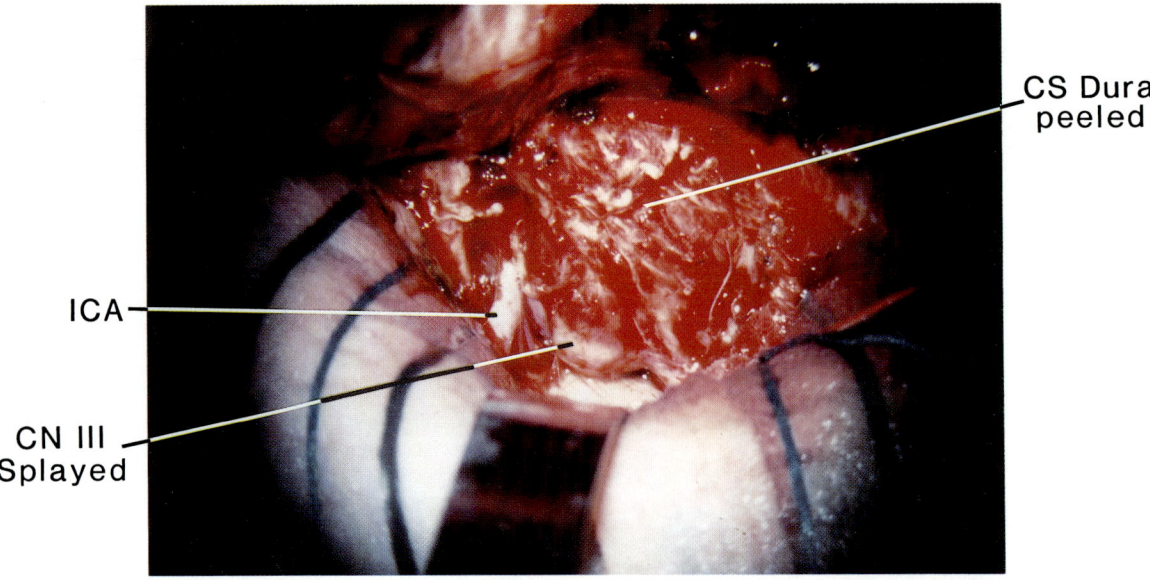

FIG. 66. The lateral wall of the cavernous sinus has been peeled away, revealing a very vascular tumor.

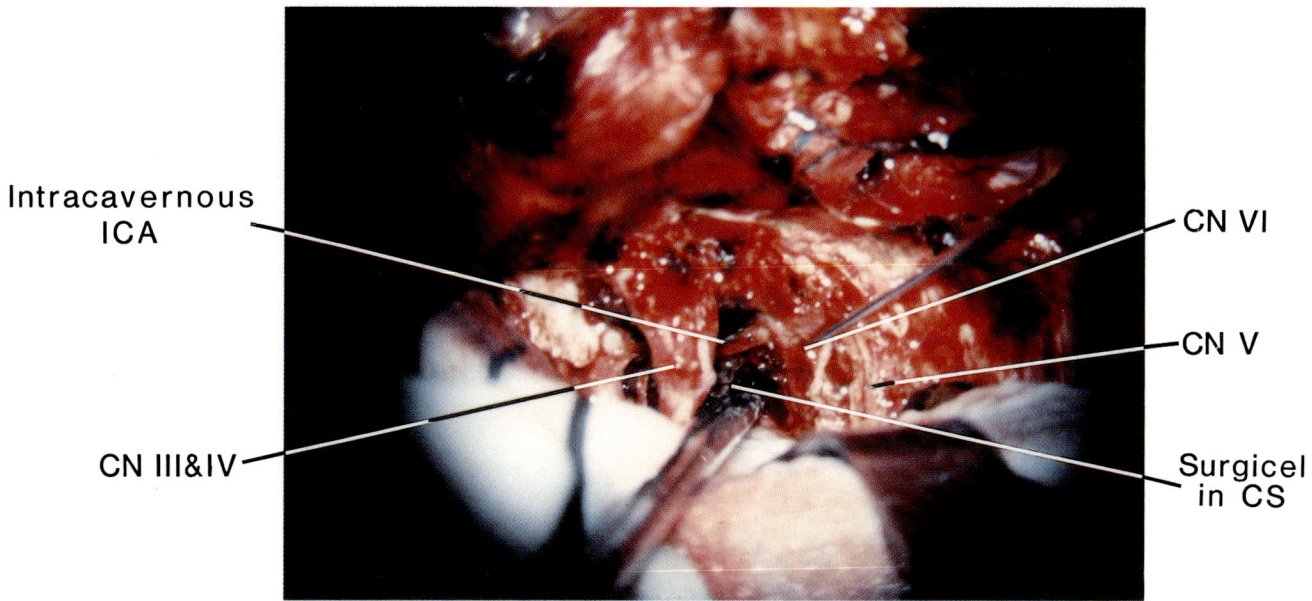

FIG. 67. Considerable tumor removal has been accomplished within the cavernous sinus. Despite the vascular nature of the tumor, its soft consistency enabled the surgeon to easily peel it off the encased internal carotid artery. The various neurovascular structures are seen.

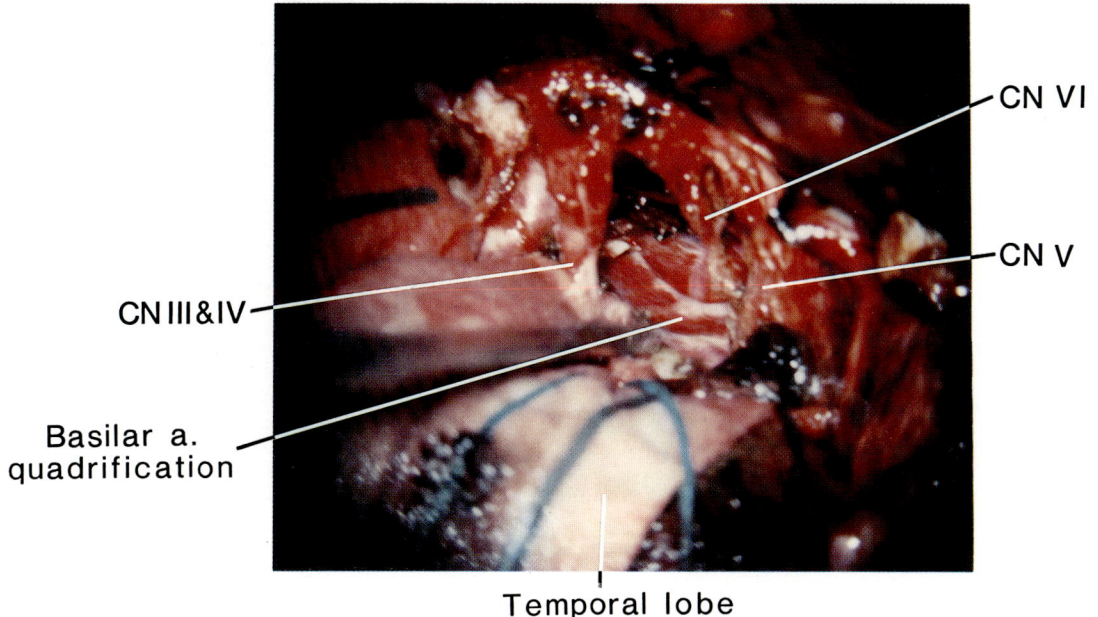

FIG. 68. After removal of the intracavernous tumor, the upper clival tumor could be more easily removed. The basilar artery quadrification, brain stem, and CNs III–VI are clearly visible.

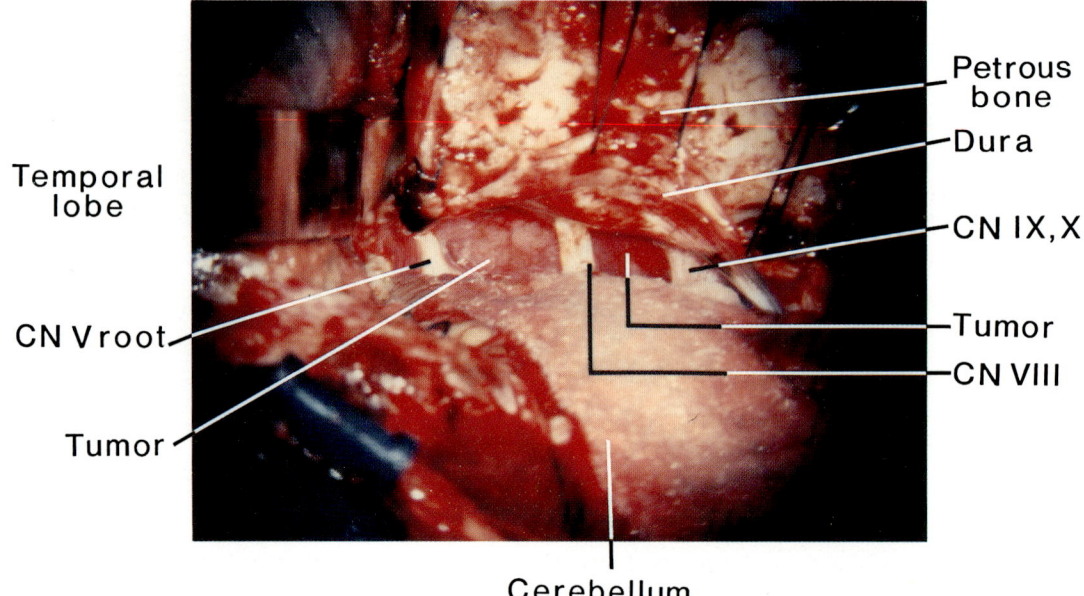

FIG. 69. In order to remove the lower half of the tumor, a retrosigmoid posterior subtemporal and transpetrosal approach with division of the sigmoid sinus was used. CNs V, VIII, IX, and X are clearly seen along with the tumor.

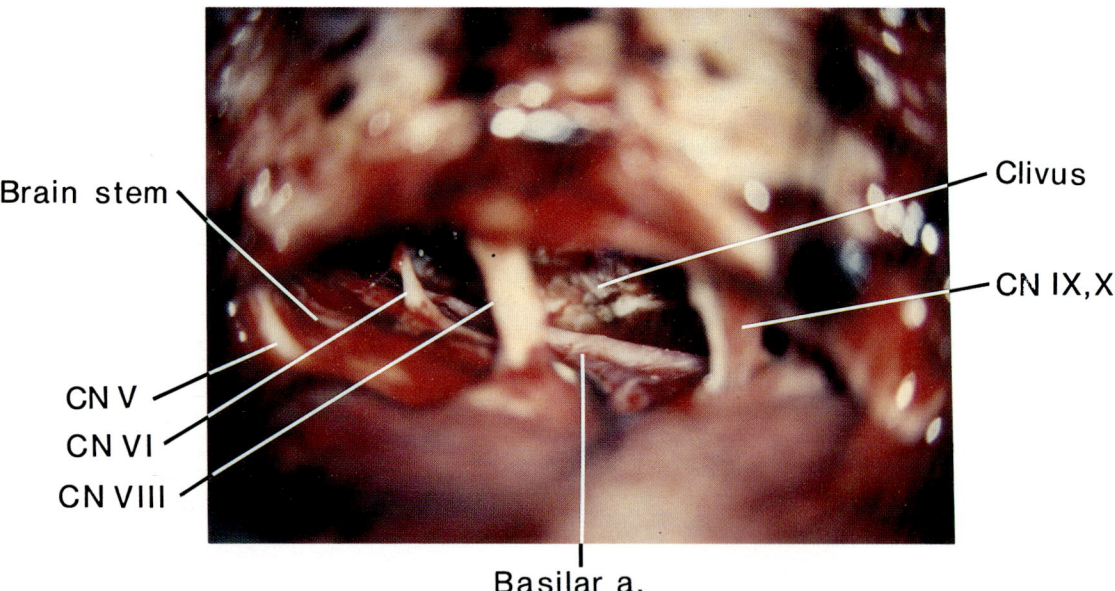

FIG. 70. CN VI was markedly encased by tumor for a great distance. At the conclusion of tumor resection, the brain stem, basilar artery, CNs V, VI, VIII, IX, and X, and the clivus are visible.

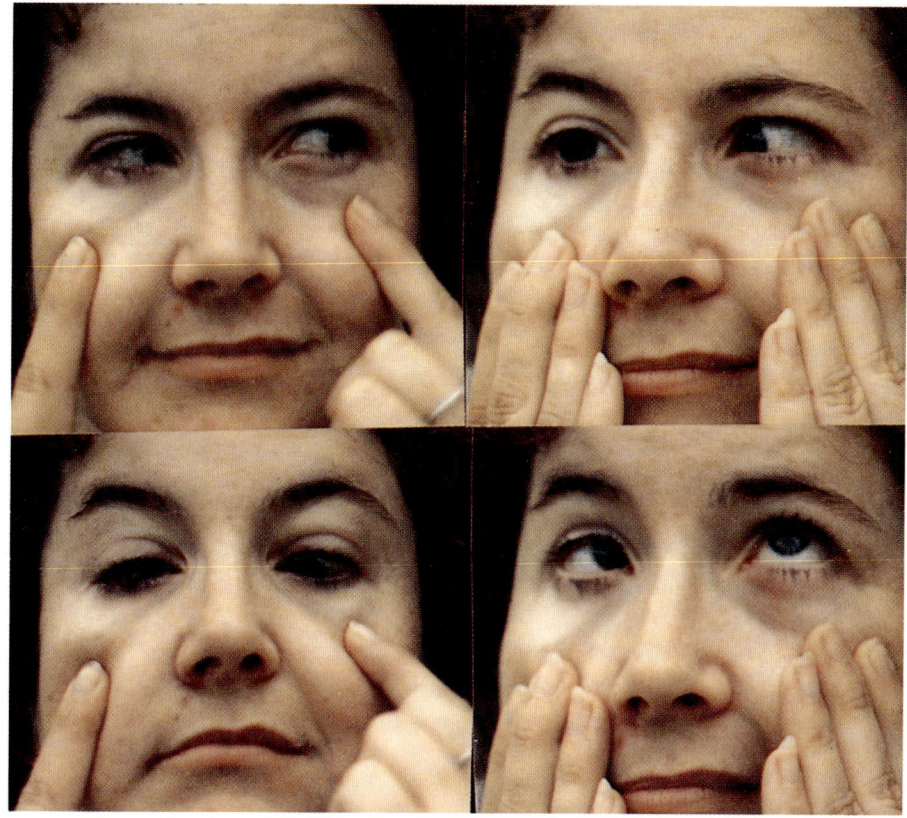

FIG. 71. Photograph 1 year postoperatively shows complete resolution of preoperative oculomotor paresis. She has a persistent abducens paresis and some reduced sensation in V_1–V_2 distribution. She has achieved binocular vision with the aid of prism glasses and has returned to full employment.

after gadolinium administration probably represents postoperative scar tissue (Fig. 72).

J.F.: Extreme Lateral Transcondylar and Subtemporal–Presigmoid Approach

This 66-year-old woman presented to her physician with a 6-month history of hearing loss and loss of equilibrium. This led to the discovery of a large petroclival meningioma. Initial treatment consisted of a ventriculoperitoneal shunt and external beam radiation of the tumor. Her symptoms continued to progress and by the time we saw her, she had right arm weakness and cerebellar signs with the patient unable to ambulate. MRI disclosed a large 4.5-cm meningioma causing considerable distortion and compression of the left anterior brain stem, with extension into the cavernous sinus and sphenoid sinus (Figs. 73 and 74). Cerebral angiogram showed severe displacement and stenosis of the basilar artery by tumor (Fig. 75). Initially, the lower third of the tumor from the foramen magnum up to the internal auditory canal (IAC) was removed through the extreme lateral transcondylar approach. The tumor was very vascular and friable. The superior aspect of the tumor was explored through a left subtemporal presigmoid approach 10 days later (Figs. 76–81). The top 1.5 cm of the basilar artery and its branches were almost totally encased within the tumor and were easily dissected free. CN III was partially encased by the tumor and dissected free. CN VI was injured during tumor removal. A subtotal resection was obtained with a small amount of tumor remaining in the anterior cavernous sinus (Fig. 82). Postoperatively, she developed recurrent aspiration pneumonia and underwent a tracheostomy. Postoperative recovery was delayed by wound infection and sepsis. She was making good progress when she died suddenly 2 months postoperatively from pulmonary complications.

M.C.: Total Petrosectomy and Frontotemporal Transsylvian Approach (Extreme Example of Petrous ICA Encasement)

This 45-year-old woman presented with paresthesia in the left side of her face, left-sided hearing loss, and unsteadiness of gait. She underwent a left temporal craniotomy with partial tumor excision in another institution. Postoperatively, she had right hemiplegia, hemianesthesia, dysphasia, and seizure disorder. At presentation to us, she exhibited global dysphasia, right CN VII paresis, and partial left CN III palsy, and the tumor was growing

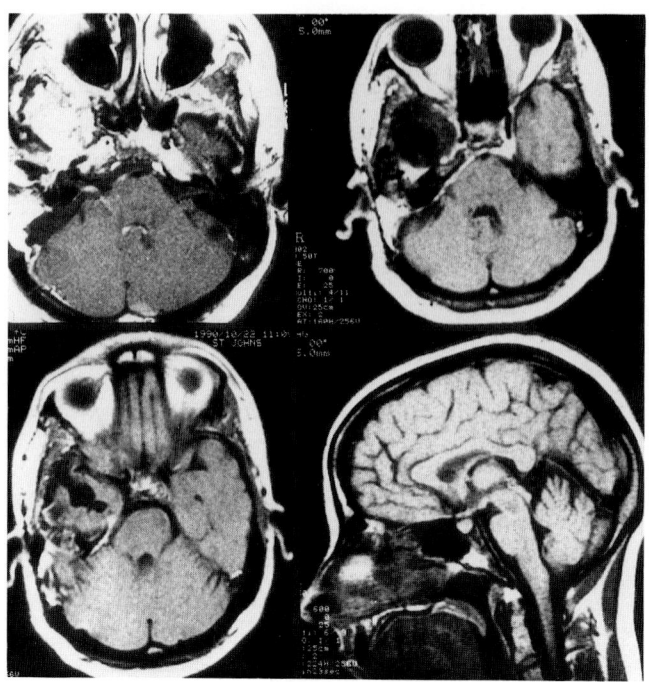

FIG. 72. Postoperative axial and sagittal MRI scans with intravenous contrast showing complete tumor resection. Enhancement around the petrous ICA is due to scar tissue.

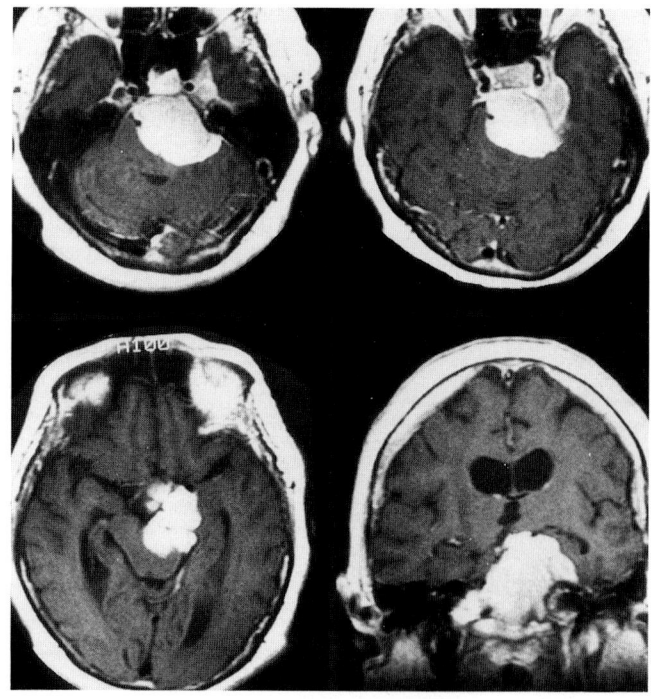

FIG. 73. (Figures 73–82 are of patient J.F.) Preoperative MRI scan with gadolinium shows a large petroclival meningioma with extension into the cavernous sinus and sphenoid sinus. There is considerable distortion and compression of the brain stem. Note encasement of the basilar artery and ICA.

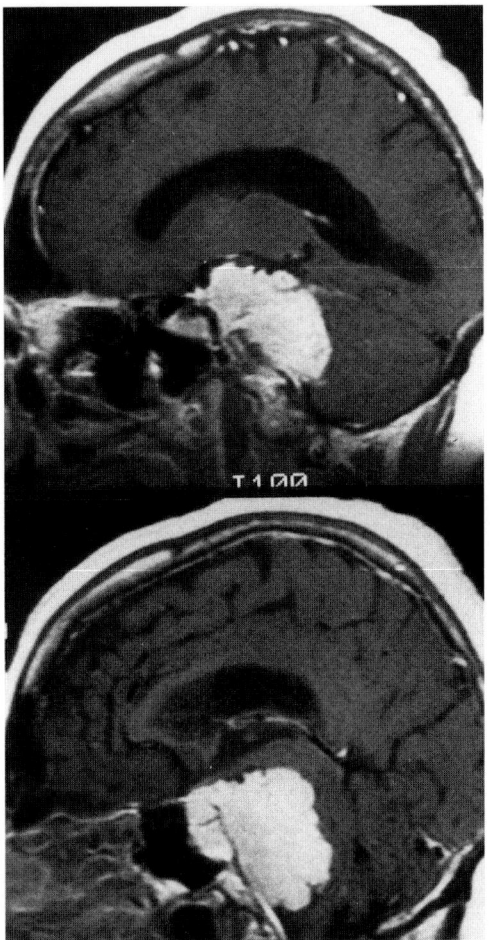

FIG. 74. Sagittal MRI scans with gadolinium contrast agent demonstrate severe brain stem compression.

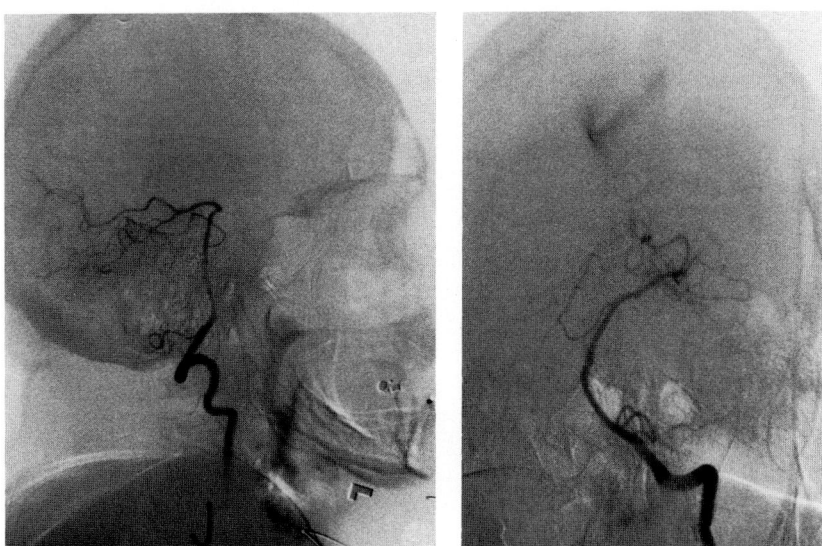

FIG. 75. Left vertebral injection lateral and AP views demonstrating severe displacement and stenosis of basilar artery.

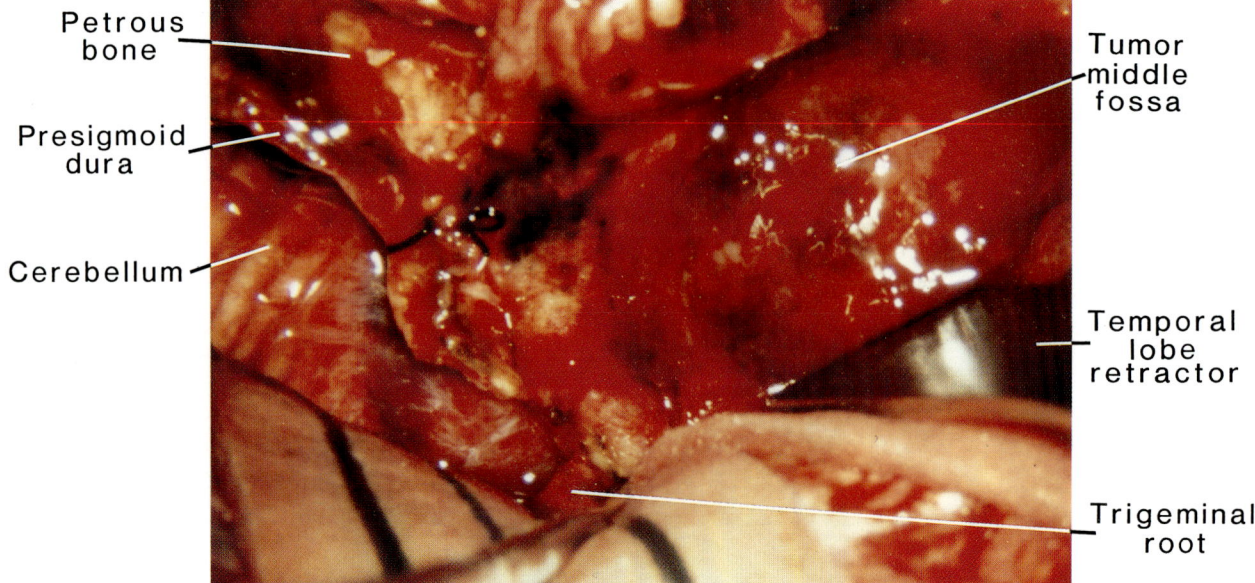

FIG. 76. Left frontotemporal craniotomy with zygomatic osteotomy has been performed. The previous retrosigmoid craniectomy and mastoidectomy approach is also opened. The dural opening is performed in the temporal and presigmoid region. Tumor is exposed in the middle cranial fossa and tentorial notch region.

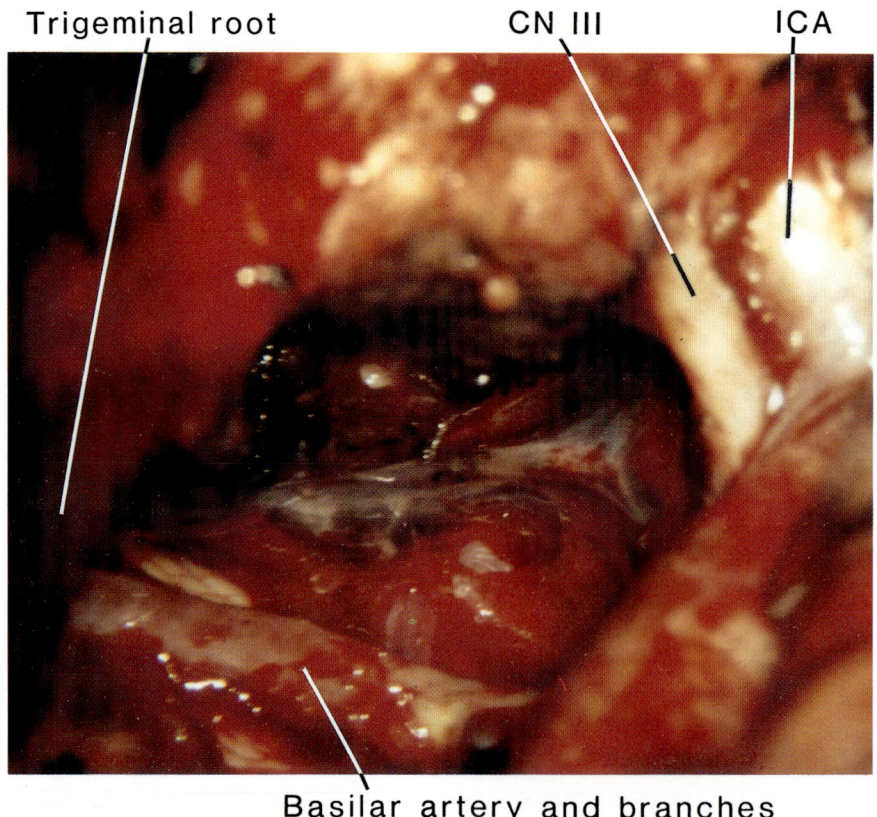

FIG. 77. Overview following complete tumor resection showing basilar artery, brain stem, internal carotid artery (ICA), CN III, and trigeminal root.

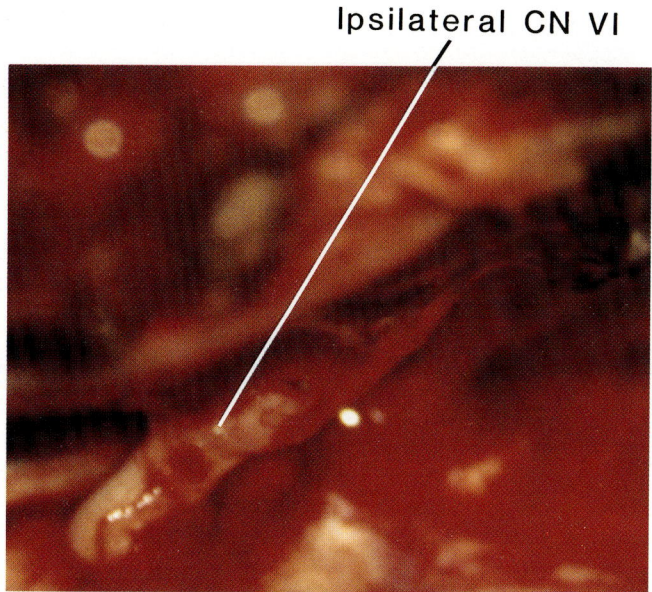

FIG. 78. Ipsilateral CN VI coming out of the brain stem, after tumor resection.

progressively. MRI showed a giant petroclival meningioma involving the left cavernous sinus and extending from the lower clivus to the body of the left ventricle superiorly and orbital apex anteriorly. There was a considerable mass effect on the brain stem and left temporal lobe (Fig. 83). Angiography showed encasement of the left anterior cerebral artery, supraclinoid ICA, and the entire basilar artery including the thalamic perforators (Fig. 84). The tumor was supplied predominantly by the meningohypophyseal artery with some external carotid artery supply via the middle meningeal and internal maxillary branches. The patient failed the balloon test occlusion of the left ICA. Initial ventriculoperitoneal shunt placement was followed by a frontotemporal–infratemporal approach with orbitozygomatic osteotomy and condylectomy. Tumor was peeled away from the supraclinoid ICA and its branches. Partial tumor resection was performed from the cavernous sinus. In a second stage, a total petrosectomy was performed and further removal was performed in the clival area. During basilar artery dissection, the left superior cerebellar artery was injured and was reapproximated by end-to-end suture anastomosis. All perforator vessels except one were preserved. The facial nerve was so badly involved with tumor that it was resected and grafted. Postoperatively, the patient had the clinical appearance of the locked-in syndrome with severe brain stem edema. CT scan showed a severe edema and a small area of hemor-

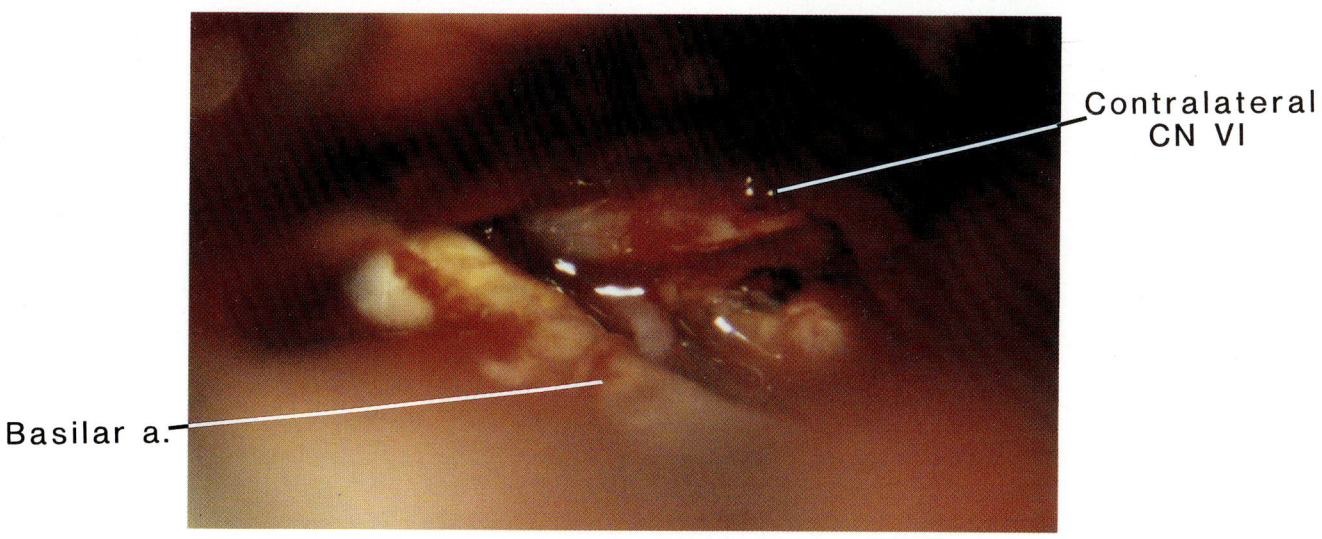

FIG. 79. Contralateral CN VI after tumor resection.

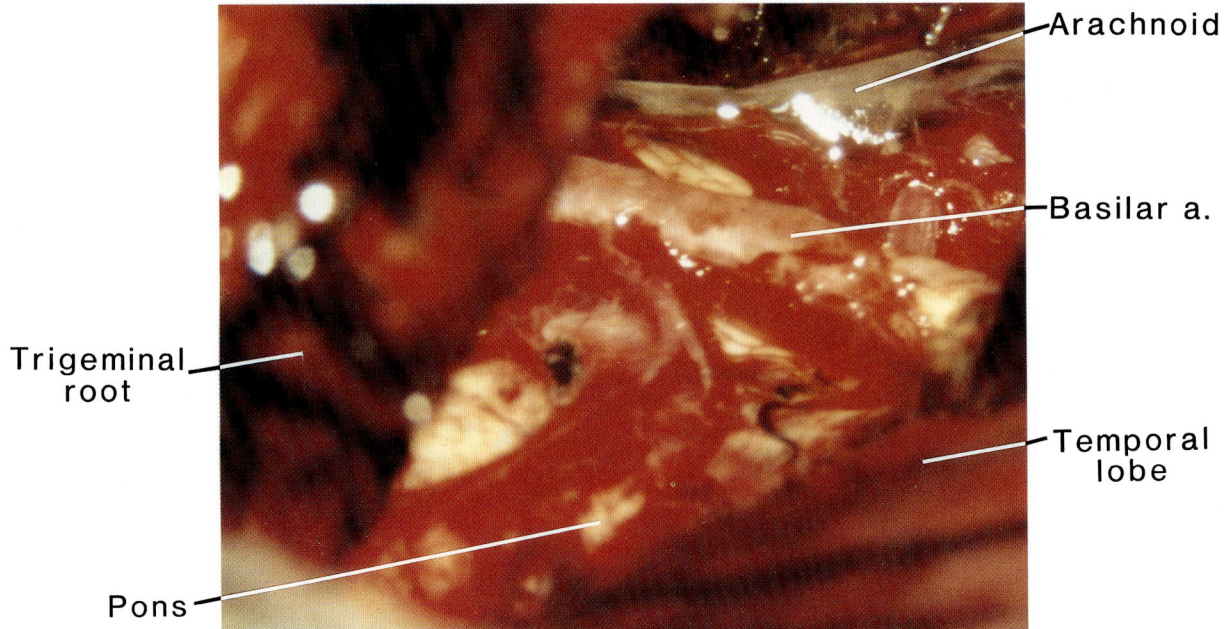

FIG. 80. View of basilar artery dissected free of tumor. Brain stem (pons) is visible, with the temporal lobe retracted out of the way. Note the arachnoid membrane between the tumor and the brain stem.

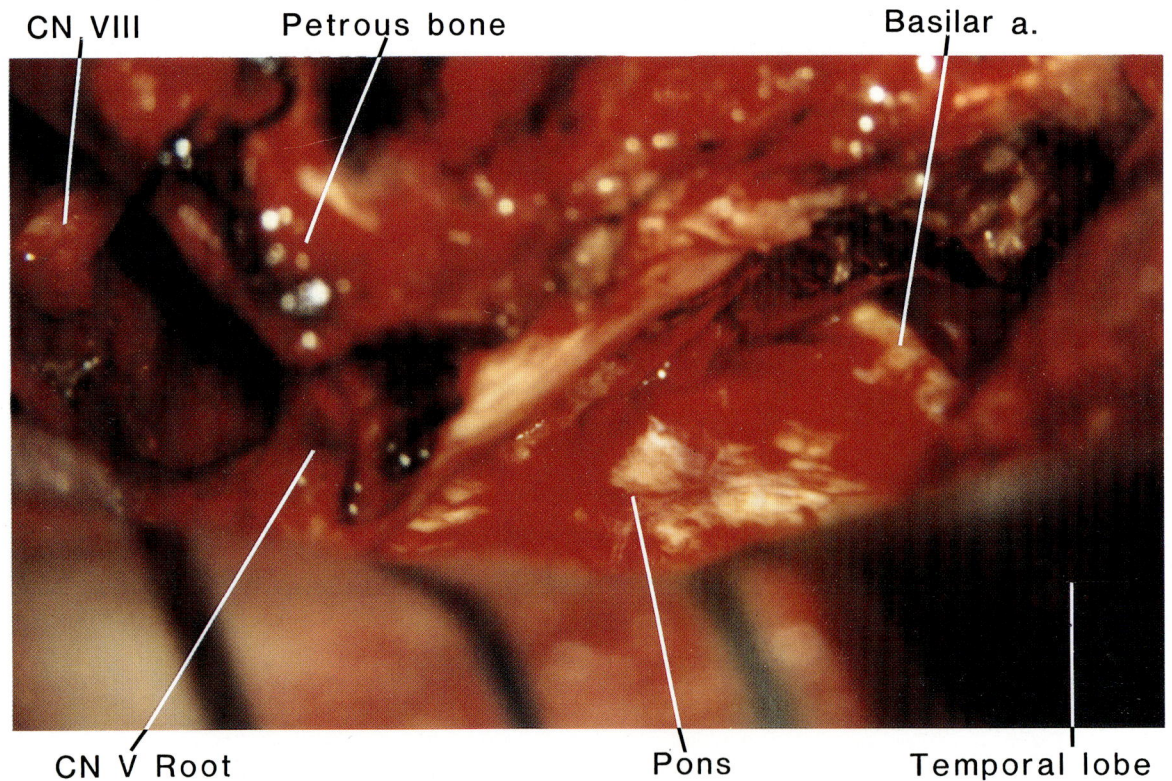

FIG. 81. View of basilar artery, trigeminal nerve, and the pons following complete tumor resection.

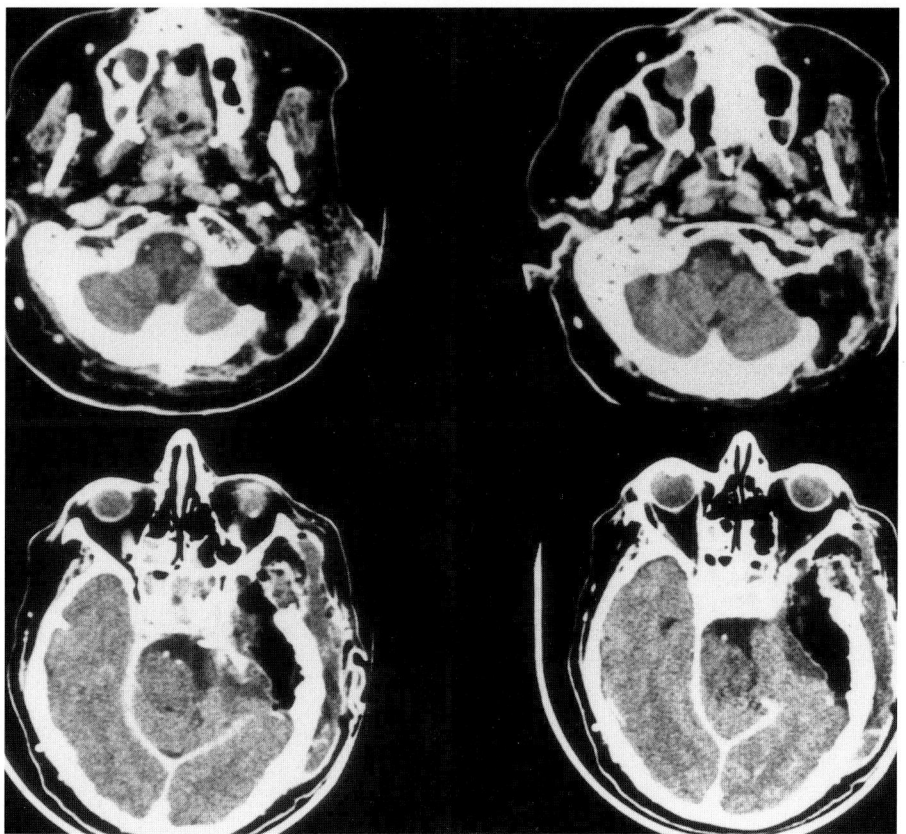

FIG. 82. Postoperative CT scan with contrast shows subtotal tumor resection. Some tumor remains in the cavernous sinus.

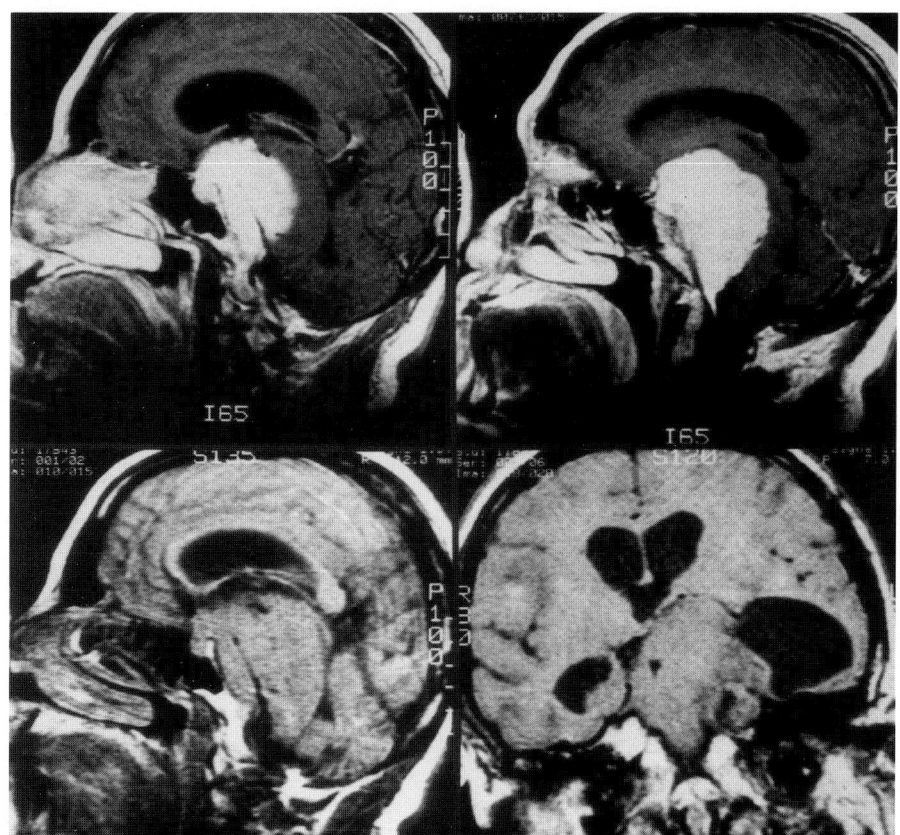

FIG. 83. (Figures 83–90 are of patient M.C.) MRI scans with and without intravenous contrast show a giant petroclival meningioma extending from the lower clivus to the body of the left ventricle superiorly and orbital apex anteriorly. The unenhanced scan (**left**) clearly demonstrates the encased basilar artery (**lower left**). Basilar artery quadrification is seen on the **lower right** MRI scan.

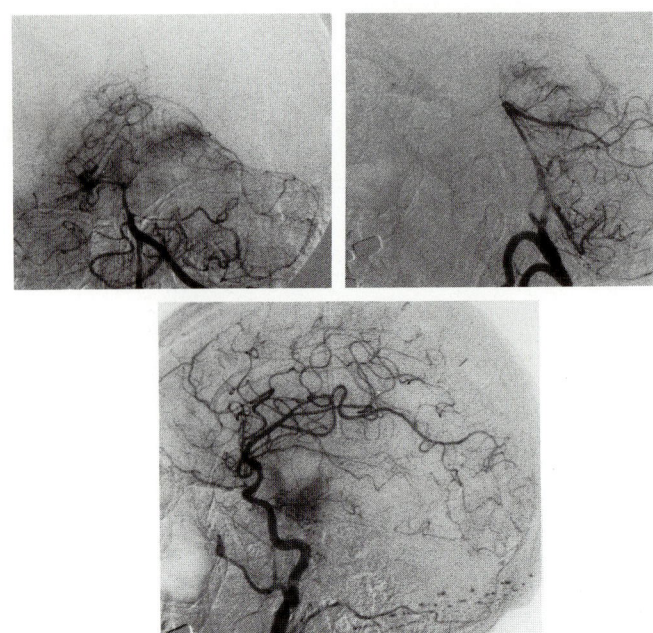

FIG. 84. Vertebral and carotid angiogram. There is stenosis of the cavernous and supraclinoid ICA and superior displacement (**bottom**). Stenosis and posterior displacement of basilar artery by tumor are apparent (**top**) on this vertebral angiogram. Tumor blood supply is mainly via the meningohyophyseal trunk.

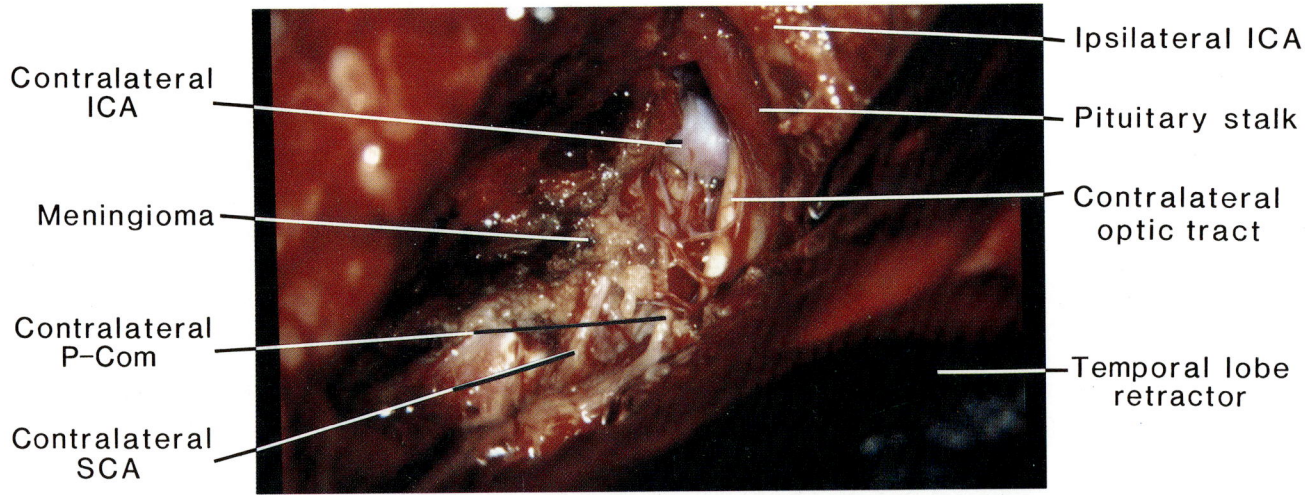

FIG. 85. During the second operation by the frontotemporal–infratemporal approach the ipsilateral ICA, pituitary stalk opposite the ICA, the opposite posterior communicating artery, and the superior cerebellar artery have been dissected free of tumor. Residual tumor is visible.

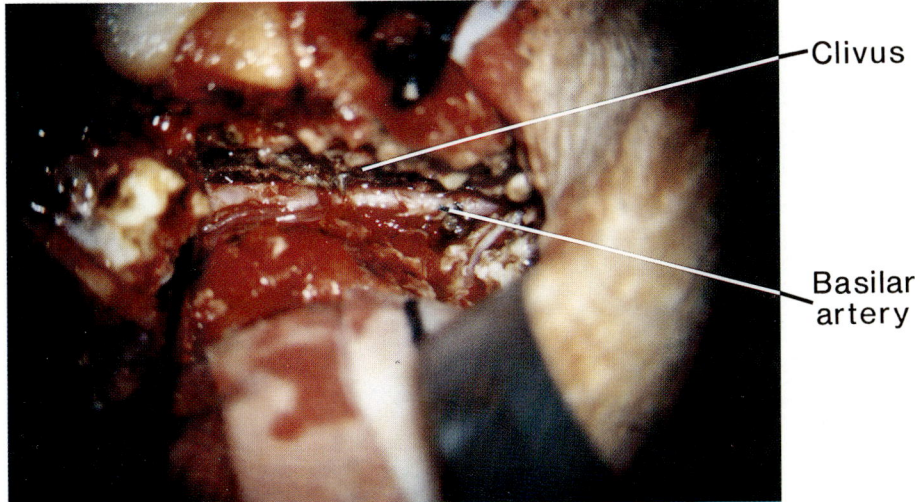

FIG. 86. The basilar artery is dissected free of tumor and is seen to be lying on the clivus.

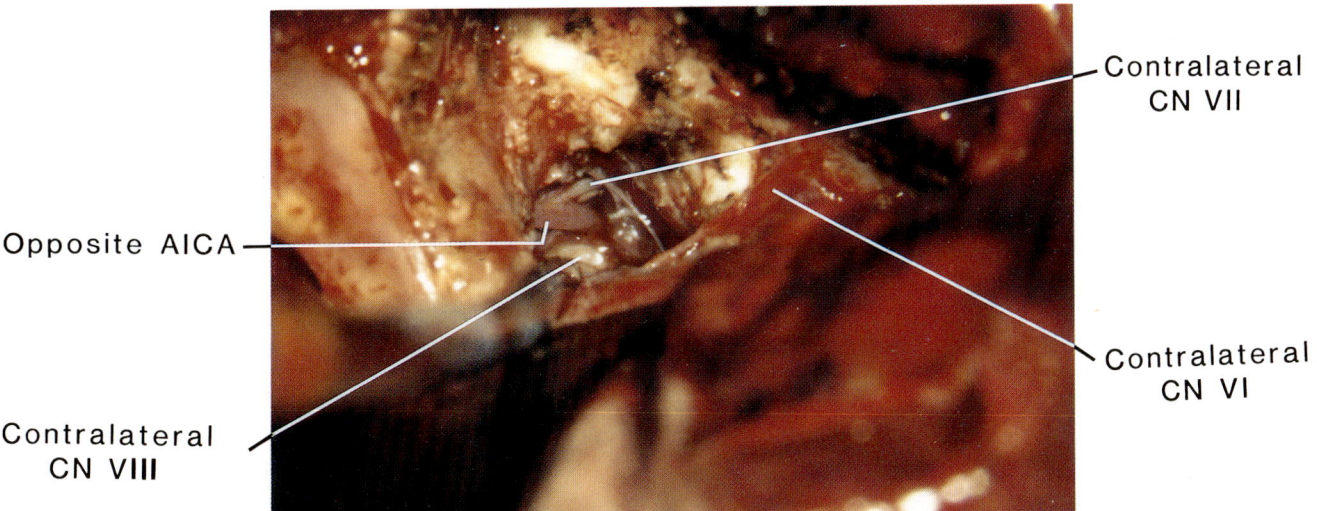

FIG. 87. Opposite CNs VI, VII, VIII and opposite AICA are well demonstrated.

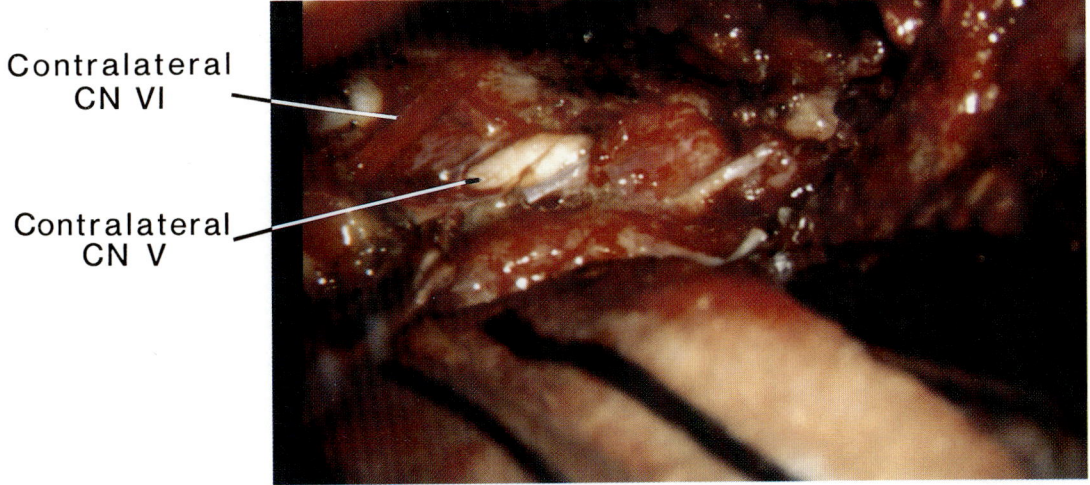

FIG. 88. At the end of the operation, contralateral CN VI and contralateral CN V are visible.

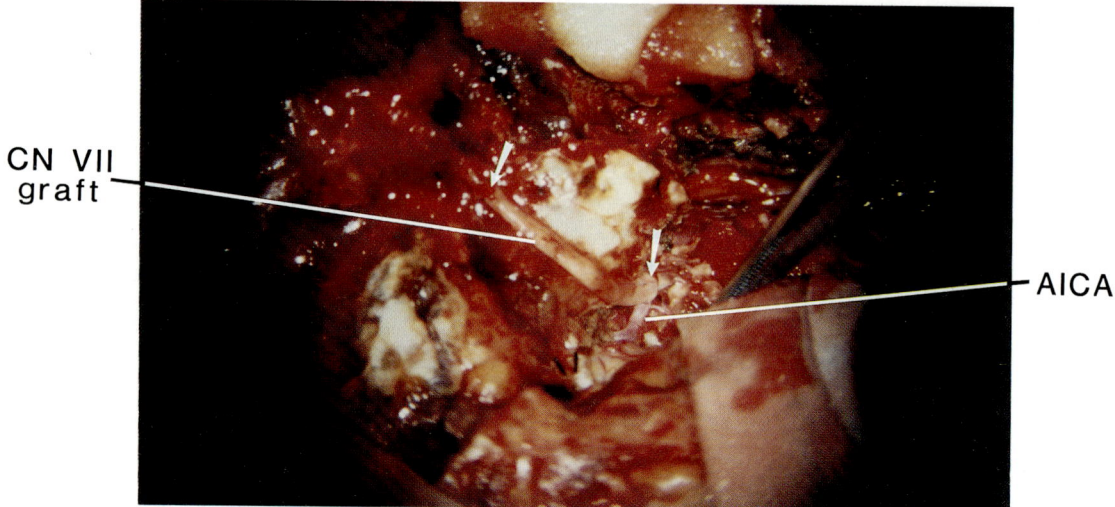

FIG. 89. View of the greater auricular nerve graft used to reconstruct the damaged facial nerve. The *arrow* points to the anastomotic site.

rhage in the midbrain. On follow-up, 12 months later, she had regained normal function of the left side but remained dysphasic and hemiparetic on the right, as before the operation (Karnofsky 50). Her facial nerve function is recovering and is at present House grade II. Further tumor resection was performed (Figs. 85–89) and the patient was given external beam radiation therapy for residual tumor (Fig. 90).

This patient represents our current limitation of surgical therapy. Had this patient been treated before her previous operations (with resulting scar), a better resection might have been possible.

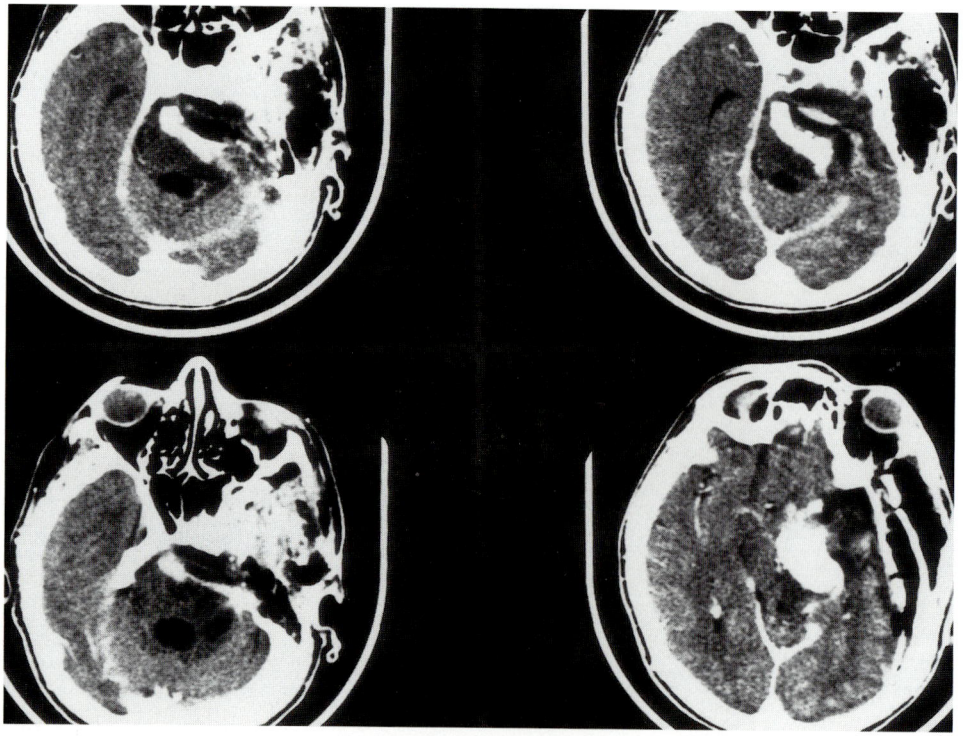

FIG. 90. Postoperative CT scans with intravenous contrast show residual tumor, which was treated with external beam radiation.

TABLE 3. Operative approaches used for tumor resection

Approaches	Number of cases	Percentage
Simple approaches		
Frontotemporal transsylvian or subtemporal/transzygomatic	10	19
Frontotemporal/orbitozygomatic/transcavernous	19	36
Retrosigmoid approach (suboccipital)	23	44
Extreme lateral transcondylar–C1 laminectomy	7	13
Complex approaches		
Subtemporal–preauricular infratemporal approach	10	19
Posterior subtemporal transzygomatic and presigmoid transpetrous approach		
With sigmoid sinus division	3	6
Without sigmoid sinus division	5	10
Total petrosectomy	6	12
Number of stages for tumor resection		
Single operation	28	54
Two or more operations	24	46

OPERATIVE RESULTS

Operative approaches and results are summarized in Tables 3–5. Of the 52 patients in our series, there were 44 women and 8 men aged 24–73 years (average 51). As one can see from Table 3, an array of different approaches were used, with the retrosigmoid (44%) and frontotemporal–orbitozygomatic transcavernous approach (36%) being the most common. Just under half (46%) of the cases required two or more operations. Patients with giant or more complex tumors (vascular encasement or scarring from previous surgery) generally required more than one operation. Eleven patients (21%) had encasement of the vertebrobasilar artery and its branches. Extent of tumor resection was based on operative findings and MRI and CT scans (with and without contrast) obtained 2–3 months postoperatively. On this basis, total tumor excision was achieved in 38 cases (73%), subtotal excision in 11 (21%), and partial excision in 3 (6%). In the patients with vertebrobasilar artery encasement, six had gross total resection, four subtotal resection, and one partial resection. The total excision rate might have been higher if two additional patients had undergone a second-stage operation to remove tumor (one elected to forego any further surgery, and surgery was postponed for medical reasons in the other case).

The follow-up period has ranged from 4 months to 83 months. To date, two recurrences have been observed in patients who had an apparent total tumor excision. One had a small recurrence at the margin of prior resection and was reoperated. The other patient had a very aggressive, probably radiation-induced tumor. He had a sizable recurrence that was treated by reoperation and external beam radiation. He eventually died of uncontrolled tumor growth.

COMPLICATIONS

Postoperative complications are noted in Table 5. Postoperative deaths occurred in two patients. One patient with a large middle and lower clival tumor developed ipsilateral CN IX, X, and XII paralysis postoperatively and required tracheostomy for airway protection. She developed massive pneumonia and died suddenly (patient M.H.). The second patient with a giant petroclival meningioma with basilar artery encasement had a rather complicated postoperative course, including wound infection and sepsis. She had recovered from local wound problems when she died suddenly 2 months postoperatively of pulmonary complications (patient J.F.). Three patients sustained probable brain stem infarction: in one patient, occlusion of a tumor-encased superior cerebellar artery was felt to be responsible for temporary hemiparesis and obtundation, with eventual mild worsening of preoperative hemiparesis (Karnofsky preop 70; postop 60). In a second case of recurrent me-

TABLE 4. Extent of tumor resection, treatment of residue and recurrence

Procedure	Number of cases	Percentage
Total excision	38	73
Subtotal excision (90% of tumor volume)	11	21
Partial excision (second planned operation refused)	3	6
Location of residual tumor (in more than one area in some patients)		
Clivus	10	19
Cavernous sinus	7	13
Treatment of residual tumor		
Observation (some awaiting second stage of surgery)	10	19
Gamma knife	4	8
Recurrence treatment		
Reoperation	2	4
+ External radiation	1	2

TABLE 5. Major complications of surgery

Complications[a]	Number of cases	Percentage
Death	2	4
Cerebral infarction (hemiparesis/worsening mental status)	3	6
Cerebral edema (hematoma)[b]	4	8
Subdural hygroma/hematoma (operative drainage)[b]	3	6
Temporary hemiparesis (recovered)[b]	7	13
Locked in syndrome, temporary (recovered)[b]	1	2
Cerebral abscess (resolved)[b]	1	2
CN IX and X palsies requiring tracheostomy[b]	10	19
Aspiration pneumonia[b]	7	13
CSF leaks (resolved)[b]	5	10
Meningitis (resolved)[b]	2	4
Wound infection (resolved)[b]	1	2
Diabetes insipidus (resolved)[b]	3	6
Hydrocephalus (VP shunt)[b]	3	6

[a] More than one complication occurred in each individual patient.
[b] Complications which resolved with treatment.

ningioma, a perforator occlusion was felt to be responsible for postoperative dementia and hemiparesis (Karnofsky preop 70, postop 40). The third patient had five previous operations and radiation therapy and sustained superior cerebellar artery occlusion at operation. This patient sustained a worsened hemiparesis (Karnofsky preop 50, postop 40).

There were a number of additional significant complications which resolved with treatment. One patient sustained temporal lobe and cerebellar contusion after a posterior–subtemporal and presigmoid transpetrous approach to the tumor. Reoperation to remove contused brain was followed by a prolonged convalescence (Karnofsky preop 90, postop 70). Another patient with a giant-sized tumor encasing the basilar artery had had a progressively worsening preoperative neurological condition. Postoperatively, she developed a delayed temporal lobe hematoma and abscess related to pulmonary embolism, anticoagulation, and systemic sepsis. She made an eventual recovery from these complications (Karnofsky preop 60, postop 60). The most frequent complications were related to dysfunction of CNs IX and X and associated pulmonary problems. This has increased the use of temporary tracheostomy to prevent aspiration pneumonia and to improve pulmonary toilet. Most of these patients on follow-up are able to discontinue the tracheostomy and regain swallowing function.

With increasing surgical experience and careful selection of operative approach, it has become progressively easier to obtain complete tumor resection of petroclival meningiomas and reduce morbidity to an acceptable level, even with some extraordinarily difficult cases seen in our institution. However, many cases remain wherein total resection may result in considerable patient morbidity, such that residual tumor is left behind. In such patients, the combination with gamma knife or LINAC radiosurgery may provide effective tumor control.

It is quite apparent to us that the first set of operations to remove tumor is the most important to both the patient and the surgeon, since the ability to resect tumor completely without major complications is the greatest. Both resectability and complications are worse in patients who have had prior operations or radiation therapy.

REFERENCES

1. Al-Mefty O, Fox JL, Smith RR. Petrosal approach for petroclival meningiomas. *Neurosurgery* 1988;22:510–517.
2. Campbell E, Whitfield RD. Posterior fossa meningiomas. *J Neurosurg* 1948;5:131–153.
3. Cherington M, Schneck SA. Clivus meningiomas. *Neurology* 1966;16:86–92.
4. Crockard HA, Sen CN. The transoral approach for the management of intradural lesions at the craniovertebral junction: review of 7 cases. *Neurosurgery* 1991;28:88–98.
5. Cushing HW, Eisenhardt L. *Meningiomas. Their classification, regional behaviour, life history and surgical end results.* Springfield, IL: Charles C. Thomas, 1938;3–387.
6. Hakuba A, Nishimura, Jang BJ. A combined retroauricular and preauricular transpetrosal–transtentorial approach to clivus meningiomas. *Surg Neurol* 1988;30:108–116.
7. House WF, De la Cruz A, Hitselberger WE. Surgery of the skull base: transcochlear approach to the petrous apex and clivus. *ORL J Otorhinolaryngol Relat Spec* 1978;86:770–779.
8. House W, Hitselberger W. The transcochlear approach to the skull base. *Arch Otolaryngol* 1976;102:334–342.
9. Long DM. Surgical approaches to tumors of skull base: an overview. In: Wilkins RH, Rengachary SS, eds. *Neurosurgery update I: diagnosis, operative technique, and neuro-oncology.* New York: McGraw-Hill, 1990;266–276.
10. Malis LI. Surgical resection of tumors of the skull base. In: Wilkins RH, Rengachary SS, eds. *Neurosurgery;* Vol 1. New York: McGraw Hill, 1985; 1011–1021.
11. Mayberg MR, Symon L. Meningiomas of the clivus and apical petrous bone. Report of 35 cases. *J Neurosurg* 1986;65:160–167.
12. Moller AR. Electrophysiological monitoring of cranial nerves in operations in the skull base. In: Sekhar LN, Schramm VL, eds: *Tumors of the cranial base: diagnosis and treatment.* Mount Kisco, NY: Futura Publishing Company, 1987;123–132.

13. Russell JR, Bucy PC. Meningiomas of the posterior fossa. *Surg Gynecol Obstet* 1953;96:183–192.
14. Samii M, Ammirati M, Mahran A, et al. Survey of petroclival meningiomas: report of 24 cases. *Neurosurgery* 1989;24:12–17.
15. Sekhar LN, Estonillo R. Transtemporal approach to the skull base: an anatomical study. *Neurosurgery* 1986;19:799–808.
16. Sekhar LN, Jannetta PJ. Petroclival and medial tentorial meningiomas. In: Sekhar LN, Schramm VL, eds. *Tumors of the cranial base: diagnosis and treatment.* Mount Kisco, NY: Futura Publishing Company, 1987;623–640.
17. Sekhar LN, Jannetta PJ, Burkhart L, et al. Meningiomas involving the clivus: a six-year experience with 41 patients. *Neurosurgery* 1990;27:764–781.
18. Sekhar LN, Jannetta PJ, Maroon JC. Tentorial meningiomas: surgical management and results. *Neurosurgery* 1984;14:268–275.
19. Sekhar LN, Samii M. Petroclival and medial tentorial meningiomas. In: Scheunemann H, Schurmann K, Helms J, eds. *Tumors of the skull base: extra- and intracranial surgery of skull base tumors.* Berlin: Walter de Gruyter, 1986;141–158.
20. Sekhar LN, Schramm VL, Jones NF. Subtemporal–preauricular infratemporal fossa approach to large lateral and posterior cranial base neoplasms. *J Neurosurg* 1987;67:488–499.
21. Sekhar LN, Sen CN, Jho HD, Janecka IP. Surgical treatment of intracavernous neoplasms: a four-year experience. *Neurosurgery* 1989;26:18–30.
22. Sekhar LN, Sen CN, Jho HD. Saphenous vein bypass of the cavernous internal carotid artery. *J Neurosurg* 1990;72:35–41.
23. Sen CN, Sekhar LN. An extreme lateral approach to intradural lesions of the cervical spine and foramen magnum. *Neurosurgery* 1990;27:197–204.
24. Yasargil MG, Mortara RW, Curcic M. Meningiomas of basal posterior cranial fossa. In: Krayenbuhl H, ed. *Advances and technical standards in neurosurgery,* vol. 7. Wien: Springer-Verlag, 1980;1–115.

CHAPTER 39

Combined Supra- and Infra-Parapetrosal Approach for Petroclival Lesions

Takanori Fukushima

Petroclival tumors present the neurosurgeon with extreme difficulty for radical resection. These tumors are located deep at the base of the brain, mostly hypervascular with broad attachment to the petrous, clival, and tentorial regions, often invading into the cavernous sinus and involving or adherent to the vital perforating arteries, multiple cranial nerves, and the brain stem. A number of operative approaches or combined surgical techniques have been described to achieve access to the petroclival area (Table 1). The routine frontotemporal pterional approach has been used by many neurosurgeons, particularly in cases with large suprasellar or parasellar extension of the tumor. When the tumor is widely invading the frontal skull base or the cavernous sinus, Derome's frontal transbasal techniques or Dolenc's cavernous procedures can be used. The author has been using a special operative approach of the anterior temporopolar trans-cavum Meckeli posterior transcavernous technique to some of the trigeminal neurinomas and petroclival meningiomas. The conventional subtemporal transtentorial approach has been performed in many neurosurgical centers; however, one must be extremely careful because this approach carries the risk of postoperative temporal contusion hemorrhage. Large temporal hematoma can occur even if all veins are preserved and the brain is retracted minimally. Particularly, some elderly patients have an extremely nonresistant fragile brain and unexpected contusion can be encountered with the least operative manipulation. When the subtemporal approach is used, the lateral part of the temporal bone must be drilled away completely to make a flat access to the tentorial hiatus with minimal temporal lobe retraction, and resection of the tumor should be limited to the supratentorial portions. If the infratentorial mass is resected via the transtentorial route, there will be a significant risk of postoperative temporal lobe problems. The retromastoid suboccipital approach has been used as one of the most standard operative techniques for petroclival tumors. This retromastoid approach allows a simple and rapid opening and is still my favorite technique to treat many of the petrous and clival tumors. In particular, for cases whose tumor mass is mainly located in the infratentorial space, the retromastoid approach is indicated.

After performing many retromastoid trigeminal approaches to petroclival tumors, such as meningiomas, neurinomas, and epidermoids, I developed a special operative technique—the retromastoid upper CP angle trigeminal upward-transtentorial exposure—in 1984. As Fig. 1 demonstrates, a modest amount of the supratentorial extension of the tumor can be easily resected by incising the tentorium from below and exposing the medial temporal lobe, posterior cerebral artery, cranial nerve III, and the chiasm. Also, the petrous apex can be drilled away from below and the superior petrosal sinus can be resected in the paratrigeminal area to expose Meckel's cave from below. This suboccipital upward-transtentorial technique has been used in a number of

TABLE 1. *Operative approaches to petroclival tumors*

Frontotemporal pterional ⟨ transbasal (Derome)
⟨ transcavernous (Dolenc)
Temporopolar posterior transcavernous (Fukushima)
Subtemporal transtentorial
Retromastoid suboccipital (upward transtentorial, Fukushima)
Combined subtemporal and suboccipital
Combined petrosal (see Table 2)

T. Fukushima: Department of Neurosurgery and USC-Skull Base Center, University of Southern California, Los Angeles, California 90033.

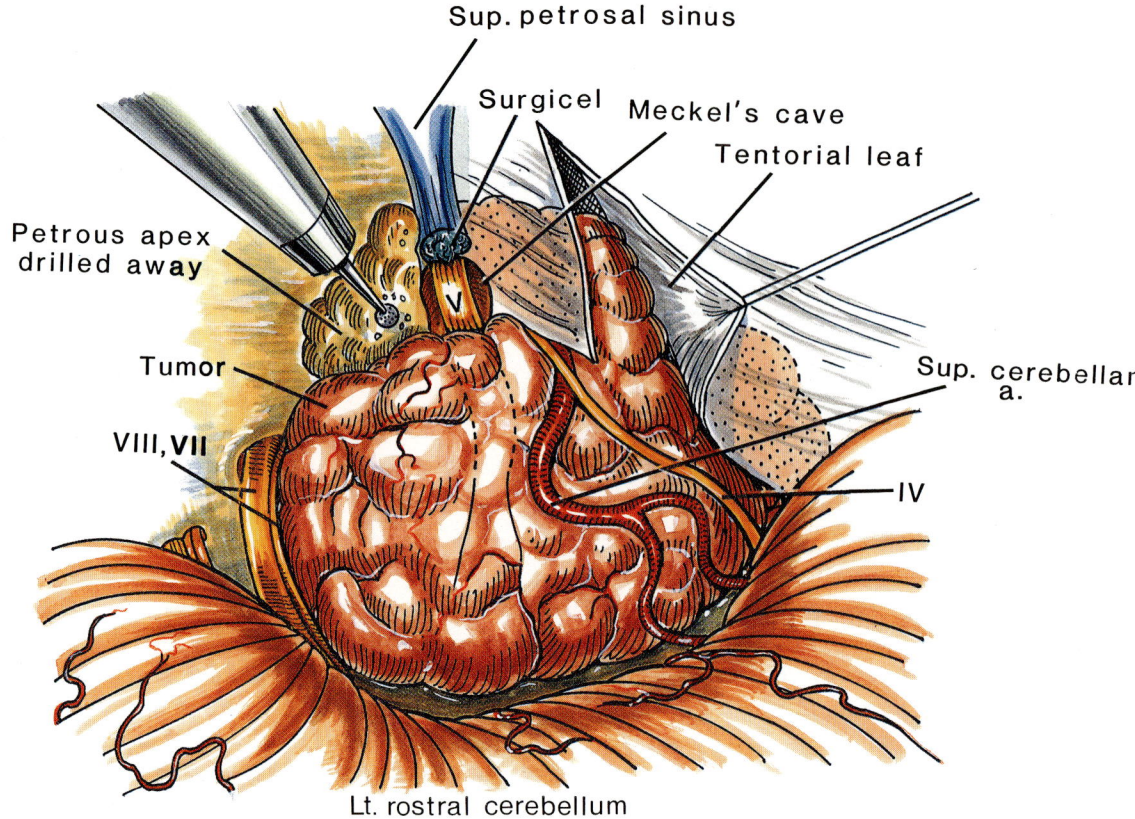

FIG. 1. An artist's drawing to illustrate the surgical technique of the retromastoid suboccipital upward-transtentorial approach.

cases and found to be extremely useful for radical tumor resection.

COMBINED PETROSAL APPROACH

The microsurgical combined petrosal approach was first described by Hitselberger and House (4) in 1966, and since then various modification techniques have been reported (Table 2) (1). Morrison and King (5) de-

TABLE 2. *Various modifications of combined approach*

1. Hitselberger–House (combined suboccipital–petrosal)	1966
2. Morrison–King (presigmoid translabyrinthine)	1970
3. Malis (retrolabyrinthine, sinus division, preserve Labbé's vein)	1970
4. Hakuba (extensive petrous drilling, transpetrosal)	1977
5. Fukushima (minimal drilling, presigmoid, preserve sinus and Labbé's vein)	1982
6. Total or subtotal petrosectomy for deaf cases	

scribed a presigmoid translabyrinthine approach to the large acoustic neuromas in 1970. Malis (6) stated that he started to use his combined approach in 1970. Malis stressed that the sigmoid sinus should be transected to obtain wide surgical exposure while preserving Labbé's vein. Hakuba (2) learned the Malis technique in New York and extended the procedure with extensive drilling and mastoidectomy. Hashi et al. (3) used less drilling technique than Hakuba and reported their approach applied to the clipping of vertebrobasilar aneurysms in 1982. In my experience with these petrosal procedures, extensive drilling had the disadvantages of cosmetic deformity, risk for CSF leak, and risks for damage to otological structures. In the majority of petroclival tumors, patients present with minimal symptoms like dizziness, ataxia, diplopia, and trigeminal neuropathy. Therefore surgeons should perform a retrolabyrinthine exposure to preserve the semicircular canals and the endolymphatic duct. As Fig. 2 shows, retrolabyrinthine drilling or even translabyrinthine drilling will not help the surgeon's keyhole access to the petrous apex and the clivus. A small parallel space is needed along the petrous ridge above and below the tentorium to resect the petroclival masses, with 1-cm brain retraction. Therefore, since 1982, I have

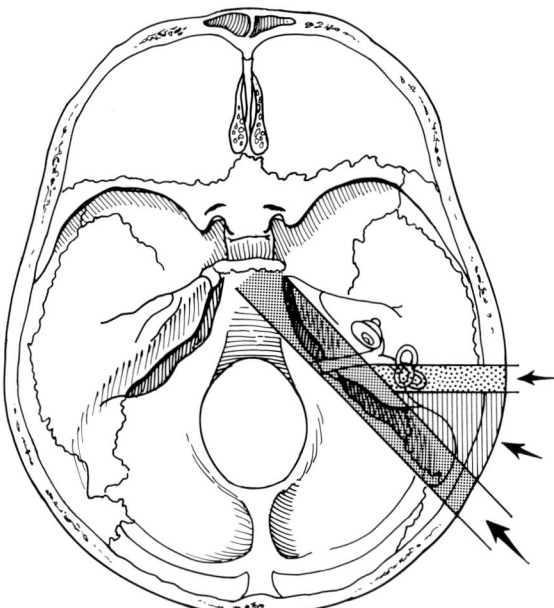

FIG. 2. A scheme of the skull base illustrating the concept of the 1-cm parapetrosal approach along the petrous ridge. Extensive mastoidectomy or retrolabyrinthine drilling is totally unnecessary to make a keyhole access to the petrous apex and the clivus.

established a combined *parapetrosal* technique with minimal drilling presigmoid exposure and preservation of both sinuses and Labbé's vein.

This approach provides excellent surgical exposure of both infratentorial and supratentorial spaces with direct access to the petroclival region along the petrous ridge. Because the transverse and sigmoid sinuses and Labbé's vein are preserved, the incidence of occipital or posterior temporal contusion swelling is very low and not significant if it does exist. The cavum Meckeli can be opened and the whole petrous and clival areas and the basilar trunk are satisfactorily exposed with minimal brain retraction.

INDICATION FOR THE COMBINED PARAPETROSAL APPROACH

Table 3 demonstrates the selection of operative approaches to the various petroclival tumors treated in my neurosurgical service during the period between 1982 and 1989. As already mentioned, the retromastoid approach was the most popular one (58 cases out of 103, 56%), and the pterional transcavernous approach was performed in ten cases. The subtemporal transtentorial approach was done earlier in the cases of 11 patients. The combined retromastoid and subtemporal approach was tried in two cases as two-stage operations.

The combined parapetrosal approach is much simpler and less time-consuming compared to other extensive petrosal procedures, but it still requires a larger craniotomy, drilling, presigmoid dural incision, division of the superior petrosal sinus, and retraction of both the cerebellum and the posterior temporal lobe. Therefore the combined parapetrosal approach carries more complicated surgical exposures than the simple and easy retromastoid exposures. This combined approach is best indicated for petroclival tumors with both large supratentorial and infratentorial extensions and with wide involvement of the petrous apex, clivus, and the tentorial region. The parapetrosal approach is better indicated in younger patients below 60 years of age. For elderly patients, the retromastoid or two-stage procedure with nearly total resection is indicated.

OPERATIVE TECHNIQUE OF THE COMBINED PARAPETROSAL APPROACH

Microsurgical Instrumentation

To conduct rapid and efficient exposure of the presigmoid dura, a high-speed air drill is crucial. Various sizes of cutting burrs and diamond burrs are necessary with various lengths (short, medium, and long) and straight

TABLE 3. *Selection of approaches to petroclival tumors (1982–1989)*

Tumor	Retromastoid suboccipital	Pterional cavernous	Subtemporal transtentorial	Two-stage retromastoid subtemporal	Combined parapetrosal
Meningioma	50	5	9	2	12
V-neurinoma	8	2	—	—	4
Chordoma	—	3	2	—	1
Sigmoid AVM					3
Giant acoustic					1
Giant cavernoma					1
					22

and angled hand pieces. A pair of black nonreflecting tapered brain retractors are useful for retraction of the brain. A pair of straight and curved microscissors, thick blades for dura, tentorium, and tumor, and thin blades for arachnoid dissection are necessary. Several microprobes and skull base dissectors are also necessary. Malleable monopolar coagulating probes are extremely useful to detach the tumor origin from the skull base and coagulate bony bleeding. Microcurettes and 2.5-mm as well as 3-mm microring curettes are useful to eradicate the mass from the meatus and from Meckel's cavity. Laser apparatus is usually of no help, while the ultrasonic aspirator is useful in some cases. High-power bipolar forceps are most helpful to dissect and resect fibrous and vascular tumors.

Patient Positioning

The patient is placed in a lateral decubitus position with the torso elevated about 20° (Fig. 3). The patient's knees are comfortably bent with a large pillow between the two legs. An adequate soft mattress is inserted under the lower axilla to avoid chest compression. The patient's upper shoulder is slightly rotated toward the anesthesia side and gently pulled toward the legs. The head is held in the exact lateral horizontal position and flexed moderately and fixed with a three-point Mayfield–Portenoy skull clamp.

During the operative procedure, the surgeon's view can be altered quickly by maneuvering a Contraves microscope in all directions and also by rotating the operating table from side to side and up or down.

Scalp Incision and Craniotomy

A small question mark incision is made around the posterior temporal and retromastoid area, as illustrated

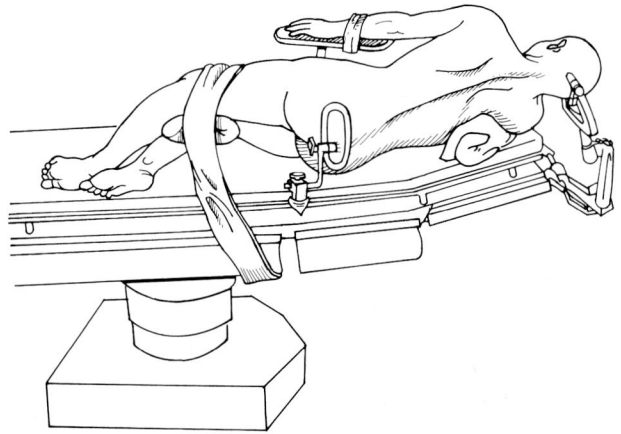

FIG. 3. Patient positioning for the combined parapetrosal approach.

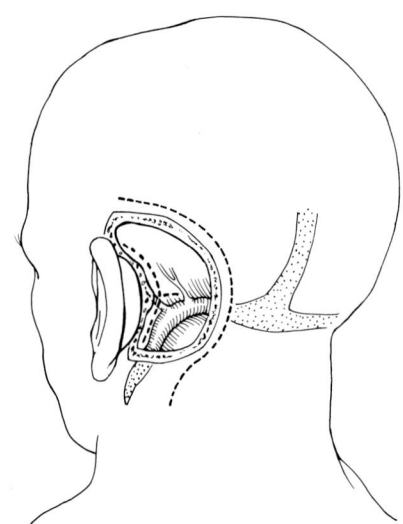

FIG. 4. Scalp incision, L-shaped craniotomy, and dural incision.

in Fig. 4. The scalp flap is turned anteriorly using special large blunt hooks (Fig. 5A,B). The suboccipital fascia and the temporal pericranium are carefully preserved for later use at closure to cover the opened mastoid air cells and to make a dural patch graft. An L-shaped bone flap is turned to expose the posterior temporal dura, the upper half of the retromastoid dura, and the transverse and sigmoid sinuses. The outer dura covering the sigmoid sinus is extremely thin and adherent to the bony groove, so the craniotomy should be performed with extreme care over this portion. A right angle dural elevator is helpful to dissect the dura from the bony adhesion. Then a small portion of the posterior petrous bone is drilled away just enough to expose a 4 × 10 mm area of the presigmoid dura. All semicircular canals and the endolymphatic duct must be preserved to maintain normal 8th nerve functions postoperatively. After initial rapid drilling with cutting burrs, the presigmoid dura is exposed with various sizes of diamond burrs. It is not necessary to perform a mastoidectomy or extensive drilling, as already explained (Fig. 2). A small amount of drilling limited to exposing the presigmoid dura is sufficient.

Dural Incision and Access to the Tumor

The posterior temporal dura and the presigmoid dura are incised near the bone edge (Fig. 4) and CSF is gradually aspirated to obtain slack brain. The superior petrosal sinus (Fig. 6, arrow) is ligated with two sutures and divided between the sutures. After division of the superior petrosal sinus, the superior surface of the cerebellum and the posterior temporal lobe base are retracted gently using a pair of 2.2-mm black retractors (Fig. 6). The brain surface is protected with collagen sheets and cottonoids.

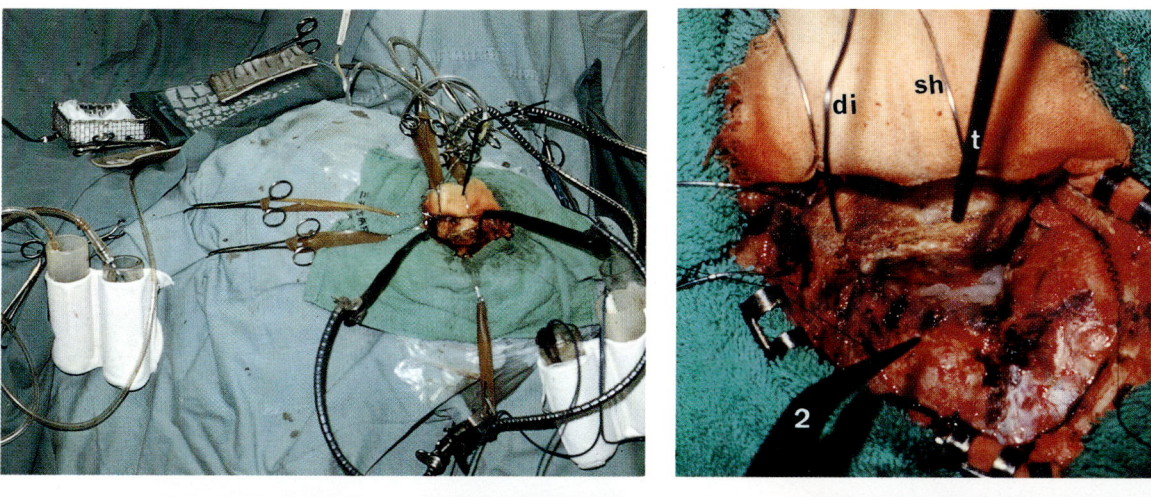

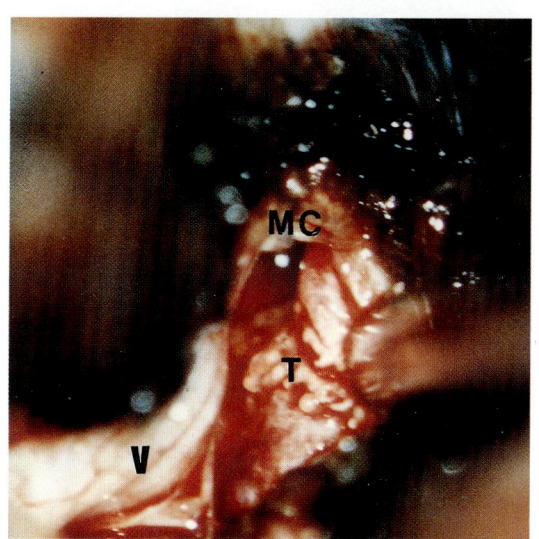
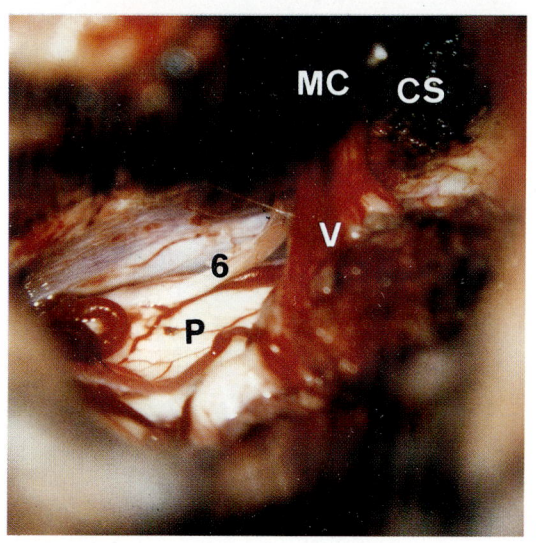

FIG. 5. A: Operative arrangements for left combined parapetrosal approach. The left instrument pocket contains a couple of pressure-adjustable suckers. The right pocket has bipolar forceps and a monopolar cautery. A small C-clamp (developed in 1980) is attached to the side arm of the Mayfield headholder and provides two lightweight titanium snakes. The other side of the snake holders will hold a serrated tumor retractor and a continuous saline drip irrigating malleable needle. All sizes of Surgicel pieces and cottonoids are readily available. **B:** Appearance after parapetrosal craniotomy. The scalp is turned with large blunt hooks (sh). The operative area can be continuously irrigated with a malleable blunt needle held on a snake holder (di). The posterior temporal dura, suboccipital area, transverse-sigmoid sinuses, and presigmoid dura are all well exposed by minimal drilling of the petrous bone. A pair of nonreflecting malleable retractors (2 and 4) and a serrated tumor retractor (t) are in place. **C:** Microscope photograph from surgery on patient O.M. Exposure is along the petrous ridge. The porus trigeminus is entirely dissected and Meckel's cave is opened to remove the invading tumor. MC, Meckel's cave; V, trigeminal nerve root; T, meningioma. **D:** Operative photograph of patient O.M., after radical total resection. Meckel's cave is opened completely to remove the tumor while preserving the flattened trigeminal root (V) and the abducens nerve (VI). The posterior cavernous sinus is also opened and packed with Surgicel (CS). The brain stem and pons (P) are intact.

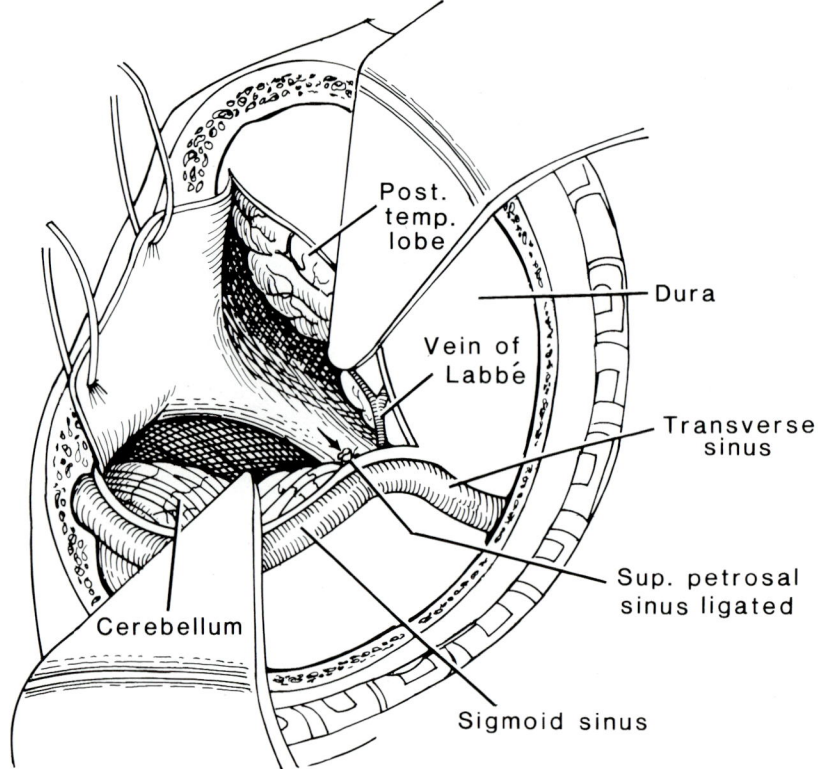

FIG. 6. Dural incision and retraction of the cerebellum and the posterior temporal lobe. The superior petrosal sinus is divided with two sutures (*arrow*). Labbé's vein (VL) is preserved inside the dura and the transverse sigmoid sinuses are kept intact. A pair of 2.2-mm nonreflecting black spatulas are useful.

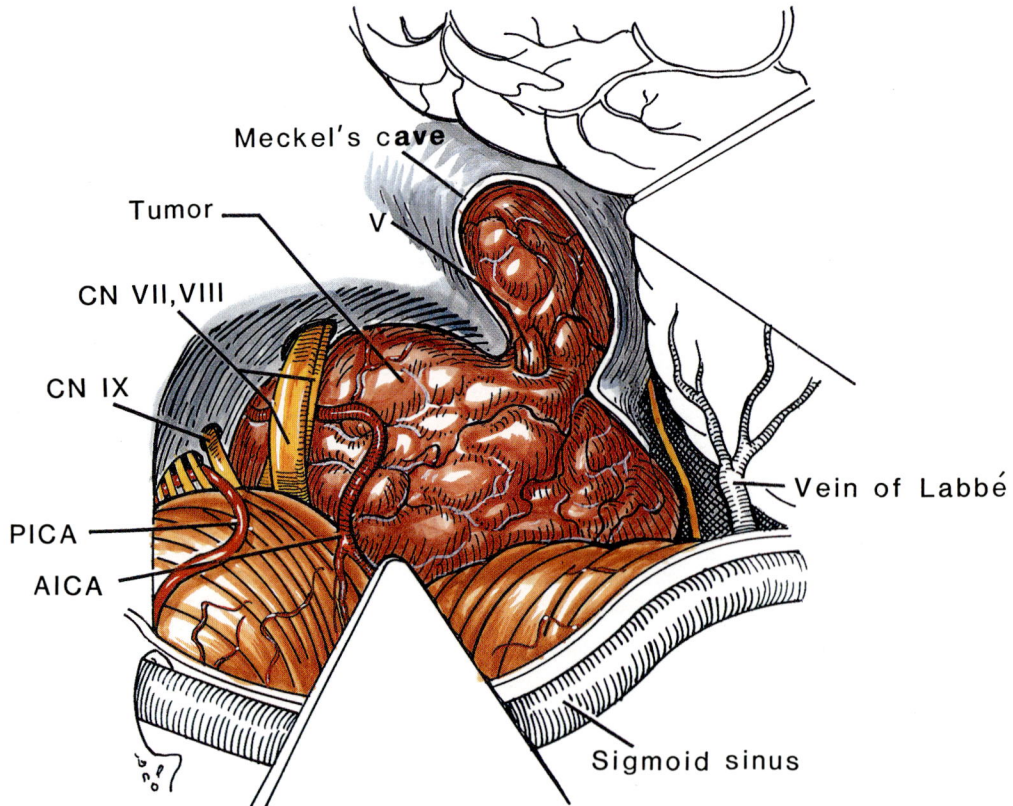

FIG. 7. Exposure and resection of a petroclival meningioma through a combined parapetrosal approach. The entire tumor can be exposed through a beautiful supra- and infratranstentorial approach along the petrous ridge. The tumor is easily detached from the skull base with drilling of the petrous apex, monopolar coagulating dissectors, and high-power bipolar techniques. Meckel's cave is also opened to eradicate the mass completely.

Labbé's vein is preserved inside the posterior temporal dura (Fig. 6, VL). While retracting the brain and aspirating CSF, the tentorium is detached along the petrous ridge toward the free edge by means of monopolar coagulating probes and bipolar forceps. When the free edge of the tentorium is divided and the arachnoid membrane is incised, the tumor surface is already observed and cranial nerve IV is visible. The tumor can be exposed from both the supratentorial and infratentorial directions along the petrous bone. Precise microsurgical–anatomical knowledge is required to appreciate all displaced locations of cranial nerves and vessels. The tumor surface is carefully exposed toward the depth and the surface is coagulated. Then the tumor origin or attachment is dissected, coagulated, and detached from the base. First, the tumor is elevated from the temporal base toward the dura of Meckel's cave and second, the tumor is detached from the petrous dura at the suboccipital space. It is most important, particularly in cases of meningioma, to detach the tumor origin and to devascularize the mass. The dural and bony bleeding is controlled by monopolar coagulation, Surgicel packings with or without cyanoacrylate glue, and bone wax.

Resection of Tumor

After the tumor attachment is divided off the petrous ridge and off the basal dura, the tumor is cored with high-power bipolar forceps. Debulking of the tumor mass is very important to elevate the tumor capsule from the nerves and from the brain stem. After sufficient internal decompression, the tumor capsule is retracted using a special serrated tumor retractor (see Fig. 5A,B). Cranial nerves VIII and IX are dissected while monitoring the auditory brain stem response (ABR). The dura over Meckel's cave (Fig. 7, MC) is opened and the tumor mass inside Meckel's cave is removed while preserving the trigeminal rootlets. The dura at the tumor origin is resected as much as possible or coagulated in older patients. The petrous apex bone can be drilled off with tumor invasion and the porus trigeminus is widely opened for radical tumor resection. The trigeminal nerve root can be dorsal to the tumor mass, or ventral, or engulfed within the mass. Extreme care should be paid to preserve CN VI at the tumor bed. When the tumor has involved the basilar perforators or cranial nerves with tough fibrous adhesion, that portion of the tumor capsule must be left with the brain stem to avoid serious postoperative sequelae (see Fig. 10). When the tumor invades the cavernous sinus, that portion of the mass should be left untouched when using the parapetrosal approach. The cavernous portion of the tumor should be operated on later using the Dolenc technique as the second-stage operation.

Closure

After confirming complete hemostasis, the wound is closed in anatomical approximation. The dura must be closed watertight using fascia graft and additional fibrin glue. Mastoid air cells are packed with muscle or covered with pericranium. The bone flap is replaced and fixated with wires. A small amount of bioresin may be used for cosmetic skull reconstruction. Postoperative lumbar drainage may be used to prevent CSF leak. Intraoperative and perioperative antibiotic administration is recommended to prevent possible infection.

ILLUSTRATIVE CLINICAL CASES

Left Petroclival Meningioma

This 57-year-old female presented with diplopia, CN III paresis, and trigeminal dysesthesia. Figures 8a and 8b show preoperative MRI films visualizing a 4-cm dumbbell-shaped tumor. Figure 8c demonstrates a preoperative CT scan and Fig. 8d shows a postoperative CT scan after the combined parapetrosal total resection. Figure 5C shows the exposure of the trigeminal nerve root and removal of the meningioma from the incised Meckel's cave. Figure 5D demonstrates Meckel's cave, the trigemi-

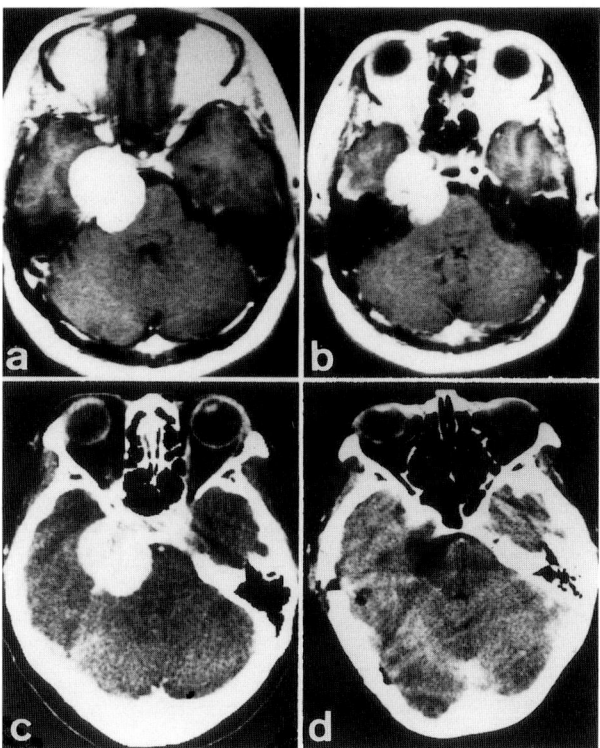

FIG. 8. Left petroclival meningioma.

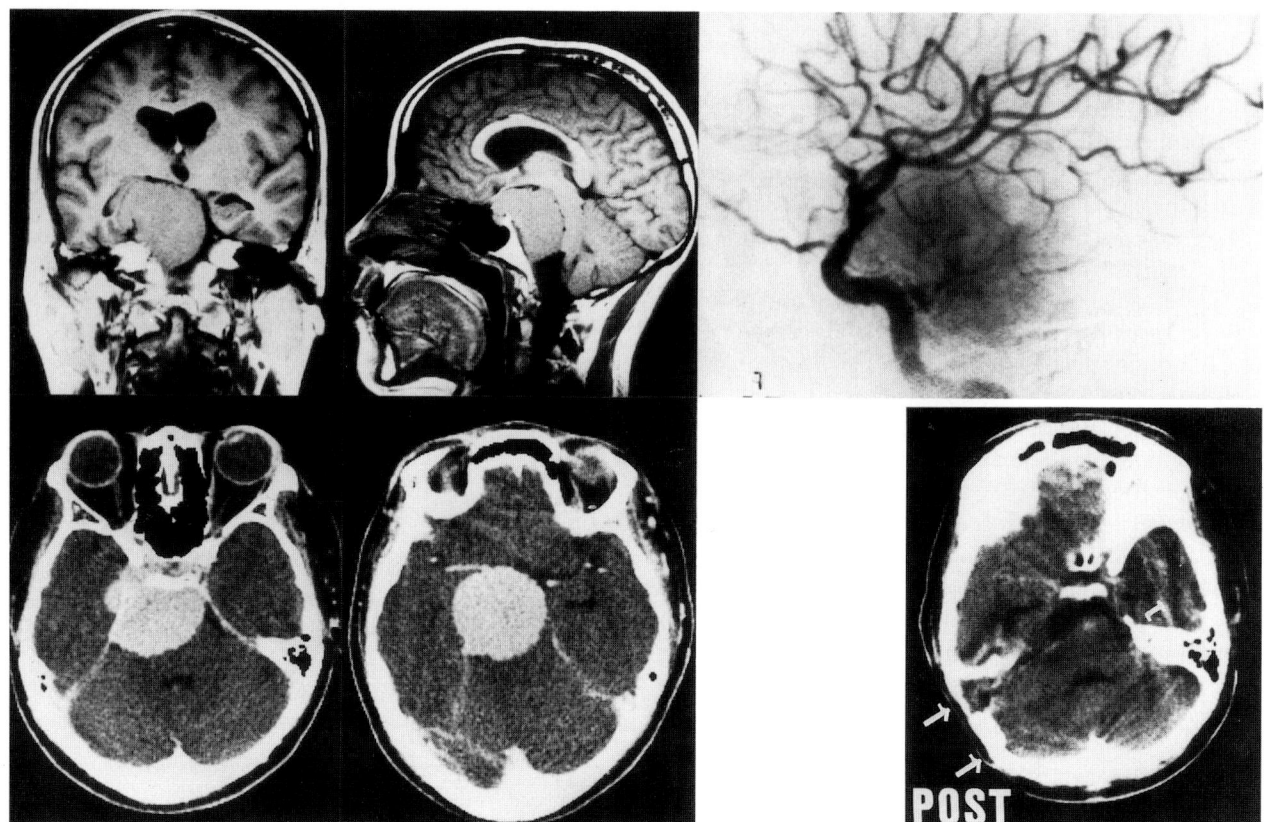

FIG. 9. Large left petroclival meningioma.

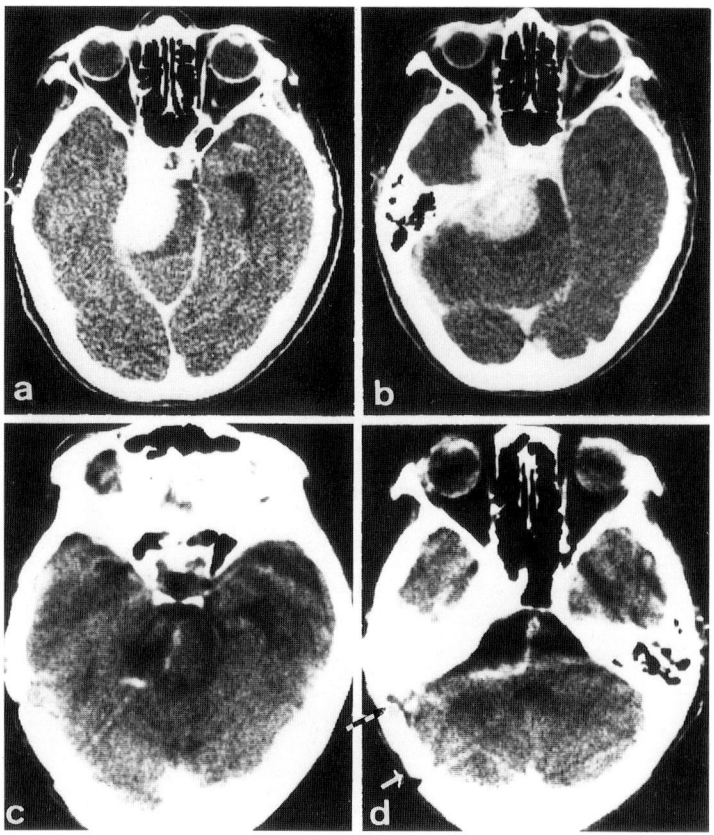

FIG. 10. Large invasive meningioma.

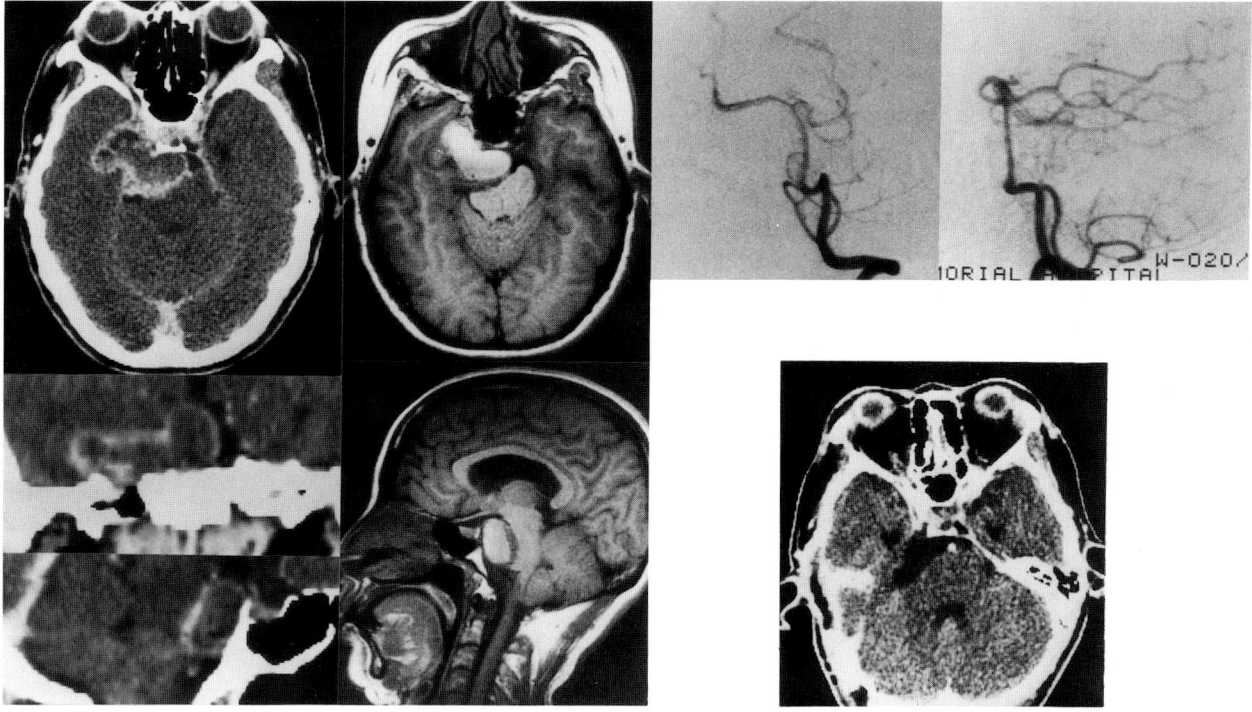

FIG. 11. Large dumbbell-shaped trigeminal neurinoma.

nal root, CN VI, and the brain stem after total resection of the tumor in this patient.

Large Left Petroclival Meningioma

This 29-year-old female presented with headache, trigeminal hypoesthesia, and left oculomotor paresis. Figure 9 illustrates preoperative MRI, CT, and angiogram and postoperative CT scan. A 5-cm large meningioma was resected in a radical fashion, leaving a bit of tumor invasion in the cavernous sinus. Postoperative CT demonstrates radical tumor resection through a small parapetrosal opening (white arrows).

Large Invasive Meningioma

This 71-year-old female was admitted with symptoms of ataxia, diplopia, and facial hypoesthesia. Figure 10 shows preoperative (a,b) and postoperative (c,d) enhanced CT scans. Because of the invasive and adherent nature of the tumor and the patient's advanced age, radical subtotal removal was performed, leaving some portion of fibrous adherent capsules with the brain stem. Arrows indicate the area of parapetrosal craniotomy.

Large Dumbbell-Shaped Trigeminal Neurinoma

This 51-year-old female presented with facial hypoesthesia, mastication weakness, and CN VI paresis. Figure 11 demonstrates preoperative MRI and CT scan, vertebral angiograms, and postoperative film. The tumor was successfully and totally removed through a combined parapetrosal approach.

REFERENCES

1. Al-Mefty O, Fox JL, Smith RR. Petrosal approach for petroclival meningiomas. *Neurosurgery* 1988;22:510–517.
2. Hakuba A, Nishimura S, Tanaka K, Kishi H, Nakamura T. Clivus meningioma: six cases of total removal. *Neurol Med Chir (Tokyo)* 1977;17:63–77.
3. Hashi K, Nin K, Shimotake K. Transpetrosal combined supratentorial and infratentorial approach for midline vertebro-basilar aneurysms. *Mod Neurosurg* 1982;1:442–448.
4. Hitselberger WE, House WF. A combined approach to the cerebellopontine angle. *Arch Otolaryngol* 1966;84:267–285.
5. King TT. Combined translabyrinthine–transtentorial approach to acoustic nerve tumors. *Proc R Soc Med* 1970;63:30–32.
6. Malis LI. Surgical resection of tumors of the skull base. In: Wilkins RH, Rengachay SS, eds. *Neurosurgery.* New York: McGraw-Hill, 1985;1011–1021.

CHAPTER 40

Transcondyle Approach for Foramen Magnum Meningiomas

Akira Hakuba and Takeshi Tsujimoto

The foramen magnum is a short tunnel with walls of varying height, ranging about 4 mm anteriorly to roughly 1 cm laterally, and narrowing posteriorly to 4–6 mm. Just in front of its transverse axis, the foramen magnum is encroached upon by the medial aspects of the occipital condyles so that it is somewhat ovoid in shape and narrow in front. This narrow anterior part lies above the dens of the axial vertebra; its wider, posterior part communicates below with the spinal canal, and through it the medulla oblongata becomes continuous with the spinal cord.

Foramen magnum tumors show bizarre symptoms and signs and are difficult to diagnose.

They were divided into two anatomical classes: craniospinal and spinocranial lesions.

SPECIFIC DIAGNOSTIC CONSIDERATIONS

The pyramidal decussation begins just below the obex and ends some distance below the exit of the first cervical nerve root. The more medial fibers in the pyramidal tract cross superior to the more lateral fibers. The former carries impulses relating to movements of the upper limbs, and the latter to ones of the lower limbs. The medial lemniscus decussates more cranially to the pyramidal tract. Within the lemniscus, fibers mediating impulses from the lower extremities are ventrally and caudally located, and those carrying impulses from the upper extremities are dorsally and laterally situated. A tumor at this level can produce confusion when attempting to attribute signs and symptoms to a single lesion. Because this subarachnoid space is capacious, a foramen magnum tumor may be asymptomatic until it has reached a considerable size capable of compromising the neuraxis (3).

Often these tumors present ill-defined symptoms, such as neck pain and varying dysesthesia in the ipsilateral upper limb (2,5,8). Weakness of the ipsilateral upper limb followed by paresis of the ipsilateral lower limb is recognized and then motor disturbance of the contralateral upper limb appears. Decreased pain sensation on the contralateral side and decreased deep sensation, more on the ipsilateral side, accompanied by slow athetosis-like movements of the upper limbs (pseudo-athetotic or piano playing fingers) (1,5) are commonly observed. Neurological examination sometimes fails to demonstrate signs that are easily referable to pathology at the foramen magnum. Sometimes they are diagnosed as other clinical entities, such as cervical spondylosis and amyotrophic lateral sclerosis (2,5,6,9,10).

Recent developments in MRI will provide very useful noninvasive means of evaluating the foramen magnum lesions.

INDICATION

There is no specific selection for the operation.

OPERATIVE TECHNIQUE

When the tumor is located either posteriorly or posterolaterally to the foramen magnum, the operation is relatively easily accomplished. However, when the main portion of the tumor is situated in the anterior part of the foramen magnum, the operation is thought to be difficult. In the latter situation we prefer to use a lateral suboccipital transcondyle approach. In this approach, 30–50%

A. Hakuba and T. Tsujimoto: Department of Neurosurgery, Osaka City University Medical School, Osaka 545, Japan.

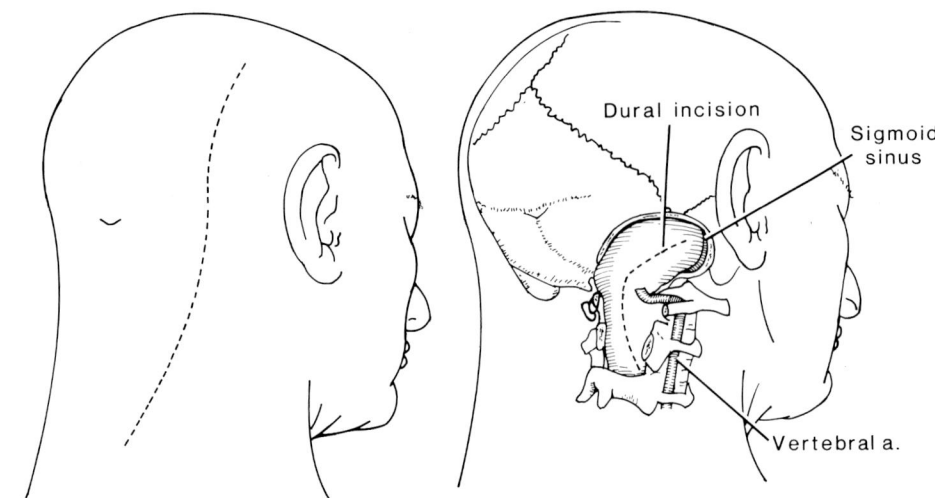

FIG. 1. Suboccipital transcondyle approach. Skin incision (**left**) and extent of craniotomy and laminectomy (**right**). (From ref. 13, with permission.)

of the condyle process is removed in order to gain access to the anterior part of the foramen magnum easily without retraction of the cerebellum and medulla oblongata (Fig. 1) (13).

Anesthesia Considerations and Patient Position

The anesthesia is selected by the anesthesiologist in charge and is usually a controlled anesthesia with a respirator. Either the upright or the park-bench position is employed. In either position, in order to prevent air embolism during the operation, a 16-gauge argyle medicut catheter is inserted into the subclavian vein and the tip of the catheter is placed in the superior vena cava; a pediatric Doppler cardiac monitor is placed in the precordial region.

Surgery

The patient is placed in either the sitting or park-bench position with the head kept in maximal flexion at the craniovertebral junction and rotated about 45° toward the side of lesion with a Mayfield three-pin head-holder so that the condyle process on the side of the lesion is brought out backward in a posteriorly subluxated position (Fig. 2A). A paramedian skin incision is made, starting about 1.5 cm above the posterior end of the crista supramastoidea, running in a line through the lateral two-thirds between the tip of the mastoid process and the inion, and extending down to the level of the C5 spinous process 1 cm lateral to it (Fig. 1 left). The lateral part of the mastoid process is drilled away and the midline half of the sigmoid sinus is exposed as low as the jugular foramen. Then a lateral suboccipital craniotomy from the posterior end of the condyle to the suboccipital bone 4 cm above the posterior margin of the foramen magnum is made. A laminectomy of the C1 and hemilaminectomy of the C2 are added (Fig. 1 right and Fig. 2).

The posterolateral part of the foramen magnum is further removed with removal of the medial third condyle process. During this procedure, care is taken to avoid injuring the jugular bulb and the vertebral artery. The dura mater is opened (Fig. 1 right) and dural fringes are retracted by fish hooks. The arachnoid membrane between the tumor capsule and cerebellum is divided. The exposed tumor capsule is opened. After internal decompression of the tumor and coagulating feeders passing through the ventral dural attachment at the foramen magnum, the dorsomedial wall of the tumor is separated from the ventrolateral wall of the upper cervical cord. The adhesion of the inferolateral part of the tumor capsule with the vertebral artery is sharply separated. The deep portion of the tumor ventral to the medulla oblongata is removed without retraction of the cerebellum and lower brain stem. The last piece of the tumor is removed. The dura mater is closed and made watertight. The bone flap is replaced and fixed to the bone edges through small drill holes at multiple points. The wound is closed, leaving a epidural drain.

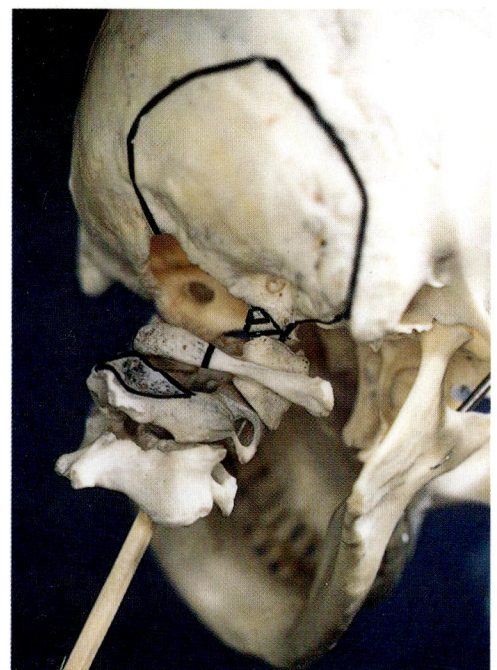
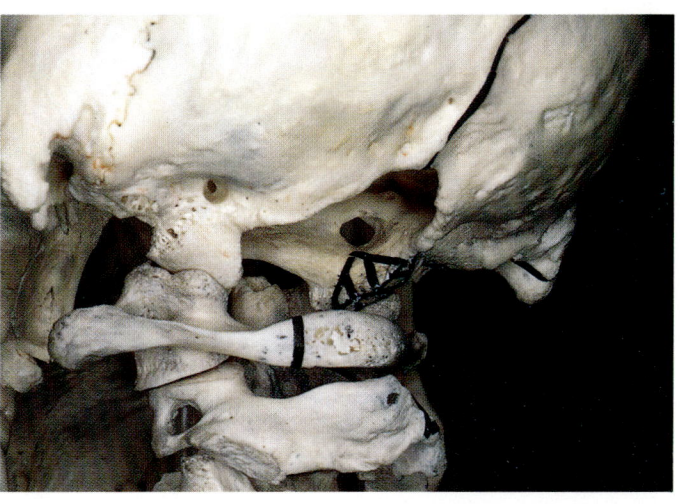

FIG. 2. A,B: Suboccipital transcondyle approach. *Black lines* indicate the suboccipital craniotomy and laminectomy; *shaded area* indicates removal of the condyle process. (Fig. 2A from ref. 13, with permission.)

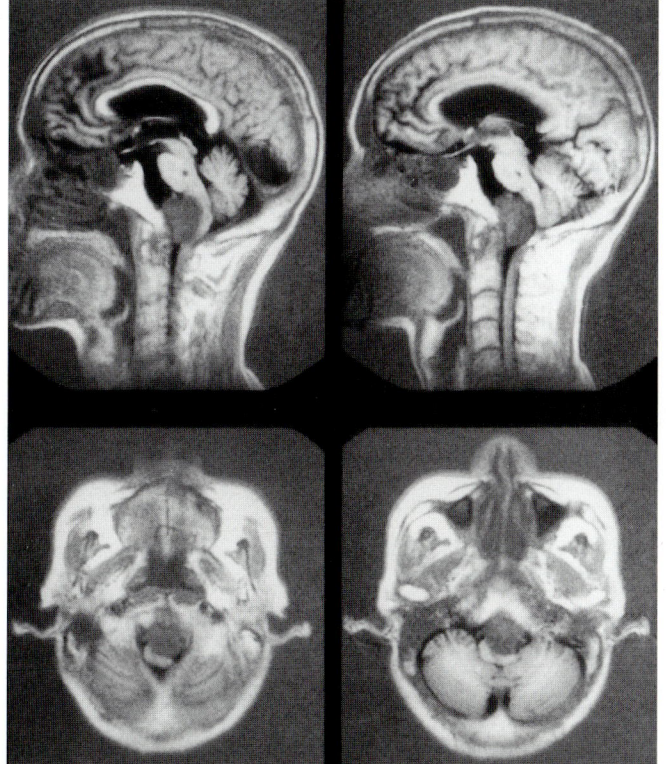
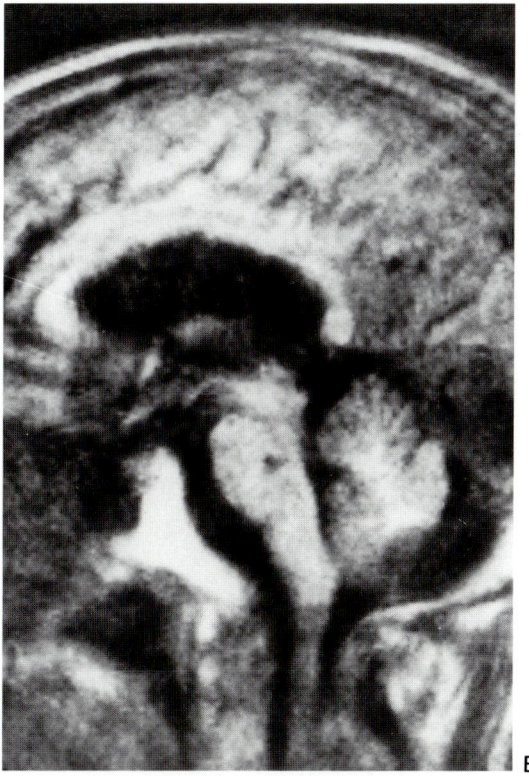

FIG. 3. Case 1. **A:** Preoperative MRI scans in T1-weighted image showing a slightly low-intensity mass at the foramen magnum. **B:** Postoperative MRI scan (sagittal view) in T1-weighted image showing no residual tumor.

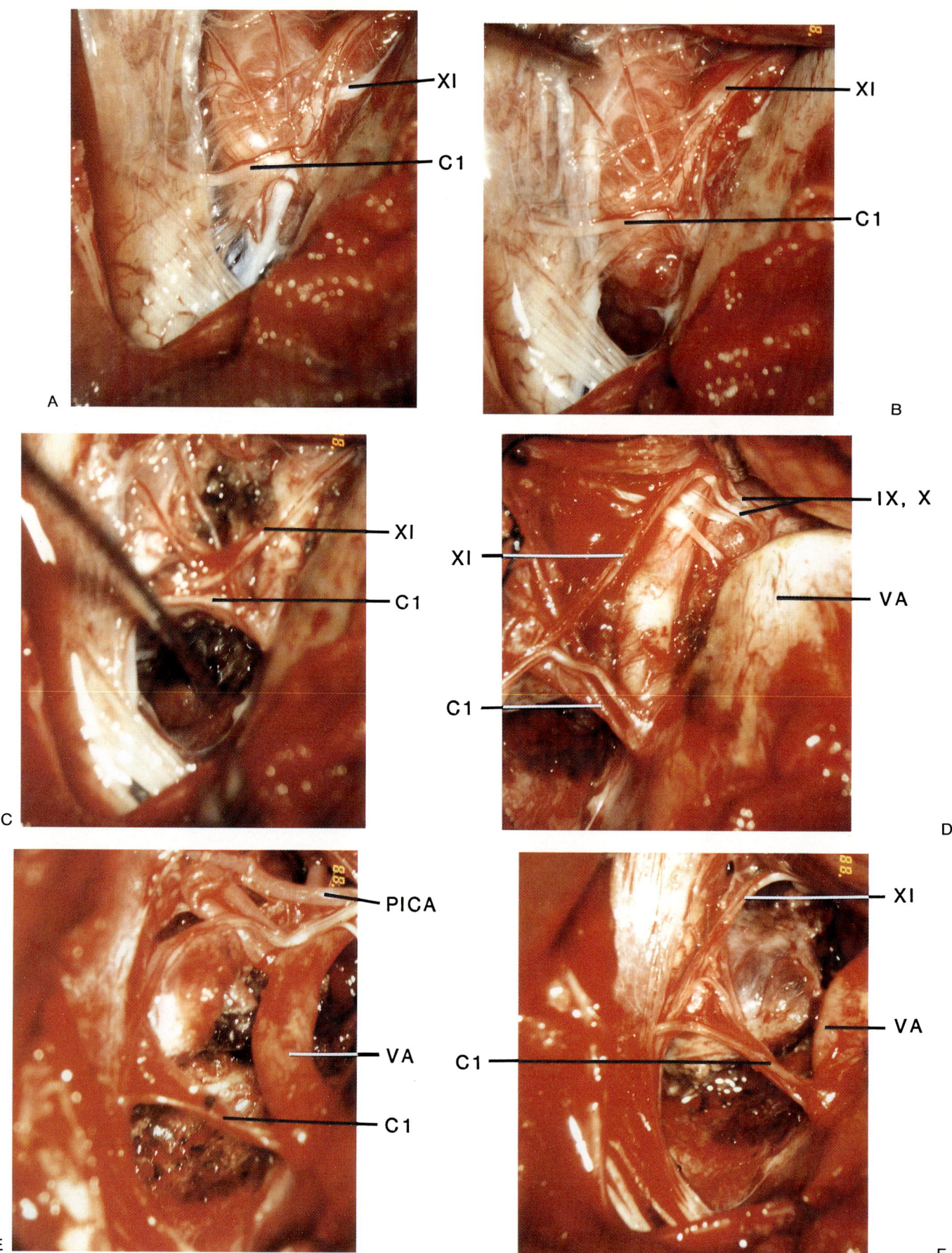

FIG. 4. Intraoperative photograph of case 1 via a right transcondyle approach. **A:** The tumor is well exposed without retraction of the cerebellum and the medulla oblongata. **B:** The dentate ligament below the first cervical nerve root (C1) has been divided. **C:** The inferior pole of the tumor has been removed. **D:** The right vertebral artery (VA) is partially denuded with removal of the engulfed tumor.

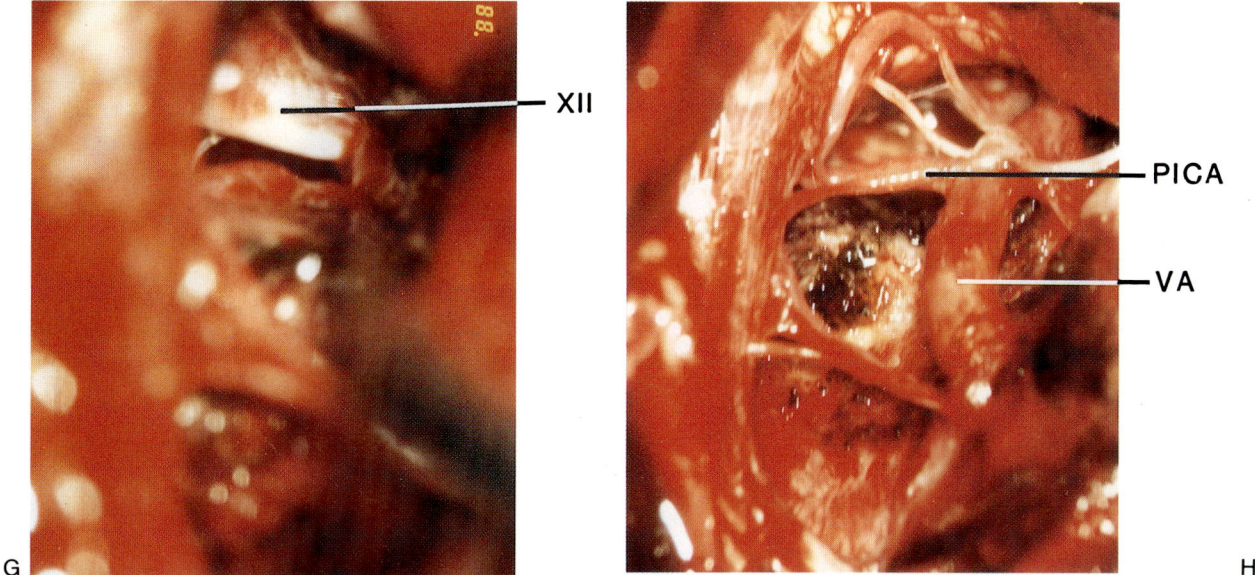

FIG. 4. *Continued.* **E:** The entire vertebral artery has been denuded. The right posterior inferior cerebellar artery (PICA) is well preserved. The tumor ventral to the medulla oblongata is partially separated. **F:** More dissection of the dorsal wall of the tumor has been accomplished after internal decompression of the tumor. **G:** The hypoglossal nerve (XII) is dissected out with removal of the tumor ventral to it. **H:** The tumor has been totally resected. The attachment of the tumor to the dura mater at the anterior rim of the foramen magnum has been coagulated by a YAG laser beam. IX, X, XI represent the glossopharyngeal, vagal, and accessory nerves. (Fig. 4B from ref. 13, with permission.)

POSTOPERATIVE MANAGEMENT

On a few occasions, a respirator is kept ready postoperatively in our series. A large dose of corticosteroid is given intravenously every 6 hr during a few days and tapered off within 2 weeks after the operation. Preventive antibiotics are also given during the same period.

COMPLICATIONS AND MANAGEMENT

Respiratory problems are frequent (2,5) and were also seen in our series. Tracheostomy may be essential for the maintenance of an adequate airway and for better evacuation of secretion after the operation.

ILLUSTRATIVE CASES

Case 1: Spinocranial Type

A 68-year-old male patient with a 1-year history of progressive weakness of both lower extremities was admitted to our hospital in July 1988. Neurological exami-

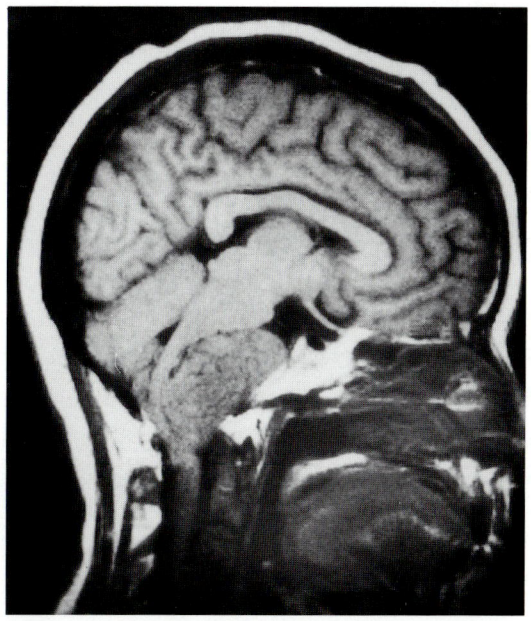

FIG. 5. Case 2. MRI scan (sagittal view) in T1-weighted image before the first operation, showing a huge isointensity mass occupying the retroclival and ventral upper cervical regions.

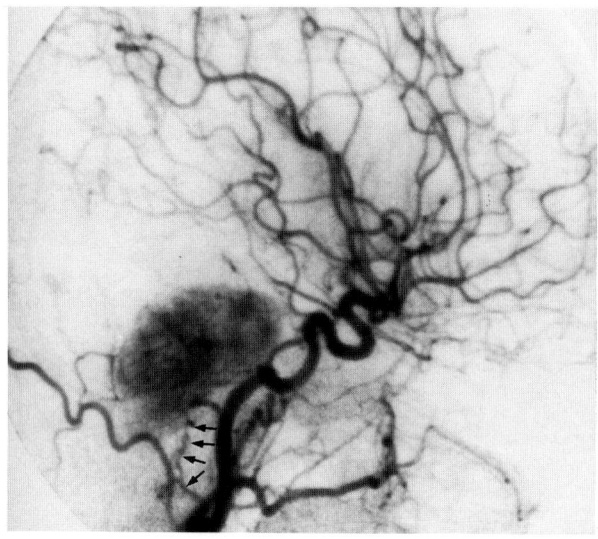

FIG. 6. Case 2. Right common carotid arteriogram before the first operation, showing a huge vascular tumor fed by branches off the ascending pharyngeal artery (arrows).

nation on admission showed absent gag reflex and paresis of the sternocleidomastoid muscle on the right side. There was positive Babinski's signs bilaterally. His sensation to pin prick was impaired more on the left side up to the fourth dermatome. Deep sensation was also decreased bilaterally more on the left side. His gait was unsteady.

MRI scans disclosed a well demarcated mass, 3.5 × 2 × 2 cm in size, which displaced the medulla oblongata and upper cervical cord backward (Fig. 3A). A right common carotid arteriogram showed tumor feeders off the right ascending pharyngeal artery with a vascular tumor shadow at the ventral part of the foramen magnum. Right vertebral arteriogram also showed that tumor feeders off the radicular branch of the right vertebral artery originated at the C2–C3 level. On August 8, 1988, total removal of the tumor was made via a right suboccipital transcondyle approach (Fig. 4). Postoperatively, temporary dysphagia was seen. The patient was improved and had very minimal weakness of his right upper limb without other neurological deficit at 6-months postoperative follow-up clinic. A MRI scan showed no residual tumor (Fig. 3B).

Case 2: Craniospinal Type

A 46-year-old woman suffered from headache almost once per month since March 1988. An unsteady gait and dizzy feelings were also noticed during almost the same period. Since February 1989 she had difficulty in swallowing, associated with cough and sputum. Her gait became more unsteady and tended to go toward her left side. She was admitted to hospital on April 8, 1989. MRI scans disclosed a mass, 6 × 4 × 4 cm in size, occupying the retroclival and ventral upper cervical regions with a low-density peritumor between the tumor and the brain stem. The pons, medulla oblongata, and upper cervical cord were markedly displaced backward by the mass (Fig. 5). A right carotid arteriogram showed a highly vascular, huge mass occupying the same regions (Fig. 6). She had VP shunt for acute hydrocephalus on April 11, 1989. External decompression via a right temporosuboccipital craniotomy and C1 laminectomy with a dural plasty were done on April 25, 1989. On May 16, 1989

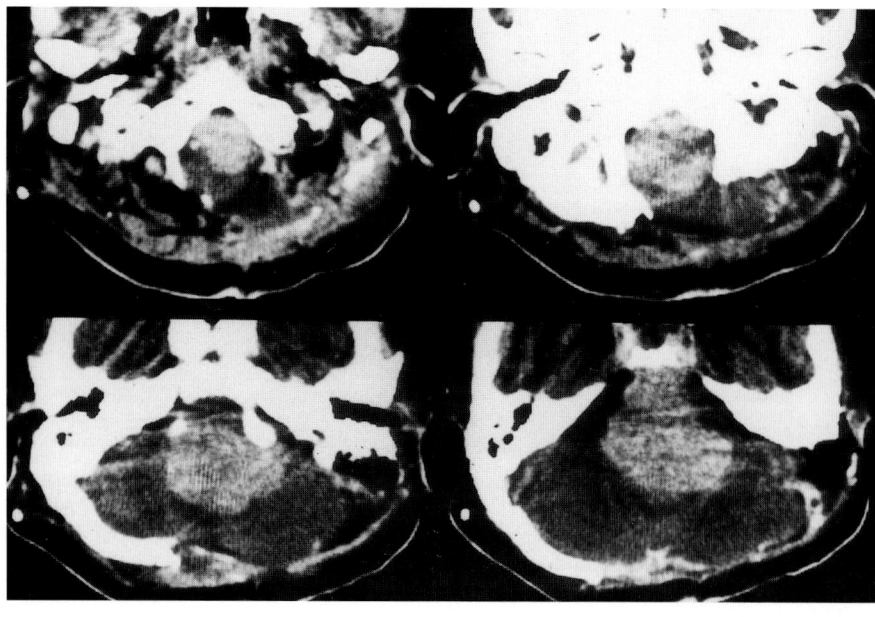

FIG. 7. Case 2. CT scans after partial removal of the tumor via a transpetrosal transtentorial approach, revealing a diffusely enhanced mass in the retroclival and ventral high cervical regions.

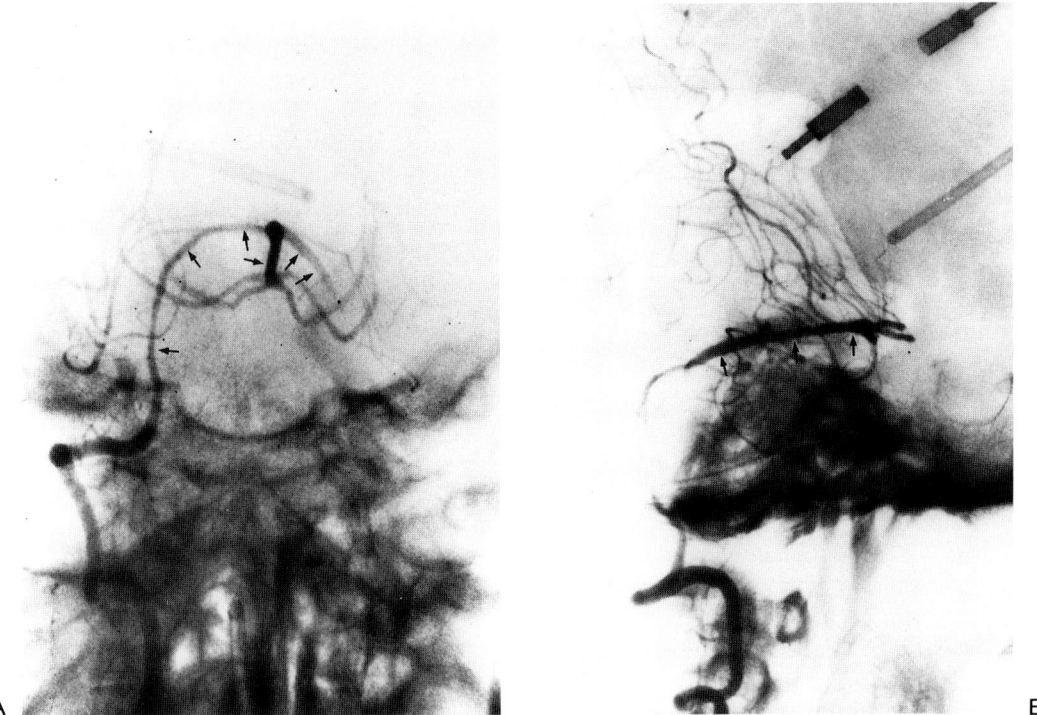

FIG. 8. Case 2. Right ventral arteriograms after partial removal of the tumor via a transpetrosal transtentorial approach. **A:** Town's view showing round and posterolateral displacement of both vertebral arteries (*arrows*) and elevation of the basilar artery. **B:** Lateral view showing marked posterior displacement of the vertebrobasilar system (*arrows*).

she had a partial removal of the tumor via a right transpetrosal transtentorial approach (4). Neurological examination in June 1989 showed right cranial nerve VI, VII, VIII (deaf), IX, and X paresis, but there was no weakness, ataxia, or dysmetria, and she was mentally alert. CT scans demonstrated a very large residual tumor at the same regions (Fig. 7). A right vertebral arteriogram showed marked elevation and lateral displacement of both vertebral arteries and marked posterior displacement of the basilar artery (Fig. 8). On June 6, 1989, a right suboccipital transcondyle approach was taken and total removal of the tumor was made.

Postoperatively, she improved greatly, and CT scan showed no residual tumor (Fig. 9).

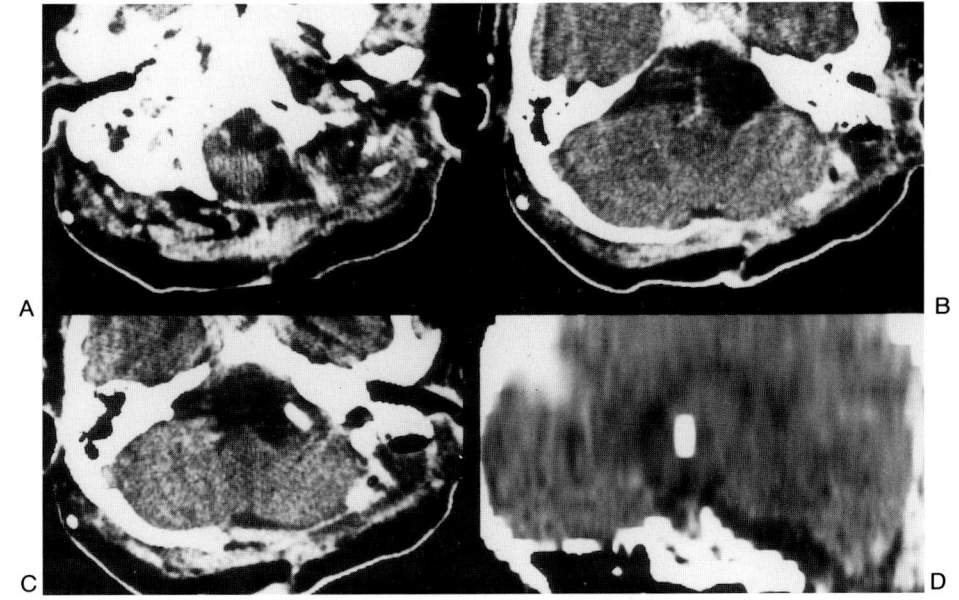

FIG. 9. Postoperative enhanced CT scans of case 2. **A–C:** Axial views. **D:** Sagittal reconstruction. The tumor is totally removed.

AUTHORS' EXPERIENCE AND SERIES

We have surgically treated 45 cases of foramen magnum tumors during the last 19 years, 11 of which were meningiomas (24%). [This incidence is much less than reported by others: 78 out of 102 cases (78%) in Meyer's series (9) were diagnosed to be meningiomas.] Six of our cases were spinocranial; the remaining five were craniospinal. The tumor attached to either the ventral or ventrolateral rim of the foramen magnum in ten cases, and at the dorsolateral rim in the remaining one.

The ratio of males to females was 3:8, and the age of the patients ranged widely from 36 to 74 years, with a mean of 52.8 years.

The most frequent initial symptoms of the craniospinal type tumors were headache and vomiting, exhibited in four out of five cases. Other symptoms of the craniospinal patients were noted in small percentages.

Suboccipital or neck pain were the most common initial symptoms of the spinocranial type, noted in four out of six cases and numbness or weakness of the extremities was found in all cases. Among neurological findings, motor weakness was the most prevalent, recorded in all the patients. Also common were sensory disturbances and increased deep tendon reflexes. A wide variety of sensory disturbance patterns were recorded in all six spinocranial meningiomas. In regard to hypalgesia, disturbances below the C2 level were most common.

Posterior fossa syndrome (lower cranial nerve palsy or cerebellar sign) was detected in all cases of craniospinal meningiomas. Papilledema and nystagmus were seen in four out of five cases. One case exhibited signs in the spinal cord area, suggesting existence of tumor in the foramen magnum and upper spinal canal.

With the recent introduction of MRI, a more precise picture can be obtained, and the anatomical relationship between the tumor and the neighboring structures can be defined (7,11,12). MRI is also very useful in analyzing the postoperative state.

Total removal of tumor was accomplished in five out of six spinocranial cases. A large meningioma originating from the anterior rim of the foramen magnum, which was the earliest case in this series, could not be resected, and the patient died of respiratory arrest on the seventh postoperative day (5). Four cases had remarkable neurological improvement and were good to excellent in condition. There was no recurrence.

Of the craniospinal meningiomas, total removal was accomplished in four cases and subtotal removal was achieved in one case. Three cases demonstrated neurological improvement after surgery and were found to be in good condition without recurrence. Two cases with recurrent clivus meningiomas extending into the upper cervical spinal canal became neurologically worse after surgery.

As postoperative complications, respiratory difficulty was frequent, especially in the cases of large tumors that were located anterior to the spinal cord. Intensive care following surgery must be stressed. Tracheostomy was performed in eight cases, while four patients required a respirator.

With early diagnosis, early removal with microsurgical techniques, and appropriate postoperative care, excellent results can be obtained.

REFERENCES

1. Blom S, Ekbom KA. Early clinical signs of meningiomas of the foramen magnum. *J Neurosurg* 1962;19:661–664.
2. Dodge HW Jr, Love JG, Gottlieb CM. Benign tumors at the foramen magnum: surgical considerations. *J Neurosurg* 1956;13:603–617.
3. Fujimoto K, Ikuno H, Hakuba A, Mishima Y, Kondou M, Maeno T. Foramen magnum neurinomas. Report of 5 cases. *Central Jpn J Orthop Traumatic Surg* 1976;19:1159–1163 (in Japanese).
4. Hakuba A. Total removal of cerebellopontine angle tumors with a combined transpetrosal–transtentorial approach. *Neurol Surg* 1978;6:347–354 (in Japanese).
5. Hakuba A, Nishimura S, Mishima Y, Kawano K. Foramen magnum tumors—report of 21 cases. *Neurol Med Chir (Tokyo)* 1982;22:563–576.
6. Howe JR, Taren JA. Foramen magnum tumors. Pitfalls in diagnosis. *JAMA* 1973;225:1061–1066.
7. Komiyama M, Yagura H, Baba M, Yasui T, Hakuba A, Nishimura S, Inoue Y. MR imaging: possibility of tissue characterization of brain tumors using T1 and T2 values. *AJNR* 1987;8:65–70.
8. Krayenbühl H. Special clinical features of tumors of the foramen magnum. *Schweiz Arch Neurol Neurochir Psychiatry* 1973;112:205–218.
9. Meyer FB, Ebersold MJ, Reese DF. Benign tumors of the foramen magnum. *J Neurosurg* 1984;61:136–142.
10. Stein BM, Leeds NE, Taveras JM, Pool JL. Meningiomas of the foramen magnum. *J Neurosurg* 1963;20:741–750.
11. Takemoto K, Matsumura Y, Hashimoto H, et al. MR imaging of intraspinal tumors—capability in histological differentiation and compartmentalization of extramedullary tumors. *Neuroradiology* 1988;30:303–309.
12. Yagura H, Komiyama M, Fu Y, et al. Diagnosis of meningioma in magnetic resonance imaging. *CT Kenkyu* 1986;8:675–682 (in Japanese).
13. Hakuba A. Foramen magnum meningiomas. *Clin Neurosci* 1990;8:78–81 (in Japanese).

CHAPTER 41

Clivus Chordomas

Edward R. Laws, Jr.

Chordomas are uncommon tumors, presumably of congenital origin. They are thought to arise from remnants of the primitive notochord and can occur anywhere along the spinal axis but are most frequently located at either end, the clivus rostrally and the sacrum caudally. About 35% occur at the base of the skull, arising from the clivus. Although usually midline, the notochord may have distal projections that extend to the clinoid processes or the petrous bones. The location of a chordoma within the clivus determines the nature and path of its growth, the associated anatomic structures involved, the clinical symptomatology, and the approach for surgical management.

Chordomas arising near the inferior tip of the clivus, the basion, usually produce lower brain stem compression as they expand and present clinically with hypoglossal nerve palsy and tongue atrophy, weakness, and fasciculation. Tumors arising from the body of the clivus are the most common. They may expand ventrally and produce a nasopharyngeal mass with obstruction, or they may expand dorsally where they stretch the sixth cranial nerve as it runs along and penetrates the clival dura. This accounts for the typical clinical presentation with side-by-side diplopia and abducens nerve palsy, usually bilateral. Tumors arising at the rostral end of the clivus involve the sella turcica and may present with hypopituitarism or, with suprasellar extension, a chiasmal syndrome with bitemporal hemianopsia. Lateral extensions of rostral clival chordomas may produce a parasellar mass or extend into the cavernous sinus, affecting other cranial nerves. Posterolateral extensions of midclival chordomas can produce tinnitus, hearing loss, or facial weakness.

It is evident that the clinical presentation and neurologic examination offer significant clues as to the diagnosis and the anatomic extent of the lesion. The definitive study for anatomic diagnosis and planning of surgical approach is the MRI scan. If the visual system is involved, a formal neuro-ophthalmologic examination is advisable. If there are symptoms or signs of endocrinopathy, or if the sella turcica is involved, an endocrine evaluation should be performed. If pituitary replacement therapy is indicated, it should be started prior to surgery, and steroid coverage through the stress of surgery and subsequent therapy should be planned.

It is difficult to cure a chordoma with surgical resection alone. The origin of the tumor from the bone at the base of the skull often precludes "total" removal, and the recurrence rate even after radical surgical removal remains high. These considerations are important in formulating a surgical plan of management.

A number of standard surgical approaches may be entirely satisfactory for a clival chordoma. Rostral lesions may be exposed though a unilateral subfrontal or frontotemporal (pterional) craniotomy. The bifrontal approach may be preferable for some midline lesions, and Derome's bifrontal radical approach provides excellent access to the entire midline base of the skull (Fig. 1). Tumors in the midclivus can be attacked by a number of lateral approaches leading to the midline. The infratemporal fossa and transcochlear routes may be suitable, as may Malis' subtemporal transtentorial approach. Tumors located inferiorly in the clivus or at the craniocervical junction may be exposed posteriorly through a suboccipital approach or ventrally using a transoral or submandibular approach. We have used a mandible splitting transoral approach when extensive exposure of the ventral midline has been required. A midfacial degloving approach had also been described and is useful for some ventrally placed chordomas.

The transseptal transsphenoidal approach has many virtues. Because it is suitable for the management of so many chordomas, it is the focus of this chapter. This

E. R. Laws, Jr.: Department of Neurological Surgery, George Washington University Medical Center, Washington, DC 20037.

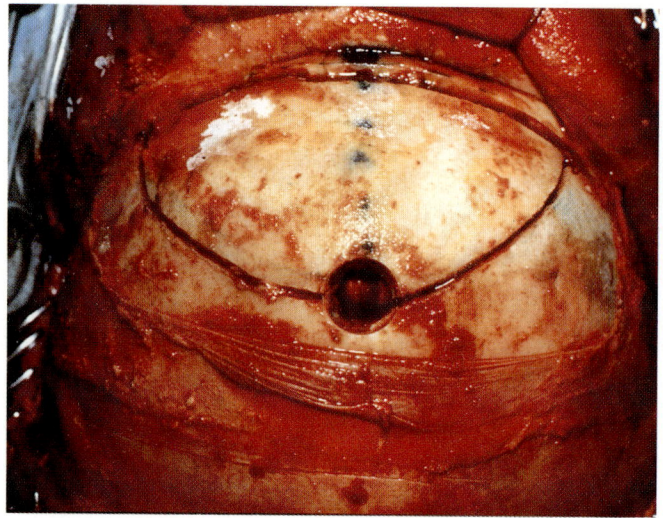 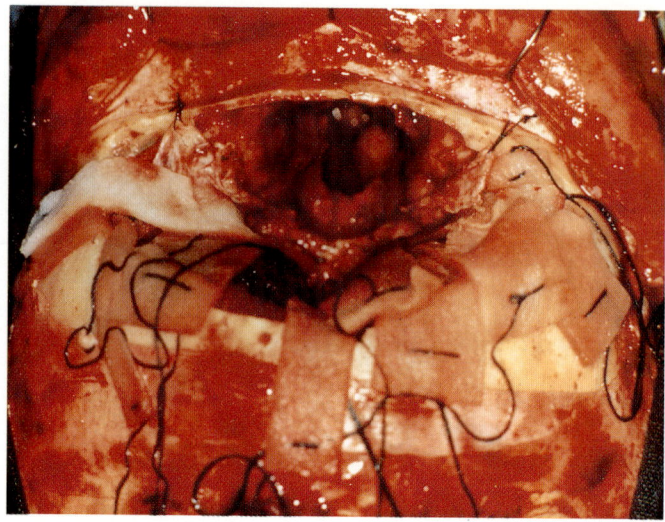

FIG. 1. **A:** Bifrontal craniotomy for removal of clivus chordoma through the base of the frontal fossa between the orbits. **B:** Derome's procedure.

approach is logical for those midline tumors that extend into the sphenoid sinus and, for those tumors, effective radical resection can be accomplished. Other clivus chordomas, primary and recurrent, can often be treated for effective palliation using this approach (Fig. 2).

The patient is prepared with steroids and prophylactic antibiotics in the usual fashion. The endotracheal tube is positioned at the left side of the mouth and secured with tape in a manner that does not restrict movement of the upper lip. The oropharynx is packed with moist gauze to prevent blood and secretions from the operative site from reaching the stomach and causing postoperative nausea and vomiting. The head is positioned on the horseshoe of an adjustable headrest and tilted laterally so that the left ear is close to the left shoulder. The table is placed in a semirecumbent position with the thorax elevated 15°, and the right lower quadrant of the abdomen is prepared for harvesting of a fat graft if necessary. A lumbar catheter is frequently used for the injection of air, if necessary, to visualize the brain on fluoroscopy or to manipulate it with pressure differentials. The nasal mucous membranes are decongested with Afrin spray and pledgets in Afrin or 4% cocaine solution. The nose and face are cleansed with soap and aqueous solutions and the nasal mucosa is then infiltrated with 0.5% xylocaine in 1:200,000 epinephrine solution. Injection is carefully done and raises the mucosal flaps away from the nasal septum. Injection is extended to the premaxilla and the upper buccogingival border, with a total of 18–20 ml used, if tolerated without cardiovascular side effects. The operative fields are draped, and the initial exposure is carried out using a headlight and loupes.

The initial exposure is directed toward the caudal end of the cartilaginous nasal septum. The columella is retracted to the patient's left and an incision is made through the right nostril directly along the caudal border of the septum. Careful sharp dissection with fine scissors or the Cottle knife defines a plane against the cartilage, and the nasal mucosa is carefully elevated from the left side of the septum, avoiding tears if possible. The mucosa of the premaxilla and nasal spine is carefully elevated and the mucosal plane below the pyriform aper-

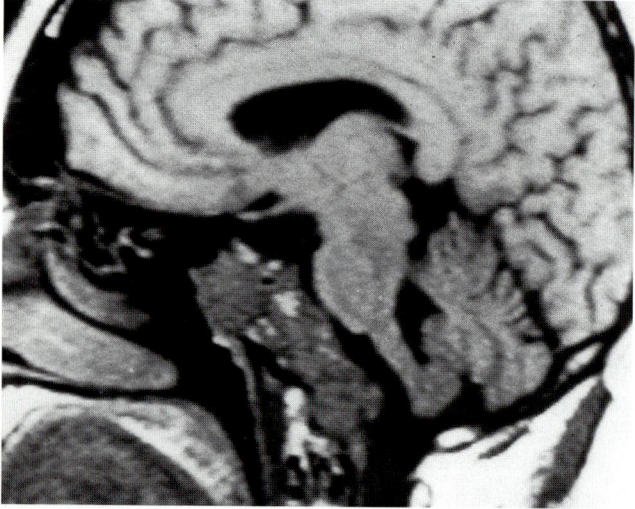

FIG. 2. Sagittal MRI of extensive clivus chordoma. This patient had three procedures: transsphenoidal, suboccipital, and transcochlear.

ture and the maxillary roof is developed. Then left anterior and bilateral inferior mucosal tunnels are made.

The upper lip is elevated and a transverse incision is made in the buccogingival fold from one canine tooth to the other, leaving an ample cuff for closure. Excessive use of cautery is discouraged, as it can devitalize the upper teeth. The mucosa is elevated away from the face of the maxilla, and the pyriform aperture is carefully dissected from lateral to medial, further developing the right and left inferior tunnels. Using sharp dissection, the caudal end of the cartilaginous septum is dissected free from below and the left anterior and inferior tunnels are joined (Fig. 3A).

Dissection along the septum defines the junction of the cartilaginous septum with the bony septum, the perpendicular plate of the ethmoid. The posterior nasal mucosa on the right and the left is elevated, thus creating the two posterior tunnels.

Careful dissection is then employed to detach the inferior border of the cartilaginous septum from its attachment to the maxillary ridge, and the cartilaginous septum is reflected to the right, hinged superiorly, taking the right sided nasal mucosa with it. Further dissection of the posterior mucosal tunnel defines the vomer inferiorly and the rostrum of the sphenoid superiorly, two excellent midline landmarks.

Careful pressure with dissectors crushes the turbinates, and the transsphenoidal speculum is inserted. The bony septum is resected, with the pieces carefully preserved in saline solution for later use of reconstruction of the sella, sphenoid face, or septum, as required.

The opened retractor exposes the face of the sphenoid and one or both sphenoid ostia can usually be seen. At this point a lateral image on x-ray or videofluoroscopy is obtained for confirmation of landmarks and direction of approach. The operating microscope is used for the remainder of the procedure (Fig. 3B).

The face of the sphenoid is resected with heavy forceps, exposing the clivus and the sella, and the sphenoid mucosa is stripped away and resected. Wide exposure allows for maximal opening of the retractor. The tumor is usually readily visualized and may be carefully removed with curettes and rongeurs. A radical tumor removal is desirable but may be difficult to accomplish because of the extent of involvement of the bone and the base of the skull. Chordomas often penetrate dura, and CSF leakage during the procedure is common, as is venous bleeding.

Once the resection is complete, the resection cavity can be obliterated with a fat graft taken from the abdomen. If there is no CSF leak, Gelfoam may suffice. If a major leak is present, fibrin glue may be helpful, and fat should be used to pack the entire sphenoid sinus.

Packing and closure must be accomplished carefully, as it is possible to transmit excessive pressure against intracranial structures through the exposed dura.

Postoperative care is similar to that given to pituitary tumor patients, with replacement therapy as necessary if the sella turcica has been involved by the chordoma and if postoperative endocrine determinations show deficiencies (Fig. 4).

For extensive chordomas of the clivus, particularly those that begin ventrally in the body of the clivus and extend superiorly and inferiorly, a transoral approach

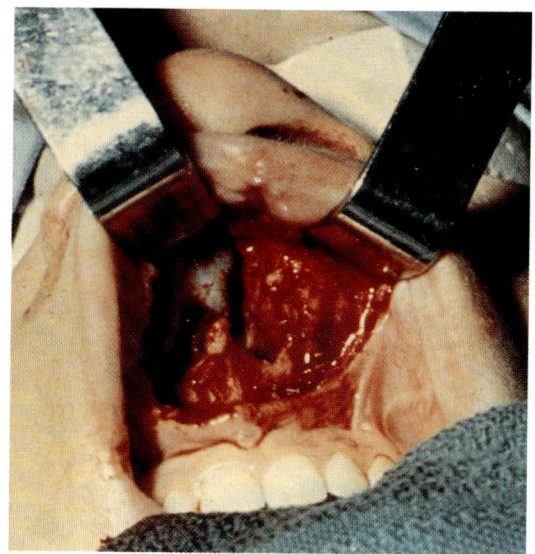
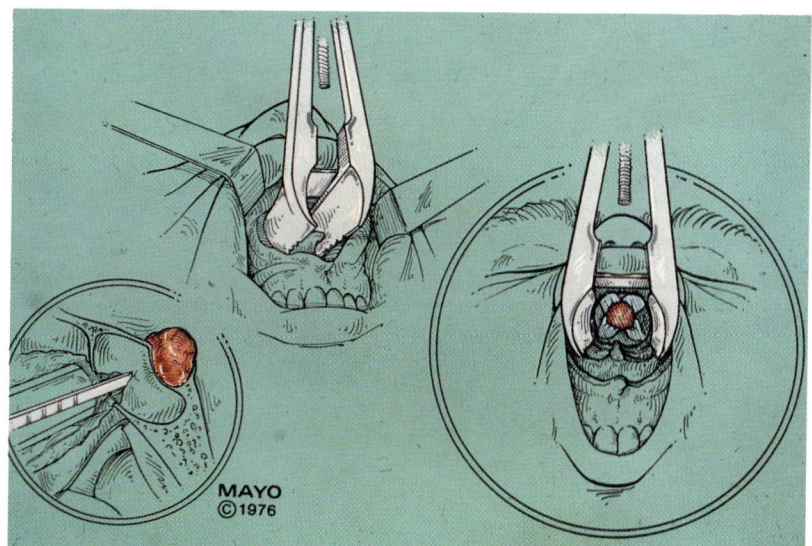

FIG. 3. Sublabial transseptal transsphenoidal approach.

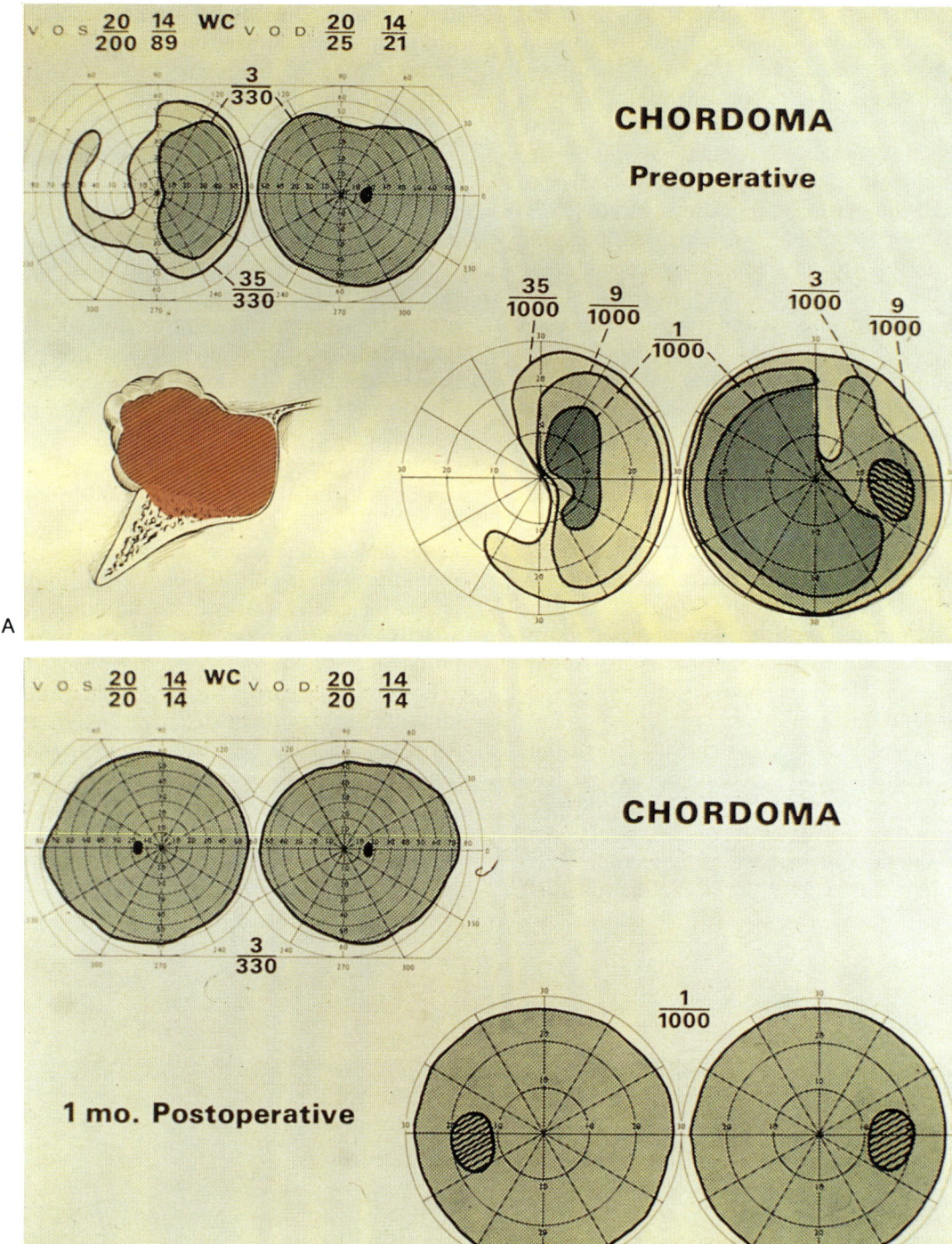

FIG. 4. Visual fields before (**A**) and after (**B**) transsphenoidal removal of a chordoma of the clivus.

may be quite satisfactory (Fig. 5). The disadvantage of the transsphenoidal route is the lateral limitation to exposure produced by the walls of the pyriform aperture, and also the inferior limitations provided by the roof of the hard palate. A transoral approach can be taken more widely and gives excellent exposure of the inferior clivus, making it suitable for tumors that are primarily centered at the basion or C1–C2. A transoral approach through the mouth is limited by the jaw, which may obstruct lateral, inferior, and even superior transpharyngeal exposure. Splitting the mandible allows for very wide exposure in all directions, and in some cases it is worth the additional discomfort and inconvenience to the patient. This method usually requires tracheostomy, often requires a period of tube feeding (nasal, oral, or gastric), and always requires wiring of the teeth and jaw for proper healing of the mandible.

The incision divides the lower lip and skin of the chin in the midline and then is taken laterally in the submandibular plane much as described initially by Stevenson (Fig. 6A,B). Using a sagittal saw, the mandible is split between the incisors and the split is purposely made jagged so as to strengthen the subsequent bony repair (Fig. 6C). The oral mucosa is divided anterolaterally and the incision is carried backward lateral to the tongue so that the entire tongue can also be reflected laterally. The lingual artery and nerve are identified and dissected as a pedicle, which remains attached to the tongue (Fig. 6D). The mandibular segments then can be opened like a book, exposing the oropharynx overlying the clivus and craniocervical junction. Superior exposure, if necessary, can be achieved by mobilizing the soft palate and uvula and by resecting the posterior portion of the hard palate.

Removal of tumor can proceed under direct vision of the entire extent of the ventral clivus, and videofluoroscopic control can also be used. Removal of chordomas can result in CSF leaks that must be repaired with grafts of fat or fascia and fibrin glue. Repairs of the mucosal flaps and the paralingual incision are straightforward. The mandible split is wired and the teeth are wired for support. The dental wires can be removed 6 weeks postoperatively. Tracheostomy and feeding tubes are managed appropriately.

This technique is radical but may provide the means for removal of an otherwise unresectable lesion.

In the usual case, where a radical but subtotal resection has been accomplished, postoperative radiotherapy is generally recommended. Although chordomas are thought to be radioresistant, several studies attest to the efficiency of adjunctive radiation therapy, particularly with fractionated proton beam therapy.

The prognosis of patients with clivus chordomas is variable but generally is favorable in about 50% of cases. Pathologic analysis may be important, with suggestions that the chondroid chordoma and those lesions found to be low grade chondrosarcomas may have a more optimistic outlook.

The surgeon must be prepared to be versatile in the management of clivus chordomas. Many patients require more than one surgical procedure, and familiarity with indications and techniques for a variety of approaches is desirable.

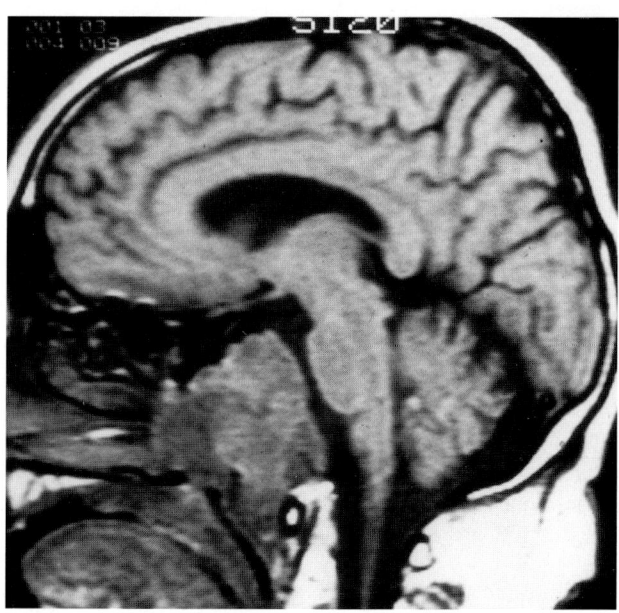

FIG. 5. Sagittal MRI of clivus chordoma. This tumor was removed by a mandible-splitting approach.

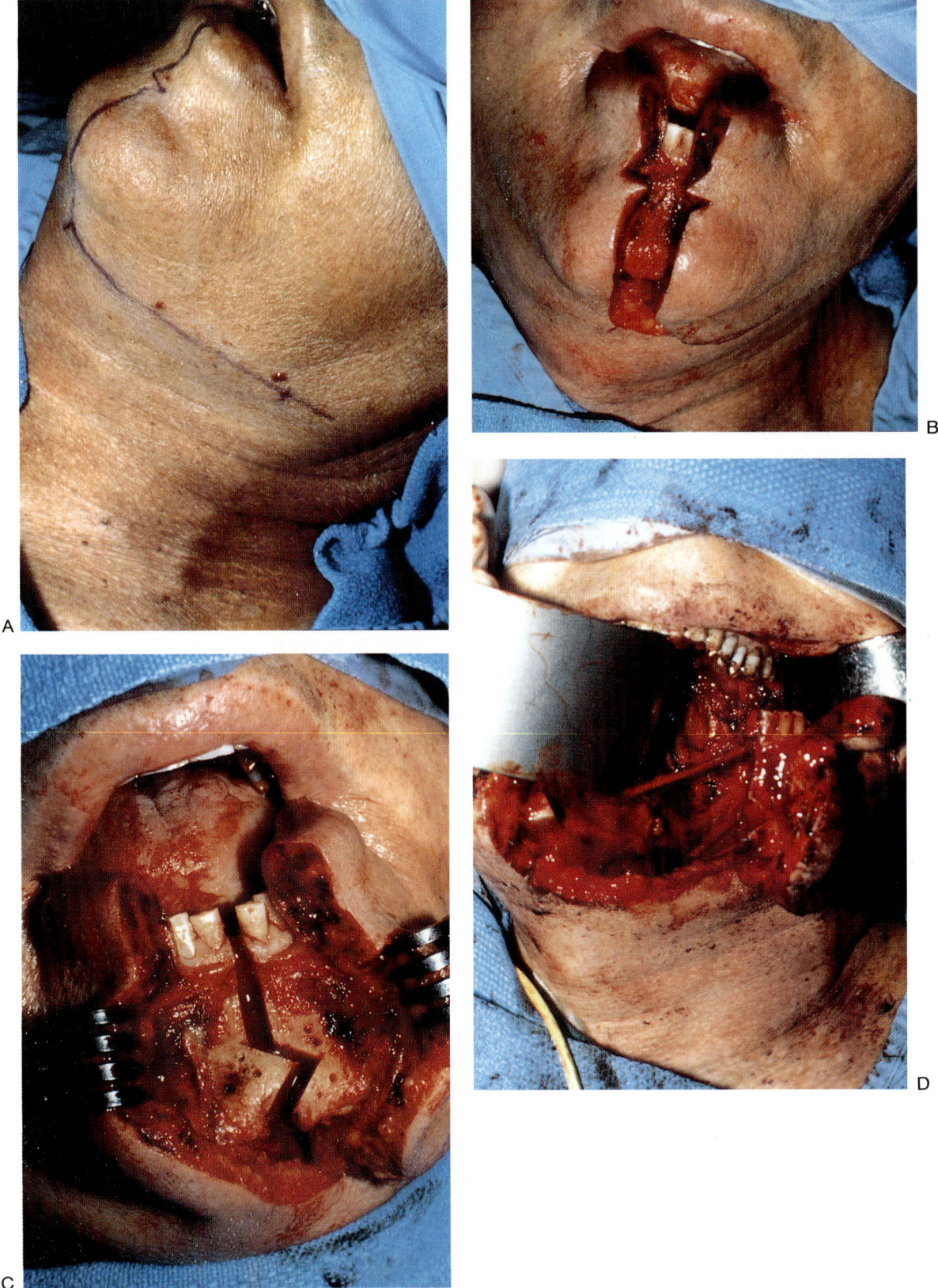

FIG. 6. The mandible-splitting transoral approach. **A:** Skin incision. **B:** Exposure of mandible. **C:** Division of mandible. **D:** Retraction of mandible and displacement of the tongue to the right on a neurovascular pedicle, which is preserved.

SUGGESTED READINGS

1. Biller HF, Shugar JMA, Krespi YP. A new technique for wide field exposure of the base of the skull. *Arch Otolaryngol Head Neck Surg* 1981;107:689–702.
2. Delgado TE, Garrido E, Harwick RD. Labiomandibular transoral approach to chordomas in the clivus and upper cervical spine. *Neurosurgery* 1981;8:675–679.
3. Derome PJ. The transbasal approach to tumours invading the skull base. In: Schmidek HH, Sweet WH, eds. *Operative neurosurgical techniques,* vol 1. New York: Grune & Stratton, 1988;619–633.
4. Fisch U, Pillsbury HC. Infratemporal fossa approach to lesions in the temporal bone and base of the skull. *Arch Otolaryngol Head Neck Surg* 1979;105:99–107.
5. House WF, Hitselberger WE. The transcochlear approach to the skull base. *Arch Otolaryngol Head Neck Surg* 1976;102:334–342.
6. Laws ER Jr. Cranial chordomas. In: Wilkins RH, Rengachary SS, eds. *Neurosurgery,* vol 1. New York: McGraw-Hill, 1985;927–929.
7. Malis LI. Surgical resection of tumours of the skull base. In: Wilkins RH, Rengachary SS, eds. *Neurosurgery,* vol 1. New York: McGraw-Hill, 1985;1011–1020.
8. Price JC. The midfacial degloving approach to the central skull base. *Ear Nose Throat J* 1986;65:46–53.
9. Price JC, Holliday MT, Kennedy DW, et al. The versatile midface degloving approach. *Laryngoscope* 1988;98:291–295.
10. Stevenson GC, Stoney RJ, Perkins RK, et al. A transcervical transclival approach to the ventral surface of the brain stem for removal of a clivus chordoma. *J Neurosurg* 1966;24:544–551.

CHAPTER 42

Microsurgical Anatomy of Acoustic Neuromas

Albert L. Rhoton, Jr.

Acoustic neuromas, as they expand, may involve a majority of the cranial nerves and cerebellar arteries, and the midbrain, pons, and medulla. An understanding of microsurgical anatomy of the cerebellopontine angle and internal acoustic meatus provides the basis for optimizing surgical results with these tumors. This chapter reviews this anatomy and my technique for removing acoustic neuromas.

MICROSURGICAL ANATOMY

Neural Relationships

An understanding of microsurgical anatomy is especially important in preserving the facial and vestibulocochlear nerves, which are the neural structures at greatest risk during acoustic neuroma removal. A widely accepted operative precept is that a nerve involved by tumor should be identified both proximal and distal to the tumor, where its displacement and distortion are least, before the tumor is removed from the involved segment of nerve. This operative principle has received only limited application in operations for acoustic neuroma removal. Considerable attention has been directed to the early identification of the facial and vestibulocochlear nerves distal to the tumor at the lateral part of the internal acoustic canal (12–18), but less attention has been directed to identification at the brain stem on the medial side of the tumor. The neural considerations are divided into sections dealing with the relationships at the lateral end of the tumor in the meatus, and those on the medial end of the tumor at the brain stem.

A. L. Rhoton, Jr.: Department of Neurological Surgery, University of Florida Medical Center, Gainesville, Florida 32610.

Meatal Relationships

The four nerves in the lateral part of the internal acoustic meatus are the facial, the cochlear, and the inferior and superior vestibular nerves (Fig. 1). The position of the nerves is most constant in the lateral portion of the meatus, which is divided into a superior and an inferior portion by a horizontal ridge, the transverse or falciform crest. The facial and the superior vestibular nerves are superior to the crest. The facial nerve is anterior to the superior vestibular nerve and is separated from it at the lateral end of the meatus by a vertical ridge of bone, called the vertical crest. The cochlear and inferior vestibular nerves run below the transverse crest with the cochlear nerve located anteriorly. Thus the lateral meatus can be considered to be divided into four portions, with the facial nerve being anterior–superior, the cochlear nerve anterior–inferior, the superior vestibular posterior–superior, and the inferior vestibular nerve posterior–inferior.

Because acoustic neuromas most frequently arise in the posteriorly placed vestibular nerves, they usually displace the facial and cochlear nerves anteriorly (Fig. 2). The facial nerve is stretched around the anterior half of the tumor capsular. Variability in the direction of growth of the tumor arising from the vestibular nerves may result in the facial nerve being displaced, not only directly anteriorly, but also anterior–superiorly or anterior–inferiorly. Because the facial nerve always enters the facial canal at the anterior–superior quadrant of the lateral margin of the meatus, it is usually easiest to locate it here after the posterior lip of the meatus has been removed, rather than at a more medial location where the degree of displacement of the nerve is more variable. The cochlear nerve also lies anterior to the vestibular nerve and will be stretched around the anterior margin of the tumor.

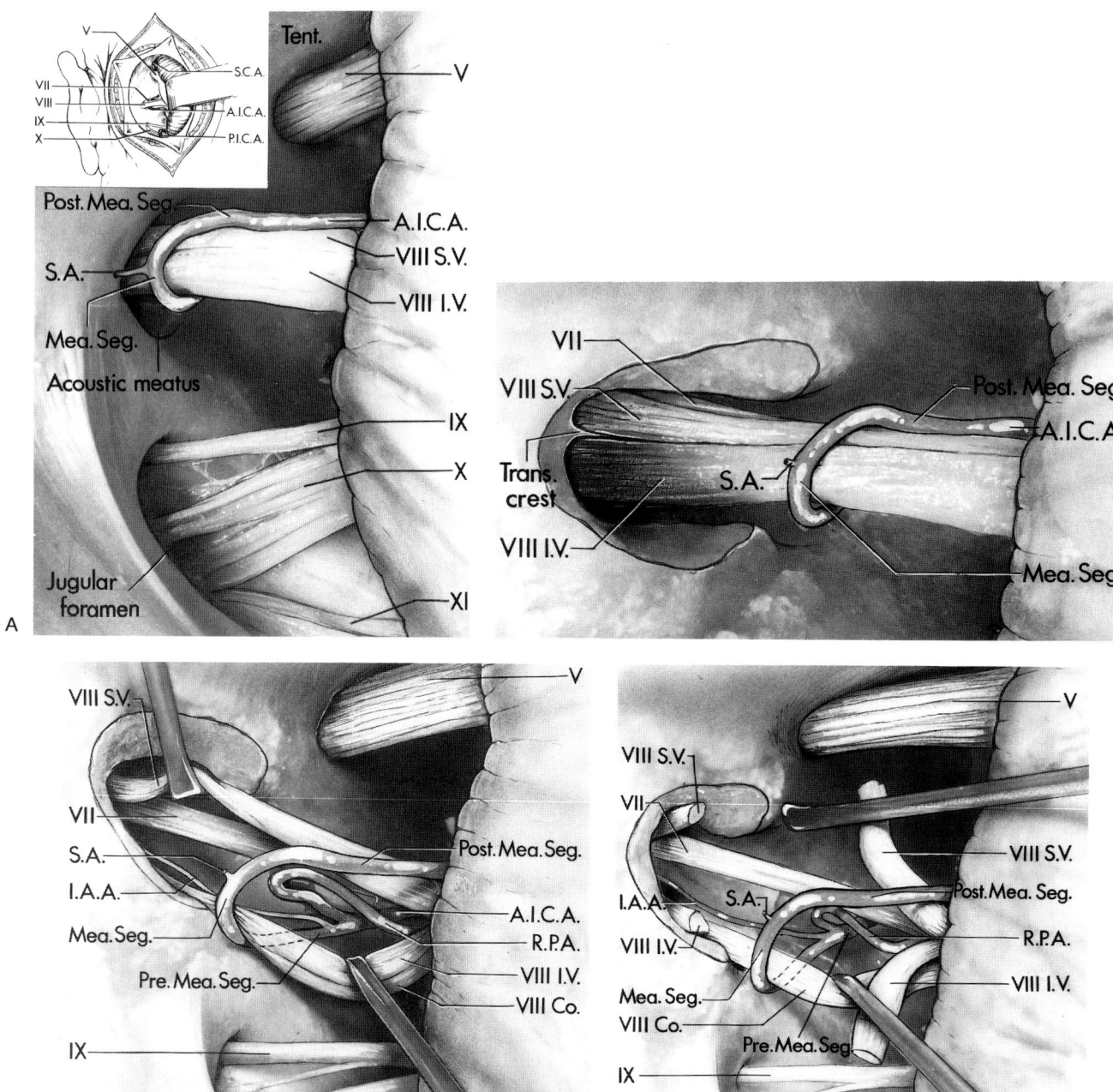

FIG. 1. Posterior view into the left cerebellopontine angle. The **insert** shows the orientation. **A:** The tentorium (Tent.) is above the trigeminal nerve (V). The facial and vestibulocochlear nerves enter the internal acoustic meatus. The posterior surface of the vestibulocochlear nerve is formed by the inferior (VIII I.V.) and superior vestibular (VIII S.V.) nerves. The glossopharyngeal (IX), vagus (X), and spinal accessory nerves (XI) enter the jugular foramen. The premeatal segment of the anterior inferior cerebellar artery (A.I.C.A.) is not visible because it is anterior to the nerves. The meatal segment (Mea. Seg.) passes posterior to the nerves and gives rise to the subarcuate artery (S.A.). The postmeatal segment (Post. Mea. Seg.) passes above the nerves. The **insert** shows the superior cerebellar artery (S.C.A.) above the trigeminal nerve, and the posterior inferior cerebellar artery (P.I.C.A.) below the glossopharyngeal nerve. **B:** The posterior wall of the internal acoustic canal has been removed. The facial nerve (VII) is anterior to the superior vestibular nerve. The subarcuate artery had to be divided to gain access to the posterior wall of the acoustic canal. The transverse crest (Trans. Crest) separates the superior and inferior vestibular nerves at the lateral end of the canal. **C:** The superior vestibular nerve has been elevated to expose the facial nerve. The inferior vestibular and cochlear (VIII Co.) nerves have been depressed to show the premeatal segment (Pre. Mea. Seg.) of the anterior inferior cerebellar artery. The premeatal segment gives origin to the internal auditory (I.A.A.) and recurrent perforating (R.P.A.) arteries. The initial segment of the recurrent perforating artery loops toward the meatus before turning medially to reach the side of the brain stem. **D:** The superior and inferior vestibular nerves have been divided to expose the facial and vestibulocochlear nerves and to show the relationship of the premeatal, meatal, and postmeatal segments and their branches to the nerves. (From ref. 8, with permission.)

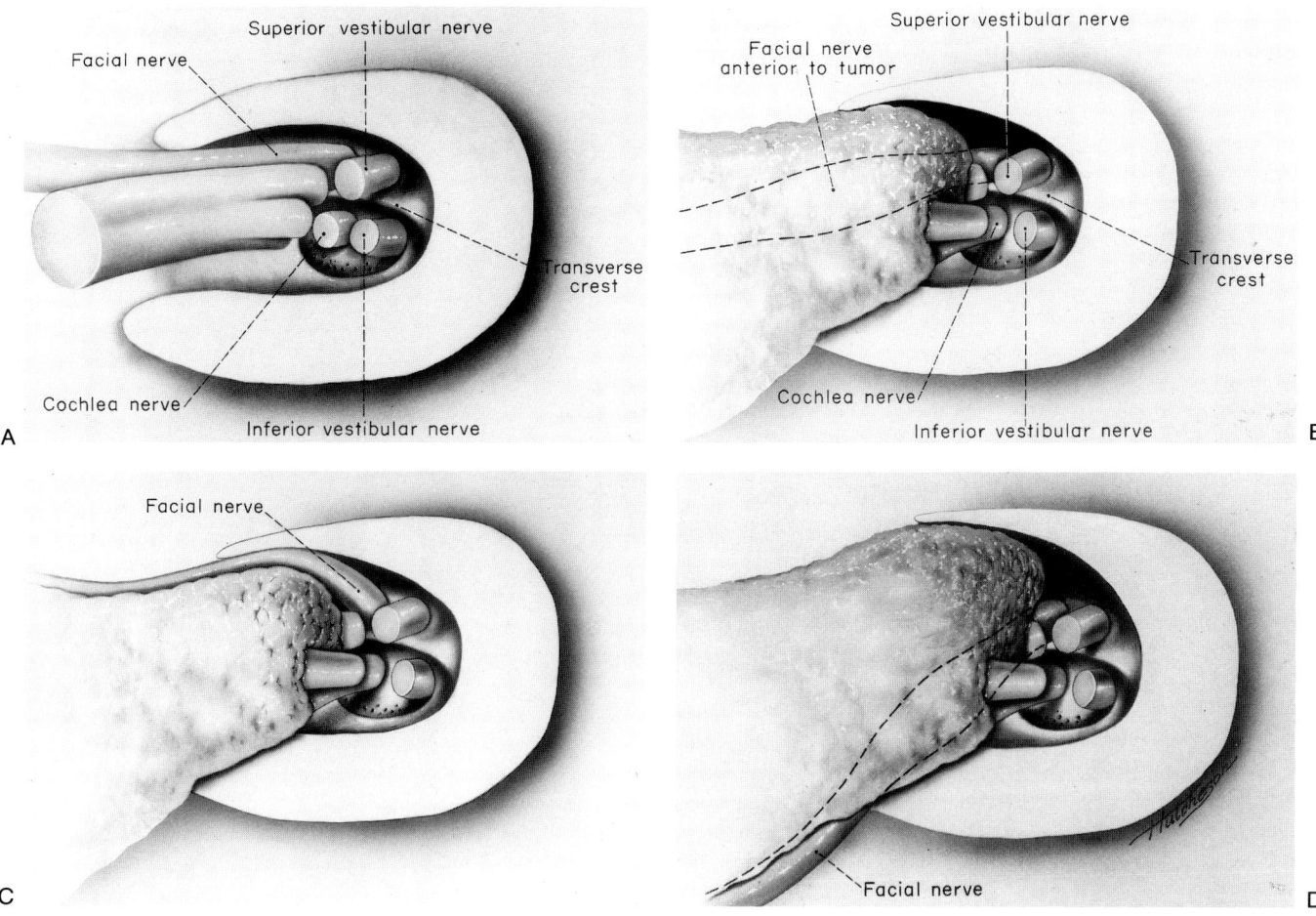

FIG. 2. View of right internal acoustic meatus with the posterior lip removed to show variable direction of facial nerve displacement by acoustic neuroma. **A:** Normal neural relationships with eighth nerve dividing into its three parts in the lateral meatus. The facial and superior vestibular nerves are above the transverse crest and the cochlear and inferior vestibular nerves are below. The facial nerve occupies the anterior–superior quadrant of the lateral meatus. **B:** The facial nerve is displaced directly anteriorly. This is a frequent direction of displacement with acoustic neuroma. **C:** Another frequent direction of displacement of the facial nerve is anterior and superior. **D:** The facial nerve is displaced anteriorly and inferiorly by tumor, which erodes the superior wall of the meatus above the nerves and grows into the area above the nerves, displacing them inferiorly. (From ref. 14, with permission.)

Brain Stem Relationships

The importance of early identification of the facial nerve proximal to the tumor at the brain stem has received less attention, even though there is a consistent set of relationships at the brain stem that facilitates identification of the facial nerve on the medial side of the tumor (19).

The neural structures most intimately related to the medial side of an acoustic neuroma are the pons, medulla, and cerebellum (Figs. 3A, 4A, and 5A). The landmarks on these structures that are helpful in guiding the surgeon to the junction of the facial nerve with the brain stem are the pontomedullary sulcus; the junction of the glossopharyngeal, vagus, and accessory nerves with the medulla; the foramen of Luschka; and flocculus; and the inferior olive.

Pontomedullary Sulcus

The facial nerve arises from the brain stem near the lateral end of the pontomedullary sulcus. This sulcus extends along the junction of the pons and the medulla, and ends just medial to the foramen of Luschka and the lateral recess of the fourth ventricle. The facial nerve arises in the pontomedullary sulcus 1–2 mm anterior to the point at which the vestibulocochlear nerve joins the

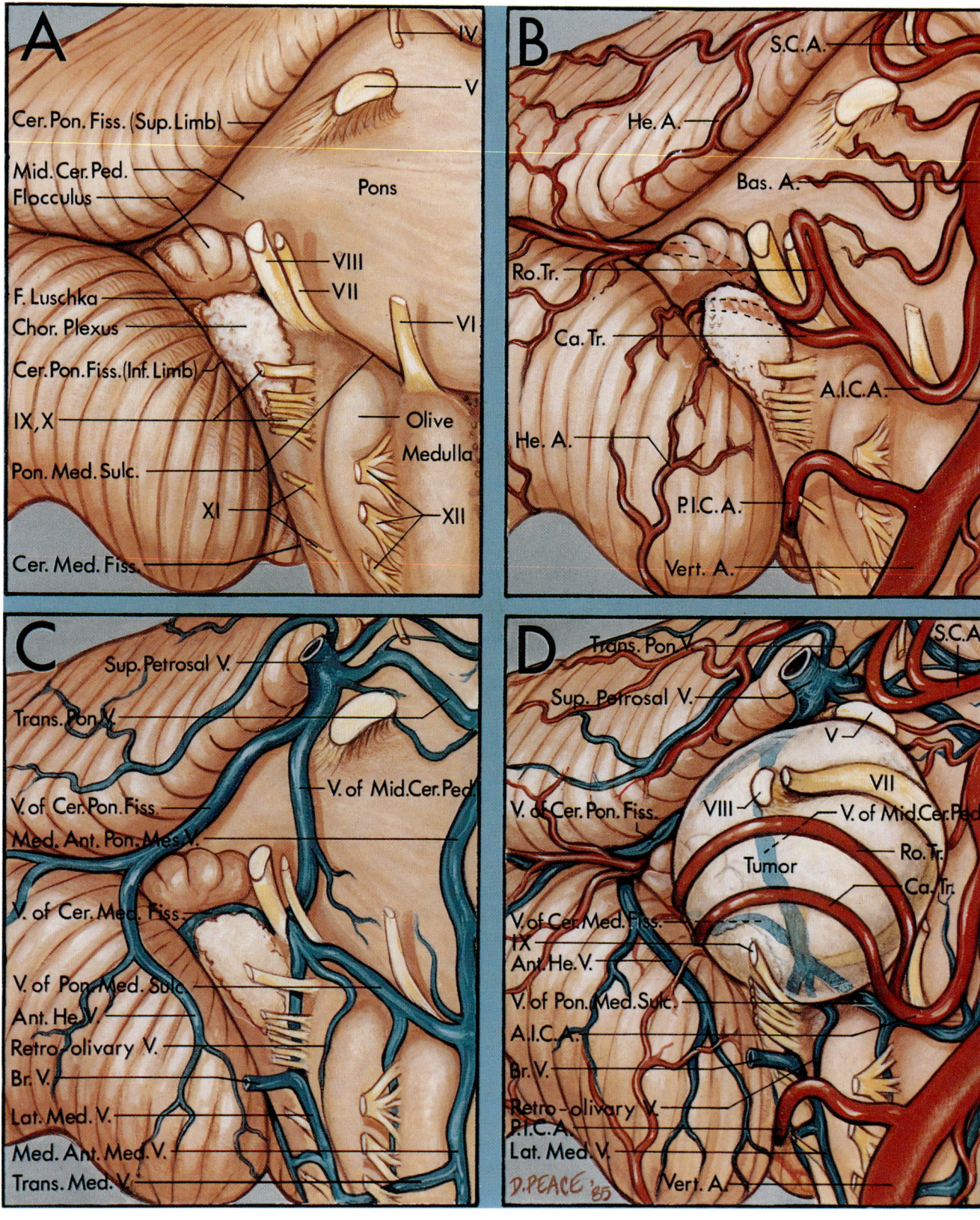

brain stem at the lateral end of the sulcus. The interval between the vestibulocochlear and facial nerves is greatest at the level of the pontomedullary sulcus and decreases as these nerves approach the meatus. In an erect man, the pontomedullary sulcus is roughly horizontal. In the exposure provided by a retrosigmoid craniectomy, the junction of the facial nerve with the pontomedullary sulcus will be hidden directly anterior to the vestibulocochlear nerve, and in some cases the facial nerve can be seen only by gently elevating or depressing the vestibulocochlear nerve.

Glossopharyngeal, Vagus, and Accessory Nerves

The facial nerve enjoys a consistent relationship to the junction of the glossopharyngeal, vagus, and accessory nerves with the lateral side of the medulla. The facial nerve arises 2–3 mm above the most rostral rootlet contributing to these nerves. In the suboccipital operative exposure, the rootlets of these three nerves are seen entering the brain stem below the tumor. A helpful way of visualizing the point where the facial nerve will exit from the brain stem, even when displaced by tumor, is to project an imaginary line along the medullary junction of the rootlets forming the glossopharyngeal, vagal, and accessory nerves, and upward through the pontomedullary junction. This line, at a point 2–3 mm above the junction of the glossopharyngeal nerve with the medulla, will pass through the pontomedullary junction at the site where the facial nerve exits from the brain stem.

Cerebellar–Brain Stem Fissures

Acoustic neuromas are closely related to the cerebellopontine and cerebellomedullary fissures, the clefts formed by the folding of the cerebellum around the pons and medulla. The cerebellopontine fissure is a V-shaped fissure formed by the folding of the petrosal surface of

FIG. 3. Neurovascular relationships on the brain stem side of an acoustic neuroma. Anterolateral view of the right cerebellopontine angle. **A:** Neural relationships. The facial (VII) and vestibulocochlear (VIII) nerves arise from the brain stem near the lateral end of the pontomedullary sulcus (Pon. Med. Sulc.), anterior–superior to the choroid plexus (Chor. Plex.) protruding from the foramen of Luschka (F. Luschka), anterior to the flocculus, rostral to a line drawn along the junction of the rootlets of the glossopharyngeal (IX), vagus (X), and accessory (XI) nerves with the brain stem, and slightly posterior to the rostral pole of the inferior olive. The abducent nerve (VI) arises in the medial part of the pontomedullary sulcus. The hypoglossal rootlets (XII) arise anterior to the olive. The cerebellopontine fissure (Cer. Pon. Fiss.) formed by the cerebellum wrapping around the lateral side of the pons and middle cerebellar peduncle (Mid. Cer. Ped.) has a superior limb (Sup. Limb) that passes above the trigeminal nerve (V) and an inferior limb (Inf. Limb) that extends below the foramen of Luschka. The cerebellomedullary fissure (Cer. Med. Fiss.), which extends superiorly between the medulla and cerebellum, communicates in the region of the foramen of Luschka with the cerebellopontine fissure. The trochlear nerve (IV) is above the trigeminal nerve. **B:** Arterial relationships. The anterior inferior cerebellar artery (AICA) arises from the basilar artery (Bas. A.) and divides into rostral (Ro. Tr.) and caudal (Ca. Tr.) trunks. The rostral trunk, which is usually the larger of the two trunks, courses below the facial and vestibulocochlear nerves, and then above the flocculus to reach the surface of the middle cerebellar peduncle. The posterior inferior cerebellar artery (PICA) arises from the vertebral artery (Vert. A.) and passes first between the hypoglossal rootlets, and then between the vagus and accessory nerves on its way to the cerebellar hemisphere. The superior cerebellar artery (S.C.A.) passes above the trigeminal nerve. The cerebellar arteries give rise to hemispheric branches (He. A.). **C:** Venous relationships. The veins that converge on the junction of the facial and vestibulocochlear nerves with the brain stem are the veins of the pontomedullary sulcus (V. of Pon. Med. Sulc.), cerebellomedullary fissure (V. of Cer. Med. Fiss.), middle cerebellar peduncle (V. of Mid. Cer. Ped.), and the retro-olivary (Retro-olivary V.) and lateral medullary veins (Lat. Med. V.). The vein of the cerebellopontine fissure (V. of Cer. Pon. Fiss.), which passes above the flocculus on the middle cerebellar peduncle, is formed by the anterior hemispheric veins (Ant. He. V.) that arise on the cerebellum. Transverse pontine (Trans. Pon. V.) and transverse medullary (Trans. Med. V.) veins cross the pons and medulla. The median anterior medullary (Med. Ant. Med. V.) and median anterior pontomesencephalic veins (Med. Ant. Pon. Mes. V.) ascend on the anterior surface of the medulla and pons. The veins of the middle cerebellar peduncle and the cerebellopontine fissure and a transverse pontine vein join to form a superior petrosal vein (Sup. Pet. V.), which empties into the superior petrosal sinus. A bridging vein (Br. V.) passes below the vagal rootlets toward the jugular foramen. **D:** Neurovascular relationships of an acoustic neuroma. The tumor arises from the vestibulocochlear nerve and displaces the facial nerve anteriorly, the trigeminal nerve superiorly, and the vagus and glossopharyngeal nerves inferiorly. The facial nerve, even though displaced by the tumor, enters the brain stem along the lateral margin of the pontomedullary sulcus, rostral to the glossopharyngeal and vagus nerves, anterior to the flocculus, and rostral to the choroid plexus protruding from the foramen of Luschka. The rostral trunk of the anterior inferior cerebellar artery, after passing below the tumor, returns to the surface of the middle cerebellar peduncle above the flocculus. The veins displaced around the medial side of the tumor are the veins of the middle cerebellar peduncle, cerebellomedullary fissure, cerebellopontine fissure and pontomedullary sulcus, and the retro-olivary and lateral medullary veins. (From ref. 19, with permission.)

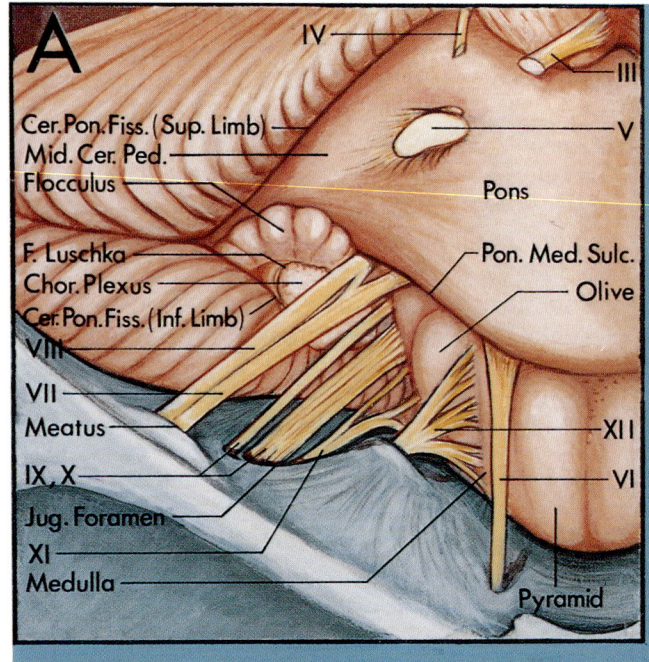
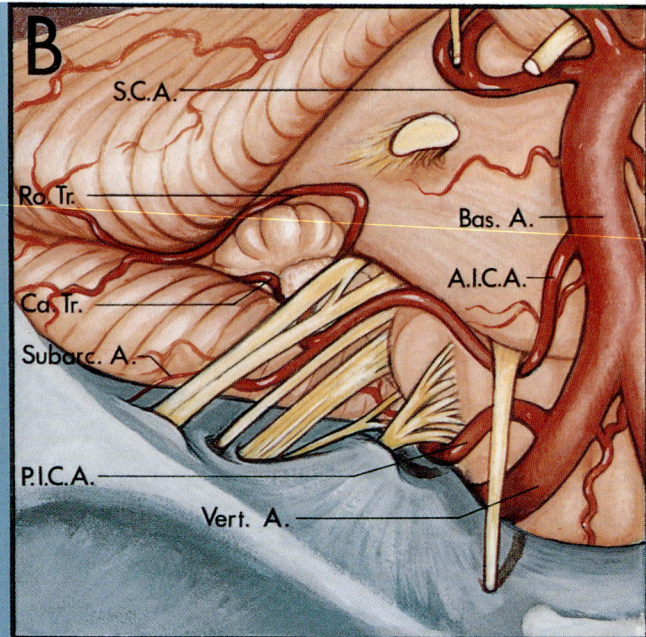
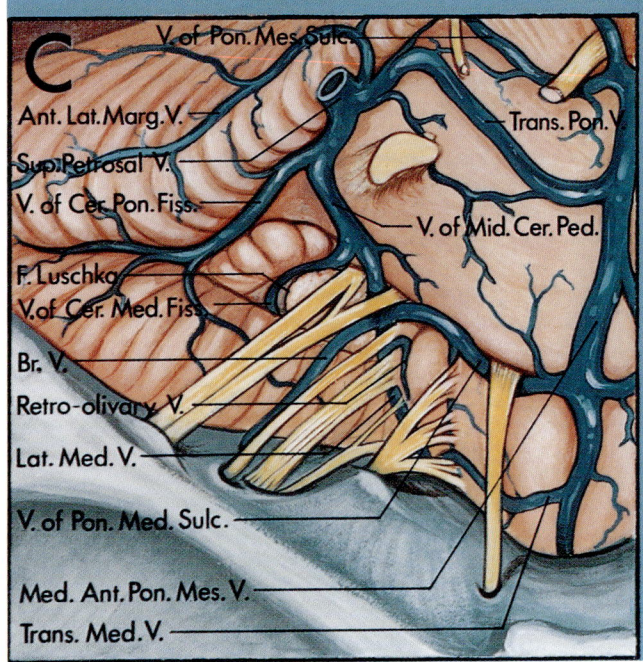
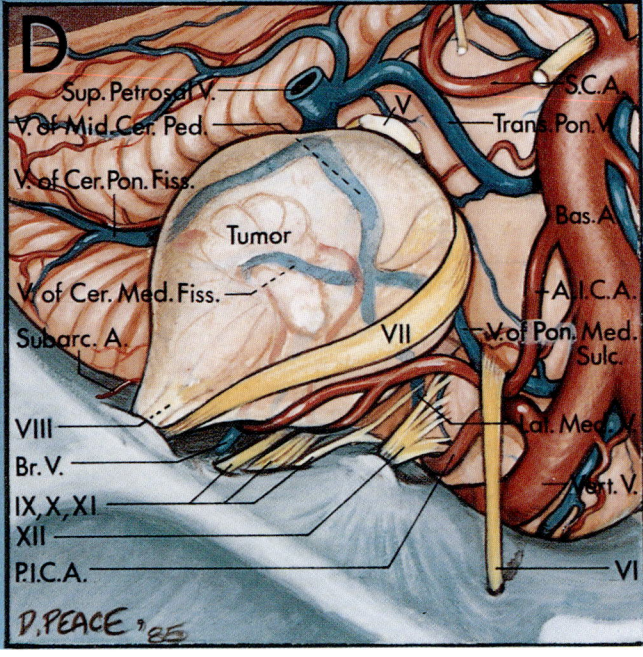

the cerebellum around the lateral side of the pons and middle cerebellar peduncle. The petrosal surface is the cerebellar surface that faces the posterior surface of the petrous bone and is retracted to expose the nerves entering the internal acoustic meatus. The cerebellopontine fissure has a superior limb situated between the rostral half of the pons and the superior part of the petrosal surface, and an inferior limb located between the caudal half of the pons and the inferior part of the petrosal surface. The apex of the fissure is located laterally where the superior and inferior limbs meet. The V-shaped area between the superior and inferior limbs, which has the middle cerebellar peduncle in its floor, corresponds to the area that is referred to as the cerebellopontine angle. The trigeminal, abducent, facial, vestibulocochlear, and glossopharyngeal nerves arise between the superior and inferior limbs of the fissure. The facial and vestibulocochlear nerves arise just anterior to the inferior limb of the fissure, and just below the middle cerebellar peduncle. The trigeminal nerve arises near the superior limb of the fissure.

The cerebellomedullary fissure—the cleft between the cerebellum and medulla, which extends upward between the cerebellar tonsil and the medulla—communicates with the inferior limb of the cerebellopontine fissure near the lateral recess of the fourth ventricle. Several structures related to the lateral recess project into the cerebellopontine angle near the facial and the vestibulocochlear nerves.

Foramen of Luschka, Choroid Plexus, and Flocculus

The structures related to the lateral recess of the fourth ventricle that have a consistent relationship to the facial and vestibulocochlear nerves are the foramen of Luschka, the choroid plexus projecting from it, and the flocculus (Fig. 6). The foramen of Luschka is situated at

FIG. 4. Neurovascular relationships on the brain stem side of an acoustic neuroma. Anterosuperior views. **A:** Neural relationships. The cerebrum and tentorium cerebelli have been removed, and the trigeminal (V), trochlear (IV), and oculomotor (III) nerves have been divided to allow the brain stem to be displaced posteriorly in order to expose the cerebellopontine angle from above. The facial (VII) and vestibulocochlear (VIII) nerves arise at the lateral end of the pontomedullary sulcus (Pont. Med. Sulc.) anterior to the flocculus, rostral to the glossopharyngeal (IX), vagus (X), and accessory (XI) nerves, and anterosuperior to the choroid plexus (Chor. Plex.) protruding from the foramen of Luschka (F. Luschka). The hypoglossal nerve (XII) arises anterior to the inferior olive. The abducent nerve (VI) arises from the medial part of the pontomedullary sulcus and ascends to pierce the dura mater on the clivus. The facial and vestibulocochlear nerves pass laterally to enter the internal acoustic meatus. The glossopharyngeal, vagus, and accessory nerves converge on the medial side of the jugular foramen (Jug. Foramen). The cerebellopontine fissure, formed where the cerebellum wraps around the lateral side of the pons and middle cerebellar peduncle (Med. Cer. Ped.) has superior (Sup. Limb) and inferior (Inf. Limb) limbs. The foramen of Luschka opens into the inferior limb near the facial and vestibulocochlear nerves. **B:** Arterial relationships. The anterior inferior cerebellar artery (AICA) arises from the basilar artery (Bas. A.), passes below the facial and vestibulocochlear nerves, gives rise to the subarcuate artery (Subarc. A.), and divides into a rostral (Ro. Tr.) and a caudal (Ca. Tr.) trunk. The rostral trunk passes above the flocculus to course on the middle cerebellar peduncle, and the caudal trunk supplies the area below the flocculus. The posterior inferior cerebellar artery (PICA) arises from the vertebral artery (Vert. A.) and passes below the hypoglossal nerve. The superior cerebellar artery (S.C.A.) passes above the trigeminal nerve. **C:** Venous relationships. The veins converging on the junction of the facial nerve with the brain stem are the lateral medullary (Lat. Med. V.) and retro-olivary (Retro-olivary V.) veins, and the veins of the pontomedullary sulcus (V. of Pon. Med. Sulc.), cerebellomedullary fissure (V. of Cer. Med. Fiss.), and middle cerebellar peduncle (V. of Mid. Cer. Ped.). The median anterior pontomesencephalic vein (Med. Ant. Pon. Mes. V.) ascends on the anterior surface of the brain stem, and the transverse pontine (Trans. Pon. V.) and transverse medullary (Trans. Med. V.) veins cross the pons and medulla. The vein of the cerebellopontine fissure (V. of Cer. Pon. Fiss.) passes above the flocculus. The transverse pontine vein and the veins of the middle cerebellar peduncle and cerebellopontine fissure join to form one of the superior petrosal veins (Sup. Pet. V.) that empty into the superior petrosal sinus. A bridging vein (Br. V.) passes from the side of the brain stem to the jugular foramen. The anterolateral marginal vein (Ant. Lat. Marg. V.) crosses the anterolateral margin of the cerebellum. The vein of the pontomesencephalic sulcus (V. of Pon. Mes. Sulc.) courses in the pontomesencephalic sulcus below the oculomotor nerve. **D:** Neurovascular relationships of an acoustic neuroma. The tumor arises from the vestibulocochlear nerve and displaces the facial nerve anteriorly, the trigeminal nerve superiorly, and the glossopharyngeal and vagus nerves inferiorly. The vestibulocochlear nerve disappears into the tumor. The facial nerve enters the brain stem along the lateral margin of the pontomedullary sulcus, rostral to the glossopharyngeal nerve, anterior to the flocculus, and rostral to the choroid plexus protruding from the foramen of Luschka. The anterior inferior cerebellar artery is usually displaced around the lower margin of the tumor. The veins displaced around the medial side of the tumor are the veins of the pontomedullary sulcus, middle cerebellar peduncle and cerebellomedullary fissure, and the lateral medullary and retro-olivary veins. (From ref. 19, with permission.)

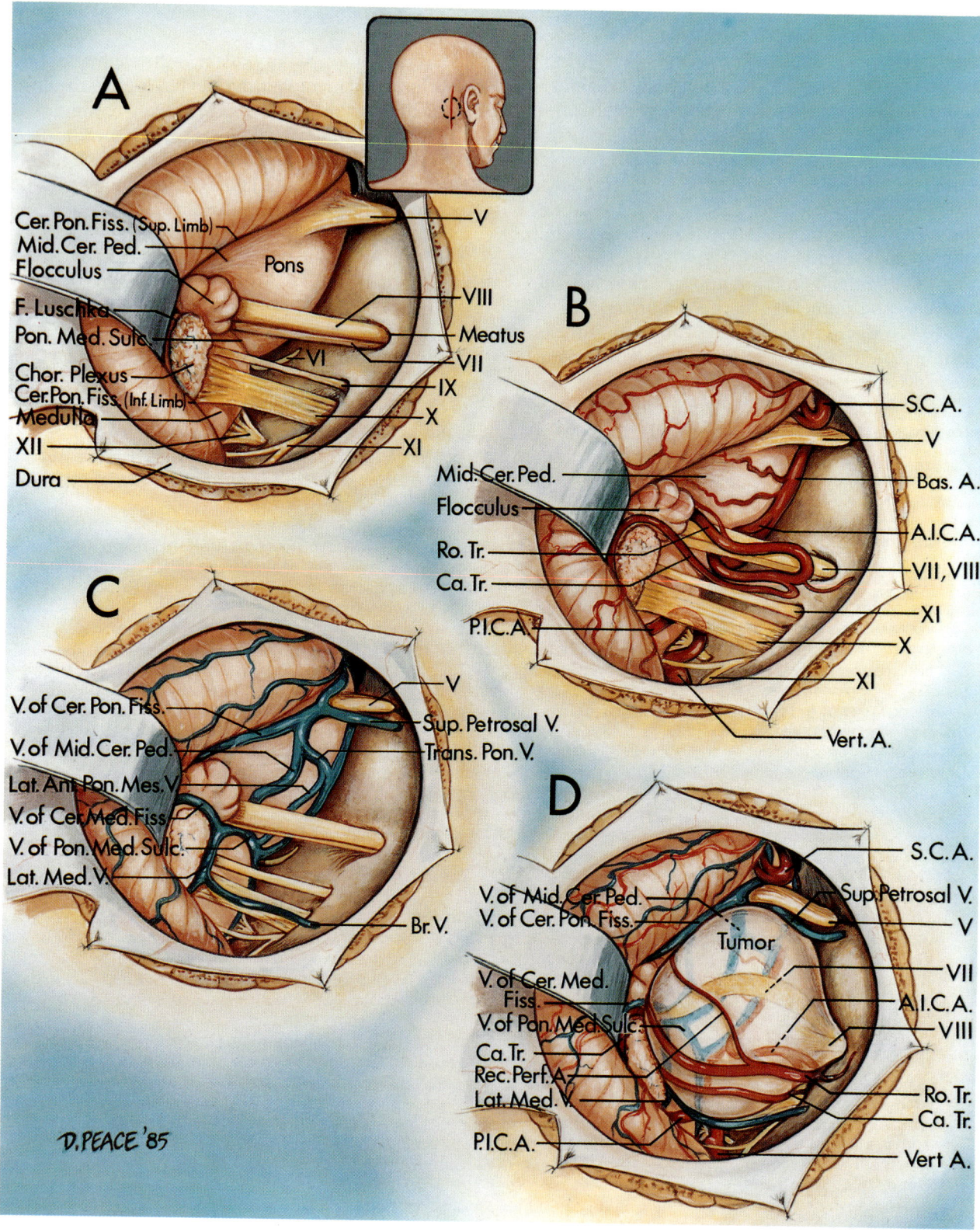

the lateral margin of the pontomedullary sulcus, just dorsal to the junction of the glossopharyngeal nerve with the brain stem, and immediately posteroinferior to the junction of the facial and vestibulocochlear nerves with the brain stem. The foramen of Luschka is infrequently seen from the view provided by the retrosigmoid operative exposure. However, there is consistently identifiable tuft of choroid plexus that hangs out of the foramen of Luschka and sits on the posterior surface of the glossopharyngeal and vagus nerves just inferior to the junction of the facial and vestibulocochlear nerves with the brain stem.

Another structure related to the lateral recess is the flocculus. It is a fan-shaped cerebellar lobule that projects from the margin of the lateral recess into the cerebellopontine angle. The flocculus, together with the nodule of the vermis, forms the primitive flocculonodular lobe of the cerebellum. The flocculus is attached to the rostral margin of the lateral recess and foramen of Luschka. The flocculus is continuous medially with the inferior medullary velum, a butterfly-shaped sheet of neural tissue that forms on the surface of the nodule and sweeps laterally above the tonsil to form part of the inferior half of the roof of the fourth ventricle. The lateral part of the inferior medullary velum narrows to a smaller bundle, the peduncle of the flocculus, which fuses to the rostral margin of the lateral recess and foramen of Luschka. The flocculus projects from the peduncle of the flocculus into the cerebellopontine angle just posterior to where the facial and vestibulocochlear nerves join the pontomedullary sulcus.

Arterial Relationships

The arteries crossing the cerebellopontine angle, especially the anterior inferior cerebellar artery (AICA), enjoy a consistent relationship to the facial and vestibulocochlear nerves, foramen of Luschka, and the flocculus (Fig. 1, 3B, 4B, 5B, and 7) (1,4,5,7,8). The AICA originates from the basilar artery and encircles the pons near the pontomedullary sulcus. After coursing near, and sending branches to the nerves entering the acoustic meatus and the choroid plexus protruding from the foramen of Luschka, it passes around the flocculus to reach the surface of the middle cerebellar peduncle and terminates by supplying the lips of the cerebellopontine fissure and the petrosal surface of the cerebellum. The AICA may pass around the brain stem either above, below, or between the facial and vestibulocochlear nerves; but

FIG. 5. Neurovascular relationships on the brain stem side of an acoustic neuroma. Posterior view through a retrosigmoid craniectomy. **A:** Neural relationships. The orientation, skin incision (*solid line*), and craniectomy site (*interrupted line*) are shown in the **insert**. The retractor is on the petrosal surface of the cerebellum. The facial (VII) and vestibulocochlear (VIII) nerves arise at the lateral end of the pontomedullary sulcus (Pon. Med. Sulc.), anterior to the flocculus, rostral to the glossopharyngeal (IX), vagus (X), and accessory (XI) nerves, and anterosuperior to the choroid plexus (Chor. Plexus) protruding from the foramen of Luschka (F. Luschka). The hypoglossal nerve (XII) arises anterior to the olive. The abducent nerve (VI) arises from the medial part of the pontomedullary sulcus. The trigeminal nerve (V) arises in the upper part of the exposure. The cerebellopontine fissure, formed where the cerebellum wraps around the lateral side of the pons and middle cerebellar peduncle (Mid. Cer. Ped.) has superior (Sup. Limb) and inferior (Inf. Limb) limbs. **B:** Arterial relationships. The anterior inferior cerebellar artery (AICA) arises from the basilar artery (Bas. A.) and divides into a rostral trunk (Ro. Tr.), which passes above the flocculus to reach the surface of the middle cerebellar peduncle, and a caudal trunk (Ca. Tr.), which supplies the area below the flocculus. The posterior inferior cerebellar artery (PICA) arises from the vertebral artery (Vert. A.) and passes dorsally between the vagus and accessory nerves. The superior cerebellar artery (S.C.A.) courses above the trigeminal nerve. **C:** Venous relationships. The veins that join near the junction of the facial and vestibulocochlear nerves with the brain stem are the lateral medullary (Lat. Med. V.) veins and the veins of the cerebellomedullary fissure (V. of Cer. Med. Fiss.), pontomedullary sulcus (V. of Pon. Med. Sulc.), and middle cerebellar peduncle (V. of Mid. Cer. Ped.). The vein of the cerebellopontine fissure (V. of Cer. Pon. Fiss.) passes above the flocculus along the superior limb of the cerebellopontine fissure and joins the vein of the middle cerebellar peduncle and a transverse pontine vein (Trans. Pon. V.) to form a superior petrosal vein (Sup. Pet. V.), which empties into the superior petrosal sinus. A bridging vein (Br. V.) passes behind the vagus nerve. The lateral anterior pontomesencephalic vein (Lat. Ant. Pon. Mes. V.) ascends on the pons. **D:** Neurovascular relationships of an acoustic neuroma. The tumor arises from the vestibulocochlear nerve and displaces the facial nerve anteriorly, the trigeminal nerve superiorly, and the glossopharyngeal and vagus nerves inferiorly. The vestibulocochlear nerve disappears into the tumor. The facial nerve enters the brain stem at the lateral margin of the pontomedullary sulcus, anterior to the flocculus and rostral to the choroid plexus protruding from the foramen of Luschka. The rostral trunk of the anterior inferior cerebellar artery courses below the tumor and above the flocculus to reach the surface of the middle cerebellar peduncle. The veins displaced around the medial side of the tumor are the lateral medullary veins and the veins of the middle cerebellar peduncle, cerebellomedullary fissure, and pontomedullary sulcus. The vein of the cerebellopontine fissure passes above the tumor. A recurrent perforating branch (Rec. Perf. A.) of the anterior inferior cerebellar artery passes across the tumor and supplies the brain stem. (From ref. 19, with permission.)

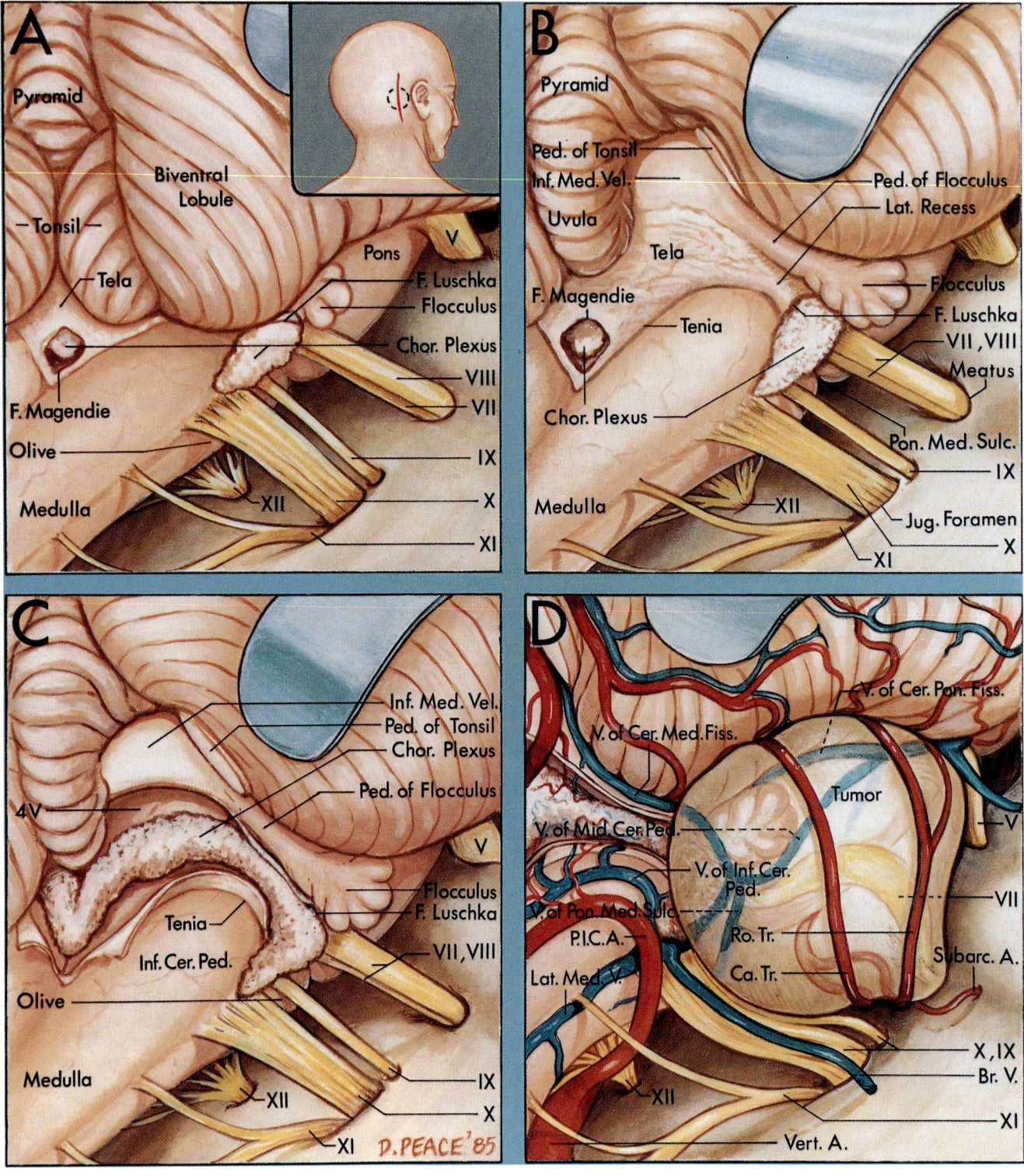

after passing these nerves, the artery consistently passes back to the surface of the middle cerebellar peduncle above the flocculus. The AICA usually bifurcates near the facial and vestibulocochlear nerves to form a rostral and a caudal trunk. The rostral trunk courses along the middle cerebellar peduncle to supply the upper part of the petrosal surface, and the caudal trunk passes near the lateral recess and supplies the lower part of the petrosal surface. If the AICA bifurcates into rostral and caudal trunks prior to reaching the region of the flocculus, it is the rostral trunk that can be followed above the flocculus to the surface of the middle cerebellar peduncle.

In most cases, the AICA passes below the facial and vestibulocochlear nerves as it encircles the brain stem, but it may also pass above or between these nerves in its course around the brain stem (Fig. 7). In the most common case, in which the AICA passes below the nerves, the tumor would displace the artery inferiorly. If the AICA courses between the facial and vestibulocochlear nerves, a tumor arising in the latter nerve will displace the AICA forward. Tumor growth would displace the AICA superiorly if the artery passes above the nerves. In each case, once the flocculus is identified below the suprafloccular segment of the AICA, the site of entry of the facial nerve into the brain stem can be predicted because of its relationship to the AICA. The branches of the AICA that arise near the facial and vestibulocochlear nerves are the internal auditory arteries, which supply the facial and vestibulocochlear nerves and adjacent structures; the recurrent perforating arteries, which may initially pass toward the meatus but subsequently turn medially and supply the brain stem; and the subarcuate artery, which enters the subarcuate fossa—a small depression on the posterior wall of the meatus.

The superior cerebellar artery, which is separated from the tumor by the trigeminal nerve, is displaced rostrally

FIG. 6. Relationship of the foramen of Luschka and the lateral recess of the fourth ventricle to the junction of the facial and vestibulocochlear nerves with the brain stem as seen through a suboccipital craniectomy. **A:** The orientation, skin incision (*solid line*), and craniectomy (*interrupted line*) are shown in the **insert**. The foramen of Magendie (F. Magendie) opens in the midline between the cerebellar tonsils and the foramen of Luschka (F. Luschka) opens into the cerebellopontine angle. The choroid plexus (Chor. Plexus) is attached to the inner surface of the tela choroidea (Tela) and protrudes from the foramen of Luschka slightly below and behind the facial (VII) and vestibulocochlear (VIII) nerves, and behind to the glossopharyngeal (IX) and vagus (X) nerves. The flocculus protrudes into the cerebellopontine angle above the foramen of Luschka. The accessory nerve (XI) arises below the vagus nerve. The hypoglossal rootlets (XII) arise ventral to the olive. The trigeminal nerve (V) crosses in the upper part of the exposure. **B:** The right cerebellar tonsil has been removed by dividing the tonsillar peduncle (Ped. of Tonsil) to show the relationship of the lateral recess (Lat. Recess) to the facial and vestibulocochlear nerves. The flocculus and choroid plexus protrude in the cerebellopontine angle behind the junction of the facial and vestibulocochlear nerves with the brain stem. The inferior medullary velum (Inf. Med. Vel.) stretches from the lateral side of the vermis to the flocculus and is all that remains of the connection between the flocculus and the nodulus, which form the flocculonodular lobe of the cerebellum. The inferior medullary velum stretches laterally to form the peduncle of the flocculus (Ped. of Flocculus). The tela choroidea forms the caudal part of the roof of the fourth ventricle and has the choroid plexus attached to its inner surface. Small ridges called the tenia are the site of attachment of the tela choroidea to the edge of the floor of the fourth ventricle. The glossopharyngeal, vagus, and accessory nerves pass through the jugular foramen (Jug. Foramen). The facial and vestibulocochlear nerves enter the brain stem at the lateral end of the pontomedullary sulcus (Pon. Med. Sulc.). **C:** The tela choroidea has been opened, but the choroid plexus, which arises on the inner surface of the tela in the fourth ventricle (4V), has been preserved. The fringelike choroid plexus extends through the foramen of Luschka slightly below and behind the junction of the facial and vestibulocochlear nerves with the brain stem. The inferior cerebellar peduncle (Inf. Cer. Ped.) ascends on the dorsolateral margin of the medulla. **D:** Relationships of an acoustic neuroma. The facial nerve is displaced anteriorly and superiorly in the cerebellopontine angle and enters the brain stem at the lateral end of the pontomedullary sulcus, anterosuperior to the choroid plexus protruding from the foramen of Luschka, and near where the flocculus is attached along the margin of the lateral recess. The tumor displaces the trigeminal nerve upward and the glossopharyngeal and vagus nerves downward. The anterior inferior cerebellar artery (AICA) gives rise to a subarcuate artery (Subarc. A.), which enters the subarcuate fossa in the posterior wall of the internal acoustic meatus and bifurcates into a rostral (Ro. Tr.) and a caudal trunk (Ca. Tr.). The rostral trunk courses above the flocculus to reach the surface of the middle cerebellar peduncle. The posterior inferior cerebellar artery (PICA) arises from the vertebral artery (Vert. A.) and passes around the lateral surface of the medulla. The lateral medullary vein (Lat. Med. V.) and the veins of the inferior cerebellar peduncle (V. of Inf. Cer. Ped.) and cerebellomedullary fissure (V. of Cer. Med. Fiss.) join in the area below where the facial nerve enters the brain stem to form the vein of the middle cerebellar peduncle (Mid. Cer. Ped.). A bridging vein (Br. V.) passes from the lateral surface of the medulla to the jugular foramen. The vein of the cerebellopontine fissure (V. of Cer. Pon. Fiss.) ascends along the superomedial margin of the tumor. (From ref. 19, with permission.)

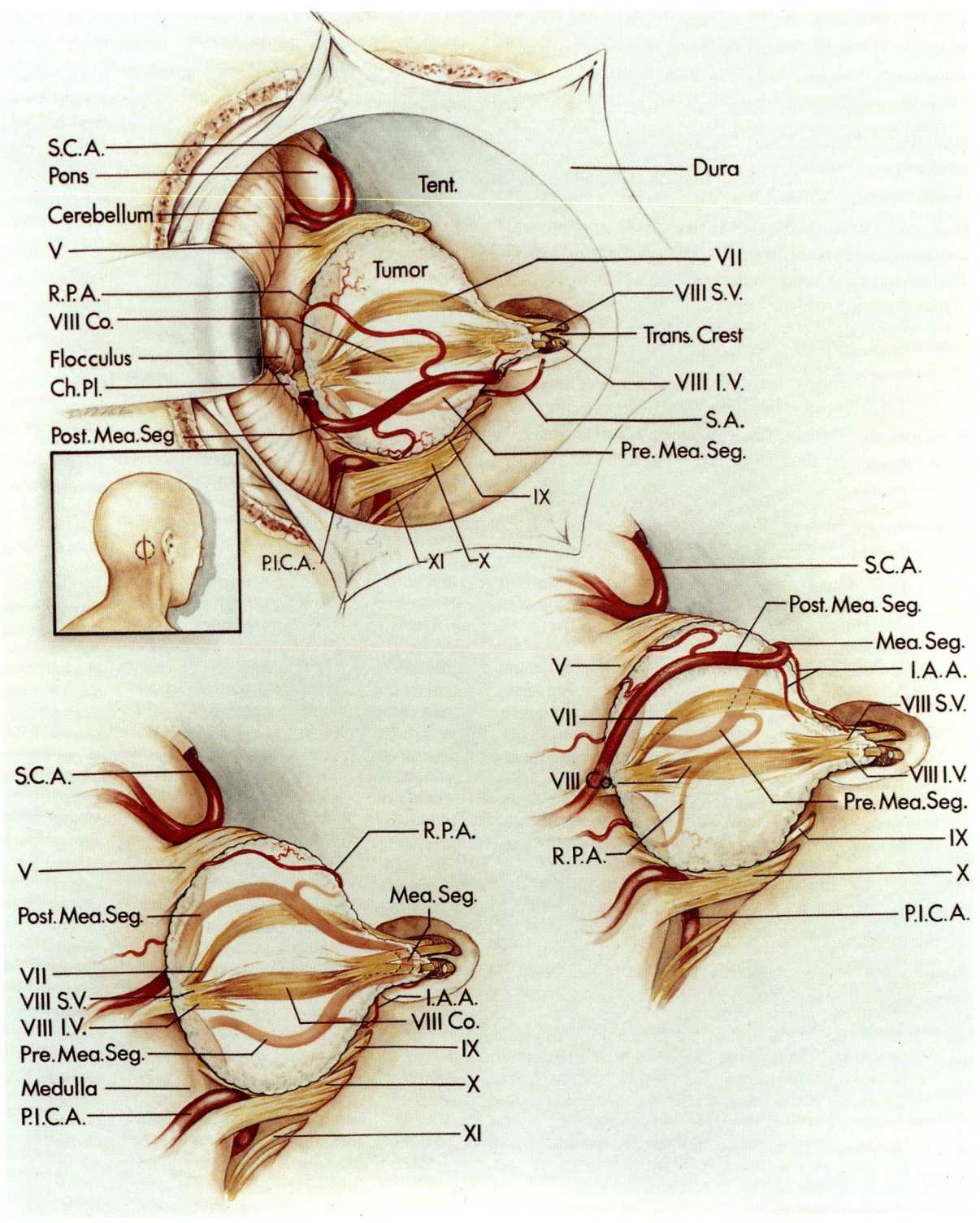

by the tumor, and the posterior inferior cerebellar artery is displaced caudally with the glossopharyngeal and vagus nerves by the tumor.

Venous Relationships

The veins on the side of the brain stem that have a predictable relationship to the facial and vestibulocochlear nerves are those draining the petrosal surface of the cerebellum, the pons and medulla, and the cerebellopontine and cerebellomedullary fissures (Fig. 3C, 4C, and 5C) (9,10). The identification of any of these veins during removal of the tumor makes it easier to identify the site of the junction of the facial and vestibulocochlear nerves with the brain stem. These veins on the medial side of the tumor are the vein of the pontomedullary sulcus, which courses transversely in the pontomedullary sulcus; the lateral medullary vein, which courses longitudinally, dorsal to the olive, along the line of origin of the rootlets of the glossopharyngeal, vagus, and accessory nerves; the vein of the cerebellomedullary fissure, which courses above the cerebellar tonsil on the inferior medullary velum and passes dorsal or ventral to the flocculus before joining the other veins in the cerebellopontine angle; the vein of the middle cerebellar peduncle, which is formed by the union of the lateral medullary vein and the vein of the pontomedullary sulcus and ascends on the middle cerebellar peduncle to join the vein of the cerebellopontinue fissure; and the vein of the cerebellopontine fissure, which is formed by the union of the veins that arise on the petrosal surface of the cerebellum and converge on the apex of the cerebellopontine fissure. All these veins course near the lateral recess and the junction of the facial and vestibulocochlear nerves with the brain stem. The vein of the cerebellomedullary fissure may pass either dorsal or ventral to the flocculus before joining the other veins. If it passes ventral to the flocculus, it joins the vein of the pontomedullary sulcus and the lateral medullary vein to form the vein of the middle cerebellar peduncle; if it passes dorsal to the flocculus, it joins the vein of the cerebellopontine fissure.

The veins surrounding an acoustic neuroma terminate by forming bridging veins, called petrosal veins, which empty into the superior petrosal sinus. These veins crossing the cerebellopontine angle to reach the superior petrosal sinus are the ones most frequently occluded in the course of operations in the cerebellopontine angle. Bridging veins are more frequently exposed and sacrificed in the rostral part of the cerebellopontine angle during operations near the trigeminal nerve than during operations near the nerves entering the internal acoustic meatus. Exposure of the trigeminal nerve through a suboccipital craniectomy commonly requires the sacrifice of one or more bridging veins. However, exposure of the nerves entering the internal acoustic meatus infrequently requires sacrifice of a bridging vein. The exposure of an acoustic neuroma in the central part of the cerebellopontine angle near the lateral recess, by retracting the petrosal surface of the hemisphere away from the sigmoid sinus, can usually be completed without sacrificing a bridging vein. If a vein is obliterated during acoustic tumor removal, it is usually one of the superior petrosal veins, which is sacrificed near the superior pole of the tumor during the later stages of the removal of a large tumor. Small acoustic neuromas are usually removed without sacrificing a petrosal vein. The largest vein encountered around the superior pole of an acoustic neuroma is the vein of the cerebellopontine fissure, which passes from the petrosal surface of the cerebellum above the facial and vestibulocochlear nerves to join other tributaries of the superior petrosal sinus.

FIG. 7. Posterior views of the direction of displacement of the anterior inferior cerebellar artery (A.I.C.A.) around an acoustic neuroma. **Top left:** The **insert** shows the skin incision (*vertical line*) and the site of the craniectomy (*broken line*). Both the premeatal (Pre. Mea. Seg.) and the postmeatal (Post. Mea. Seg.) segments are in their most common location around the lower margin of the tumor. The premeatal segment approaches the meatus from anteroinferior, and the postmeatal segment passes posteroinferior to the tumor. The superior cerebellar artery (S.C.A.) and trigeminal nerve (V) are above the tumor, and the posterior inferior cerebellar artery (P.I.C.A.) and the glossopharyngeal (IX), vagus (X), and accessory (XI) nerves are below the tumor. The choroid plexus (Ch. Pl.) protrudes into the cerebellopontine angle medial to the tumor. The posterior wall of the internal acoustic canal has been removed to expose the transverse crest (Trans. Crest) and the superior vestibular (VIII S.V.) and inferior vestibular (VIII I.V.) nerves. The vestibular nerves disappear into the tumor; however, the cochlear (VIII Co.) and facial nerves (VII) are displaced around the anterior margin of the tumor. A subarcuate artery (S.A.) arises from the premeatal segment, and a recurrent perforating artery (R.P.A.) arises from the postmeatal segment. **Center right:** A less common pattern of displacement of the anterior inferior cerebellar artery in which the premeatal and postmeatal segments are above the tumor. The internal auditory arteries (I.A.A.) arise from the meatal segment (Mea. Seg.). A recurrent perforating artery arises from the premeatal segment. **Bottom left:** Both the premeatal and the postmeatal segments are displaced anterior to the tumor. This occurs if the anterior inferior cerebellar artery courses between the vestibulocochlear and facial nerves. The tumor arises in the vestibular nerves, and the tumor growth displaces both the premeatal and the postmeatal segments anteriorly. (From ref. 8, with permission.)

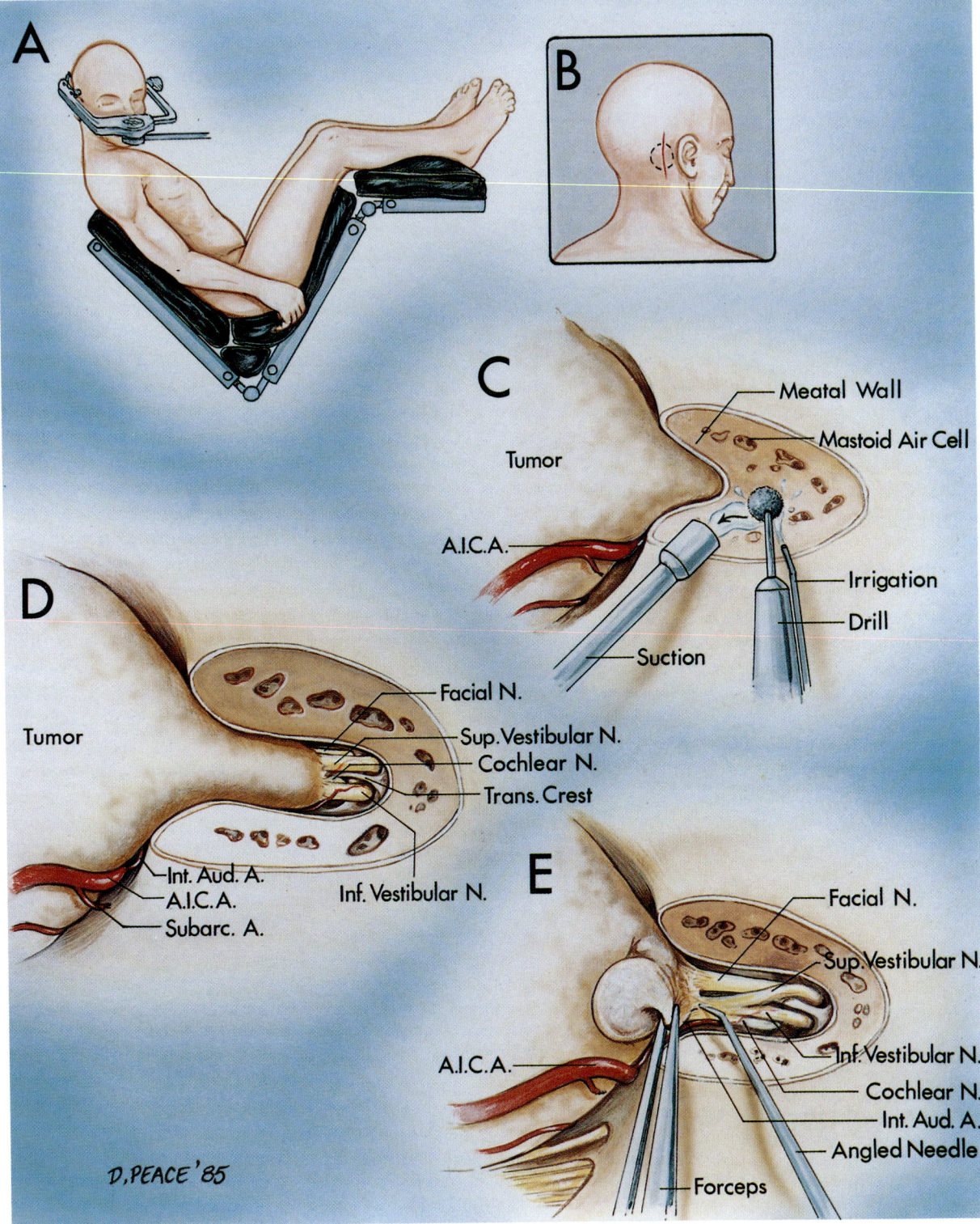

FIG. 8. A–E: See detailed description on p. 702.

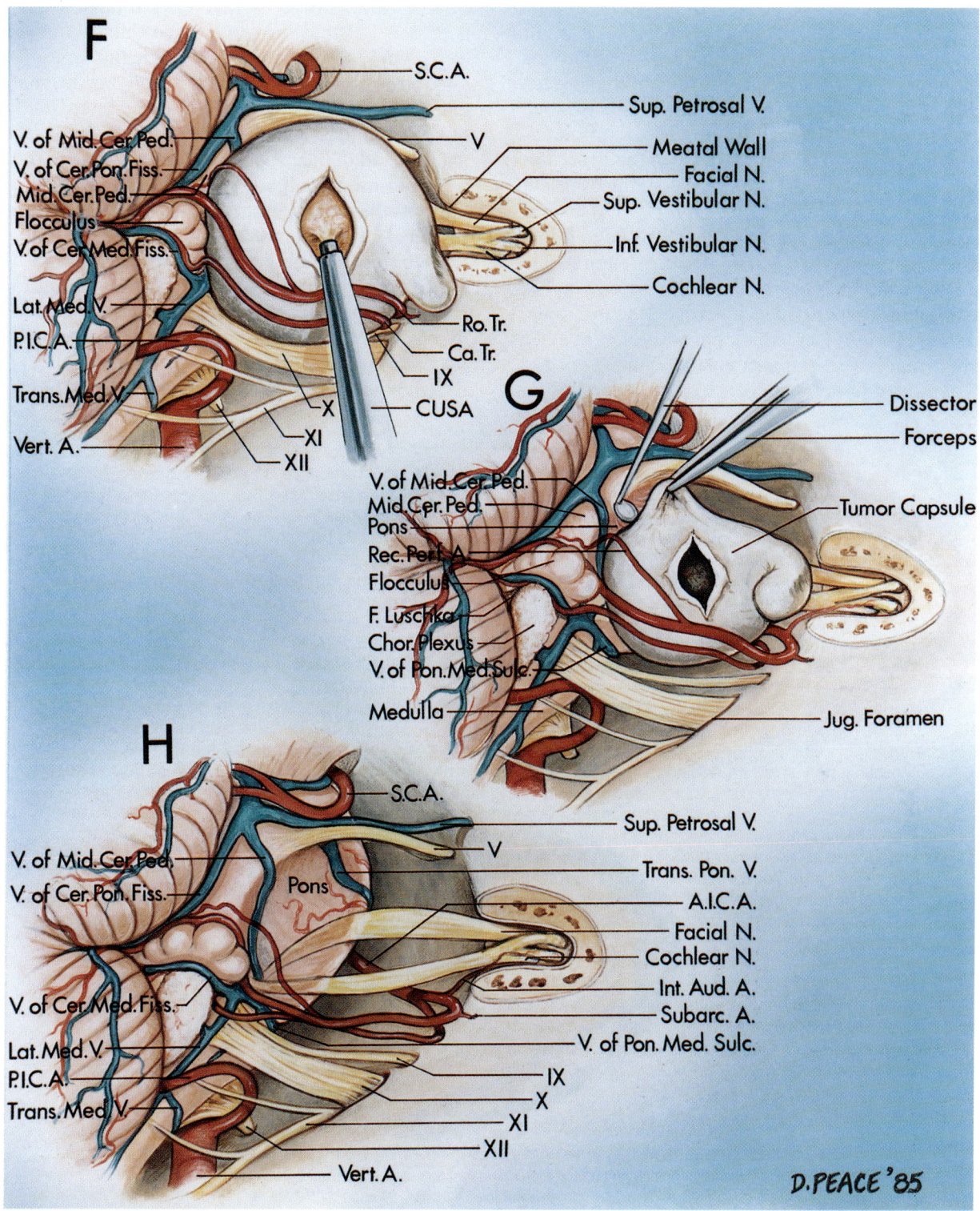

FIG. 8. F–H: See detailed description on p. 702.

OPERATIVE TECHNIQUE

This section reviews my technique for removing acoustic neuromas (17–21). The retrosigmoid approach is used because it is suitable for the removal of both small and large tumors (Figs. 8 and 9). It does not automatically lead to the loss of hearing because of the structures transgressed in reaching the tumor, as does the translabyrinthine approach, which is directed through the vestibule and semicircular canals. The retrosigmoid approach is directed through a vertical paramedian suboccipital scalp incision situated in the lateral half of the middle third of the distance between the inion and the mastoid process. The semisitting position is selected for tumors that have a diameter greater than 2.5 cm and the three-quarter prone (park bench) position is used for smaller tumors (Figs. 8 and 9). We have found, with large tumors, that the tendency of blood and cerebral spinal fluid to pool in the area where the tumor is being separated from the brain stem and nerves markedly lengthens the operative procedure and increases the risk of neural injury. The drainage of blood and cerebrospinal fluid out of the incision, with the patient in the semisitting position, facilitates the identification and preservation of the neural and vascular structures that are stretched around the margin of the tumor.

With the semisitting position, the patient is positioned so that the feet and legs are as high as the heart. The knees are flexed in order to release tension on the sciatic nerves. The arms are not allowed to hang freely at the patient's side since this may produce brachial plexus stretch but are positioned with the hands and forearms in

FIG. 8. (See figures on previous page.) Retrosigmoid approach for removal of large acoustic neuromas. **A:** The operation for a large tumor is done with the patient in the semisitting position with the head turned toward the side of the tumor. The alternative position is shown in Fig. 9. **B:** The vertical scalp incision (*solid line*) and suboccipital craniectomy (*interrupted line*) are located posterior to the ear and sigmoid sinus. **C:** The tumor is exposed in the right cerebellopontine angle, where it protrudes from the internal acoustic canal into the cerebellum and brain stem. An irrigating drill removes the posterior wall of the meatus to exposure the intracanalicular part of the tumor. The mastoid cells that extend into the meatal lip must be closed carefully in order to prevent a cerebrospinal fluid leak. The anterior inferior cerebellar artery (AICA) loops around the lower margin of the tumor. **D:** The transverse crest (Trans. Crest) divides the meatus into upper and lower compartments. The facial (Facial N.) and superior vestibular (Sup. Vestibular N.) nerves are above the crest, and the cochlear (Cochlear N.) and inferior vestibular (Inf. Vestibular N.) nerves are below the crest. The anterior inferior cerebellar artery gives off the subarcuate (Subarc. A.) and internal auditory (Int. Aud. A.) arteries. **E:** The tumor, which arises in the vestibular nerves, is being separated from the posterior aspect of the facial and vestibulocochlear nerves using a fine dissector called an angled needle. **F:** The orientation is shown in (**B**). The tumor within the meatus has been removed. The ultrasonic aspirator is being used to evacuate the content of the tumor. Alternative methods of removing the intracapsular contents are to use a laser or the suction and cup forceps. The tumor compresses and indents the side of the pons and medulla. The trigeminal nerve (V) and the superior cerebellar artery (S.C.A.) are above the tumor. The facial and cochlear nerves are anterior to the tumor, and the glossopharyngeal (IX), vagus (X), and accessory (XI) nerves are below the tumor. The anterior inferior cerebellar artery divides into rostral (Ro. Tr.) and caudal (Ca. Tr.) trunks, which pass below the tumor. The rostral trunk courses above the flocculus to reach the surface of the middle cerebellar peduncle (Mid. Cer. Ped.). The posterior inferior cerebellar artery (P.I.C.A.) arises from the vertebral artery (Vert. A.) and passes around the medulla between the rootlets of the vagus and accessory nerves. The lateral medullary vein (Lat. Med. V.) joins the vein of the cerebellomedullary fissure (V. of Cer. Med. Fiss.) to form the vein of the middle cerebellar peduncle (V. of Mid. Cer. Ped.). The latter vein ascends medial to the tumor and joins the vein of the cerebellopontine fissure (V. of Cer. Pon. Fiss.) to form a superior petrosal vein (Sup. Pet. V.), which empties into the superior petrosal sinus. A transverse medullary vein (Trans. Med. V.) courses around the medulla. **G:** The intracapsular removal of the tumor has been completed, and the tumor capsule is being separated from the side of the pons and medulla. The capsule has already been separated from the inferior margin of the trigeminal nerve, the upper margin of the glossopharyngeal nerve, and the posterior margin of the facial and vestibulocochlear nerves. The choroid plexus (Chor. Plexus) protrudes from the foramen of Luschka (F. Luschka) just posterior to where the glossopharyngeal and vagus nerves join the medulla. The junction of the lateral medullary vein with the veins of the pontomedullary sulcus (V. of Pon. Med. Sulc.) and middle cerebellar peduncle comes into view as the tumor is removed. The anterior inferior cerebellar artery gives rise to a recurrent perforating branch (Rec. Perf. A.), which crosses the tumor capsule to reach the brain stem. The nerves entering the jugular foramen (Jug. For.) course below the tumor. **H:** The tumor removal has been completed. The tumor indents the side of the brain stem and flattens the facial and cochlear nerves. A transverse pontine vein (Trans. Pon. V.) courses in the tumor bed. The facial and vestibulocochlear nerves join the brain stem at the lateral end of the pontomedullary sulcus, above the glossopharyngeal nerve, anterosuperior to the choroid plexus hanging out of the foramen of Luschka, anterior to the flocculus, near where the anterior inferior cerebellar artery passes above the flocculus, and at the junction of the lateral medullary vein with the veins of the pontomedullary sulcus, middle cerebellar peduncle, and cerebellomedullary fissure. (From ref. 19, with permission.)

the patient's lap. The head is turned toward the side of the operation so that the surgeon seated behind the patient can look directly into the plane between the posterior surface of the petrous bone and the anterior surface of the cerebellum. Doppler precordial and end tidal CO_2 monitoring to detect air emboli and a right atrial catheter to aspirate air if it is detected are instituted prior to starting operations. With the three-quarter prone position the patient is reclining on the operating table with the head elevated slightly higher than the feet.

Brain stem auditory evoked potentials, if intact prior to surgery, are monitored during operations in the cerebellopontine angle (Figs. 10 and 11) (3,11). Recording electrodes are placed in the ipsilateral facial muscles prior to beginning the operation in order to monitor the response of the facial nerve to electrical and even mechanical stimulation. Exploration of the tumor capsule with a nerve stimulation may locate a thinned facial nerve before it is visible under the operating microscope.

Enough hair is removed to allow placement of a parietal burr hole and tapping of the ventricle if necessary because of tightness of the cerebellum. However, it is rarely necessary to tap the ventricle at the time of removing a cerebellopontine angle tumor. The muscle opening is carried inferiorly to just lateral to the foramen magnum. Care is taken to avoid injury to the vertebral artery as it courses behind the atlanto-occipital joint and the arch of the atlas. The craniectomy should extend to the lower margin of the transverse sinus and the medial margin of the lateral sinus. The mastoid air cells entered in the lateral part of the craniectomy are carefully closed with bone wax.

The dura is opened with the pedicle medially. In order to minimize the need for cerebellar retraction, the dural cuff bordering the transverse and lateral sinuses is tacked up with sutures to the muscles and fascia bordering the craniectomy margin. Decadron therapy is instituted at the beginning of the operation and is tapered over several days after the operation. Mannitol is given during the exposure. The cerebellum, which commonly bulges outward upon opening the dura, usually relaxes after opening the arachnoid membrane over the cisterna magna and allowing cerebrospinal fluid to escape. Cerebellar resection is rarely needed even when removing large tumors.

All of the intradural part of the procedure is done using the operating microscope. The surface of the cerebellum facing the posterior surface of the petrous bone is gently elevated to expose the tumor. Self-retaining rather than hand-held retraction is used. A wide brain spatula that covers most of the lateral margin of the cerebellum and that does not need to be moved as the operation progresses causes less damage than one or two smaller brain spatulas that must be repeatedly shifted. A tapered spatula 20–25 mm wide at its base and 15–20 mm at its tip is commonly used. Care is taken to prevent the brain spatula from drifting inferiorly and damaging the glossopharyngeal and vagus nerves, which may be situated a few millimeters below the edge of the spatula.

I commonly remove the posterior wall of the internal auditory canal prior to opening the arachnoidal membrane around the tumor. The posterior meatal wall is removed using an irrigating drill. The preservation of the arachnoid membrane that lies posterior to an acoustic neuroma and that extends into the internal acoustic meatus during the removal of the posterior meatal wall with a drill prevents bone dust from entering the subarachnoid space. In addition, if the tumor capsule is opened prior to drilling away the posterior meatal lip, there are often cottonoids packed within the tumor capsule or tags of tumor capsule that may become enmeshed in the drill. The semicircular canals should be preserved in exposing the internal acoustic meatus if there is the possibility of preserving hearing because hearing will be lost if they are damaged by the drill (4). The semicircular canals are situated just posterior to the lateral end of the internal acoustic meatus. Care is required to avoid injury to the anterior inferior cerebellar artery if it is adherent to the dura covering the posterior wall of the internal auditory meatus.

After removing the posterior wall of the meatus, the dura that lines the meatus is opened to expose its contents. The facial nerve is identified near the origin of the facial canal at the anterior–superior quadrant of the meatus rather than in a more medial location where the direction of displacement is variable. The tumor within the meatus is separated from the posterior surface of the facial and vestibulocochlear nerves. It is easy to expose the labyrinth if the tumor extends into the vestibule of the labyrinth by drilling through the bone posterior to the lateral end of the internal auditory canal.

After exposing the nerves in the lateral end of the canal, the capsule of the part of the tumor in the cerebellopontine angle is opened and the intracapsular contents are removed. The most dependent portion of the exposed tumor is approached first. If the dissection is begun on the upper part of the exposure, removal of the more dependent parts may be made more difficult by blood running down from above. If the patient is in the sitting position, the intracapsular removal begins in the area just above the ninth and tenth cranial nerves, which are protected by moist cottonoids.

There are landmarks that are helpful in identifying the facial and vestibulocochlear nerves at the brain stem on the medial side of the tumor. These nerves, although distorted by tumor, can usually be identified on the brain stem side of the tumor at the lateral end of the pontomedullary sulcus, just rostral to the glossopharyngeal nerve, and just anterior–superior to the foramen of Luschka, flocculus, and choroid plexus protruding from the foramen of Luschka. After the facial and vestibulocochlear nerves are identified on the medial and lateral

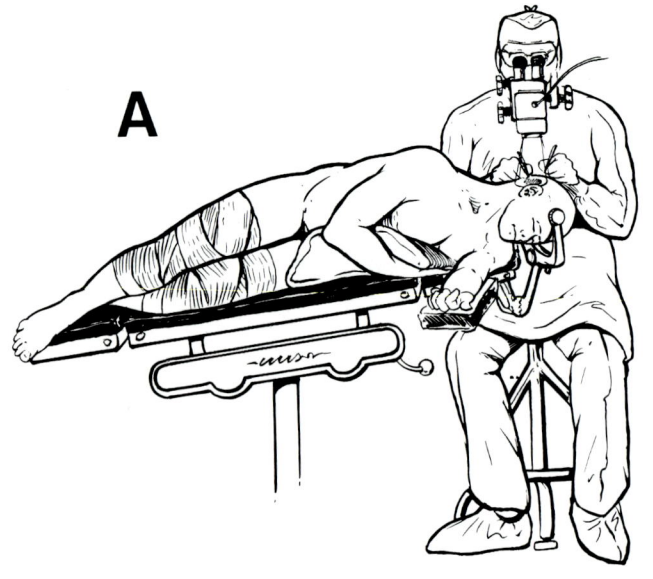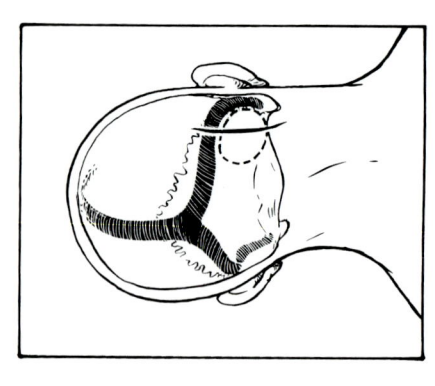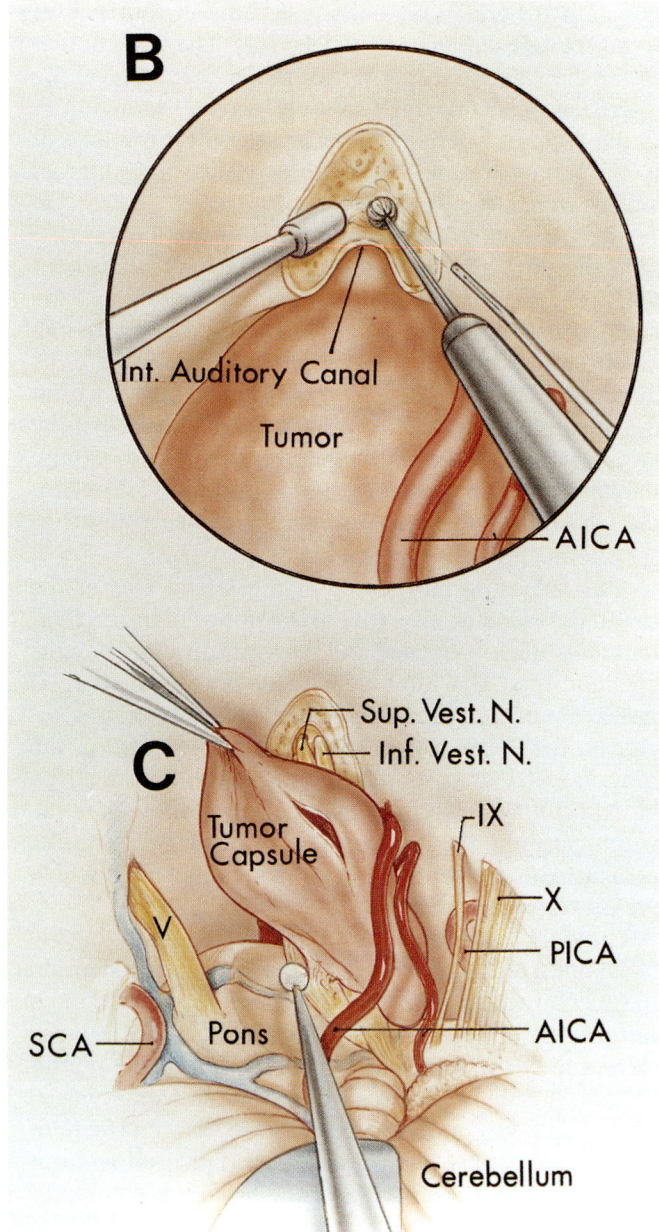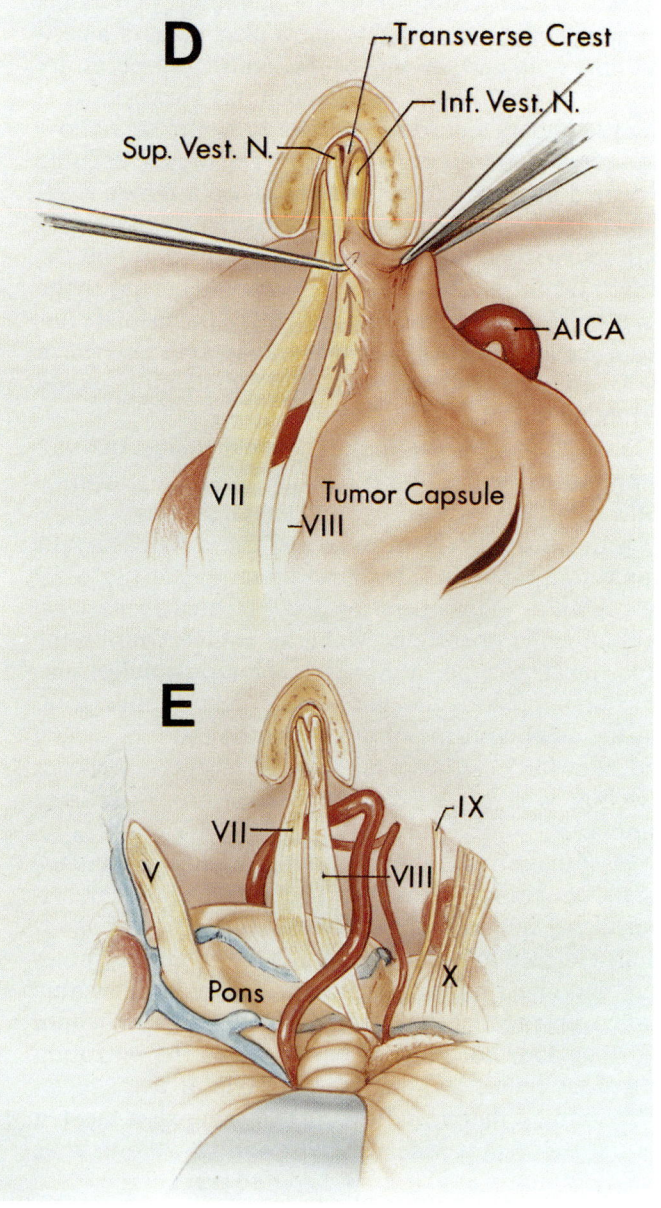

sides of the tumor, the final remnants of the tumor are separated from the intervening segment of the nerves.

The operation for a cerebellopontine angle tumor should be planned so that the tumor surface is allowed to settle away from the neural tissue rather than the neural structures being retracted away from the tumor. If the tumor is cystic, the initial step is aspiration with a needle. No attempt is made to see the whole tumor upon initial retraction of the cerebellum. The surface of the tumor is then opened and biopsied, and the intracapsular contents are removed. As the intracapsular contents are evacuated by means of a cup forceps, suction, ultrasonic aspirator, or laser, the tumor shifts laterally. This shift allows more of the tumor to be removed through the small exposure. The ultrasonic aspirator is preferred for debulking large tumors. Carefully applied fine bipolar coagulation is preferred to control bleeding and to shrink small deposits of tumor.

In the final step, the last thin sheet of tumor capsule is removed from the neural and vascular structures by the use of fine dissecting instruments (Fig. 12). The strokes of the fine dissecting instruments along the vestibulocochlear nerve should be directed from medial to lateral rather than from lateral to medial, because traction medially may tear the tiny filaments of the cochlear nerve at the site where these filaments penetrate the lateral end of the meatus to enter the cochlea.

The most common reason for tumor appearing to be tightly adherent to the neural structures is not adhesions between the capsule and surrounding tissue but rather the residual tumor within the capsule wedging the tumor into position. As the intracapsular contents are removed, the tumor capsule folds inward, thus making it possible to remove more tumor through the small exposure. Only rarely are tumors so densely adherent that they defy easy removal after their intracapsular contents are removed. If the tumor does not separate easily from neural tissue after the intracapsular contents have been removed, a brief wait often allows the pulsation of the brain to dislodge the tumor into the exposure, and then more tumor frequently can be removed within the capsule. Under magnification, individual adhesions between vital structures and tumor can be divided with microinstruments. A thin remnant of tumor capsule may be left if it is so firmly adherent to vital neural or vascular structures that removing it would damage these structures.

If the pia-arachnoid is adherent to the tumor capsule or if a mass of tumor within the capsule prevents collapse of the capsule away from the pia-arachnoid, there is a tendency to apply traction to both the capsule and the pia-arachnoid and to tear vessels running on the neural structures. Prior to separating the pia-arachnoid from the capsule, it is important that all of the tumor is removed so that the capsule is so thin that it is almost transparent. If one is uncertain about the margin between the capsule and the pia-arachnoid, irrigation of the area and several sweeps of a fine dissector through the area often will clarify the appropriate plane for dissection. The intracapsular removal may be completed using laser or ultrasonic dissection, or with other microsurgical instruments. After evacuating the intracapsular contents, the remaining tumor capsule is gently separated from the side of the brain stem and the margins of the involved cranial nerve using gentle microsurgical techniques (7).

It is especially important that the segment of the cerebellar arteries adherent to the tumor capsule be preserved because a major cause of operative mortality and morbidity is loss of perforating arteries and branches of the cerebellar arteries, which may be adherent to and displaced by the tumor (1). Any vessel that stands above or is stretched around the tumor capsule should be dealt with initially as if it were a vessel that runs over the tumor surface to supply the brain. After the tumor has been removed from within the capsule, an attempt should be made to displace the vessel off the tumor capsule using a small dissector. When dissected free of the capsule, vessels that initially appeared to be adherent to the capsule often prove to be neural vessels. The cerebellar, basilar, and vertebral arteries may be exposed in re-

FIG. 9. Retrosigmoid approach for removal of small or medium size acoustic neuromas. **A:** The patient is positioned in the three-quarter prone position with the surgeon behind the head. The **insert** (right) shows the site of the scalp incision (*continuous line*) and the bony opening (*interrupted line*). **B:** The posterior wall of the internal auditory canal is removed using an irrigating drill. The anterior inferior cerebellar artery (AICA) courses around the lower margin of the tumor. **C:** The intracapsular contents of the tumor have been removed. The capsule of the tumor is being separated from the pons and the posterior surface of the part of the facial (VII) and vestibulocochlear nerves adjacent to the brain stem. The superior (Sup. Vest. N.) and inferior vestibular nerves (Inf. Vest. N.) are seen at the lateral end of the internal auditory canal. The trigeminal nerve (V) and superior cerebellar artery (SCA) are above the tumor and the glossopharyngeal (IX) and vagus (X) nerves and the posterior inferior cerebellar artery (PICA) are below the tumor. **D:** The dissection along the eighth nerve (VIII) is done in a medial to lateral direction (*arrows*) in order to avoid tearing the tiny filaments of the nerve in the lateral end of the canal where they pass through the lamina cribrosa. The transverse crest separates the superior and inferior vestibular nerves in the lateral end of the canal. **E:** Cerebellopontine angle and internal auditory canal after tumor removal. The facial and vestibulocochlear nerves have been preserved.

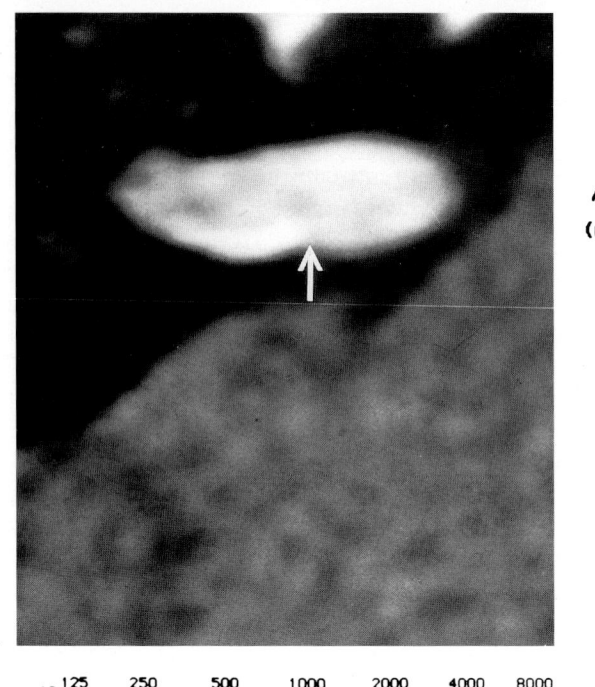
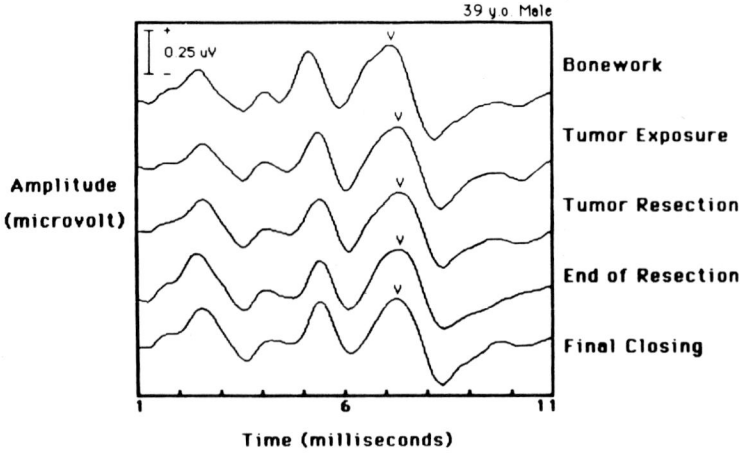
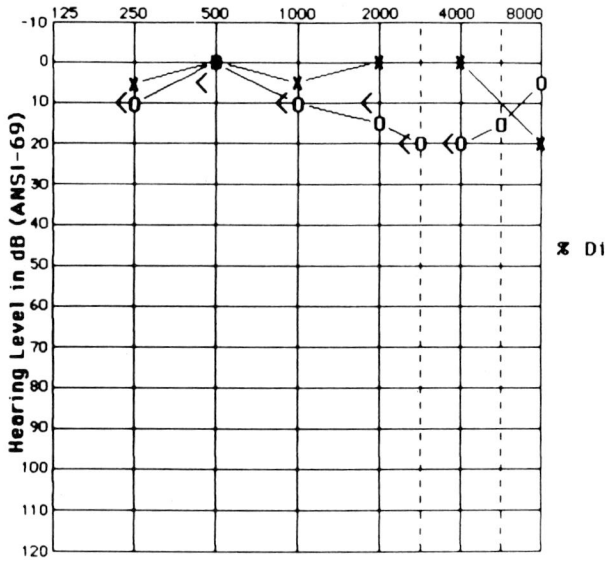
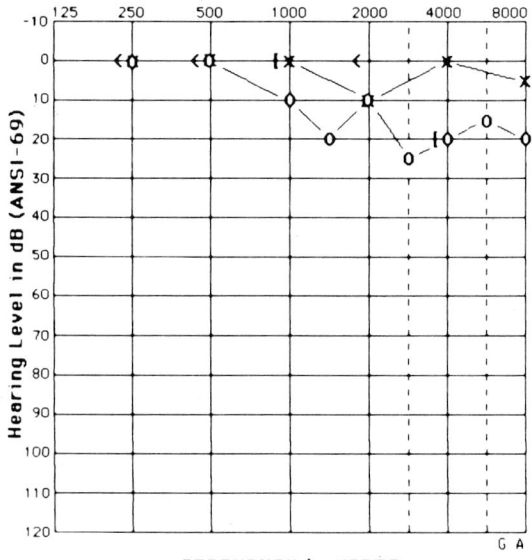

FIG. 10. Retrosigmoid approach to an acoustic neuroma with hearing preservation. MRI, pre- and postoperative audiograms, and intraoperative auditory evoked potentials. **A:** Axial MRI of a small right acoustic neuroma. The *arrow* is located at the level of the porus acusticus. **B:** Preoperative audiogram. **C:** Postoperative audiogram. **D:** Auditory evoked potentials during each step of the tumor removal. The patient had excellent hearing and word discrimination in the involved ear following surgery.

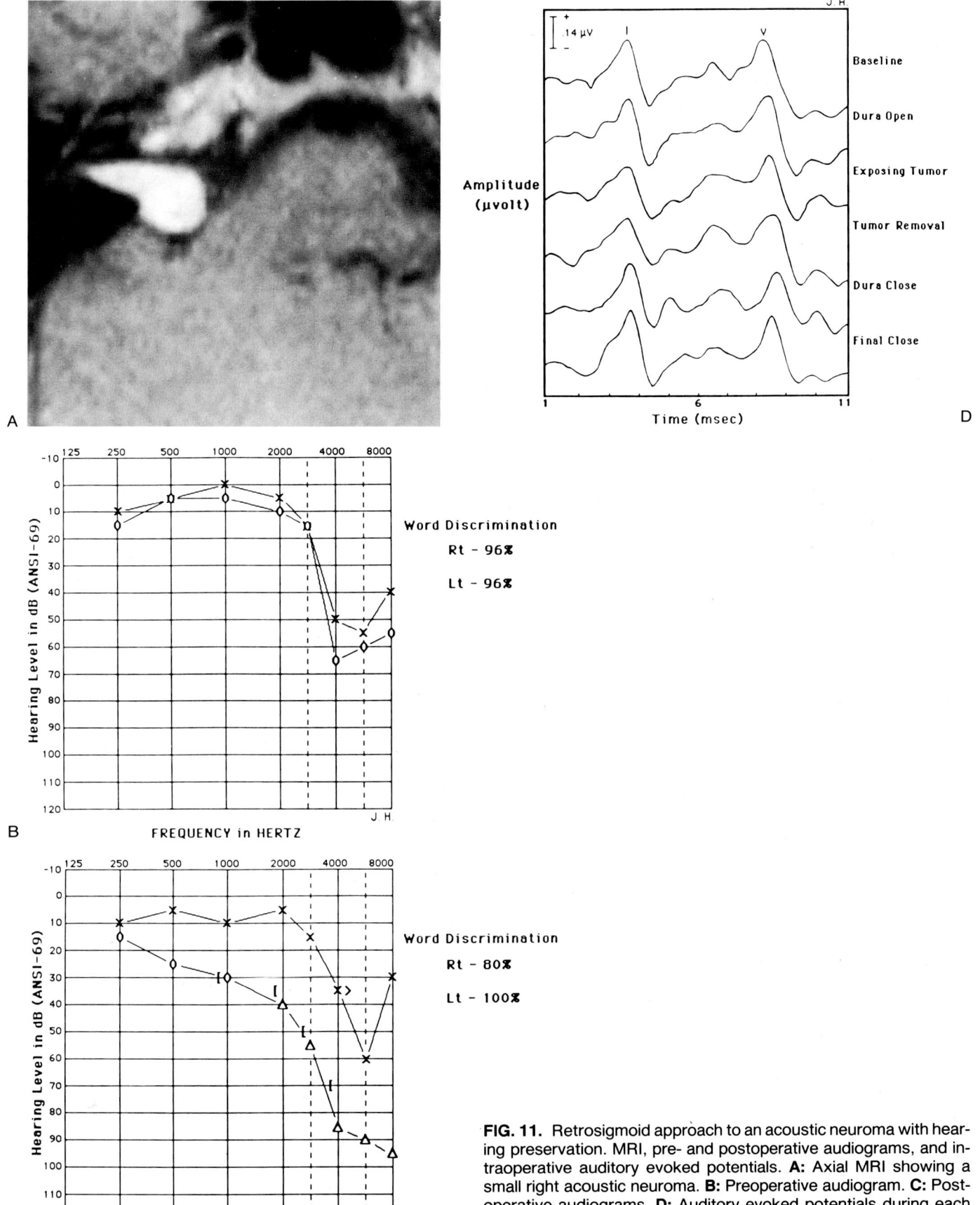

FIG. 11. Retrosigmoid approach to an acoustic neuroma with hearing preservation. MRI, pre- and postoperative audiograms, and intraoperative auditory evoked potentials. **A:** Axial MRI showing a small right acoustic neuroma. **B:** Preoperative audiogram. **C:** Postoperative audiograms. **D:** Auditory evoked potentials during each step of the tumor removal. The patient had useful hearing and speech discrimination in the involved ear following surgery.

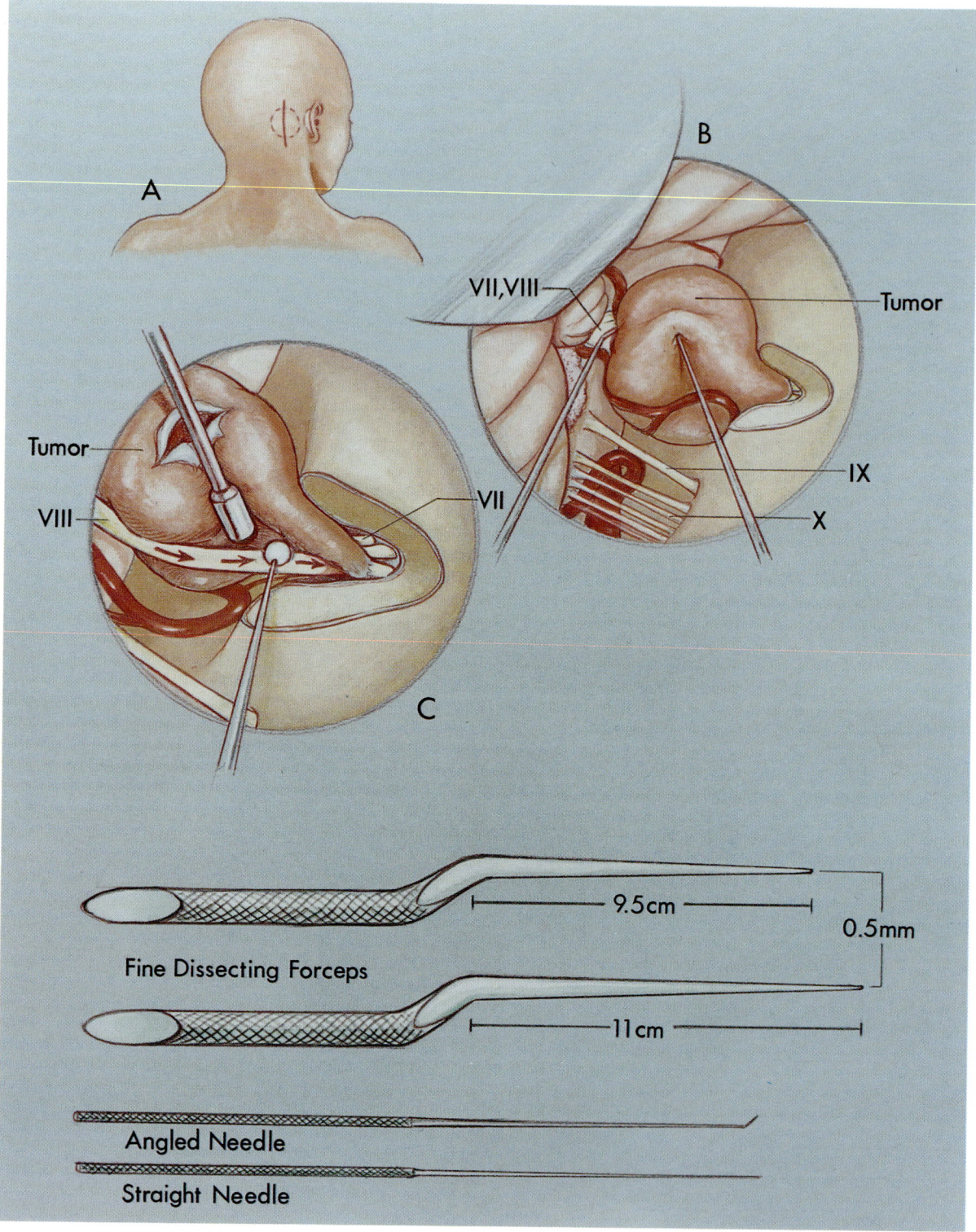

FIG. 12. Technique and selection of instruments for dissection of tumor from cochlear nerve when the goal is to preserve hearing. **A:** Site of scalp incision (*solid line*) and craniectomy (*interrupted line*). **B:** The medial side of the tumor is being elevated with a straight needle and the capsule is being separated from the posterior surface of the facial (VII) and vestibulocochlear nerve (VIII) with an angled needle. The glossopharyngeal (IX) and vagus nerves (X) are below the tumor. **C:** The residual tumor capsule is being elevated with a blunt-tip 5 french suction tube. The capsule is being separated from the cochlear nerve with a small round dissector using strokes directed from medial to lateral (*arrows*) along the nerve. Fine dissecting forceps with 0.5-mm tips are also used to separate the surface of the tumor capsule from delicate neural structures. Forceps having 9.5-cm shafts are needed to comfortably grasp tissue in the deep location in the cerebellopontine angle. Forceps with 11.5-cm shafts are needed for work in an extra-deep location, as in the area medial to the cerebellopontine angle in front of the brain stem.

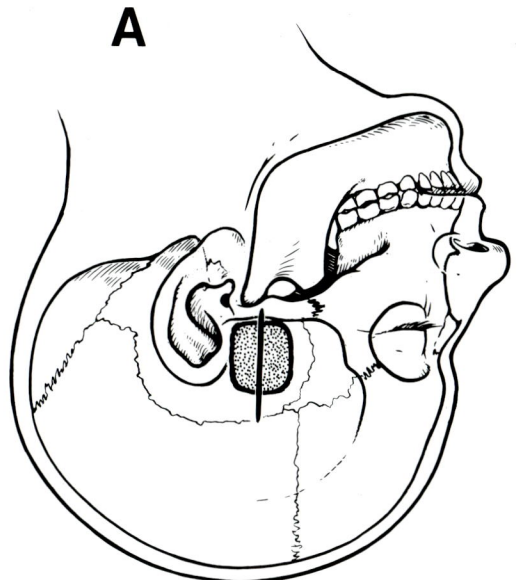
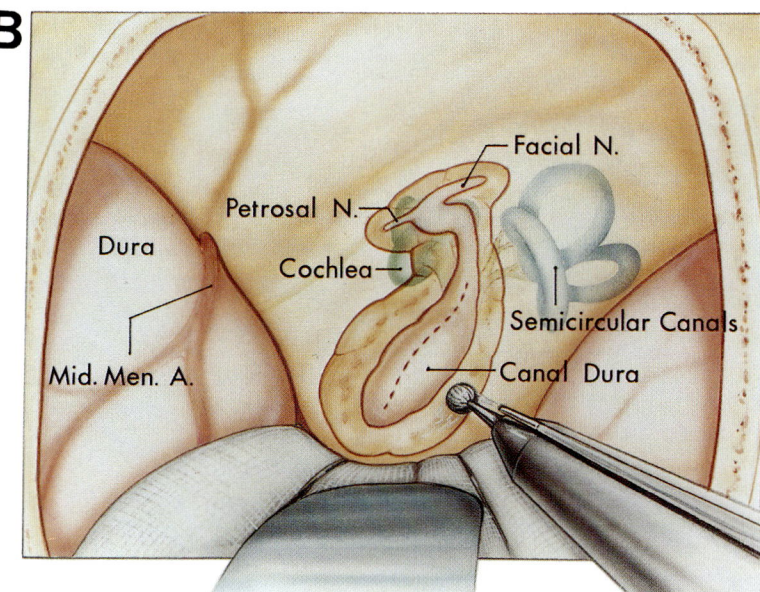
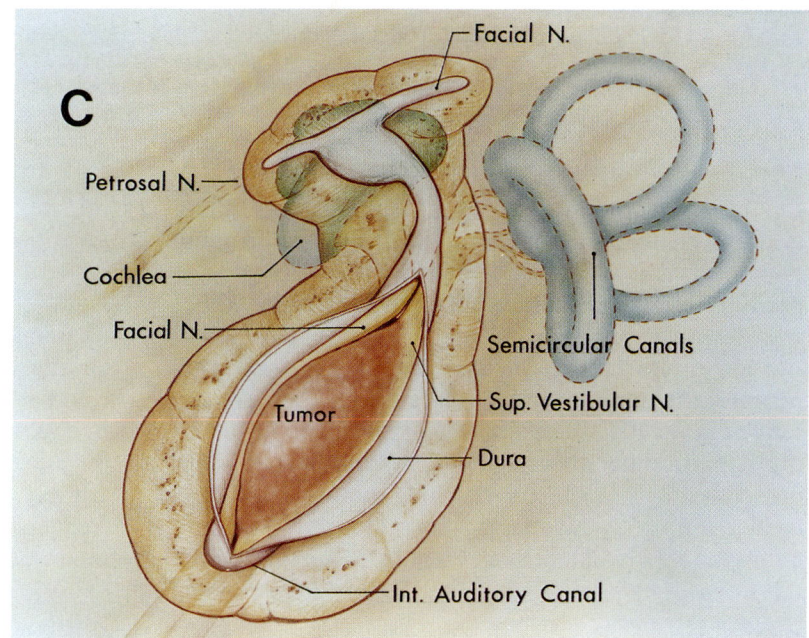

FIG. 13. Middle fossa approach for removing very small acoustic neuromas. **A:** The vertical skin incision is located anterior to the ear and the craniotomy is situated with its base on the floor of the middle cranial fossa (*stippled area*). **B:** The dura is elevated from the floor of the middle cranial fossa to identify the greater petrosal nerve (Petrosal N.). The middle meningeal artery (Mid. Men. A.) courses on the dura. Bone is removed over the greater petrosal nerve (Petrosal N.) to expose the facial nerve (Facial N.), which is followed proximally by removing bone to expose the superior wall of the internal auditory canal. Extreme care must be taken to avoid injuring the semicircular canals located in the bone at the posterior margin of the exposure and the cochlea situated in the bone just anterior and deep to the facial nerve. **C:** Enlarged view of the area of bone removal. The dura has been opened to expose the tumor in the internal auditory canal (Int. Auditory Canal). The tumor arises in the superior vestibular nerve (Sup. Vestibular N.) and displaces the facial nerve anteriorly.

moving tumors of the cerebellopontine angle. Occlusion of a cerebellar artery is one of the most common causes of morbidity and mortality in removing cerebellopontine angle tumors. The anterior inferior cerebellar artery is the artery most commonly involved by an acoustic neuroma (1).

The number of veins sacrificed should be kept to a minimum because of the undesirable consequences of their loss. Obliteration of the petrosal veins, which pass from the surface of the cerebellum and brain stem to the superior petrosal sinus, is inescapable in reaching and removing some cerebellopontine angle tumors. Occlusion of these veins, which drain much of the cerebellum and brain stem, may infrequently cause hemorrhagic edema of the cerebellum and the brain stem. Some of these veins may need to be sacrificed if the tumor extends into the area above the internal acoustic meatus. However, small acoustic neuromas and other tumors in the lower part of the cerebellopontine angle may frequently be removed without sacrificing a petrosal vein.

At the time of the craniectomy and the removal of the posterior meatal lip, the mastoid air cells may be opened and must then be sealed to prevent cerebrospinal fluid leakage and meningitis. The air cells that are opened in removing the posterior meatal lip are carefully closed with bone wax, after which a patch of suboccipital mus-

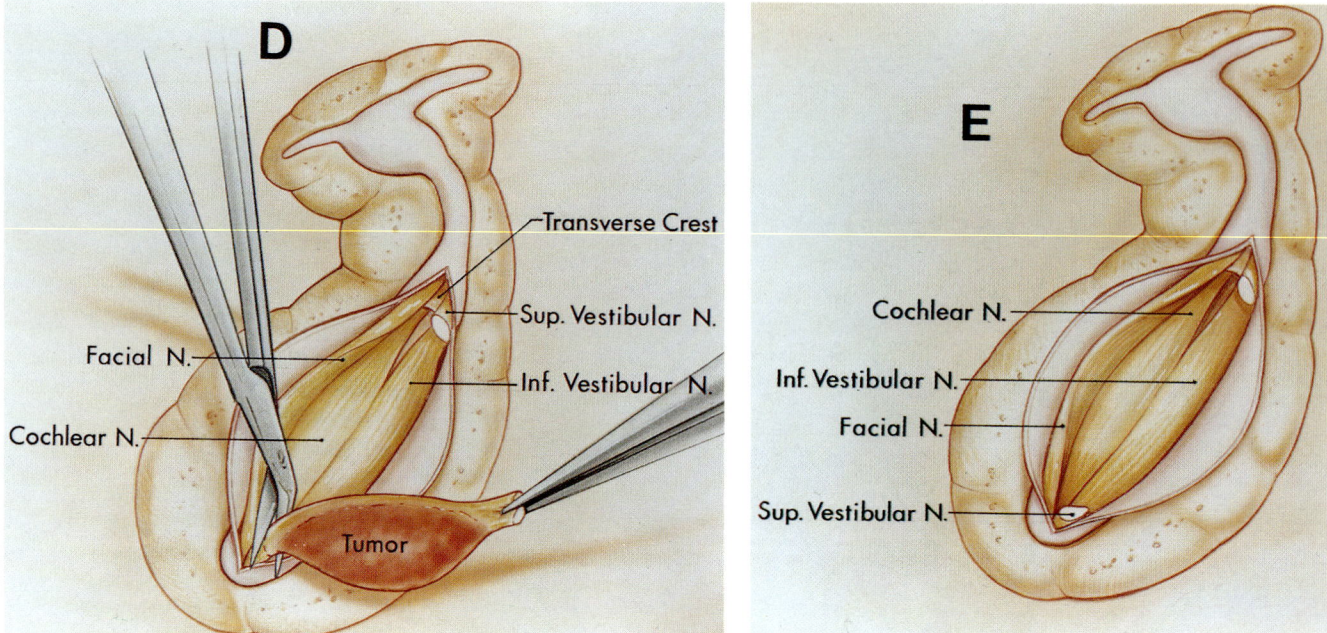

FIG. 13. *Continued.* **D:** The superior vestibular nerve has been divided above the transverse crest and elevated with the tumor. The superior vestibular nerve is being divided medial to the tumor. The facial, cochlear (Cochlear N.), and inferior vestibular (Inf. Vestibular N.) nerves are preserved. **E:** View of nerves after removal of the tumor.

cle that settles into the depression created by the drilling is laid over the posterior meatal wall. The craniectomy margin is carefully closed with bone wax. The dura is carefully closed with interrupted sutures and a dural graft if needed.

There are two other operative approaches to acoustic neuromas in addition to the retrosigmoid approach described in detail earlier. These are the middle fossa and translabyrinthine approaches. The middle fossa approach is only suitable for very small tumors (Fig. 13). It is done through a small temporal craniotomy. The dura under the temporal lobe is elevated from the floor of the middle cranial fossa until the greater petrosal nerve is identified. Bone is removed over the greater petrosal nerve to expose the genu of the facial nerve. The facial nerve is followed proximal by drilling away bone. In the final stage of bone removal, the upper wall of the internal auditory canal is removed to expose the dura lining the internal auditory canal. The dura of the canal is opened to expose and remove the tumor. This approach is used only for removing very small tumors that are located entirely within the internal auditory canal. It is the least frequently performed operative approach to an acoustic neuroma. The technique is useful for removal of small

---

FIG. 14. Translabyrinthine approach to removal of acoustic neuromas. **A:** The operation is done with the patient in the supine position with the face turned toward the side opposite the tumor. Site of the retromastoid skin incision. **B:** The *stippled area* shows the site of the bony opening through the mastoid. **C:** The mastoid air cells are being exenterated and the semicircular canals have been exposed. The drilling will be carried medially through the semicircular canals. The sigmoid sinus is in the posterior part and the facial nerve (Facial N.) is in the anterior part of the exposure. **D:** The bone surrounding and including the semicircular canals has been removed to expose the dura lining the internal auditory canal. The dura between the superior petrosal (Sup. Petrosal Sinus) and sigmoid sinuses has been exposed. The *interrupted lines* show the site of the dural opening. **E:** The intracapsular contents of the tumor are being removed with cup forceps. The superior (Sup. Vestibular N.) and inferior vestibular (Inf. Vestibular N.) nerves are seen lateral to the tumor, where they are separated by the transverse crest. The anterior inferior cerebellar artery (AICA) courses around the lower margin of the tumor. The facial nerve is anterior to the tumor. The trigeminal nerve (V) is above and the glossopharyngeal (IX) and vagus nerves (X) are below the tumor. **F:** The final fragments of tumor are being removed from the surface of the facial nerve. The superior and inferior vestibular and cochlear nerves (Cochlear N.) have been removed along with the tumor since there is no chance of saving hearing or vestibular function because the operation is directed through the semicircular canals, which leads to loss of hearing. The central stump of the eighth nerve (VIII) is exposed at the brain stem.

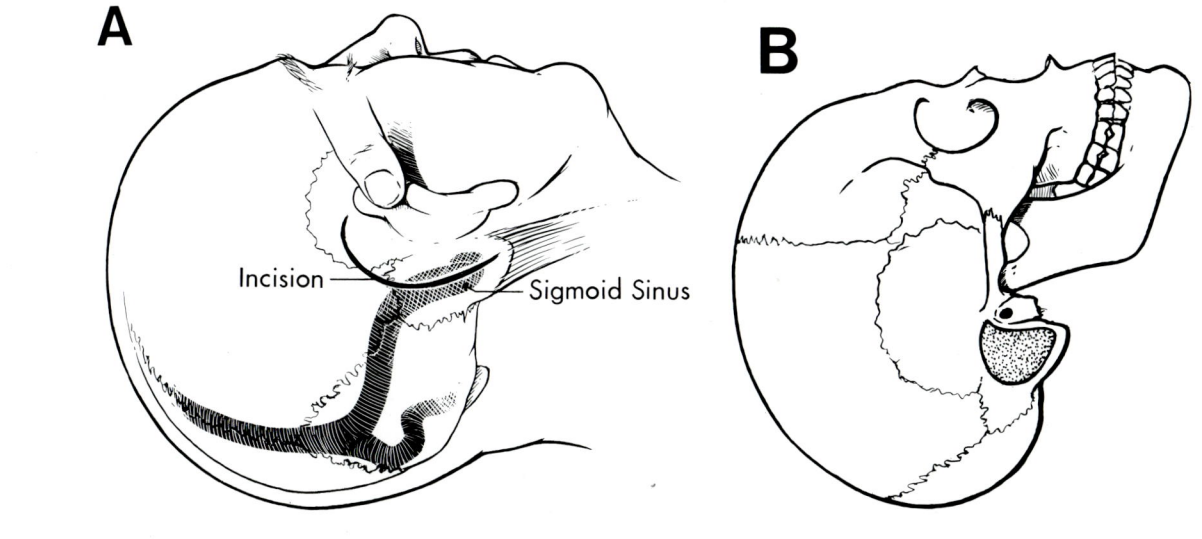
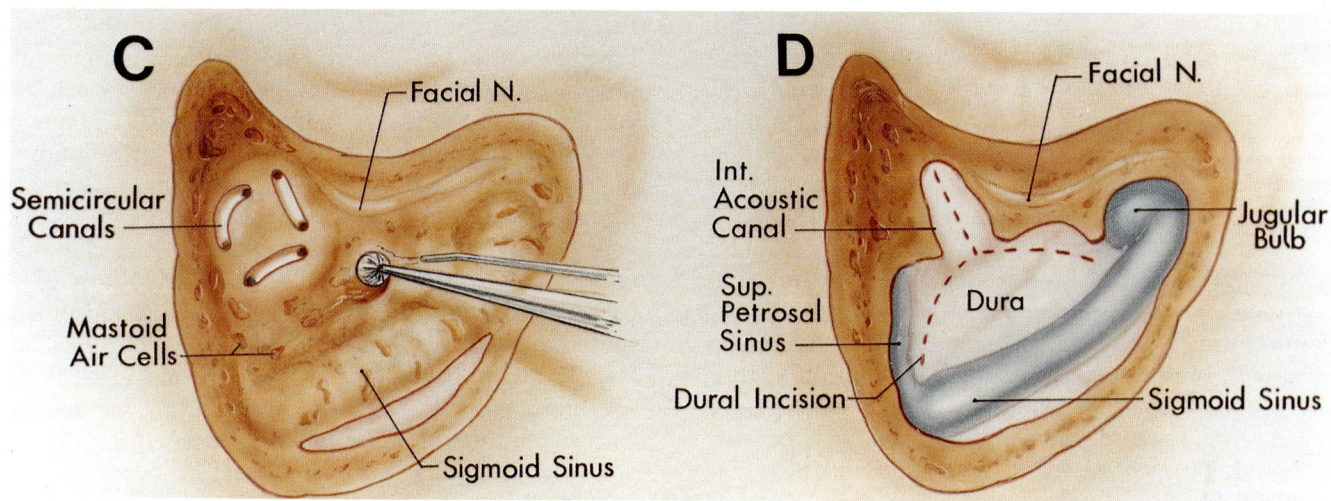
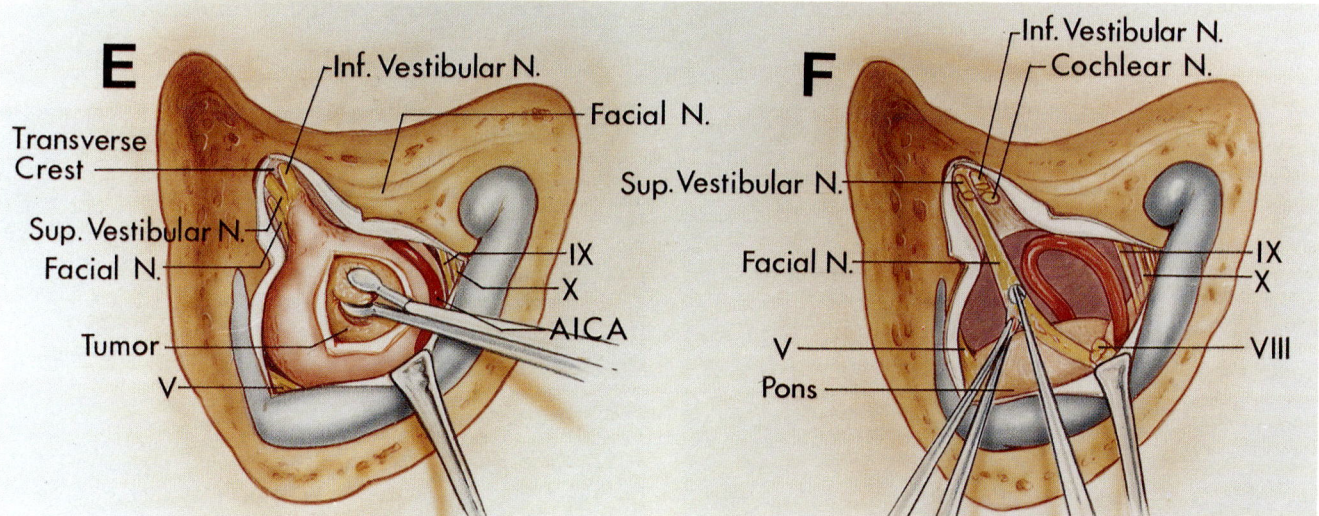

tumors in which there is useful hearing that may be preserved. I prefer the retrosigmoid approach for these small tumors because it provides a better exposure of the involved structures while allowing the preservation of hearing. During the middle fossa approach, care must be taken to avoid injury to the cochlea, which sits only a few millimeters anterior to the site of bone removal, and the semicircular canals, which are located a few millimeters behind the area of bone being removed. Entering either the cochlea or the semicircular canals will result in a loss of hearing.

The translabyrinthine approach is directed through the mastoid air cells and vestibular portion of the labyrinth (Fig. 14). A skin incision located behind the ear is used to expose the mastoid bone. The mastoid air cells are exenterated and the semicircular canals, which are located behind the lateral end of the internal acoustic meatus, are removed. The removal of these canals results in the loss of hearing in the involved ear. The approach is carried through the posterior wall of the internal auditory canal. This approach automatically destroys hearing and is suitable only for the removal of small or medium sized tumors in which there is no chance of preserving hearing. Another disadvantage of this route is that the limited exposure makes complete removal of the tumor more difficult. Surgeons that operate by this route commonly combine the approach with a retrosigmoid craniectomy for the removal of large tumors. A final disadvantage of this approach is the large communication that is established between the subarachnoid space and the mastoid, so there is a significant risk of postoperative CSF leak through the eustachian tube and nose and meningitis.

Another technique used to manage acoustic neuromas is stereotactic radiosurgery. Stereotactic radiosurgery refers to the stereotactically directed destruction of an intracranial lesion by ionizing beams of radiation (2,6). The ionizing radiation is directed precisely to the intracranial target using computer tomography or magnetic resonance imaging. The current systems use the photons from a stereotactically directed linear accelerator or the radiation from a cobalt-60 gamma unit. Treatment is commonly done in one sitting as an outpatient and has the advantage of being performed completely without a major surgical incision. The major value of radiosurgery is that it arrests the growth of these tumors in patients who are not candidates for surgery. Although most tumors are not cured by this technique, the tumors do shrink and often remain dormant through the lifetime of the patient. It should prove most valuable in patients who are elderly or have significant medical problems that increase the risk of surgery. It has also been proposed for use in patients who have a tumor in their only hearing ear (have bilateral tumors), who refuse open surgery, or who have tumors larger than 3 cm. The rate of loss of hearing with radiosurgical treatment is approximately the same as with operative treatment using microsurgical techniques.

Acoustic neuromas infrequently recur after complete removal. In the past, when making the diagnosis of recurrent tumor required painful or risk-bearing diagnostic studies, no attempt was made to define a recurrence unless the patient had symptoms and findings suggesting a recurrence. Today, the ease of diagnosing recurrences with gadolinium enhanced MRI makes it reasonable to do a scan 1–2 years following surgery in order to have a baseline study should a question of recurrence arise (Fig. 15). These postoperative studies commonly show some

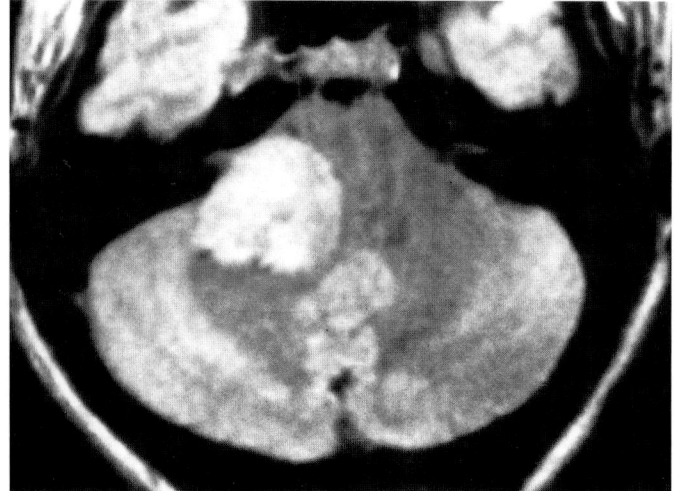
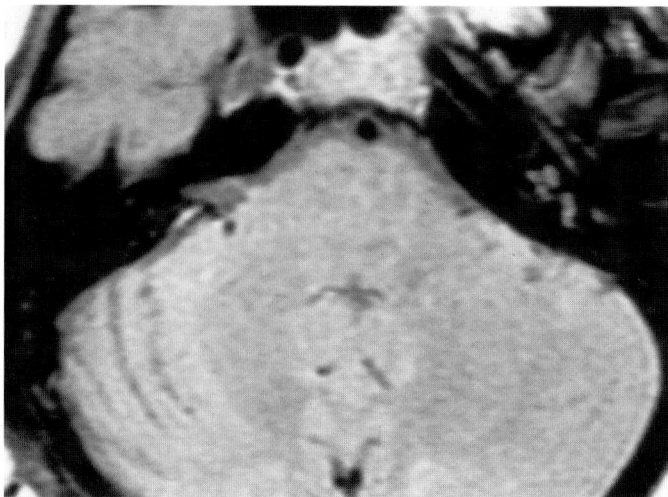

FIG. 15. Pre- and postoperative MRI. **A:** Preoperative MRI showing a large acoustic neuroma in the right cerebellopontine angle. **B:** Postoperative MRI with gadolinium enhancement done 1 year after total removal of the tumor. Facial nerve function following tumor is fully intact. There is a small amount of dural enhancement behind the internal auditory canal.

abnormality in the region of the operation, especially thickening and enhancement of the dura, or abnormalities related to the muscle plug or other materials used to close the openings in the mastoid air cells. The common abnormalities, found routinely on postoperative gadolinium enhanced MRI, should not lead to early reoperation or to the physician making the patient unduly apprehensive about recurrence. Abnormalities suspicious of a recurrence should be evaluated with scans done annually. Only progressive abnormalities demonstrated over a period of time should lead to consideration of reexploration. If the early scans show only the expected postoperative change, no additional scan is done. If there are any symptoms to suggest recurrence in the future this initial scan will serve as a baseline for future comparison.

The Acoustic Neuroma Association, P.O. Box 398, Carlisle, PA 17013, through its chapter meetings and publications can play a valuable role in helping patients adjust and cope with residual symptoms that may follow treatment of an acoustic neuroma.

REFERENCES

1. Atkinson WJ. The anterior inferior cerebellar artery. *J Neurol Neurosurg Psychiatry* 1949;12:137–151.
2. Friedman WA, Bova FJ. The University of Florida Radiosurgery System. *Surg Neurol* 1989;32:334–342.
3. Friedman WA, Kaplan BJ, Gravenstein D, Rhoton AL Jr. Intraoperative brain-stem auditory evoked potentials during posterior fossa microvascular decompression. *J Neurosurg* 1985;62:552–557.
4. Fujii K, Lenkey C, Rhoton AL Jr. Microsurgical anatomy of the choroidal arteries: fourth ventricle and cerebellopontine angles. *J Neurosurg* 1980;52:504–524.
5. Hardy DG, Peace DA, Rhoton AL Jr. Microsurgical anatomy of the superior cerebellar artery. *Neurosurgery* 1980;6:10–28.
6. Linskey ME, Lunsford LD, Flickinger JC. Radiosurgery for acoustic neuromas, neurinomas: early experience. *Neurosurgery* 1990;26:736–745.
7. Lister JR, Rhoton AL Jr, Matsushima T, Peace DA. Microsurgical anatomy of the posterior inferior cerebellar artery. *Neurosurgery* 1982;10:170–199.
8. Martin RG, Grant JL, Peace D, Theiss C, Rhoton AL Jr. Microsurgical relationships of the anterior inferior cerebellar artery and the facial–vestibulocochlear nerve complex. *Neurosurgery* 1980;6:483–507.
9. Matsushima T, Rhoton AL Jr, de Oliveira E, Peace D. Microsurgical anatomy of the veins of the posterior fossa. *J Neurosurg* 1983;59:63–105.
10. Matsushima T, Rhoton AL Jr, Lenkey C. Microsurgery of the fourth ventricle: part I. Microsurgical anatomy. *Neurosurgery* 1982;11:621–667.
11. Ojemann RG, Levine RA, Montgomery WM, McGaffigan P. Use of intraoperative auditory evoked potentials to preserve hearing in unilateral acoustic neuroma removal. *J Neurosurg* 1984;61:938–948.
12. Pait TG, Zeal A, Harris FS, Paullus WS, Rhoton AL Jr. Microsurgical anatomy of dissection of the temporal bone. *Surg Neurol* 1977;8:363–391.
13. Rhoton AL Jr. Microsurgery of the internal acoustic meatus. *Surg Neurol* 1974;2:311–318.
14. Rhoton AL Jr. Microsurgical removal of acoustic neuromas. *Surg Neurol* 1976;6:211–219.
15. Rhoton AL Jr. *Microsurgery of the temporal bone and of acoustic neuromas.* Tryon, NC: Paul C. Bucy & Associates, 1977.
16. Rhoton AL Jr. Microsurgical anatomy of the posterior fossa cranial nerves. *Clin Neurosurg* 1979;26:398–462.
17. Rhoton AL Jr. Suboccipital–retrolabyrinthine removal of acoustic neuromas. *J Fla Med Assoc* 1983;70:895–901.
18. Rhoton AL Jr. Microsurgical anatomy of acoustic neuromas. *Neurol Res* 1984;6:3–21.
19. Rhoton AL Jr. Microsurgical anatomy of the brainstem surface facing an acoustic neuroma. *Surg Neurol* 1986;25:326–339.
20. Rhoton AL Jr. Meningiomas and other cerebellopontine angle tumors. In: Long D, ed. *Current therapy in neurological surgery.* Toronto: B.C. Decker Publishers, 1989:14–19.
21. Rhoton AL Jr. Acoustic neuromas and other tumors of the cerebellopontine angle. In: Kassell NF and Vollmer DG (eds). *Advances in neurosurgery.* Philadelphia: F. A. Davis Company, 1992.

CHAPTER 43

Acoustic Neurilemoma

Otological Approaches

Jean-Marc Sterkers

The main object of the otological approaches is to expose and remove acoustic neuromas through the temporal bone without any displacement of the cerebellum and the brain stem, regardless of whether the size of the tumor is small or giant.

To perform these approaches, the otological surgeon and the neurosurgeon need a thorough knowledge of the anatomy and surgery of the temporal bone, which is in fact an extension of middle ear surgery. They must also have acquired a specific knowledge of the anatomy and pathology of the cerebellopontine angle.

SPECIFIC DIAGNOSTIC CONSIDERATIONS

Initial symptoms of acoustic neuromas may include fullness of the ear, progressive or sudden deafness, fluctuating hearing loss, speech discrimination problems, recruitment, tinnitus, and any sort of vertigo, brief or episodic, and rotary or positional. In other patients, otalgia, trigeminal neuralgia, facial palsy mimicking Bell's palsy, dysgeusia, or dryness of the mouth have been the presenting symptoms, with or even without hearing loss. Headache or vomiting can also be presenting symptoms.

Examination of hearing, balance, trigeminal function, and facial function is first carried out. Brain stem evoked potentials (BSEPs) are performed next. A retrocochlear type of BSEP is obtained in 97% of the cases. It is followed by CT scan with intravenous contrast or MRI with gadolinium enhancement. These studies are also performed in patients with a total unilateral deafness and a labyrinthine hyporeflexia, and in young patients who have a normal or endocochlear type of BSEP response without any explanation. The most typical case of Ménière's disease can be mimicked by a tumor interfering with the cochleovestibular functions.

PATIENT SELECTION

Most acoustic neuromas need to be removed since these tumors grow into the posterior fossa and have a potential for patients' infirmity and death. In a few patients, the operation may be postponed or not performed, according to the size of the tumor, the functional deficit, the growth rate of the tumor, and the general state and age of the patient.

In older patients with an intracanalicular tumor, or with a tumor measuring less than 15 mm in the CP angle and without any other deficit than a unilateral deafness (no vestibular deficit, normal facial function), a reevaluation at 1 year by CT or MRI may show no measurable growth. In the case of a tumor involving the only functional ear, we postpone the operation until the hearing is lost. In all other patients, surgery is performed.

OPERATIVE APPROACHES

Anesthetic Considerations

One of the advantages of the otological approach is that the patient may be placed in the supine position, which eliminates the risk of air embolism. The endotracheal tube is connected to a volume regulated respirator. The patient is under fentanyl, droperidol, isoflurane, and nitrous oxide anesthesia. Electrocardiogram, blood

---

J.-M. Sterkers: O. R. L. Paris Hospital, College of Medicine, 75016 Paris, France.

pressure, and pulse monitoring are continuously performed. Prophylactic antibiotic therapy with ampicillin (2 g intravenous) is started during the operation and continued for 2 days. A preoperative intravenous infusion of mannitol (250 ml of 25% solution) is administered when the operation is done by the middle fossa approach or by the mastoid and retrosigmoid approach.

While using the translabyrinthine approach, no ventricular or spinal drainage is performed. An area about four fingers large is shaved behind and above the ear 1 hr before the operation and the skin preparation with Betadine is carried out. The same preparation is done on the lateral side of the thigh or the abdomen where the free grafts will be extracted at the end of the operation. The legs are wrapped with elastic gauze to prevent deep venous thrombosis.

Patient Position

The patient is placed in the supine position with the head rotated toward the side opposite to the tumor and maintained by an adhesive strip to the table, unless preoperative ultrasound has shown an abnormality of the carotid flow. In the middle fossa approach, the patient lies horizontally. In the translabyrinthine approach, the head is slightly lowered until the mastoid lies in a horizontal plane. In the mastoid and retrosigmoid approach, the head is lowered to place the retrosigmoid area at an angle of 20° to the horizontal plane.

Operative Technique

The otological approaches are the translabyrinthine approach and the middle fossa approach. We also describe the mastoid and retrosigmoid approach, which is a flexible approach, as it can be converted into a translabyrinthine approach.

Translabyrinthine Approach

First Step: The Approach

A curved skin incision approximately 8 cm long is made about two fingers behind the ear, ending inferiorly behind the mastoid tip (Fig. 1). The skin is elevated to expose the temporal fascia and the mastoid periosteum.

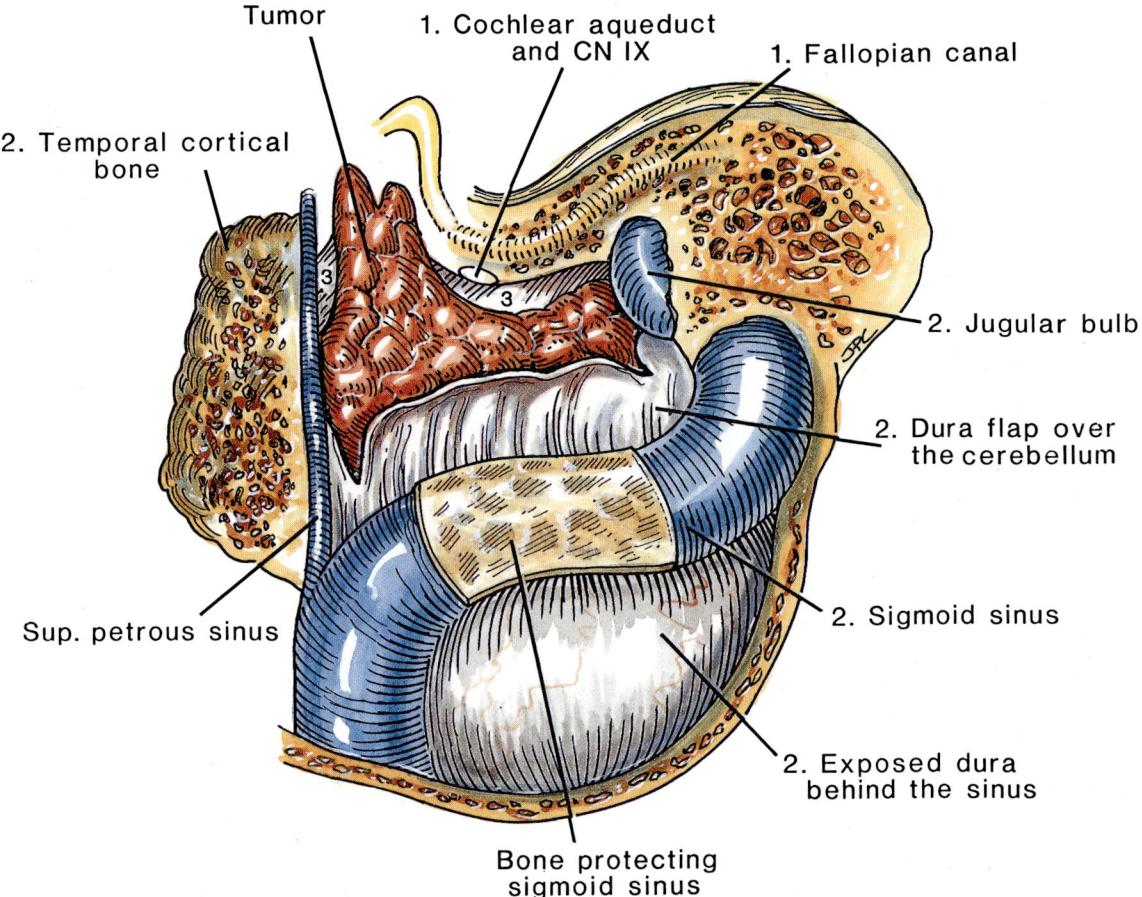

FIG. 1. Limits of the translabyrinthine approach: 1, impassable; 2, movable; 3, in cross lines, drilling of the superior and inferior walls of the internal auditory canal.

The mastoid periosteum is dissected from the mastoid bone to form a superiorly pedicled flap. An enlarged mastoidectomy is carried on under constant suction irrigation, with conical metallic burrs and diamond burrs. The retrosigmoid dura is widely exposed, removing 1 or 2 cm of cortical bone behind the sinus. This is the important aspect of the enlarged translabyrinthine approach to the angle. The emissary vein is coagulated with bipolar cautery and then divided. If a perforation of the emissary vein or the sinus occurs, a strip of Oxycel mixed with wax is applied on it. In the case of a larger perforation of the sinus, it may have to be closed with a small free-muscle graft threaded on a silk suture and sutured across the margins of the perforation. The sigmoid sinus is kept protected by an island of bone, and the dura anterior to the sinus is exposed. Anteriorly, the drilling is stopped when the body of the incus appears. The atticoatrial isthmus is closed by two small fascia and free-muscle grafts, which are inserted laterally and medially to the body of the incus. This provides a tight closure of the eustachian tube orifice against a cerebrospinal fluid (CSF) leakage.

The fallopian canal is exposed in its mastoid segment and inferior to the lateral semicircular canal. It is first recognized on its lateral face and then on its posterior one. It is the anterior border of the approach. Then the labyrinth, which lies posterosuperiorly, is drilled away, recognizing successively the lateral canal, the posterior canal, and the superior canal. The vestibule is opened, the vestibular aqueduct is seen, and at the junction of the superior and lateral canal, the fibers of the superior vestibular nerve are identified. It is the landmark for the superior vestibular fossa of the internal auditory canal (IAC). The fibers lie medial to the wall of the vestibule.

The wall of the petrous bone between the posterior fossa and the IAC dura is drilled away until the porus is reached. This drilling is done with a metallic conical burr, which is replaced by a diamond burr when the surgeon approaches the dura. During this drilling, one will recognize superiorly the subarcuate artery, which is the only artery encountered in this area, and inferiorly the jugular bulb. If the jugular bulb is in a high position, the bulb is depressed and maintained by an island of bone. If a perforation of the bulb occurs, Oxycel mixed with wax is applied on it and pressure is maintained for several minutes. It can be sealed to the bone by Histoacryl. To enlarge the approach, it may also be necessary to elevate the temporal cortical bone and to flatten the posterosuperior borders of the mastoidectomy. During this enlargement, the superior petrous sinus is exposed; it is the superior border of the approach.

At this stage of the operation, the dura of the IAC is completely exposed on its posterior wall. It is now necessary to drill away half of the inferior wall and the superior wall of the IAC until a vertical plane is obtained. This is done first with a very small metallic burr, making a groove that is widened with a diamond burr until the dura is reached. Between the IAC and the jugular bulb lies the cochlear aqueduct. It is the anteroinferior limit of the drilling. The dura is punctured at this site, a small gush of CSF appears, and CN IX is visible (Fig. 2).

Second Step: Removal of Tumor

The cerebellar dura is now opened as a U-shaped flap, with its base posteriorly, the incision being made initially at the inferior border. Then a small dissector is introduced tangential to the inferior pole of the tumor, to open the arachnoid of the cistern. The arachnoid is opened with a small hook above the ninth nerve in a small tumor, or more posteriorly in a larger tumor. Care is taken not to injure the vagal vein, which is posterior, or the anterior inferior cerebellar artery (AICA), which makes a loop beneath the arachnoid and above the ninth nerve. Immediately, a huge gush of CSF appears, and the posterior fossa is progressively decompressed (Fig. 2). In the case of very large tumors, this decompression is done after debulking the inferior pole of the tumor. When the decompression is achieved, a very good exposure is ob-

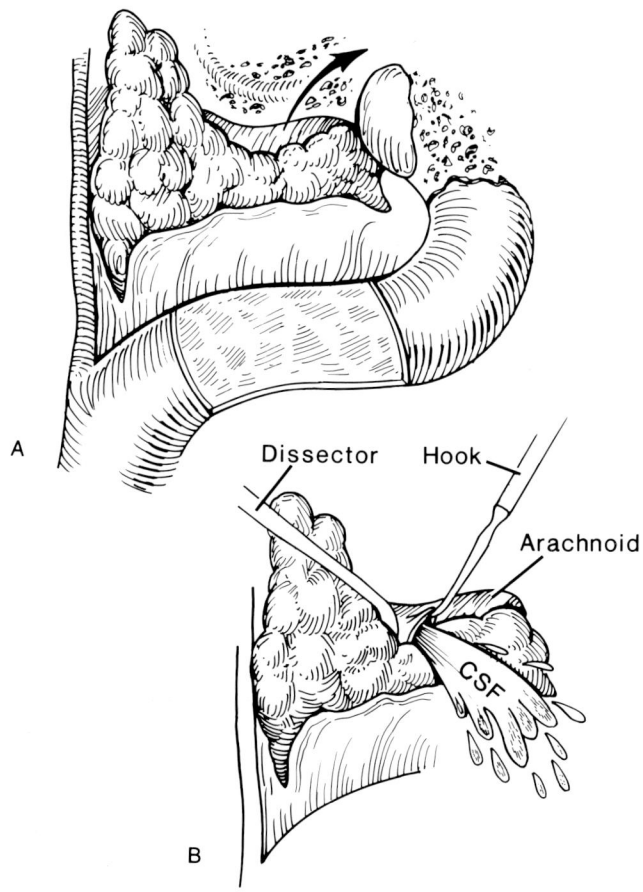

FIG. 2. Translabyrinthine approach. **A:** CSF decompression before removal of the tumor or after debulking the inferior pole of the tumor. **B:** Issue of CSF after opening of the great cisterns.

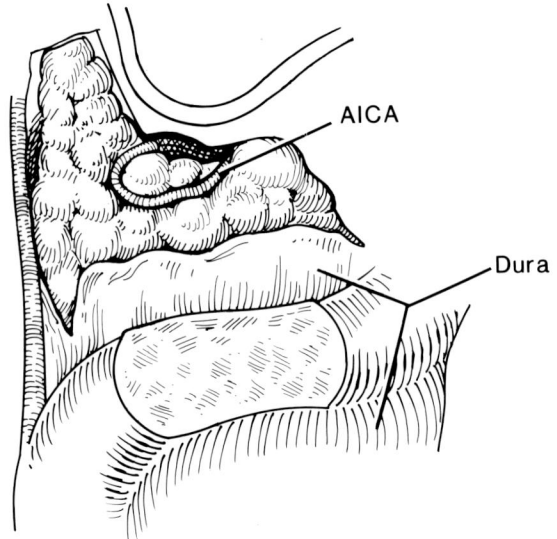

FIG. 3. Translabyrinthine approach. A loop of the anterior/inferior cerebellar artery (AICA) crossing between the dura and the tumor or inserted in the dura is encountered on occasion and must be dissected with the arachnoid sheath.

tained, which can be enlarged much further as needed by retracting the sigmoid sinus. The U-shaped dural flap is then incised on its superior and medial part, taking care not to damage a possible loop of the AICA, located between the dura and the tumor (Fig. 3). At this point, the dura of the IAC is opened, first on its inferior border and then at the fundus, until the lateral extremity of the superior vestibular fossa is reached.

The removal of the tumor begins by identification of the facial nerve at the fallopian foramen. The fibers of the superior vestibular nerve or the root of the tumor are avulsed and, just anteriorly, the greyish facial nerve will be seen before it enters the fallopian foramen (Fig. 4).

The dissection of the facial nerve from the tumor is done with a small hook, under constant suction irrigation with the Brackmann cannula. All the root of the tumor is removed close to the seventh nerve. It is necessary to make a very precise dissection around the nerve, as small tongues of tumoral tissue are adjacent to the seventh nerve. The dissection of the facial nerve needs to be very smooth. Mechanical stimulation of the nerve can be recorded by neurophysiological monitoring or more simply by the fingers of the assistant recording twisting of the face. When the dissection reaches the porus, the facial nerve disappears from view, making an anterior curve. To see the nerve again, it is necessary to remove all the anterior parts of the tumor. The removal is first done inside the neuroma. It is done with fenestrated curettes, which remove the tissue piece by piece, or more easily by the ultrasonic apparatus (Cavitron or Surgitron). The anterior pole and the center of the neuroma are debulked. Then the anterior pole of the tumor can be retracted, and the dissection of the seventh nerve is continued until the brain stem is reached. Most often, there are some great adhesions about 1 cm medial to the porus, and the nerve is not visible. In such a case, the part that is adherent to the seventh nerve is removed at the end of the dissection. The inferior pole is then removed. Around the inferior pole, great care is necessary to avoid injuring the AICA, which makes a loop. Its preservation is essential as its interruption could produce a catastrophic brain stem hemorrhagic infarction (Atkinson syndrome). Also, if its small branches are divided before sufficient coagulation, severe hemorrhage may result (Figs. 5–8).

When the inferior pole is debulked, the caudal cranial nerves are dissected from the tumor, especially the ninth nerve. Bradycardia occurs if one exerts some traction on the tenth nerve. Then the eighth nerve is seen and, just in front of it, the facial nerve and intermediate nerve of Wrisberg, at their exit from the brain stem. The dissection of the seventh nerve is then done medial to lateral, until the peripheral part of the nerve, which has been previously dissected, is reached. This last part of the dissection can be dreadfully difficult as a result of the adhesions of the neuroma (Fig. 9). If an interruption of the nerve happens, it is usually in this segment of the nerve. When the anterior part of the tumor has been removed, the fifth nerve, sixth nerve, and the pons are in view, and it is possible to remove the rest of the tumor, first making a central cavity and then debulking the superior and pos-

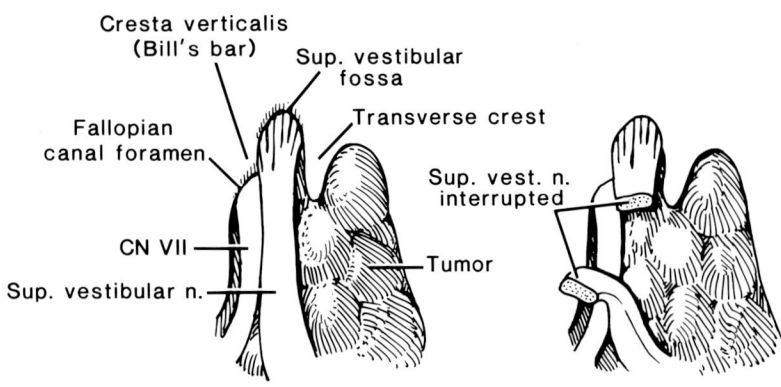

FIG. 4. Translabyrinthine approach. Identification of the facial nerve in the internal auditory canal. (In this case, the neuroma has grown from the inferior vestibular nerve.)

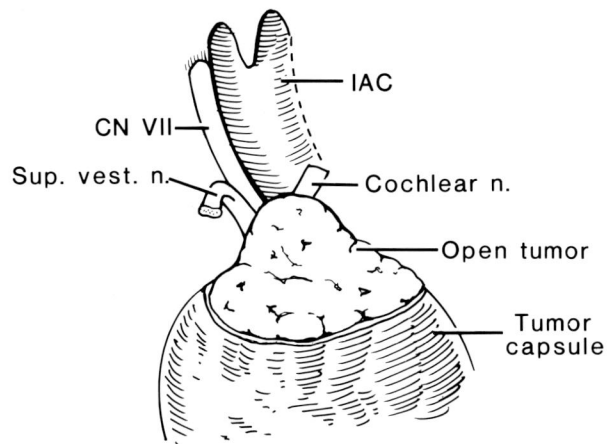

FIG. 5. First step: dissection of the seventh nerve in the IAC and removal of the root of the tumor.

terior pole, which are separated from the cerebellum, from the choroid plexus inferiorly, from the superior petrosal vein superiorly, and with variable difficulties from the brain stem and the middle cerebellar peduncle. Bipolar coagulation of all the vessels is done during this last dissection of the capsule of the tumor. The arachnoid sheath that surrounds the tumor, vessels, and nerves is pushed back with the AICA and the superior petrosal vein.

When the removal of the tumor is total, hemostasis is achieved, and the operative site is washed with physiologic saline. If the seventh nerve has been interrupted and the central part has been identified, an anastomosis is performed, either end-to-end or with a cable graft from the auricular branch of the cervical plexus. Fibrin glue is used to seal the ends of the nerves.

A tight closure of the translabyrinthine approach is obtained by superposition of multiple grafts. The barrage is built first with the application of a small fat graft placed in the IAC, then a large fascia is draped over the gap. The fascia is maintained by apposition of adipose grafts, and the mastoid periosteal flap is sutured over it. The skin is closed in two layers. A bandage is wrapped tightly over the wound and kept for a fortnight. Any physical effort should be avoided for 3 weeks.

Middle Fossa Approach

A 4-cm-long vertical or S-shaped incision is made, beginning at the zygomatic root in front of the helix. The temporal muscle is incised and a craniotomy of 3 × 3 cm is performed with the burr. Under mannitol infusion, and after making a 1-cm incision of the dura to decompress the brain, the temporal lobe is elevated extradurally on the arcuate eminence, until the superior petrosal sinus is seen; the dura is then elevated in front of the eminence, and the greater superficial petrosal nerve appears (Fig. 10).

To find the IAC, several techniques have been described. William House exposes the labyrinthine segment of the facial nerve from the geniculate ganglion to the fallopian foramen. Ugo Fisch finds the blue line of the superior semicircular canal (SSCC) and finds the fundus of the IAC at a 60° angle to the line of the SSCC. P. Narcy unroofs the middle ear and takes the head of the malleus as a landmark of the axis of the IAC. We locate the IAC 3 cm deep to the external border of the craniotomy on the biauricular axis and drill with a diamond burr until we find the dura. The neuroma appears under the dura, and we drill away the roof of the IAC medially to the porus and laterally to the fundus. It must be remembered that the vulnerable structures are concentrated at the fundus of the IAC, namely, the cochlea in front and the SSCC behind. The dura is opened posteriorly; the facial nerve is identified on top of the tumor, lying against the anterior wall of the IAC.

The neuroma is removed piece by piece. A small neuroma growing from the inferior vestibular nerve can be hidden by the facial and superior vestibular nerves. The Bill's bar is a vertical crest that separates the fallopian foramen from the superior vestibular fossa, which is more lateral than the fallopian foramen. When the superior part of the tumor has been partially removed, it is possible to remove its inferior part and its lateral pole, which lies between the cochlear and the facial nerves. At the medial extremity of the neuroma, great care must be taken not to injure the loop of the AICA, which may also be encountered in the IAC itself, under the dura or between the nerves and the tumor.

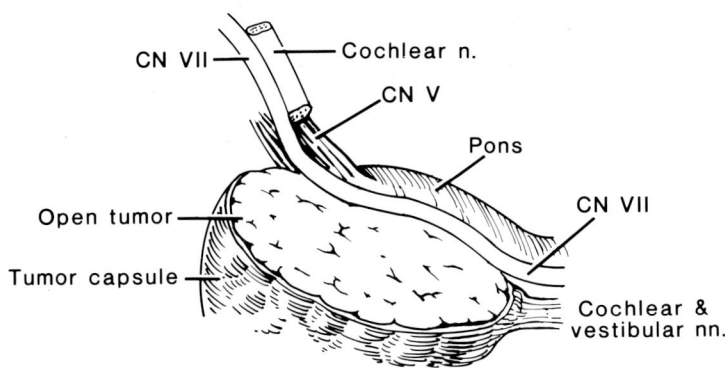

FIG. 6. Second step: debulking the anterior pole of the tumor until the brain stem appears.

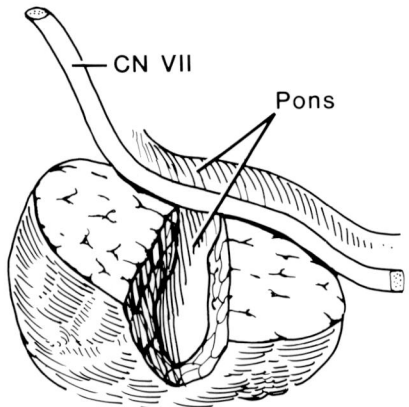

FIG. 7. Third step: debulking the medial pole to mobilize the superior and inferior poles; the brain stem appears between the two parts of the tumor. The seventh nerve is in an anterior situation visible from the brain stem to the IAC.

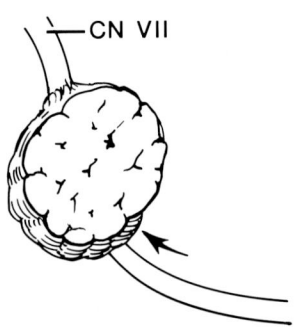

FIG. 8. Difficult case. The seventh nerve runs around the superior and medial pole of the tumor, adheres to the dura at the porus, and is almost inseparable from the tumor between the porus and the fifth nerve. After debulking the inferior pole, and dividing the eighth nerve at its origin, the seventh nerve is identified and dissected from medial to lateral until the distal part of the seventh nerve is rejoined.

The IAC is closed with a fascia graft and a free-muscle graft from the temporal muscle. The dura of the temporal lobe is sutured to the temporal muscle, and the temporal muscle and skin are closed by interrupted sutures. A suction drainage is left.

During this approach, the patient is in the supine position, the head being placed in such a way that the biauricular axis is almost vertical. To get a good view of the fundus of the IAC, it is necessary to incline the operating table in procubitus, and to drill a small groove in the arcuate eminence following the biauricular axis.

Mastoid Retrosigmoid Approach

The mastoid retrosigmoid approach is a posterior approach and the dura is opened behind the sigmoid sinus. A large mastoidectomy is first performed, the sinus is exposed, and the dura posterior to the sigmoid sinus is exposed, making a 3-cm-large craniotomy between the superior and inferior nuchal lines after dividing the muscles and the occipital artery. In this approach, the head must be placed inferior to the chest, the patient lying in the supine position.

The mastoidectomy is an adjunct to the retrosigmoid approach. It has three aims: first, an initial decompression of the CSF is made by a small retrolabyrinthine incision; second, if the removal of the tumor is abandoned by the retrosigmoid approach, conversion to a translabyrinthine approach is greatly facilitated; third, in case of postoperative hemorrhage, it will allow decompression without damage to the cerebellum, via a translabyrinthine approach.

The retrosigmoid dura is incised in a U-shaped flap based posteriorly; the sigmoid sinus is retracted anteriorly (Fig. 11). A lyophilized dura graft is inserted between the cerebellum and temporal bone, and the tumor

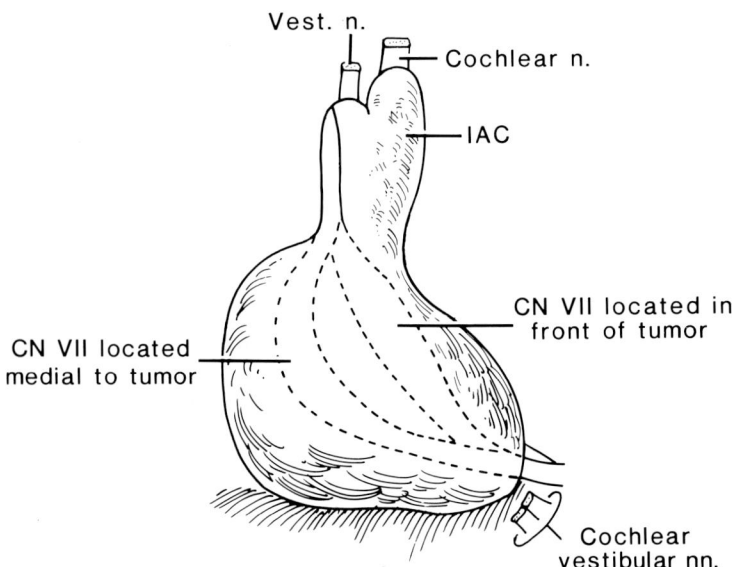

FIG. 9. Translabyrinthine approach. The two locations of the facial nerve in front or medial to the tumor.

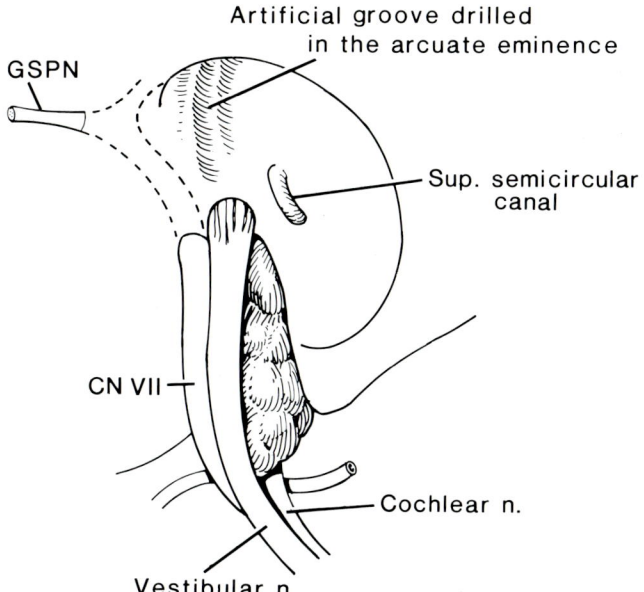

FIG. 10. Middle fossa approach. It is necessary to drill a small groove in the arcuate eminence, in the axis of the IAC, to see the fundus of the IAC and remove the root of the tumor (in this case, the neuroma has grown from the inferior vestibular nerve). Note the AICA crossing at the medial pole of the tumor. In other cases, the loop of the AICA can be encountered between the nerves and the tumor, inside the IAC.

will appear when the arachnoid of the great cistern is opened and the CSF is decompressed. Dissection around the tumor is then performed to expose the brain stem, the cochlear nerve, and the facial nerve in front of the cochlear nerve. The neuroma is debulked from within to allow better delineation of the nerves and is also dissected toward the internal auditory meatus. When debulked up to the IAC, the intracanalicular portion is removed by drilling away the posterior wall of the internal auditory canal, taking care to avoid damaging the superior semicircular canal. For this reason, it is not possible to fully expose the fundus by this route. The two factors that generally result in the abandoning of this approach are dense adhesions between the neuroma and the cochlear nerve, and failure to expose the end of the intracanalicular portion of the neuroma; although the facial nerve is at risk, this is also an indication for conversion to a translabyrinthine approach (Fig. 12). This approach is used only if the case fulfills the following criteria:

1. A tumor size of less than 20–25 mm.
2. Subnormal, but useful, hearing in the affected ear.
3. Nuclear magnetic resonance imaging showing the fundus to be clear of tumor.
4. A BSEP response that is not flat.
5. Favorable operative findings (Fig. 13).

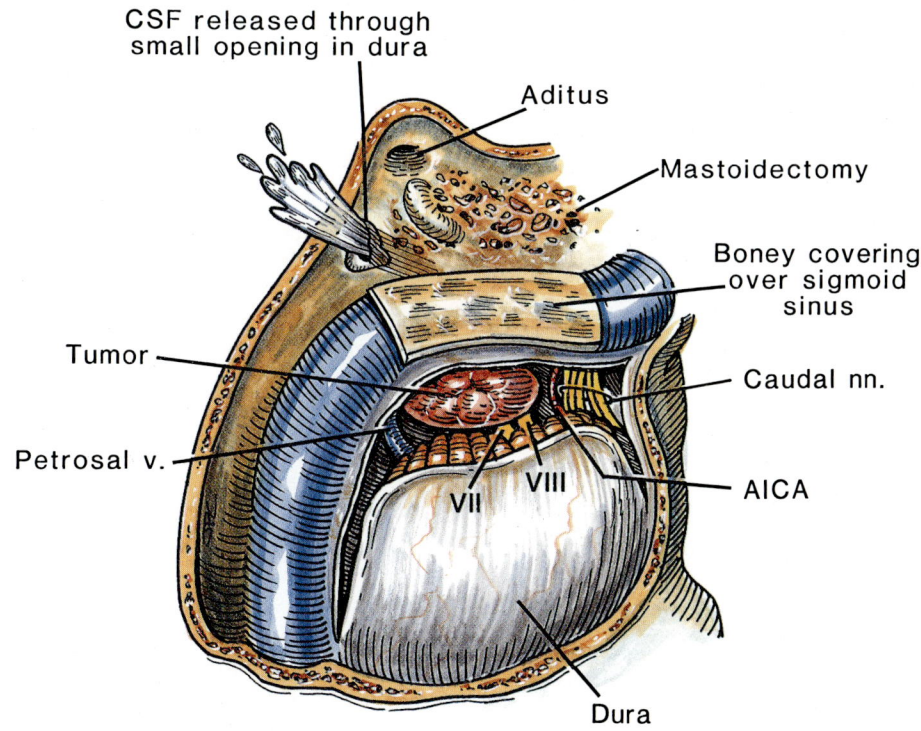

FIG. 11. First step: mastoidectomy. Retrosigmoid craniotomy.

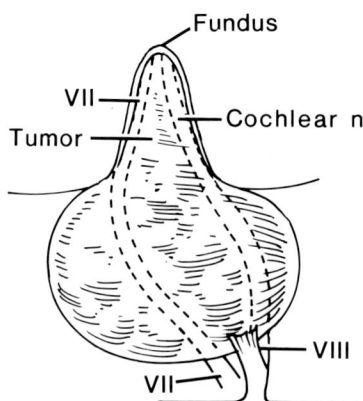

FIG. 12. Second step: upon drilling the IAC, the tumor completely fills the IAC; the cochlear and facial nerves are separated by the tumor. The approach is transformed to a translabyrinthine approach.

These criteria are not absolute, but, when they are not fulfilled, the possibility of successful hearing preservation is diminished. Each patient should be warned that there is a significant chance that conversion to a translabyrinthine approach will be required with subsequent loss of hearing in that ear.

During the closure of the mastoid and retrosigmoid approach, the mastoid has to be filled with adipose tissue, and the dura must be closed behind the sigmoid dura, also covering it with a free adipose graft. The skin is sutured without drainage.

POSTOPERATIVE MANAGEMENT

Extubation is done at the end of the operation, and the patient will stay in the intensive care unit for 2 days, with a constant monitoring of the pulse, respiration, and alertness. The patient stays for 15 days in the hospital, during which time a bandage is kept on the head.

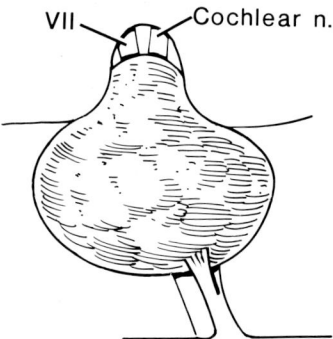

FIG. 13. Second step: upon drilling the IAC, the tumor partially fills the IAC; when fundus is free of tumor, the cochlear and facial nerves are contiguous. The cochlear nerve and the hearing might be preserved by the retrosigmoid approach.

COMPLICATIONS AND MANAGEMENT

Death during the procedure is a rarity. One patient died in a series of 1000 cases, which was due to hemorrhage and brain stem infarction.

In the immediate postoperative period, if the patient fails to arouse from anesthesia, or, if after awakening, the patient suddenly loses consciousness and presents alterations in the pulse and respiratory rates, rise of blood pressure, hyperpyrexia, and possibly extensor spasms, one of the following events is occurring: *primary tracheobronchial–pulmonary dysfunction, intracranial hemorrhage, or brain stem swelling and softening.* If after reintubation the patient fails to respond to a clear airway, bleeding into the tumor site is the most likely cause, particularly if the patient is in immediate distress. Because it is the most lethal of all complications, treatment is of great urgency.

Immediately, in the intensive care unit, the wound is reopened to decompress the brain stem. By the translabyrinthine approach, this can be done very rapidly by pulling out the fat and fascia plugs that closed the angle. Then the patient is transferred to the operating room, and, with the operative microscope, the clot is very carefully evacuated and the bleeding vessel is coagulated. The branches of the AICA or the AICA itself, or the branches of the extracranial arteries can be the cause of the hematoma.

During the operation, the prevention of secondary bleeding relies on an adequate hemostasis. It must be emphasized that after section of a vessel between two points of bipolar coagulation, it is essential to coagulate again each end of the interrupted vessel. If this is not done, it could bleed again a few hours later, or even in one of our cases, 28 hr after the operation. Death or severe neurologic sequelae are the result of hemorrhage, despite prompt evacuation of the clot. Some fortunate cases can be saved without severe sequelae.

Other complications can be swelling of the pons, of the cerebellum, or elevated cerebrospinal fluid pressure. In these situations, the symptoms of distress are progressive, and there is time to make the diagnosis by a CT scan, which can also show a hematoma of the bed of the tumor or the presence of blood in the ventricles.

During the intermediate period, another lethal complication can occur—the AICA syndrome. Preservation of this artery is essential to avoid the eventuality of a catastrophic brain stem hemorrhagic infarction. This artery is at risk during the dissection of both small tumors and large ones.

With the use of the microscope and bipolar coagulation, this complication is now extremely rare.

Cerebrospinal fluid leaks and meningitis can occur after the otological approaches. The leak presents either in the postauricular wound or via the eustachian tube in the pharynx or the nose. If acetazolamide, a low fluid diet, spinal taps, or lumbar subarachnoid drainage are not effective rapidly, a reparative procedure is needed. More plugs with adipose tissue and fascia are inserted in the fistula, which generally lies behind the fallopian canal.

It may also be located in the medial wall of the middle ear, and the closure will be successful when the site of the fistula is seen and closed with fascia and a chip of bone is inserted in the hole.

Meningitis can be the cause or the consequence of the CSF leakage. It can also be iatrogenic. The symptoms can be typical or latent. It must be systematically suspected, a lasting fever over 3 or 4 days needs a spinal tap and bacteriological exam of the CSF.

Thrombosis of the lateral sinus and of the superior sagittal sinus with seizure or neurological deficit is an extremely rare complication.

Cranial Nerve Dysfunction

Trigeminal Nerve. Irreparable keratitis may develop in the case of combined facial palsy and cornea anesthesia: proper corneal protection during and after the operation is necessary. An immediate prophylactic tarsorrhaphy is frequently indicated postoperatively.

Abducens Nerve. Temporary sixth nerve palsy with associated diplopia may occur in large tumors.

Facial Nerve and Wrisberg Nerve. Prevention of facial palsy is one of the greatest advantages of early surgery of acoustic neuromas using microsurgery. Since the majority of patients do not have a facial paralysis prior to surgery, the preservation of facial nerve function is dependent on the surgical technique, the size of the tumor, and the adhesions between the tumor and the nerve, which vary from one case to another. It is very important to preserve normal facial function immediately or at 1 month postoperatively, and in such cases no facial weakness or synkinesis will be present. This can be obtained even in the largest tumors, but most frequently in the middle size tumors and almost always in intracanalicular tumors.

In the case of long-lasting facial palsy, the recovery is of variable degree, achieving 50–70% of the normal with synkinesis and abnormal movements. Facial exercises are recommended when the face starts functioning. Artificial tears and ophthalmic vitamin A and liquid paraffin cure the corneal ulceration. Protection of the eye by glasses or a tarsorrhaphy may be necessary.

When the facial nerve is interrupted or does not recover function after reanastomosis or graft repair, a hypoglossal–facial anastomosis can be performed later, which gives a much better result than plastic surgery.

Acoustic Nerve. Sparing the cochlear nerve gives good functional result when all the criteria required to save this function are present. This is rarely achieved. Sparing the vestibular nerve is exceptional and may be the cause of difficulties in vestibular compensation.

Glossopharyngeal and Vagus Nerves. Dysphagia and depressed cough and gag reflexes might be bulbar, nuclear, or peripheral. They may necessitate tracheotomy and nasogastric tube feedings. Paralysis of a vocal cord with hoarseness will compensate. These complications are very rare.

Cerebellar Dysfunction. This dysfunction includes ipsilateral extremity ataxia, tendency to fall to that side, and dysarthria. These complications occur in removal of large tumors when traction is applied to the middle cerebellar peduncle. The syndrome will recover after several months. It can also be seen after a hemorrhage in the site of the tumor; after thrombosis of the AICA it may be permanent.

Long Tract Deficits. These may occur when a very adherent tumor is being separated from the brain stem.

In the Later Period. Seizures and dysphasia can be complications of the middle fossa approach. Their incidence is very low.

Disturbances in CSF Circulation. The diagnosis is confirmed by changes in ventricular size demonstrable on the CT scan. Postoperative bleeding and aseptic and low-grade septic meningitis may produce these disturbances. Mental deterioration, trunkal ataxia, and urinary incontinence are the symptoms of communicating hydrocephalus. A CSF shunt is indicated.

Recurrence. After partial tumor removal, a recurrence that can be very rapid happens in 80% of the cases. After total tumor removal, a recurrence occurs in 6% of patients from tumoral tissue hidden in the porus in front of the nerves, or from the fundus of the IAC, if the removal has not been done by the translabyrinthine approach or the middle fossa approach. It is necessary to do a CT scan 1 year after the removal, and every year or two for 6 years. If there is a recurrence, a second operation will be done without waiting for a large regrowth.

In bilateral acoustic tumors, we operate only on the side of the greatest hearing loss; to preserve at least one facial nerve, the operation is done on the other side when the hearing is lost. This can happen only after many years of evolution. We have tried stereotactic surgery in a few patients who have lost hearing immediately or gradually.

AUTHOR'S EXPERIENCE

From 1966 to December 1991, 1300 patients have been operated on, by myself alone or with a neurosurgical team (R. Billet, M. Desgeorges, R. Grob). Twenty percent of the tumors measured 3–7 cm, 75% measured 1–3 cm, and 5% were intracanalicular tumors. The mean age of the patients was 50 years: the youngest was 11 years old, the eldest was 85 years old.

The choice of the approach, according to our experience, varied during the last decades. Presently, the translabyrinthine approach is used in 85% of the cases; the other approaches (middle fossa or retrosigmoid) are used in approximately 9% and 6%, respectively. During several years, we used the retrosigmoid approach almost exclusively to try to preserve hearing, but the result was not satisfactory (10% kept a functional hearing). Additionally, this approach, in the supine position, was not suitable for removal of the largest tumors. It also presented more risks for preservation of the facial nerve function than the translabyrinthine approach.

The mastoid–retrosigmoid approach as described is now used only in cases that fulfill the precise criteria; hearing preservation is obtained at 1 year in 20%.

In our entire series, the facial nerve has been preserved in 89%, the facial function being active immediately or after 1 month of the operation in 65% (45% for the largest tumors, 3 cm or more).

An immediate or subsequent repair of the seventh nerve was necessary in 11%. The removal was total in 91%, subtotal in 6%, and partial in 3%. Presently, the removal is total in 95%. It is subtotal in 5%, which means that a few millimeters of tumoral tissue are left adherent to the seventh nerve. However, it must be recalled that even after total removal a recurrence has been found in 6%.

The overall mortality was 0.7% and severe cerebellar disability occurred in 0.4%.

All these progresses achieved in the surgery of the acoustic neuroma by otological approaches are due to the original work of William House and William Hitselberger, who described this new subspeciality devoted to the treatment of the disease of the temporal bone and pontocerebellar angle.

BIBLIOGRAPHY

1. House WF. Transtemporal bone microsurgical removal of acoustic neuromas. *Arch Otolaryngol* 1964;80:597.
2. House WF, Luetje CM. *Acoustic tumors,* vols I and II. Baltimore: University Park Press, 1979.
3. Horowitz NH, Rizzoli HV. *Postoperative complications of intracranial neurological surgery.* Baltimore: William & Wilkins, 1982.
4. Rhoton AL Jr. Microsurgical anatomy of the brain stem surface facing an acoustic neuroma. *Surg Neurol* 1986;25:326–339.
5. Sterkers JM, Billet R. Petites tumeurs de l'acoustique. Diagnostic et cure précoces. *Ann Otolaryngol* (Paris) 1972;89:323–339.
6. Sterkers JM, Desgeorges M, Corlieu P, Sterkers O. Ablation par voie translabyrinthique des volumineux neurinomes de l'acoustique. *Ann Otolaryngol* (Paris) 1984;101:9–14.
7. Sterkers JM, Desgeorges M, Sterkers O, Corlieu P. Our present approach to acoustic neuroma surgery. *Adv Otorhinolaryngol* 1984;34:160–163.

CHAPTER 44

Facial Nerve Neurilemomas

Ivo P. Janecka and Laligam N. Sekhar

Primary tumors of the facial nerve are quite rare. When they do occur they can be found along the nerve's entire course (Fig. 1). However, most frequently they are found within the temporal bone (Fig. 2) or extracranially. Intracranial isolated facial nerve neurilemomas are exceedingly rare. They originate from the Schwann cells of the nerve sheath, and thus their occasional finding within the internal auditory canal or intracranially may be explained on the basis of embryonic rests of ganglionic cells from the geniculate ganglion region. The vast majority of facial nerve neurilemomas are benign, but several malignant schwannomas have been reported, primarily in the parotid region.

DIAGNOSIS

A patient's symptomatology leading to a diagnosis of facial nerve neurilemoma varies depending on the site of tumor origin along the course of the facial nerve. The neurilemomas found along the extracranial course of the facial nerve present primarily as parotid masses (may be multiple and/or cystic). The accompanying facial paralysis is also quite rare (about 20%). Statistically, therefore, a preoperative diagnosis of a facial nerve neurilemoma in the parotid region is seldom made. If the tumor originates within the temporal bone, and that may be anywhere from the geniculate ganglion to the stylomastoid foramen, such tumor usually produces otological symptoms. However, facial weakness frequently accompanies these tumors. This seems to be due to the nerve compression within a tight bony canal within the temporal bone. Intracranially, the facial nerve neurilemomas give mostly symptomatology of a retrolabyrinth lesion similar to other cerebellopontine angle (CPA) tumors.

Current imaging modality (CT, MRI) offers precision of our differential diagnosis by demonstrating bony erosion or soft tissue mass enlarging the fallopian canal or one adjacent to the labyrinthine course of the facial nerve. The lesion is enhancing with a contrast medium. Electrodiagnostic tests seldom can pinpoint the etiology and, in most cases, just document a clinically apparent facial weakness without specifying the etiology. An open biopsy is seldom performed as a separate procedure and is usually done as a frozen section during surgical exploration.

PLANNING

Any neoplasm of or in the vicinity of the facial nerve should include detailed explanation to the patient of the likelihood of direct facial nerve involvement and the options of tumor resection and nerve rehabilitation. With the presumptive diagnosis of facial nerve neurilemoma, a specific focus of the preoperative planning is on ultimate facial nerve grafting. That includes preparation of the nerve graft donor site as well as anticipation for the need for eye protection (see Janecka et al., Facial Nerve Management and Reconstructive Techniques).

PROCEDURES

The goals of our procedures are as follows:

1. To establish a diagnosis.
2. To attempt to preserve continuity of the facial nerve.
3. Complete tumor resection.
4. Facial nerve reconstruction/facial paralysis rehabilitation.

I. P. Janecka: Center for Cranial Base Surgery, University of Pittsburgh School of Medicine, Presbyterian University Hospital, and Department of Otolaryngology, Eye and Ear Institute, Pittsburgh, Pennsylvania 15213.
L. N. Sekhar: Department of Neurosurgery, Center for Cranial Base Surgery, University of Pittsburgh School of Medicine, and Presbyterian University Hospital, Pittsburgh, Pennsylvania 15213.

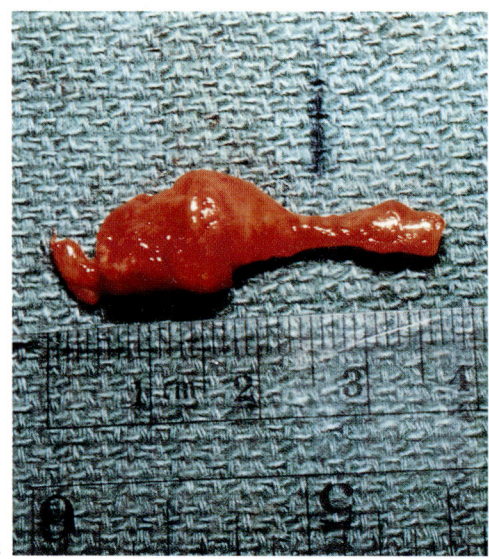 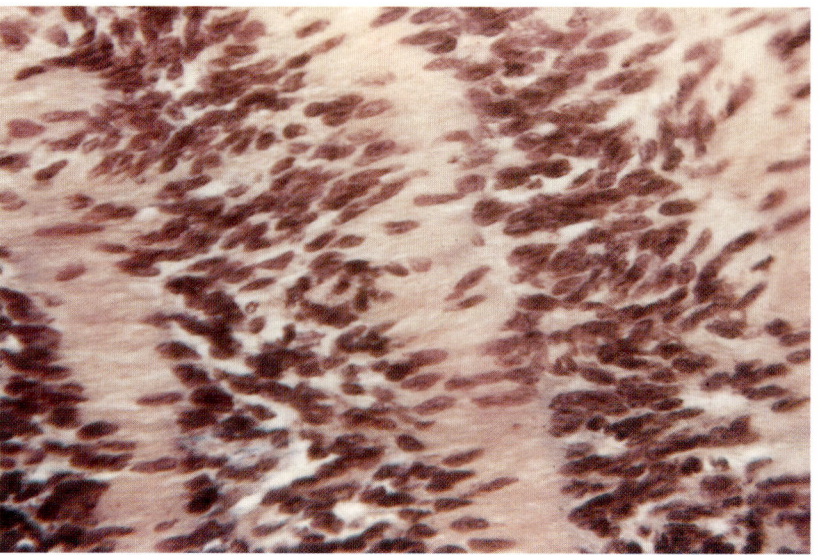

FIG. 1. A: Surgical specimen demonstrating a diffuse enlargement of main trunk of a facial nerve. **B:** Histological appearance of facial nerve neurilemoma.

Tissue diagnosis is seldom available preoperatively when operating on patients with neurilemoma of the facial nerve. In temporal bone neurilemomas, with the current state of imaging, a high degree of probability exists. Usually tissue diagnosis is obtained as a frozen section at the time of surgery.

Because of the cell of origin (Schwann cells) within the nerve sheath, it is theoretically possible to consider tumor removal without a nerve transection. However, practically speaking, this is usually feasible only in very small lesions. In the vast majority of cases, nerve transection has to be performed.

The complete tumor removal should include adequate proximal and distal nerve margin. The tumor-free margins should be verified by frozen section. This is important not only for oncological reasons but also for the reassurance of unhindered growth of axons through a nerve graft.

Facial nerve reconstruction usually includes a nerve graft (Fig. 3). If this is not feasible, a second option often is hypoglossal crossover (Fig. 4). If neither one of the two options is available, rehabilitation of the facial paralysis can be done with regional muscles and an adjunctive procedure for the eyelids.

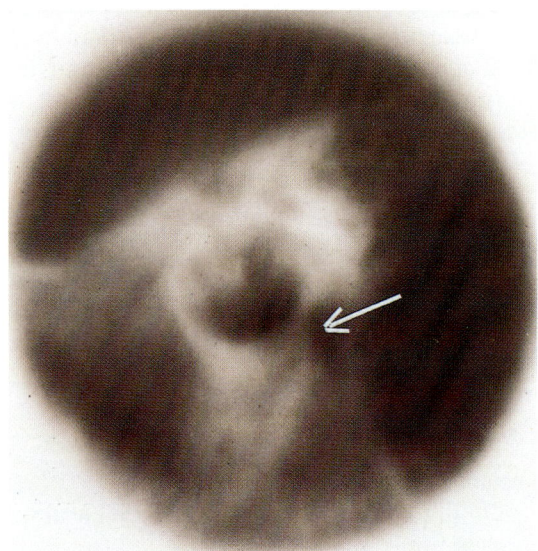

FIG. 2. Lateral temporal bone tomogram with erosion of fallopian canal.

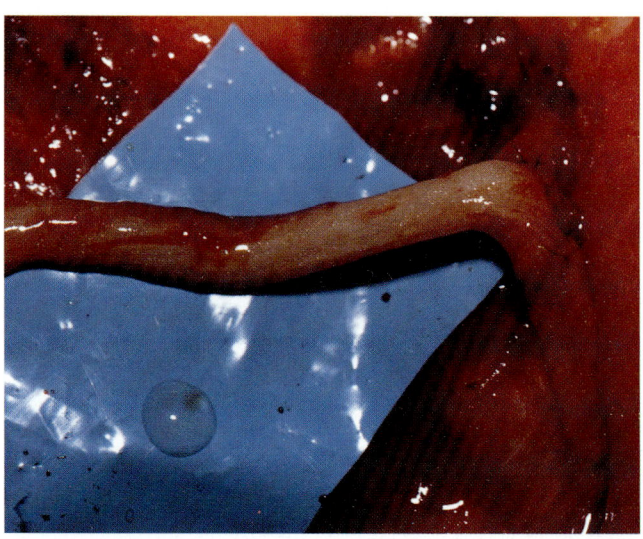

FIG. 3. Facial nerve graft from temporal bone to nerve's pes anserinus in right parotid region.

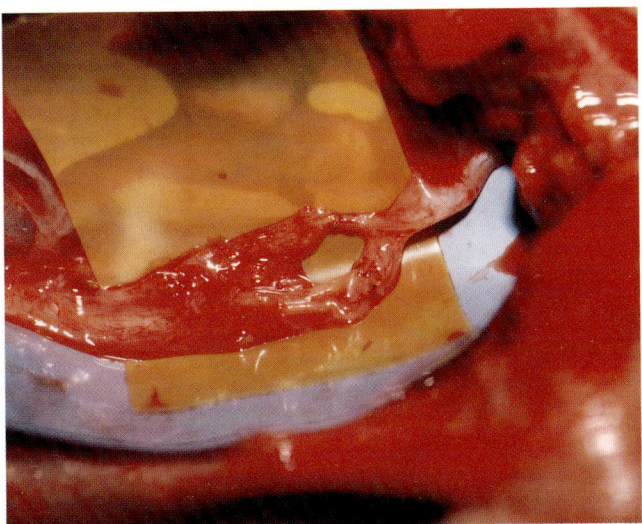

FIG. 4. Hypoglossal–facial nerve crossover demonstrating separate neurorrhaphies of hypoglossal nerve branches to upper and lower division of left facial nerve.

CASE PRESENTATIONS

Case 1. M.S. is a 24-year-old patient who underwent left parotidectomy for a suspected tumor. Cystic tumor was reportedly removed but facial nerve was not found during surgery. Postoperatively, she had a complete facial paralysis. Histology of the removed cyst revealed it to be a facial nerve neurilemoma. Since then, we have treated her with removal of the remaining tumor, necessitating a subtotal temporal bone resection and a nerve graft (Fig. 5A) placed over the rotated temporalis muscle. One year postoperatively she had House grade IV functioning in her left face (Fig. 5B).

Case 2. S.O. is a 27-year-old patient with complete left facial paralysis. CT scan revealed a destructive lesion of left temporal bone (Fig. 6A) involving the fallopian canal and jugular foramen.

Surgical exploration revealed tumor originating in the facial nerve (Fig. 6B). Following tumor resection, a nerve graft was used for facial nerve reconstruction from the internal auditory canal to the peripheral segment of the facial nerve (Fig. 6C).

Case 3. K.C. is a 30-year-old patient who developed isolated weakness of her left lower lip (Fig. 7A). The rest of her facial nerve function appeared clinically to be symmetrical with the other side.

Contrast enhanced CT revealed enhancing tumor involving the superior aspect of the left temporal bone and extending into the middle fossa (Fig. 7B).

Surgical exploration via low temporal craniotomy revealed an extradural tumor (Fig. 7C) that could be removed with preservation of the continuity of the facial nerve. Removed specimen had a multilobular appearance with origin at the geniculate ganglion (Fig. 7D). Postoperatively, this patient regained some function of the lower lip.

POSTOPERATIVE

In the postoperative period, the focus is usually on compensating for the ipsilateral facial paralysis. This involves eye protection as well as assistance with speech and swallowing. The wound care is identical to those of parotid, temporal bone, or posterior fossa surgical procedures.

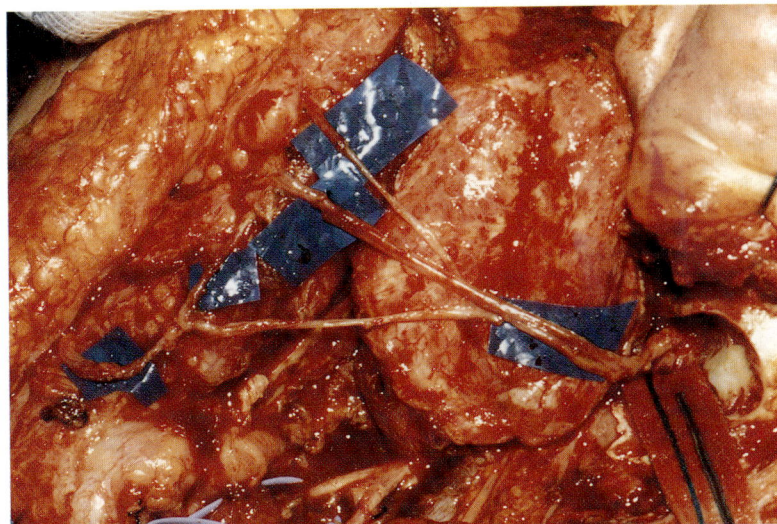
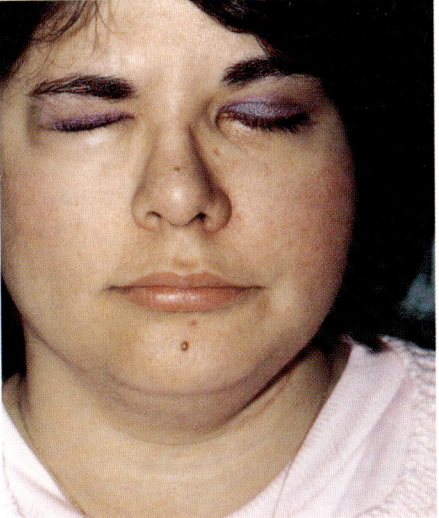

FIG. 5. A: Clinical photograph of left temporal and parotid region with facial nerve graft (greater auricular nerve) from the internal auditory canal to peripheral branches of the facial nerve coursing over transferred temporalis muscle. **B:** One year postoperative result with good eye closure and movement of oral commissure.

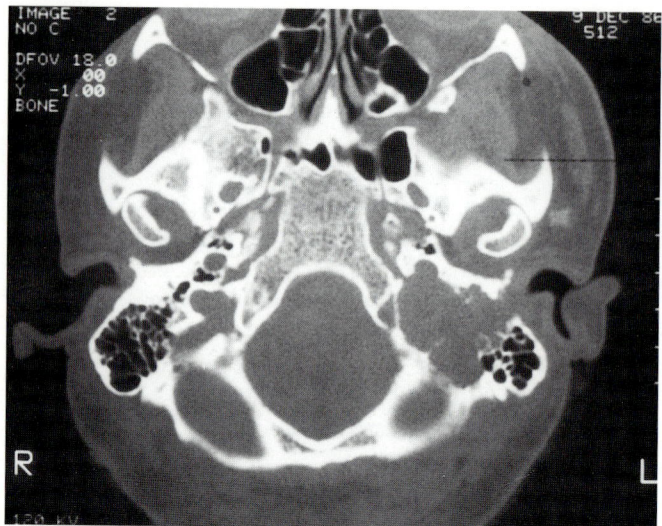
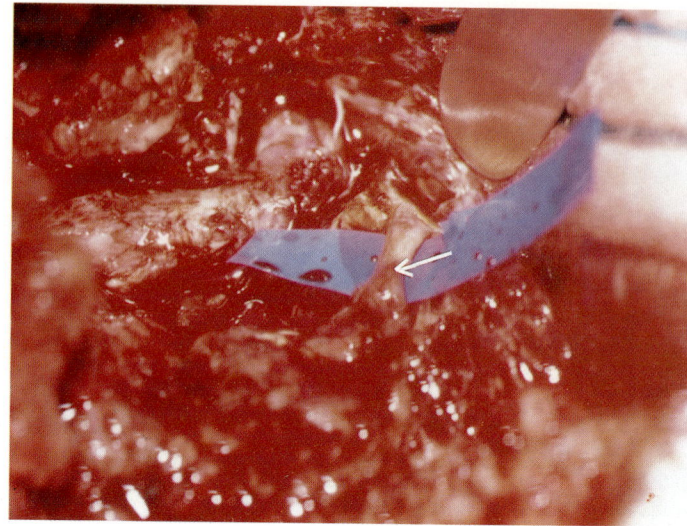
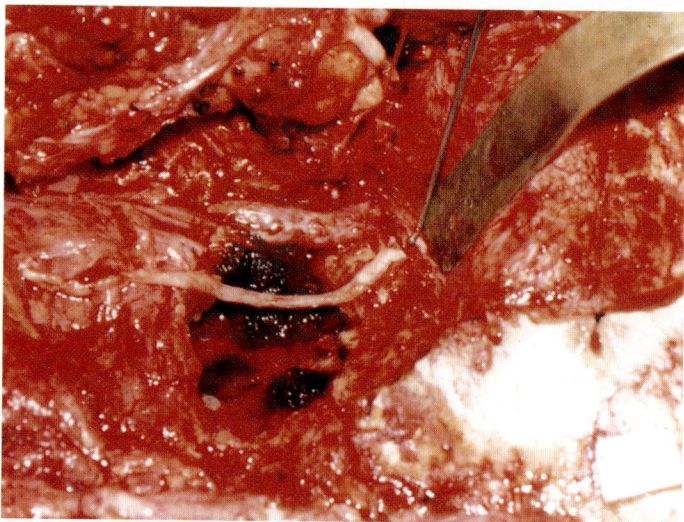

FIG. 6. A: Axial CT scan with bone algorithm demonstrating a destructive lesion of left temporal bone including fallopian canal and jugular foramen. **B:** Facial nerve neurilemoma involving the facial nerve up to the left geniculate ganglion. **C:** Nerve graft courses from internal auditory canal to facial nerve periphery.

COMPLICATIONS

Facial paralysis following removal of a facial nerve neurilemoma is an expected development and not a surgical complication. In posterior fossa and temporal bone facial nerve neurilemomas, the intraoperative focus should be to prevent injuries to other cranial nerves or the labyrinth.

FOLLOW-UP

Complete resection of a facial nerve neurilemoma results, in most cases, in a cure. The follow-up focuses on oncological concerns and the recovery of facial nerve function. It is anticipated that following a nerve graft (depending on the level of nerve transection) the facial nerve function should recover within 9–12 months. The degree of recovery varies with the level of nerve transection, the duration of preoperative paralysis, and the vascularity of the nerve graft recipient bed. The length of the nerve graft does not appear to significantly affect the duration or the quality of recovery. According to the broad grading of facial nerve recovery (House–Brackman), the quality of recovery falls in grades III–V with the majority of them in grade IV.

STATISTICS

Only a few authors have reported on a series of 20–30 facial neurilemomas. Most reports in the literature are on sporadic tumors.

1. *Statistically significant correlations.* Tumor resection with free margins equals the best tumor-free follow-up.
2. *"Better trend" but no statistical significance.* When we compared the duration of preoperative facial weakness with postoperative recovery of facial nerve function,

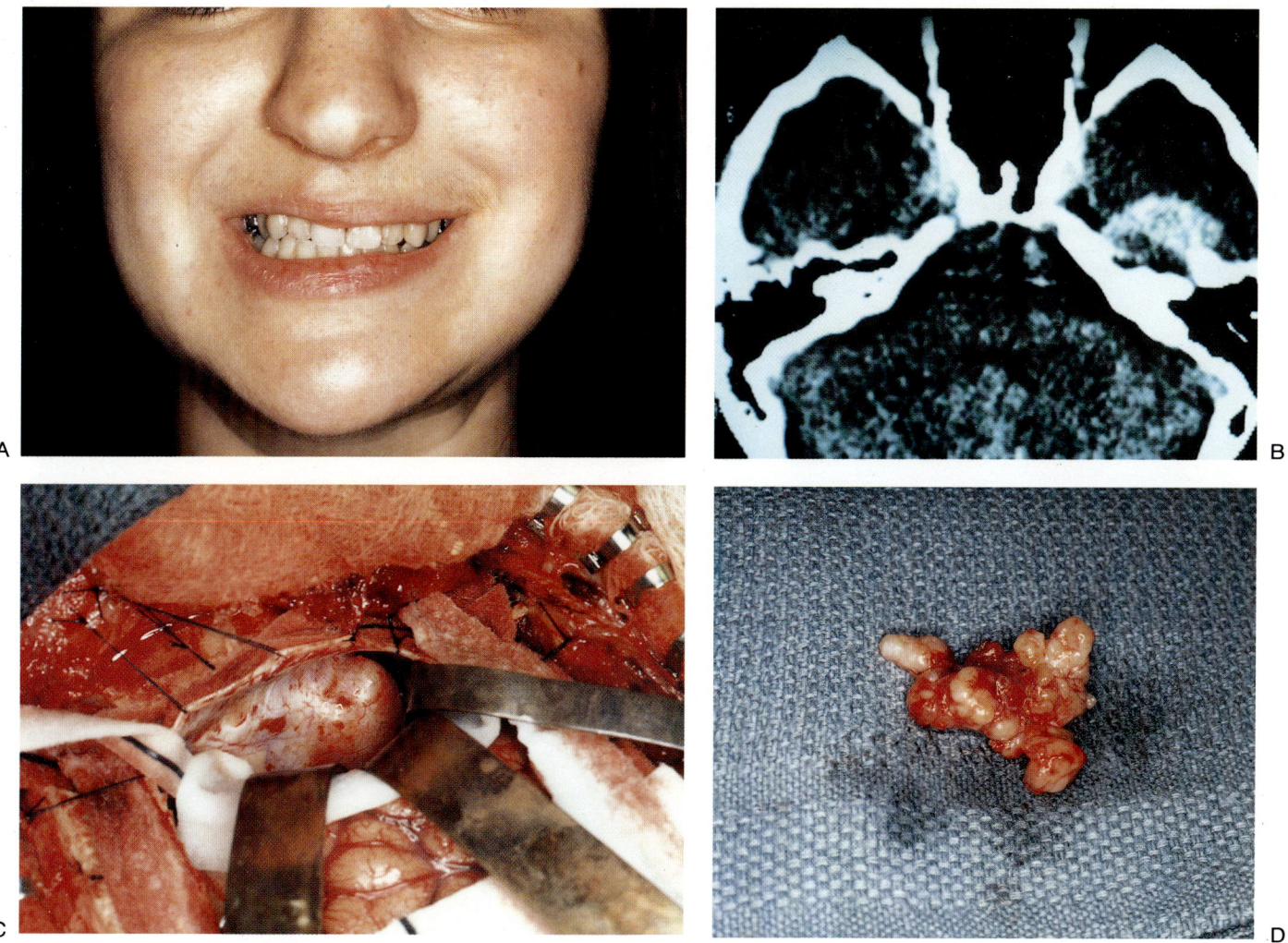

FIG. 7. A: Clinical photograph of a patient with asymmetry of lower lips secondary to left lower lip weakness. **B:** Axial CT with contrast demonstrating an enhancing mass in left middle fossa with erosion of the superior aspect of temporal bone. **C:** Intraoperative view of the floor of the left temporal fossa with an extradural bulging tumor. **D:** Surgical specimen of multilobulated neurilemoma, which originated at the geniculate ganglion of the left facial nerve.

we found that a shorter preoperative facial paralysis indicates a better function recovery. Preoperative facial paralysis is predominant (+80%) in intratemporal tumors. Both intracranial and extratemporal tumors rarely present with facial paralysis. They demonstrate neurootological as well parotid mass symptomatology, respectively. The average duration of preoperative symptomatology is 2 years.

3. *No statistical significance.* The length of the facial nerve graft has no significant bearing on the potential recovery of facial nerve function. Here the major obstacle to facial nerve recovery with nerve graft is the need to overcome two neurorrhaphies with each graft. Once the proximal neurorrhaphy is overcome, the segment of the nerve graft should easily be transgressed by the growing axons, providing it has become vascularized. The second hurdle then comes at the distal neurorrhaphy.

RECOMMENDATIONS

1. Minimal asymptomatic facial nerve neurilemomas may be observed with careful follow-up with MRI and CT scans.
2. Treatment of facial nerve neurilemomas consists of surgical resection with frozen section for verification of tumor-free margins and then a nerve graft (great auricular or sural nerve).
3. Microsurgical techniques should be used.
4. Recovery is expected in most patients. However, the quality of recovery will likely range from House grade III to grade V.

SUGGESTED READING

1. Dort JC, Fisch U. Facial nerve schwannomas. *Skull Base Surg* 1991;1(1):51–56.

2. Janecka IP, Conley J. Primary neoplasms of the facial nerve. *Plast Reconstr Surg* 1987;79:177.
3. Conley J, Janecka IP. Schwann cell tumors of the facial nerve. *Laryngoscope* 1974;84:958–962.
4. Pulec J. Facial nerve tumors. *Ann Otol Rhinol Laryngol* 1969;78:962–982.
5. Nelson RA, House WF. Facial nerve neuroma in the posterior fossa: surgical considerations. In: Graham MD, House WF, eds. *Disorders of the facial nerve.* New York: Raven Press, 1982;403–406.
6. Burres S, Fisch U. The comparison of facial grading systems. *Arch Otolaryngol Head Neck Surg* 1986;112:755–758.
7. May M. *The facial nerve.* New York: Thieme, 1986.
8. Jackson CG, Glassrock M, Hughes G, Sismanis A. Facial paralysis of neoplastic origin: diagnosis and management. *Laryngoscope* 1980;90:1581–1595.
9. Neely JG, Nebett CR. Differential facial nerve function in tumors of the internal auditory meatus. *Ann Otol Rhinol Laryngol* 1983;92:39–41.
10. Horn K, Crumley R, Schindler R. Facial neurilemmomas. *Laryngoscope* 1987;91:1326–1331.
11. Conley J, Baker DC. Hypoglossal–facial anastomosis for reinnervation of the paralyzed face. *Plast Reconstr Surg* 1979;63:63–72.

CHAPTER 45

Jugular Foramen Neurilemoma

Sam E. Kinney

The jugular foramen neurilemoma is a rare tumor of the skull base. A review of the literature by Maniglia et al. (1) in 1979 reported 56 cases. In 1984, Kaye et al. (2) reported 13 cases operated at the Cleveland Clinic Foundation. Smaller series have been reported that confirm the jugular foramen neurilemoma is an unusual skull base tumor (3–6). It would be unusual for a skull base surgery center to treat more than one or two of these cases per year.

The patient usually presents with a unilateral lesion of cranial nerves IX, X, or XI or a combination of the three nerves. Occasionally, the patient will present with a retrocochlear finding similar to a cerebellopontine angle tumor, such as an acoustic neuroma or meningioma. The patients do not have pulsatile tinnitus, which is commonly seen with glomus jugulare tumors.

The physical examination includes a complete head and neck evaluation and neurologic evaluation of the cranial nerves. One patient in the Cleveland Clinic series had been treated for 2 years by an orthopedic surgeon for severe shoulder pain. The patient was found to have paralysis of cranial nerve (CN) IX from a jugular foramen neurilemoma. The pain was similar to that described by patients following CN IX sacrifice during a radical neck dissection.

The diagnosis is made from an imaging study, either high resolution CT scan with bone algorithm or a MRI scan. The CT scan usually demonstrates a smooth edged enlargement of the jugular foramen, with extension inferiorly into the neck, posteriorly into the posterior fossa, or directly into the skull base, usually the clivus. MRI scans will show a mass lesion similar to the CT scan. Digital subtraction angiography (DSA) may be useful for a differential diagnosis. The DSA scan may show an external compression of the jugular vein, in contrast to the intraluminal involvement seen in glomus jugulare tumors. The internal carotid artery may be displaced anteriorly on the angiogram. The carotid is more likely to be displaced by a neurilemoma, while a glomus tumor may surround the carotid artery. The vascular blush seen on angiogram will be much less prominent with a neurilemoma, as opposed to a glomus tumor. The neurilemoma will have fewer major feeding blood vessels than the glomus tumor. The glomus tumor has a 10% incidence of multiple tumor sites. The neurilemoma is unlikely to be multicentric; however, a patient with neurofibromatosis may develop a lesion associated with CNs IX, X, and XI.

As noted by Kaye et al. (2), the jugular foramen neurilemoma can be categorized into types A, B, and C, depending on its growth pattern. The type A tumor presents with primary involvement of the posterior fossa, as shown in Fig. 1. The type B tumor remains confined to the skull base, often with extension into the soft center of the clivus (Fig. 2). The type C tumor begins in the jugular foramen and extends inferiorly below the skull base (Fig. 3). It is felt that the presentation of the tumor is determined by the point of origin of the tumor from the cranial nerve as it passes into the skull base, along the jugular vein, or passes through the pars nervosa compartment of the jugular foramen, or directly from the nerve in the posterior fossa.

The decision to recommend surgery to a patient with a jugular foramen neurilemoma is similar to that made with other benign lesions of the skull base. Little is known about the natural history of the growth of this rare tumor. Similar to glomus tumors, the patient could anticipate losing more cranial nerve function as the tumor grows. The major problem with an unoperated tumor would be the mass effect of the tumor in the posterior fossa.

Age and general medical health would be important factors in a recommendation to offer surgical treatment. There is most often either temporary or permanent addi-

---

S. E. Kinney: Section of Otology and Neurotology, Department of Otolaryngology, Cleveland Clinic Foundation, Cleveland, Ohio 44195-5034.

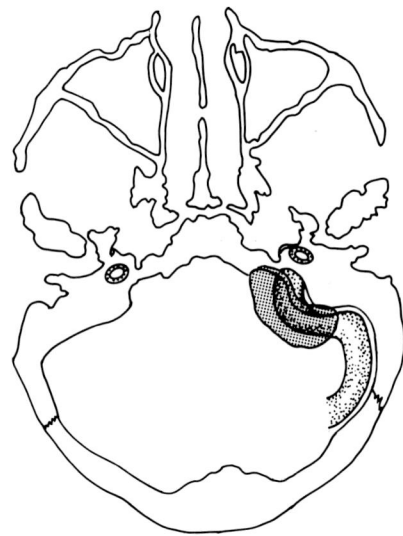

FIG. 1. Type A tumor. Note primary involvement of the posterior fossa.

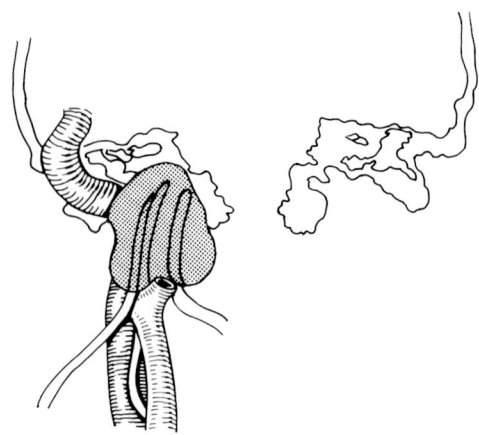

FIG. 3. Type C tumor, coronal view. Note extension of tumor inferiorly into the neck.

tional cranial nerve deficits with surgery. Older patients and patients with other medical problems do not tolerate the rapid change in cranial nerve function that often accompanies surgical removal of a jugular foramen neurilemoma. In general, surgery is not recommended for those lesions in patients over 65 years of age.

OPERATIVE TECHNIQUE

Anesthetic requirements for surgery of a jugular foramen neurilemoma are not unlike any major head and neck procedure with the patient in the supine position. General endotracheal anesthesia is used with appropriate monitoring techniques. This usually includes a central venous pressure line and an arterial line. The arterial line may not be as important in a jugular foramen neurilemoma as with a glomus tumor, where rapid blood loss may be encountered. Recently, the addition of a facial nerve monitor has been helpful in preserving facial nerve function in those cases where the facial nerve must be transposed to gain exposure.

The patient is placed on the operating room table in a supine position, with the head rotated away from the affected side. The surgery requires the expertise of an otologic surgeon, a head and neck surgeon, and a neurosurgeon. For this reason, the patient is placed on the table backward, as for ear surgery, which allows the surgeons to work in either the sitting or standing mode. This also allows access to the operating room table controls, so that the patient may be rotated as needed for exposure. The scalp is shaved to allow for a wide postauricular incision and possible posterior fossa craniotomy. The skin preparation is standard; the drapes are sutured or stapled into position to allow for exposure of the head, face, occiput, and the entire neck. It is useful to include a large craniotomy irrigation collection drape. During the otologic portion of the procedure, large quantities of irrigating fluid are used.

Intraoperative antibiotics are generally not used unless there is a large portion of tumor in the posterior fossa. In these cases, an antibiotic is given preoperatively, intraoperatively, and 48 hr postoperatively that will cross the blood–brain barrier.

The surgery is performed in three phases. The head and neck surgeon will make the incision and expose the high cervical region of the neck. The great vessels are identified and controlled with umbilical tapes. Cranial nerves IX, X, XI, and XII are identified and followed to the skull base. The otologic surgeon defines the structures of the temporal bone and develops the superior aspect of the tumor in the skull base. The neurosurgeon

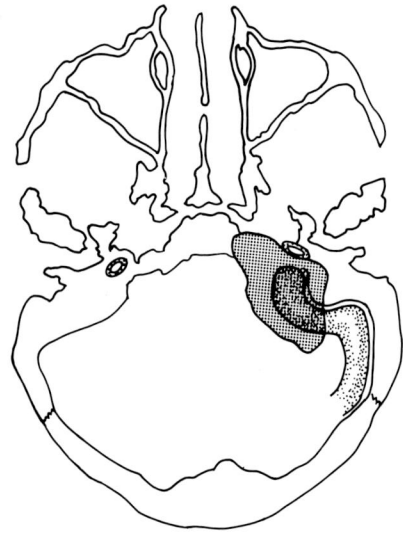

FIG. 2. Type B tumor. Primary involvement is in the skull base with extension into the clivus.

may open the dura of the posterior fossa to expose the intracranial portion of the tumor. If the tumor is very large, both in the skull base and intracranially, a decision may be made to remove the tumor in two stages. The skull base portion is removed first to the posterior fossa dura. At some later date the posterior fossa portion is removed with a separate craniotomy.

The incision is a wide postauricular incision, approximately four finger widths behind the auricle (Fig. 4). The superior limb is kept fairly high to preserve the blood supply to the auricle. The inferior incision is made along the anterior border of the sternocleidomastoid muscle to expose the structures of the neck. The flap is elevated across the mastoid to the external auditory canal. The posterior canal skin is elevated and transected close to the annulus. The anterior canal is transected at the bony cartilaginous junction. This stepwise canal cut helps prevent stenosis of the canal postoperatively. The flap is elevated forward over the parotid gland.

The common carotid artery, its bifurcation, and the external and internal branches are isolated. Cranial nerves IX, X, XI, and XII are identified and traced up to the skull base. The sternocleidomastoid muscle is detached from the mastoid tip, and the posterior belly of the digastric muscle is detached. The digastric muscle may be rotated forward or elevated with the facial nerve and the contents of the stylomastoid foramen. The facial nerve is identified at the stylomastoid foramen and traced to its bifurcation in the parotid gland.

The otologist now begins the exposure of the superior aspect of the tumor. Figure 5 shows the relationship of the facial nerve to a jugular foramen tumor. The otologist must decide how to gain access to the tumor, with the least risk to facial nerve function. If the tumor is a type C, the top of the tumor may be identified by working around the nerve in its normal anatomic position. If the tumor does not extend into the internal auditory canal, the facial nerve may be elevated out of the stylomastoid foramen and rerouted around the skeletonized external auditory canal, as shown in Fig. 6. In this manner, the external auditory canal and middle ear transformer mechanism may be preserved.

If the tumor is a type B, with involvement of the petrous apex and clivus, the facial nerve must be elevated to the geniculate ganglion and rerouted anteriorly (Fig. 7), in order to gain access to the superior limit of the tumor. This necessitates the removal of the external auditory canal and middle ear transformer. If the tumor also extends intracranially, the conductive mechanism may need to be sacrificed in order to prevent a cerebral spinal

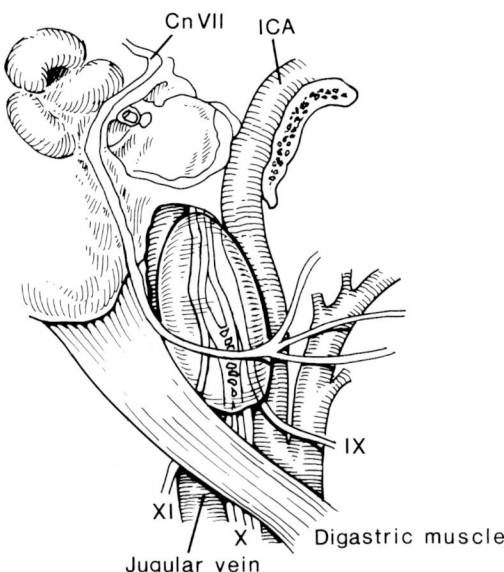

FIG. 5. The normal position of the facial nerve crosses over the tumor, limiting exposure.

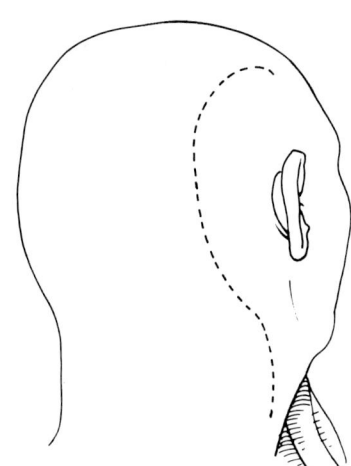

FIG. 4. Incision for combined head and neck, otologic, and neurosurgical removal of jugular foramen tumor.

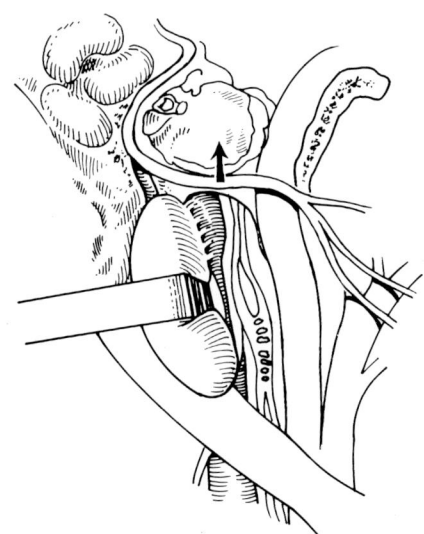

FIG. 6. The facial nerve has been rotated around the external auditory canal to expose the top of the tumor.

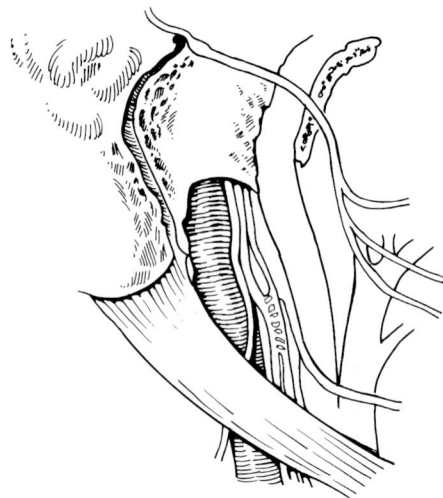

FIG. 7. The facial nerve has been rerouted anteriorly from the geniculate ganglion. Note the external canal and middle ear transformer has been removed.

fluid leak. In this case, the external auditory canal is closed, and the eustachian tube is plugged with muscle or removed surgically.

The external auditory canal is best closed by dissecting the canal skin from the cartilage in a medial to lateral direction. The cartilage of the ear canal is trimmed flush to the concha. The sleeve of canal skin is everted out at the meatus and oversewn externally. In this manner, all squamous epithelium is exteriorized.

A complete mastoidectomy is performed and the facial nerve identified. The mastoid tip is removed, and all bone lateral to the facial nerve and inferior to the external canal is removed. If the facial nerve is to be elevated from the stylomastoid foramen, a 180° decompression of the nerve is accomplished to the first genu. The elevation of the nerve can be accomplished without creating paresis if a facial nerve monitor is used and care is taken to completely decompress the nerve before attempting elevation.

After rotation of the facial nerve, the sigmoid sinus is followed to the jugular bulb. The sigmoid sinus and jugular vein may be preserved; however, in some cases, the sigmoid sinus must be occluded, and the jugular vein tied. The sigmoid sinus may be sutured using a neurosurgical pass-through needle or by external and internal packing with Surgicel gauze.

The bone of the skull base over the jugular foramen and carotid artery must be removed. All soft tissue over the jugular vein and carotid artery must be removed. In this manner, the otologic dissection and the head and neck dissection are joined.

At this point, the tumor can be identified in the jugular foramen. A biopsy may be taken to confirm the diagnosis. As with other forms of neurilemoma, tumor removal is performed by debulking the center of the tumor and then removing the capsule. This is unlike the procedure for a glomus tumor, where the dissection is best performed in an extracapsular dissection.

The most important feature of the removal of the jugular foramen neurilemoma, or any skull base tumor, is to have constant control of the internal carotid artery. As shown in Fig. 6, the carotid artery is followed from the neck into the skull base. The tumor is then rotated posteriorly off the carotid artery, cranial nerves, and jugular bulb.

It is a goal of this surgery to try to leave cranial nerve function intact. Clearly, the nerve of origin will be resected as the tumor is removed. The space where CNs IX, X, and XI pass through the pars nervosa becomes very tight, and injury to all three nerves at this point is possible. The widest possible exposure of the jugular foramen and careful dissection of the vessels and nerves into the skull base give the best chance of preservation of these nerves.

In a type B tumor, once the inside of the tumor has been debulked, the tumor capsule will direct the medial dissection. It is helpful to have the CT scans in view of the surgeon, as well as a dry skull in the operating room for reference. The capsule is removed easily and leaves a smooth surface in the skull base. The tumor may elevate the dura of the middle fossa, but it rarely traverses this dura. The tumor may elevate the dura of the posterior fossa, but it may also penetrate the dura, usually through the pars nervosa.

If there is a limited extension of the tumor into the posterior fossa, the neurosurgical service may elect to open the dura posterior to the sigmoid sinus, as seen in Fig. 8. The craniotomy bone removal is accomplished starting at the sigmoid sinus and working posteriorly.

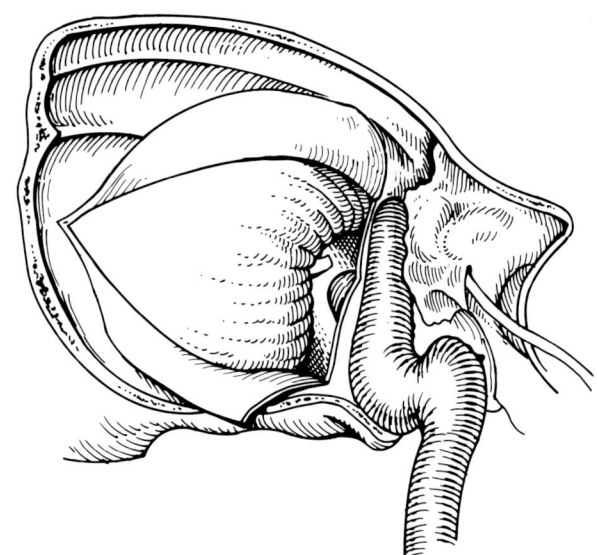

FIG. 8. Posterior fossa retrosigmoid exposure of intracranial portion of the tumor.

The dura is opened, and the cerebellum is gently retracted to expose the intracranial portion of the tumor.

After the intracranial portion of the tumor is removed, care must be taken to obtain a watertight seal to prevent cerebral spinal fluid leakage. Direct suture closure is most effective if possible. This can be supplemented by a fascia graft or lyophilized dural graft. If the eustachian tube has been blocked, and the external canal closed, autologous abdominal fat may be used to obliterate a dural defect. The closure may be supplemented with control of cerebral spinal fluid pressure with a temporary lumbar cerebral spinal fluid drain.

The wound is closed in layers, and suction drains are placed in the neck. Care must be taken not to create a CSF leak with the suction catheters. If the external auditory canal is retained, it must have the edges reapproximated and stented for 7–10 days to prevent stenosis.

The postoperative management of the patient with a jugular foramen neurilemoma is complicated by cranial nerve deficits. A patient may have compensated for a preexisting cranial nerve deficit before surgery; however, the postoperative swelling of the area may break down the level of compensation acutely. A nasogastric tube may be used to control secretions. Careful intensive care nursing may be necessary to suction secretions and maintain the airway. Occasionally, a patient may need to be reintubated, or a tracheotomy may need to be performed. The patient must be monitored carefully for a CSF leak, for this complication may lead to a life-threatening infection. If a lumbar spinal fluid drain is used, the patient should be kept in a neurosurgical intensive care unit until the drain is removed.

Swallowing may need to be retrained with the help of a speech pathologist or other swallowing therapist. If glottic incompetence complicates swallowing or allows aspiration, a vocal cord injection may be performed. The injection material used, Gelfoam, glycerin, or Teflon, will be determined by the expectation of return of vocal cord function.

Fourteen cases of jugular foramen neurilemoma have been managed by the Otolaryngology and Neurosurgery Departments of the Cleveland Clinic Foundation since 1976. There was a nearly equal distribution of male and female patients, with an average age of 43 years. The type A tumors presented with retrocochlear findings of hearing loss, vertigo, or ataxia. The type B and C tumors more frequently presented with involvement of cranial nerves IX, X, and XI.

Five tumors were removed entirely by a posterior fossa craniotomy. Six tumors were removed using a combined infralabyrinthine–posterior fossa approach, and four tumors were removed by the infralabyrinthine approach alone.

All patients experienced some swallowing difficulty postoperatively; however, only six required injection of the vocal cord. Four patients had a transient weakness of the facial nerve. One patient developed a CSF collection under the flap, but there were no cases of meningitis and no operative mortality. All patients were able to return to their presurgery lifestyle. One patient was operated at the Cleveland Clinic Foundation for a recurrence of tumor. At this writing, no patients operated in this series have had a recurrence of tumor.

SUMMARY

A jugular foramen neurilemoma is a rare tumor of the skull base. The patient presents with the symptoms of involvement of CNs IX, X, and XI or with retrocochlear CN VIII findings. The diagnosis is made using imaging and angiography techniques.

The treatment of the lesion is surgical, with a good prognosis for total tumor removal, and return to usual life activities. There is a high incidence of transient or permanent involvement of the cranial nerves of the jugular foramen.

REFERENCES

1. Maniglia A, Chandler J, Goodwin W, Parker J. Schwannomas of the parapharyngeal space and jugular foramen. *Laryngoscope* 1979;89:1405–1414.
2. Kaye A, Hahn J, Kinney S, Hardy R, Bay J. Jugular foramen schwannomas. *J Neurosurg* 1984;60:1045–1053.
3. Clemis J. Neurogenic tumors of the skull base. *Otolaryngol Head Neck Surg* 1980;88:511–518.
4. Call W, Pulec J. Neurilemmoma of the jugular foramen, transmastoid removal. *Ann Oto Rhinol Laryngol* 1978;87:313–317.
5. Crumley R, Wilson C. Schwannomas of the jugular foramen. *Laryngoscope* 1984;94:772–778.
6. Horn K, House W, Hitselberger W. Schwannomas of the jugular foramen. *Laryngoscope* 1985;95:761–765.

CHAPTER 46

Trigeminal Neurilemoma

Ian F. Pollack and Laligam N. Sekhar

Neurilemomas of the trigeminal nerve account for approximately 0.2% of intracranial tumors and 2% of intracranial neurilemomas. These tumors can originate in any section of the fifth cranial nerve from the root to the distal extracranial branches; as a result, a variety of symptoms and signs may develop, depending on the direction and extent of tumor growth. Accordingly, the operative approaches necessary to remove these lesions also vary significantly. Neurilemomas arising from the trigeminal ganglion can remain localized to the middle fossa and present solely with symptoms of trigeminal dysfunction, although, more commonly, these lesions extend along the course of the nerve into the posterior fossa and/or the cavernous sinus and extracranial structures. Neurilemomas arising from the trigeminal root often remain strictly infratentorial and present as a cerebellopontine angle mass. Tumors originating from the intracranial branches of the trigeminal nerve commonly present a diagnostic dilemma, growing extracranially through the superior orbital fissure, foramen rotundum, or foramen ovale, and manifesting as an orbital, paranasal sinus, or nasopharyngeal mass with only subtle associated neurological deficits.

DIAGNOSTIC CONSIDERATIONS

Fifty percent of all intracranial trigeminal neurilemomas arise from the trigeminal ganglion and remain predominantly localized to the middle fossa. Patients typically complain of pain and/or paresthesias in a trigeminal nerve distribution, which may spread from one to all three divisions of the nerve, often followed by progressive sensory loss and, less commonly, by atrophy of the masticatory muscles. Although loss of a corneal reflex is not uncommon, total trigeminal anesthesia and severe masticatory muscle wasting are more typical of a malignant process than a benign neurilemoma. The fact that, on presentation, 15% of patients with middle fossa neurilemomas have no objective evidence of trigeminal dysfunction is explained by displacement, rather than actual destruction, of trigeminal nerve fibers by tumor. Involvement of the cavernous sinus, manifested by impairment of third, fourth, and, less commonly, sixth nerve function is seen in 25% of patients. Proptosis resulting from rostral extension of tumor into the superior orbital fissure and unilateral visual loss from compression of the optic nerve in the optic foramen also are occasionally seen.

Approximately 20% of intracranial trigeminal neurilemomas arise from the trigeminal root and remain primarily infratentorial. These lesions commonly present with a combination of ataxia, hearing loss, tinnitus, nystagmus, and facial nerve dysfunction. Although facial pain was once felt to be uncommon with infratentorial trigeminal neurilemomas, in our own experience and in several other recent series, atypical trigeminal neuralgia has been a fairly frequent presenting symptom. Lower cranial nerve palsies and signs of increased intracranial pressure are found in about 30–50% of patients. Pyramidal tract signs are seen in 30–40% of patients and frequently are ipsilateral, presumably resulting from compression of the cerebral peduncle against the contralateral tentorial edge by slowly growing tumor.

"Hourglass" tumors arising from the trigeminal ganglion or distal roots and growing both above and below the tentorium account for 25% of all intracranial trigeminal neurilemomas. These lesions produce an often confusing combination of clinical findings, reflecting involvement of supratentorial and infratentorial struc-

---

I. F. Pollack: Department of Neurosurgery, University of Pittsburgh School of Medicine, Presbyterian University Hospital, Pittsburgh, Pennsylvania 15213.
L. N. Sekhar: Department of Neurosurgery, Center for Cranial Base Surgery, University of Pittsburgh School of Medicine, and Presbyterian University Hospital, Pittsburgh, Pennsylvania 15213.

tures. Long tract signs are particularly common, owing to the presence of brain stem compression at the tentorial hiatus.

In a small subgroup of patients, neurilemomas arise from the distal intracranial branches of the fifth nerve and extend extracranially, often exhibiting signs of extracranial mass effect. These lesions most commonly originate from the ophthalmic division of the nerve (owing to the comparatively long intracranial course of V_1) and present with proptosis and oculomotor palsies with or without visual loss. Maxillary and mandibular division lesions, which grow into the pterygopalatine fossa, sphenoid sinus, or nasopharynx, may produce nasal obstruction, chronic serous otitis media, and hearing loss from eustachian tube obstruction with relatively mild associated neurological deficits.

Another small subgroup of patients have tumors that arise from the extracranial branches of the fifth nerve, progressively erode the skull base, and subsequently extend intracranially. Although this pattern of growth is most typically seen with orbital neurilemomas, which present with a combination of oculomotor paralysis, proptosis, and visual loss, intracranial extension of neurilemomas arising in the infratemporal fossa also has been described.

At present, the imaging modalities of choice for delineating the location and extent of these lesions are computed tomography (CT) and magnetic resonance imaging (MRI). On CT, trigeminal neurilemomas are usually isodense or slightly hyperdense in comparison to surrounding brain and enhance homogeneously after administration of intravenous contrast medium. Although this appearance superficially resembles that of a meningioma, bone erosion rather than hyperostosis generally is seen with a trigeminal neurilemoma. Rarely, trigeminal neurilemomas are hypodense with irregular or ring enhancement, resembling a malignant glioma, metastatic tumor, or abscess.

The improved resolution in the region of the petrous bone and the ease of multiplanar reconstruction make MRI an invaluable adjunctive study in evaluating and following patients. Neurilemomas generally appear well circumscribed and, in comparison to surrounding brain, show decreased signal intensity on T1-weighted images, increased signal on T2-weighted images, and homogeneous enhancement after the administration of gadolinium.

In patients with large lesions, angiography is useful for demonstrating vascular displacement. Additionally, a balloon test occlusion of the ipsilateral internal carotid artery (ICA) provides valuable information in patients with tumors near the ICA. During test occlusion, cerebral blood flow is measured and serial neurologic examinations are performed to assess the adequacy of collateral circulation in the event that temporary or permanent ICA occlusion is required intraoperatively.

PATIENT SELECTION

Since trigeminal neurilemomas displace rather than invade adjacent structures, tumor removal can generally be accomplished without significant permanent neurological injury provided an appropriate operative approach is chosen. In elderly patients and those with severe medical problems that would make a lengthy intracranial procedure unduly hazardous and who have severe, progressive neurological deterioration resulting from tumor growth, intracapsular debulking of the tumor may provide several years of symptom-free survival. The value of adjunctive radiotherapy for such patients has not been adequately determined.

OPERATIVE TECHNIQUE

In recent years, improvements in imaging techniques have led to earlier detection of these tumors while they are still relatively small and before they have caused significant neurological impairment. This factor and the widespread use of the operative microscope and neurophysiological monitoring techniques have contributed to an overall improvement in postoperative outcome among patients with trigeminal neurilemomas. In most recent reports, the major factors that have led to incomplete tumor removal have been involvement of the cavernous sinus, adherence of tumor to the ICA, and inadequate exposure. With an adequate preoperative evaluation and a suitable operative approach, however, none of these factors should categorically rule out the possibility of complete excision. In view of the high rate of symptomatic regrowth of tumor in patients with incompletely resected trigeminal neurilemomas, we have favored a more aggressive stance toward the management of these lesions during the last several years.

At our institution, these procedures are performed under endotracheal inhalation anesthesia. For extradural infratemporal fossa procedures, a lumbar catheter is placed for intraoperative cerebrospinal fluid (CSF) drainage. For intradural procedures, CSF drainage is accomplished by opening the basal cisterns. In general, furosemide, 40 mg, and/or mannitol, 50 mg, are administered before exposing dura.

Intraoperative monitoring of brain stem auditory evoked potentials and often somatosensory evoked potentials are routinely employed. When clinically indicated, third, fourth, sixth, and seventh nerve functions are also monitored by electromyography of the extraocular and facial muscles.

The surgical approach to these tumors depends on the location of the neurilemoma and the direction and extent of tumor spread. Tumors that are predominantly supratentorial or infratentorial can virtually always be excised using a single approach. Lesions arising from the trigeminal root that are predominantly infratentorial are removed via a retromastoid craniectomy and paracerebellar approach. Likewise, smaller (<3 cm) middle fossa lesions are best managed by a temporal or frontotemporal craniotomy and subtemporal approach.

In patients with large hourglass neurilemomas extending above and below the tentorium, both supratentorial and infratentorial procedures, performed in either one or two stages, should be employed to achieve total tumor resection. With meticulous microsurgical dissection, trigeminal sensation and motor function often can be partially preserved. Because the trigeminal nerve lies in the lateral wall of the cavernous sinus, a large hourglass neurilemoma may extend into the sinus and must be dissected medially from the intracavernous ICA and the abducens nerve in order to achieve a total excision. In such patients, a preoperative balloon occlusion study is needed to determine whether the patient will tolerate carotid occlusion should this prove necessary. In tumors with a large intracavernous component, proximal and distal control of the ICA should be obtained before the intracavernous tumor is exposed. To minimize the risk of injury to the third and fourth cranial nerves, the dura overlying the intracavernous tumor is opened well beneath these nerves. With these precautions, the tumor generally can be dissected from the wall of the cavernous sinus with minimal morbidity.

Trigeminal branch neurilemomas extending into the orbit, pterygopalatine fossa, and infratemporal fossa frequently require a combined intracranial and extracranial approach performed by a surgical team consisting of a neurosurgeon working in conjunction with an otolaryngologist, an ophthalmologist, and/or a plastic surgeon. Despite the often large size of these lesions, complete excision frequently can be achieved.

COMPLICATIONS AND THEIR MANAGEMENT

The principal complications resulting from attempted excision of these tumors consist of injury to the fifth cranial nerve as well as adjacent nerves. In our own experience, such deficits are frequently partial and transient; not uncommonly, fifth nerve function actually improves after surgery. Postoperative CSF leakage is most often encountered with large trigeminal branch lesions that have required combined intracranial and extracranial approaches. The incidence of this complication can be minimized by reconstructing the skull base with bone, fascia, muscle, and pericranial tissue, as needed, and obtaining a "watertight" dural closure; if a leak does develop, serial lumbar punctures or lumbar drainage and head elevation are almost uniformly effective in stopping the leak. If, however, the leak persists, reexploration is required. More serious complications such as injury to the cerebellum or temporal lobe from excessive retraction and damage to the ICA in a situation where inadequate proximal and distal exposure of the vessel and no preoperative assessment of collateral flow have been obtained can be minimized by obtaining adequate exposure and by performing a thorough preoperative evaluation.

ILLUSTRATIVE CASES

Case 1: Hourglass Neurilemoma

This 31-year-old male presented with a 4-month history of progressive right facial numbness, dysphagia, dysarthria, right-hand paresthesias, left upper extremity weakness and dysmetria, and gait ataxia. Examination showed diminished sensation in the right V_2 and V_3 distributions, a right peripheral seventh nerve paresis, bilateral (right greater than left) end-gaze nystagmus, left upper extremity monoparesis, prominent hyperreflexia with sustained ankle clonus and bilateral extensor plantar responses, spasticity of gait, and a positive Romberg sign. CT scan showed a large, hypodense, uniformly enhancing hourglass-shaped lesion arising from and eroding the petrous apex and extending rostrally to the region of the suprasellar cistern and caudally through the tentorial hiatus into the posterior fossa. MRI confirmed these findings and clearly demonstrated invasion of the cavernous sinus and compression of the adjacent brain stem (Fig. 1). Angiography showed a relatively avascular mass lesion with small feeding vessels arising from the meningohypophyseal branch of the ICA and the ascending pharyngeal branch of the external carotid artery. Balloon occlusion of the right ICA was well tolerated. Because of the large size and considerable extent of the patient's neurilemoma, the tumor was removed in a staged fashion. Initially, the infratentorial component was excised via a retromastoid, paracerebellar approach (Fig. 2). One week later, the supratentorial portion of the tumor was exposed through a right frontotemporal craniotomy with a transsylvian–subtemporal approach (Fig. 3A, B). Upon retracting the temporal lobe, the tumor was seen to extend extradurally along the middle fossa floor into the lateral wall of the cavernous sinus. The tumor capsule was incised in a cruciate fashion well beneath the third and fourth cranial nerves (Fig. 3C). Tumor from within the cavernous sinus and beneath the temporal lobe was then completely removed (Fig. 3D). Caudally, tumor extending through Meckel's cave and the tentorial hiatus into the posterior fossa was exposed by dividing the tentorium from Meckel's cave backward toward the superior petrosal sinus. Tumor was then carefully dissected off the brain stem. Although several fascicles of the fifth nerve were sacrificed during the tumor removal, the bulk of the nerve remained intact. Complete tumor resection was achieved. Postoperatively, the patient had

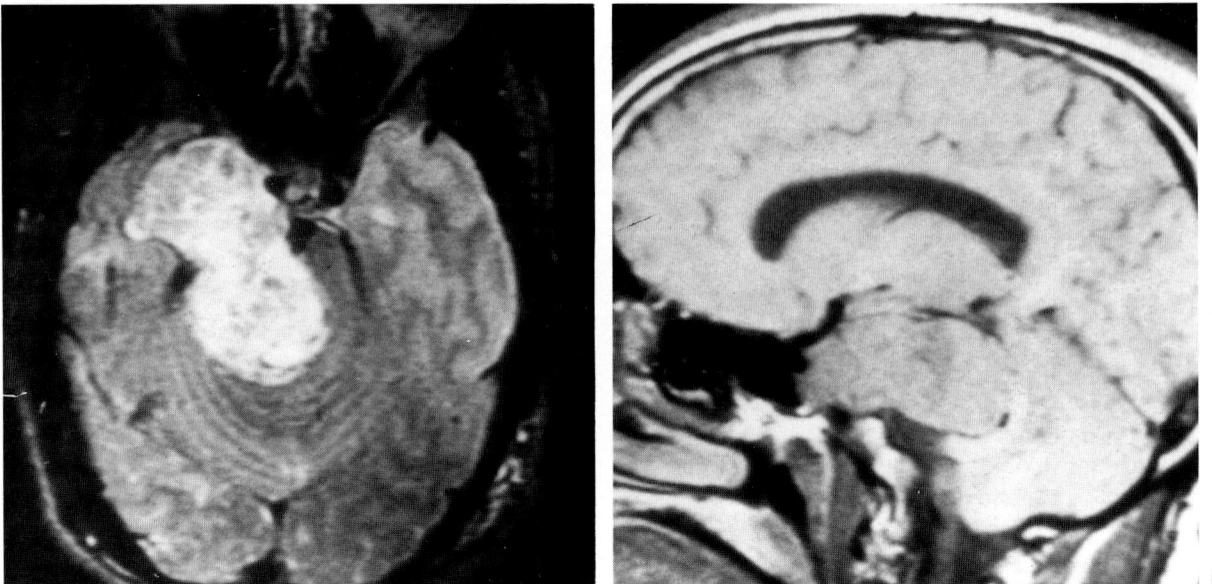

FIG. 1. Case 1. **A:** T2-weighted (TE 2500 msec, TR 120 msec) sagittal MR image showing a large, well circumscribed dumbbell-shaped mass arising from the right petrous apex and extending into both the posterior and middle fossae. **B:** T1-weighted (TE 800 msec, TR 20 msec) sagittal MR image.

transient right sixth and seventh nerve palsies, which resolved during the subsequent 6 weeks, and persistent right $V_{2,3}$ sensory loss. Serial CT and MRI studies have shown no evidence of tumor recurrence during a 3-year follow-up.

Case 2: Hourglass Neurilemoma

This 47-year-old woman presented with a 2-year history of ataxia, dysarthria, and dementia. Examination demonstrated left sensorineural hearing loss, a partial left vocal cord paresis, left trapezius weakness, mild right hemiparesis, hyperreflexia with extensor plantar responses, truncal ataxia, and a positive Romberg sign. CT scan demonstrated a hypodense, ring-enhancing lesion extending from the posterior fossa at the level of the medulla through the tentorial hiatus into the middle fossa and cavernous sinus (Fig. 4A). As in the first case, tumor removal was attempted in two stages with an initial infratentorial approach followed by a subsequent supratentorial procedure. In this case (which was treated early in our series), residual tumor was left in the lateral wall of the cavernous sinus. Postoperatively, the patient's neurological deficits largely resolved; however, 1 year later, she developed recurrent right hemiparesis and worsening dementia. Repeat CT and MRI studies demonstrated a large recurrence of her tumor in the middle fossa, arising from the cavernous sinus and extending upward and posteriorly with compression of the posteromedial temporal lobe and brain stem (Fig. 4B, C). After tolerating a balloon test occlusion, the patient underwent a subtemporal approach to the neurilemoma with complete tumor resection as outlined in Case 1. She remains recurrence-free 43 months after this procedure. This case emphasizes the importance of achieving complete tumor resection in patients with these lesions. In our experience, virtually all patients who are left with residual tumor after attempted resection develop symptomatic regrowth of tumor within 3 years of surgery.

Case 3: Extracranial–Intracranial V_2 Neurilemoma

This 41-year-old woman presented with a 3-month history of right nasal obstruction. She was initially evaluated by an otolaryngologist who biopsied what was felt to be a nasal polyp; however, on microscopic examination of the tissue obtained, the lesion proved to be a neurilemoma. CT and MRI studies were subsequently performed and demonstrated a large middle fossa lesion growing through the skull base with enlargement of the foramen rotundum, and extending into the right cavernous sinus, sphenoid sinus, pterygopalatine fossa, infratemporal fossa, and parapharyngeal space (Fig. 5). A detailed neurological examination demonstrated only

TRIGEMINAL NEURILEMOMA / 741

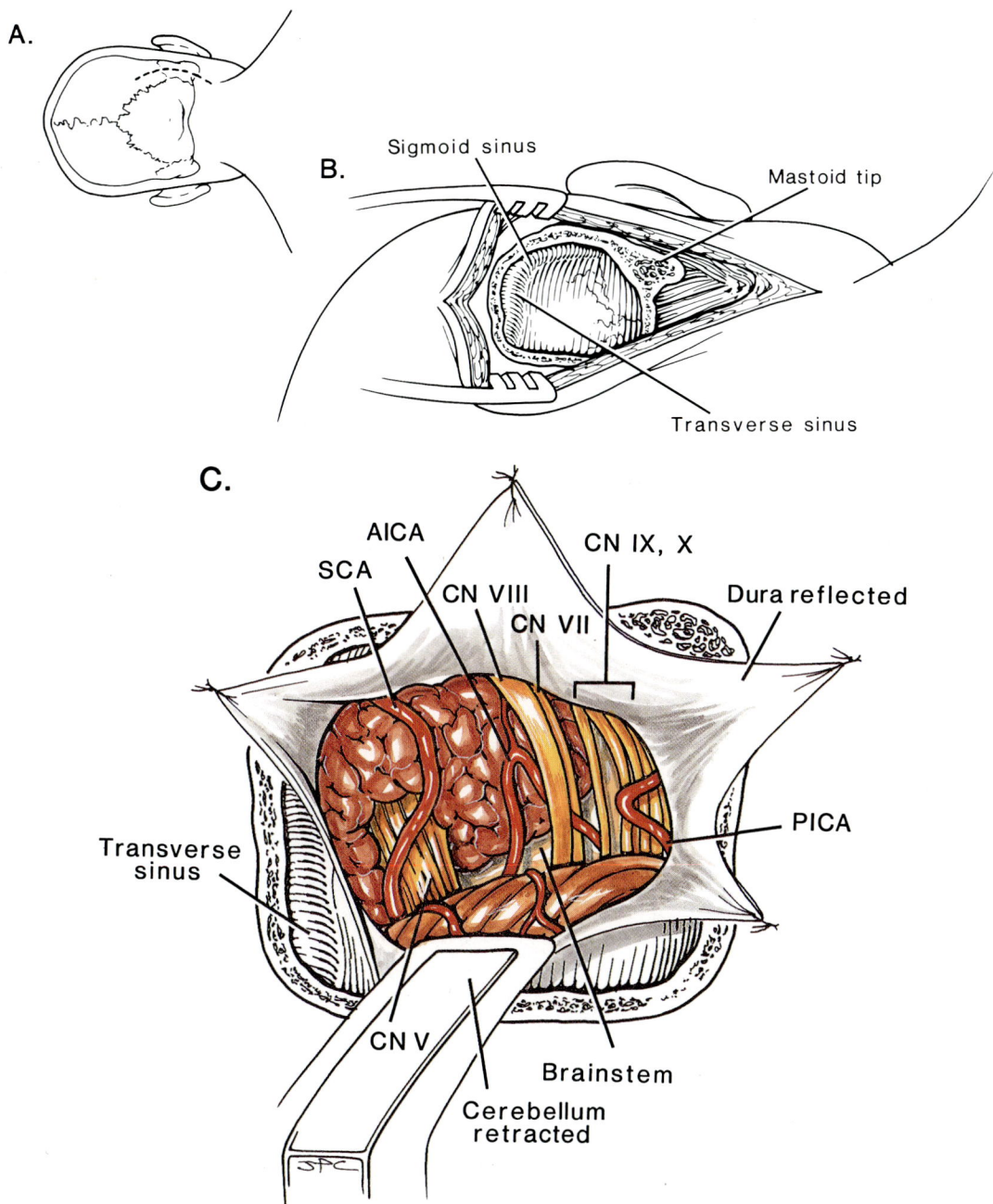

FIG. 2. Case 1. First stage removal of the infratentorial component of the tumor. **A:** Retromastoid skin incision. **B:** Suboccipital bone is removed exposing the transverse sinus superiorly, the sigmoid sinus laterally, and the basal portion of the occipital bone as it curves toward the foramen magnum inferiorly. **C:** Intradural exposure of the tumor showing the large posterior fossa component displacing the seventh through tenth nerves dorsally and the brain stem and basilar artery contralaterally. Tumor is seen extending through the tentorial hiatus and into Meckel's cave.

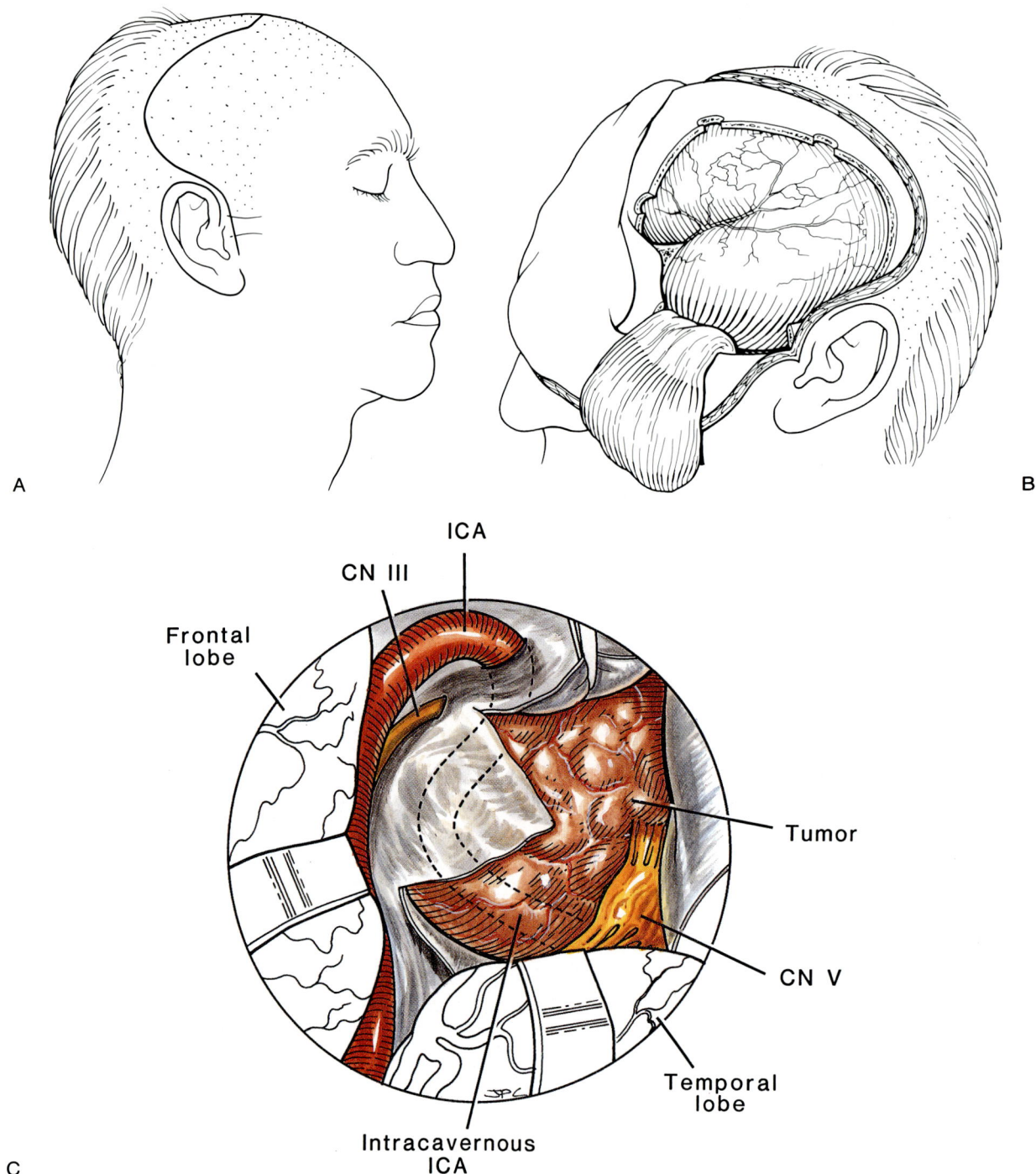

FIG. 3. Case 1. Second stage removal of the supratentorial component of the tumor. **A:** Skin incision. **B:** A frontotemporal craniotomy has been performed; the temporal bone is rongeured down to the middle fossa floor. A zygomatic osteotomy has been done. **C:** The capsule over the tumor has been incised below the third and fourth cranial nerves, exposing extradural tumor extending medially along the middle fossa floor into the cavernous sinus region.

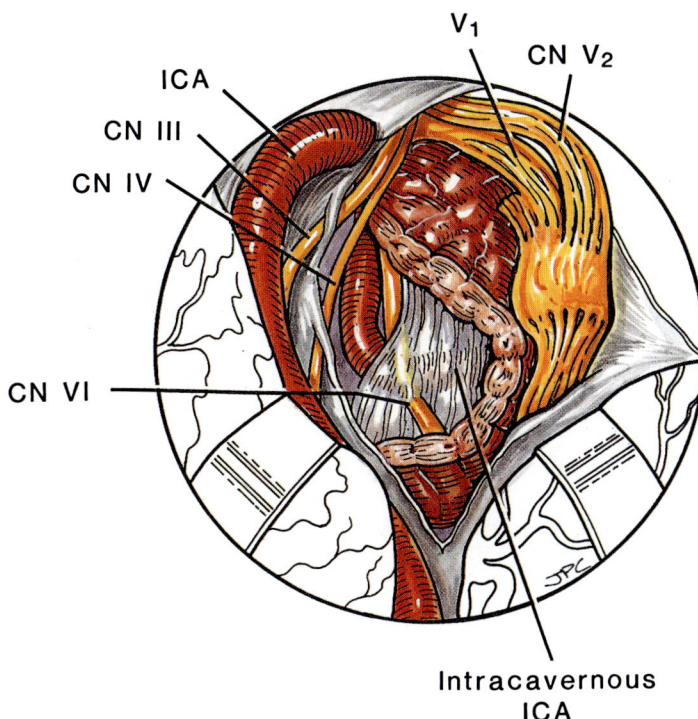

FIG. 3. *continued* **D:** View of the middle fossa floor and cavernous sinus region after tumor excision. The trigeminal ganglion and proximal branches are markedly stretched, but the bulk of the nerve remains intact.

partial right V_2 sensory loss. Balloon occlusion of the right carotid artery was well tolerated. A staged extradural–intradural approach to the tumor was planned. Initially, the extradural component was removed via a right frontotemporal craniotomy with a subtemporal and infratemporal fossa approach. This technique is well illustrated elsewhere in this volume. To minimize temporal lobe retraction, the orbital roof, superolateral orbital wall, and attached zygomatic process were removed as a unit, thus improving exposure of the subtemporal and cavernous sinus regions. After exposing V_3 and the petrous carotid artery, tumor was removed from the maxillary sinus, infratemporal fossa, and sphenoid sinus. A large portion of the middle fossa extension of tumor was removed extradurally, leaving a small portion medially in the cavernous sinus region. After tumor removal, small tears of the basal dura were closed primarily, and the infratemporal region was covered with temporalis muscle to reinforce the closure. Two weeks later, the intracavernous component of the tumor was removed via a subtemporal, intradural approach. After exposing the petrous and supraclinoid segments of the ICA to achieve proximal and distal control of the vessel, the lateral wall of the cavernous sinus was opened beneath the third and fourth nerves; the remaining intracavernous portion of the tumor was then completely excised. Postoperatively, the patient had no new neurological deficits and remains recurrence-free at 1 year follow-up (Fig. 6).

SUMMARY OF THE EXPERIENCE AT THE UNIVERSITY OF PITTSBURGH

Twenty-two patients with trigeminal neurilemomas were treated during the last 17 years; four had middle fossa tumors arising from the trigeminal ganglion, four had posterior fossa tumors arising from the trigeminal roots, ten had hourglass lesions with growth both above and below the tentorium, and four had tumor arising from the trigeminal branches and extending through the superior orbital fissure, foramen rotundum, or foramen ovale. Thirteen patients had tumors that also invaded the cavernous sinus. Complete tumor excision was achieved in 18 patients; all 18 remain free of recurrence at 9–190 months follow-up. In contrast, all four patients who had incomplete resections became symptomatic from regrowth of residual tumor within 3 years of initial surgery. Subsequently, two of these four patients underwent total tumor excision; both are disease-free 55 and 67 months after the secondary procedures. Major morbidity consisted of a CSF leak in two patients, meningitis and herpes simplex uveitis in one patient, and a symptomatic temporal lobe contusion in one patient. There were no operative deaths. Ten patients had impairment of fourth, sixth, seventh, or eighth nerve function postoperatively; in all but three patients, these deficits resolved within several months of surgery. Despite the often large size of these lesions, 12 patients had preserved or improved trigeminal function after treatment.

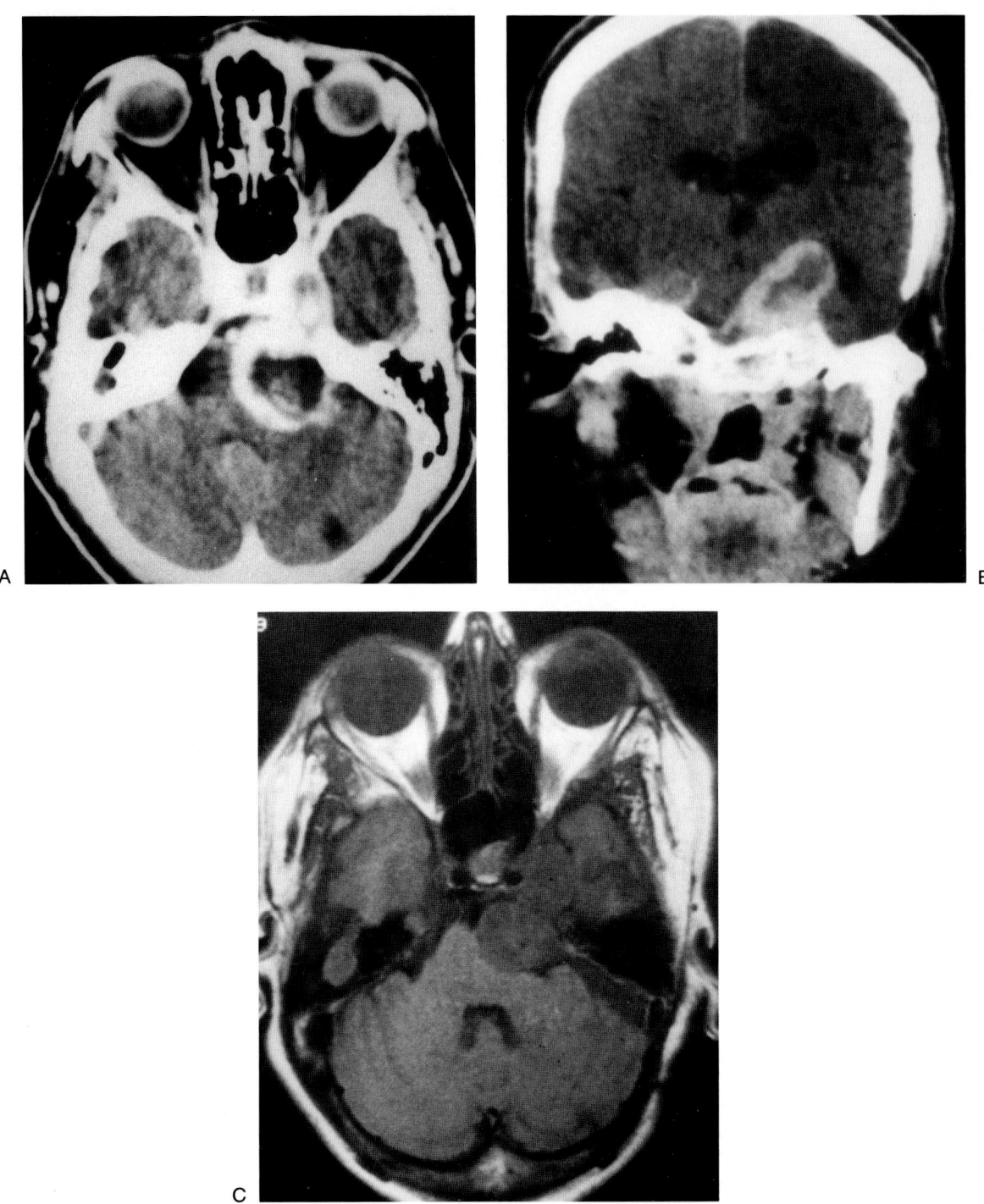

FIG. 4. Case 2. **A:** Preoperative axial CT image after administration of intravenous contrast showing a left-sided ring-enhancing mass extending from the posterior fossa through the tentorial hiatus and porus trigeminus into Meckel's cave and rostrally into the cavernous sinus. **B:** Coronal CT obtained 1 year postoperatively, showing a large middle fossa recurrence of tumor elevating the inferomedial temporal lobe and compressing the brain stem. **C:** Axial T1-weighted MR image, showing growth of tumor in the tentorial region with a large intracavernous component.

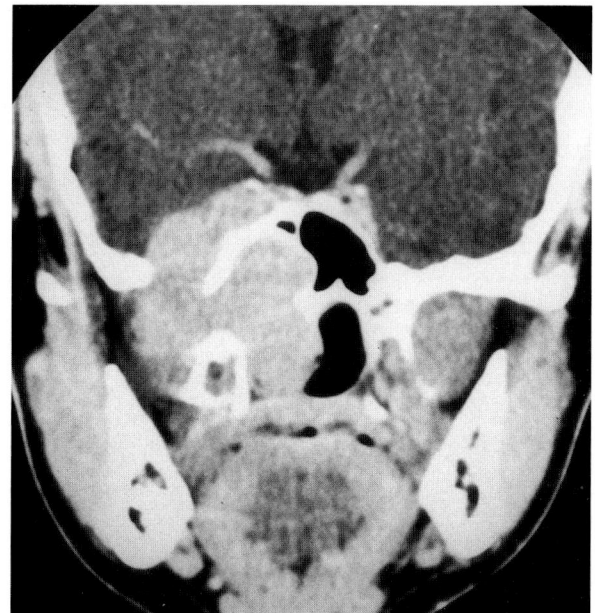
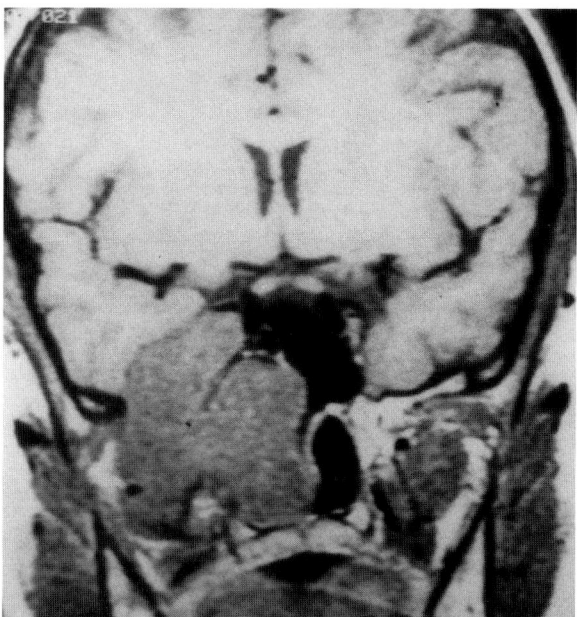

FIG. 5. Case 3. **A:** Coronal contrast-enhanced CT scan showing a V_2 neurilemoma elevating the inferomedial temporal lobe and growing medially into the cavernous sinus and inferiorly through the temporal fossa floor into the pterygopalatine fossa, infratemporal fossa, sphenoid sinus, and nasopharynx. **B:** Coronal T1-weighted MR image demonstrating the extent of subtemporal and infratemporal spread of tumor.

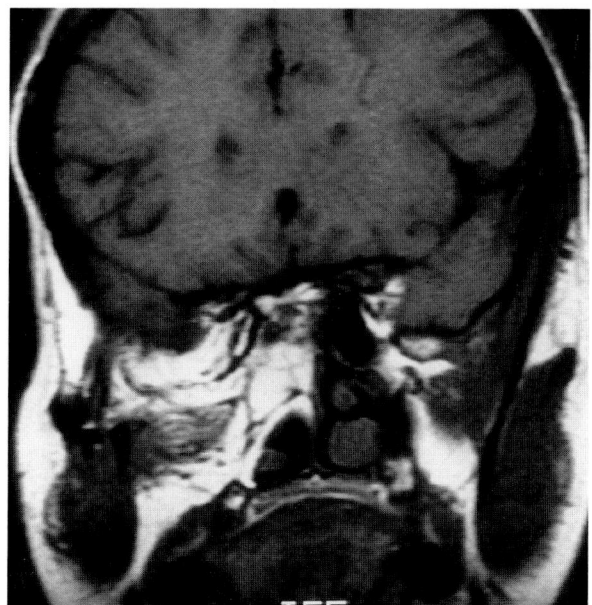
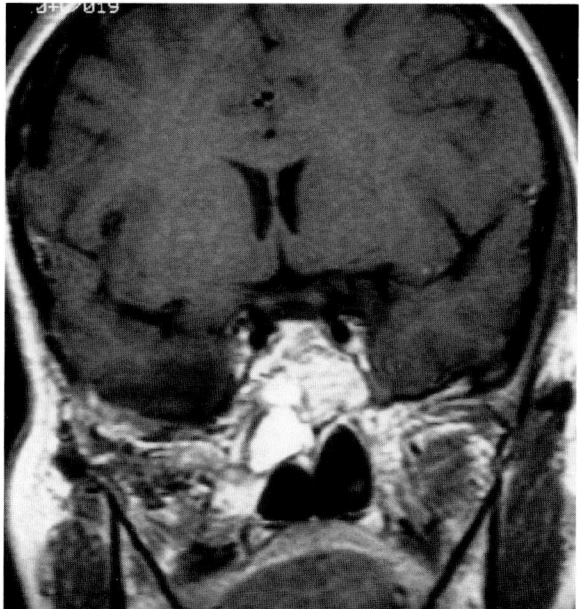

FIG. 6. Case 3. Coronal T1-weighted MR images obtained 12 months postoperatively, demonstrating complete tumor removal with no evidence of recurrence.

BIBLIOGRAPHY

1. Arseni C, Dumitrescu L, Constantines CUA. Neurinomas of the trigeminal nerve. *Surg Neurol* 1975;4:497–503.
2. de Benedittis G, Bernasconi V, Ettore G. Tumors of the fifth cranial nerve. *Acta Neurochir (Wien)* 1977;38:37–64.
3. Goldberg R, Byrd S, Winter J, et al. Varied appearance of trigeminal neuromas on CT. *AJR* 1980;134:57–60.
4. Jefferson G. Trigeminal neurinomas with some remarks on malignant invasion of the gasserian ganglion. *Clin Neurosurg* 1955;1:11–54.
5. Karyenbuhl H. Primary tumors of the root of the fifth cranial nerve: their distinction from tumors of the gasserian ganglion. *Brain* 1936;59:337–352.
6. Lesoin F, Rousseaux M, Villette L, et al. Neurinomas of the trigeminal nerve. *Acta Neurochir (Wien)* 1986;82:118–122.
7. McCormick PC, Bello JA, Post KD. Trigeminal schwannoma. Surgical series of 14 cases with review of the literature. *J Neurosurg* 1988;69:850–860.
8. Nager GT. Neurinomas of the trigeminal nerve. *Am J Otolaryngol* 1984;5:301–333.
9. Olive I, Svien HJ. Neurofibromas of the fifth cranial nerve. *J Neurosurg* 1957;14:484–505.
10. Pollack IF, Sekhar LN, Jannetta PJ, Janecka IP. Neurilemmomas of the trigeminal nerve. *J Neurosurg* 1989;70:737–745.
11. Schisano G, Olivecrona H. Neurinomas of the gasserian ganglion and trigeminal root. *J Neurosurg* 1960;17:306–322.
12. Sekhar LN, Moller AR. Operative management of tumors involving the cavernous sinus. *J Neurosurg* 1986;64:879–889.

CHAPTER 47

Glomus Jugulare Tumors

C. Gary Jackson, Charles I. Woods, and Philip N. Chironis

Disputed for so many years, the management of glomus jugulare tumors has been standardized. Advances in radiographic diagnosis, microsurgical technique, anesthesia, and reconstructive surgery have resulted in an ability to successfully treat these patients surgically. Surgical removal is the current preferred management. The surgery is reliable, its consequences now predictable and controlled.

Current technical concepts of unresectability are virtually noncxistent, modified only by individual considerations, tumor multiplicity, and tumor biology. Tumors complicated by intracranial extension (ICE), internal carotid artery (ICA) involvement, clivus or cavernous sinus extension, and so on no longer frustrate our technology. Even for these exceptional cases morbidity and mortality statistics are predictable and markedly reduced over those of the past.

The elaboration of our current concept of glomus jugulare management constitutes the objective of this chapter. Also presented is a cursory look at the senior author's experience in the treatment of these usually benign, but often devastating, lesions.

DIAGNOSTIC CONSIDERATIONS

Approximately 80% of patients with glomus jugulare tumors present with progressive unilateral hearing loss while 70% complain of pulsatile tinnitus. A mesotympanic mass is usual with TM erosion and bleeding being late symptoms. Various permutations of cranial neuropathies can occur. Related symptoms are generally minimal owing to slow neural degeneration, allowing for ongoing simultaneous compensation. Loss of airway protection and swallowing dysfunction occur with aggregate nerve loss.

The clinical picture of glomus jugulare is characteristic and the diagnosis usually readily suspect. The clinical findings alone, however, are not adequate for the purposes of surgical planning. The mainstay of glomus tumor diagnosis is radiologic.

Table 1 lists the objectives of the diagnostic inquiry for glomus jugulare tumors. Tumor identification depends on imaging the soft tissue mass and/or resultant bone destruction. The radiographic preoperative evaluation of choice is magnetic resonance imaging (MRI) using the agent gadolinium (GDTA). MRI provides unsurpassed information concerning disease extent and the relationship of the tumor to surrounding structures both neural and vascular. MRI generates data useful in differentiating glomus tumors from other skull base disease and is the modality of choice for identifying multiple lesions. ICE is best identified by MRI. Computerized tomography (CT) is obtained when further evaluation of bony detail is warranted.

Bilateral carotid angiography is considered essential to the evaluation of a surgical candidate. The size and extent of the lesion are determined by MRI. Little effort is directed toward this task angiographically. Angiography is used to determine ICA involvement and collateral blood flow to the brain, that is, the circle of Willis. Cross compression and intraluminal balloon occlusion generate data regarding collateral blood flow useful in planned or unplanned disruption of ICA flow. In general, preoperative intraluminal detachable balloon occlusion has not been embraced. As a result of the difference in hemodynamic circumstances governing flow preoperatively and in the anesthetized patient, the outcome of abrupt ICA flow disruption is not completely predictable. We have taken the position therefore that when ICA sacrifice is decided upon, interposition grafting is done in all cases.

Glomus tumors possess the histochemical machinery

C. G. Jackson and P. N. Chironis: The Otology Group, Nashville, Tennessee 37203.
C. I. Woods: State University of New York Health Science Center, Syracuse, New York 13204.

TABLE 1. *Glomus tumor diagnosis objectives*[a]

1. Determine size and extent of the disease.
2. Determine presence of associated lesions.
3. Determine CNS collateral circulation.
4. Determine extent of ICE.
5. Determine degree of involvement of major vasculature.

[a] From *The Laryngoscope,* with permission.

to produce complex neuropeptides as well as vasoactive amines (1). In addition to multiple lesions, this paraneoplastic phenomenon must be identified prior to anesthesia and differentiated from pheochromocytoma. Preoperative catecholamine screens are routinely performed. Selective renal vein catheterization may be required. The evaluation of complex neuropeptide elaboration is of potential great clinical importance (1) but is of little practical value at this time.

Table 2 outlines our diagnosis algorithm.

PATIENT SELECTION

Every patient with a glomus jugulare tumor is a potential candidate for the preferred course of management: surgery. The critical question to be asked, however, to individualize a treatment plan must be: Is this disease likely to cause the patient serious problems in the natural course of his/her remaining years? More appropriately, then, is the question: Who is *not* a surgical candidate?

In general, the elderly are not candidates for this surgery. At great risk, we'll define "elderly" as age 65. This concept is modified by physiologic considerations and tumor size. It is unlikely that a small tumor in a 69-year-old would, in the natural course of his/her remaining life, cause severe clinical problems or be life threatening. The same logic—slow growth rate—does not apply to the 30-year-old. The morbidity of this surgery in the "elderly" also exceeds the potential benefits offered. Radiation therapy with or without planned selective subtotal resection is an appropriate form of palliation. Radiation therapy is reserved for those patients with aggressive tumor biology confirmed by serial MRI or in these complicated by cranial neuropathy. Medical infirmity likewise precludes a curative direction in treatment plan.

The rare occurrence of bilateral cranial base tumors has definitively managed risks—both laryngeal denervation as well as laryngeal and hypopharyngeal deafferentation, a condition mandating tracheal diversion and/or alternate artificial methods for alimentation. Palliative therapy of the least dangerous lesion may be reasonable in this precarious situation.

TABLE 2. *Diagnostic protocol for glomus tumors: sequential algorithm*[a]

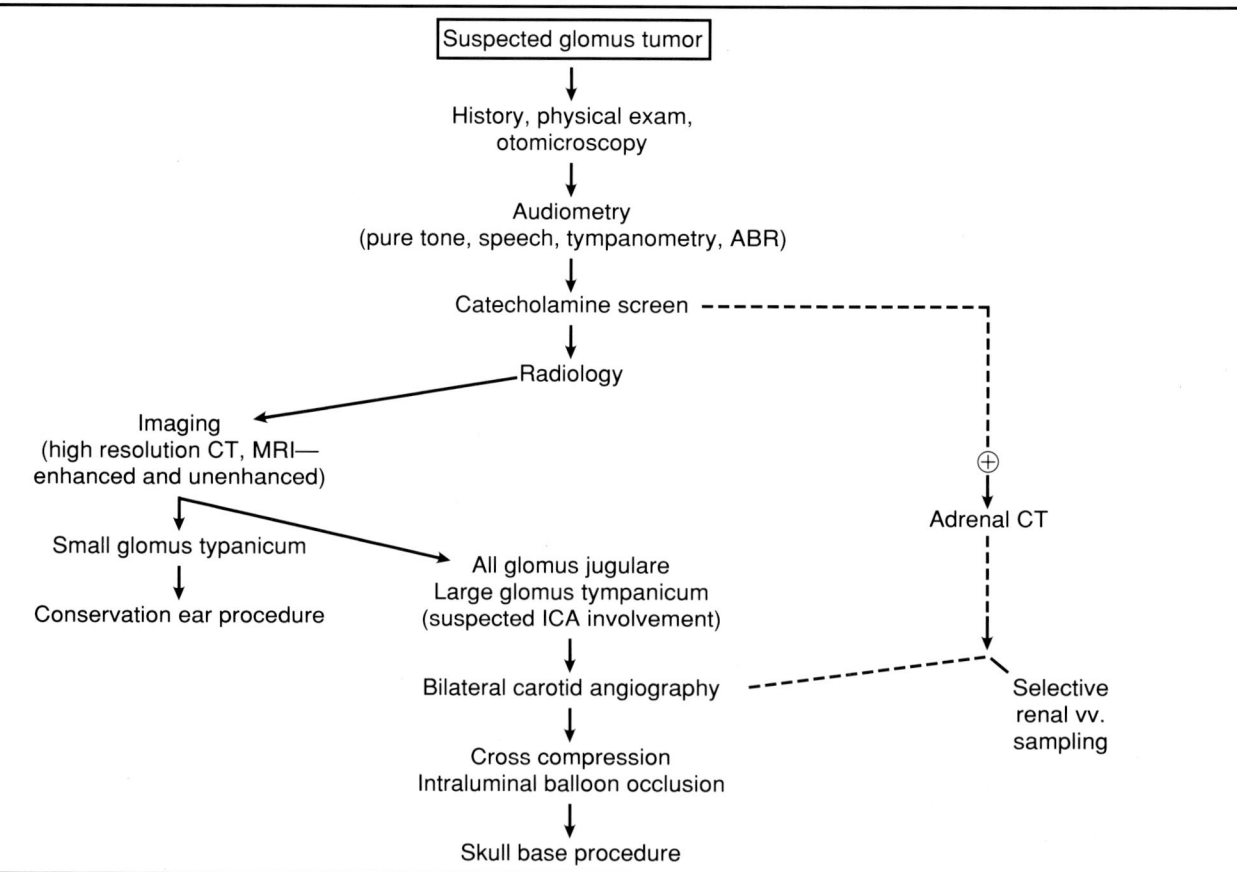

[a] From ref. 13, with permission.

OPERATIVE TECHNIQUE

Anesthetic Considerations

Anesthetic management of patients undergoing resection of glomus jugulare tumors primarily concerns close monitoring and management of the patients hemodynamic condition (2–9). Invasive monitoring (arterial line, CVP, and/or Swan–Ganz catheterization) alerts the operative team to often abrupt and wild fluctuation in pulse, blood pressure, and perfusion associated with vagal manipulation or catecholamine release consequent to tumor manipulation.

Special considerations arise when the tumor is a catecholamine "secretor." Catecholamine levels can be as high as 1000-fold normal! Preoperative preparation proceeds as for pheochromocytoma and involves both alpha- and beta-pharmacologic control for 2 weeks prior to surgery. The risks attendant to venous stasis must be acknowledged. Sequential compression stockings can be used preoperatively and are routine on all cases intraoperatively. Substitution for morphine by meperidine is done to minimize the risk of morphine-sulfate-stimulated histamine release from these tumors.

Patient Position

The patient is positioned supine with the head turned. The hemihead, ear, and neck are prepared. Also prepared are the abdomen for free flap or fat donation, the thigh for potential vein graft donation, and, possibly, the chest or back for regional flap donation as needed. Tracheostomy is not routinely performed, but when the need is obvious, anesthesia is best administered via the tracheostomy site. A facial nerve monitor is used.

The operating room is arranged so that anesthesia is cross-table from the surgeon at the foot of the OR table. The scrub nurse is positioned directly across from the surgeon at the table's head. Another assistant is stationed at the foot of the table to operate the motor-driven table, the only way in which patient "position" is altered.

Operative Approach and Technical Problems

The objective of surgical removal of these tumors is twofold:

1. Total tumor removal in a single stage.
2. Total tumor removal preserving as much normal anatomy and function as possible.

To accomplish this objective the approach must:

1. Allow access to all tumor margins.
2. Allow proximal and distal control of related major vascular and neural structures.
3. Allow access to all margins of ICE.

TABLE 3. *Facial nerve management alternatives in glomus jugulare surgery*

1. Simple exposure
2. Mobilization
   A. Short—external genu
   B. Long—geniculate ganglion
3. Division with reanastomosis
   A. With/without rerouting
4. Segmental resection
   A. Interposition graft
   B. End-to-end anastomosis
      (i) With/without rerouting
   C. Nerve substitution (rare)
   D. Alternate reanimation (rare)
      (i) Static
      (ii) Dynamic

Tumor growth from its hypotympanic origin is highly variable. No one single approach is appropriate for all patients. Surgery must be individualized based on considerations of two primary cofactors: tumor size and distal control of the ICA. All glomus jugulare tumors, save the smallest, are to some extent attached to the ICA from which they must be dissected. The basic principle of proximal and distal control must be served. Necessary exposure of the ICA in the tympanic segment proximal to the eustachian tube or in the intrapetrous portion distal to its tympanic genu determines the exposure necessary: standard skull base preserving ear anatomy or infratemporal fossa with external auditory canal (EAC) overclosure and mandibular dislocation. It is rare that the intracranial ICA must be isolated for glomus jugulare tumor removal.

The facial nerve in cranial base surgery is an anatomic exposure impediment—an unfamiliar perspective for the neuro-otologist. Its disposition is determined by the fundamental cofactors of tumor size and distal ICA control. Table 3 outlines various facial nerve management alternatives.

BASIC TRANSTEMPORAL SKULL BASE APPROACH

For small to medium size glomus jugulare tumors largely limited to the jugular foramen and infralabyrinthine chamber, involving the ICA no higher than the tympanic segment, the basic transtemporal approach, which preserves the EAC and ear anatomy, is preferred.

An incision is designed which permits access to the temporal bone, the neck, and the parotid area (Fig. 1). The upper cervical region and parotid areas are dissected to identify and delineate cranial nerves (CNs) VII, IX, XI, and XII. The lower cranial nerves are dissected to the cranial base. The common internal and external carotid arteries with the internal jugular vein (IJV) are identified. The IJV is doubly tied and suture ligated. Proximal

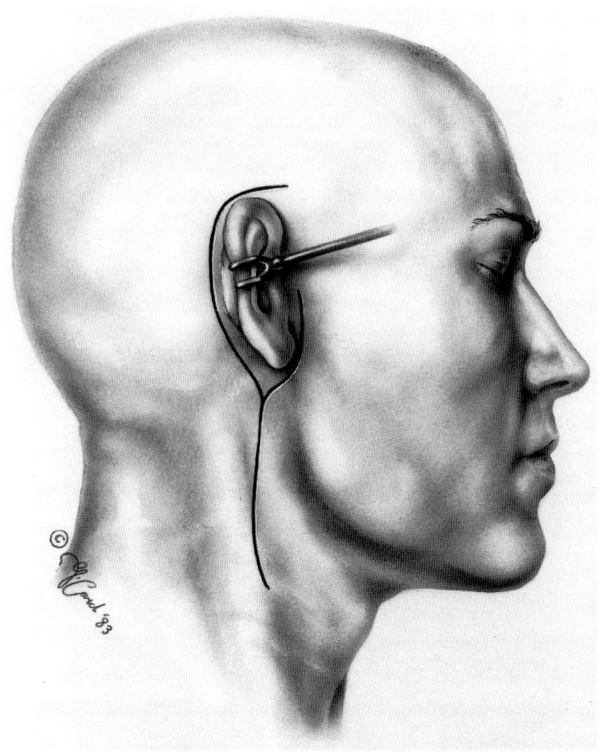

FIG. 1. A parotidectomy incision is modified to allow postauricular exposure. The ear should be left on as broad a pedicle as possible. (From refs. 8 and 13, with permission.)

arterial control of the ICA is obtained by placing a control suture of umbilical tape. A complete mastoidectomy is then performed. The extended facial recess approach is executed, removing tympanic bone and the styloid process. The facial nerve is exposed from the external genu to the previously performed intraparotid dissection. The lateral venous sinus (LVS) is exposed at least from the superior petrosal sinus distally. The tumor in its lateral extent should be visible (Fig. 2).

Proximal control of the LVS is achieved by intraluminal packing with Surgicel. The superior petrosal sinus is preferably left patent as the LVS is occluded as far distally, yet above the tumor, as tumor extent will allow (Fig. 3).

In the unusually small jugular bulb tumor, tumor removal can occur working between the undisturbed facial nerve and the lateral process of C1. This opportunity is rare. In most cases, CN VII must be mobilized. A "short mobilization" from the external genu up against the intact EAC permits unrestricted exposure to the jugular foramen region (Fig. 4). The tumor is usually attached to the undersurface of CN VII from which it must be, usually successfully, dissected. To allow as much extrinsic blood supply to CN VII as possible, as much soft tissue at the stylomastoid foramen (SMF) is left intact as exposure will allow to preserve the stylomastoid artery. Facial nerve recovery is better when this can be accom-

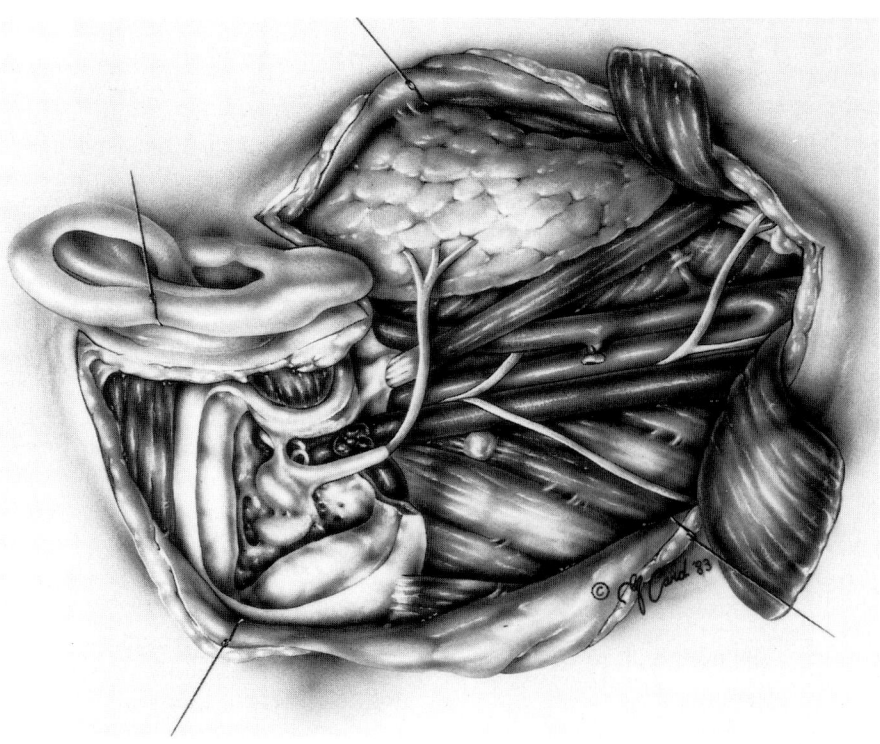

FIG. 2. The tumor is visible through the extended facial recess. Temporal bone and neck contents are identified. The EAC is preserved. (From refs. 13 and 14, with permission.)

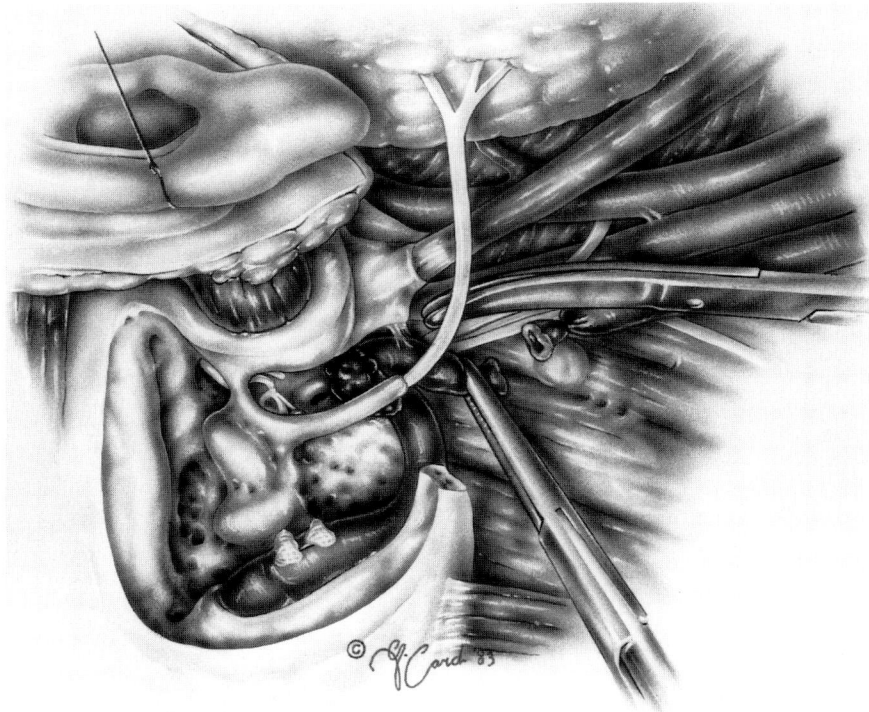

FIG. 3. Proximal and distal control of IJV/LVS is accomplished. Here CN VII is not mobilized—a rare occurrence for small tumors. (From refs. 8 and 13, with permission.)

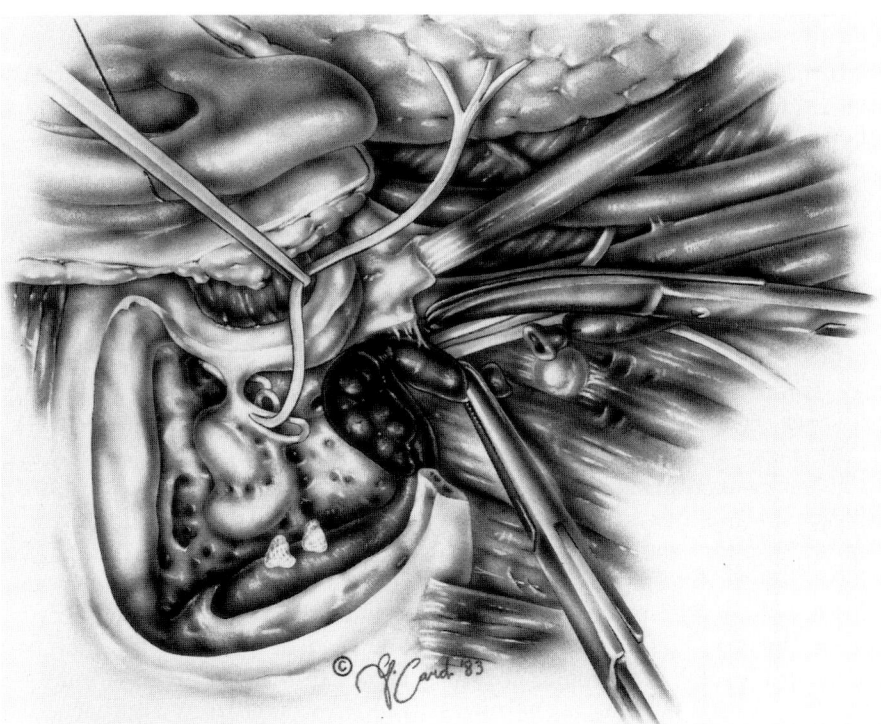

FIG. 4. "Short" mobilization of CN VII against EAC wall generates unobstructed exposure to the jugular foramen and the infralabyrinthine chamber. Dissection off ICA is sharp. Distal control is achieved at the level of the eustachian tube. (From refs. 8 and 13, with permission.)

plished. To avoid CN VII trauma, the tympanic bone dissection, extending the facial recess around the inferior and anterior EAC to the eustachian tube for distal ICA exposure *for control,* is often best done *before* the facial nerve is mobilized. With both proximal and distal control of the ICA, the tumor can now be dissected from this vital structure unobstructed by CN VII (Fig. 4).

Once free of the ICA, the IJV with the tumor can be resected. Preservation of the lower cranial nerves is tumor size dependent. Working from below, anterior and posterior, under direct vision, the pars nervosa region in the anterior–inferior medial jugular foramen can be identified. This is best done after the inferior petrosal sinuses are managed.

With total tumor removal achieved, CN VII can be replaced, any tympanoplastic work done, and the incision closed in layers. ICE is not consistent with conductive hearing preservation because the middle ear and eustachian tube must be obliterated to prevent CSF otorrhea or rhinorrhea.

INFRATEMPORAL FOSSA APPROACH

For medium to large glomus jugulare tumors generally extensive beyond the temporal bone or invading the ICA above the tympanic segment, a procedure of larger scope is required. The infratemporal fossa approach modified after that described by Fisch (10) is done. Modified extensions are described. This procedure provides exposure of the intrapetrous ICA, nasopharynx, clivus, infratemporal fossa (IFTF), and cavernous sinus.

In general, these tumors are large and are associated with cranial nerve deficits preoperatively. Intraoperative cranial nerve loss or substantive trauma is the rule. Tracheostomy is performed prior to the incision. Lumbar drains are placed at this time for tumors with substantial ICE.

The incision is C-shaped and outlines an anteriorly based flap, allowing access to the temporal bone, suboccipital, infratemporal, and temporal fossae as well as the neck (Fig. 5). The EAC is transected and oversewn inverted. The posterior aspect extends approximately 8.0 cm postauricularly. The neck dissection, mastoidectomy, and extended facial recess exposure are carried out as before. The EAC is dissected circumferentially anterosuperiorly and inferoanteriorly into the temporomandibular joint (TMJ) fossa. The incudostapedial joint is disarticulated and the EAC with middle ear contents lateral to the stapes removed (Fig. 6).

To access the intrapetrous ICA, the mandibular condyle must be displaced. Prerequisite is "long mobilization" of CN VII. With the EAC gone, CN VII can be dissected proximal to the geniculate ganglion at the distal labyrinthine segment. The superficial petrosal nerve complex is sharply divided and CN VII is mobilized out

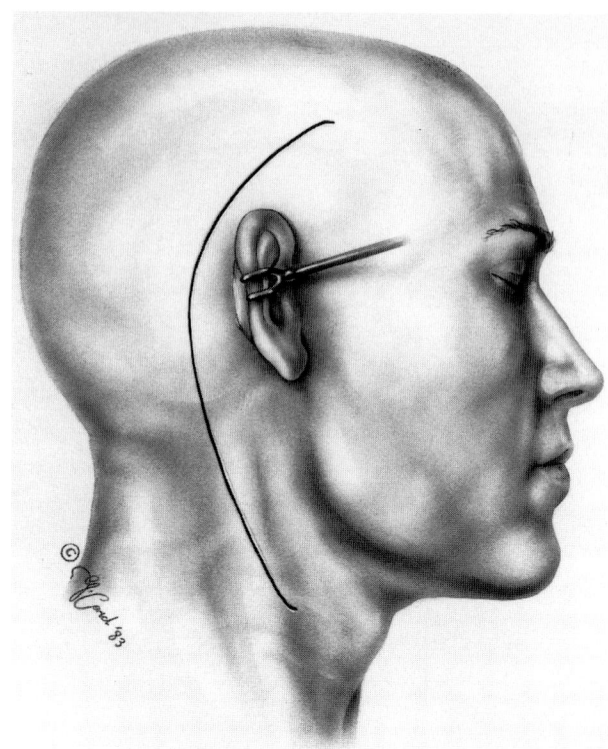

FIG. 5. Extending 5–8 cm postauricularly, this anterior based flap affords IFTF access. (From refs. 8 and 13, with permission.)

of its fallopian canal (Fig. 6). Once free of the TMJ capsule and its medial ligamentous attachments, the mandibular condyle can be anteriorly and inferiorly displaced to access the IFTF. This exposure is difficult to maintain. The most efficient device, in our experience, has been the Fisch Infratemporal Fossa Retractor (see Fig. 31). The facial nerve is reflected superiorly and anteriorly in a convenient manner, often in its own groove created superiorly. Mandibular condyle resection is now only necessary for the most extreme exposure needs.

The intrapetrous ICA can be exposed using the eustachian tube and semicanal of the tensor tympani as guides over 180° of its circumference, a maneuver necessary for *control,* not just exposure (Fig. 7). Tumor can then be dissected from it (Fig. 7).

When the tumor requires more anterosuperior exposure for margin delineation or distal ICA exposure, the IFTF exposure can be extended. The zygoma is reflected inferiorly with the temporal muscle and the IFTF opened (Fig. 8). The contents of the foramen spinosum are divided, V_3 in the foramen ovale managed and the region of the pterygoids, foramen rotundum (V_2), and the cavernous sinus approached. The ICA can be exposed to the cavernous sinus (Fig. 9). The middle cranial fossa is readily accessed via this route. This exposure for glomus jugulare tumors is not ordinarily required. Intrapetrous ICA exposure and dissection anterior to the fora-

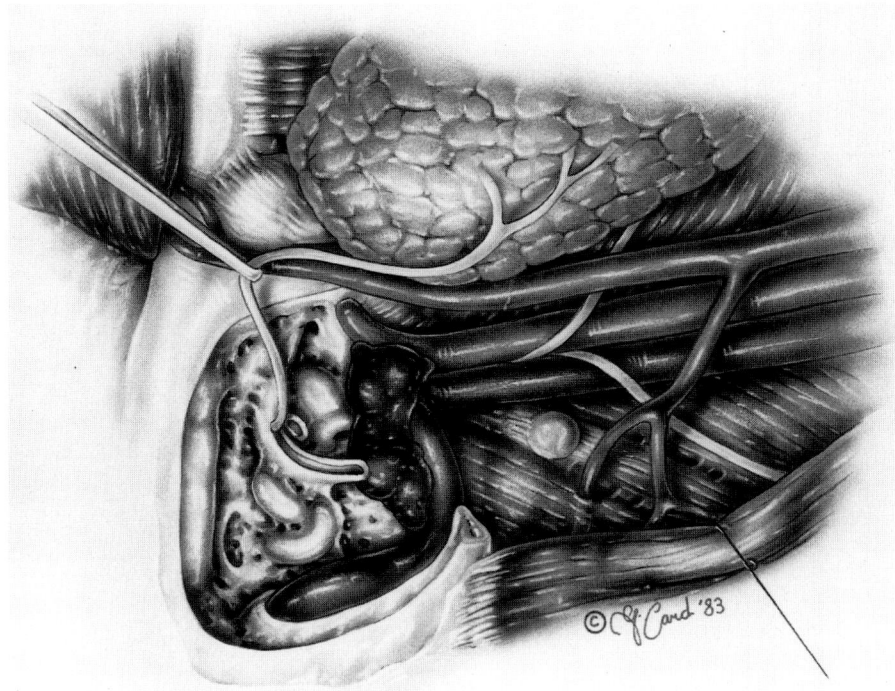

FIG. 6. The EAC has been removed with middle ear contents lateral to the stapes. "Long" CN VII mobilization allows anterior mandible dislocation. (From refs. 13 and 14, with permission.)

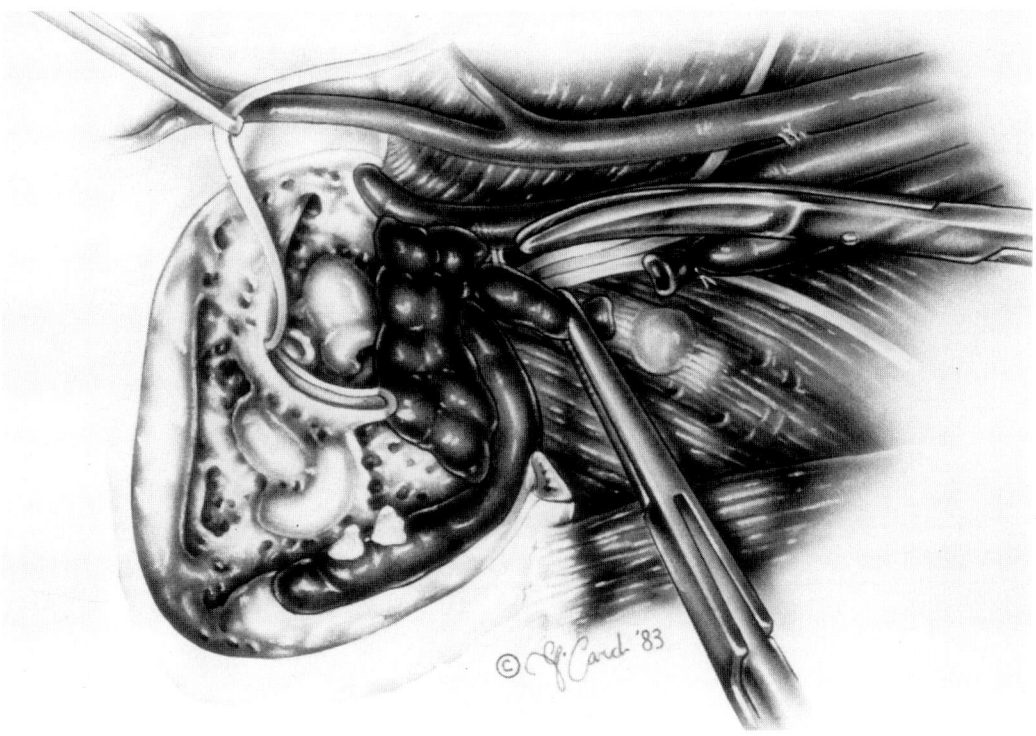

FIG. 7. Tumor dissection off ICA is the initial step in total removal. Note distal ICA exposure for control. (From refs. 13 and 14, with permission.)

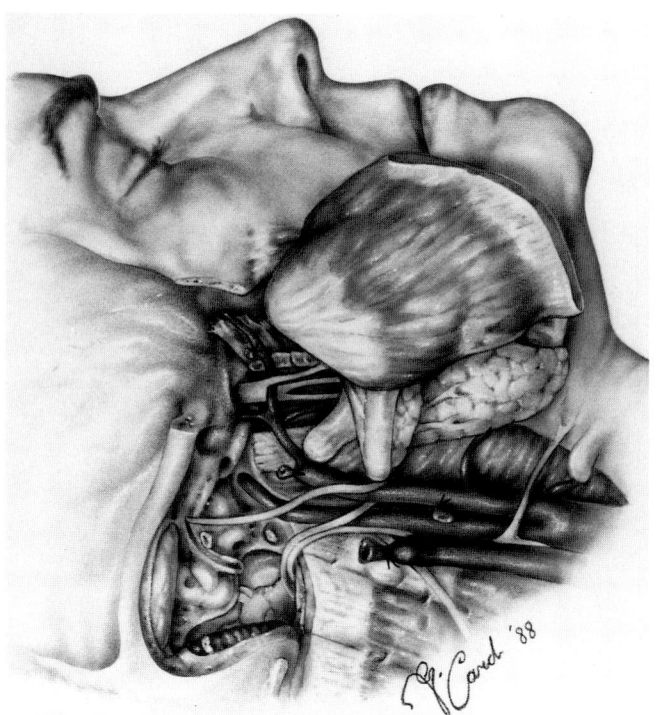

FIG. 8. Inferior zygoma reflection opens the extended IFTF exposure. (From refs. 8 and 13, with permission.)

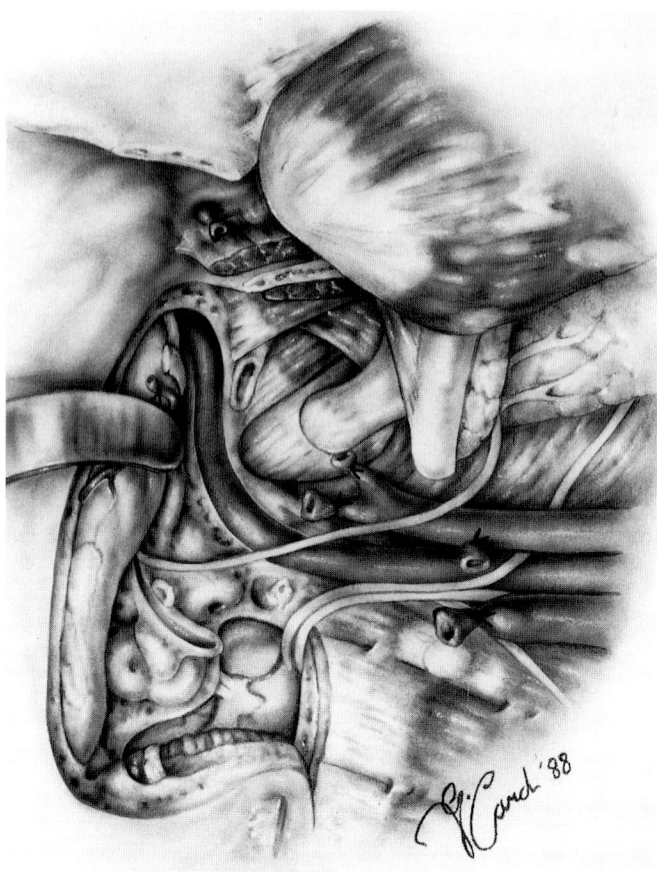

FIG. 9. The extended IFTF approach exposes more distal reaches of ICA as well as gives broader middle cranial fossa access. (From ref. 13, with permission.)

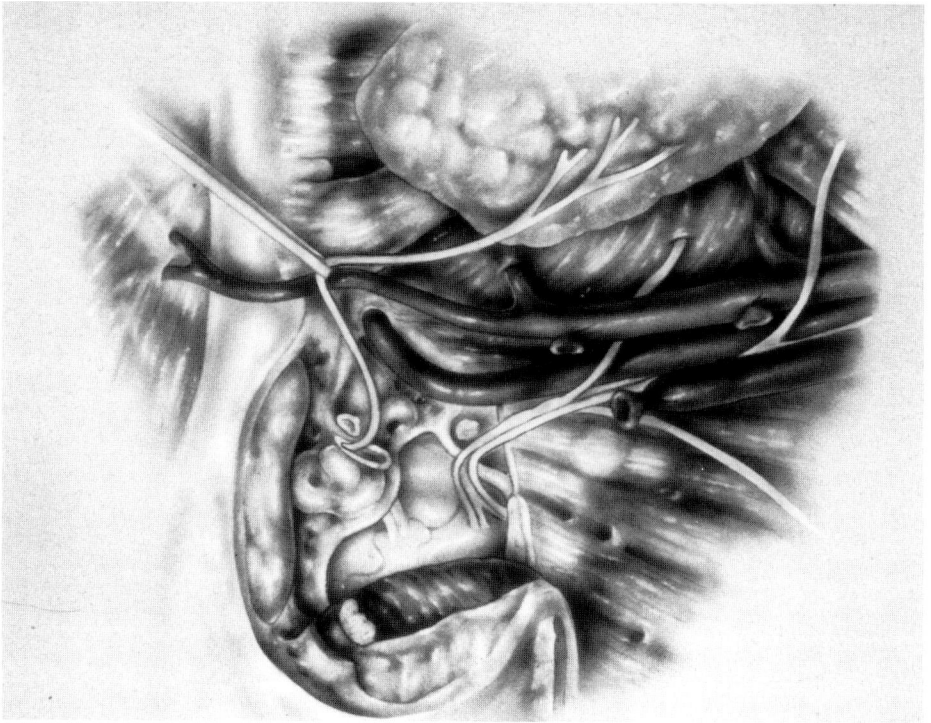

FIG. 10. A small–medium sized dural defect with an intact labyrinthine. (From refs. 8 and 13, with permission.)

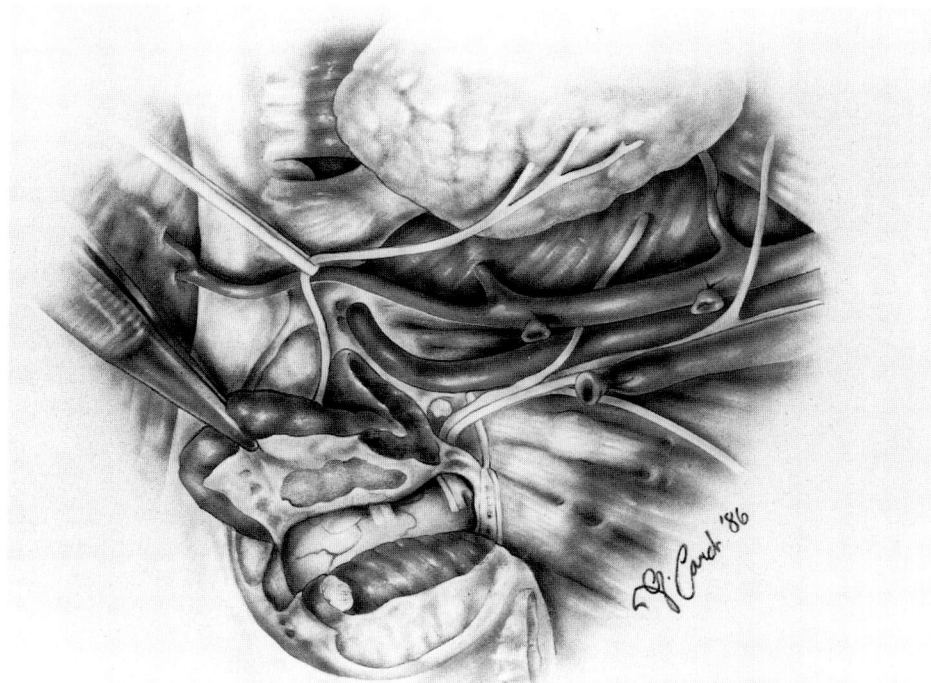

FIG. 11. Combined approach to ICE.

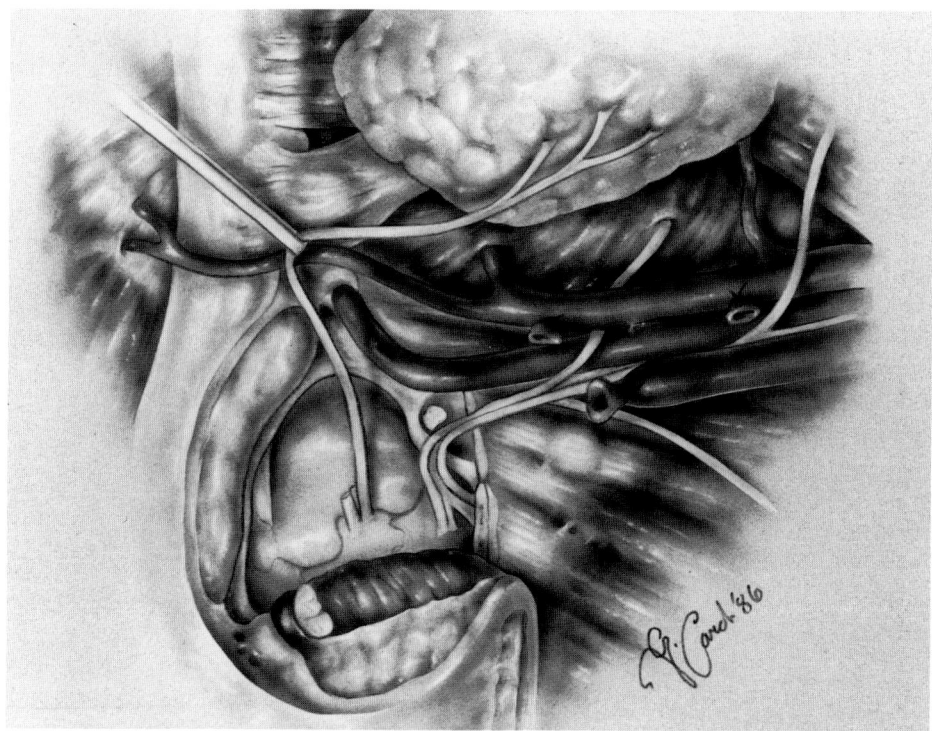

FIG. 12. A large dural defect results from transcochlear and suboccipital exposures for extensive ICE removal. (From refs. 8 and 13, with permission.)

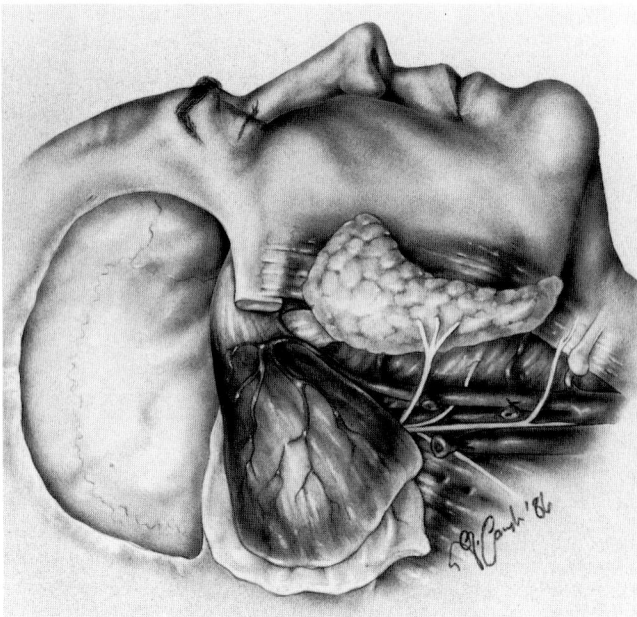

FIG. 13. A small defect reconstruction by fascia and temporal muscle flap. Temporal muscle is poor "bulk." Fat may be added between fascia and muscle. (From ref. 13, with permission.)

men spinosum, yet short of the foramen ovale, however, are frequent.

The glomus jugulare tumor is then removed from the temporal bone and/or clivus. Translabyrinthine or transcochlear exposures are not unusual to eliminate disease anterior and medial to the ICA toward the clivus.

Tumor dissection proceeds as before once the tumor is freed from the ICA.

Intracranial Extension

Our management preference is the unstaged removal of ICE (5). To manage ICE, the operative sequence is as follows:

1. Exposure.
2. Dissection of tumor from the ICA.
3. Debulking of tumor from the temporal bone.
4. Posterior fossa craniotomy and ICE removal.

ICE usually occurs initially along cranial nerves IX, X, and XI, entering the posterior fossa through the jugular foramen pars nervosa. When limited, circumferential dural resection with tumor results in a small-medium dural defect (Fig. 10). The larger glomus tumors will involve the posterior fossa dura and the temporal bone and extend into the CPA. This ICE is best approached via a formal suboccipital approach, much like the combined approach to acoustic tumors (11). With the LVS resected, exposure into the CPA is very wide (Fig. 11). The labyrinth is usually removed as well. A large dural defect results (Fig. 12).

Reconstruction of the dural defect is size dependent. All reconstructions are augmented by indwelling lumbar drain placement for 5–7 days under antibiotic coverage. Small defects are reconstructed with temporal fascia and buttressed by abdominal fat and/or temporal muscle

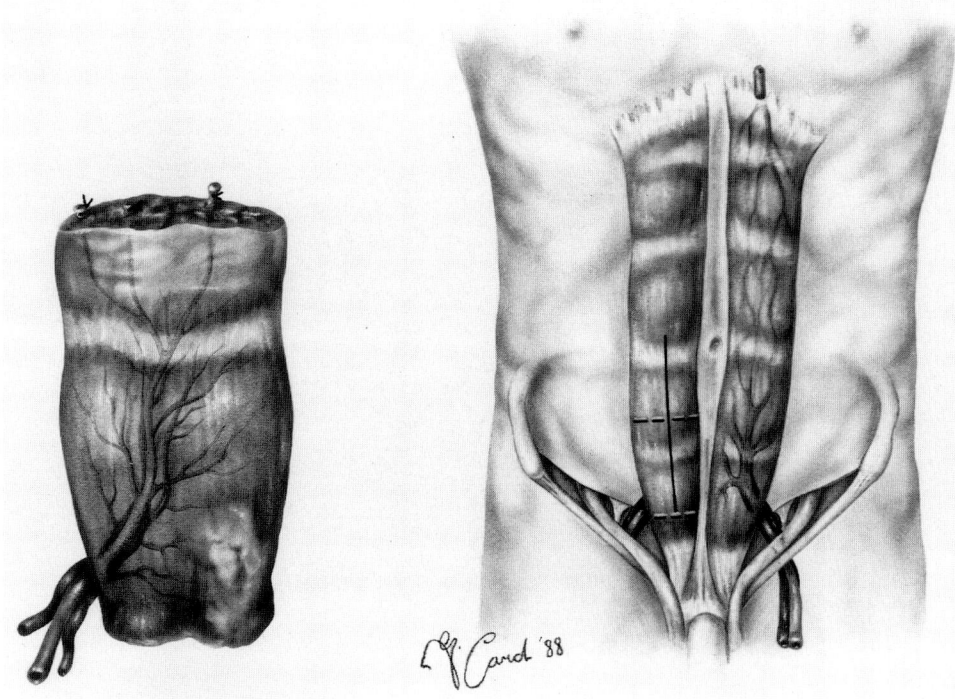

FIG. 14. The rectus abdominus free flap donor design. (From refs. 8 and 13, with permission.)

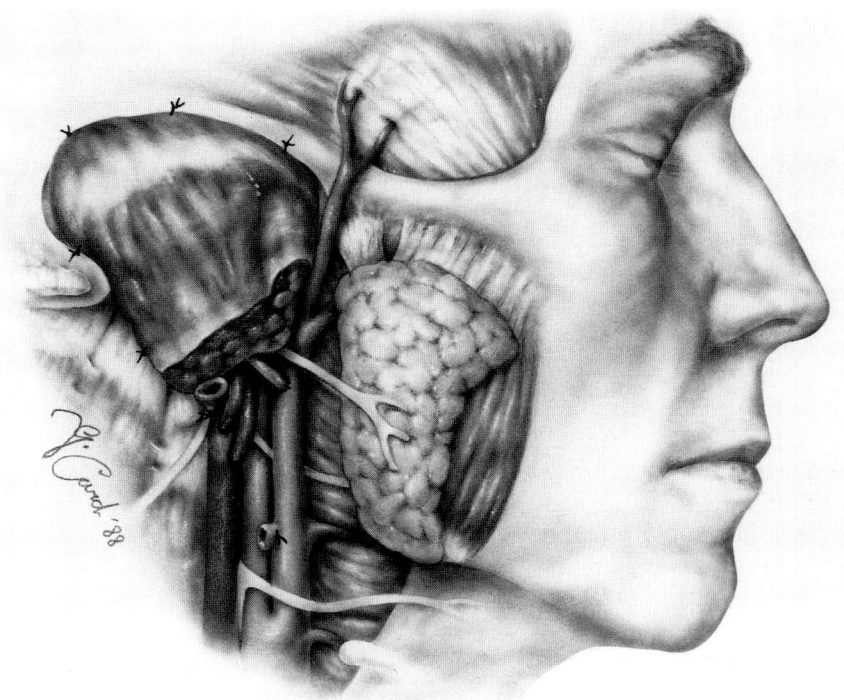

FIG. 15. The free flap adds vital tissue not only for bulk but for ICA coverage in irradiated areas as well. (From refs. 8 and 13, with permission.)

flap for containment (Fig. 13). This flap is not successful as "bulk." Larger defects, commonly occurring in patients previously irradiated in "curative" dosages, require vital tissue over temporal fascia or fascia lata. Rectus abdominus free flap pedicled on branches of the ECA and IJV adds 3 hr to the surgery time but has been effective (Figs. 14 and 15).

POSTOPERATIVE MANAGEMENT COMPLICATION PROPHYLAXIS

From the operating room the patient is taken directly to a neurosurgical ICU for monitoring observation. In addition to careful neurologic status monitoring, hemodynamic status is observed by contemporary technology. All glomus tumors secrete some level of vasoactive amine, and postoperatively blood pressure may be labile. The lumbar drain, when managed by the inexperienced, can unnecessarily be a monumental problem. Sequential compression stockings are preferred.

Postoperative complications are best managed by their prevention. The most common potential problems involve aggregate cranial nerve palsy. Routine eye care is liberal in face of the CN VII palsy often complicated by CN V paresis. Expected long-term palsies are aggressively managed by an ophthalmologic plastic surgeon using gold weighting. Tarsorrhaphy is not preferred. Airway protection is afforded by tracheostomy when necessary and GI decompression via NG intubation. When CN X is sacrificed, primary thyroplasty is performed for cord medialization at the procedure's close. Vocal cord injection is individualized and done postoperatively. Aspiration is rare. Nutrition is paramount. Negative nitrogen balance is avoided by intravenous hyperalimentation until tube feedings can be begun. Irrespective of the status of the vagus nerve, this surgery is accompanied by prolonged ileus thought to be the result of primary neuropeptide secretion by the tumor (CCK) (1). GI alimentation is conservatively begun by tube feeding only when clinical signs of GI activity are identified. A dysphagia team is involved from the outset and swallowing rehabilitation begins when it is felt that the patient is able to coordinate the passage of a food bolus. It is rare that a discharged patient needs either tracheal or nasogastric support.

CSF leakage, if it is to occur, will do so usually within the first week. Reoperation is usually necessary. Accumulation of CSF under the flap is unsightly, but of little danger. It usually resorbs over time. If the CSF accumulation is substantial enough to cause incisional compromise, aspiration and pressure dressing usually fail. Reoperation for defect reclosure usually is necessary.

Most dangerous and most unpredictable are ICA catastrophes. Most occur in irradiated patients. Adequate ICA coverage must be assured intraoperatively. Hemodynamic lability is pharmacologically controlled by ICU medical specialists. Close observation and angiography with embolectomy or repair are reserved for those instances in which prompt response is indicated. The patient is not heparinized in any dosages.

AUTHORS' EXPERIENCE: AN OVERVIEW

Between September 1970 and June 1989, 165 glomus tumors were managed by The Otology Group, PC. There were 63 glomus tympanicum lesions, 21 glomus vagale tumors at the skull base, and 84 glomus jugulare tumors on which this brief review is focused.

Table 4 generates an age breakdown of these 84 jugulare patients. There were 37 right-sided lesions and 47 on the left. Females predominated in a ratio of 3.7:1 (18 males and 66 females). Twenty percent exhibited multiple lesions: 13 carotid bodies, 1 jugulare, 2 vagales, and 1 tympanicum. Four cases (5%) were "secretor" type tumors. Two were malignant.

Various presenting symptoms were exhibited. Most common were pulsatile tinnitus (80%), some type of hearing loss (65%), aural fullness (32%), and hoarseness (14%). Dysphagia was seen in 6%; vertigo in 23%.

No physical findings were seen in 5.9% (5 patients). Cranial nerve neuropathy was absent in 35.7% (30 patients). Presenting cranial neuropathies were as follows: CN V, 4.7%; CN VI, 2%; CN VII, 18%; CN IX, 9.5%; CN X, 27%; CN XI, 13%; and CN XII, 17%. Preoperative CN VII palsy is a grave prognostic sign. All 15 patients had tumor involvement of CN VII at surgery requiring nerve resection.

Postoperatively all cranial nerves were saved in 23.8% (20 cases). This is misleading in that CN IX is often sacrificed in the course of ICA dissection. Excluding CN IX, then, yielded preservation rates of 62%! Table 5 lists postoperative neuropathies adjusted for the presence of preoperative deficits: that is, the number of nerves sacrificed that were not paralyzed preoperatively.

Fifty-six percent (56%) presented with a history of previous surgery. Total tumor removal was achieved in 87%. Subtotal excision was planned in three early in the series when distal ICA involvement was a problem; five additional cases were incompletely resected.

Skull base exposure preserving EAC was achieved in 43%. Modified IFTF approaches were performed in another 38%.

Facial nerve mobilization was the most common form of nerve management. CN VII was divided and reanastomosed in seven cases, all early in the series. Resection was necessary in 16 cases (19%). Interposition grafting was the most common form of facial reanimation.

ICE was encountered in 20% (17 cases), while CSF leak at surgery was encountered in an additional 11 cases (CSF leak encountered intraoperatively totaled 28 cases, or 33%). Repairs of defects varied as outlined, with fat/fascia and temporalis flap with lumbar drain most common. In this population rectus abdominis free flap was used only once. VA or VP shunt was employed in three cases and has been abandoned.

Tracheostomy was performed in 36%.

Table 6 lists the complications encountered.

One case fatality was found to have a "secretor" type tumor. Massive and fatal pulmonary embolus resulted in her death. This complication is thought to be related to the hemodynamic stasis of α- and β-blockade. Pulmonary embolus was thought to claim the life of a 49-year-old male on the third day postoperatively. Yet a third patient succumbed to a CVA on his first postoperative day. Aspiration pneumonia has not been seen in 3 years! The last CSF leak was reported in 1985. Results in the long term are gratifying (12).

ILLUSTRATIVE CASE 1

S.K. is a 41-year-old female who gave a 2-year history of pulsatile tinnitus, hearing loss, and aural fullness—all right sided.

Physical exam revealed a right hypotympanic vascular mass and no cranial nerve deficits. MRI revealed a medium glomus jugulare tumor with suspected ICE along the lower cranial nerves. The ICA was thought to be involved high into the tympanic segment.

Surgical plan. Even though the tumor size was medium, IFTF surgery was planned to access distal ICA control. Planned single stage removal of ICE was anticipated (Figs. 16–23).

TABLE 4. *Glomus jugulare patients (N = 84) age distribution*

Age	0–20	21–30	31–40	41–50	50+
N	1	13	31	18	21

TABLE 5. *Postoperative cranial neuropathies adjusted for preoperative deficits[a]*

Nerve	Cases (N)
V	—
VI	—
VII	24
VIII	2
IX	32
X	21
XI	23
XII	21

[a] From ref. 13, with permission.

TABLE 6. *Glomus jugulare surgical complications (N = 84)*

Complication	Percentage
Wound infection	4.7%
ICA blowout	1.0%
Aspiration	10.7%
Meningitis	2.4%
Pulmonary embolus	1.0%
ARDS	1.0%
CSF leak	8.1%
Death	3.5%

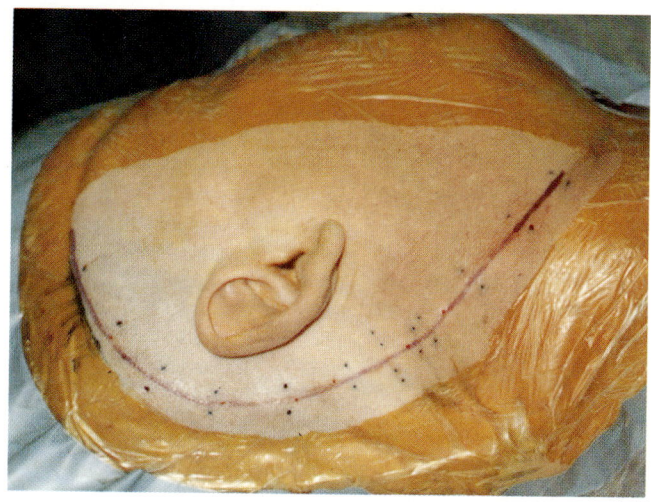

FIG. 16. Skin tattoos will aid reapproximation.

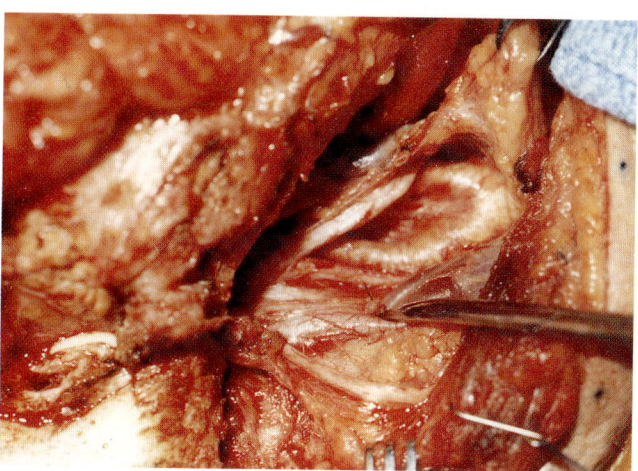

FIG. 18. Vital neck anatomy is controlled.

ILLUSTRATIVE CASE 2

R.M. is a 51-year-old female with a history identical to case 1. Physical findings were similar, again, with no cranial nerve deficits. MRI suggested a small lesion confined to the temporal bone without ICE and minimal involvement of the ICA. A small carotid body tumor is incidental.

Surgical plan. This patient was a candidate for EAC preservation (Figs. 24–26).

ILLUSTRATIVE CASE 3

R.S. is a 33-year-old female with a large skull base tumor previously irradiated. A full jugular foramen syndrome was present. MRI suggests circumferential involvement of the ICA.

Surgical plan. Proximal and distal ICA control was planned. ICA resection and vein interposition graft were probable (Figs. 27 and 28).

ILLUSTRATIVE CASE 4

N.N. is a 61-year-old female with a large tumor and extensive ICE. All lower cranial nerves are paretic.

Surgical plan. Extended IFTF approach was planned with ICE at primary stage. Rectus free flap dural defect reconstruction was also done (Figs. 29–31).

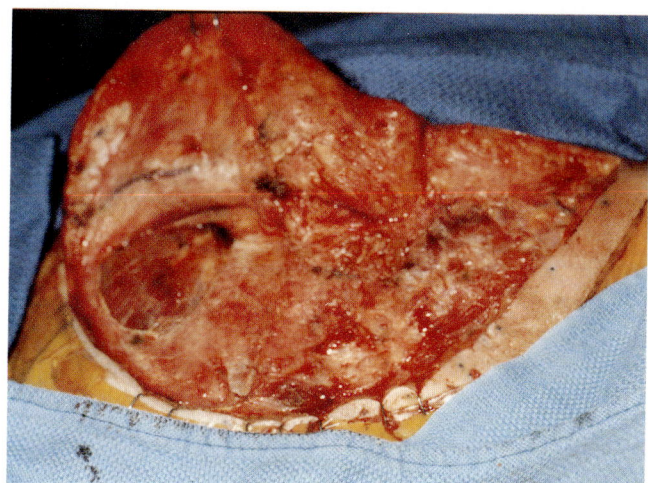

FIG. 17. The anterior based flap is elevated. The EAC is oversewn once transected.

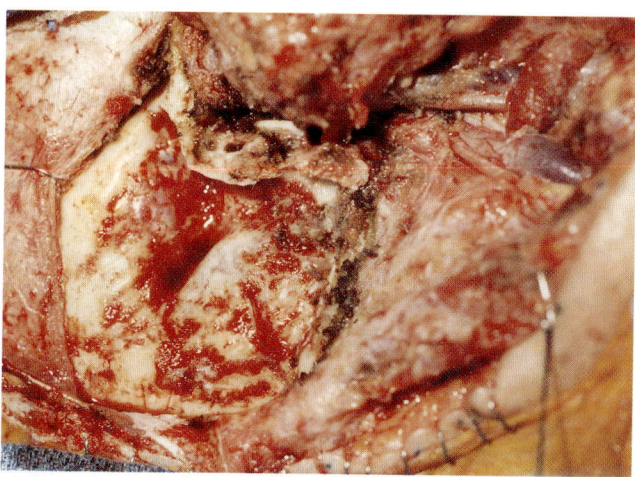

FIG. 19. A complete single mastoidectomy with EFR skeletonizes the EAC.

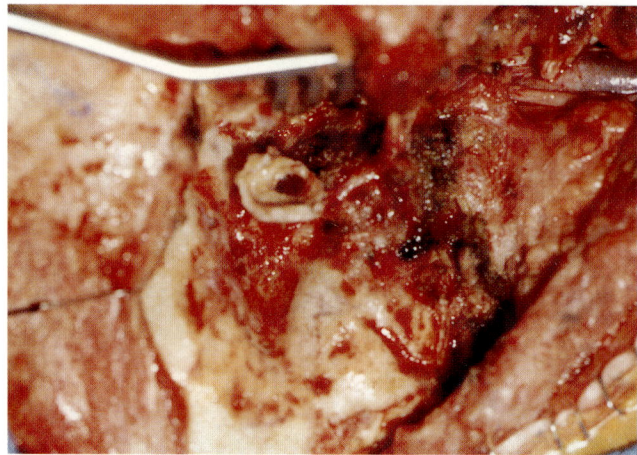

FIG. 20. After the method of partial temporal bone resection, the EAC is skeletonized.

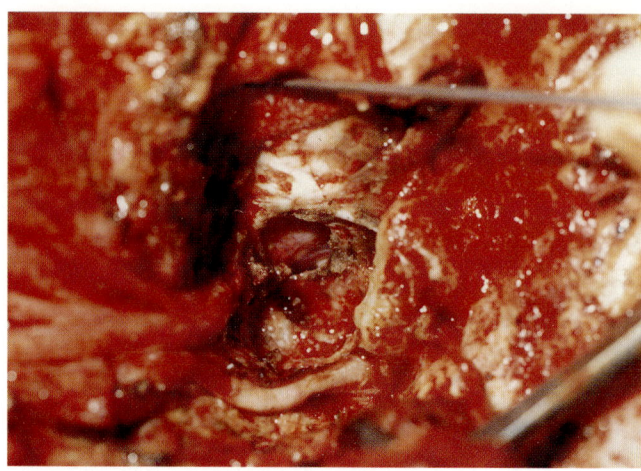

FIG. 23. ICE has been removed. A small dural defect results.

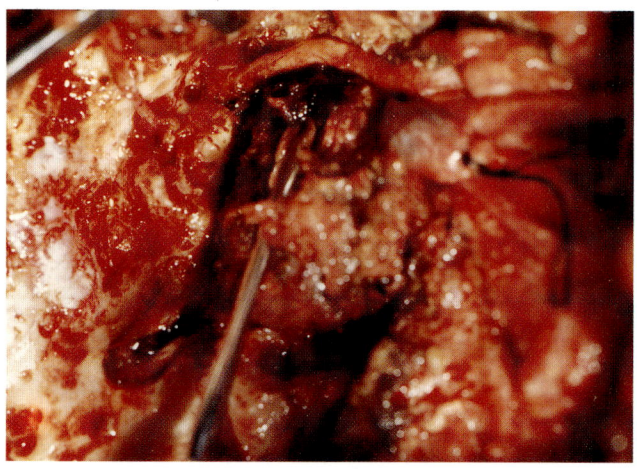

FIG. 21. Tumor has been dissected free of ICA.

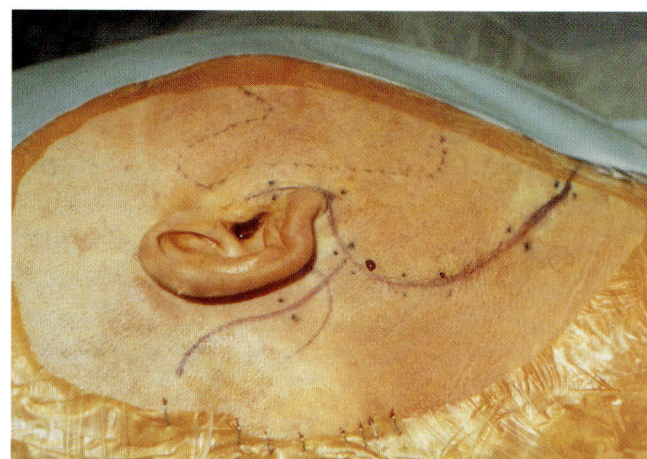

FIG. 24. Note the wide vascular pedicle for the auricle. The mandible has been "ghosted in."

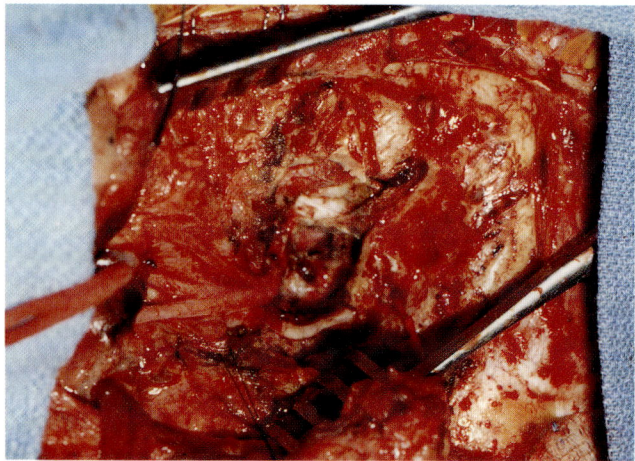

FIG. 22. Tumor has been debulked from the temporal bone down to posterior fossa dura.

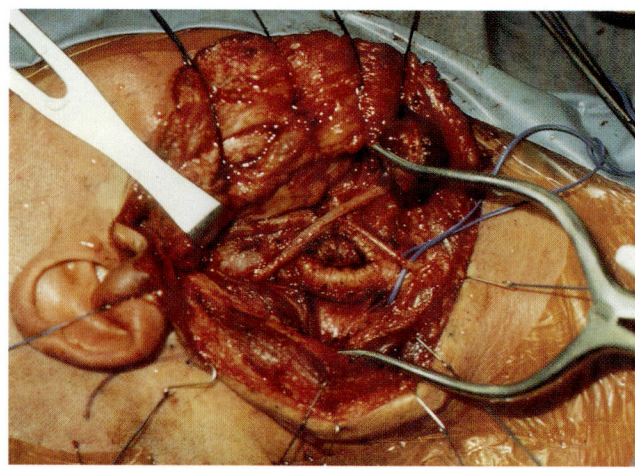

FIG. 25. Neck exposure is consistent to identify vital anatomy. A small carotid body tumor is incidental.

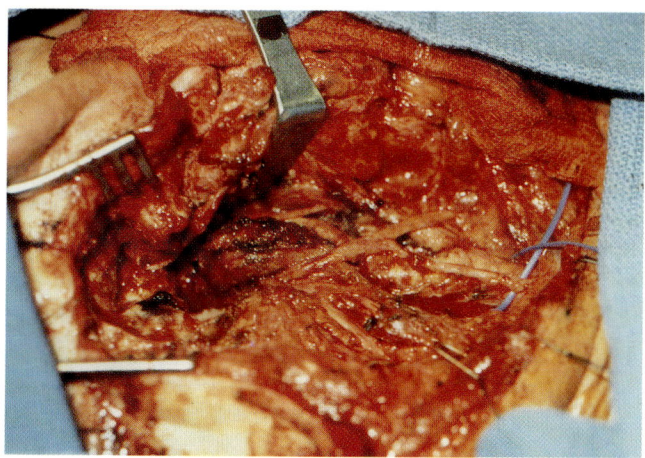

FIG. 26. Exposure of the tumor is aided by short CN VII mobilization against the preserved EAC.

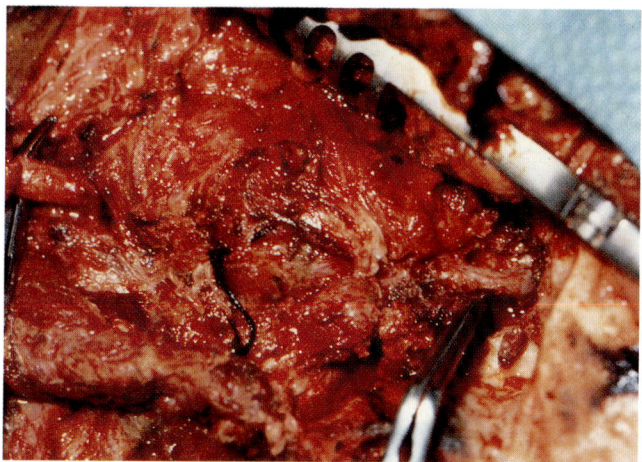

FIG. 27. Proximal and distal ICA control around the margins of this large tumor.

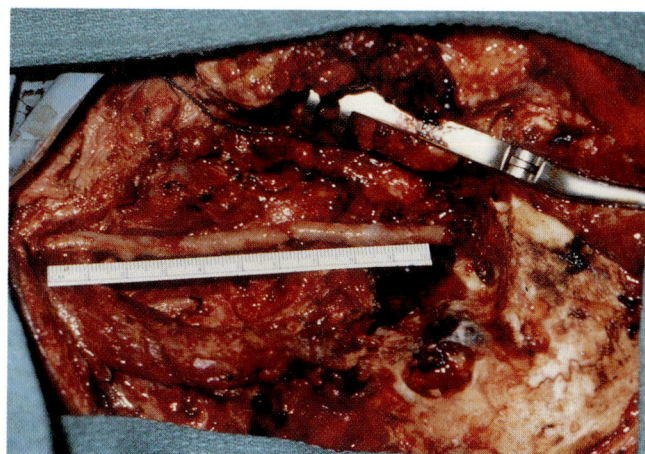

FIG. 28. This tumor fortunately was dissected free of the ICA. Interposition grafting with ICA resection was the alternative.

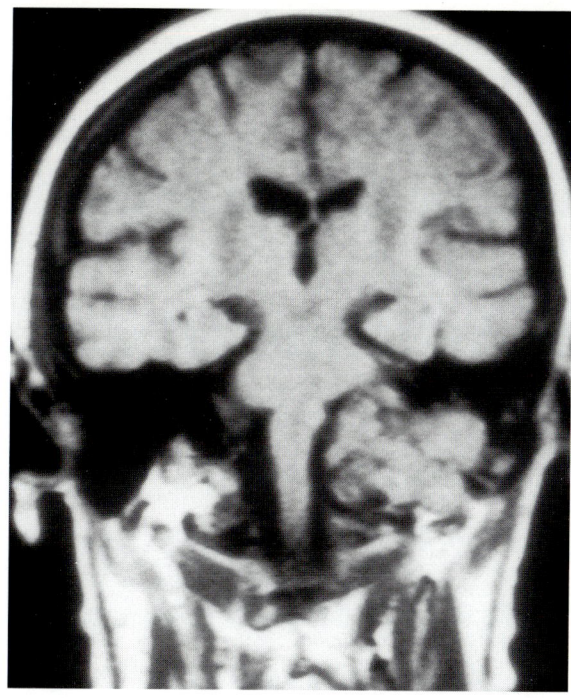

FIG. 29. Substantial ICE documented by URI.

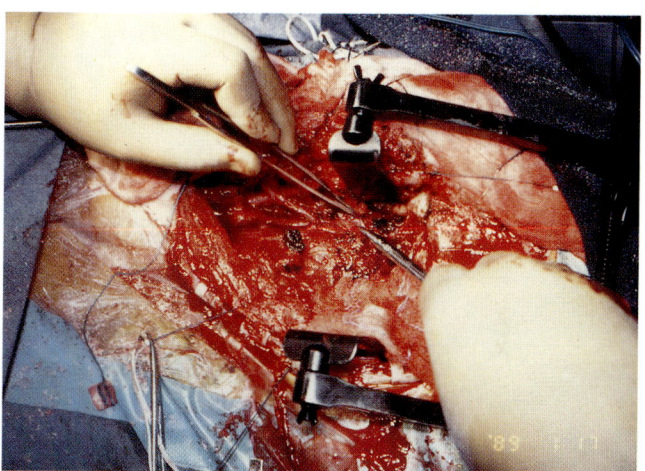

FIG. 30. Extended IFTF exposure is aided by the Fisch retractor. Tumor dissection from the ICA is proceeding. (From ref. 13, with permission.)

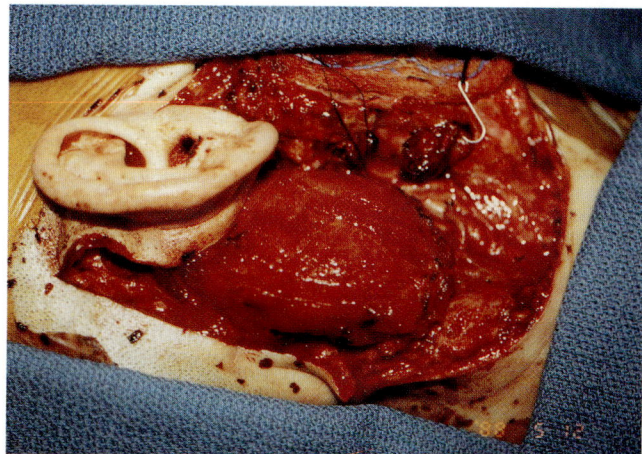

FIG. 31. A rectus abdominis free flap is in place. Note its bulk. This example is from another patient with similar ICE.

REFERENCES

1. Jackson CG, Gulya AJ, Knox GW, Glasscock ME, Pensak ML, Poe DS, Johnson GD. A paraneoplastic syndrome associated with glomus tumors of the skull? Early observations. *Otolaryngol Head Neck Surg* 1989;100:583–587.
2. Jackson CG, Glasscock ME, Harris PF. Glomus tumors. Diagnosis, classification and management of large lesions. *Arch Otolaryngol* 1982;108:401–406.
3. Jackson CG, Glasscock ME, Nissen AJ, Schwaber MK. Glomus tumor surgery: the approach, results and problems. *Otolaryngology Clin North Am* 1982;15:897–916.
4. Jackson CG, Glasscock ME. Glomus jugulare surgery. In: Wiet RJ, Causse JB, eds. *Complications in otolaryngology head and neck surgery.* Ontario, Canada: B.C. Decker, 1986.
5. Jackson CG, Glasscock ME, McKennan KX, Hoopman CF Jr, Levine SC, Hays JW, Smith HP. The surgical treatment of skull base tumors with intracranial extension. *Otolaryngol Head Neck Surg* 1987;96(2):175–185.
6. Johnson GD, Jackson CG, Fisher J, Matar SA, Poe DS. Management of large dural defects in skull base surgery: an update. *Laryngoscope* 1990;100:200–202.
7. Jackson CG, Welling DB, Chironis PI, Glasscock ME, Woods CI. Glomus tympanicum tumors: contemporary concepts in conservation surgery. *Laryngoscope,* 1989;99(9):875–884.
8. Jackson CG, Johnson GD, Poe DS. Surgical treatment of glomus tumors. In: Pillsbury H, Goldsmith MM, eds. *Operative challenges in otolaryngology–head and neck surgery.* Chicago: Year Book Medical Publishers, 1990;514.
9. Jackson CG, Poe DS, Glasscock ME, Johnson GD, Ragheb S. Diagnosis and management of glomus tumors of the temporal bone. In: *Proceedings of the Sixth International Symposium of Neurologic Surgery of the Ear and Skull Base.* Amstelveen, The Netherlands: Shimon Kugular Medical Publications, 1989.
10. Fisch U. Infratemporal fossa approach to tumors of the temporal bone and base of skull. *J Laryngol Otolaryngol* 1978;92:949–967.
11. Glasscock ME, Hays JW, Jackson CG, Steenerson RL. A one-stage combined approach for the management of large cerebellopontine angle tumors. *Laryngoscope* 1978;88:1563–1576.
12. Poe DS, Jackson CG, Glasscock ME, Johnson GD. Long-term results after lateral cranial base surgery. *Laryngoscope* 1991;101:372–378.
13. Jackson CG, Johnson GD, Poe DS. Lateral Transtemporal approaches to the skull base. In: *Surgery of Skull Base Tumors.* New York, Churchill Livingstone, 1990;141–196.
14. Glasscock ME, Kveton JF. Surgical methods: therapy of glomus tumors of the ear and base of skull. In: Thawley SE, Panje, eds. *Comprehensive Management of Head and Neck Tumors.* Philadelphia, W. B. Saunders, 1987;222–246.

CHAPTER 48

Glomus Vagale Tumors

Eugen J. Dolan and Patrick Gullane

Glomus vagale tumors, a rare subset of the nonchromaffin paragangliomas, are associated with afferent parasympathetic fibers. These tumors arise from paraganglionic tissue thought to be derived from the neural crest. Glomus vagale tumors comprise about 5% of all paragangliomas (6) seen in the head and neck regions, and most are associated with paragangliomas elsewhere. The multicentric characteristic of paragangliomas is of importance when evaluating patients with these tumors.

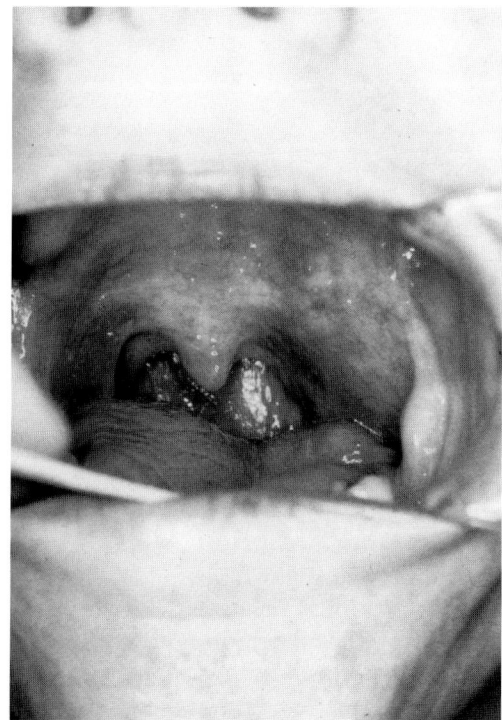 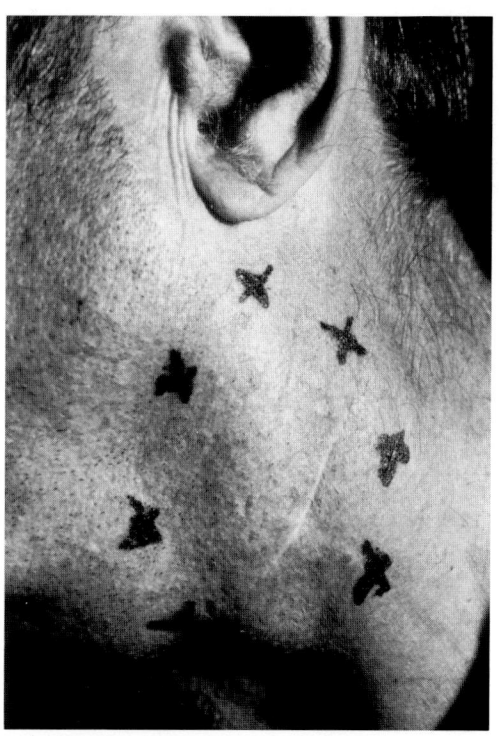

FIG. 1. A: A view showing a mass protruding into the left side of the oropharynx. **B:** Lateral view of neck showing mass.

E. J. Dolan: Division of Neurosurgery, The Billings Clinic, Billings, Montana 59107-5100.
P. Gullane: Department of Otolaryngology, Toronto General Hospital, University of Toronto, Toronto, Ontario, Canada M5G 1L7.

DIAGNOSTIC CONSIDERATIONS

Most patients present with a neck or pharyngeal mass (Fig. 1). The mass is generally more cephalad than with carotid body tumors and often extends to the base of the

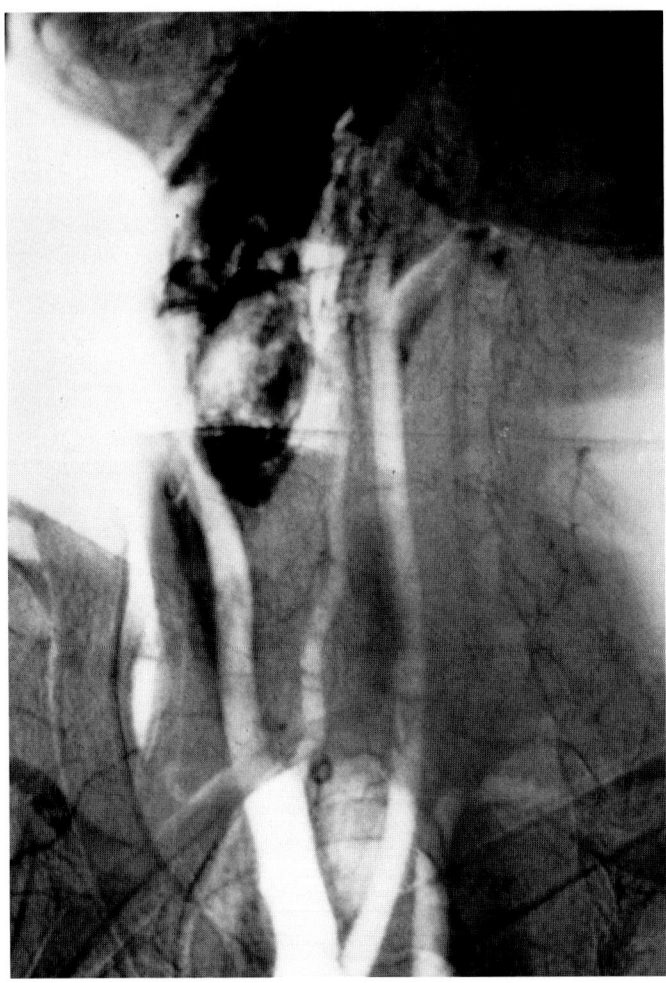 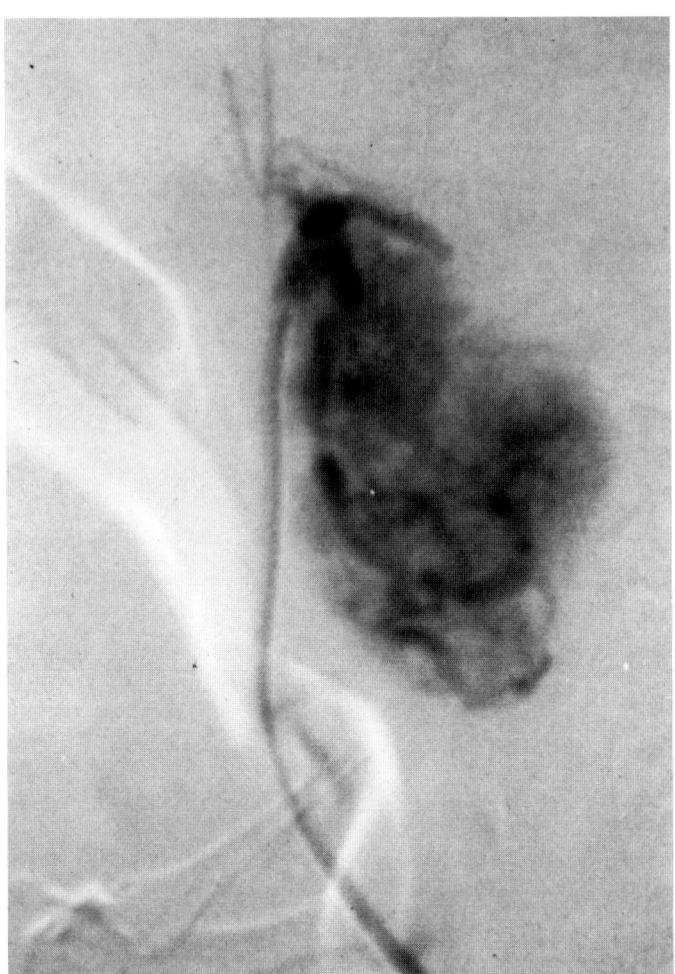

FIG. 2. A: Carotid angiogram showing a glomus vagale tumor extending to the base of the skull. **B:** Selective angiography of glomus vagale tumor.

skull. Rarely, they extend intracranially with a dumbbell component. Although some patients may complain of pain at presentation, none of our six cases had pain, but all presented with a neck mass. None had symptoms referable to the vagus nerve or any other cranial nerve at the time of presentation.

Family history is important in all paragangliomas as they can be multicentric in up to 35% of the familial paragangliomas, and in up to 5% of the nonhereditary group (4).

Paraganglionic tumors are frequently multicentric in origin (2, 4, 6), and although glomus vagale tumors themselves are rarely functional [only one case (7) of just over 75 reported cases], some of the associated tumors may function actively. These considerations therefore demand that particular studies be undertaken. Thorough examination of both cervical areas, measurement of catecholamine production (24-hr urine collection), and ultrasound examination of the abdomen, especially of the paraspinous areas, are mandatory.

All patients undergo both CT and MRI scanning to delineate the boundaries of the lesion and to detect any related lesions. To date, we have had no experience with gadolinium enhanced MRI for the investigation of either carotid body or glomus vagale tumors.

Angiography is performed in all cases to demonstrate the angioarchitecture of these vascular tumors (Fig. 2). Ideally, selective bilateral carotid angiography is performed 48–72 hr prior to surgery. This allows embolization of the lesion with Ivalon sponge particles at the same session as the angiography.

The anatomic extent of the lesion and its angioarchitecture provide the information needed to formulate the surgical approach to the lesion.

PATIENT SELECTION

Age

Most glomus vagale tumors are slow growing, nonfunctional, and rarely metastasize. They can be well controlled with radiation (5). For this reason, most elderly patients should not be considered for surgery unless the mass itself presents a significant symptomatic problem.

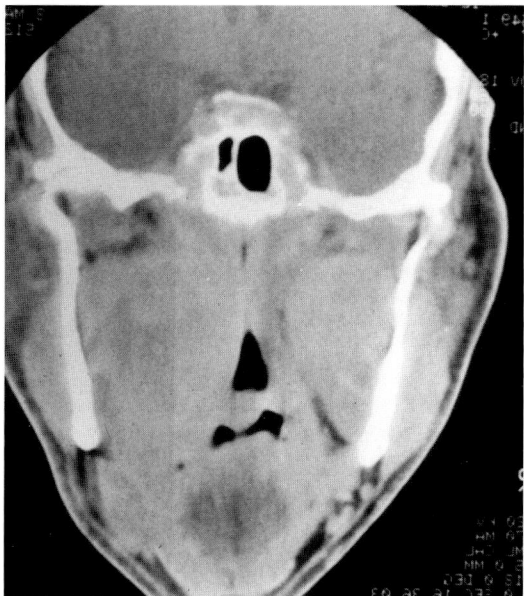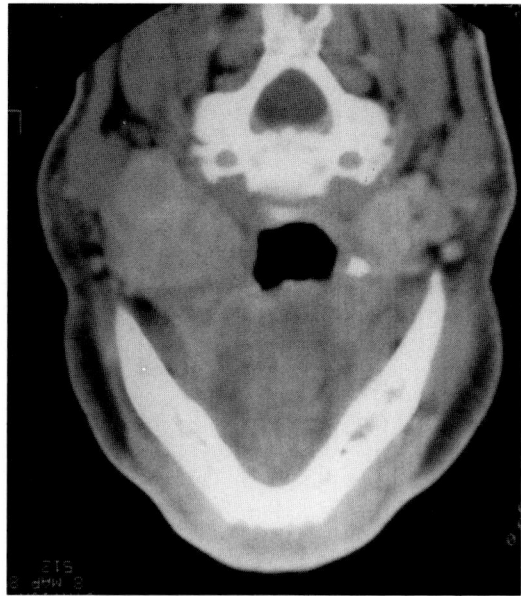

FIG. 3. CT scan of a patient with bilateral glomus vagale tumor.

Bilateral Glomus Vagale Tumors

Bilateral glomus vagale tumors pose the risk of loss of both vagus nerves, possibly resulting in a fatal outcome (1). There has been but one case reported of functional preservation of the vagus nerve when glomus vagale tumors are removed surgically (3). For this reason, when one of the lesions is very large and symptomatic (Fig. 2), and the contralateral vocal cord is functional, we would treat the larger symptomatic lesion surgically and follow with radiation therapy to the second lesion. In other cases when the glomus vagale tumors are bilateral, our recommendation would be for treatment primarily with radiation (Fig. 3).

Paragangliomas in Addition to the Glomus Vagale Tumor

If a functional paraganglioma is discovered, this should be dealt with first. With respect to carotid body tumors, an ipsilateral carotid body tumor presents little difficulty, and both this and the glomus vagale tumor can be dealt with during the same operation. A significant contralateral carotid body tumor should be treated after dealing with the glomus vagale tumor. Glomus tympanicum tumors are a special case of the above. If asymptomatic they need not be treated immediately but should be removed surgically when indicated.

For example, in our series, three patients had unilateral glomus vagale tumors. One patient had an asymptomatic contralateral glomus tympanicum that was not treated. One patient with a very large glomus vagale tumor (Fig. 2) was treated surgically; later, the patient was found to have a small glomus vagale tumor on the contralateral side and is presently being followed for this. One patient had bilateral glomus tumors and is presently being followed (Fig. 3).

OPERATIVE TECHNIQUE

A lateral approach was used in all our cases. Nonetheless, we would consider a midline approach, involving the splitting of the symphysis and hinging the jaw laterally as an alternative approach to lesions that extend to the skull base with no intracranial component. The present work describes the lateral approach.

Anesthetic Considerations

Fluothane anesthesia is used in all our cases. An arterial vascular catheter and a central venous pressure line are used. Six units of blood are on hand at the start of the procedure, because of the risk of significant blood loss with these vascular tumors.

During the initial exposure of the tumor, the blood pressure is kept slightly below the patient's normal blood pressure. During the actual dissection of the tumor, particularly from the major vessels, the mean blood pressure is maintained at about 80 mm Hg in younger patients, but somewhat higher in older patients. The blood pressure was regulated pharmacologically with a continuous nitroglycerine infusion. This allowed rapid reversal of hypotension if needed.

Patient Position

Patients are placed supine with a sandbag under the ipsilateral shoulder to elevate it, and the head is turned to the contralateral side (Fig. 4). The operating table is flexed, to elevate the patient's head and maintain good venous drainage.

Surgery

As mentioned previously, all patients undergo preoperative embolization of their tumors with Ivalon particles 48–72 hr prior to the operative procedure. A curvilinear skin incision begins at the mastoid process and follows the natural skin lines anteroinferiorly (Fig. 4). If necessary, the incision can be extended anterior to the ear for mobilization of the parotid gland and upper mandible as required.

The incision is carried down through the platysma and along the anterior border of the sternocleidomastoid muscle. The great auricular nerve is mobilized and, if possible, spared. Dissection is then carried along the jugular vein, mobilizing it, usually with ligation of the common facial vein, and the common carotid artery is mobilized inferiorly. Plastic vessel loops are placed around the common carotid artery for vascular control. The dissection then mobilizes all the structures in the carotid triangle, including the hypoglossal, accessory, and vagus nerves (Fig. 5), the internal carotid artery (ICA), and the external carotid artery (ECA) and its branches. Plastic vessel loops are placed around all major structures as shown in Figs. 5 and 6, and in particular double loops are used around the common, internal, and external carotid arteries. Only those branches of the jugular vein and ECA necessary to expose the tumor are ligated. Occasionally, the ECA must be ligated to control bleeding. After the tumor is dissected from its surroundings, the vagus nerve is identified at its entry into the tumor and carefully, with the aid of magnifying loops or the operating microscope, freed from the tumor (Fig. 5). The tumor is then dissected from the underlying carotid artery (Fig. 6). At this stage hypotension to 80 mm Hg mean arterial pressure is a significant benefit to control bleeding. A combination of sharp and blunt dissection is used to remove the tumor. It has not been found necessary to use the operating microscope for the tumor resection.

Following tumor resection, the platysma layer is closed with 3-0 Dexon and the subcutaneous tissue with 4-0 Dexon. A $\frac{1}{8}$-inch hemovac drain is left in place. Skin is closed with staples.

Technical Considerations

Excessive internal carotid artery bleeding can be controlled by carefully tightening the loops around the internal and common carotid arteries to temporarily occlude them. A Javid or Imodex vascular shunt is then inserted into the ICA through a small arteriotomy. The shunt helps to preserve cerebral perfusion while bleeding is being controlled. This was required in one case. After removal of the shunt, the arteriotomy and any tears in the ICA are closed with 6-0 Prolene. If the jugular bulb at the skull base presents a problem in the dissection, the surgeon should be prepared to ligate the sigmoid sinus.

Despite the difficulty of isolating and preserving the function of the vagus nerve (one reported case of functional preservation of the vagus nerve after removal of a glomus vagale tumor), every effort should be made to preserve the nerve in all cases (Fig. 5). If the lesion is near the skull base, the accessory and glossopharyngeal nerves

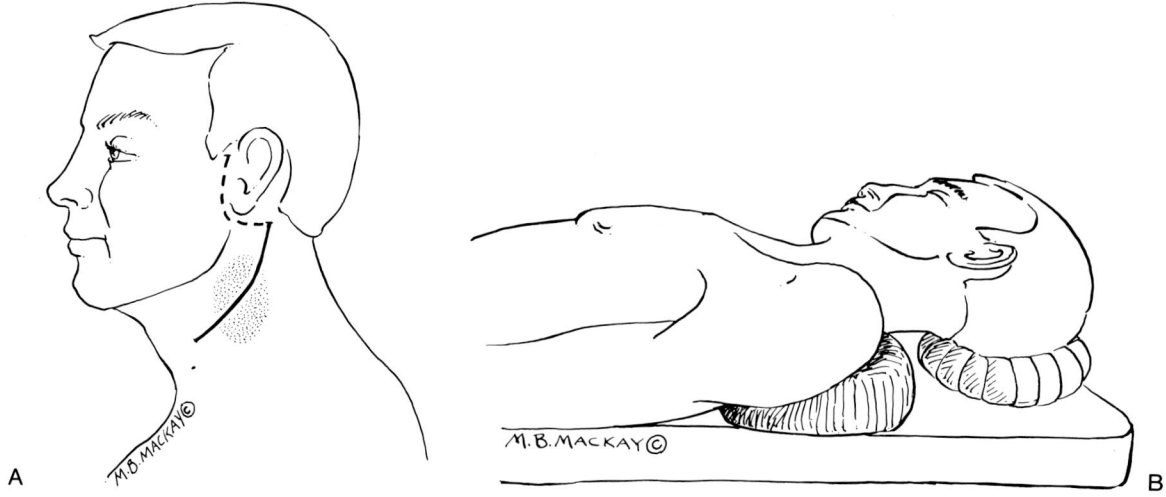

FIG. 4. A: Diagram showing the incision used for the lateral approach to glomus vagale tumors. The *dotted line* is the extension anterior to the ear used when the parotid requires mobilization. **B:** Position of the patient.

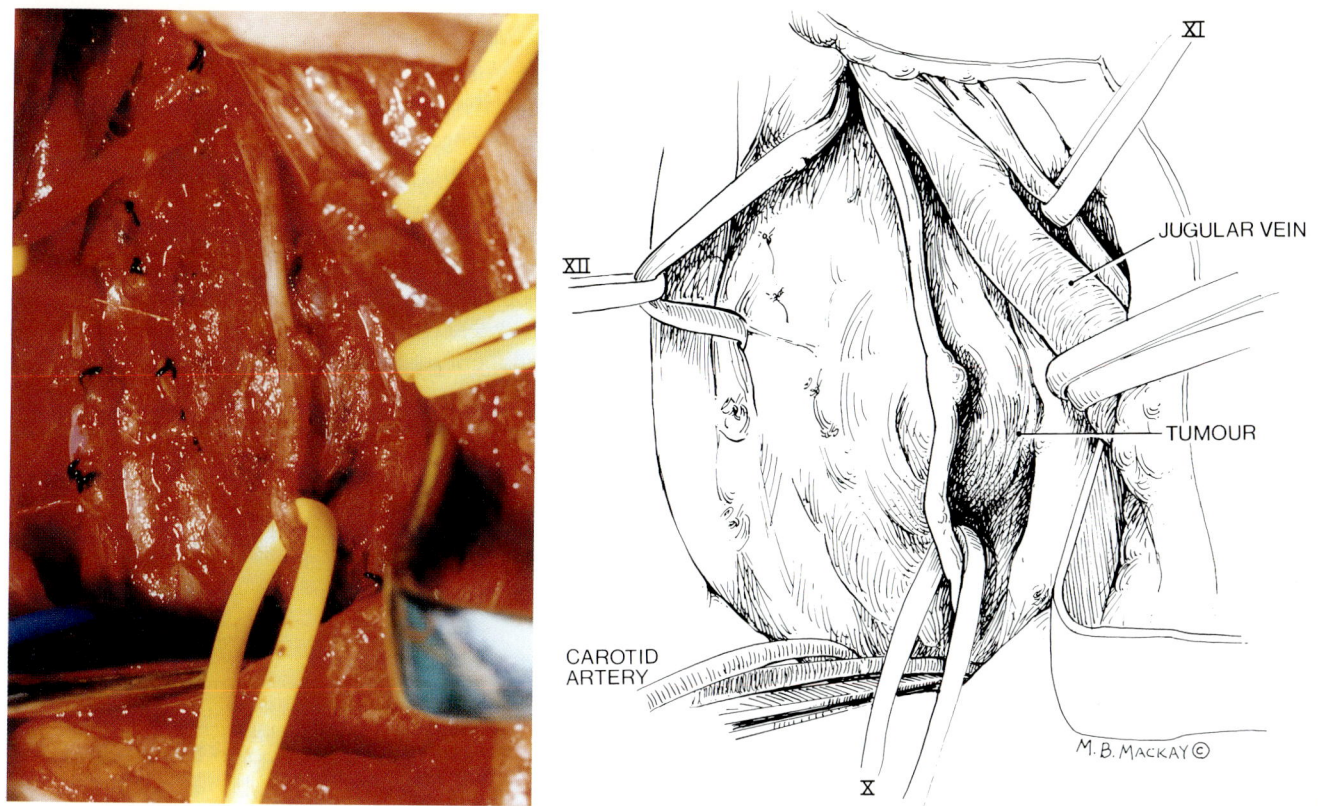

FIG. 5. A: Intraoperative exposure of the glomus vagale tumor showing the common carotid artery, and cranial nerves X, XI, and XII. The vagus nerve has been dissected free of the tumor. **B:** Artist's drawing of the surgical field shown in (**A**).

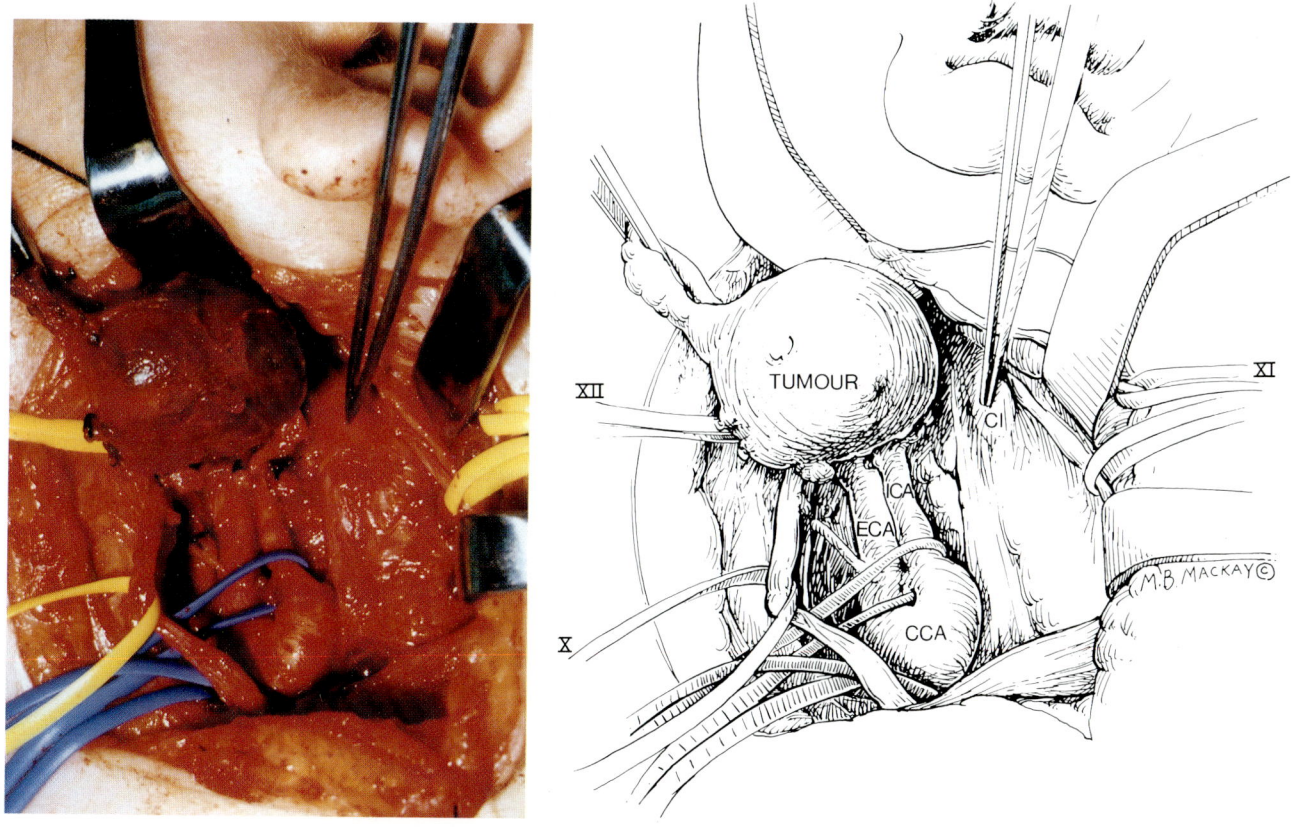

FIG. 6. A: Operative photograph showing the tumor removal. Internal (ICA) and external (ECA) carotid arteries can now be seen. **B:** Artist's drawing of the surgical field in (**A**).

are also at significant risk. If these nerves cannot be spared, consideration should be given to either primary anastomotic repair or grafting (using the great auricular nerve).

POSTOPERATIVE MANAGEMENT

All patients receive Ancef 1 g every 8 hr, beginning immediately preoperatively and continued for 24 hr postoperatively. All patients are closely monitored in the intensive care unit for 24 hr following surgery. Drains may be removed in 48 hr. The patient is mobilized on the second day. All patients are expected to have some degree of hoarseness and dysphagia, and if the dissection was near the head of the mandible a degree of trismus may also be present.

Feeding is begun after 48 hr, but only after ensuring good function of the contralateral pharynx. Soft foods (e.g., gelatins) are given initially, graduating to solid foods as tolerated.

COMPLICATIONS AND MANAGEMENT

The complications of glomus vagale tumor removal relate to injury to the nerves or vessels in the surgical field. Vagus nerve palsy will result in all cases, producing hoarseness, dysphagia, and possible cardiac dysrhythmias. The hypoglossal and accessory nerves may also be injured depending on the extent of the resection.

In our series of five surgical patients, all but one had a permanent vagus nerve palsy on the operated side. Nevertheless, none developed problems with aspiration or airway compromise, and none required Teflon injection of the vocal cords. Vagus nerve dysfunction was the only permanent sequela.

REFERENCES

1. Brodal A. *Neurological anatomy in relation to clinical medicine.* New York: Oxford University Press, 1981;466–470.
2. Conley JJ, Clairmont AA. Glomus intravagale. *Laryngoscope* 1977;87:2096–2100.
3. Davidson J, Gullane P. Glomus vagale tumors. *Otolaryngol Head Neck Surg* 1988;99:66–70.
4. Parkin JL. Familial multiple glomus tumors and pheochromocytomas. *Ann Otol* 1981;90:60–63.
5. Sharma PD, Johnson AP, Whitton AC. Radiotherapy for jugulotympanic paragangliomas. *J Laryngol Otol* 1984;98:621–629.
6. Sykes JM, Ossoff RH. Paragangliomas of the head and neck. *Otolaryngol Clin North Am* 1986;19:755–767.
7. Tannir NM, Cortas N, Allam C. A functioning catecholamine secreting vagal body tumour. *Cancer* 1983;52:932–935.

CHAPTER 49

Orbital Surgery

Jack Rootman and Felix Durity

PRESENTATION

The abnormal changes brought about by disease in the orbit can be divided into four basic categories of clinical manifestation. These categories are not necessarily independent but provide a working framework for characterization of a particular orbital problem. The changes seen consist of inflammatory signs, mass effect, infiltration, and vascular change. Mass effect consists of displacement with or without signs of involvement of sensory or neuromuscular structures. Displacement of orbital structures may point to the location of the disease and help define its nature. Inflammation is characterized by, and can be inferred from, signs and symptoms of pain, warmth, loss of function, and mass effect. The degree to which one categorizes the process as either acute or chronic is related to the severity of the signs and symptoms as well as the rapidity of onset. Infiltrative changes are usually associated with evidence of destruction, entrapment, or both, which may lead to effects on ocular movement or neurosensory function (e.g., diplopia, muscle restriction or fibrosis, optic neuropathy, pain, or paresthesia). Alterations in the character, size, and structural integrity of vessels may imply an underlying vascular process. The major features suggesting vascular changes consist of venous dilatation, tissue exudation, hemorrhage, infarction, and structural alterations of vascular components.

In our experience, the most common manifestation brought about by neoplasia is the mass effect. Secondarily, infiltration is a significant feature in neoplasia, usually implying a more malignant process. Clinically apparent inflammatory features and vascular phenomena were extremely rare signs at onset in neoplastic disorders.

PROFILE OF DISEASE

In order to provide a contextual framework for understanding surgical indications and approaches to the orbit, it is worthwhile to divide orbital disorders into six major categories (Table 1). These processes can occur either independently or together, in or around the orbit, and all fit within the differential diagnosis of "orbital tumors" insofar as they produce mass and functional effects based on displacement or infiltration of the structures. In the UBC Orbital Clinic, 45.6% of patients presenting had thyroid orbitopathy. The most common nonthyroid orbital disorders encountered were neoplasia, accounting for close to 18.7% of primary orbital disease processes in the overall group. Neoplasia may present as either benign or malignant disorders demonstrating either infiltrative or noninfiltrative behavior. Next in order of occurrence were structural disorders, constituting 15.8% of our experience. Structural processes can be divided into congenital or acquired disorders and include within the group bony abnormalities, cysts, ectopias, and traumatic lesions. In particular, the cysts and ectopias behave very similar to many noninfiltrative tumor masses, thus constituting an important part of the differential diagnosis of neoplasia. Inflammation was the fourth most common disorder (11% of cases). Chronic inflammatory conditions, in particular, may mimic infiltrative or noninfiltrative orbital mass lesions. Vascular lesions, which were much less common (4.1%), include a large number of diseases, the character of which are governed primarily by their hemodynamic associations. These can be divided into nonobstructive lesions on the arterial side—including tumors (hemangiomas and lymphangiomas), malformations, and fistulas —and venous lesions, which were either distensible or

---

J. Rootman: Department of Ophthalmology and Pathology, University of British Columbia; and Orbital Clinic, Vancouver General Hospital, Vancouver, British Columbia, Canada V5Z 3N9.

F. Durity: Division of Neurosurgery, University of British Columbia, and Vancouver General Hospital, Vancouver, British Columbia, Canada V5Z 4E9.

TABLE 1. *Distribution of orbital disease processes: UBC Orbital Clinic, 1976–1988*

Category	Number	Percentage (%)
Thyroid orbitopathy	860	45.6
Neoplasia	353	18.7
Structural	297	15.8
Inflammatory	208	11.0
Vascular	77	4.1
Degenerative, atrophy, and deposition	30	1.6
Functional or normal	59	3.1
Total	1884	

nondistensible varices. All the vascular lesions in some way or another can behave as masses within the orbit and thus fit into the differential diagnosis of orbital neoplasia. In some instances, there can be a relatively acute onset due to hemorrhage within the tumor. Finally, the least common category of disease consisted of degenerations, atrophies, and depositions (1.6%). These include such disorders as facial and orbital atrophy, amyloidosis, myopia, and linear scleroderma. All these may lead to mass effect by deposition of material or by atrophy with loss of orbital substance and thus may enter into the differential diagnosis of disorders causing proptosis or pseudoproptosis due to asymmetry.

INDICATIONS FOR SURGICAL INTERVENTION

The approach and timing of surgical intervention depend on the nature of the disease as defined by clinical and laboratory investigation (Table 2). The primary indications for intervention were decompression for thyroid orbitopathy, biopsy, excision of a cyst or mass, repair and reconstruction, drainage of an abscess, and removal of a foreign body.

Orbital mass lesions can be divided into two broad categories in terms of the indications for surgery:

1. Well defined, slow growing, or nonprogressive lesions whether they are cystic, neoplastic, or structural, which do not lead to functional deficit can generally be observed. Intervention is based on the size, location, rate of progression, or functional deficit produced by the lesion and is usually extirpative.
2. Progressive, poorly defined, or infiltrative lesions that cause functional deficits or entrapment of orbital structures generally require incisional biopsy prior to definitive management. Management is then based on the appropriate and specific histopathologic diagnosis. Biopsy, in particular, requires meticulous care and a preoperative consultation with pathologists in order to define the most appropriate means of acquisition and treatment of tissues for pathologic investigation.

The other broad indications for orbital intervention noted earlier do not generally involve neoplastic lesions except in the case of debulking, exenteration, and supraexenteration for malignant disorders of the orbit and periorbital structures.

Special Considerations

In the category of neurogenic tumors there are some special considerations for surgical intervention. We would excise an optic nerve glioma only if it is anterior to the chiasm, resectable, and has demonstrated growth. Diffuse, chiasmal, or bilateral optic nerve gliomas are managed nonsurgically in our center. Meningiomas of the optic nerve are also resected only if they cause severe functional visual loss, or are of significant size, or evidence progression into the intracranial space. In our experience optic nerve meningiomas are best completely excised along with the nerve except for rare incidences of exophytic and anterior optic nerve meningiomas, which may be resected locally without removal of the optic nerve. Sphenoid wing meningiomas are approached in our clinic by a combined orbitotomy craniotomy approach in instances of large lesions that cause progressive, functional deficit and/or severe proptosis.

INVESTIGATION: ORBITAL IMAGING

Since the emphasis in this chapter is on disorders of the orbit that require, on the whole, combined or complicated approaches to the orbit, we restrict our discussion to the major masses that would affect this group of patients. These include patients with large orbital tumors, optic nerve masses, and tumors that extend between the boundaries of the orbit and the adjacent orbital structures intracranially or into the nasopharynx and face. Broadly speaking, the investigations of these diseases should be based on the clinical analysis of the patient, which would define the structural and functional changes as well as location of the orbital lesions. The categories of investigation are careful clinical examination, ocular and visual function assessment, orbital

TABLE 2. *Indications for orbital surgery: UBC Orbital Clinic, 1976–1988*

Indication	Number
Decompressions	131
Biopsy	129
Excision	180
Repair and reconstructions	40
Exenteration	17
Debulking	20
Aspiration needle biopsy	13
Drainage	9
Foreign body removal	5
Nerve sheath decompression	4
Total	548

imaging, systemic survey, and pathologic study. The ocular and psychophysical investigations include visual field assessment, oculomotor examination, psychophysical studies, such as color vision and contrast sensitivity, and electrophysiologic investigations that provide the information to assess the functional damage brought about by disease. In addition, careful oculomotor assessment would also delineate functional damage. Systemic investigation is particularly important in the assessment of these patients. The purely ocular and functional examination of the orbit is beyond the context of this chapter and requires careful and complete ophthalmic assessment.

Orbital imaging has undergone an explosive growth in the last 20 years and is providing detailed pictures that allow localization and suggest features of inflammatory, mass, infiltrative, vascular, and structural changes. This information, combined with clinical and ophthalmic investigation, allows increasing specificity in terms of defining the position, nature, and progress of lesions. These modalities can provide useful information on relationships to adjacent structures, evidence of infiltration, capsular definition, tissue characteristics, and the relationship to the vascular system, which will aid in determining both the need for and the approach in surgery. In addition, changes with time on follow-up can aid in diagnosis or assessment of a treatment modality.

Routine radiographic methods have limited use but can outline dense tumors such as osteomas and the bony changes associated with both expansive and destructive lesions. In our experience, the mainstay of the common orbital imaging investigation remains accurate computed tomographic (CT) studies both with and without contrast. The CT scan can define the margin of the lesions (smooth, nodular, or infiltrative) and demonstrate contrast enhancement in the case of inflammatory, vascular, and some solid tumors. Density differentiation may help in defining fat and calcium and delineate adjacent soft tissues. The sites of lesions as well as their extensions into either the nasopharyngeal or intracranial spaces can also be studied both with soft tissue and bone settings.

Vascular studies, both arterial and venous, are really only useful in selected aspects of orbital tumors. Magnified and subtracted views of the arterial supply can aid in defining the location and character of the blood supply of tumors preoperatively. Some vascular tumors can be treated with preoperative embolization and occlusion. Venography is rarely used now except for specific indications in the case of varices of the orbit. Orbital echography can provide useful information on location, size, shape, tissue characteristics, and vascular features of many lesions.

Magnetic resonance imaging (MRI) may give additional information regarding the structural nature of orbital lesions and is particularly useful in the study of optic nerve masses wherein the normal nerve structures can be defined separately from adjacent tumor masses, thus differentiating between intrinsic and extrinsic optic nerve tumors. In addition, it is a modality that has been found useful in demonstrating some vascular lesions and delineating the anatomy of and relationship to intracranial structures in lesions that have extended beyond the orbit into the adjacent cavities.

Pathologic assessment of both extirpated and biopsied tissue has become increasingly sophisticated and it is important to emphasize that the appropriate management and processing of these tissues should be clearly outlined in advance of surgery to maximize the diagnostic yield. Preoperative consultation with the pathologist is important in this regard.

SURGICAL APPROACHES TO THE ORBIT

The three major surgical approaches to the orbit are anterior, lateral, and superior (Table 3). The structures can be approached by any one or combinations of these routes as defined by the location and character of the lesion prior to surgery. Combined neurosurgical, otorhinolaryngologic, and reconstructive teams may be necessary for the more complicated lesions involving the intracranial or sinus cavities. Fine needle aspiration biopsy may circumvent the need for open biopsy in some cases, particularly in suspected malignancies and some lymphomas.

The majority of orbital procedures can be carried out through an anterior incision either via conjunctiva or skin. Incision sites can be superior, inferior, in the various quadrants, or directly over a palpable lesion.

Lateral orbitotomy with variation in the amount and location of bony removal can be customized to include more of the superior lateral orbital rim or even the zygomatic arch when necessary depending on the size and location of the lesion being attacked.

The superior approach to the orbit is either by a transfrontal or a frontotemporal–orbitozygomatic approach. The majority of lesions in this category are apical or combined apical–intracranial lesions, or represent aggressive malignancies requiring en bloc exenteration or orbitectomy.

All of the above approaches can be used in combination or with variations. In order to access any of these

TABLE 3. *Surgical approaches to the orbit: UBC Orbital Clinic, 1976–1988*

Approach	Percentage (%)
Anterior	63.9
Lateral	17.5
Cranial	8.4
Anterior + otolaryngological	5.7
Aspiration biopsy	3.1
Anterior and lateral	1.0
Cranial + otolaryngological	0.4

surgical spaces of the orbit, widening bony incisions or removal of adjacent bony structures may be necessary to facilitate the approach to more complex lesions.

TECHNIQUE

The operative principles in the orbit are similar to neurosurgery and require the meticulous maintenance of a bloodless field by appropriate patient positioning, hypotensive anesthesia (when no systemic contraindications exist), and careful local control of bleeding with fine bipolar coagulators, microvascular clips, bone wax, vacuum suction, neurosurgical patties, and chemical coagulators. Adequate exposure and visualization are maximized by the use of careful retraction, periosteal elevation, excellent lighting, multiple incisions when necessary, wide bony cuts, and operative magnification. Fixed orbital retractors have been designed by ourselves and by Kennerdell and Maroon (Fig. 1).

Tissue manipulation should be minimized, particularly in the orbit. The technique for retracting fat in a nontraumatic way is important in identifying and excising orbital masses. We use both specially designed rigid and malleable retractors with dry neurosurgical patties to expose lesions and retract fat. Appropriate planes of dissection should be established by entering through nonpathologically involved tissues in order to define the boundaries between the normal and abnormal structures. Because the orbit is a small, rigidly confined space, postoperative drainage is extremely important and we generally use vacuum drains following major orbital procedures to reduce postoperative edema. The Rootman orbital instruments (Downs Surgical Ltd.) are specially designed for the orbit. Many are modifications of the fine microsurgical instruments used in intracranial surgery.

SPECIFIC ORBITAL APPROACHES

Anterior Orbitotomy

The three anterior orbital approaches are transconjunctival, extraperiosteal, and transeptal. The transeptal approach can be accessed through a number of incisions made in the relaxation lines surrounding the eye (Fig. 2).

Transconjunctival Approach

Many anterior, periocular, and intraconal lesions can be approached by a direct transconjunctival incision and dissection (Fig. 3). A rectus muscle may be detached in order to enter the intraconal space and retractors are placed between the muscle and the globe. This is a useful approach in accessing the anterior portion of the optic nerve for nerve sheath decompression, wherein the medial rectus muscle is detached and the globe is rotated laterally and distracted anteriorly to expose the anterior optic nerve sheath (Fig. 3B).

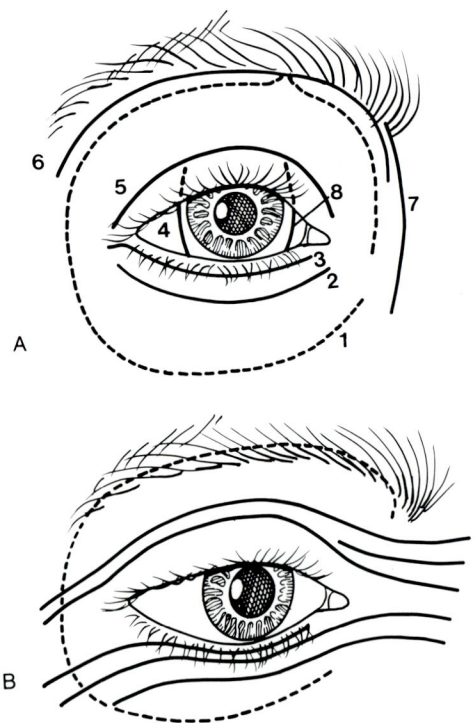

FIG. 2. A: Schematic demonstrating various incision sites for anterior orbitotomy. 1, This line defines the position of the orbital margins; 2, lower lid; 3, subciliary; 4, lateral conjuctiva; 5, lid crease; 6, supraorbital; 7, medial (Lynch); and 8, medial conjunctival. **B:** The relaxation lines around the eyes are useful sites for line of incision. (Redrawn from ref. 19.)

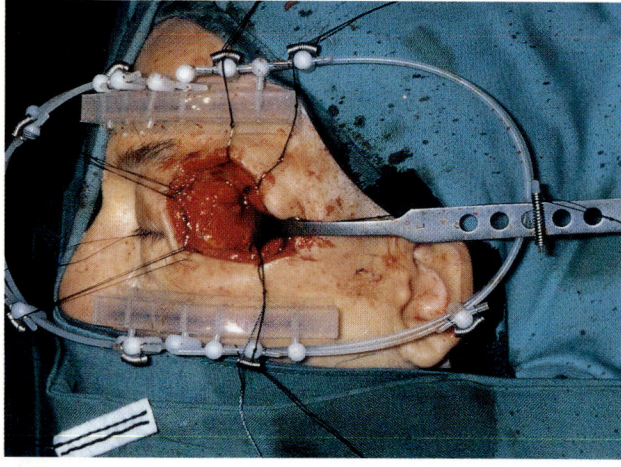

FIG. 1. A fixed orbital stage-type retractor is attached to the face with surgical adhesive. The temporalis fossa is retracted by a temporalis retractor, and the skin and subcutaneous tissues by silk sutures and nonbarbed fish hooks. (From ref. 19, with permission.)

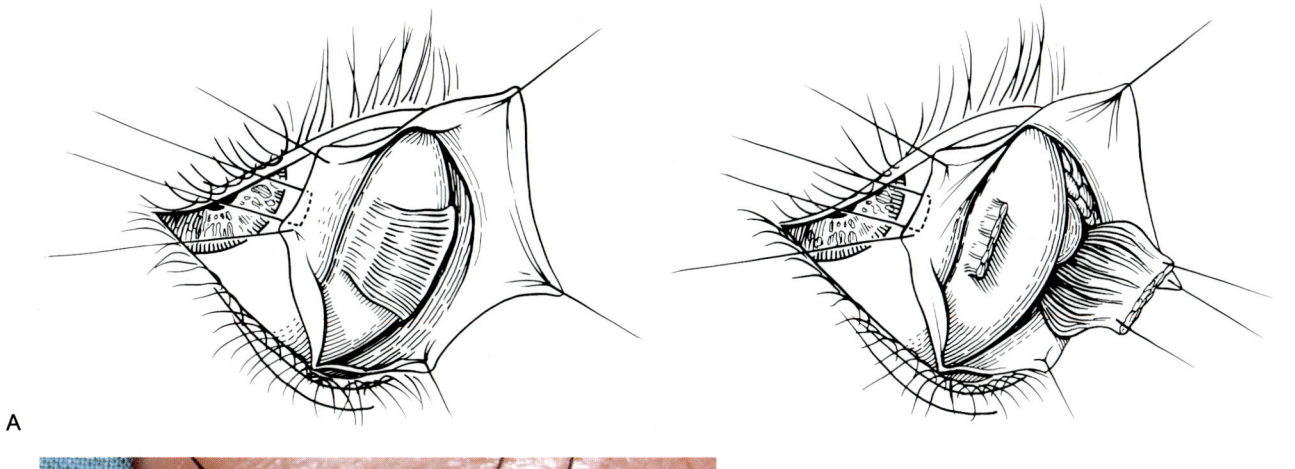

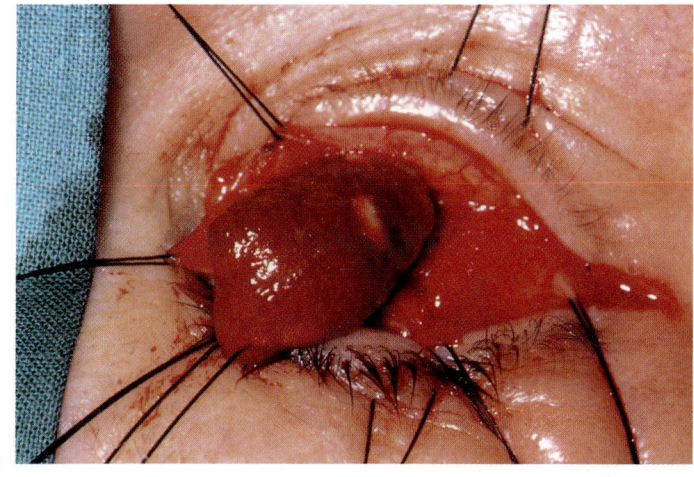

FIG. 3. A: A medial conjunctival incision for removal of an orbital tumor. Note the limbal suture placed for rotation of the eye and suture retraction of conjuctiva with exposure of the medial rectus muscle. **B:** Disinsertion of the muscle with rotation of the globe, and identification of the optic nerve in deeper orbital space for surgery. **C:** Removal of a medially located cavernous hemangioma of the orbit through a conjunctival incision. (Redrawn from ref. 19.)

Extraperiosteal Approach

This approach is most useful for anterior lesions occurring in the peripheral orbital space adjacent to the periosteum or those arising from and involving bone. Such lesions as dermoid cysts and mucoceles are readily approached this way. The skin may be incised at the orbital rim and the subcuticular tissues dissected down to the level of the periosteum so that the extraperiosteal space can be explored (Fig. 4A). Inferiorly, the same space can be accessed through a subciliary incision.

Some large anterior lesions may be removed more readily by a temporary removal of orbital margin particularly superiorly (Fig. 4B). The supraorbital nerve may be dissected free and distracted in order to access the space. The extraperiosteal approach should be avoided in biopsy of malignant lesions since maintenance of this barrier may be important for later management.

Transseptal Approach

The transseptal incisions are based on the natural contours and folds of the lid as well as the site of the lesion being approached (Fig. 2B). Generally, the orbicularis can easily be split between the contours of the muscle fibers and the levator palpebrae superioris can be distracted in order to identify structures behind it. Incision through the levator can be made, but it should be made in the vertical plane and resutured after tumor removal to avoid permanent damage. A remarkable number of procedures can be carried out through wisely placed and expanded anterior orbital incisions. These dissections can be enhanced by using traction sutures to distract structures during surgery.

Lateral Orbitotomy

Lateral orbitotomy with various modifications can provide access to the overwhelming majority of orbital lesions not accessible anteriorly. Modification of bony excision to include the anterior superior rim, inferior rim, zygomatic arch, and even the wing of the sphenoid can allow for wide and deep access to the orbital structures.

The incision for this procedure will depend on the location of the lesion. Generally, when lesions are primarily lateral or superior in location, a lazy "S" incision is favored, and for lesions of the inferior and inferolateral

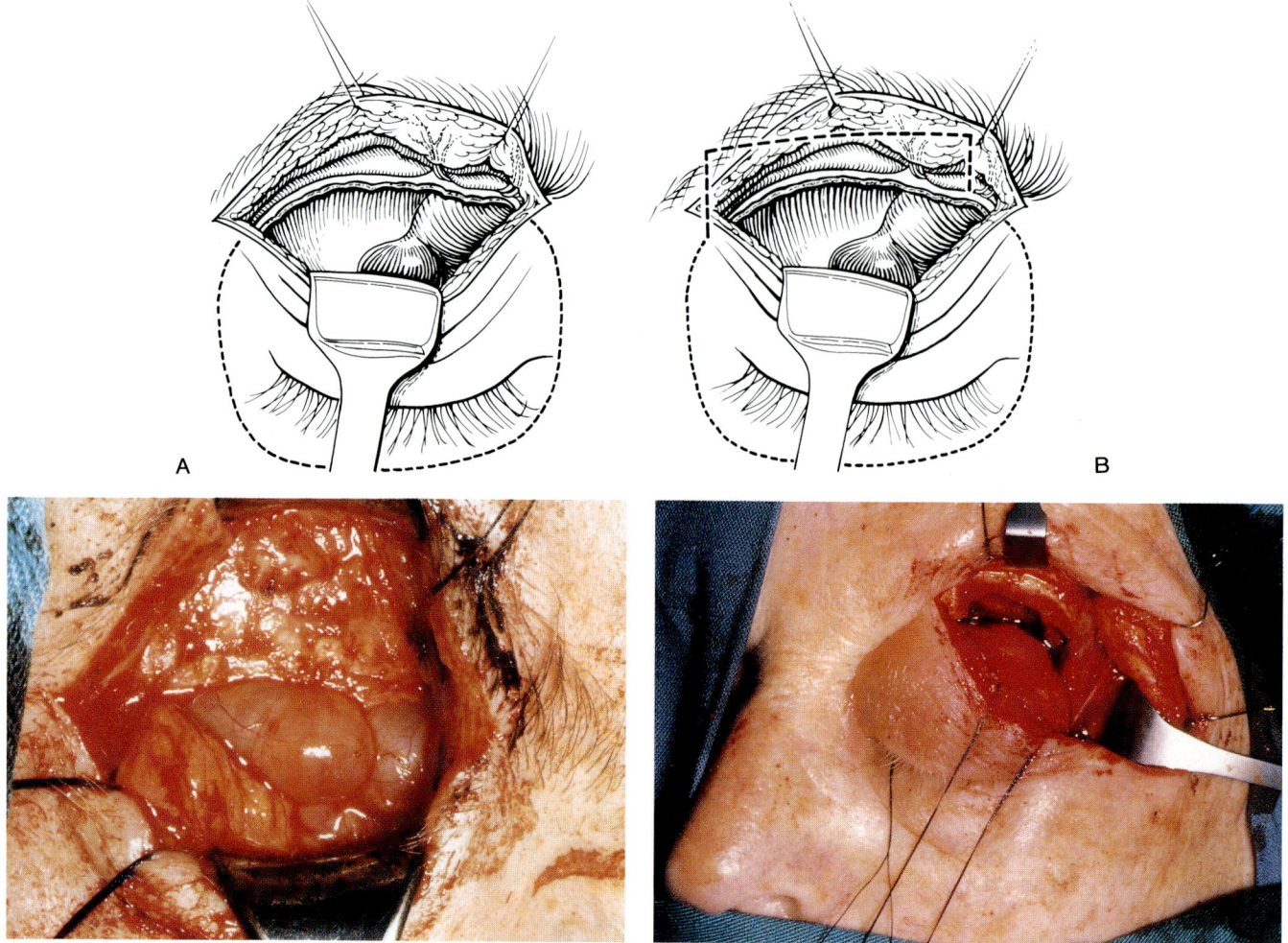

FIG. 4. A, upper: Schematic demonstrating a superior orbital extraperiosteal incision for removal of a tumor. Note distraction of the subcuticular tissues in periorbita with exposure of the supraorbital space and the supraorbital notch. When necessary, it is possible to distract the supraorbital nerve and dissect it free of the orbital contents while removing the tumor, thus avoiding transecting it. **A, lower:** A superior orbital schwannoma being removed by such an incision. **B, upper:** Schematic demonstrating the bony incision site to expand access to the superior orbital space. The supraorbital nerve can be distracted at the time of bony incision. **B, lower:** Clinical photograph demonstrating a patient with a bone temporarily excised, allowing greater access to the superior orbital space. (Redrawn from ref. 19.)

orbit, a lower swinging eyelid flap through the lateral canthus and inferior conjunctiva. The lazy "S" incision is made at the supralateral orbital margin and the zygomaticofrontal process (Fig. 5A) extending along the superior margin of the zygoma approximately 3–4 cm. Prior to incision, a 4-0 silk suture is usually placed in the insertion of the lateral, inferior, or superior rectus muscles, depending on the location of the underlying orbital lesion. The incision is deepened and the subcuticular tissues are dissected to the level of the fascia overlying the temporalis, where they are then separated by means of blunt dissection to minimize damage to critical overlying tissues (Fig. 5B). This subcuticular dissection gives adequate mobility to the tissues and is carried forward over the orbital margin in a plane that avoids branches of the seventh nerve. The degree of mobilization is customized depending on the intrinsic elasticity of the tissue and the size and location of the necessary bony opening. The tissues are then retracted using nonbarbed fish hooks or skin sutures.

The fascial and periosteal incision includes a superior relaxing incision at the inferior temporal line as well as an inferior relaxing incision along the zygomatic arch (Fig. 5C). This allows for mobilization of the temporalis muscle. The periosteum is elevated to the anterior orbital rim and posteriorly the temporalis muscle is detached (Fig. 5D,E). The lateral periorbita is carefully elevated and the frontozygomatic nerves and vessels are identified, clipped, and cauterized. A temporalis retractor is inserted into the temporalis fascia, allowing a clear view to complete the dissection (Fig. 5F).

The usual bony incision is made at the superolateral

margin just above the zygomaticofrontal suture line and inferiorly along the line of the superior margin of the body of the zygoma (Fig. 5F). The bony incision is then extended with rongeurs and when necessary the posterolateral orbital walls are removed using diamond drills, wherein the dura of the temporal lobe is exposed providing wider access to the very apex of the orbit when necessary.

The periorbita is then incised, generally in an H-shaped fashion, usually by means of scissors with careful dissection (Fig. 5G). It is worthwhile to identify at this point the lateral rectus muscle by pulling on the previously placed lateral rectus suture (Fig. 5H). The lateral rectus is then noted, dissected free of its surrounding septa, and distracted usually using moist umbilical tape (Fig. 5I).

Orbital exploration is carried out using fine blunt microsurgical dissectors (Figs. 5J). Dissection of orbital tumors is facilitated by remaining close to the capsule of well defined masses, in a sense freeing them away from the orbital contents rather than dissecting into the adjacent structures. The orbital dissection is generally started by exposing the most accessible part of the tumor and gradually freeing it from surrounding structures, which usually leads to a spontaneous extrusion of the mass. The bulk of the surgery can usually be carried out with blunt microdissecting instruments. However, some fine bands may be freed with microscissors. Careful identification prior to incision of any of these bands is important to avoid cutting important neural structures. Traction may be placed on solid benign tumors by using sutures or alternatively a cryoprobe. Occasionally, after careful dissection of benign cystic lesions, they may be decompressed by draining them and then they are excised.

The wound closure is usually fairly loose, using interrupted, absorbable sutures (Fig. 5K). The bone is reinserted using drill holes and 3-0 neurolon (Fig. 5L). We no longer use wire because of its interference with postoperative imaging. As stated, we usually use a vacuum drain extending through an abexterno site (Fig. M,N). The drain should be anchored to the skin to avoid accidental tugging on it in the postoperative period. The periosteum and fascia overlying the temporalis muscle are closed with interrupted, absorbable sutures and generally subcutaneous running sutures are used to close the wound.

Both during and after surgery we avoid significant pressure on the orbit itself and disparage the common use of lid sutures during orbital surgery, which we consider a dangerous method since it provides a very tight closed space. The same applies postoperatively. We generally leave the drain in for 24–48 hr. The wound is redressed within 12 hr postoperatively, at which time ocular function is evaluated by assessment of visual acuity, ocular movements, pupillary functions, and orbital edema. Swelling can be minimized by the use of cold packs, elevation of the head of the bed, and ambulation, which is immediate postoperatively. Careful operative planning, compulsive and meticulous technique, and vigilant postoperative care will minimize complications, which are rare in our experience. The major complications are tissue damage, inflammation, and hemorrhage.

Operative tissue damage may lead to excessive postoperative edema and compression may thus contribute to direct injury to orbital structures or their blood supply. Excessive trauma and traction to extraocular muscles may produce a postoperative neuropraxia, which is usually transient and avoidable. In rare circumstances, extensive posterolateral orbitotomies may lead to small dural tears that can be directly repaired or patched using temporalis fascia fixed with a biologic glue such as Tisseal.

Postoperatively, excessive noninfectious inflammation can be modified by the use of systemic steroids. Infection should be handled by appropriate systemic antibiotics, drainage, and decompression when necessary.

Postoperative hemorrhage is rare in our experience but may occur and threaten ocular function as defined by a decrease in vision or limitation of movement. Prompt relief of severe orbital pressure may be necessary and requires reexploration of the orbit.

Combined Frontotemporal–Orbitozygomatic Approach for Tumors of the Sphenoid Wing and Orbit

Group A: Surgery for Sphenoid Wing, Orbit, and Middle Fossa Tumors

The patients are premedicated with dexamethasone 10 mg p.o. or i.m. 10 hr and 2 hr preoperatively. A lumbar subarachnoid drain is inserted and furosemide 1 mg/kg and mannitol 1 g i.v. are administered before the incision and continued for 24 hr postoperatively. With the patient supine, the head is placed in three-point pin fixation and rotated 30° to the opposite side. Fine (4-0) silk sutures are placed under the tendons of the lateral rectus, superior rectus, and levator complex for later identification during the orbital dissection. A bicoronal scalp incision is fashioned and may be extended to just below the tragus for tumors that extend into the pterygopalatine or infratemporal fossa (Fig. 6A upper). In these cases, the facial nerve is protected by dissecting the skin flap and fascia over the upper parotid gland. The upper cervical spaces can be explored by extension of the incision if needed (Fig. 6A lower) as described by Sekhar et al.

Once the scalp flap has been turned, the superficial temporalis fascia is incised along the frontozygomatic process, down onto the body of the zygoma and posteriorly along the zygomatic arch. With a periosteal elevator, the origin of the masseter muscle is removed from the

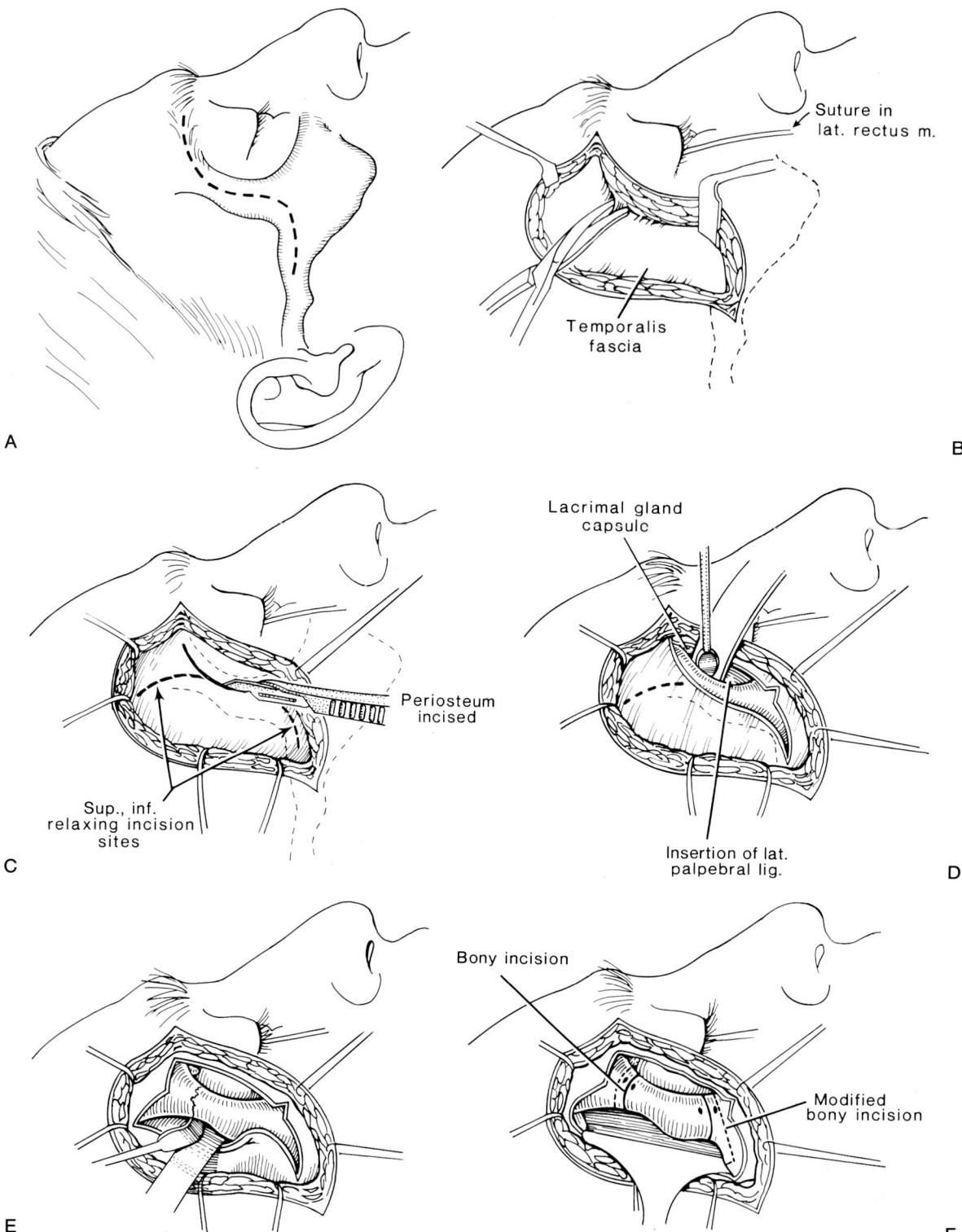

FIG. 5. The lateral orbitotomy procedure.

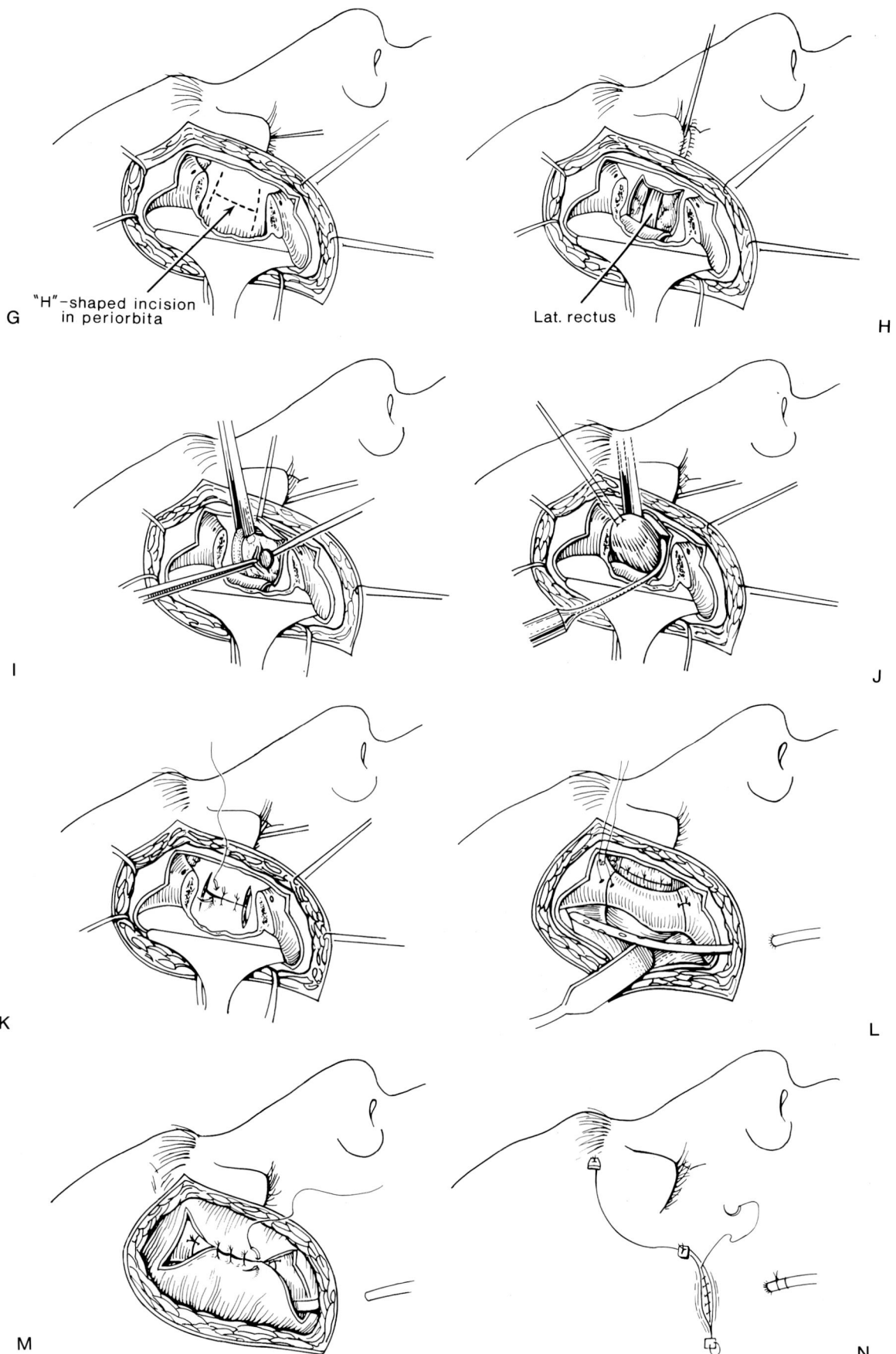

FIG. 5. *Continued.*

undersurface of the arch and back to the body of the zygoma. The temporalis muscle is incised along the superior temporal line and posteriorly in front of the skin incision; the muscle is then dissected from the temporal fossa and retracted inferiorly with fish hooks.

The pericranium is reflected down over the supraorbital margin and the supraorbital nerve is dissected free of its notch or foramen in standard fashion. The orbital surgeon then dissects the periorbita off the superior and lateral walls of the orbit to the superior orbital fissure and lateral aspect of the inferior orbital fissure, or to the anterior limit of bone and soft tissue involvement by tumor. This allows one surgeon to protect the periorbita during creation of the second bone flap, hence avoiding troublesome herniation of orbital fat.

The extradural component of the procedure begins with the creation of two bone flaps: a free frontotemporal–sphenoidal craniotomy and en bloc removal of the superior and lateral orbital walls with attached zygomatic arch (Fig. 6B). By using a high-speed air craniotome, only a single burr hole at the pterion is required for the first bone flap. Then, working from above, one surgeon reflects the frontal dura off the orbital roof while the orbital surgeon protects the periorbita as the roof and lateral orbital walls are cut (Fig. 6C). The lateral end of the inferior orbital fissure marks the medial and inferior limits of the lateral wall bony incision. Using this point as a landmark, the body of the zygoma is cut through its midportion, along a line directed toward the lateral end of the inferior orbital fissure (Fig. 6D). By using this technique, the maxillary sinus is rarely entered. The zygomatic arch is then cut posteriorly above, and just anterior to the temporomandibular joint, and the complex of the superior and lateral orbital margins, with zygomatic arch, is removed en bloc. With the temporalis muscle retracted further inferiorly, the resulting exposure provides access to the orbital contents, orbital apex, pterygopalatine, and infratemporal fossa (Fig. 6E).

The remaining roof of the orbit and the lesser and greater wings of the sphenoid can then be removed with rongeurs and a high-speed drill, exposing the superior orbital fissure. The optic canal is opened with a drill in those cases where the optic nerve is to be removed or when the apical periorbita or annulus zinnii is involved with tumor. Tumor invading the greater wing of the sphenoid along the floor of the middle cranial fossa can be removed medially to the foramina rotundum and ovale, posteriorly to the foramen spinosum, and laterally to the squamous temporal bone anterior to the temporomandibular joint (Fig. 6F). The sphenoid sinus and the outer wall of the cavernous sinus can be reached if necessary.

At this point in most cases, removal of all extradural tumor in bone, pterygopalatine, and infratemporal fossa proceeds. Thereafter the intradural and intraorbital removal is begun. When the intradural tumor is bulky, however, and retraction of this mass would increase pressure on the surrounding brain, the intradural component is debulked or removed as the first step. All dissection of the periorbita and removal of the intraorbital portion of the tumor are carried out by the orbital surgeon. The extent of the involvement of the periorbita is delimited, the involved periorbita is then resected, and the dissection is extended into the orbital soft tissues. The superior rectus–levator complex and lateral rectus are identified and retracted in order to dissect out and remove tumor. Any excised periorbita or dura is replaced with pericranium or cadaver dura.

Following replacement of the superior and lateral orbital margins and zygomatic arch, the roof and lateral wall of the orbit are reconstructed with autologous inner table split thickness frontal bone graft (Fig. 6G). Two triangular pieces of bone are wired or sutured together at their apices and then secured in place to the orbital rim segment previously removed.

This reconstruction prevents enophthalmos and orbital pulsation and provides a useful plane of dissection if repeat surgery becomes necessary (Fig. 6H,I). The

FIG. 6. A, upper: Bicoronal incision extending just below tragus on involved side. **A, lower:** Extension of incision into neck for exposure of upper cervical reaches if needed. **B:** Outline of two bone flaps used **(upper left)** and relationship of incisions in roof and lateral wall of orbit to the inferior orbital fissure **(lower right)**. **C:** Frontotemporal sphenoidal bone flap removed as dura and frontal lobe is retracted for incision in the roof of the orbit. Note dissection and protection of periorbita. **D:** Body of zygoma cut through its midportion, directed toward the anterolateral end of the inferior orbital fissure. (Redrawn from ref. 21) **E:** Removal of bone flaps in superior and lateral walls of orbit provides exposure of orbit, anterior and middle skull base, and infratemporal fossa. **F:** *Hatched area* of greater wing of sphenoid and temporal bone can be removed to expose infratemporal fossa. Optic canal (*arrow*) can be opened through superior and lateral aspects.

ORBITAL SURGERY / 779

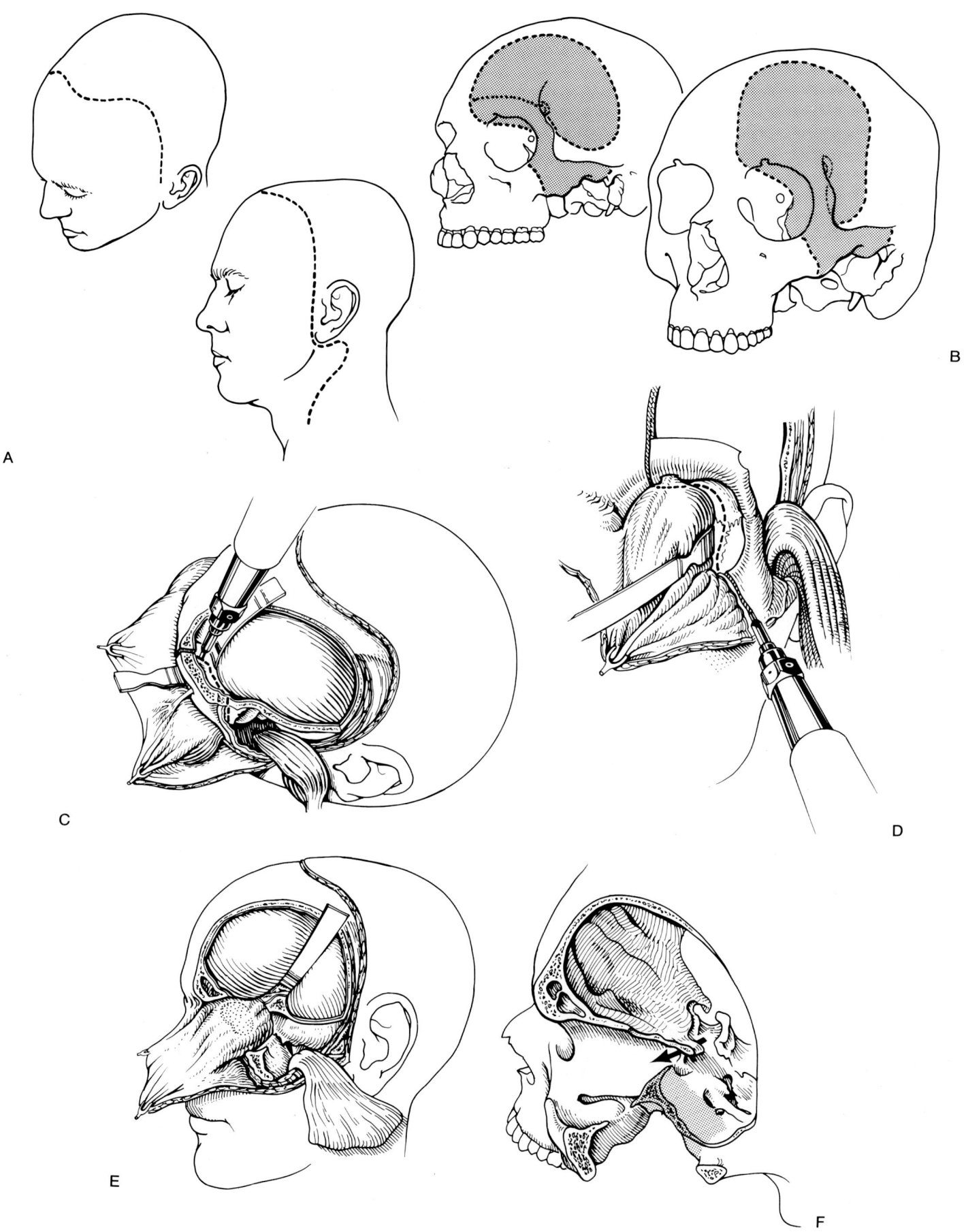

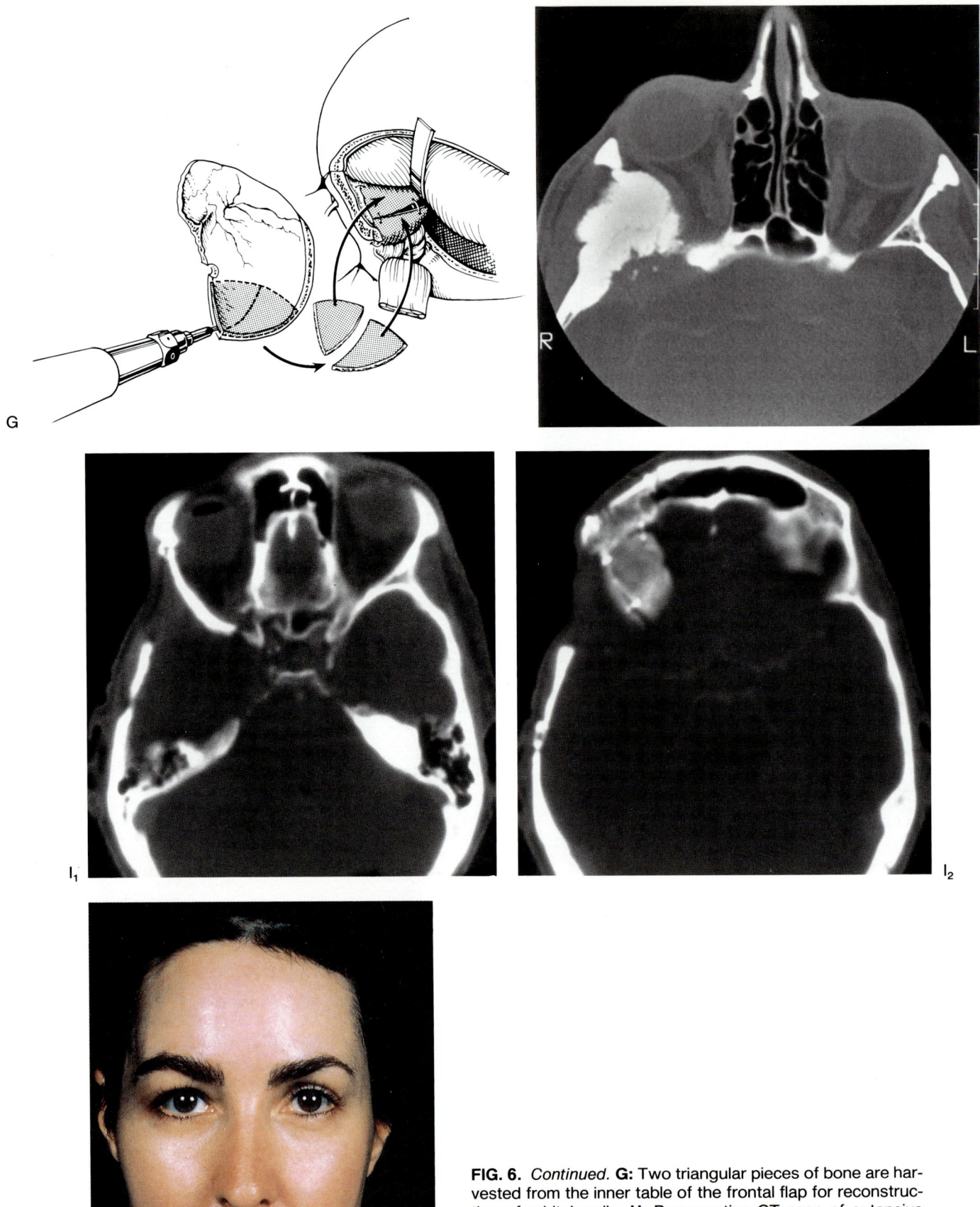

FIG. 6. *Continued.* **G:** Two triangular pieces of bone are harvested from the inner table of the frontal flap for reconstruction of orbital walls. **H:** Preoperative CT scan of extensive hyperostosing sphenoid wing meningioma. **I:** Postoperative CT scan appearance following resection of the greater wing of sphenoid and reconstruction of the lateral ($6I_1$) and superior orbital walls ($6I_2$). **J:** Postoperative appearance following resection of the sphenoid wing meningioma shown above. (Redrawn from ref. 21.)

floor of the middle cranial fossa is not reconstructed, however.

With the orbital reconstruction complete, the free pterional flap is repositioned and if no sinuses have been opened acrylic is used to fill the bony defect at the pterion prior to resuturing the temporalis muscle. A subgaleal hemovac drain is placed and the galea and skin are closed in standard fashion. A good cosmetic result is achieved (Fig. 6J).

Group B: Surgery for Complicated Intraorbital Tumors with and Without Intracranial Extension

Apical or orbitocranial lesions are approached initially as described previously with the exception that the inferior limit of the lateral orbital wall removal is at the level of the orbital floor (usually the base of the frontozygomatic process). The bone incisions involve an en bloc removal of the roof and lateral wall, leaving them entirely intact for later reconstruction. This approach allows a panoramic view of the orbit with a wide access to the superior and lateral contents.

Removal of an optic nerve for tumor is illustrated (Fig. 7). The preplaced sutures in the superior rectus, lid, and lateral rectus insertions allow identification of the muscles through the periorbita, which is incised between the lateral rectus and superior rectus laterally, and between the superior rectus–levator complex and the superior oblique medially (Fig. 7A). The periorbita is reflected and using blunt microdissectors the orbital contents are dissected carefully in order to identify the optic nerve, posterior emissarial vessels, and ciliary nerves. The emissarial vessels and ciliary nerves are dissected free of the sheath of the optic nerve (Fig. 7B).

Attention is then turned to the fourth nerve, which is also mobilized apically (Fig. 7C). The optic nerve is sectioned at the globe with serial placement of 4-0 silk sutures to close the distal end and prevent spillage of tumor. From a superior view between the superior rectus and levator complex and the superior oblique, the nerve is identified, distracted, and dissected free to the apex (Fig. 7C,D). The annulus zinnii is incised (Fig. 7D) apically in order to mobilize that portion of the optic nerve. Intracranially, the proximal nerve is cut and the ophthalmic artery identified and either dissected free or clipped. The roof of the optic canal has been previously removed. The entire optic nerve is now free and it can be removed by distracting it anteriorly (Figs. 7E,F) or, using the previously placed distal sutures, it can be pulled superiorly behind the dissected fourth nerve, which is thus preserved.

En Bloc Orbitectomy

Patients requiring en bloc orbitectomy usually have malignancies of the lacrimal gland or orbit. These require a multidisciplinary procedure involving a neurosurgeon, orbital surgeon, and facial reconstructive surgeon. We proceed by first making the periorbital skin incision. In the case of adenoid cystic carcinoma of the lacrimal gland, the skin incision should be carried out laterally beyond the zygomaticofacial and zygomaticotemporal nerves because they pass through the lacrimal gland and may be involved by carcinoma. With this carcinoma the excision should also include the anterior portion of the temporalis muscle, which relates immediately to the zygomaticotemporal nerve and vessel. A coronal skin flap is prepared (Fig. 8A). A frontotemporal sphenoidal craniotomy is carried out (Fig. 8B,C). The subfrontal dura is mobilized and retracted extradurally to just behind the lesser wing of the sphenoid and the tip of the anterior clinoid and adjacent tuberculum sellae, and the anterior temporal dura is mobilized posterior to the greater wing of the sphenoid so that the superior orbital fissure and its contents are well exposed. Only the medial portion of the orbit is entered in the case of lacrimal tumors where the periorbita is elevated to guide the bony incision superomedially. The bone is then incised from above and below in the superomedial orbit. In other malignant tumors in the medial or central orbit requiring en bloc orbitectomy, the medial incision includes the medial wall and thus is through the cribriform plate superiorly (Fig. 8D–F). The inferomedial orbit is then dissected free of the periorbita and en bloc bony excision is carried out including the floor of the orbit through the upper portion of the zygomatic arch. The posterior roof of the orbit is incised to the region of the superior orbital fissure and connected to a bony cut deep through the temporalis fossa into the middle cranial fossa beyond the most posterior reaches of the lateral wall of the orbit, just anterior to the foramen rotundum. The incision is carried superiorly just anterior to the tip of the anterior clinoids and laterally into the temporalis fossa to avoid entering the orbit or damaging the carotid artery. The orbit then is completely free for en bloc excision.

After replacement of the frontal bone (Fig. 8G) there are a number of reconstructive options for repairing the defect. We have usually used bone from the posterior plate of the frontal craniotomy or occasionally a rib graft to perform a primary bone reconstruction of the orbit. The orbitectomy cavity can either be filled with a deltopectoral myocutaneous vascularized flap or an extended trapezius musculocutaneous flap. If the superficial temporal artery has been preserved, a free latissimus dorsi myocutaneous vascular flap may potentially be obtained and used (Fig. 9).

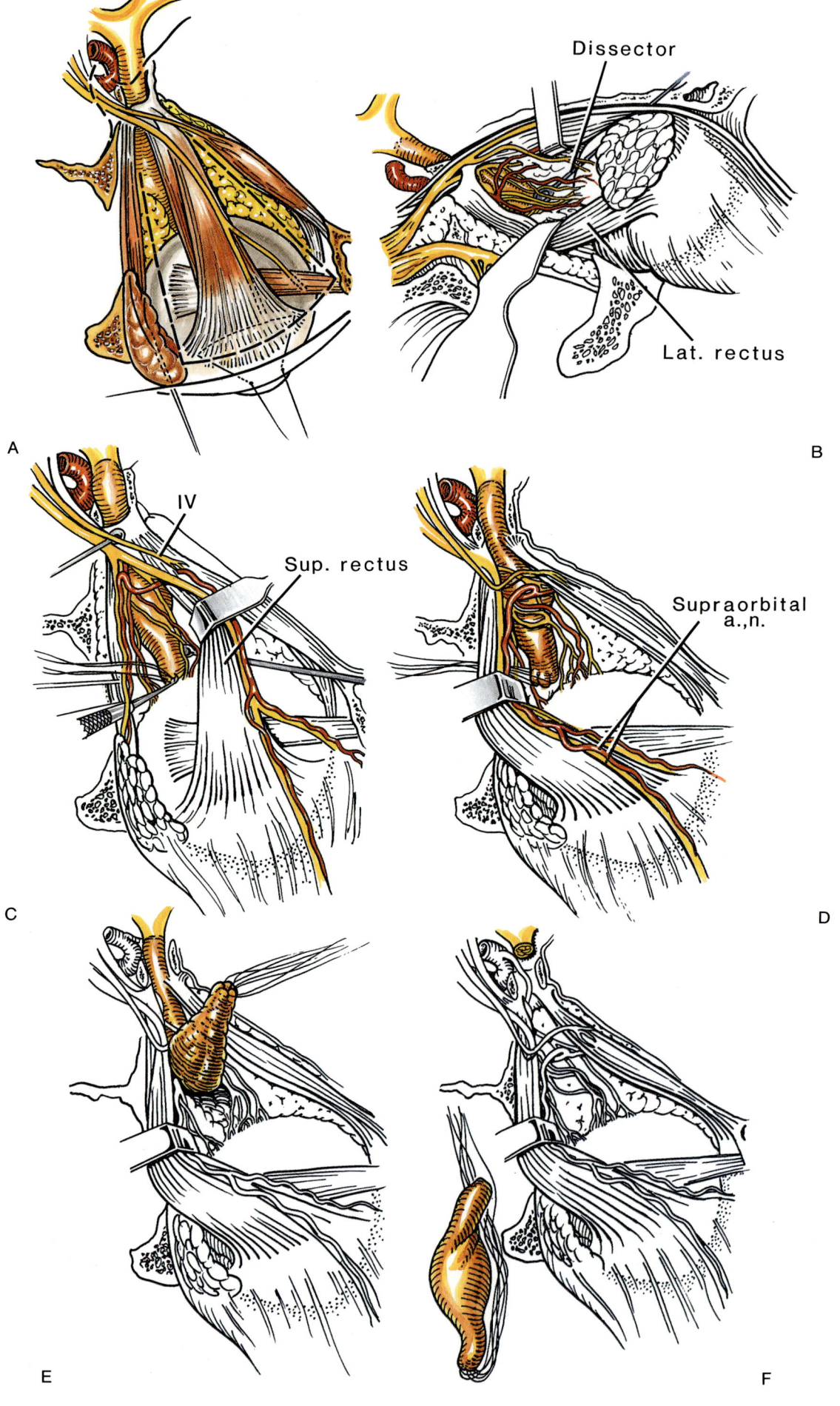

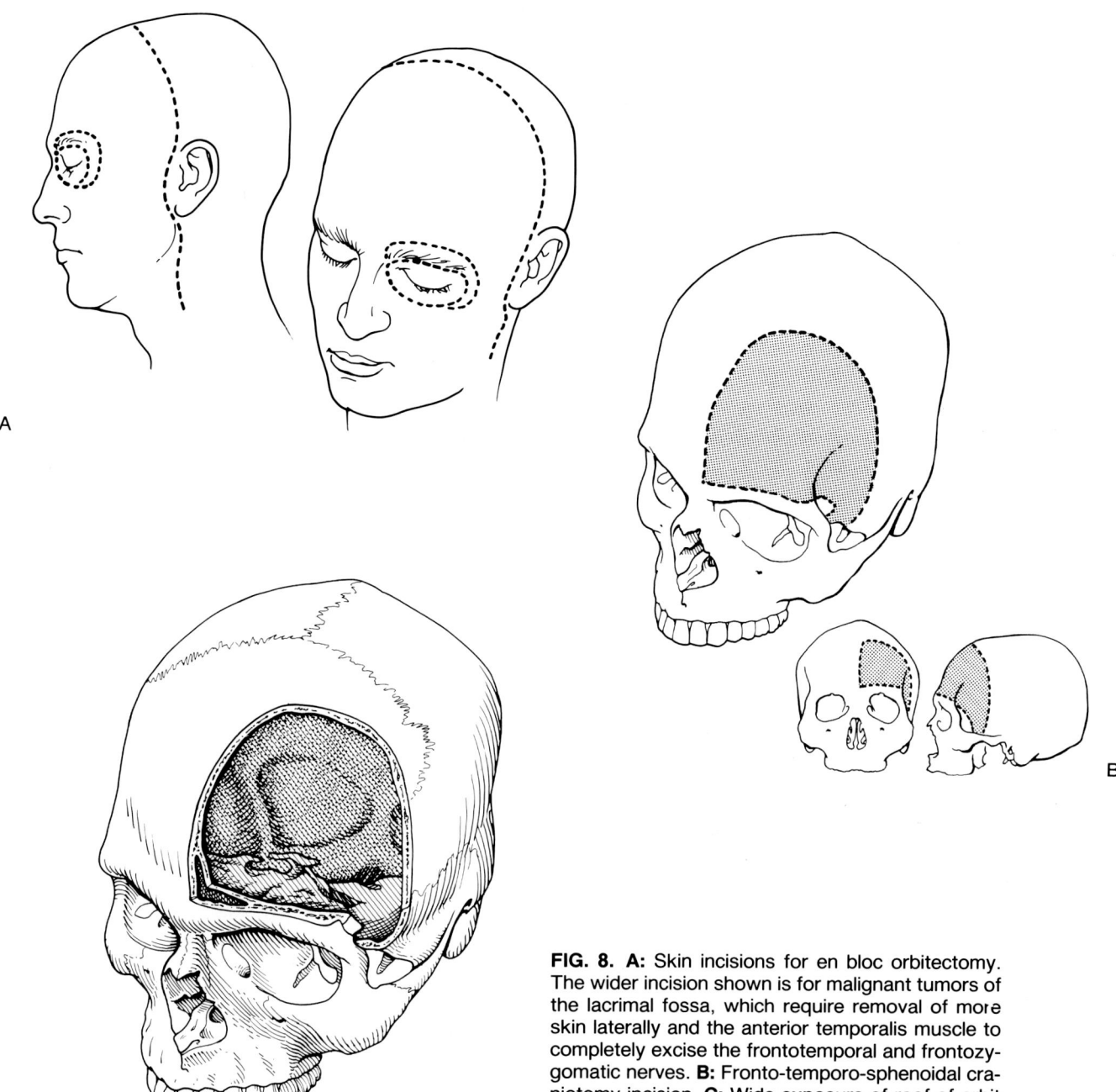

FIG. 8. A: Skin incisions for en bloc orbitectomy. The wider incision shown is for malignant tumors of the lacrimal fossa, which require removal of more skin laterally and the anterior temporalis muscle to completely excise the frontotemporal and frontozygomatic nerves. **B:** Fronto-temporo-sphenoidal craniotomy incision. **C:** Wide exposure of roof of orbit following removal of craniotomy bone.

FIG. 7. The illustrations demonstrate removal of the optic nerve with preservation of the fourth nerve. (Redrawn from ref. 21.)

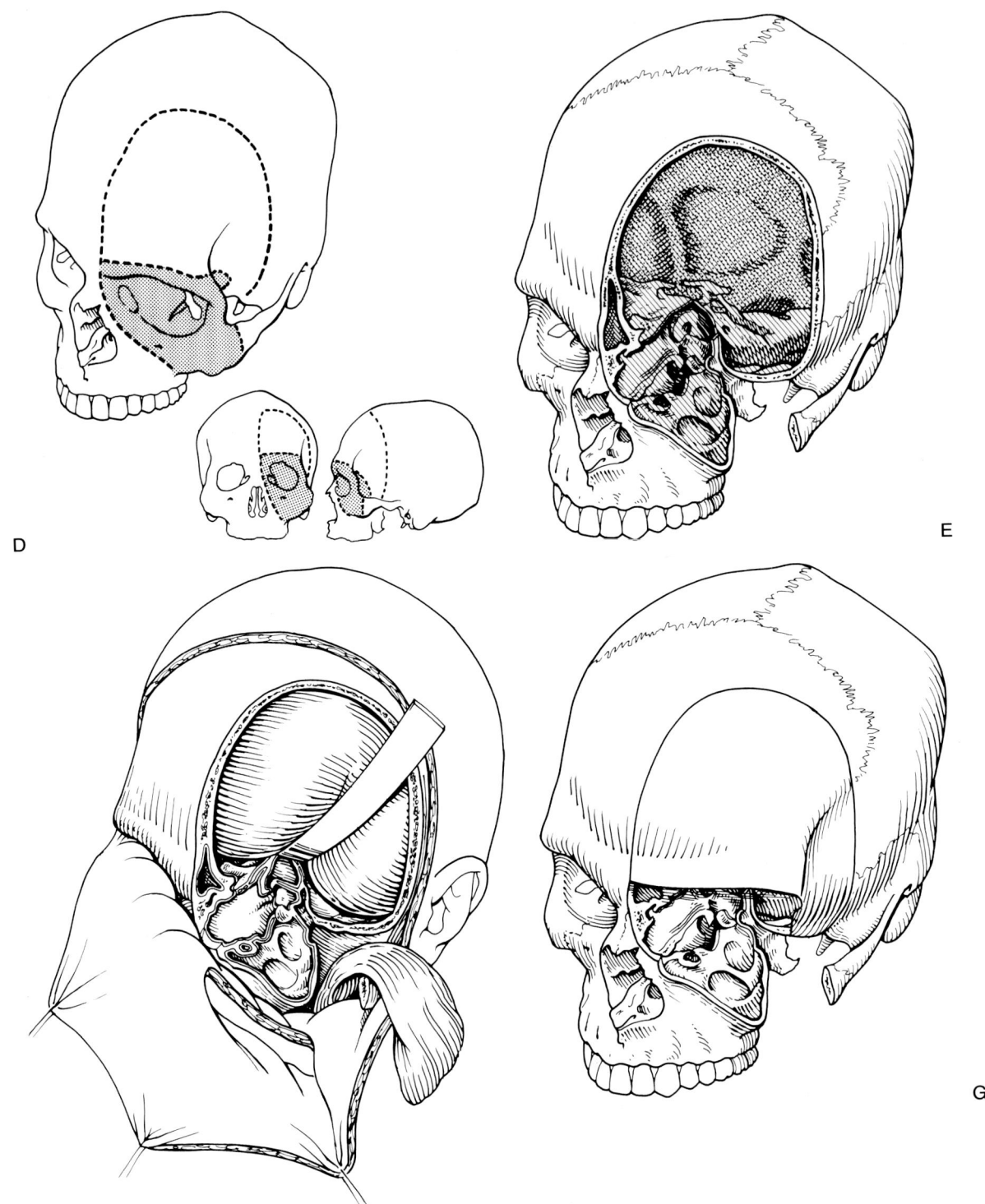

FIG. 8. *Continued.* **D, E:** Outline of bony excision for a complete en bloc orbitectomy. **F:** The operative site after removal of the entire orbit en bloc. Note floor of maxillary sinus and nasopharynx. **G:** Reinsertion of the craniotomy bone.

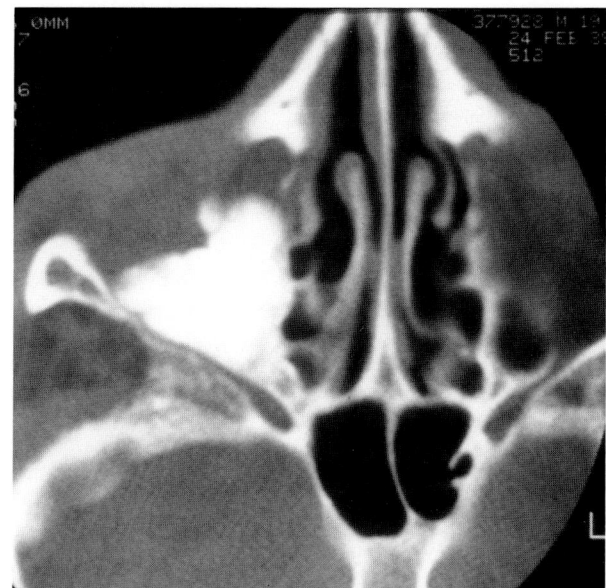 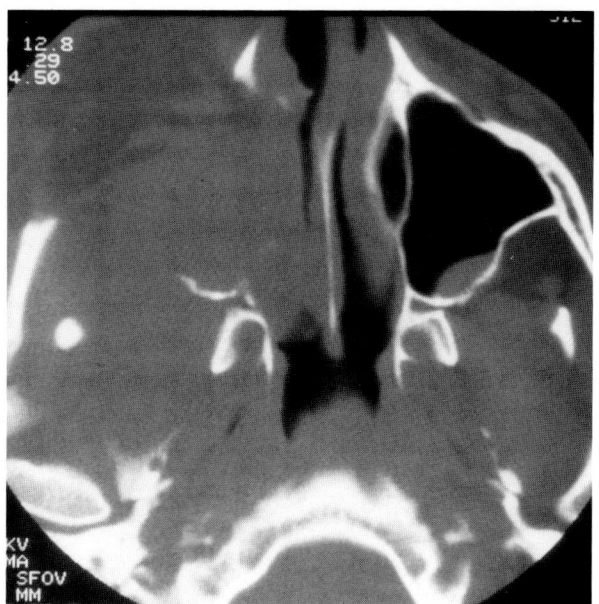

FIG. 9. A: Axial CT scan of an osteogenic sarcoma of the orbit, which was removed by en bloc orbitectomy. **B:** Postoperative axial CT scan just below the orbital excision showing that only the posteroinferior maxillary sinus wall remains. Reconstruction was carried out using a free anastomosis of a myocutaneous flap.

BIBLIOGRAPHY

1. Berke RN. A modified Kronlein operation. *Arch Ophthalmol* 1954;51:609.
2. Henderson JW, Farrow GM. *Orbital tumours.* New York: Thieme-Stratton, 1980;567.
3. Housepian EM, Trokel SL, Jakobiec FO, et al. Tumours of the orbit. In: Youmans JR, ed. *Neurological surgery,* 2nd ed, vol 5. Philadelphia: Saunders, 1982;3024.
4. Jones IS. Deep orbital surgery. In: Soll DB, ed. *Management of complications in ophthalmic plastic surgery.* Birmingham, AL: Aesculapius, 1976;259.
5. Jones BR. Surgical approaches to the orbit. *Trans Ophthalmol Soc UK* 1970;90:269.
6. Kennerdell JS, et al. Fine needle aspiration biopsy. *Arch Ophthalmol* 1979;97:1315.
7. Kennerdell JS, Maroon JC. Microsurgical approach to intraorbital tumours. *Arch Ophthalmol* 1976;94:133.
8. Kennerdell JS, Maroon JC, Dekker A, et al. Microsurgery and fine needle aspiration biopsy. *Trans Pa Acad Ophthalmol Otolaryngol* 1979;32(2):147.
9. Krohel GB, Stewart WB, Chavis RM. *Orbital disease: a practical approach.* New York: Grune & Stratton, 1981.
10. Leone CR. Surgical approaches to the orbit. *Ophthalmology* 1979;86:930.
11. Linberg JV, Orcutt JC, VanDyk HJL. Orbital surgery. In: Duane TD, Jaeger EA, eds. *Clinical ophthalmology,* vol 5. New York: Harper & Row, 1985.
12. Maroon JC, Kennerdell JC. Microsurgical approach to orbital tumours. *Clin Neursurg* 1979;26:479.
13. Maroon JC, Kennerdell JS. Surgical approaches to the orbit: indications and techniques. *J Neurosurg* 1984;60:1226.
14. McCord CD. Surgical approaches to orbital disease. In: McCord CD, ed. *Oculoplastic surgery.* New York: Raven Press, 1981;285.
15. Wright JE. The role of surgery in the management of orbital tumours. *Mod Probl Ophthalmol* 1975;14:553.
16. Wright JE. Orbital surgery. In: Silver B, ed. *Ophthalmic plastic surgery,* 34d ed. San Francisco: American Academy of Ophthalmology, 1977;213.
17. Wright JE, Steward WB. Orbital surgery. In: Tenzel RR, ed. *Ocular plastic surgery. Int Ophthalmol Clin* 1978;18(3):149.
18. Wright JE. Surgical exploration of the orbit. *Trans Ophthalmol Soc UK* 1979;99:238.
19. Rootman J. Orbital surgery. In: *Diseases of the orbit: a multidisciplinary approach.* Philadelphia: Lippincott, 1988;579–612.
20. Sekhar LN, Schramm VL, Jones NF. Subtemporal–preaurical infratemporal fossa approach to large and posterior cranial base neoplasms. *J Neurosurg* 1987;67:488–499.
21. McDermott MW, Durity FA, Rootman J, Woodhurst WB. Combined frontotemporal–orbitozygomatic approach for tumours of the sphenoid wing and orbit. *J Neurosurg* 1990;26(1):107–116.

CHAPTER 50

Surgical Management of Craniopharyngioma

Dachling Pang

Craniopharyngiomas are unique lesions among childhood brain tumors. They are histologically benign yet so located that their radical excision is fraught with difficulties and great potential hazards. Their intimate adherence to the infundibular stalk and hypothalamus predisposes to a gamut of endocrinological and neurobehavioral problems seldom seen in other brain tumors. They are slow growing but recalcitrant lesions in that a residual fleck of tumor almost guarantees a recurrence. Yet, they are occasionally so responsive to radiation that specialized radiotherapy modalities lately offer a number of nonsurgical options that are useful in selective circumstances but may also at times confound an already complex therapeutic decision. In general, the management of craniopharyngioma remains in the domain of the neurosurgeon, and a thorough knowledge of the surgical anatomy and techniques involved is vital to choosing the optimal treatment.

INCIDENCE

Craniopharyngiomas are relatively rare tumors, constituting between 2.5 and 4% of all intracranial tumors (19,35). They are much more common among children, forming 9% of Matson's series of childhood brain tumors (50), and making up 54% of neoplasms in the sella-chiasmal region in children. There is a bimodal age distribution with the first peak at 5–10 years (14,37), and the second peak between 55 and 65 years (10), but the tumor may become symptomatic at any age.

Recent large series show equal sex distribution (15,28).

D. Pang: Department of Pediatric Neurosurgery, Children's Hospital of Pittsburgh, University of Pittsburgh School of Medicine, Pittsburgh, Pennsylvania 15213.

EMBRYOLOGIC ORIGIN

For several decades, the origin of craniopharyngioma was thought to be related to the embryogenesis of the anterior pituitary lobe. At the end of the third gestational week, the stomodeal ectoderm invaginates toward the diencephalon and eventually meets the downwardly projecting infundibular bud. As the sphenoid bone forms ventral to this complex, the stomodeal cleft is pinched off from the pharyngeal epithelium, and the cleft becomes a pouch (of Rathke) whose wall later thickens to form the various parts of the anterior pituitary lobe. Ectoblastic cell rests have been found in the pars distalis and tuberalis and along the dorsal migration path of the stomodeal cleft, known as the hypophyseopharyngeal duct. The frequent occurrence of craniopharyngiomas around the infundibular stalk, their occasional presence along the ventral hypophyseopharyngeal duct (e.g., within the sphenoid bone), and the striking histologic similarities between some craniopharyngiomas and tumors of known ectoblastic origin, such as adamantinoma, led Erdheim (21) and others (25,56,67) to propose that craniopharyngiomas are all derived from ectoblastic remnants.

During the 1950s, the embryonic origin of craniopharyngioma was challenged when it was discovered that the pituitary squamous cell rests were rarely present in children under 10 years but were found with increasing frequency in each succeeding decade, even though the peak incidence of craniopharyngiomas are from age 5 to 10 years (47). It was then postulated that these squamous cell nests, from which craniopharyngiomas originate, are products of metaplasia of the mature cells of the anterior pituitary, and not embryonic remnants.

There is evidence to suggest that craniopharyngiomas may indeed have dual origins. The so-called childhood type, which occurs in all ages and has a more aggressive growth pattern, contains palisading columnar cells reminiscent of the ameloblasts of fetal tooth buds (adamantinomatous craniopharyngioma) and may be of embryonic origin (32,68). The adult type, which occurs mostly in adults and has less aggressive growth propensity, consists of mature stratified squamous cells and may be of metaplastic origin.

SURGICAL PATHOLOGY

Most craniopharyngiomas are located in the suprasellar cistern. Approximately one-third of cases are retrochiasmatic; the tumor displaces the pituitary stalk forward, and the chiasm forward and upward, making the optic nerve appear falsely prefixed (pseudoprefixity). Another one-third of cases are subchiasmatic; the tumor displaces the pituitary stalk backward and the chiasm upward, stretching the optic nerves. Both the retro- and subchiasmatic types are usually solid tumors that slowly distort and elevate the hypothalamus until the third ventricle or the foramen of Monro is obstructed. The third ventricular floor is thus severely attenuated so that the tumor dome frequently appears on computerized tomography (CT) or magnetic resonance imaging (MRI) to be inside the third ventricle. In reality, the tumor is seldom truly intraventricular, and a transventricular approach to the tumor from above will risk injuring the hypothalamus. About 20% of craniopharyngiomas are prechiasmatic. These tumors are frequently cystic and, by burrowing under and expanding within the basal frontal lobes, may reach enormous sizes. The tumors sometimes extend laterally into the sylvian fissure and then may severely compress the temporal lobe to cause complex psychomotor seizures. Intrasellar craniopharyngiomas are least common (10–15%) (53,62) but because they expand within the sella and compress the pituitary gland early to cause endocrinopathies long before the optic nerves are injured, they are often diagnosed when still relatively small and thus may be removed by the transsphenoidal route.

Craniopharyngiomas may be primarily solid, primarily cystic, or cystic with a large solid component that may in turn contain small cysts. The solid part is usually smooth, rubbery firm, and pinkish gray, resembling fish flesh. The cyst wall may be diaphanous or a thick shell of solid tumor. The fluid is typically dark green with suspended birefringent cholesterol crystals.

Either the solid part or the cyst wall, or both, may be calcified. Calcification marks the site of regressive changes in the epithelial cells; calcium is deposited within the laminated whorls of dead cells, especially in the adamantinomatous (childhood) tumor type. This explains why calcium is detected on CT in almost all childhood craniopharyngiomas and only in slightly over 50% of adult craniopharyngiomas (14). Small foci of calcium may become confluent to form large stones, and actual bone formation has been demonstrated. It is important not to mistake a large stone as a sign of "burnt-out" tumor. Within the stone, thin layers of live tumor cells are sandwiched between thick lamellae of calcium; indeed a craniopharyngioma stone grows by concretions actively laid down after *live* cells undergo regressive changes. In fact, reappearance of calcium after tumor excision is a reliable sign of recurrence of actively growing tumor cells.

The anterior, inferior, and lateral walls of the capsule of a large tumor are normally separated from surrounding structures by a single layer of arachnoid; the posterior wall is separated from the basilar artery and midbrain by the double-layered membrane of Lilliquist. However, the dome of the tumor is almost always adherent to the infundibular stalk and basal hypothalamus due to an intense glial reaction in this region of the brain where most craniopharyngiomas arise. This tenacious glial sheath frequently contains pseudopods of tumor extending beyond the capsule. Contrary to some opinions, firmly teasing and separating tumor capsule off this glial sheath ensures total removal and actually protects against injury to the functional neural tissue. Occasionally, the inferior pole of the tumor grows toward the sella and the capsule fuses tightly with the sellar dura and the medial walls of the cavernous sinus.

As embryologic remnants of Rathke's pouch, craniopharyngiomas share the same blood supply as the anterior diencephalon (39,41,56). The anterior portion of the tumor thus receives perforators from the anterior communicating artery and the A-1 segment of the anterior cerebral arteries, and its lateral portion receives branches from the posterior communicating artery. If the tumor involves the sella, it will also pick up arterial twigs from the capsular meningohypophyseal arteries. It is important to realize that the tumor virtually never receives blood supply from the posterior cerebral or basilar artery, no matter how far posterior it extends (54,56), since these vessels do not normally irrigate the diencephalon. This fact is basic to the removal of the retrosellar portion of the tumor.

CLINICAL FEATURES

The clinical presentation of craniopharyngioma differs between children and adults. Even though the optic chiasm and nerves are affected first by enlargement of this tumor, only 20–30% of children will present with visual symptoms. This is because children tolerate progressive visual failure amazingly well, and they seldom complain until one eye is totally blind and the other barely able to count fingers (10,14,54,56). Subtle clues of progressive visual failure in young children include inexplicable deterioration in school performance, frequent stumbling, and the child's insistence on situating closer and closer to the television.

Other early symptoms of an enlarging intracranial mass such as headaches and personality changes are also easily overlooked in a young child. Diagnosis is often delayed until intracranial hypertension is significant and sustained, usually when there is already severe hydrocephalus due to third ventricular or foramen of Monro obstruction. Thus 75–80% of children with craniopharyngiomas present with severe headache and vomiting, without focal neurologic deficits.

The most frequent endocrinopathic manifestation in children are short stature and diabetes insipidus (DI) (10,19). Sexual development is often delayed in adolescents, but symptoms of hypothyroidism and hypercortisolemia are unusual. The most common hypothalamic dysfunction is central hyperphagia and obesity, which is sometimes disproportionate to the food intake and may be partially due to metabolic derangement. Sleep and temperature regulations are rarely affected. Neurobehavioral abnormalities probably related to injury to the hypothalamus or its constituent pathways occur in 20% of children (10,14,19). Affected children show psychomotor retardation, flattening of affects, and loss of enthusiasm toward the environment (abulia minor) as well as significant recent memory deficits (54). Thus the typical child with a craniopharyngioma is short, obese, dull, half-blind, and with a poor school record.

Unlike children, most adults are very sensitive to visual disturbance, and 80% of adults in Banna's series (9) presented with assorted combinations of field deficits, scotomas, and decreasing visual acuity. In contrast, less than one-third of adults have signs of increased intracranial pressure (ICP). Nevertheless, neurobehavioral syndromes unrelated to raised ICP are much more common in adults than in children (14,19,56). These include intermittent confusion, hypersomnia, dementia, a Korsakoff-like amnesia, and occasionally severe depression and apathy (11,31,57,58). The most common endocrinopathy in adults is gonadal failure (37%) presenting as secondary amenorrhea in woman and loss of libido in men (56).

RADIOLOGIC DIAGNOSIS

Craniopharyngioma is one of few intracranial tumors that can be accurately diagnosed with a skull x-ray. Two-thirds of the adults and 95% of children with this tumor have an abnormal skull x-ray. The usual findings are erosion of the anterior clinoids and dorsum sellae, expansion of the upper part of the sella, and suprasellar calcification. Intrasellar extension of a craniopharyngioma may produce a "ballooned" sella that mimics a pituitary adenoma, but a calcified adenoma is exceedingly rare.

CT and MRI are both important, but for different reasons. CT is less ambiguous than MRI in distinguishing the solid from the cystic parts of the tumor; the MR signal intensity of the cystic fluid varies widely depending on the lipid, protein, and methemoglobin contents and may be confused with that of the solid tumor. The CT density of the fluid is usually between that of brain and cerebrospinal fluid (CSF), so that the cyst is always hypodense compared to the enhanced solid part. The most important function of CT is thus to classify the tumor according to its solid/cyst ratio: a primarily solid tumor has more than 70% solid component, whereas a primarily cystic tumor has the reverse ratio. This aspect has great therapeutic implications, for the management may be different for the two tumor types.

CT is also better in identifying calcium deposits in the tumor than MRI. For the same reason, properly angled thin coronal CT cuts (1.5-mm thickness) often display the bony anatomy of the sella, the frontal skull base, and the sphenoid sinus to great advantage. Such information is essential in planning a transsphenoidal or frontobasal approach to the tumor.

On the other hand, MRI is better than CT in identifying the interphase between tumor and brain. Where CT may not distinguish between solid craniopharyngioma and a calcified hypothalamic glioma, MRI will show the extra-axial nature of the former, and the intra-axial blending of tumor with hypothalamic tissue in the latter. In addition, the sagittal imaging capabilities of the MRI enable a graphic display of neuroanatomy unachievable by CT: for example, the minute hypothalamic and brain stem details in their distorted configuration, or the delicate relationship of the lamina terminalis and other peri-third-ventricular structures with the tumor. Such MRI details allow the surgeon to select the surgical approach most likely to achieve total resection. With improving MRI technology in visualizing blood vessels (MRI angiography), conventional angiography is seldom necessary and should only be performed if an aneurysm is strongly suspected.

MODALITIES AND OPTIONS OF TREATMENT: PATIENT SELECTION

Primary Tumor, Predominantly Solid

Four treatment options are available for predominantly solid tumors diagnosed for the first time. The clinician must remain flexible in exercising these options and be prepared to change them at different points of the treatment course, guided by the following factors: (a) the experience of the surgeon; (b) the accessibility to specialized technology in radiation therapy; (c) the age and medical condition of the patient; (d) the size of the tumor; and (e) the surgical anatomy, the degree of adherence, and the textural characteristics of the tumor capsule at surgery.

Total Resection

In skilled and experienced hands, total resection of solid craniopharyngiomas is feasible with low mortality and morbidity. The achieved/attempted ratio for total resection, composed of the number of cases in which total resection was accomplished by radiographic standards versus the number in which total resection was attempted, varies between 30 and 90% among experienced surgeons using modern microsurgical techniques (14,28,33,59,63,64,65). The realistic expectation for total resection is probably around 70–80%. A CT should be performed 1–2 days postoperatively to eliminate cases of "false cure" because even experienced surgeons may inadvertently leave behind tumor fragments that are adherent to the underside of the chiasm or hypothalamus, or within the sella. Resectability depends on many factors, chief among them the tumor size [tumors larger than 3 cm in diameter are less likely to be totally resectable (59,63)], the degree of adherence of the capsule to the chiasm and great vessels, and the extent of rambling of the tumor within the basal cisterns and deep brain structures.

The overall operative mortality is probably around 2–3%, and the best reported serious postoperative morbidity is probably below 10%.

In spite of meticulous technique, a number of tumors will nonetheless recur after what has been deemed "complete" resection. This is probably due to regrowth of deeply rooted tumor pseudopods that have been broken off from the dissection plane. Recurrences are usually detected within 5 years of the surgery (14,63), but late recurrences after 20 years have been reported (15). Thus follow-up of shorter than 10 years is probably meaningless for this disease. A long-term review by Katz (33) of Matson's original series (51) reported recurrences in 25% of patients 4–19 years after "total" resection, and most other series recorded similar recurrence rates of 15–25%, with a mean of 20% (15,28,59,63,65). With further refinement of microtechniques, this number will likely prove to be even smaller in future series. In any case, the 10-year survival rate of patients who have undergone total resection is well over 85% in spite of these recurrence rates. Thus the overall results of total resection for solid craniopharyngiomas are excellent, and it is the treatment of choice in children and young adults. Obviously, the associated mortality and morbidity and, to a certain extent, the recurrence rate are commensurate with the experience of the surgeon. Total resection should thus be considered only in institutions where a large number of these tumors are managed.

Subtotal Resection, with Postoperative Radiation

When only subtotal resection of the tumor was achieved, the recurrence rate is unacceptably high if postoperative radiation (RT) is not given. The combined recurrence rate from several large series for subtotal resection alone is about 75% (13,14,27,28,44,48,52,63), with a 10-year survival of only 25%. Postoperative RT significantly improves the outcome. Recent results show a 10-year survival of 75–80% with subtotal resection and postoperative RT (48,59,67). Thus some surgeons are adopting a planned subtotal resection followed by postoperative conventional external beam radiation.

External radiotherapy is usually delivered by a three- or four-field technique over a field size of 6×7 cm, with a total dose of 50–60 Gy fractionated over 6–7 weeks, with the daily dose not exceeding 2 Gy. Even with these precautions, conventional radiation is not without hazard. Visual failure, hypopituitarism, organic brain syndrome, dementia, and sensorimotor deficits have all been reported (7,26,38,49,64). Frontal lobe dysfunction resulting in severe learning disabilities is especially troublesome in children (17), and RT has also been etiologically implicated in mesenchymal tumors occurring within the radiated brain (18,71). Furthermore, recent long-term follow-up studies (19,27) are beginning to reveal that subtotal resection and RT only delay and do not prevent eventual recurrence of the tumor. This treatment option is therefore not ideal for children and healthy young adults with potentially long life spans but may be recommended for older patients with large tumors. It is also a wise option if a piece of the tumor capsule is obstinately adherent to the underside of the chiasm or to the great vessels at the time of attempted total resection.

Biopsy and Radiation

Most workers now believe that simple tumor biopsy and postoperative RT are inferior to either total resection or subtotal resection and RT. Shapiro et al. (59) reported 5- and 10-year survival rates of only 62% and 50%, respectively, for biopsy and RT. The figures from Sung et al. (61) and Manaka et al. (48) are comparable. Thus this option is only endorsed for the very old, the very infirm, or those patients refusing more radical approaches. Because the biological effects of RT may take 6–9 months to occur, patients suffering from imminent compression symptoms to the optic structures or hypothalamus will not benefit from this treatment method. If a cyst contributes significantly to the mass effect, an indwelling catheter connected to a subcutaneous reservoir may be implanted in the cyst to permit percutaneous aspiration as a means of mass control during the waiting period.

Primary Stereotactic Radiosurgery

Recently, stereotactic radiosurgery using the gamma irradiation unit (8,40,42,43) has been showing some promise in controlling growth of small solid tumors and solid recurrences following aspiration of tumor cysts. The principle of radiosurgery is based on the fact that the biological effects produced by a single radiation dose are greater than that produced by the same dose fractionated. Thus if the radiation is delivered as a single dose to sharply circumscribed and precisely targeted areas of tissue, tumor necrosis may be achieved with comparative low morbidity to surrounding brain tissues. In solid craniopharyngiomas, approximately 50 Gy are intended for the main parts of the tumor.

To date, only a small number of patients who had undergone this treatment modality are available for analysis, and Backlund's 15-year follow-up results are encouraging for tumor-shrinkage accomplished with a low morbidity (5). A much larger series is needed to ascertain the long-term value and late adverse effects of stereotactic radiosurgery. At the moment, it is tantalizing as a nonsurgical alternative for small to moderate sized solid craniopharyngiomas, as well as for tumor remnants found to be too hazardous to excise.

Primary Tumor, Predominantly Cystic

Approximately 30% of craniopharyngiomas are predominantly cystic (48,59). If the wall of the cyst is relatively thick and the maximum tumor diameter does not exceed 5 cm, total resection should probably be attempted. However, if the cyst wall is very thin, it cannot be used as a "handle" during tumor dissection and may fragment into little pieces behind collapsing cisterns, indistinguishable from thickened arachnoid. Cystic tumors also tend to be very large and rambling within expanded subarachnoid spaces and within brain. In these circumstances, total excision is difficult to achieve and may even be associated with unacceptable surgical trauma to the brain.

An alternative is to instill beta-emitting radionuclide into the cyst cavity in order to deliver a high dose to the cyst wall so that tumor cell necrosis can be induced and fluid accumulation arrested. The radiation dose planned for the cyst wall is from 200 to 400 Gy, depending on the wall thickness. Pure beta-emitting isotopes such as yttrium−90 and phosphorus−32 are preferred because beta-rays have short tissue penetration and can exert tumoricidal activity at the cyst wall without injuring the adjacent hypothalamus and optic chiasm.

Preliminary results reported by Backlund (6) and Kobayashi (36) are encouraging. The cyst shrinkage rate is around 90%, and the complication rate is low, but not zero. Partial blindness, endocrinopathies, third nerve palsy, and mild psychiatric disturbances have been documented. There are also pitfalls to this treatment. Most thin-walled cystic craniopharyngiomas have thickened portions of the wall not affected by the intracavitory beta radiation. These thickened parts will continue to grow as solid tumors. They may be independently treated with stereotactic radiosurgery, or by microsurgical removal. Currently, I am evaluating the efficacy of a two-stage treatment protocol for tumors with large, rambling cystic parts, first using intracystic irradiation to collapse the cyst toward the solid part, which is usually within the suprasellar cistern, and then removing the cyst–solid composite by elective microsurgery.

SURGICAL MANAGEMENT

Preoperative Evaluation and Management

As soon as the diagnosis is made, complete endocrinological evaluation should be made to establish a baseline against which the effect of therapy can be gauged. More importantly, preoperative testing may uncover hypocortisolemia and hypothyroidism that will contribute to intra- and postoperative morbidity unless promptly treated. Subtle hormonal deficiencies may require challenging tests using arginine infusion, insulin-induced hypoglycemia, and thyrotropin releasing hormone and LHRH administration. An 8-hr partial water deprivation test may be used to stress the pitressin axis if symptoms of diabetes insipidus (DI) are mild, although this information is only of academic value, since DI is almost a certainty in the immediately postoperative period.

Adequate thyroid replacement takes several days to 2 weeks with oral L-thyrosine and should be started immediately. Intravenous L-thyroxine may be given if the patient's condition demands immediate surgical intervention, but it must be infused extremely carefully in elderly patients lest it produce arrhythmias and acute myocardial ischemia.

Corticosteroid replacement can be done rapidly. All except the smallest craniopharyngiomas with proven preserved ACTH axis should be given preoperative stress steroid doses. The first crisis of physiologic stress requiring stress levels of circulating corticosteroids is during the induction of general anesthesia. Patients should therefore be given stress doses before the morning of surgery equivalent to three times the physiologic daily cortisol production [the mean physiologic cortisone requirement is 13 mg/m^2/day for normal individuals over 4 months of age (34)]. For adults, this can be given by infusing intravenous Solu-Cortef beginning the night before, but for children it is simpler to give a single intramuscular injection of the daily stress dose of cortisone acetate both the night before and the morning of surgery, followed by a slow Solu-Cortef intravenous drip during the operation.

Detailed neuro-ophthalmological assessment is also important to follow the patient's postoperative and post-radiation visual status. Because of the recent interest in neurobehavioral syndromes following treatment of craniopharyngiomas (17,23), I routinely obtain detailed preoperative neuropsychological testing (54). The test results are especially important for monitoring a child's intellectual and psychosocial progress following therapy and are helpful in identifying specific cognitive deficits for which remedial strategies may be constructed.

Management of Hydrocephalus

Over 60% of children with craniopharyngiomas have obstructive hydrocephalus at diagnosis. If the symptoms of raised ICP are not disabling, it is preferable to perform all preoperative evaluations and preparations expeditiously without preresection shunting, and then put in an external ventricular drain (EVD) at the time of tumor resection to assist in brain relaxation. The drip chamber of the EVD is set at physiologic levels after surgery for 3–4 days and then gradually raised to test the patient's CSF absorption capacity. The majority of hydrocephalus resolves after total or subtotal excision of the tumor, and the EVD is removed. Only rarely will the EVD "Chamber test" indicate permanently impaired CSF resorption requiring shunting.

If the patient presents with dangerously high ICP due to hydrocephalus at the time of diagnosis, a temporary EVD is still preferable to preresection shunting. A temporary EVD is just as effective in allowing time for the proper preoperative tests and preparation but does not carry the risk of shunt infection, which is not insubstantial considering the long exposure time of the CSF during the radical resection operation.

Surgical Approaches and Technical Considerations

Subfrontal Approach

This is the approach I prefer because it affords total excision of most craniopharyngiomas except for those eccentric large tumors that require staged procedures from diverse angles. Unilateral frontal lobe retraction is almost always adequate for exposure, and it minimizes the disastrous prospect of bifrontal damage with bilateral frontal retraction. The right side is usually used by the right-handed surgeon, unless there is significant lateral extension of tumor into the left sylvian fissure or temporal lobe. The head is fixed by a pin-type headholder in a midline neutral position so that the anterior fossa floor is approximately perpendicular to the floor. The back of the table is slightly elevated and the body is well padded and securely strapped to the table to allow for 20°–25° of rotation of the head to either side during extreme lateral exposures of the tumor bed.

A bicoronal scalp flap is fashioned just behind the hairline. Making the incision too far back incurs unnecessary dissection and interferes with subsequent incisions for a CSF shunt if that becomes necessary (Fig. 1A). A hinged periosteal flap 1.5 cm wide is elevated from the skull over the frontal sinuses to be used later as a vascularized covering for the frontal sinus openings. A right osteoplastic frontal craniotomy is made so that the medial extent crosses the midline by 1.5 cm to expose the superior sagittal sinus. The lowest extent is flush with the orbital roof, and the lateral–posterior margin may be extended posteriorly to the sphenoid ridge if the pterional approach is to be used for certain parts of the tumor (Fig. 1B).

The anterior-most portion of the superior sagittal sinus is doubly ligated and transected (Fig. 2A,B). The anterior falx is then completely detached from the crista galli to expose the interhemispheric fissure (Fig. 2C). For larger tumors, it is usually necessary to divide the right olfactory tract (Fig. 3A). Deep subfrontal retraction along the proximal olfactory tract will bring the right optic nerve and chiasm into view, at which time the prechiasmatic cistern is quickly opened to allow egress of CSF. Time is well spent to patiently aspirate as much CSF as possible, for this allows the brain to sag backward and reduces retraction pressure on the vital subfrontal deep nuclei. The arachnoid incision is then carried laterally to the right carotid cistern and part of the proximal sylvian cistern, medially along the front of the chiasm, and contralaterally over the left optic nerve and internal carotid artery (Fig. 3B). The frontal lobe is thus "untethered" from the optic structures and carotid arteries and may be further retracted to expose the entire anterior–superior surface of the chiasm, and usually also the A-1 segment of both anterior cerebral arteries. With the medial brain retractor now on the left gyrus rectus, and the lateral retractor over the right parolfactory lobules, all the major "surgical spaces" through which tumor extraction is to occur are widely exposed: namely, the interoptic, left and right carotico-optic, and carotico-sylvian spaces.

The anterior lower aspect of the tumor is now visible behind dense arachnoid adhesions between the optic nerves (interoptic space) and between the nerve and the carotid artery (carotico-optic space). Tumor with lateral extension beyond the carotid is seen in the proximal sylvian fissure after gentle retraction of the temporal lobe. It is at once obvious that the surgical exercise involves extracting a large, but (fortunately) usually soft, bulk through a series of relatively small holes (the surgical spaces). The tactic thus consists of debulking and collapsing the center of the bulk, pulling in and freeing the peripheral capsule from surrounding structures, and finally grabbing and pulling out the morsellated capsule through these small holes. It is advisable to follow a drilled sequence of maneuvers because each preceding step makes the next one easier and safer. The recom-

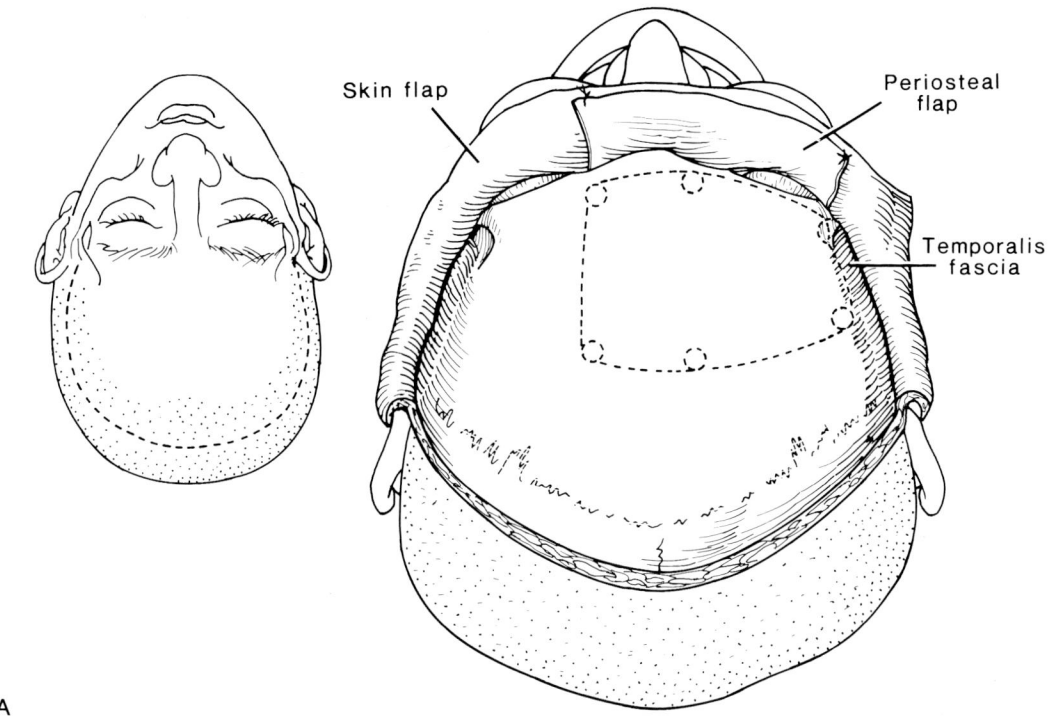

FIG. 1. Initial exposure of the right subfrontal approach. **A:** Bicoronal scalp flap. **B:** Right osteoplastic frontal bone flap hinging on temporalis muscle. Medial extent crosses midline by 1.5–2 cm; inferior extent flush with anterior fossa floor. Note periosteal flap for later coverage of opened frontal sinuses.

mended sequence goes as follows: interoptic debulking; separation from optic structures; right lateral dissection; left lateral dissection; detaching upper pole from the hypothalamus, basilar tip dissection; and, finally, dorsum sellae–intrasellar dissection.

Tumor reduction begins with aspiration of cyst fluid and excision of a generous piece of capsule for biopsy in the interoptic space (Fig. 4). This space is usually quite large, but a retrochiasmatic tumor occasionally pushes the chiasm forward to make it appear prefixed. This "pseudoprefixity" is lost as soon as further debulking causes the chiasm to fall back, thereby widening the interoptic space for further debulking.

Arterial feeders to the tumor from the anterior communicating and anterior cerebral arteries can be taken with impunity as long as the vascular supply to the chiasm and optic nerves is preserved.

Collapse of the center causes the capsule to pull away from the underside of the optic nerves and anterior chiasm. There is often an arachnoid plane between capsule and the optic structures which should be carefully exploited to peel the capsule off intact, the peeling motion always proceding from brain to tumor (Fig. 5). Occasionally, the capsule obliterates this subarachnoid space and becomes adherent to the underside of the optic nerves, a blind spot that not infrequently harbors residual tumor.

In accordance with its embryologic origin from anterior diencephalic and stomodeal structures, the tumor receives its blood supply anteriorly from the anterior communicating and anterior cerebral arteries (anterior feeders already taken), laterally from medial branches of the posterior communicating arteries, and inferiorly from the meningohypophyseal vessels around the pituitary gland. Except when the tumor is enormous, it does not usually parasitize feeders from the basilar–posterior cerebral complex. Thus one of the main objectives of the lateral dissection is eliminating the lateral blood supply of the tumor. Right lateral dissection is best done through the carotico-optic space. The lateral capsule is manipulated medially toward the collapsed central cavity of the tumor, thereby putting the lateral feeders from the posterior communicating artery on stretch. Usually the arachnoid plane is very clear here, and the posterior communicating artery can be seen in its entirety from carotid to posterior cerebral artery. Its medial tumor branches are cauterized and divided while its important superior (thalamotuberal) and lateral branches are preserved (Fig. 6). The third cranial nerve is usually seen lateral to the artery and is seldom involved in tumor. In tumors with lateral extension, the carotico-sylvian space lateral to the carotid may have to be used, but dissection of capsule from the proximal sylvian fissure is usually straightforward. Once these lateral feeders are divided and lateral adhesions to the sylvian veins are detached, the lateral capsule is basically free and can be grasped through the large interoptic space and resected in large pieces.

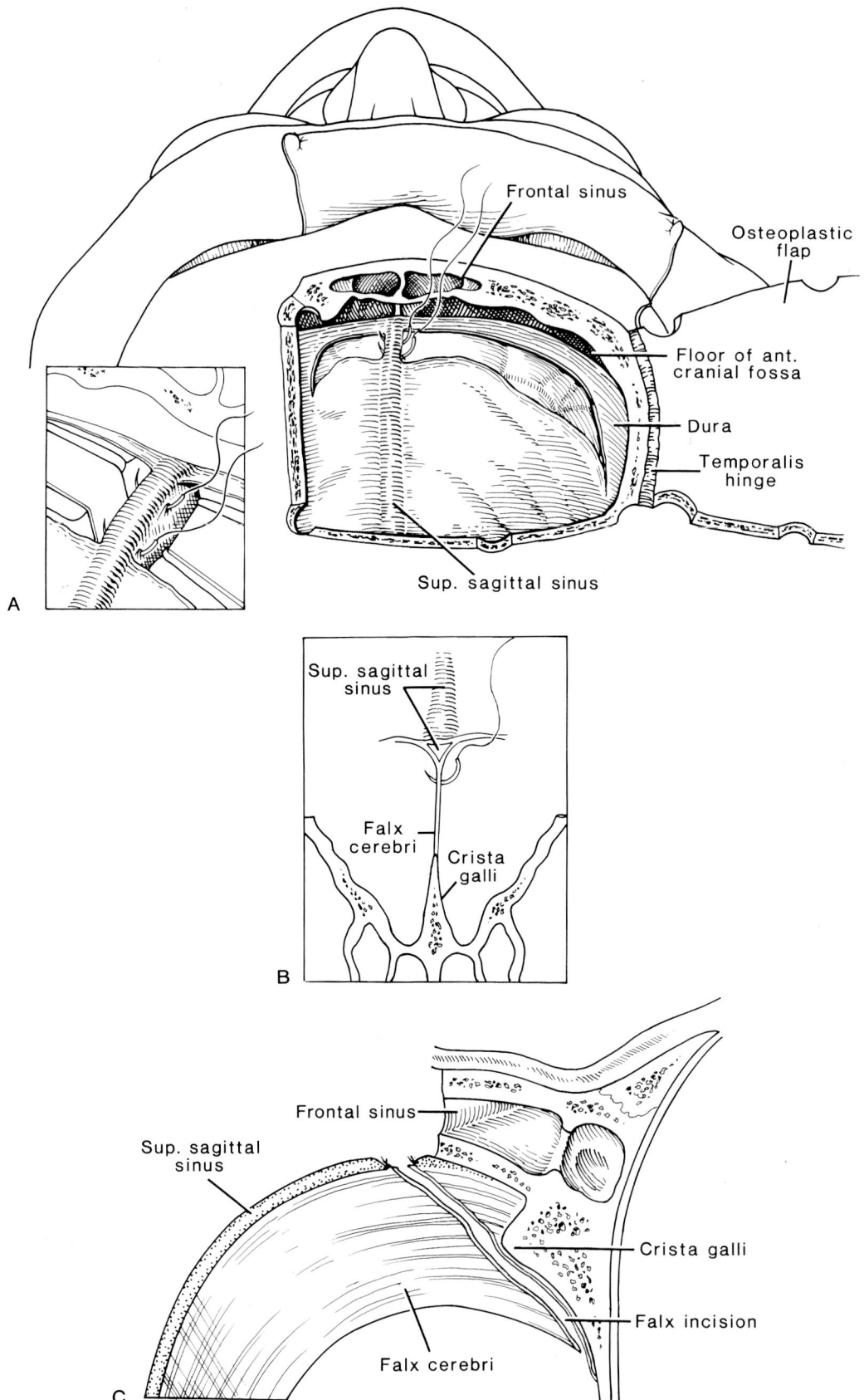

FIG. 2. Dural opening, superior sagittal sinus ligation, and incision of the anterior falx. **A:** Bilateral J-shaped dural incisions. **Insert** shows double suture ligation of the anterior extreme of the superior sagittal sinus. **B:** Coronal view shows the suture ligation needle passing beneath the superior sagittal sinus. **C:** Sagittal view shows anteriorly oblique incision of the falx along its attachment to the crista galli.

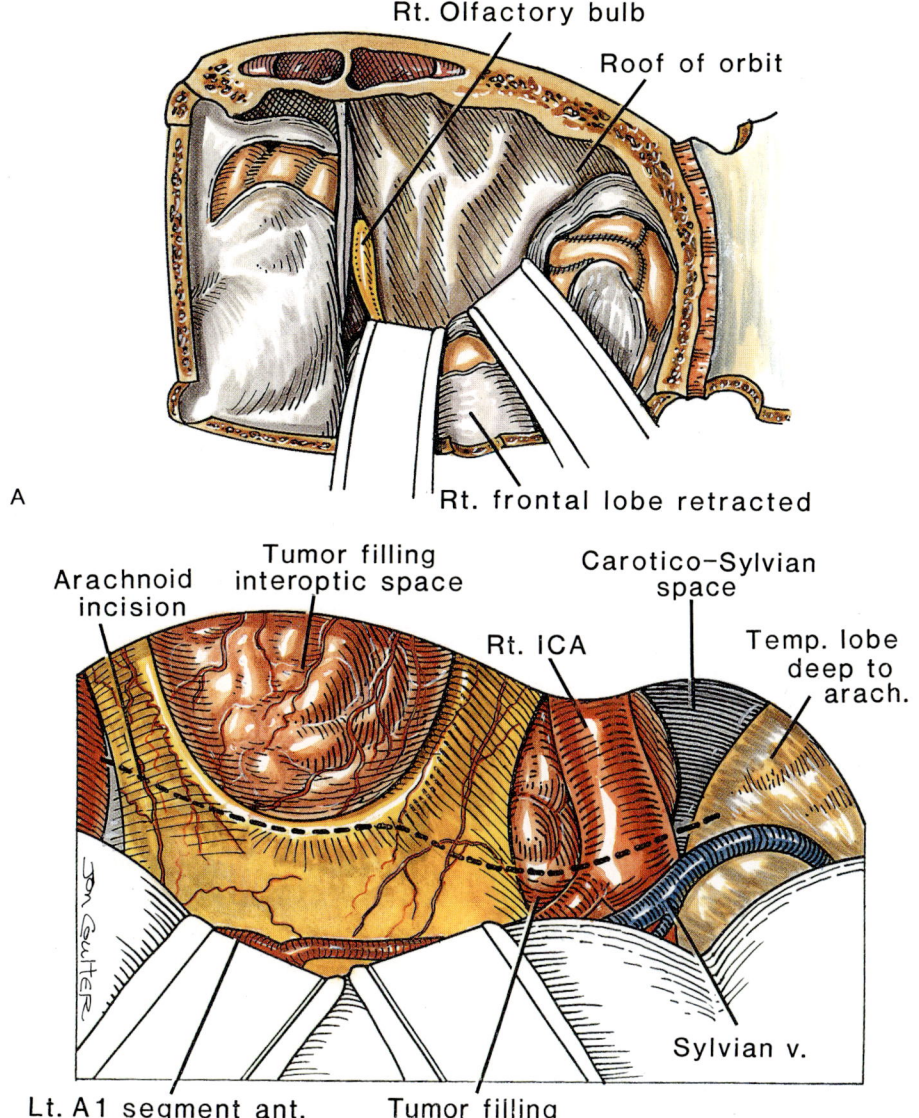

FIG. 3. Right subfrontal exposure. **A:** Initial retraction of right frontal lobe exposes the right olfactory bulb and tract. **B:** Deeper right frontal lobe retraction exposes both optic nerves, the anterior upper surface of the chiasm, the right internal carotid artery (ICA), and the A-1 segment of the anterior cerebral artery. The three surgical spaces are well seen. Tumor fills the interoptic space and is visible within the carotico-optic and carotico-sylvian spaces. *Dotted line* shows line of arachnoid incision.

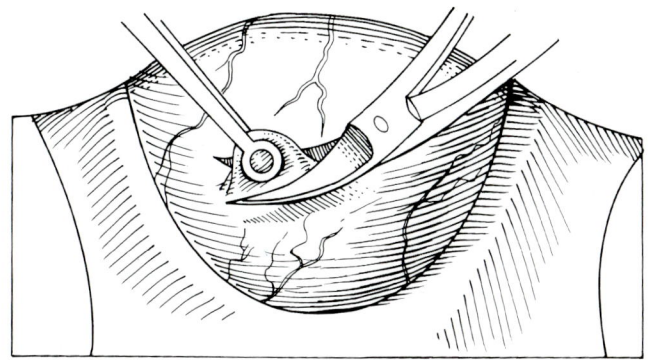

FIG. 4. Debulking tumor through the interoptic space.

Because of the convenient microscope angle for the right-handed surgeon, the left lateral dissection may be accomplished through the large intraoptic space (Fig. 7). Lateral tumor extension may be handled by rotating the operating table to the left, which allows the surgeon to see as far lateral as the proximal sylvian fissure.

Once the lateral capsule is removed from both sides, there is enough room in the suprasellar cistern to detach the upper pole of the tumor from the hypothalamus. At this point, most of the upper part of the tumor has already descended to the level visible through the interoptic space. The downward CSF pulsation within the third ventricle helps in this regard. The capsule can usually be

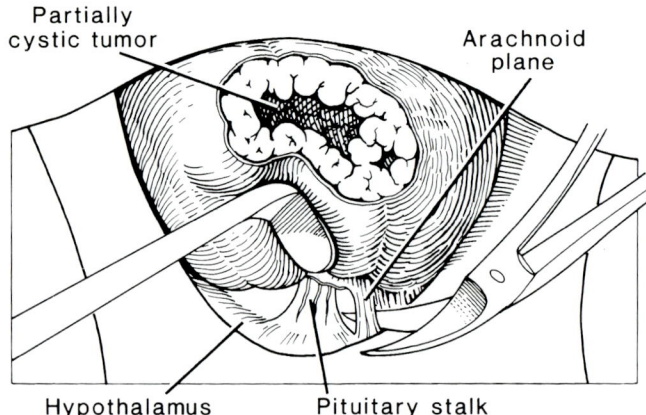

FIG. 5. Separation of tumor from optic structures. Relatively intact arachnoid plane between tumor capsule and the medial surface of the optic tracts and the anterior surface of the chiasm can be exploited by pulling tumor away from the brain surface. The pituitary stalk is sometimes visible with more posterior exposure, identified by its straight portal vessels.

ensures that the tumor pseudopods are avulsed from the surrounding gliotic rim rather than being left behind. The distorted pituitary stalk is usually encountered at this stage of the dissection and is recognized by its longitudinal striation due to the straight, parallel arrangement of the long portal vessels (Fig. 5) (14–16). It can occasionally be preserved by sharply dissecting tumor off it, but in large lesions the stalk is hopelessly encased in tumor and will have to be divided. Most often the stalk is pushed anteriorly by the tumor and will be identified early. The posteriorly displaced stalk is much more vulnerable to injury, since it is obstructed from view by the tumor bulk.

The posterior pole or retrosellar portion of the tumor can now be rolled forward and often detached from the basilar and proximal posterior cerebral arteries with surprising ease, since these do not usually supply the tumor and are more than likely separated from the capsule by the intact, double-layered membrane of Liliequist. Thus even a large posterior piece extending behind and below the dorsum sellae, by right invisible through the subfrontal approach, can be pulled up and forward into view, and removed by cutting the tethering arachnoid bands. Afterward, cranial nerves III and IV and sometimes even the distal VI nerve are visible in front of the midbrain.

peeled off the underside of the chiasm and the anterior floor of the third ventricle along a well defined arachnoid plane, but as the attachment nears the infundibular stalk, the capsule almost always becomes seemingly fused with the hypothalamus. This unique part of the tumor is usually more tenacious than brain tissue and can literally be torn away from the brain by firmly grasping and pulling it downward using the alternating right and left tumor microforceps (Fig. 8A–C). This technique may be likened to pulling a large rag out of a deep bag with two hands. The tear usually occurs conveniently within the gliotic layer between functional hypothalamus and capsule, and the tearing and pulling motion

The last remaining part of the tumor is its inferior pole relating to the diaphragma sella and the pituitary gland. If the CT or MRI scan shows only widening of the upper sella but not ballooning or inferior expansion of the sella toward the sphenoid sinus, the inferior capsule is usually free from attachment with the intrasellar dura and can be pulled upward without problem (Fig. 9A–C). Bleeding from meningohypophyseal feeders within the sella can be easily controlled with tamponade. Posteriorly, the

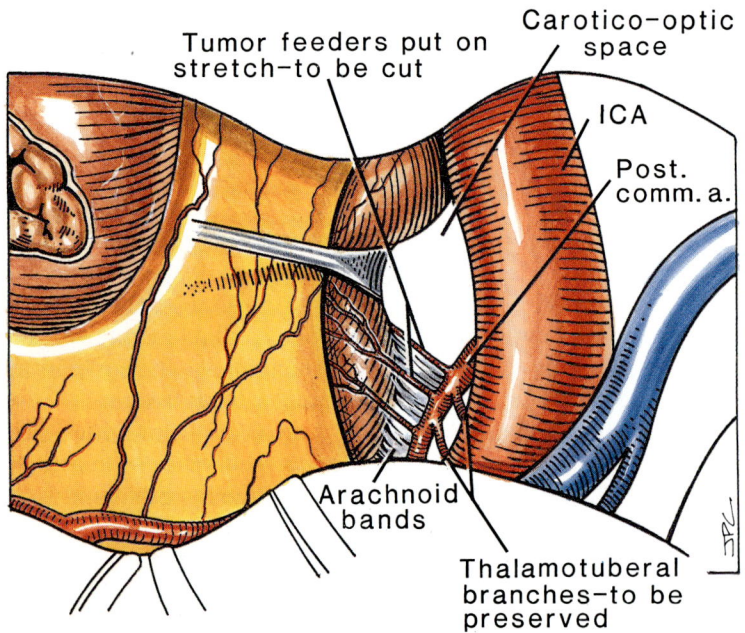

FIG. 6. Right lateral dissection within carotico-optic space. The right lateral surface of the tumor capsule is pulled away from the internal carotid (ICA) and posterior communicating arteries (post. comm.a.), putting stretch on the lateral tumor feeders from the medial surface of the posterior communicating artery. The superiorly coursing thalamotuberal branches to the hypothalamus and thalamus are preserved.

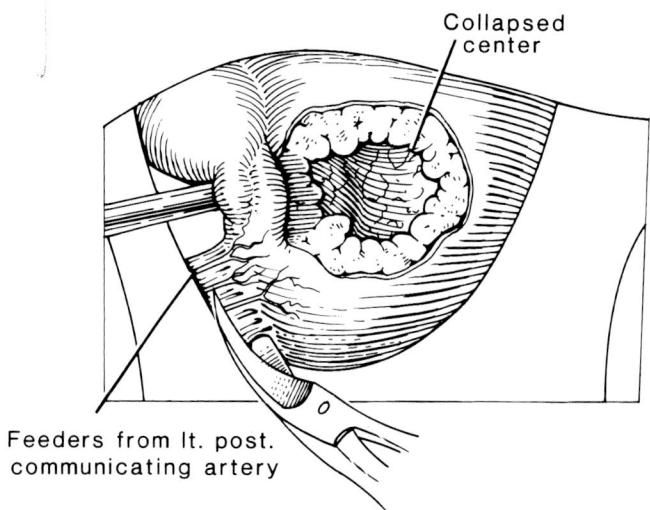

FIG. 7. Left lateral dissection through the interoptic space. The microscope is angled severely to the left. The left lateral tumor capsule is retracted medially to expose lateral tumor feeders from the left post communicating artery.

inferior capsule may be adherent to the dorsum sella dura, but this can be peeled off under direct vision (Fig. 10).

Translamina Terminalis Approach

In patients with prefixed chiasm, the interoptic space is too small for the extensive maneuvers needed to remove a large craniopharyngioma. Also, some childhood tumors are very large and their solid upper poles often push the third ventricular floor so far up as to reach the level of the foramen of Monro. In these situations, the lamina terminalis may be traversed to gain access to the tumor done. Normally this is one way of entering the anterior third ventricle, but with large suprasellar tumors, the tuberal portion of the basal hypothalamus, from the mamillary bodies to the chiasm, is often stretched very thin and may actually be coapted with the lamina terminalis to form a single membrane (Fig. 11). Both the infundibular and supraoptic recesses are obliter-

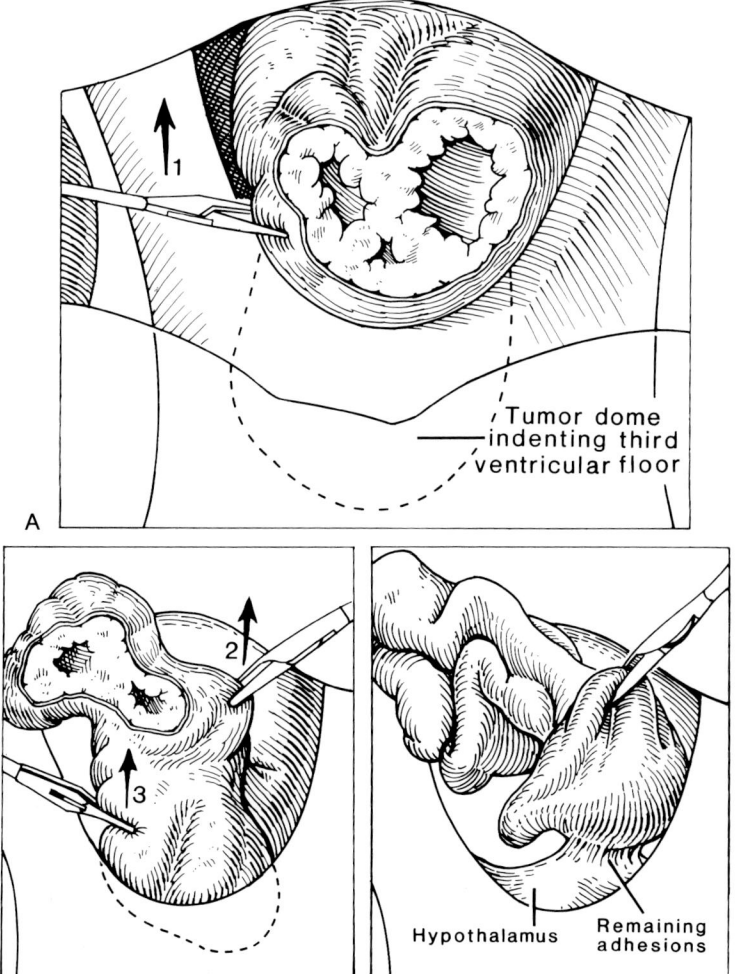

FIG. 8. Detaching the upper pole of tumor from the hypothalamus. A: After considerable reduction of tumor volume through interoptic debulking, the base of the upper tumor piece (indenting third ventricular floor) is firmly grasped by the left microforceps and pulled down toward the suprasellar cistern (grasp 1). B: When more tumor appears in the upper interoptic space, it is, in turn, grasped by the right microforceps, which continues the pull (grasp 2), alternating with the left hand (grasp 3). C: The entire upper pole is pulled down, and the previously severely elevated hypothalamic floor is now visible through the interoptic space.

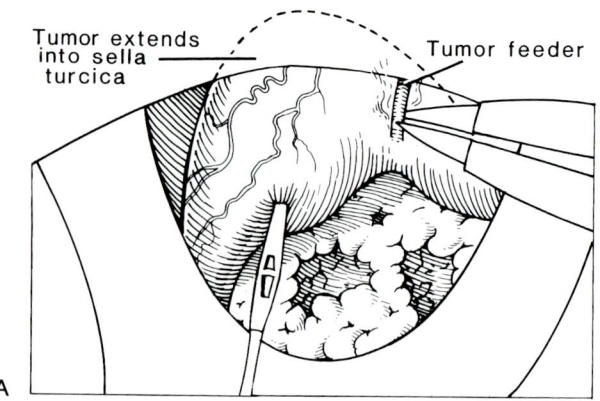
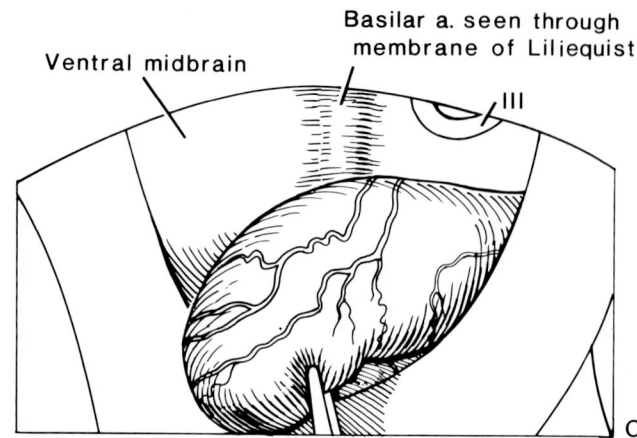
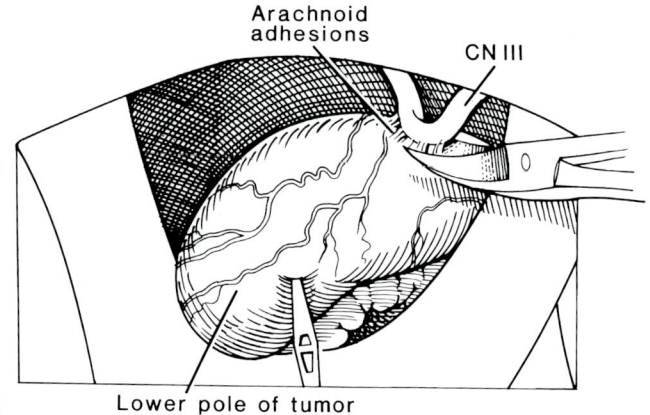

FIG. 9. Removal of the lower pole of the tumor. **A:** The sellar part of the tumor (lower pole) is often easily lifted upward from its loose attachment with the dura over the dorsum sellae and sella. Inferior feeders from capsular and meningohypophyseal vessels are cauterized. **B:** Cranial nerve III is often attached to the lower capsule. **C:** Extracting the last remaining piece away from its loose attachment with the membrane of Liliequist, through which can be seen the basilar artery and its terminal branches.

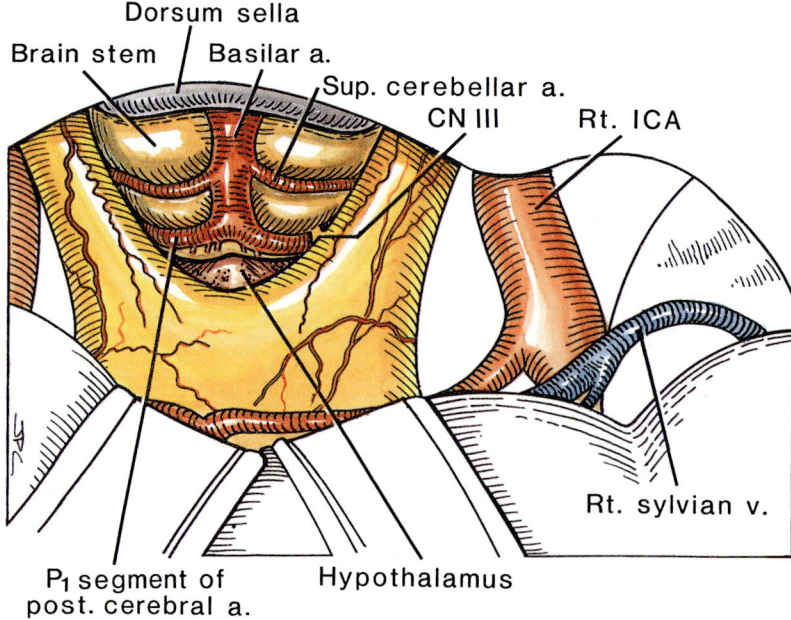

FIG. 10. View after total resection of tumor.

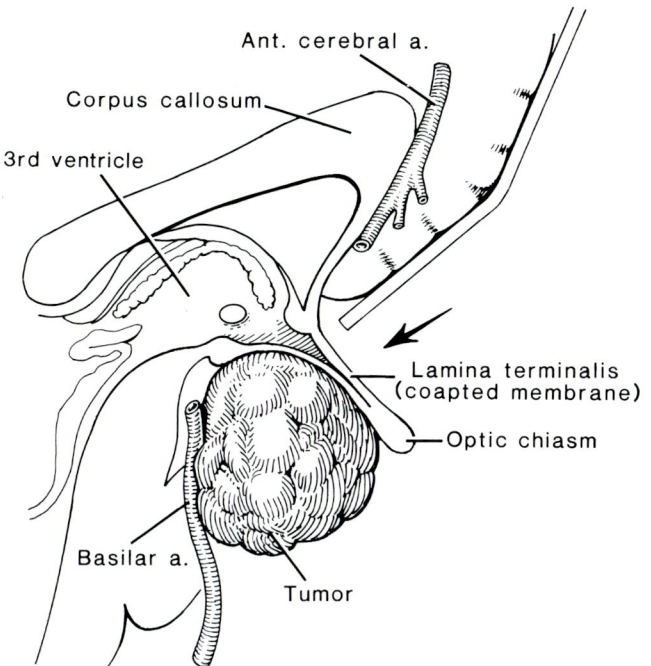

FIG. 11. Schematic view of the tumor pushing the third ventricle floor upward and coapting the attenuated midline basal hypothalamus with the lamina terminalis.

ated, so that traversing this coapted membrane instantly gains access to the tumor below the hypothalamus without actually entering the third ventricle. It appears likely that the basal hypothalamic nuclei have been displaced laterally in the presence of chronic compression by large tumors, and using the translamina terminalis route does not usually produce hypothalamic deficiency.

In most large solid craniopharyngiomas with prominent domes, the lamina terminalis is widely expanded behind the chiasm, and the yellowish gritty tumor can easily be seen through the diaphanous coapted membrane in-between the splayed-out optic tracts (Fig. 12). This membrane may be opened widely over the bulging tumor, but the posterior margin of the chiasm must be carefully protected since it contains the crossing macular fibers. An excellent view is obtained of the tumor dome, which can be dissected under direct vision from the hypothalamic floor and manipulated downward to be removed either behind or in front of the chiasm (Figs. 13–15).

Subfrontal-Transsphenoidal Approach

When the tumor possesses a large intrasellar part, especially if the preoperative imaging studies show a grossly

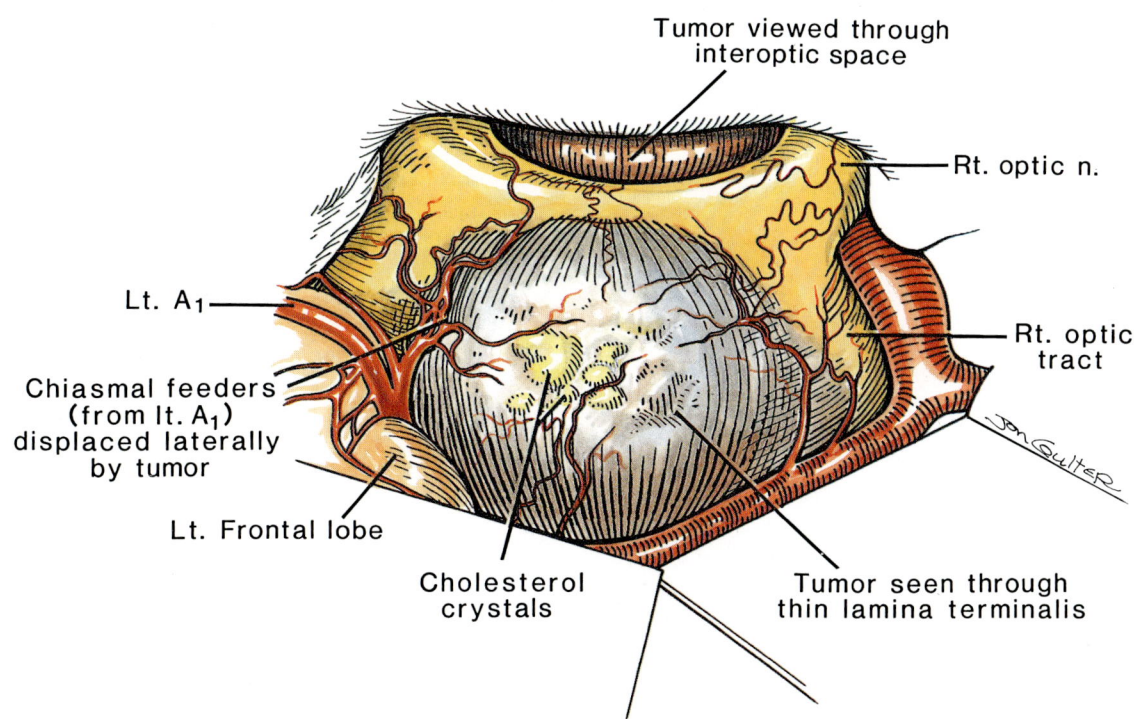

FIG. 12. Tumor and prefixed chiasm. Only the most posterior segments of the optic nerves are seen; the small interoptic space is inadequate for tumor extraction. Tumor is seen bulging through the thin (coapted) lamina terminalis, splaying open the optic tracts. The chiasmal feeders from the anterior surface of the A−1 are displaced laterally by the bulging tumor.

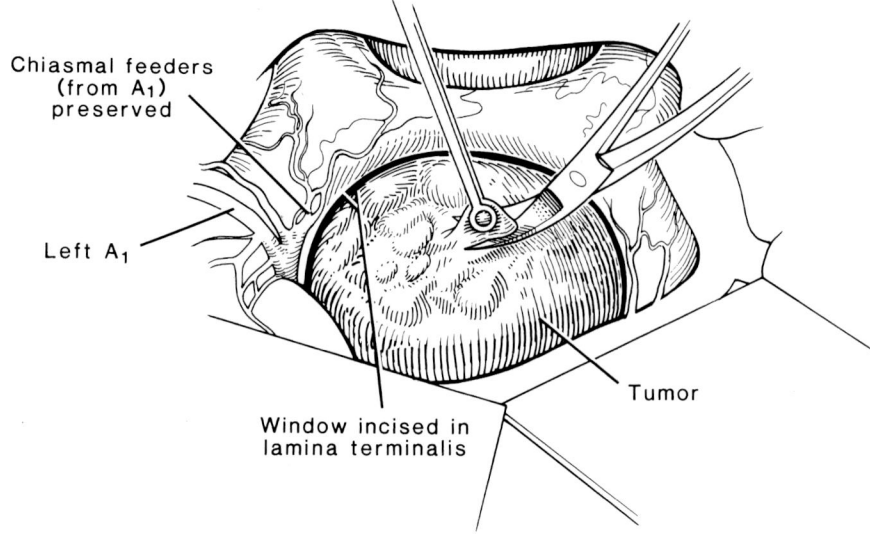

FIG. 13. The thin lamina terminalis has been excised along margin of the optic tracts and posterior chiasmal surface. Tumor is being debulked, and tumor capsule can be dissected from optic structures.

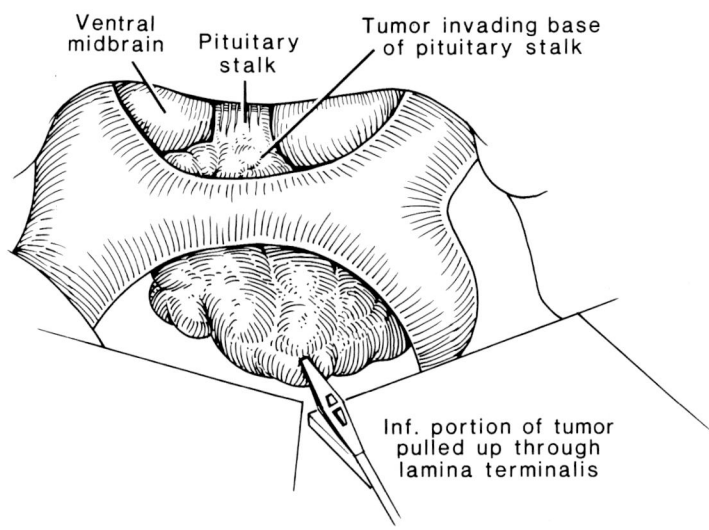

FIG. 14. Inferior portion of tumor pulled up from the sellar region through the large opening in laminar terminalis.

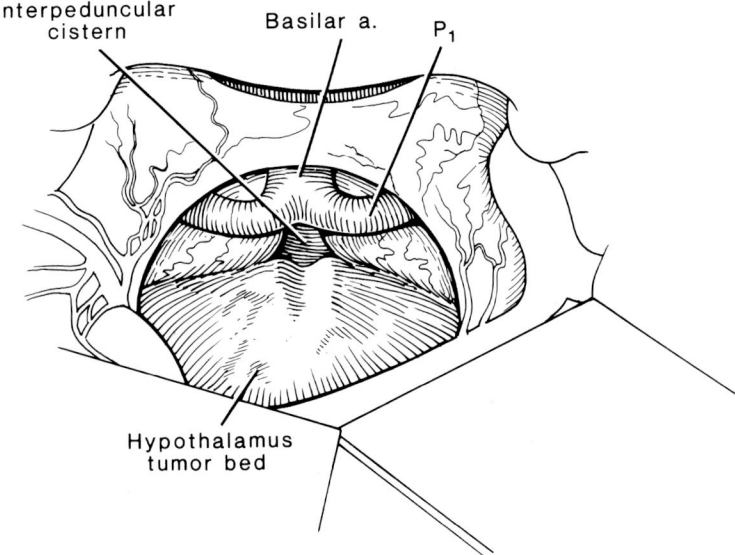

FIG. 15. After total excision of tumor, basal hypothalamus (tumor bed), basilar artery, ventral midbrain, and interpeduncular cistern are all well seen through lamina terminalis opening.

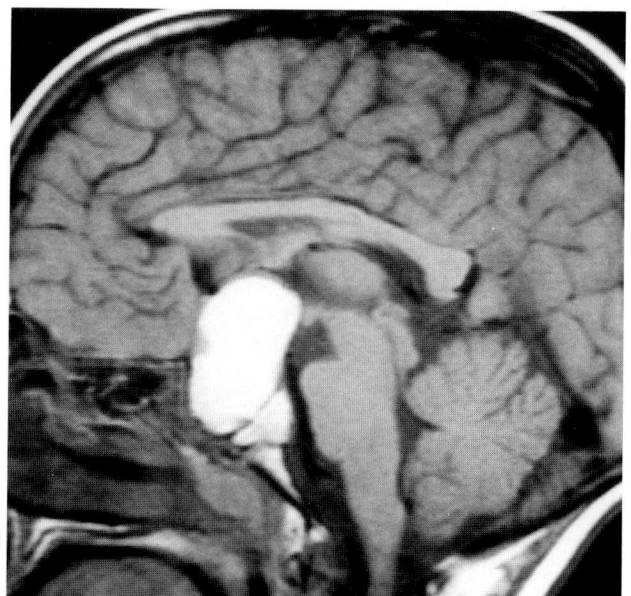
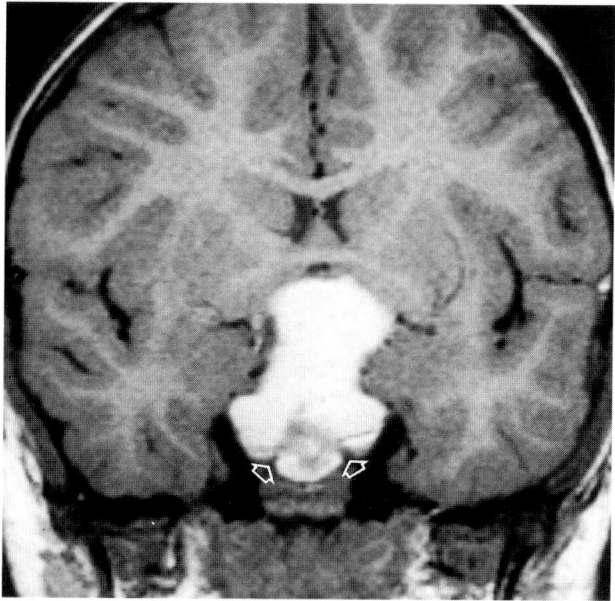

FIG. 16. MRI scan of a 15-year-old boy with large partially cystic craniopharyngioma. **A:** Sagittal image without gadolinium injection shows wide expansion of the sella and encroachment of the sphenoid sinus. Upward extension of the tumor elevates hypothalamus almost to the level of foramen of Monro. Note mamillary bodies just behind the posterior surface of the tumor. **B:** Coronal image without gadolinium shows expansion of the sella, wide lateral displacement of the intracavernous internal carotid arteries and cavernous sinuses, and a defect in the sella floor (*arrows*) through which tumor extends into the sphenoid sinus.

expanded sella and/or an invaded sphenoid sinus (Fig. 16), the inferior capsule of the tumor is often tightly adherent to the dura of the dorsum sellae and sella, and to the sphenoid mucosa. If the sella floor is eroded, the capsule is also adherent to the medial and superior walls of the cavernous sinus. The sellar and infrasellar portion can no longer be extracted satisfactorily or safely through the standard subfrontal approach. In these situations, direct access to the inferior pole of the tumor can be gained by the subfrontal–transsphenoidal route (Fig. 17). A dural flap is raised over the tuberculum sellae, through which a window is made by the microdrill to enter the superior–anterior chamber of the sphenoid sinus (Fig. 18). The sinus mucosa is preserved but pushed downward to expose the anterior wall of the sella (Fig. 19). This is often paper thin, and breaking through it reveals the sella dura and the sella tumor (Fig. 20). A thin shell of pituitary gland is often sandwiched between the tumor capsule and the dura and is frequently indistinguishable from tumor. If the pituitary stalk has already been cut, there is no point saving the gland; the sella is thus completely exenterated using curettes and cautery (Figs. 21 and 22). The circular sinus and the cavernous sinus sometimes bleed profusely, but this type of venous bleeding always stops with tamponade unless the latter sinus is opened widely. Aggressively packing the cavernous sinus occasionally produces oculomotor palsies.

Postoperatively, the confluent sella–sphenoid cavity is

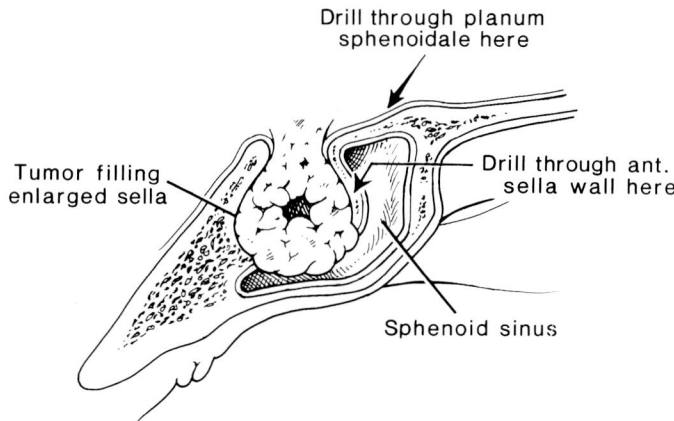

FIG. 17. Subfrontal–transsphenoidal approach. Sagittal view to show the intrasella and intrasphenoid tumor. *Arrows* show direction of drilling through the planum sphenoidale to gain entrance into the sphenoid sinus and access to the anterior sellar wall.

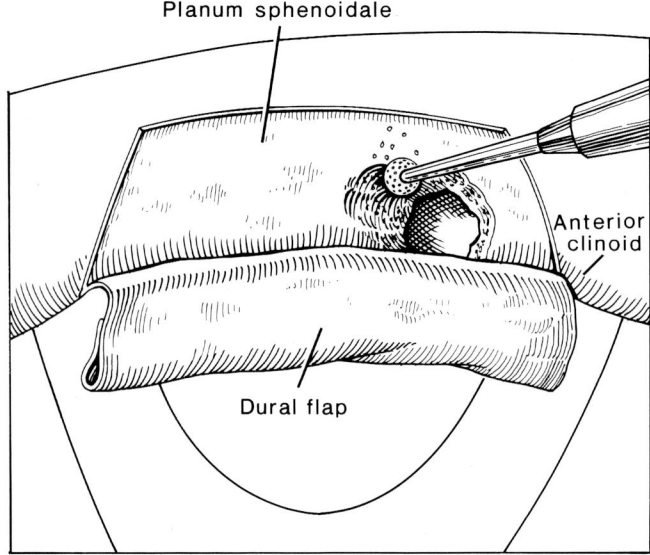

FIG. 18. Subfrontal–transsphenoidal approach. Drilling through the planum sphenoidale after dural flap was raised over the tuberculum sellae.

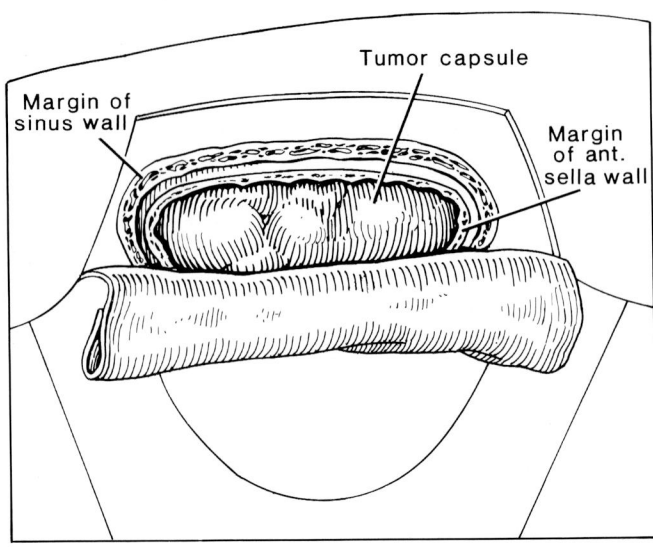

FIG. 20. Subfrontal–transsphenoidal approach. After traversing the anterior sella wall, tumor capsule is encountered; it is often fused with the sella dura and a thin rim of compressed pituitary gland.

packed with fat, and a piece of fascia lata is sutured to the edge of the tuberculum dural defect and laid over the sella (Fig. 23). If the sphenoid mucosa is accidentally perforated, a lumbar drain may be needed to prevent postoperative CSF leak (Fig. 24).

Staged Procedures

Occasionally, lateral tumor extension into the choroidal fissure cannot be adequately visualized by any of the

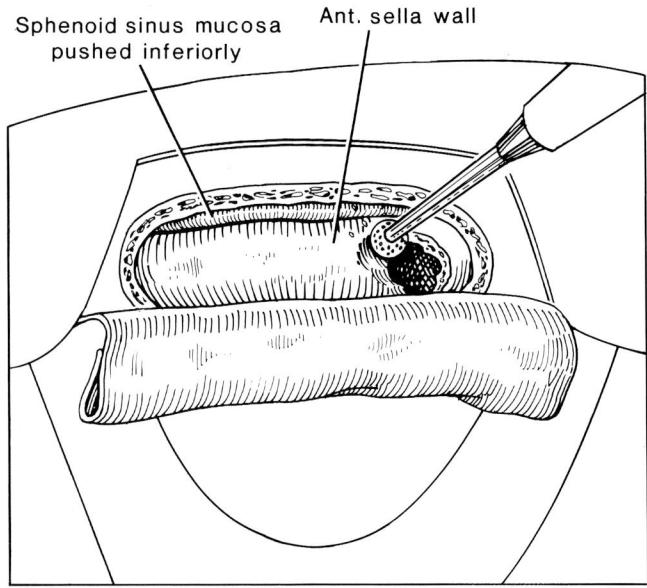

FIG. 19. Subfrontal–transsphenoidal approach. After entering sphenoid sinus, the mucosa is kept intact and swept inferiorly to expose anterior sella wall, which is, in turn, opened with drilling.

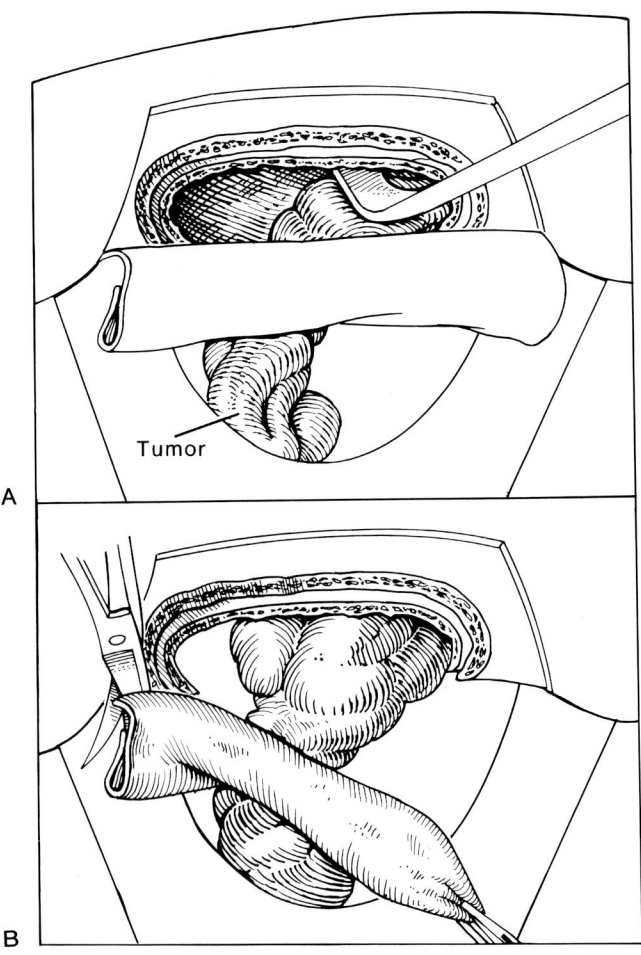

FIG. 21. Subfrontal–transsphenoidal approach. **A:** Exenteration of sella content with microcurette scraping against the anterior and inferior sella wall. **B:** Intrasellar tumor is pushed into the interoptic space. If necessary, the remaining tuberculum sellae dura may be excised to gain better exposure.

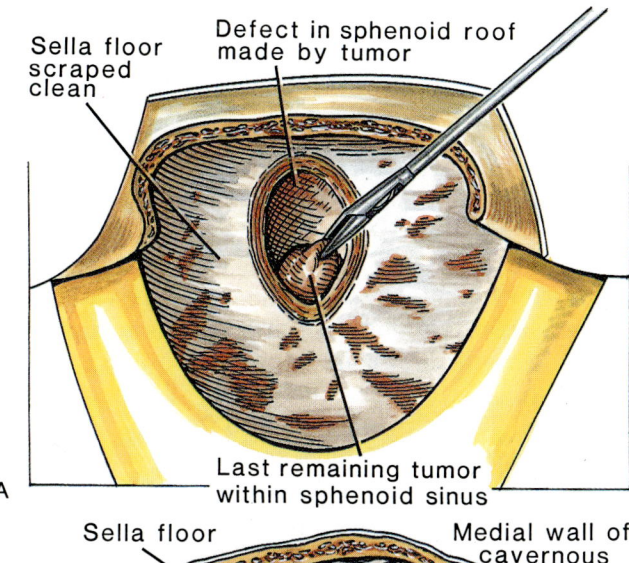
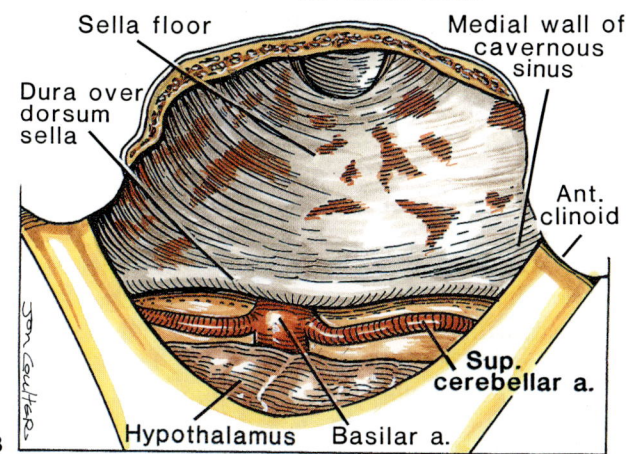

FIG. 22. Subfrontal–transsphenoidal approach. **A:** Identification of defect in the sella floor and extraction of last remaining tumor from the sphenoid sinus. **B:** View after complete excision of tumor.

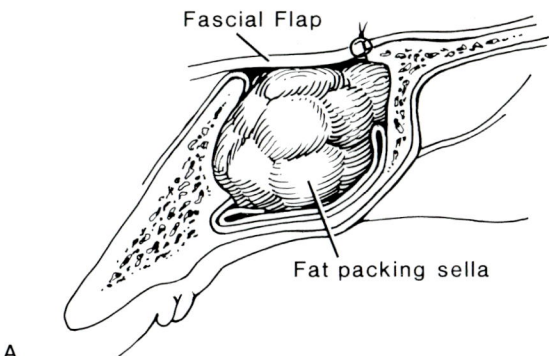
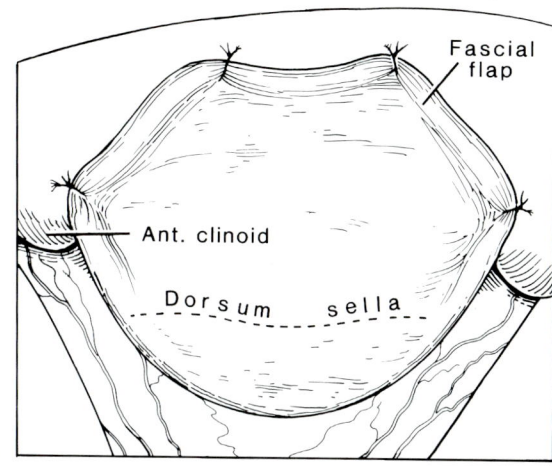

FIG. 23. Subfrontal–transsphenoidal approach. Skull base repair. **A:** Sagittal view shows that sella and upper sphenoid sinus are packed with free fat graft. A fascial flap is laid over the defect and its anterior edge is sutured to the tuberculum dural flap margin. **B:** Operative view showing fascial flap sutured in place.

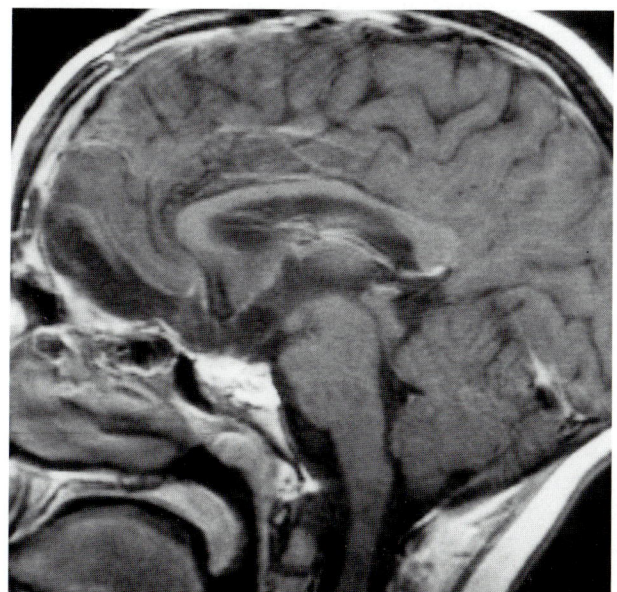
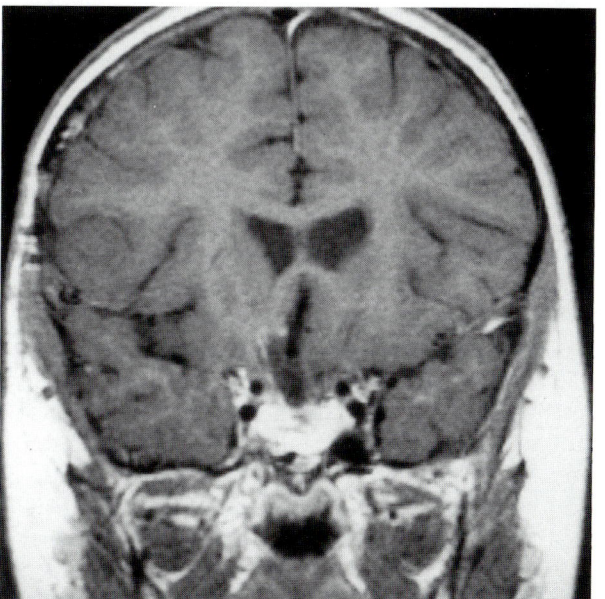

FIG. 24. Postoperative MRI of the case shown in Fig. 16. **A:** Sagittal view with gadolinium. **B:** Coronal view with gadolinium. Note the total excision of tumor by the subfrontal–transsphenoidal approach, loss of the tuberculum sellae "angle," and presence of the fat–fascia graft within the sella–sphenoid sinus complex. Note resumption of air-filling in the sphenoid sinus, indicative of mucosal preservation.

above approaches to allow total excision by a single procedure. A second procedure using the subtemporal route is then necessary to remove the lateral portion after the main bulk has been resected. By itself, the subtemporal route is not recommended as a primary approach because of the high frequency of postoperative CN III, IV, and VI palsies. Also, the intrasellar portion of the lesion below the level of the diaphragma cannot be visualized well, and the approach does not permit either a transsphenoidal or translamina terminalis option if these become necessary.

Because on coronal CT large craniopharyngiomas may appear to be completely within the third ventricle, they have been approached by the transcallosal route through the dilated lateral ventricle. This CT appearance is usually misleading because the third ventricular floor, though severely distorted and thinned, is still intact above the tumor, and a primary transventricular removal from above has been associated with significant hypothalamic damage and poor results (46,70). With the very rare exception of the truly intraventricular craniopharyngiomas, this approach is only recommended as a second procedure if after the subfrontal operation a portion of the tumor is found to have penetrated far into the third ventricle and would not descend with suprasellar debulking. In this case, the transcallosal approach offers an excellent view of the residual tumor near the foramen of Monro, where adherence to large veins may make other less direct approaches hazardous.

POSTOPERATIVE COMPLICATIONS AND MANAGEMENT

Visual loss is the most common neurological deficit after radical or subradical resection. The preoperative visual status is the most important determining factor for subsequent visual outcome (15). Patients with total or near total blindness for longer than a week do not usually regain any useful vision, but those with decreased acuity or constricted visual fields may well improve after surgery. Another important prognostic factor is the duration of visual loss before surgery. Patients with visual impairment for less than a year have greater than three times the chance of improvement than those with impairment longer than a year (3).

With the recent push for total excision, treating hormone deficiencies has become an integral part of the total management of this tumor. With the high incidence of stalk sectioning or stalk injury during tumor resection, DI is almost a universal postoperative endocrinopathy and also the one that requires immediate attention. Excessive diuresis usually begins within the first 24 h, but degeneration of the hypothalamo–hypophyseal tract and necrosis of the axon terminals in the neurohypophysis cause release of stored antidiuretic hormone (ADH) 24–96 hr after surgery, with a rebound tendency toward water intoxications (14,60). This "second phase" response of stalk sectioning must be kept in mind when administering pitressin analogs in order to avoid aggravating the postsurgical edema of the hypothalamus and frontal lobes. The initial DI is best managed with small doses of intravenous DDAVP (desmopressin), which has a therapeutic effect lasting up to 18 hr. When the patient is more alert, DDAVP can be given by nasal spray usually with 10 times the intravenous dose. It is interesting that although DI is universal after stalk sectioning, 10–15% of patients will resume partial production of ADH within 3 years, and their DDAVP requirement may lessen. This is probably due to formation of new neurovascular units in the magnocellular portion of the supraoptic and paraventricular nuclei of the hypothalamus (2).

Stress doses of corticosteroid are maintained for 3–4 days and then gradually tapered to normal daily requirement in the form of oral cortisone acetate tablets. If dexamethasone was also used prophylactically for postsurgical edema, it should be tapered off completely according to the anticipated time course of edema and not be mixed up with the tapering schedule of hydrocortisone requirement. Postoperative hypothyroidism requiring thyroxine replacement occurs in approximately 60–80% of patients with total excision. FSH and LH deficiencies are also inevitable after stalk sectioning and spontaneous puberty in children does not occur. Patients can be given synthetic estrogen and progesterone combinations at the expected age of puberty to impart secondary sexual characteristics and to mimic menstrual cycles. Male adults usually require testosterone injections to maintain libido and potency. Ovulation in adult females can be induced by a costly process of priming ovarian follicular growth with human menopausal gonadotropins (Pergonal, containing FSH and LH) and then stimulating the follicles with a burst of human chorionic gonadotropins (possessing strong LH activity) (24). Patients with a preserved pituitary stalk have been known to regain endocrine functions, but recovery of the exquisitely sensitive LHRH pacemaker function in the arcuate nucleus of the hypothalamus, vital to the induction of ovulation, has not been observed to date.

The growth rate remains low in most children following radical excision of tumors. Growth can generally be maintained with growth hormone (GH) replacement starting 6–9 months after surgery. In some children, however, the postoperative growth rate is normal despite absence of GH (4,20,22,30,34,66). In a few of these children, growth associated with marked weight gain and hyperphagia can be attributed to hyperinsulinemia (4,20), but in others with normal insulin level, the continued growth is related to normal to supranormal levels of insulin-like growth factors (IGFs)(12). IGFs are probably stimulated by increased prolactin secretion from retained pituitary tissues when the output of prolactin inhibitory factor from the injured hypothalamus is reduced.

With increasingly sophisticated microsurgical techniques, florid hypothalamic syndromes such as hypersomnia, loss of thirst sensation, temperature dysregulation, profound amnesia, and disturbances of caloric balance are very seldom seen after total excision. More likely one encounters "minor" hypothalamic disturbance such as transient recent memory deficits and appetite changes. In children and young adults, it is especially common to see some degree of central hyperphagia 1-6 months after surgery—especially if the translamina terminalis approach was used (54). The increased desire to eat is accompanied by weight gain. Severely hyperphagic children also show bizarre food finding behaviors and eating habits. Central hyperphagia is recently postulated to be due to injury to serotoninergic eating inhibition pathways originating from the anterior nucleus and preoptic area of the anterior hypothalamus. Fortunately, when the hyperphagia subsides, the weight also reduces or stabilizes, but strict behavioral modification and counseling must be enforced on children during the overeating phase to avoid morbid obesity.

Another interesting neurobehavioral syndrome following total excision is abulia minor. The affected patients have various degrees of slowness of motor action, ideation, and emotion. They lack spontaneity of action and thoughts, have slow and infrequent adventitious body motions and gesticulations, lack enthusiasm to surroundings, show little exploratory behaviors, and have flat affects (54). Children thus affected are unmotivated in play or school activities and subsequently have poor progress in learning. The neuropathological lesion causing this syndrome is not known, but abulia may be related to injury to the mesolimbic pathway by the deep subfrontal retractors during exposure of the lamina terminalis. This pathway has been linked to exploratory behaviors in animals and projects from the rostral midbrain to the medial septal nuclei, nucleus accumbens, and the anterior cingulate gyrus (29,42,43,69) by way of the medial septal area just underneath the retractors.

POSTOPERATIVE FOLLOW-UP

Postoperative CT with and without contrast should be obtained 1-2 days after surgery (when contrast enhancement of surgically traumatized brain tissue is minimal) to detect residual tumor. Even experienced surgeons are not exempt from leaving behind small pieces of tumor within operative blind spots, such as under the chiasm and in the anterior alcove of the sella. Residual specks of calcium or enhancing tumor fragments on the immediate postoperative CT are indications for reexploration before exuberant scarring makes dissection difficult. This practice should eliminate some of the cases of false cure that are reported in most large series of craniopharyngiomas (1,55,63,64). If the immediate postoperative CT shows no residual tumor, or if the second attempt at total excision accomplishes its goal, the next CT and MRI can be obtained in 3-6 months. Because gadolinium enhancement of the surgical field may still be present on MRI 2-3 months after surgery, it is fruitless to obtain a MRI before 2-3 months. Thereafter, a yearly CT and MRI should be adequate.

Complete endocrine evaluation including basal hormone levels and stimulation tests should be performed 3-6 months after surgery to determine whether thyroid replacement should be continued. Cortisone replacement will almost certainly be necessary for at least 1-2 years, but the requirement for DDAVP may decrease after 6 months if the pituitary stalk was preserved at surgery (14). At least 1 year should elapse after surgery before it can be determined whether a child requires growth hormone injections, or whether normal growth continues due to sustained IGF levels. A low growth hormone level has no bearing on the growth curve after craniopharyngioma resection (12,22,30).

Neuro-ophthalmological examinations should be done twice yearly. It is most useful for cases of known residual or recurrent tumor, when a subtle change in vision may signal a change in the growth status of the tumor before an actual increase in tumor size can be appreciated on imaging studies.

It is helpful to utilize a checklist of follow-up parameters at each 6-month clinic visit. A complete neurological and ophthalmological examination is recorded. The patient is questioned about urine output "breakthroughs" in order to assess adequacy of DDAVP dosage and to determine whether endogenous ADH has resumed production. All growth indices are measured for children. The body weight and eating habits of overweight patients are carefully evaluated to distinguish between central hyperphagia, psychogenic polyphagia, and excessive corticosteroid intake. An abridged neuropsychological battery should include a verbal recall test, complex figure duplication, and recall to assess nonlogic memory and spatial orientation, object similarities and differences, and proverb interpretation. The patient's psychomotor activity level, willingness to participate in work and recreation, enthusiasm for social interaction, and emotional tone are also recorded.

RECURRENT CRANIOPHARYNGIOMAS

Three options may be considered in the case of recurrent tumor: a second attempt at total excision, subtotal resection and postoperative radiation, and radiation alone. It has been shown that reoperation for radical excision of craniopharyngioma carries a higher morbidity and a lower probability of a curative resection (15,63). However, total excision with acceptable morbidity has been accomplished in selective cases (14), and it seems reasonable for an experienced surgeon to undertake a second attempt at total excision, with the knowledge that tumor fragments may be more adherent to vessel walls and hypothalamus than before, and that good sense must be exercised to dictate how aggressive the dissection should be. Reoperation is especially recommended for those who had already received radiation after the first operation, or if the solid component of a cystic tumor regrows following intracavitary radionuclide injection. If a total excision is thought to have been achieved, the patient is followed by the same protocol as for the primary operation. If only a subtotal excision was obtained at reoperation, conventional radiation or stereotactic radiosurgery should be given to control the residual disease. If a patient returns with recurrence after multiple attempts at radical resection, radiosurgery should also be considered to prolong symptom-free survival.

REFERENCES

1. Amacher AL. Craniopharyngioma: the controversy regarding radiotherapy. *Childs Brain* 1980;6:57–64.
2. Antunes JL, Carmel PW, Zimmerman EA, Ferin M. Regeneration of the magnocellular system of the rhesus monkey following hypothalamic lesions. *Ann Neurol* 1979;5:462–469.
3. Artero JMC, Crespo JV, Zabolgoita GB. Status of vision following surgical treatment of craniopharyngiomas. *Acta Neurochir (Wien)* 1984;73:165–177.
4. Ayral D, Talot L, David M, Lecornu M, Francois R. Etude de la croissance paradoxale de certains enfants apres chirurgie hypothalamo-hypophysaire en depit de l'absence d'hormone de croissance. *Pediatrie* 1980;35:389–401.
5. Backlund EO. Solid craniopharyngiomas treated by stereotactic radiosurgery. *INSERM Symp (#12)* 1979;340:271–277.
6. Backlund EO. Stereotactic treatment of craniopharyngiomas—15 years' experience (abstract). The 32nd Annual Meeting of the Scandinavian Neurosurgical Society, Linkoping, Sweden, September 5, 1980.
7. Backlund EO. Studies on craniopharyngiomas. III. Stereotaxis treatment with intracystic yttrium-90. *Acta Chir Scand* 1973;139:237–247.
8. Backlund EO. Studies on craniopharyngiomas. IV. Stereotaxis treatment with radiosurgery. *Acta Chir Scand* 1973;139:248–250.
9. Banna M. Craniopharyngiomas in adults. *Surg Neurol* 1973;1:202–204.
10. Banna M, Hoare RD, Stanley P, Till K. Craniopharyngiomas in children. *J Pediatr* 1973;83:781–785.
11. Bartlett JR. Craniopharyngiomas—an analysis of some aspects of symptomatology, radiology, and histology. *Brain* 1971;94:725–732.
12. Bucher H, Zapf J, Torresani T, Prader A, Froesch ER, Illig R. Insulin-like growth factors I & II, prolactin, and insulin in 19 growth hormone-deficient children with excessive, normal, and decreased longitudinal growth after operation for craniopharyngioma. *N Engl J Med* 1983;309:1142–1146.
13. Cabezudo JM, Vaguero J, Areitia E, Martinez R, DeSola RG, Bravo G. Craniopharyngiomas: a critical approach to treatment. *J Neurosurg* 1981;55:371–375.
14. Carmel PW. Craniopharyngiomas. In: Wilkins RH, Rangachary SS, eds. *Neurosurgery.* New York: McGraw-Hill, 1985;905–916.
15. Carmel PW, Antunes JL, Chang CH. Craniopharyngiomas in children. *Neurosurgery* 1982;11:382–389.
16. Carmel PW, Antunes JL, Ferin M. Collection of blood from the pituitary stalk and portal veins in monkeys, and from the pituitary sinusoidal system of monkey and man. *J Neurosurg* 1979;50:75–80.
17. Cavazzuti V, Fischer EG, Welch H, Belli JA, Winston KR. Neurological and psychophysiological sequelae following different treatment of craniopharyngioma in children. *J Neurosurg* 1983;59:409–417.
18. Chadduck WM, Roberts M. Long term survival with craniopharyngioma: report of patient in 29th year after treatment, seen for a second intracranial tumor. *J Neurosurg* 1966;25:312–314.
19. Cobb CA, Youmans JR. Brain tumors of disordered embryogenesis in adults. In: Youmans JR, ed. *Neurological surgery,* 2nd ed. Philadelphia: Saunders, 1982;2899–2935.
20. Costin G, Hogut MD, Philips LS, Daughaday WH. Craniopharyngioma: the rate of insulin in promoting postoperative growth. *J Clin Endocrinol Metab* 1976;42:370–379.
21. Erdheim J. Uber hypophysengangges chwiilste und hirncholesteatome. Sitzungsh d. k. Akad k. Wissehseh Math–Naturw Klin 113 Pt. III:1940;537–726.
22. Finkelstein JW, Kream J, Ludan A, Hellman L. Sulfation factor (somatomedin): an explanation for continued growth in the absence of immunoassayable growth hormone in patients with hypothalamic tumor. *J Clin Endocrinol Metab* 1972;35:13–37.
23. Fischer EG, Welch K, Belli JA, Wallman J, Shillito JJ, Winston KR, Cassady R. Treatment of craniopharyngiomas in children. *J Neurosurg* 1985;62:496–501.
24. Glass RH. Infertility. In: Yen SSC, Jaffe RB, eds. *Reproductive endocrinology: physiology, pathophysiology and clinical management.* Philadelphia: Saunders, 1978;398–417.
25. Goldberg GM, Eshbaugh DE. Squamous cell nests of the pituitary gland as related to the origin of craniopharyngiomas. *Arch Pathol* 1960;70:293–299.
26. Harris JR, Levene MB. Visual complications following irradiation for pituitary adenomas and craniopharyngiomas. *Radiology* 1976;120:167–171.
27. Hoff JT, Patterson RH. Craniopharyngiomas in children and adults. *J Neurosurg* 1972;36:299–302.
28. Hoffman HJ, Hendrick EB, Humphreys RP, Buncic JR, Armstrong DL, Jenkin RDT. Management of craniopharyngioma in children. *J Neurosurg* 1977;27:218–227.
29. Iversen SD, Koob GF. Behavioral implications of dopaminergic neurons in the mesolimbic system. *Adv Biochem Psychopharmacol* 1977;16:209–214.
30. Job JC, Lambertz J, Sizonenko PC, Rossier A. La croissance des enfants atteints de craniopharyngiome: vitesse de croissance et resultats des dosages d'hormone de croissance dans le plasma avant et apres intervention chirurgicale. *Arch Fr Pediatr* 1970;27:341–353.
31. Kahn EA, Cosby EC. Korsakoff's syndrome associated with surgical lesions involving the mammillary bodies. *Neurology* 1972;22:117–125.
32. Kahn EA, Gosch HH, Seeger JF, Hicks SP. Fifty-five years experience with the craniopharyngiomas. *Surg Neurol* 1973;1:5–12.
33. Katz EL. Late results of radical excision of craniopharyngiomas in children. *J Neurosurg* 1975;42:86–90.
34. Kenny FM, Preeyasombat C, Migion CH. Cortisol production rate II, normal infants, children, and adults. *Pediatrics* 1966;37:34–42.
35. Kernohan JW. Tumors of congenital origin. In: Minckler J, ed. *Pathology of the nervous system.* New York: McGraw-Hill, 1971;1927–1937.
36. Kobayashi T, Kageyama N, Ohara K. Internal irradiation for cystic craniopharyngioma, *J Neurosurg* 1981;55:896–903.
37. Koos WT, Miller MJ. *Intracranial tumors of infants and children.* Stuttgart: Thieme, 1971;188–213.
38. Kramer S, Southard M, Mansfield CM. Radiotherapy in the management of craniopharyngiomas: further experiences and late results. *Am J Roentgenol Radiat Ther Nucl Med* 1968;103:44–52.
39. Krayenbuhl H, Yasargil MC. Radiological anatomy and topography of the cerebral arteries. In: Vinken PH, Bruyn GW, eds. *Handbook of clinical neurology, volume 2. Vascular diseases of the nervous system, part I.* Amsterdam: North-Holland, 1972;65–101.
40. Larrson B, Liden K, Sarby B. Techniques for irradiation of small intracranial structures through the intact skull. Proceedings of the 9th Symposium Neuroradiologium, Gothenburg, April 11–15, 1979, pp 14–16.

41. Lazorthes G. *Vascularization et circulation cerebrales.* Paris: Masson, 1961:14–30.
42. Leksell L. *Stereotaxis and radiosurgery.* Springfield, IL: Charles C Thomas, 1981;1–69.
43. Lessell L, Backlund EO, Johansson L. Treatment of craniopharyngiomas. *Acta Chir Scand* 1967;133:345–350.
44. Lichter AS, Wara WM, Sheline GE, Townsend JJ, Wilson CB. The treatment of craniopharyngiomas. *Int J Radiat Oncol Biol Phys* 1977;2:675–683.
45. Lindvall O, Bjorklund A. The organization of the ascending catecholamine neuron system in the rat brain. *Acta Physiol Scand [Suppl]* 1974;412:1–49.
46. Long DM, Chou SN. Transcallosal removal of craniopharyngiomas within the third ventricle. *J Neurosurg* 1973;39:563–567.
47. Luse SA, Kernohan JW. Squamous-cell nests of the pituitary gland. *Cancer* 1955;8:623–628.
48. Manaka S, Teramoto A, Takakura K. The efficacy of radiotherapy for craniopharyngiomas. *J Neurosurg* 1985;62:648–656.
49. Martin AM, Johnston JS, Henry JM, Stoffel TJ, CiChico G. Delayed radiation necrosis of brain. *J Neurosurg* 1977;47:336–345.
50. Matson DD. *Neurosurgery of infancy and childhood,* 2nd ed. Springfield, IL: Charles C Thomas, 1969;544–574.
51. Matson DD, Crigler JF. Management of craniopharyngioma in childhood. *J Neurosurg* 1969;30:377–390.
52. McKissock W, Ford RK. Results of treatment of the craniopharyngiomas. *J Neurol Neurosurg Psychiatry* 1966;29:475 (abstract).
53. Olivecrona H. The surgical treatment of intracranial tumors. In: Olivecrona H, Tonnis W, eds. *Handbuch der neurochirurgie,* vol IV. Heidelberg: Springer-Verlag, 1967;1–301.
54. Pang D. Craniopharyngiomas. *Management of childhood brain tumors.* In: Deutsch M, ed. Norwell, MA: Kluwer Publishers; 1990;285–307.
55. Patterson RH, Danylevich A. Surgical removel of craniopharyngiomas by a transcranial approach through the lamina terminalis and sphenoid sinus. *J Neurosurg* 1950;7:11–117.
56. Pertuiset B. Craniopharyngiomas. In: Vinken PH, Bruyn FW, eds. *Handbook of clinical neurology, volume 19. Tumors of the brain and skull, part II.* Amsterdam: North-Holland, 1975; 530–572.
57. Rougerie J, Fardeau M. *Les craniopharyngiomes.* Paris: Masson, 1962.
58. Russel RW, Pennybacker JB. Craniopharyngiomas in the elderly. *J Neurol Psychiatry* 1961;24:1–13.
59. Shapiro K, Till K, Grant N. Craniopharyngioma in childhood. *J Neurosurg* 1979;50:617–623.
60. Shucart WA, Jackson I. Management of diabetes insipidus in neurosurgical patients. *J Neurosurg* 1976;44:65–70.
61. Sung DI, Chang CH, Harisiadis L, Carmel PW. Treatment results of craniopharyngiomas. *Cancer* 1981;47:847–852.
62. Svien HJ. Surgical experiences with craniopharyngiomas. *J Neurosurg* 1965;23:148–155.
63. Sweet WH. Radical surgical treatment of craniopharyngioma. *Clin Neurosurg* 1976;23:52–79.
64. Sweet WH. Recurrent craniopharyngiomas. Therapeutic alternatives. *Clin Neurosurg* 1980;27:206–229.
65. Symon L, Sprich W. Radical excision of craniopharyngioma. *J Neurosurg* 1985;62:174–181.
66. Thomsen MJ, Conte FA, Kaplan SK, Grumbach MM. Endocrine and neurologic outcome in childhood craniopharyngioma: a review of the effect of treatment in 42 patients. *J Pediatr* 1980;97:728–735.
67. Tiberin P, Goldberg GM, Schwartz A. Craniopharyngiomas in the aged. *Neurology* 1958;8:31–54.
68. Till K. Craniopharyngioma. *Childs Brain* 1982;9:179–187.
69. Ungerstedt U. Stereotaxic mapping of the nomamine pathways in the rat brain. *Acta Physiol Scand [Suppl]* 1971;367:1–48.
70. Van den Bergh R. The transventricular approach in craniopharyngioma of the third ventricle. Neurosurgical and neuropathological aspects. *Neurochirurgie* 1970;16:51–65.
71. Waga S, Handa H. Radiation induced meningioma: with review of literature. *Surg Neurol* 1976;5:215–219.

CHAPTER 51

Osseous Lesions of Anterior and Middle Base

Patrick J. Derome and A. Visot

Many types of osseous lesions are encountered in the anterior and middle base (4–7). Primary bone lesions include tumors of cartilaginous origin (chordomas, chondrosarcomas), tumors of true osseous origin (osteomas, osteoblastomas, osteosarcomas, dermoid or epidermoid cysts), tumors of vascular origin (hemangiomas), tumors of fibrous origin (ossifying fibromas, fibrosarcomas), or giant cell tumors. One must add lesions that are not true tumors, such as fibrous dysplasia, osteopetrosis, histiocytosis X, and the involvement or the destruction of the skull base by surrounding tumors may also be considered as osseous lesions. It occurs in meningiomas, trigeminal neurilemomas, olfactory neuroblastomas, and carcinomas.

Since the first description of the "transbasal approach" in 1972 (4), the most frequent bone tumors operated on in our series have been fibrous dysplasia, invading meningiomas, chordomas, and chondromas. Other tumors are relatively rare. Laterally, in the pterional area and middle fossa, hyperostosing meningiomas are the most common. For this reason, patients with fibrous dysplasia and hyperostosing meningioma will be chosen for the demonstrative surgical procedures.

The three goals of the surgery are the total or near-total excision of the tumor (according to its extension and type), the decompression of the cranial nerves included or surrounded by the lesion (particularly the optic nerves), and the anatomical reconstruction, which avoids postoperative complications and may include the correction of large craniofacial deformities.

The risks of this surgery are conditioned by the opening of the septic facial cavities. These risks (infection or CSF leaks) are quite different in the midline where the frontal sinus, nasal cavities, ethmoidal and sphenoidal cells, and sphenoidal cells are successively found, in contrast to the lateral area where no air sinuses are encountered except sometimes for the alar extension of the sphenoidal sinus. Therefore particular attention must be paid preoperatively to the meningeal plane for possible destruction or involvement of the dura (rare in primary bone tumors, systematic in meningiomas, frequent in the other lesions).

DIAGNOSTIC CONSIDERATIONS

MRI is particularly important in the diagnosis of dural or soft tissue involvement and gives more accurate delimitations of the lesion. But the CT scan and even plain x-rays and cranial base tomographies are very useful in the evaluation of tumors. Very often, these data are sufficient for the surgical decision. Angiography is required when the lesion appears to have a great vascular supply, and always in paracavernous localizations. According to its results, internal carotid artery balloon occlusion or embolization will be proposed preoperatively.

Biopsy may be proposed in dubious cases of sphenoidal lesions. The biopsy is performed through a rhinoseptal approach that sometimes allows a near-total removal of the tumor when its consistency is not too hard.

PATIENT SELECTION

Most of the bone lesions require a surgical removal because they are responsible for clinical symptoms that are the witnesses of a tumor evolution. Such symptoms may be cranial orbital or craniofacial evolutive deformations, exophthalmos, visual disturbances, or cranial nerve palsies. But some of them evolve very slowly, and the patient's age at the time of the diagnosis must be considered before deciding on their surgical management (e.g., hyperostosing meningioma in a relatively old patient).

P. J. Derome and A. Visot: Department of Neurosurgery, Hospital Foch, 92151 Suresnes, France.

Others are totally asymptomatic and discovered occasionally through a radiological exam. When the lesion is apparently benign and well delimited, a mere surveillance is preferred to a surgical removal, which will be proposed only in the case of obvious tumoral growth (i.e., some basal osteomas or presumed epidermoid cysts).

Fibrous dysplasia must be discussed separately (6). The disease begins in childhood, and the evolution is slow and usually stops during the third decade of life. Of course, surgery is absolutely necessary when visual disturbances are proved with unilateral or bilateral loss of visual acuity. In other cases with a mild deformity, what should be done when we consider rare cases of sudden unilateral or bilateral blindness? Our experience suggests that preventive surgery is required when the area of the optic canal is involved. Subtotal removal of the pathologic bone is probably sufficient to avoid any further visual complication. This preventive surgery is proposed during the first or second decade of life. We have never performed radical surgery after 25 years of age.

OPERATIVE TECHNIQUE

Anesthetic Considerations

Surgery of osseous lesions at the anterior and middle base does not create particular problems for the anesthesiologist. Despite the possible risk of opening the nasal cavities transbasally, nasotracheal intubation is always preferred to orotracheal intubation, except in cases where the tumor invades the entire nasal fossae. All the classic methods are used to get good brain relaxation: in truly extradural approaches, mannitol must be combined with a drainage of CSF. Rather than continuous intraoperative lumbar drainage, a small opening of the subfrontal dura (which often occurs during the dissection of olfactory grooves) is sufficient. Antiepileptic drugs are given perioperatively. Antibiotics are added when the surgical procedure will last more than 6 hr or when the septic facial cavities are opened. In such cases, broad spectrum antibiotics are started during premedication and continued for 24 hr.

Lateral Osseous Lesions (Middle Fossa and Pterional Area)

Paracavernous tumors such as chondromas, chordomas, and trigeminal neurilemomas bulging in the middle fossa are approached in most cases transdurally, after the temporal lobe has been elevated or partially resected. When the tumor extends down to the retro- or parapharyngeal area and the pterygomaxillary fossa, the removal is completed through an infratemporal and/or transzygomatic approach in one or two stages. We normally reconstruct the floor of the middle fossa at the end of the transdural approach, particularly when the removal of the infratemporal part of the lesion extends toward the lateral wall or the alar extension of the sphenoidal sinus, with a risk of CSF leak. For the infratemporal approaches, we ask the reader to refer to the proper chapters in this volume.

Hyperostosing meningioma "en plaque" is the most frequent "lateral" osseous lesion extending from the pterional area to the greater and lesser sphenoidal wings (Figs. 1 and 2). Hyperostosis (the pathological bone with meningiomatous cells in the haversian canals) must be resected, as well as the meningiomatous "plaques" that may be found around the hyperostosis in the temporal fossa, on the deep aspect of the temporal muscle, and the orbit (1,3,9,10).

The patient lies on his/her back with the head turned 30° to the opposite side. After a frontotemporal incision behind the hairline, the temporal muscle is cut along the temporal crest and dissected from the temporal fossa and retromalar area down to the zygomatic arch. The pericranial flap is turned down anteriorly (it will eventually close a possible opening of a large frontal sinus). We use a free frontotemporal flap. Its anterior edge is the supraorbital notch (some difficulties may occur during its rotation if the hyperostosis extends upward; then the osteoma must be partially resected to allow a section of the flap to fit sufficiently downward in the anterior fossa). The subfrontal dura is separated from the orbital roof to the posterior edge of the sphenoidal wing and medially to the lateral margin of the olfactory groove. This limited dissection is sufficient to give access to the homolateral optic canal. In the middle fossa, the temporal dura is separated simultaneously as the osteoma is resected.

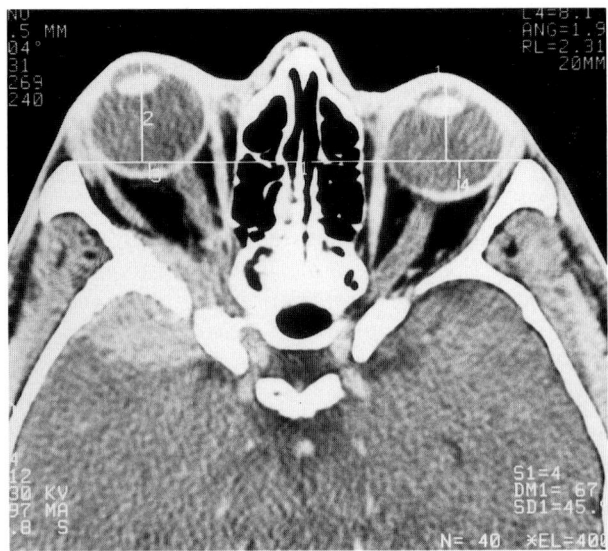

FIG. 1. Hyperostosing meningioma "en plaque" before its surgical removal.

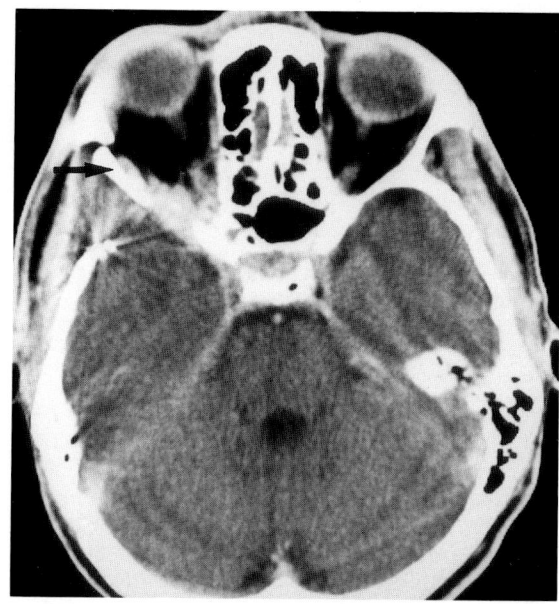

FIG. 2. Following surgical removal of meningioma in Fig. 1. Note repair of the orbital wall with a bone autograft (*arrow*).

The resection of the hyperostosis is the first stage of the operation. The pathological orbital roof is resected, going posteriorly to open the optic canal and supraorbital fissure. The anterior clinoid process is removed as far as possible, then, laterally, extensive resection will free the lower aspect of the superior orbital fissure, removing the thick external orbital wall as deeply as necessary, down to the inferior orbital fissure. In the case of trigeminal compression, the resection is carried on posteriorly and inferiorly to free the nerves in the foramen rotundum and foramen ovale. Very often the "osteoma" has the consistency of marble and requires the use of drills and rongeurs for the resection. The optic canal and superior orbital fissure are opened with small rongeurs and drills are only used to thin out the hyperostosis.

The second stage is the removal of the meningiomatous "plaques." The temporal plaque is always found in the temporal fossa around the external edge of the superior orbital fissure. It is not seen extradually and must be located intradurally. The pathologic dura will be resected and the dural defect is closed with a pericranial graft extracted posteriorly on the vault. An orbital plaque is frequent. It will be removed, using the operating microscope, as completely as possible (depending on its extension to the orbital apex). It is usually located laterally in the orbit, and it is often possible to split the plaque from the orbital dura. It is also necessary to look for a third plaque at the deeper aspect of the temporalis muscle.

The reconstruction of the orbit is not absolutely necessary, provided the dissected temporal muscle is firmly attached to the bone flap (muscle is sutured with nonre-sorbable material on the temporal crest). We repaired the orbit in only one case of large dead space; the external wall and roof of the orbit were reconstructed with autogenous grafts extracted from the bone flap, split from its deeper aspect. The free bone flap is wired, and the scalp is closed with a drain for the subcutaneous space and the dead space in the temporal fossa. When the temporal dura has been widely resected, the eyelids are closed with a mildly compressive dressing to avoid postoperative chemosis.

Medial Ethmoidosphenoidal Osseous Lesions

Illustrative Case: Fibrous Dysplasia with Bilateral Compression of Optic Nerves

The patient lies on his/her back with the head held straight in the headrest. The scalp incision is a temporo-temporal one, just behind the hairline (4,5,7). The pericranial incision is H-shaped along the temporal crests, preserving an anterior pericranial flap turned down to the upper orbital margins. A bifrontal free bone flap is elevated. Its anterior margin is strictly supraorbital, without regard for the frontal sinuses. If the frontal sinuses are widely opened, they may be sealed by the removal of their posterior wall and mucosa and closure of their ostia with bone autografts. Alternatively, they may be closed by an anterior pericranial flap sutured to their posterior wall with transosseous and nonresorbable stitches.

The subfrontal dura is dissected to the posterior limits of the anterior fossa. This dissection is fairly easy laterally on the orbital roofs and lesser sphenoidal wings except for a few adhesions at the synostosis between the frontal and sphenoidal bones. In the midline, the crista galli is resected, and the olfactory nerves are dissected from the olfactory grooves. Very often, the dura is partially opened during this dissection, allowing egress of CSF and favoring the extradural brain retraction. Then the anterior fossa is exposed.

If the dysplasia involves the whole anterior fossa, the bone resection begins as in hyperostosing meningioma en plaque with the removal of the orbital roofs, anterior clinoid processes, and the opening of the optic canals and supraorbital fissures (Figs. 3–5). If necessary, this removal is carried on laterally. When the orbital roof and lesser sphenoidal wings are not invaded, a partial resection of the roof and opening of the optic canal are still necessary for localizing the extradural part of the optic nerves. Then the ethmoidosphenoidal tumor is progressively resected between the optic nerves down to the normal ethmoidal cells (or nasal fossae) and cavum mucosa below the sphenoid body. Posteriorly, the pathologic tuberculum sellae and vertical part of the sellar floor are also removed. This vertical line in continuity with the

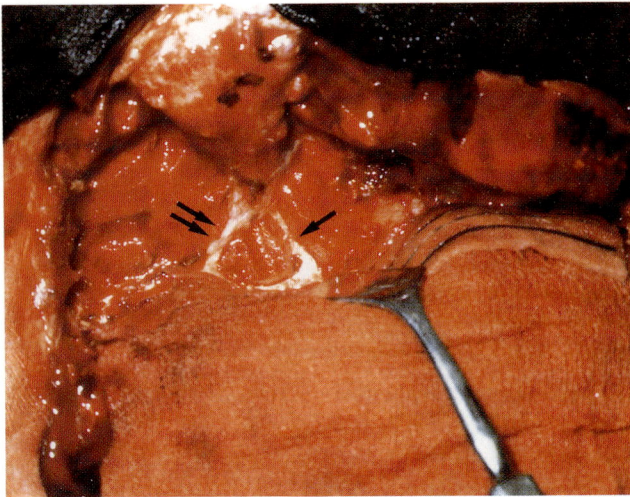

FIG. 3. Fibrous dysplasia. The frontal lobes are elevated with the subfrontal dura. The dysplasia involves the whole anterior base. The left orbital roof is removed. Between the opening of the optic canal (*single arrow*) and the superior orbital fissure (*double arrow*) the huge pathological anterior clinoid process is visible.

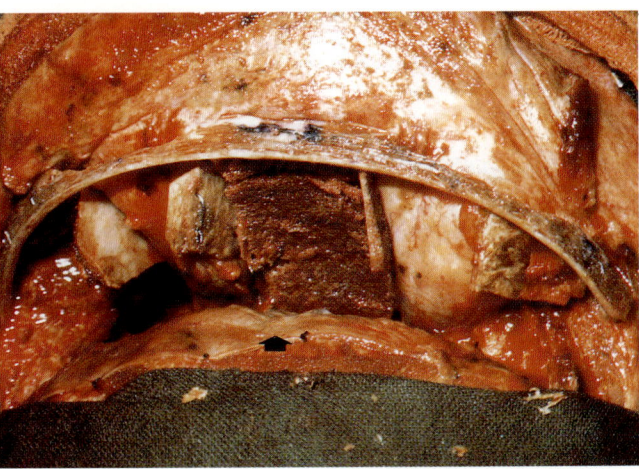

FIG. 5. Reconstruction by autogenous grafts: orbitofrontal margin with a split rib graft; lateral and medial orbital wall with cortical iliac graft and cancellous iliac grafts in the ethmoidosphenoidal area. Orbital roofs are not yet repaired and a large cortical graft will be impacted on the midline between the clivus and the root of the nose. Note the strengthening of the subfrontal dura with a free pericranial graft (*arrow*).

sellar floor is the reasonable posterior limit of basal resection through this approach (see later discussion for the possibilities of enlargement). It is very important to decompress the optic nerves at least on their lateral, superior, and medial sides. The resection of the anterior clinoid process sometimes allows the surgeon to decompress its inferior side, by removing the optic strut.

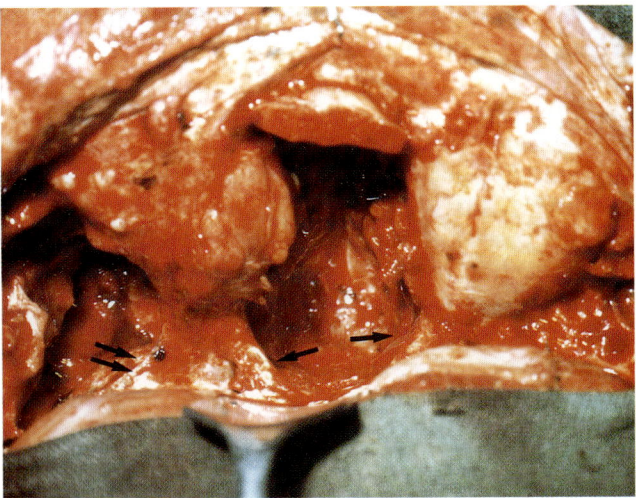

FIG. 4. After the total resection of the fibrous dysplasia, the anterior base has disappeared; between the orbits, one can see the root of the nose, the nasal fossae, and the inner face of the cavum mucosa below the sphenoid body, which has been removed. The extradural portions of the optic nerves (*single arrow*) are totally free and the superior orbital fissure is decompressed (*double arrows*).

Extensive resection may be carried on anteriorly (orbital margins or root of the nose), according to the craniofacial deformation, but mere modeling of the bone with drills is usually sufficient.

If there are tears in the subfrontal dura, they are closed, and the dura is strengthened in the midline with a pericranial graft extracted from the vault posteriorly, behind the bone flap.

The basal repair is necessary to avoid a large dead space, with resulting complications. Bone autografts are used; cancellous iliac grafts are certainly the best for the basal closure near the septic facial cavities; the orbital roofs and medial orbital walls are reconstructed and cancellous grafts are packed in the ethmoidosphenoidal area. The last graft is usually a cortical one and is impacted medially, between the clivus and anterior basal resection (root of the nose), below the sella turcica, taking care that the freed optic nerves are not compressed.

The bifrontal free flap is replaced with dural suspensions, and the scalp is sutured with an extradural drainage.

Technical Problems

Wide Opening of Nasal Fossae

Certain extensive, aggressive, and large tumors involving the nasal fossae are responsible for a large basal defect and a destruction of the mucosal layer (6,7). If such a basal defect is anticipated at the beginning of the operation, a large pericranial flap extending from the coronal suture to the upper orbital margin is dissected free laterally (along the temporal crests) and posteriorly (at the level of the coronal suture), leaving the anterior vascular supply intact (Fig. 6). After tumor removal, the flap is brought down over the nasal fossae (Fig. 7) and sutured to the subfrontal dura at its farthest limits in the anterior fossa. Then the autogenous bone grafts are inserted between this new "mucosal plane" and the subfrontal dura (or the free pericranial graft repairing the dural defect) (Fig. 8).

Dural Defect

Pathological involvement of the dura is characteristic of all meningiomas, but it is also found in other "osseous lesions," such as ossifying fibromas, chordomas, olfactory placode tumors, and carcinomas. Therefore the tumoral resection produces a dural defect. A watertight closure of the dura is absolutely necessary before the removal of the basal part of the tumor and the opening of the air-filled facial cavities because of the risk of CSF leakage and meningitis.

Rather than using foreign material or an aponeurotic graft, a pericranial graft is preferred because of its capacity to form adhesions and to revascularize quickly. It is obtained from the parietal area, immediately dorsal to the posterior edge of the bone flap. This pericranial graft must overlap widely the edges of the defect and will be stitched to adjacent normal subfrontal dura.

In some tumors (especially tuberculum sellae meningiomas), the dura cannot be sealed after resection because the dural defect extends to the suprasellar cistern, and even a very large graft cannot be sutured posteriorly. In these cases, the graft is placed with its posterior edge

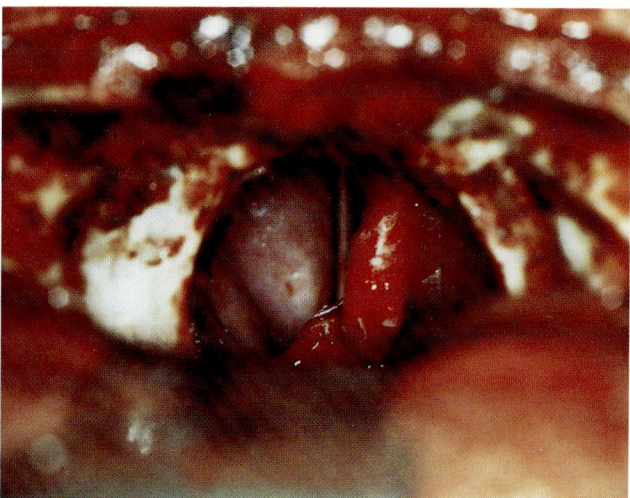

FIG. 7. Wide opening of the nasal fossae after the tumor removal. The turbinates and nasogastric tube are quite visible transbasally.

folded back to overlie the base of the skull by approximately 1 cm. The graft is then stitched anteriorly and laterally to normal dura. It will be necessary to wait 3–4 months and then perform the second-stage operation, by which time watertight closure of the dura will have occurred. There will be no risk of CSF leak or infection during the extradural approach.

To avoid a tumor involvement of the graft during the period between procedures, the dural repair is separated from the basal tumor by a sheet of foreign material such as Silastic (7), which will be removed at the time of reoperation and will make dissection and the extradural approach easier (Fig. 9). The same method is used for two-stage management of tumors in the middle fossa.

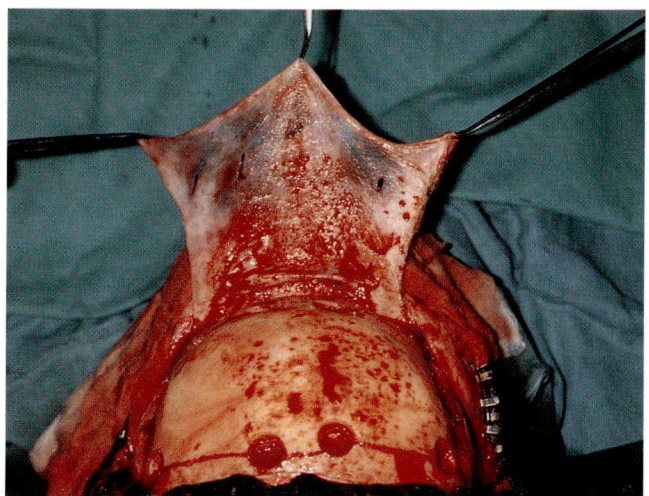

FIG. 6. A large anterior pericranial flap is raised at the beginning of the surgical procedure expected to result in a large defect of the skull base and wide opening of nasal fossae with insufficient mucosa.

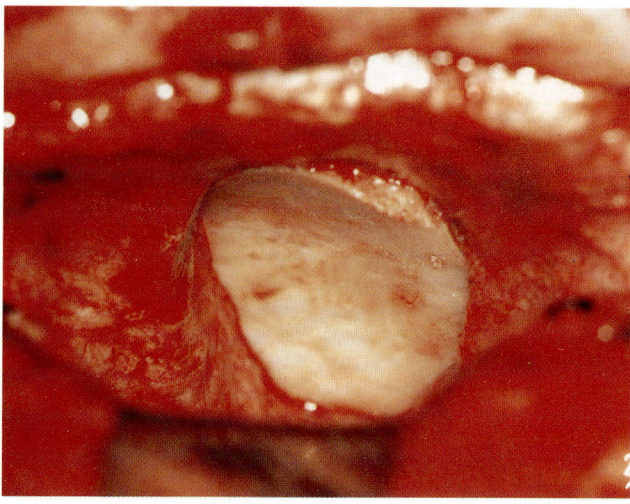

FIG. 8. The anterior pericranial flap closes the basal defect and an autogenous bone graft is fitted into the bony defect above the pericranial flap.

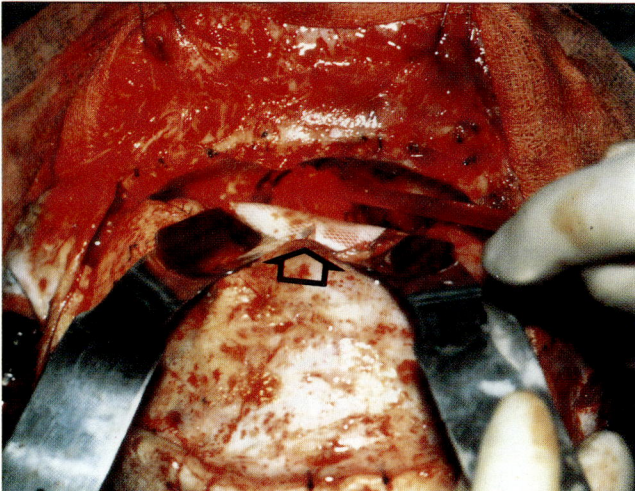

FIG. 9. A sheet of Silastic (*arrow*) is inserted between the basal tumor and the pericranial graft repairing the subfrontal dura in a two-stage operation (invasive meningioma of the anterior skull base).

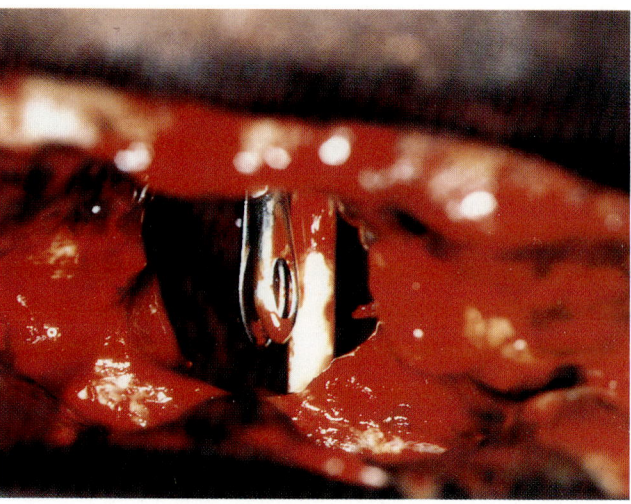

FIG. 11. One-stage combined transbasal and transsphenoidal operation. After the removal of the ethmoidosphenoidal portion of the chordoma between the periorbitum and optic nerves, one can see, through the medial defect in the anterior fossa, the instruments introduced through the nasal septum for the removal of the subsellar and retrosellar portions of the tumor.

Reconstruction Materials

Because any air-filled cavities of the face must be considered to be septic, autogenous bone grafts are recommended rather than any foreign material. At the base of the skull, cancellous bone grafts are more useful than cortical grafts because of their malleability and better resistance to infection.

Large grafts may be extracted easily from the iliac bone. In children, we prefer to use grafts from the cranial vault (split from the frontal flap or from the parietal area) rather than split rib grafts. Bone dust is very useful to complete the repair at the base of the skull.

When autogenous material is not sufficient because of the extension of the lesion to the frontal flap, bone homografts (extracted from cadavers and irradiated with gamma rays) may be used for the cranial vault reconstruction. Polymerizable cement may be also used on the vault, but this should be a few months after the basal reconstruction to avoid infectious complications.

One-Stage Multiple Approaches

Transsphenoidal

Some osseous lesions such as chordomas or chondromas may invade the anterior base and sphenoidal si-

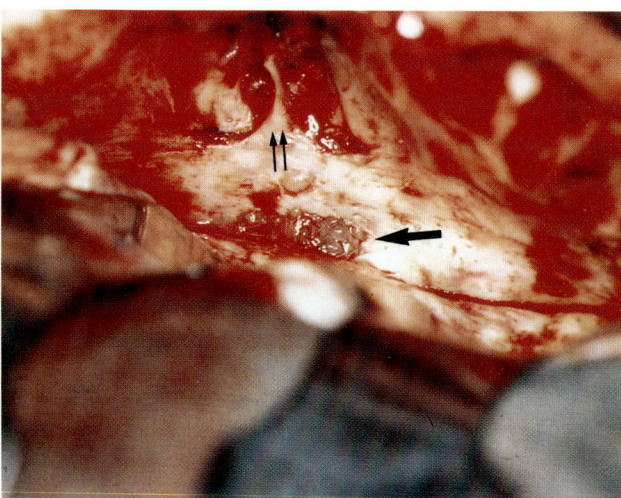

FIG. 10. Chordoma (same case as Figs. 11 and 12). Transbasal approach: the frontal lobes are elevated extradurally. The chordoma involves the anterior base on the midline (*arrow*) just behind the olfactory grooves and the crista galli apophysis (*double arrows*).

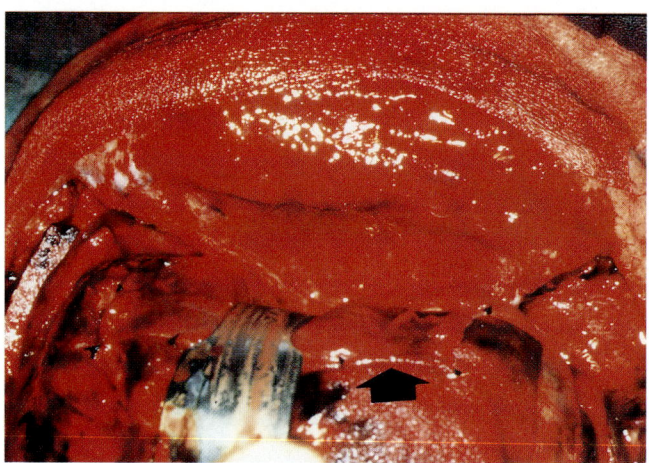

FIG. 12. Closure at the base of the skull with an anterior pericranial flap brought down over the nasal fossae and sutured to the subfrontal dura. Note the repair and strengthening of the subfrontal dura with a free pericranial graft (*arrow*).

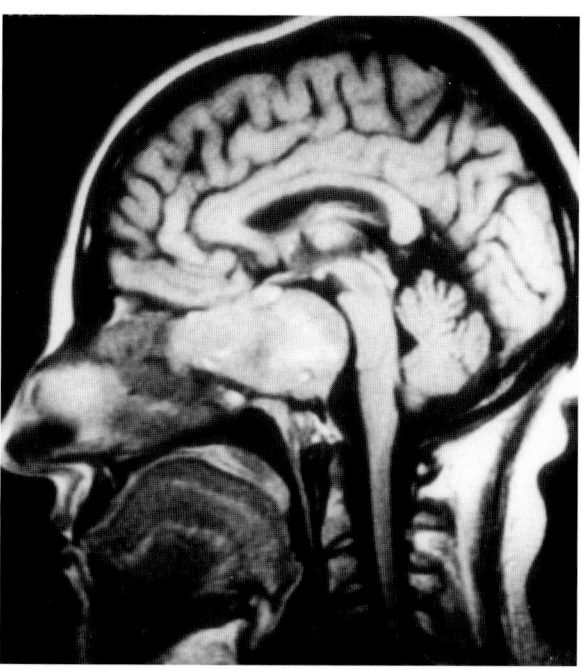

FIG. 13. Preoperative MRI scan of a chordoma.

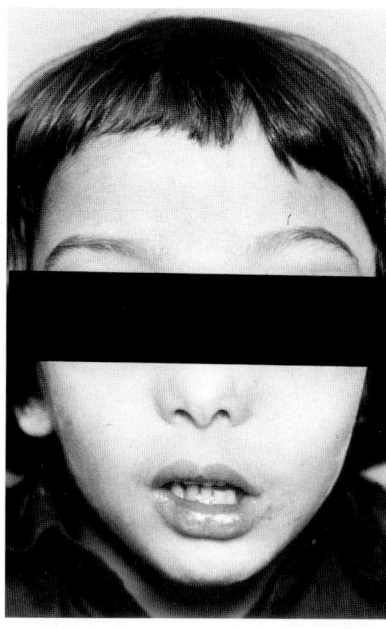

FIG. 15. Fibrous dysplasia (same case as Figs. 16–19) in a 5 year-old boy, which is responsible for visual symptomatology ($\frac{1}{10}$ of vision on the right side and light perception on the left), exorbitism, and hypertelorism.

nuses and compress extradurally the optic nerves and extend posteriorly to the clivus. Because the surgeon's view is limited posteriorly below the sellar floor, it may be useful to combine, in a one-stage procedure, the transbasal and the transsphenoidal approaches (Figs. 10–14). The transsphenoidal approach is performed when the neurosurgeon reaches the limits of tumor removal through the transbasal approach, before the basal reconstruction. It allows the resection of the posterior part of the tumor, masked by the sellar floor, from the middle of the sphenoidal body to the clival dura (8). This does not change anything in the operative technique except for the position of the patient's head (elevated 30° from the horizontal to make the transsphenoidal approach easier) and the anesthesia, which requires an orotracheal intubation.

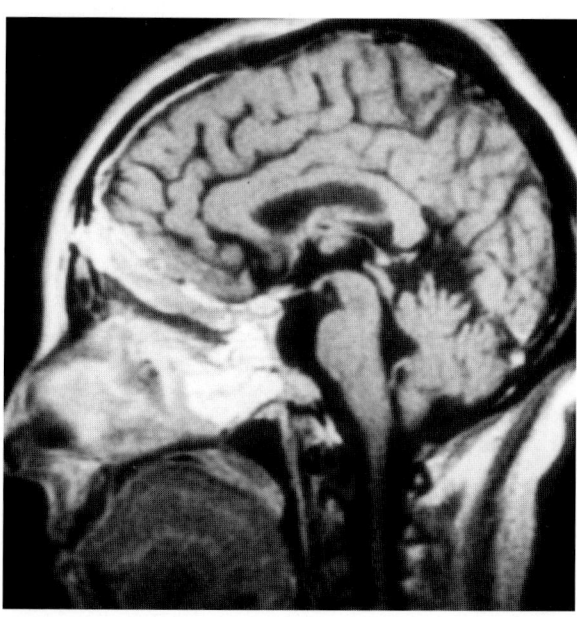

FIG. 14. Postoperative MRI scan after a combined one-stage transbasal and transsphenoidal removal of the chordoma in Fig. 13.

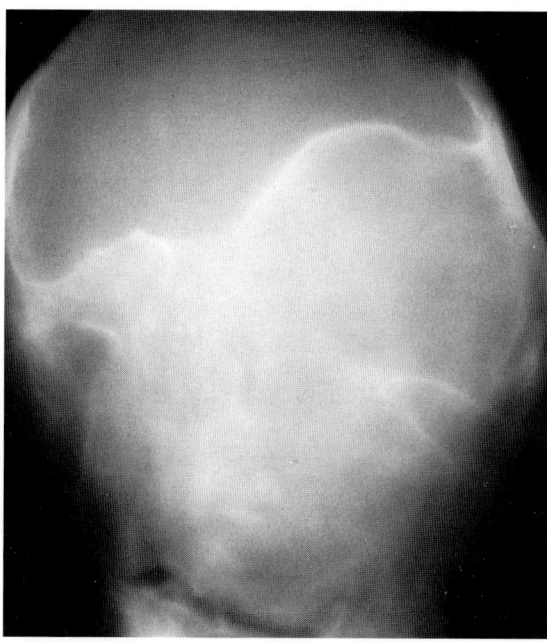

FIG. 16. Preoperative cranial base tomography. The orbits are widely separated and their volume is obviously reduced.

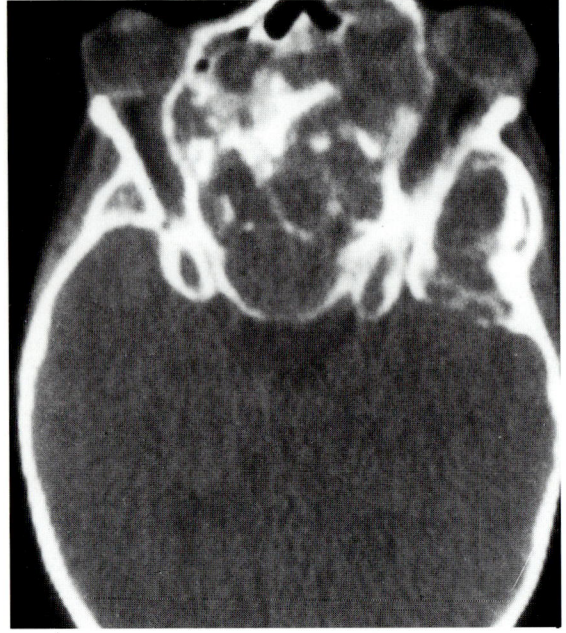

FIG. 17. Preoperative CAT scan. The optic nerves (58 mm length) are stretched by the huge medial cystic dysplasia.

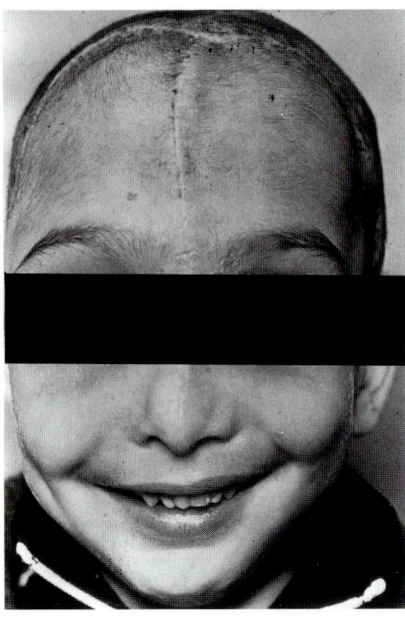

FIG. 19. Postoperative aspect. Satisfactory cosmetic result with an improvement of the visual symptomatology after 6 months ($\frac{9}{10}$ on the right side and $\frac{8}{10}$ on the left).

Resection of the anterior frontoethmoidal area has also been proposed to enlarge the transbasal approach toward the clival area (2).

Transfacial

This combination may be proposed in two instances: because of the tumoral extension toward the face, in which the inferior part of the lesion cannot be reached transbasally (e.g., nasopharyngeal fibroma), or for the correction of a huge craniofacial deformity following the osseous lesion's excision (e.g., hypertelorism in huge cystic fibrous dysplasias) (Figs. 15–19). Such combined approaches require the addition of an otolaryngological or maxillofacial surgeon to the neurosurgical team (6).

COMPLICATIONS AND MANAGEMENT

CSF Leakage

CSF leaks may occur after excision of osseous basal lesions invading the dura. If it occurs, one can wait 1 week for the frontal lobes to adhere to the dural repair and stop the leak. Contrary to the management of CSF leak following transsphenoidal surgery, we do not recommend a lumbar drainage in such cases. If the leakage does not stop, reoperation is necessary to get a watertight closure of the dura and/or to interpose between the bone graft and the dura a flap of temporalis muscle.

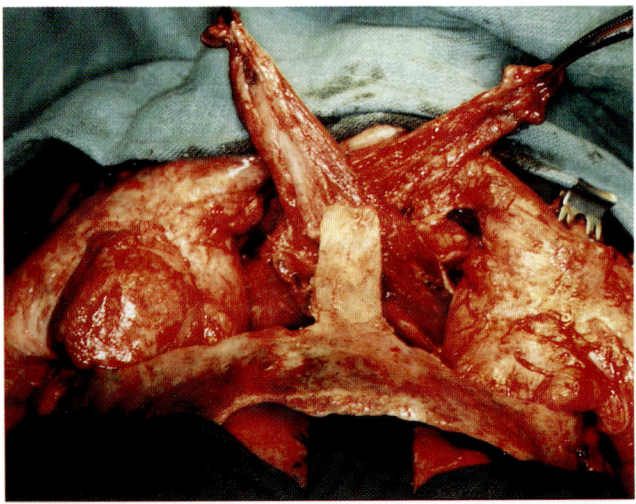

FIG. 18. Combination of transbasal and transfacial approach. The dysplasia has been removed. After reducing the hypertelorism, the dead space and the skull base are closed with the two temporal muscles transposed below the soft orbital tissues and crossed on the midline.

Extradural Pneumatoceles

In our experience, extradural pneumatoceles followed the removal of two huge basal osteomas invading the sphenoidal sinus and destroying the subfrontal dura. One disappeared in 2 weeks. The second was responsible for an extradural infection that ended with the removal of the bone flap. Improper basal reconstruction is probably the origin of this complication, which may be avoided by using the anterior pericranial flap.

Infection

Postoperative meningitis is treated with appropriate antibiotic therapy. This is why our preventive antibiotic therapy is given during the perioperative period for only 24 hr.

Extradural infections rarely stop with antibiotic therapy and require the removal of the bone flap. The same bone flap may be used again after irradiation, or a cranioplasty is performed a few months later.

Worsening of Preoperative Visual Symptoms

This occurred in 1% of cases in our series. Particular care must be taken during tumor removal around the optic nerves mainly in cases where the patient is almost blind preoperatively. In one exceptional case of fibrous dysplasia, an insufficient basal repair was responsible for a displacement of the brain with a compression of the chiasm on a residual intrasellar part of the dysplasia; the transsphenoidal removal of this residual fragment was followed by a complete visual recovery.

AUTHORS' EXPERIENCE: 1969–1989

Laterally in Middle Fossa

Hyperostosing meningioma en plaque	46
Trigeminal neurinoma	16
Chordoma	8
Chondroma and chondrosarcoma	5
Osseous angioma (of sphenoidal wings)	2
Epidermoid cyst of sphenoidal wings	2

Medially in Anterior Fossa and Ethmoidosphenoidal Area

Fibrous dysplasia	50
Meningioma	31
Chordoma	11
Olfactory neuroblastoma	6
Chondroma and chondrosarcoma	5
Osteoblastoma	4
Ossifying fibroma	4
Malignant nasopharyngeal tumor	4
Osteoma	3
Hemangioma	2
Nasopharyngeal fibroma	2
Hemangiopericytic bone tumor	1
Giant cell tumor	1

Various osseous lesions are removed using the same operative techniques. If the immediate results, particularly regarding the visual symptomatology, are usually good or fair (except in cases of preoperative blindness or atrophy of optic nerve), the late results and possibilities of recurrence depend on three conditions: the quality of the removal, the natural history of the lesion, and the degree of malignancy of the tumor. A sufficient neurosurgical experience is necessary to know the reasonable limits in the surgical removal according to the type of tumor, symptomatology, and age of the patient.

REFERENCES

1. Castellano F, Guidetti B, Olivecrona H. Pterional meningiomas "en plaque." *J Neurosurg* 1952;9:188–196.
2. Cophignon J, George B, Marchac D, et al. Voie transbasale élargie par mobilisation du bandeau fronto-orbitaire médian. *Neurochirurgie* 1983;29:407–410.
3. Cushing H, Eisenhardt L. *Meningiomas: their classification, regional behaviour, life history and surgical end results.* Springfield, IL: Charles C Thomas, 1938.
4. Derome PJ, et al. Les tumeurs sphénoethmoïdales. Possibilités d'exérèse et de réparation chirurgicales. *Neurochirurgie* 1972;18(suppl 1).
5. Derome PJ. The transbasal approach to tumors invading the base of the skull. In: Schmidek MH, Sweet WH, eds. *Current technics in operative neurosurgery.* New York: Grune & Stratton, 1977;223–245.
6. Derome PJ, Visot A, et al. Fibrous dysplasia of the skull. *Neurochirurgie* 1983;29(suppl 1).
7. Derome PJ, Visot A. Bony lesions of the anterior and middle cranial fossa. In: Sekhar LN, Schramm VL Jr, eds. *Tumors of the cranial base: diagnosis and treatment.* Mount Kisco, NY: Futura Publishing Company, 1987.
8. Derome PJ, Visot A, Monteil JP, Maestro JL. Management of cranial chordomas. In: Sekhar LN, Schramm VL Jr, eds. *Tumors of the cranial base: diagnosis and treatment.* Mount Kisco, NY: Futura Publishing Company, 1987.
9. Guiot G, Derome P. A propos des méningiomes en plaque du ptérion. Le traitement chirurgical des méningiomes osseux hyperostosants. *Ann Chir* 1966;20:C1109–C1127.
10. Pompili A, Derome PJ, Visot A, Guiot G. Hyperostosing meningiomas of the sphenoid ridge. Clinical features, surgical therapy and long-term observations: review of 49 cases. *Surg Neurol* 1982;17:411–416.

CHAPTER 52

Rehabilitation of Swallowing

Carl H. Snyderman and Jonas T. Johnson

The physiology of swallowing may be seriously disrupted in patients requiring cranial base surgery. In contrast to patients undergoing more conventional surgery of the head and neck in whom swallowing is disturbed by tumor involvement or surgery of the upper aerodigestive tract, patients with cranial base tumors often present with cranial neuropathies or develop cranial nerve deficits as a consequence of therapy. Management of the swallowing dysfunction that develops in patients with cranial base tumors is the subject of this chapter.

PHYSIOLOGY OF SWALLOWING

Mastication and deglutition are complex neuromuscular activities (1). The preliminary acts of swallowing are voluntary in nature. However, as the bolus reaches the oropharynx, a series of involuntary coordinated neuromuscular actions must take place in order to effect normal swallowing. The swallowing mechanism is mediated largely through cranial nerves V, VII, IX, X, and XII.

The oral phase of swallowing is felt to be largely voluntary. During this time, food is masticated and mixed with saliva. As the swallow is initiated in the involuntary phase of deglutition, the palate elevates to contact the posterior wall of the pharynx, completing oral-nasal separation as the stripping action of the tongue moves the bolus into the oropharynx. Simultaneously, the suprahyoid musculature draws the laryngeal complex anteriosuperiorly, causing the epiglottis to passively fold over the larynx and prevent aspiration. Closure of the glottis at the level of the false and true vocal cords also protects the larynx. Food passes posterior and lateral to the larynx as reflex relaxation of the cricopharyngeus muscle allows entry into the cervical esophagus. The bolus is then propelled by coordinated peristaltic contractions of the esophagus into the stomach.

Through innervation of the muscles of mastication, the trigeminal nerve participates in mastication and the oral phase of swallowing. The lingual nerve, a terminal branch of the mandibular division of the trigeminal nerve, also provides sensation to the anterior two-thirds of the tongue. The integrity of the facial nerve is important to allow complete lip closure and to facilitate clearance of food from the oral cavity. The oral tongue, innervated by the hypoglossal nerve, participates in the voluntary phases of mastication and the stripping motion necessary to move the bolus posteriorly. The complex involuntary activities of swallowing, including velopharyngeal closure, contraction of the constrictor muscles, relaxation of the cricopharyngeus, and the subsequent peristalsis of the esophagus, are mediated through sensory stimuli conveyed by the glossopharyngeal nerve and efferent motor pathways via the vagus nerve and pharyngeal plexus. The glossopharyngeal nerve also supplies sensation to the posterior one-third of the tongue.

SINGLE CRANIAL NERVE INJURY

The ability of a patient to cope with a neurologic deficit is dependent on the cranial nerve(s) involved, the number and combination of cranial neuropathies, and the time course of development. Isolated cranial nerve deficits rarely produce significant disability. The presence of two or more neuropathies, especially in combination with the vagus nerve, markedly impairs swallowing function. The most severely impaired patients are those with temporal bone tumors with involvement of the fa-

---

C. H. Snyderman: Department of Otolaryngology, Center for Cranial Base Surgery, University of Pittsburgh School of Medicine, and Eye and Ear Institute, Pittsburgh, Pennsylvania 15213.

J. T. Johnson: Division of Head and Neck Oncology and Immunology, Department of Otolaryngology, University of Pittsburgh School of Medicine, and Eye and Ear Institute, Pittsburgh, Pennsylvania 15213.

cial nerve, jugular foramen (CNs IX and X), and hypoglossal canal (CN XII). Patients with cranial base tumors often develop cranial nerve deficits slowly over a prolonged period and adapt well. Deficits of acute onset (postoperative) are not as well tolerated.

Unilateral injury to the trigeminal nerve may result in muscular wasting and deviation of the jaw toward the side of injury, with jaw opening. Anesthesia of the hemitongue may interfere with passage of the food bolus into the oropharynx and is frequently associated with injury to the tongue, which is not perceived by the patient during biting and chewing. Facial nerve injury produces cosmetic and ophthalmologic problems, which obviate masticatory problems when the injury is confined to the seventh nerve. Minor difficulties with drooling and clearance of food from the lingual–buccal sulcus result. In contrast, patients who have undergone major resection of oropharyngeal structures may have incomplete lip seal and drooling when injury to the marginal mandibular branch of the facial nerve accompanies these procedures. When reinnervation is not anticipated, competency of the oral commissure may be improved with static or dynamic (temporalis muscle transposition) suspension procedures or a Z-plasty.

Isolated glossopharyngeal injury is rarely detectable. Initiation of the involuntary phase of swallowing may be delayed due to the loss of afferent stimuli. The effect of injury to the vagus nerve varies according to the location of the lesion. Isolated injury to the recurrent branch of the vagus nerve results in unilateral vocal cord paralysis. Characteristically, the vocal cord remains in the paramedian position. This results in a somewhat breathy, hoarse voice. Incomplete glottic seal may result in minimal aspiration and cough. In the majority of patients, the contralateral innervated vocal cord adapts by adducting across the midline with subsequent improvement in voice. When the voice does not improve or significant aspiration persists, techniques to augment the paralyzed cord may be employed successfully. Bilateral injury to the recurrent laryngeal nerve may result in airway obstruction. However, this situation is rarely encountered in cranial base surgery.

Isolated injury to the superior laryngeal nerve may produce vocal dysfunction and aspiration. This reflects the fact that the sensory branch of the superior laryngeal nerve supplies the supraglottic larynx, while the motor branch innervates the cricopharyngeus muscle, a tensor of the vocal cords. Accordingly, the voice may lack range especially into the high frequencies and food/secretions are not sensed until they pass through the glottis and elicit reflexive coughing.

Complete section of the vagus nerve above the take-off of the superior laryngeal nerve is the injury most commonly encountered with tumors of the skull base. This injury characteristically leaves the vocal cord in the intermediate position, midway between full abduction and adduction. Additionally, there is anesthesia of the supraglottic larynx. The voice is characteristically breathy and weak. Aspiration invariably occurs. Instruction in swallowing techniques by a speech pathologist or swallowing therapist is of primary importance. Additionally, various methods currently available to bring the paralyzed vocal cord into the midline greatly facilitate these efforts.

When injury to the vagus nerve is felt to be incomplete or temporary, Gelfoam injection of the true vocal cord may be employed to temporarily restore glottic competence. Laryngeal electromyography may be useful in predicting the prognosis for recovery and aiding in the selection of Gelfoam or Teflon for injection (2).

In some patients, the profound changes associated with injury to the superior and recurrent laryngeal nerves cannot be satisfactorily managed by Teflon injection. Newer techniques of phonosurgery (3) in which the paralyzed vocal cord is displaced medially are now receiving widespread acclaim. Reinnervation of the larynx via a neuromuscular pedicle is generally considered a less reliable alternative. Similarly, reanastomosis of a severed vagus nerve rarely results in satisfactory recovery.

A high vagal injury or injury to the pharyngeal plexus may also result in palatal paresis with deviation to the contralateral side with elevation. Hypernasal speech with nasal regurgitation of liquids may result. If severe, oral–nasal separation may be augmented through the use of a palatal elevation prosthesis or by various pharyngeal flap procedures.

Isolated injury to the hypoglossal nerve results in hemiatrophy of the involved tongue and deviation of the tongue toward the injured side with protrusion. This deficit is rarely functionally detectable and most patients accommodate in a brief period of time. In combination with facial paralysis, paresis of the tongue may severely impair the oral phase of swallowing. The delivery of food directly into the oropharynx with a syringe may be necessary.

COMPLEX CRANIAL NERVE INJURY

When multiple cranial nerves are involved by tumor or injured at surgery, severe and frequently irreversible dysfunction results. Combinations of injury to the glossopharyngeal, vagus, and hypoglossal nerves result in serious swallowing dysfunction with resultant aspiration. Aspiration may result by multiple mechanisms: reduced tongue control, delayed triggering of the swallowing reflex, reduced glottic closure, reduced laryngeal sensation, reduced laryngeal elevation, and reduced pharyngeal and esophageal peristalsis (4). Swallowing function is further impaired in patients who have received preoperative radiation therapy. Untreated aspiration may be life-threatening due to airway obstruction and pneumonia. Additionally, older patients often have compromised pulmonary function with an impaired cough reflex. When these cranial nerves are injured at surgery, temporary tracheotomy is mandated. Inflation of a cuffed tracheotomy tube reduces, but will not prevent, aspiration. Additionally, the tracheotomy tube allows access to the tracheobronchial tree for frequent suctioning and pulmonary toilet. Paradoxically, a tracheostomy may contribute to aspiration by restricting laryngeal elevation during swallowing, preventing an effective cough and altering laryngeal reflexes (5). Secretions that pool above the cuff of the tracheotomy tube may be aspirated when the cuff is intermittently deflated. The tracheotomy must be maintained until the patient has convalesced enough to begin swallowing therapy. Diversion of feedings with a nasogastric tube is used in conjunction with a tracheotomy, although nasogastric tubes also interfere with normal laryngeal function and promote reflux of gastric contents.

In patients with combined injury of the hypoglossal and vagus nerves, we prefer to remove the tracheotomy tube prior to initiating oral feeding. As a first step in decannulation, the cuff of the tracheotomy tube should be deflated. The patient is then observed for 24 hr. Nutritional support is continued through an enteric tube. If aspiration of saliva is intractable, the cuff is reinflated and the patient is allowed further time to convalesce.

If tracheotomy tube cuff deflation is tolerated, the decannulation may be completed. The tracheostomy site is allowed to heal by secondary intention prior to initiation of an oral diet. At this time, the patient is instructed in chewing and swallowing techniques to minimize aspiration due to the effect of the cranial neuropathies. A modified barium swallow is often helpful in characterizing the etiology and phase of swallowing difficulties, as well as quantitating the degree of aspiration present (4). These techniques include tilting the head and chewing on the side of the remaining innervation. Thermal stimulation may also be helpful in initiating the swallowing reflex. Before voluntarily initiating the swallow, the patient is instructed to breath deeply and close the glottis. The swallow is initiated; then the patient is instructed to cough, swallow again, and cough before inhaling. This seeks to clear the glottis of potential fluid prior to inhaling.

Texture of the diet is critical to success in the severely compromised patient. Most patients function far better with a pureed, nonpourable diet. Liquids tend to be uncontrollable and easily aspirated. The patient can then be advanced to liquids and solids according to his/her progress.

Some patients cannot tolerate deflation of the tracheotomy tube cuff. In general, this group of patients lies in one or another of two extremes. In some patients, accommodation will gradually be made to the injury and the tracheotomy tube can be removed. In other patients, aspiration is intractable. This occasionally develops even with a cuffed tracheotomy tube in place. Aspiration of saliva and refluxed gastric contents may become a life-threatening problem. Under these circumstances, various alternatives exist. Removal of the nasogastric tube may reduce reflux. Nutritional support must then be undertaken with other means. Most commonly, we employ gastrostomy tube feedings. If a prolonged recovery is anticipated, a gastrostomy will be performed early in the postoperative period. If aspiration of saliva remains a serious problem, some technique of aerodigestive separation must be considered and may be life saving.

Various laryngeal closure methods have been advocated in the past (6). These can be divided into four basic techniques: (a) glottic closure, (b) supraglottic closure, (c) laryngotracheal separation, and (d) total laryngectomy. Suturing of the epiglottis over the larynx rarely accomplishes satisfactory aerodigestive separation inasmuch as constant motion tends to separate the suture line. Similarly, efforts at glottic closure tend to fail unless the larynx is denervated bilaterally. Others have described various techniques of laryngeal collapse or total laryngectomy to accomplish this goal. Of the various procedures, the technique that best meets the ideal criteria of simplicity, reliability, and reversibility is laryngotracheal separation as originally described by Lindeman (7) (Fig. 1A) and subsequently modified by Lindeman et al. (8) and Baron and Dedo (9) (Fig. 1B). Laryngotracheal separation consists of oversewing of the proximal trachea to effect complete separation of the aerodigestive tract. The "modified Lindeman" procedure is potentially reversible in patients who eventually recover neurologic function. This life-saving technique necessarily results in loss of normal speech but allows most patients to resume an oral diet. Speech employing an electrolarynx is most commonly achieved.

TECHNIQUE: LARYNGOTRACHEAL SEPARATION

Laryngotracheal separation may be performed under local or general anesthesia. With the neck in extension, a transverse skin incision is made approximately at the level of the second tracheal ring or at the level of the tracheostomy. Skin flaps are elevated deep to the platysma muscle and strap muscles are separated in the midline and retracted laterally. The thyroid isthmus is retracted inferiorly or divided and suture-ligated. Dissection is continued down to the layer of the pretracheal fascia. The trachea is mobilized laterally, taking care to dissect on the surface of the trachea to avoid injury to the recurrent laryngeal nerves. This maneuver is important to maintain the potential reversibility of laryngotracheal separation. The trachea is then transected between the second and third tracheal rings or at the level of the exist-

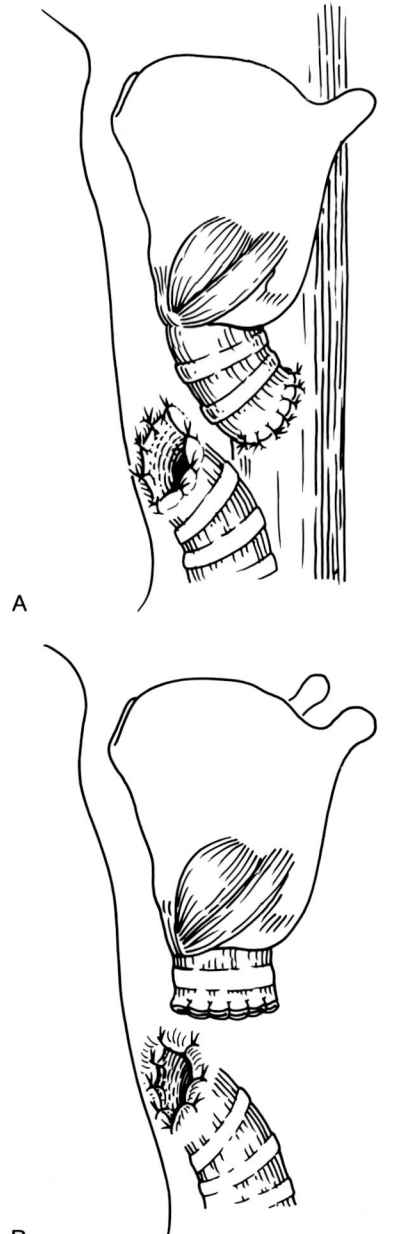

FIG. 1. A: Tracheoesophageal diversion procedure (7) consisting of proximal end-to-side tracheoesophageal anastomosis and distal tracheostomy. **B:** Laryngotracheal separation procedure (8,9).

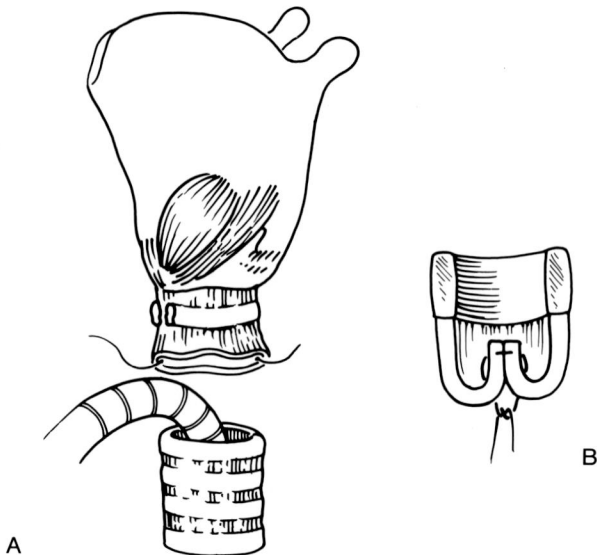

FIG. 2. Laryngotracheal separation. **A:** The trachea is transected between the second and third tracheal rings or at the level of the tracheostomy. **B:** The second tracheal ring is removed and the underlying mucosa is inverted and oversewn to close the subglottic trachea. The distal trachea is sutured to the skin edges with an overlapping "pie-crusting" technique.

ing tracheostomy (Fig. 2A). Care is taken not to perforate the esophagus. Dissection in the plane between the trachea and the esophagus allows mobilization of both ends of the trachea. The second tracheal ring is then dissected free from the underlying mucosa and removed. The subglottic mucosa is inverted with interrupted 4-0 vicryl sutures and the stump is oversewn with a running 3-0 vicryl suture (Fig. 2B). The inferior trachea is then sewn to the skin margins with an overlapping "pie-crusting" technique using 2-0 chromic sutures. A Penrose drain is inserted and remaining skin incisions are closed. After several days, the cuffed tracheotomy tube is replaced with an uncuffed laryngectomy tube. An oral diet is resumed after 5–7 days.

SUMMARY

Cranial neuropathy associated with tumors of the skull base and their subsequent removal may have a severe impact on speech and swallowing. These complex neuromuscular functions may be satisfactorily managed with a team of accomplished professionals employing intensive nursing efforts, swallowing rehabilitation training, and surgical intervention as needed. Adaptation to solitary cranial neuropathy is readily achieved by most patients. Severe, sometimes life-threatening, dysfunction with aspiration and pneumonia may accompany polyneuropathies, especially when lesions involve the hypoglossal and vagus nerves. These patients require intensive nursing care with frequent surgical intervention including tracheostomy, enteric tube feeding, and, occasionally, permanent separation of the aerodigestive tract. A clear understanding of these issues is critical for the surgeon caring for patients with cranial base tumors.

REFERENCES

1. Effron MZ, Johnson JT, Myers EN, et al. Advanced carcinoma of the tongue: management by total glossectomy without laryngectomy. *Arch Otolaryngol Head Neck Surg* 1981;107:694–697.

2. Hirano M, Nozoe I, Shin T, Maeyama T. Electromyography for laryngeal paralysis. In: Hirano M, Kirchner JA, Bless DM, eds. *Neurolaryngology. Recent advances.* Boston: Little, Brown, 1987;232–248.
3. Tucker HM. Rehabilitation of the immobile vocal fold: paralysis and/or fixation. In: Fried MP, ed. *The larynx. A multidisciplinary approach.* Boston: Little, Brown, 1988;191–201.
4. Logemann JA. Aspiration in head and neck surgical patients. *Ann Otol Rhinol Laryngol* 1985;94:373–376.
5. Motoyama EK. Physiologic alterations in tracheostomy. In: Myers EN, Stool SE, Johnson JT, eds. *Tracheotomy.* New York: Churchill Livingstone, 1985;177–200.
6. Snyderman CH, Johnson JT. Laryngotracheal separation for intractable separation. *Ann Otol Rhinol Laryngol* 1988;97:466–470.
7. Lindeman RC. Diverting the paralyzed larynx: a reversible procedure for intractable aspiration. *Laryngoscope* 1975;85:157–180.
8. Lindeman RC, Yarington CT Jr, Sutton D. Clinical experience with the tracheoesophageal anastomosis for intractable aspiration. *Ann Otol Rhinol Laryngol* 1976;85:609–612.
9. Baron BC, Dedo HH. Separation of the larynx and trachea for intractable aspiration. *Laryngoscope* 1980;90:1927–1932.

CHAPTER 53

The Central Electroauditory Prosthesis

William F. House, William E. Hitselberger, Jed A. Kwartler, and Derald E. Brackmann

Electrical stimulation of the auditory pathway by cochlear implantation has made possible the restoration of limited hearing in the totally deafened patient. Essential to the successful rehabilitation with a cochlear implant is an intact auditory nerve. Unfortunately, there is a subset of patients who are excluded from cochlear implantation due to a bilateral loss of the auditory nerve caused by conditions such as bilateral acoustic tumors/neurofibromatosis, postmeningitic calcification of the cochlea, bilateral temporal bone fractures, and congenital inner ear agenesis. From within this subset of patients we have sought to directly stimulate the cochlear nucleus to achieve an auditory perception (1,2).

Previous experience in direct stimulation of central auditory pathways has been limited. Simmons et al., in 1964, stimulated the cochlear nerve and inferior colliculus in a patient with normal hearing undergoing removal of a recurrent cerebellar tumor. While sound sensation was perceived upon stimulation of the cochlear nerve, no such response was obtained while stimulating the inferior colliculus (3).

Unlike stimulation of the cochlear nucleus, stimulation of the auditory cortex to produce hearing is difficult in humans due to the anatomic location of the auditory cortical projections. The primary auditory projections are areas 41 and 42, located on the opercular surface of the superior temporal gyrus. These areas are deep within the sylvian fissure, and to expose them adequately for placement of an auditory prosthesis, the fissure would have to be spread widely. The middle cerebral artery courses through the fissure, and excessive retraction could damage branches of this artery with subsequent devastating neurologic sequela.

The central electroauditory prosthesis (CEP) has been developed to directly stimulate the cochlear nucleus within the lateral recess of the fourth ventricle in the posterior fossa. The CEP consists of a bipolar electrode array made of platinum mounted on a Dacron mesh pad. The mesh pad measures 2.5 mm × 8.5 mm and each electrode measures 0.75 mm × 2.5 mm × 0.025 mm. Platinum wire leads welded to the electrode plates terminate either at a percutaneous plug or titanium coil (Fig. 1).

W. F. House: Hoag Memorial Hospital, Newport Beach, California 92663.
W. E. Hitselberger: 2222 Ocean View Avenue, Los Angeles, California 90057.
J. A. Kwartler: Department of Surgery, Section of Otolaryngology, UMDNJ–New Jersey Medical School, Newark, New Jersey 07103.
D. E. Brackmann: Department of Otolaryngology, University of Southern California, and Otologic Medical Group, House Ear Clinic and Institute, Los Angeles, California 90057.

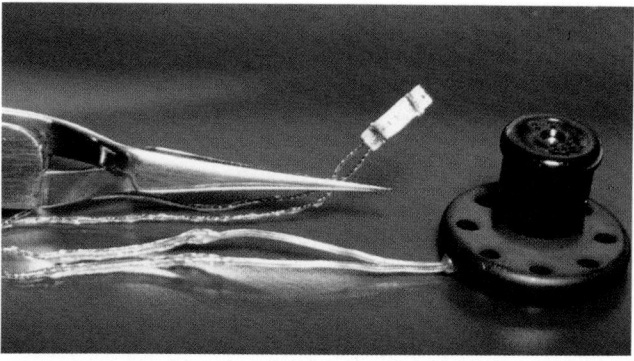

FIG. 1. CEP implant with electrode array and percutaneous pedestal.

PATIENT SELECTION

Our philosophy in the management of patients with bilateral acoustic tumors is to remove the larger tumor first, or the smaller tumor with worse hearing if no non-audiologic symptoms are referable to the larger tumor, and to follow the patient until no serviceable hearing remains in the contralateral ear. If tumor growth causes increasing nonaudiologic symptoms, then we proceed with removal even if serviceable hearing remains. The patient becomes a candidate for CEP implant at the time of the second surgery. Currently, the only other criteria for inclusion in our CEP implant program are that the patient be English speaking to facilitate rehabilitation and that the patient agree to all scheduled follow-up testing. We have not attempted to implant any patients other than those with bilateral acoustic tumors, despite the applicability and potential for rehabilitation of other types of patients. Recently, we have obtained FDA approval for CEP implantation at the time of removal of the first tumor in bilateral acoustic neuroma patients.

ANATOMY

The cochlear nucleus and its orientation to the eighth nerve root and surrounding structures have been clearly demonstrated (4–7). The cochlear nucleus complex (CNC) is a complicated formation made up of several relatively well separated divisions: the dorsal (DCN) and ventral (VCN) cochlear nuclei, the latter being further divided into an inferior (IVCN) and a superior (SVCN) component. The CNC is located on the dorsolateral surface of the brain stem, just rostral to the pontomedullary junction.

The DCN and IVCN have exposed surfaces within the confines of the lateral recess of the fourth ventricle. The exposed surface of the DCN is bordered rostrally by the floccular peduncle and by the inferior cerebellar peduncle. Its caudal border is formed by portions of the pontobulbar body, and dorsally a shallow isthmus separates the DCN from the vestibular nuclei. The exposed surface of the IVCN is bordered rostrally by the middle cerebellar peduncle and by portions of the floccular peduncle and inferior cerebellar peduncle. Caudally, it is bordered by the pontobulbar body, and dorsally the IVCN is contiguous with the DCN. Overlying the exposed surfaces of both nuclei is the roof of the lateral recess, a portion of which is formed by the tela choroidea. Within the tela choroidea is the choroid plexus. The attachment of the tela choroidea to the floor of the fourth ventricle is called the taenia, and it is this attachment that demarcates the peripheral extent of the lateral recess and the beginning of the eighth nerve root (Fig. 2).

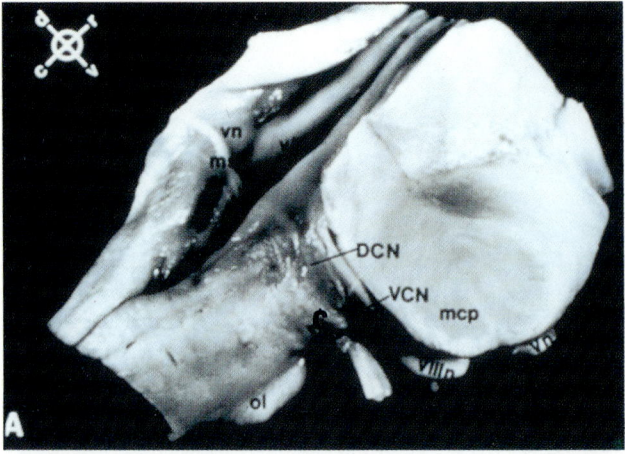
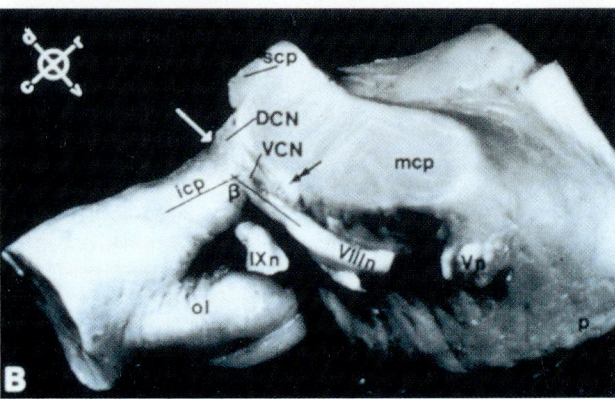

FIG. 2. Brain stem: dorsolateral view (**upper**) and ventrolateral view (**lower**). Flocculus (*double-headed arrow*), pontobulbar body, and taenia (¢) are shown. Eighth nerve (VIIIn) enters the brain stem obliquely (angle beta). *White arrow* shows groove between dorsal cochlear nucleus (DCN) and vestibular area. Also shown are inferior (icp), middle (mcp), and superior (scp) cerebellar peduncles; medullary stria (ms); olivary bodies (ol); and pons (p). Also shown are the ventral cochlear nucleus (VCN), fourth ventricle (vIV), fifth nerve (Vn), and vestibular nuclei (vn).

OPERATIVE TECHNIQUE

The translabyrinthine approach has been used to remove the majority of tumors at the Otologic Medical Group, and the one we have used exclusively in the placement of the CEP. In addition to the advantages of minimal cerebellar retraction, early identification of the facial nerve, complete tumor removal from the lateral end of the internal auditory canal, and low morbidity, the translabyrinthine approach is particularly suited for CEP placement since it provides an angle of view of approximately 70° posterior to the eighth nerve. This range of vision is considerably greater than that afforded by either the retrolabyrinthine or retrosigmoid/suboccipital approach (8).

The patient is placed supine on the operating table with the head turned away from the surgeon. The anesthesiologist is seated at the foot of the table, allowing easy access to controls for moving the table. An arterial line, Foley catheter, end tidal CO_2 monitor, and facial nerve monitor are used. Prophylactic antibiotics are given $\frac{1}{2}$–1 hr prior to surgery.

An anteriorly based temperoparietal flap is elevated. The incision should be approximately 4 cm above the ear and 7 cm behind the postauricular sulcus. This flap is turned forward and held in place by retraction sutures of 2-0 silk. Care should be taken to support the flap and not allow it to dry during the procedure. The mastoid periosteum is incised and reflected anteriorly, and the temporalis muscle is reflected superiorly. A simple mastoidectomy is performed with exposure of the middle fossa dura, the sinodural angle, the sigmoid sinus, the posterior fossa dura, and the semicircular canals. The sigmoid sinus and an adequate amount of posterior fossa dura behind the sigmoid sinus are decompressed to allow extradural retraction during the labyrinthectomy. A labyrinthectomy is performed, identifying Bill's bar and exposing the internal auditory canal. The posterior fossa dura is opened, and with the facial nerve positively identified, total tumor removal is accomplished (Fig. 3).

The surgical landmarks for the CNC include the seventh, eighth, and ninth nerves; the flocculus; the choroid plexus of the lateral recess; the eighth nerve root; and the inferior and middle cerebellar peduncles within the lateral recess.

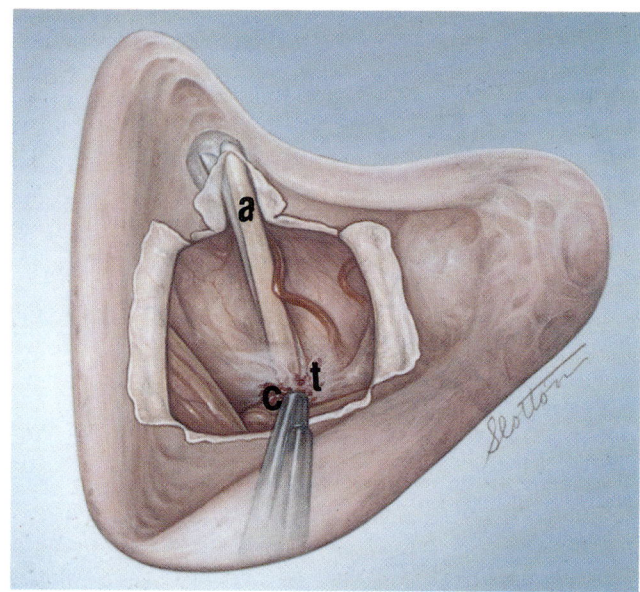

FIG. 4. Surgical view, right translabyrinthine view. The flocculus has been retracted and reveals the eighth nerve (a), the choroid plexus (c) being retracted, and the taenia (t).

Usually, the proximal stump of the eighth nerve remains after removal of the tumor. This is followed from lateral to medial, staying on the caudal side of the nerve away from the facial nerve, to the level of the brain stem and the root entry zone of the nerve. The eighth nerve is attached tangentially to the brain stem surface for several millimeters before its fibers penetrate. If a proximal stump is not readily identifiable, gentle retraction of the flocculus in a posterosuperior direction will often reveal one (Fig. 4) (9).

Continuing medially, a plane is developed between the choroid plexus and the caudal side of the eighth nerve. At the level of the ninth nerve is the taenia, a thin veil consisting of a double layer of ependymal tissue and closing the lateral recess (4,5). The taenia is often disrupted in tumor removal but when present marks the boundary between the eighth nerve root and the VCN. Even if the taenia is disrupted, the brain stem within the lateral recess has a different appearance than that which is outside. The intraventricular surface is smooth and glistening due to the ependymal covering, whereas the extraventricular surface is more whitish and dull, due to the arachnoid covering. At the level of the taenia and the ninth nerve, the VCN angles 20° superiorly from the axis of the eighth nerve root. This angulation must be accounted for in placement of the CEP to avoid implantation on the pontobulbar body.

The exposed DCN and IVCN form a bulge in the floor of the lateral recess, caused by the underlying inferior cerebellar peduncle, and encompass an area approxi-

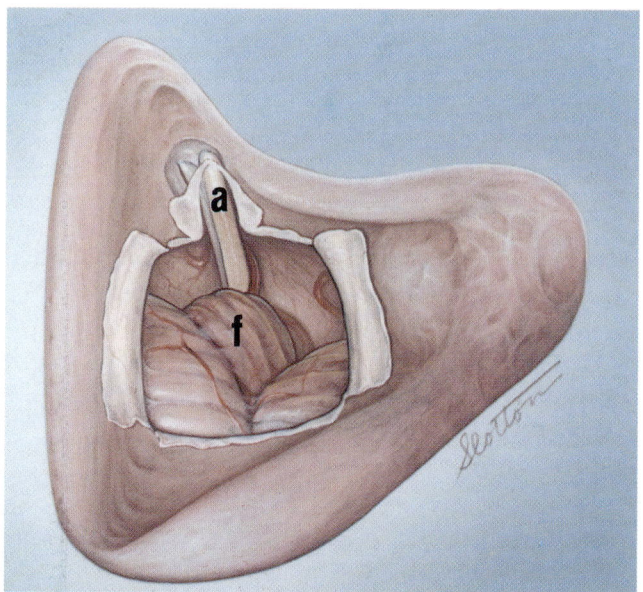

FIG. 3. Surgical view, right translabyrinthine view with eighth nerve complex (a) as it courses to the brain stem. The flocculus (f) overlies the root of the eighth nerve.

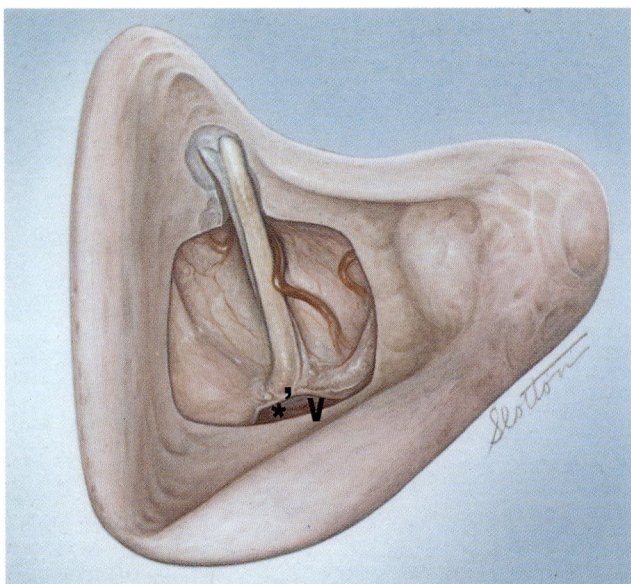

FIG. 5. Surgical view, right translabyrinthine view. The taenia has been removed, revealing the lateral recess of the fourth ventricle (v) and the intraventricular portion of the cochlear nucleus complex (*). Note the angulation of the nerve superiorly at the point where the taenia crosses the nerve root (,).

mately 3 mm × 8 mm (Fig. 5). The Dacron mesh carrier for the CEP electrodes is placed within this area and supported by abdominal fat. The lead wires are brought out through the mastoid cavity and the pedestal, with screws, or coil, with suture, is secured to the temporal/occipital bone.

The mastoid cavity is obliterated with abdominal fat and the wound is closed in layers.

POSTOPERATIVE MANAGEMENT

The postoperative care of our CEP patients does not differ from the routine care of our nonimplanted patients. They remain in the intensive care unit for 2 days or until medically stable and are then transferred to the ward. Early ambulation and activity are encouraged, and discharge from the hospital usually occurs on the eighth postoperative day.

Testing of the electrode occurs on the second postoperative day. This is done in the ICU with appropriate cardiovascular monitoring. We have not, to date, had any vital sign changes associated with initial testing of the electrode. Three months after discharge the patient is fitted with a signal processor and begins a basic orientation similar to cochlear implant patients. Follow-up testing is performed every 3 months during the first year and every 6 months thereafter.

Data collected at each test session include both electrical and audiologic measures. Electrical thresholds and uncomfortable loudness levels are obtained from 250 to 4000 Hz and at 16,000 Hz. Additionally, numerous discrimination tests are performed, including Monosyllable–Trochee–Spondee test, HEI Environmental Sound test, Speech Pattern Contrast test, and Minimal Auditory Capabilities test.

RESULTS

Since May 1979, 13 patients have had a total of 15 CEP implant procedures. Of these 15 implants, 14 have been connected with a speech processor and are available for review. Thirty-six percent (5/14) are currently in use and providing useful hearing to the patient; 28% (4/14) temporarily used the CEP ranging from 5 months to 2 years; and 36% (5/14) are nonusers. There has been one death among the implanted patients, unrelated to the CEP implant. The patient had no useful hearing with the CEP prior to death. The most common complication has been extrusion or infection of the percutaneous plug requiring explantation (6/14), followed by cut or broken wires (3/14), and nonauditory stimulation such as facial tingling, numbness, ear pain, or limb paresthesias (3/14). Of the patients with useful hearing, the mean pure tone threshold average was 65 dBHL (37–105 dBHL). Additionally, they performed comparably to a group of 75 single-channel cochlear implant patients on tests of discrimination.

CONCLUSION

Direct stimulation of the cochlear nucleus by the CEP implant provides a way to rehabilitate patients who were previously condemned to total deafness. There is no significant morbidity to the patient associated with the device, which should be considered in all patients with bilateral acoustic tumors. Research continues further to define the relationship of the cochlear nucleus complex to surrounding structures, to improve the hardware to deliver the stimulus to the cochlear nucleus, and to refine the speech processing units in the hopes of improving the overall success rate of the CEP.

REFERENCES

1. Edgerton BJ, House WF, Hitselberger WE. Hearing by cochlear nucleus stimulation in humans. *Ann Otol Rhinol Laryngol* 1982;91:117–124.
2. Eisenberg LS, Maltan AA, Portillo F, et al. Electrical stimulation of the auditory brain stem structure in deafened adults. *J Rehabil Res Dev* 1987;24(3):9–22.
3. Simmons FB, Mongeon CJ, Lewis WR, et al. Electrical stimulation

of the acoustical nerve and inferior colliculus. *Arch Otolaryngol* 1964;79:559–567.
4. Terr LI, Edgerton BJ. Surface topography of the cochlear nuclei in humans: two and three dimensional analysis. *Hear Res* 1985;17:51–59.
5. Terr LI, Edgerton BJ. Three dimensional reconstruction of the cochlear nuclear complex in humans. *Arch Otolaryngol* 1985;111:495–501.
6. Sinha UK, Terr LI, Galey FR, et al. Computer aided three dimensional reconstruction of the cochlear nerve root. *Arch Otolaryngol Head Neck Surg* 1987;113:651–655.
7. Terr LI, Sinha UK, House WF. Anatomical relationships of the cochlear nuclei and the pontobulbar body: possible significance for neuroprosthesis placement. *Laryngoscope* 1987;97(9):1009–1011.
8. Monsell EM, McElveen JT, Hitselberger WE, et al. Surgical approaches to the human cochlear nuclear complex. *Am J Otol* 1987;8(5):450–455.
9. McElveen JT, Hitselberger WE, House WF. Surgical accessibility of the cochlear nuclear complex in man: surgical landmarks. *Otolaryngol Head Neck Surg* 1987;96(2):135–140.

CHAPTER 54

Complications of Skull Base Operations

Chandranath Sen, Carl H. Snyderman, and Laligam N. Sekhar

Surgical treatment of lesions at the base of the brain situated at the border zone of the cranium, pharynx, orbit, and paranasal sinuses poses many special problems. These stem from a variety of reasons and are not routinely encountered by the neurosurgeon or the otolaryngologist individually. Their location deep underneath the brain, intimately associated with the cranial nerves and vital blood vessels and lying adjacent to the contaminated spaces of the pharynx and sinuses, produces a unique setting. Additionally, the problems of reconstruction of the considerable defect created after removal of the lesion are all potential sources of intraoperative and postoperative complications. Although these operations often are a joint venture between several disciplines, the majority of the life-threatening and disabling complications are neurological.

Prevention is definitely the most preferred course of action but this may not always be possible. Extreme vigilance during the postoperative period is important so that complications may be detected early and adequately treated to avoid permanent sequelae. Many of the potential problems can be predicted during the initial evaluation of the patient and the imaging studies that comprise the "skull base protocol" as will be evident in the following description. Table 1, listing the types of lesions and the number of operations performed by the authors (acoustic neurilemomas have not been included), forms the basis of this chapter.

Complications can be divided into broad categories:

Neurological
Cerebrospinal fluid leakage
Vascular
Infections
Systemic

TABLE 1.

Benign tumors	Number of operations
Basal meningioma	184
Neurilemoma (excluding acoustic neurilemomas)	
Trigeminal	19
Glossopharyngeal, vagus	8
Facial	5
Epidermoid cyst, cholesterol granuloma	14
Juvenile angiofibroma	7
Invasive pituitary adenoma	9
Paraganglioma	13
Spontaneous CSF leak	11
Miscellaneous	18
Vascular	
Cavernous ICA aneurysm	6
Petrous ICA aneurysm	2
Total	296

Malignant tumors	Number of operations
Chordoma	48
Chondrosarcoma	19
Esthesioneuroblastoma	8
Adenoid cystic carcinoma	18
Squamous cell carcinoma	27
Miscellaneous	22
Total	142

C. Sen: Department of Neurosurgery, Mt. Sinai Medical Center, New York, New York 10029.
C. H. Snyderman: Center for Cranial Base Surgery, University of Pittsburgh School of Medicine, Presbyterian University Hospital, Department of Otolaryngology, and Eye and Ear Institute, Pittsburgh, Pennsylvania 15213.
L. N. Sekhar: Department of Neurosurgery, Center for Cranial Base Surgery, University of Pittsburgh School of Medicine, and Presbyterian University Hospital, Pittsburgh, Pennsylvania 15213.

NEUROLOGICAL

Brain Edema and Contusion

This is a direct result of the extent and duration of brain retraction. Compromise and elimination of draining veins can further aggravate the situation.

Prevention

1. Bone removal in lieu of brain retraction must be maximally utilized. This is well illustrated by the variety of approaches that have been described earlier in the book. Such bone removal may involve drilling down the temporal bone preserving the labyrinth, temporary removal of the orbital rims and zygomatic arch, and occasionally the facial skeleton. The additional time spent in the approach is well rewarded by the working room gained and the retraction-related problems that are avoided.
2. Spinal fluid drainage can accomplish a significant amount of brain relaxation especially for extradural operations. The lumbar subarachnoid catheter is inserted after induction of anesthesia and is used to remove cerebrospinal fluid in increments of 20–40 ml as needed during the operation. During intradural operations, similar relaxation may be obtained by widely opening the subarachnoid cisterns.
3. The venous anatomy must be studied carefully on the preoperative arteriograms making note of the main draining veins and collateral drainage channels. When the draining veins at the frontal and temporal tips must be sacrificed, the posteriorly draining collaterals must be preserved. Even this is not entirely risk free. Posterior temporal veins (Labbé's vein) and veins of the posterior fossa must be greatly respected.
4. The surgical approach must be carefully considered to avoid prolonged and excessive retraction of the posterior temporal lobe and cerebellum. Hypertonic agents and diuretics are usually avoided in these long operations since along with the considerable blood loss there may be problems related to fluid and electrolyte imbalance.

Management

A CT scan is routinely performed within the first 24 hr of the operation to assess for edema, contusion, pneumocephalus, or hematoma before they assume clinical significance. If significant edema is seen, the patient is continuously observed in the intensive care setting and standard means of medical management including fluid restriction, osmotic agents, and hyperventilation are used. Temporal lobe edema is a potentially dangerous situation and a low threshold for surgical decompression to avoid uncal herniation is adopted (Fig. 1). Postoperative spinal fluid drainage is discontinued in the presence of mass effect. Serial CT scans are performed to follow the course of the pathology closely until it is resolved.

Hematomas: Intradural and Extradural

Intradural hematomas usually are encountered in the operative bed (Fig. 2). This may arise from inadequately coagulated tumor vessels especially when the surgeon attempts to reach for the tumor in blind corners. It is thus important to have excellent exposure and control of the operative area at all times so that meticulous hemostasis may be maintained. Preoperative embolization is also of significant help since it reduces intraoperative bleeding, hence providing a clearer working area. Cerebral contusions may coalesce into a hematoma and these are best detected on routine scans rather than when the patient has developed a significant deficit. The course of action is dictated by the clinical state of the patient and the size and location of the hematoma.

Extradural hematomas can arise from an inadequately coagulated middle meningeal artery, which may resume bleeding in the postoperative period (Fig. 3). These are usually of a much more acute clinical significance. Another source of an extradural hematoma or fluid collection of a subacute nature is seen in a setting where a large craniotomy has been performed, as in a bifrontal or combined anterior and lateral operation,

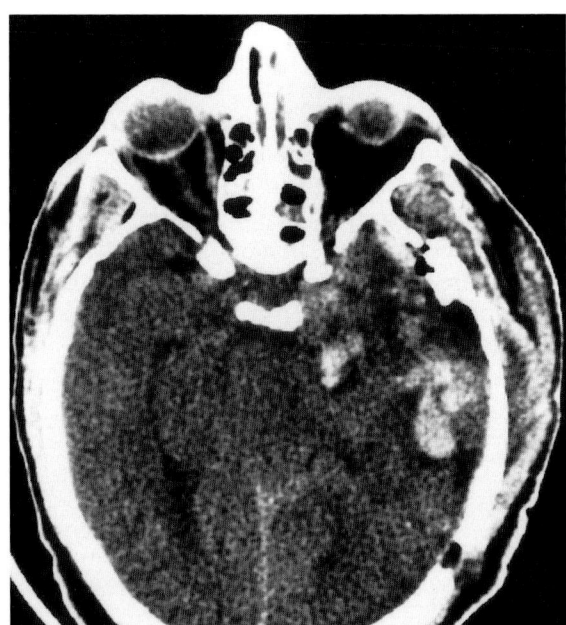

FIG. 1. Left temporal lobe contusion and edema following removal of a cavernous sinus meningioma. The patient subsequently underwent a decompressive partial temporal lobectomy.

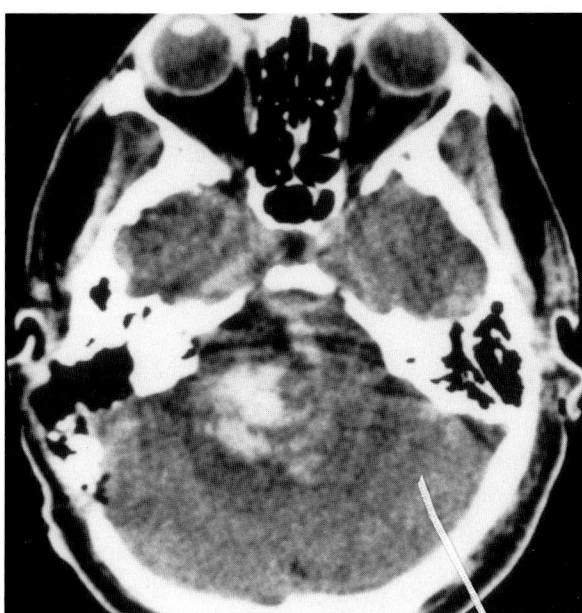

FIG. 2. A patient with acute hemorrhage in the tumor bed after resection of a large acoustic neurilemoma.

when there is persistent oozing in the epidural space and the brain does not reexpand rapidly. Under such circumstances, the dura must be secured to the overlying bone in multiple areas and an extradural drain must be used. Postoperative spinal fluid drainage in such situations must be used with caution since the risk of forming an extradural fluid collection is increased. Surgical reexploration is necessary in most circumstances since they fail to resolve otherwise. An important consideration in the situation of excessive bleeding during an operation is the presence of a coagulopathy. This may be dilutional, secondary to the replacement of packed red cells for operative blood loss. Hence the rule followed at this institution is to administer 2 units of fresh frozen plasma for every 4 units of packed cells infused. A thromboelastogram may also be performed during the operation to assess the clotting function. Disseminated intravascular coagulation, an uncommonly encountered problem, should also be kept in mind when faced with unusual bleeding.

Cranial Nerve Dysfunction

Because of the close proximity and involvement of cranial nerves (CNs) by lesions at the skull base, temporary dysfunction is a common occurrence and in some cases this can be permanent. Experience, gentle surgical technique, and intraoperative monitoring can reduce the incidence. The reversibility of cranial nerve palsies depends on the type of nerve in question; for example, olfactory, optic, and auditory nerve losses are irreversible. Motor nerves are much more resilient. The nature of the lesion is an important predictor; that is, generally neurilemomas, chordomas, and chondrosarcomas have a better outlook than meningiomas because of the extensive amount of dissection required in the latter.

Surgery in the petrous apex and cavernous sinus region risks injury to cranial nerves III, IV, V, and VI. Close association with a neuro-ophthalmologist or oculoplastic surgeon is essential for the management of patients with such tumors. As long as the nerves are in anatomical continuity, variable amount of recovery in function takes place, which compares favorably with the preoperative function of the nerve. Thus there is much less likelihood of recovery or improvement of the cranial nerve function when it was impaired prior to the operation. Since the oculomotor nerve innervates several muscles, recovery is least satisfactory when total paralysis exists immediately after surgery. If there is even a slight amount of residual extraocular motion from CN III seen at the time of discharge from the hospital, the outlook for complete recovery is greatly improved. Synkinesis from aberrant regeneration of CN III fibers is a significant limitation with regard to this cranial nerve.

Cranial nerves IV and VI are much easier to manage since they innervate single muscles. If continuity of these nerves is lost during the operation, a cable graft using the greater auricular or the sural nerve is recommended especially for CN VI. Results of resuture and cable reconstruction of CN VI and resuture of CN III are encouraging. Even when there is incomplete recovery of the muscle function, additional correction is much more fa-

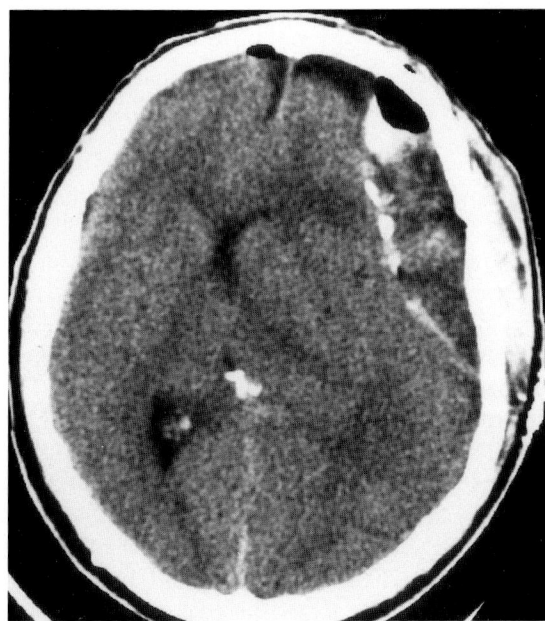

FIG. 3. A subacute epidural hematoma from a bleeding middle meningeal artery in a patient who was anticoagulated with heparin in the postoperative period for pulmonary embolism.

cilitated than in the case of total paralysis, and this can be performed by eye muscle surgery, injection of botulinum, and corrective glasses. The function of the first division of cranial nerve V is of great importance. An insensate cornea is a potential cause of blindness and the patient must be thoroughly instructed on the care of the eye. Cable graft reconstruction of the trigeminal nerve root and the first division has been carried out in five cases with partial return of corneal sensation. It is, however, difficult to state with certainty whether this resulted from the nerve graft or the natural course of recovery of the nerve. Nevertheless, any recovery of corneal sensation is desirable and all possible steps to ensure that should be taken.

Facial nerve dysfunction causes a significant functional and psychological impairment and great effort should be made to avoid injury. Lesions at the cerebellopontine angle and in and around the temporal bone put the nerve at risk. Use of facial EMG is recommended to minimize its intraoperative manipulation. If the nerve is interrupted, it should be directly anastomosed. If additional length is required, the mastoid segment can be drilled and mobilized or a cable graft using the greater auricular nerve or the sural nerve can be performed. A House–Brackmann grade II or III functional result can be expected after recovery. Coexistence of facial and trigeminal loss is a situation of great concern and a medial and lateral tarsorrhaphy should be performed immediately or soon after the surgery. When only the facial nerve is involved, a gold weight in the upper eyelid may be considered to facilitate eye closure. Anastomosis of CN XII to CN VII should be considered when the proximal stump of the facial nerve at the brain stem cannot be identified. Static slings for facial reanimation should be maintained as the last resort.

Lesions in the lower clivus and foramen magnum area expose cranial nerves IX, X, and XII to injury. Patients with preexisting cranial nerve problems usually have had time for the normal side to compensate and do not have a significant problem with the airway or swallowing postoperatively. However, those patients with intact functions before the operation should be warned about the need for a tracheostomy and/or gastrostomy in the postoperative period. The surgeon must have a low threshold for performing a tracheostomy since it is much preferable to repeated bouts of aspiration and it can make the recovery phase of the patient much smoother. Maintenance of adequate nutrition is important and a feeding gastrostomy is more comfortable and easier to manage than nasogastric tubes. The patient must be reassured that these are temporary measures and can be removed when sufficient recovery has taken place. Vocal cord augmentation may be considered early if permanent vagus nerve paralysis is expected. An occasional patient may have severe intractable aspiration requiring laryngotracheal separation. The accessory nerve responds very well to surgical repair and this should be done in all cases if it is transected. Permanent eleventh nerve palsy can lead to disabling chronic shoulder joint arthropathy. Cranial nerve palsies are perhaps the most significant causes of morbidity in cranial base operations and proper steps must be taken before the onset of serious secondary complications.

Impairment of Brain Function

This may result from brain retraction or direct manipulation of certain areas of the brain during dissection of the tumor and also from inadvertent injury to perforating vessels supplying these areas. Such problems are quite evident in surgery at the base of the brain. Temporary pituitary dysfunction is seen when a cavernous sinus meningioma is dissected away from the gland. The diabetes insipidus is usually temporary since the surgical manipulation is unilateral and care must be taken not to overtreat it. Postoperative pituitary function testing may be necessary after removal of suprasellar and cavernous sinus tumors. Hypothalamic dysfunction can be seen in third ventricular tumors and must be dealt with accordingly. It is not unusual for patients undergoing these operations to awaken slowly after termination of the procedure; this is usually related to edema or ischemia of the diencephalic region. Injury to perforating vessels may cause small focal areas of infarction and sometimes devastating neurological deficits. In patients with such impairment of brain function, proper homeostasis must be maintained in order to avoid secondary complications.

CEREBROSPINAL FLUID LEAKAGE

Incidence

There have been 39 cases of CSF leakage in the last 6 years involving the patients operated on by the authors (Table 2). The site of leakage has been as follows: the sphenoid sinus in 16 cases, frontal sinus in 2 cases, eustachian tube in 5 cases, temporal bone in 8 cases, and the incision in 4 cases. The majority of leaks presented in the immediate postoperative period while the patient was hospitalized. The surgeon can anticipate the problem if on the preoperative imaging studies there is involvement of the walls of the paranasal sinuses by the tumor itself or by hyperostotic bone (Fig. 4). The proximity of the basal CSF cisterns and the large opening in the sinuses created during the surgical resection predispose to the development of leaks. Radical resection should, however, not be compromised for the fear of a leak but instead a thorough reconstruction should be performed after such resection. Previous irradiation of the surgical area is a prime cause of postoperative leak and use of healthy

TABLE 2. *Postoperative CSF leakage*

Site of leak	Treatment	Number of cases
Sphenoid sinus	Bifrontal craniotomy	5
	Reexploration and packing	3
	Transsphenoidal repair (failed once)	2
	Spinal drain	2
	VP shunt	5
	Reexploration and free flap reconstruction (thrice)	1
	Spontaneous cessation	1
Temporal bone	Reexploration and repair	2
	Mastoidectomy and middle ear closure	2
	Spinal drain	3
	VP shunt	1
Eustachian tube	Reexploration and packing	4
	VP shunt	1
	Spinal drain	1
Surgical wound	Reexploration and repair	4
	Revision of free flap	1
	Spinal drain	1
Frontal sinus	Reexploration and packing	2
Unknown	Spinal drain	2

vascularized tissue during the initial reconstruction is an absolute must. This may be in the form of pericranial flap, galeal–pericranial flap, or temporalis flap.

Diagnosis

Suspicion is the first requisite and direct inquiries must be made of the patient during the daily rounds. Presence of CSF in the drainage can be positively confirmed by β_2-transferrin assay. Radioisotope cisternography can also detect a CSF leak but the test most frequently used at this institution is a CT cisternogram with intrathecal contrast along with elevation of CSF pressure to provoke the leak if needed. This test is much more sensitive and is useful in accurately localizing the site of the leakage. Even when the site of the leak may be suspected clinically, it is advisable to perform the test in order to confirm it and to eliminate any other concomitant sites.

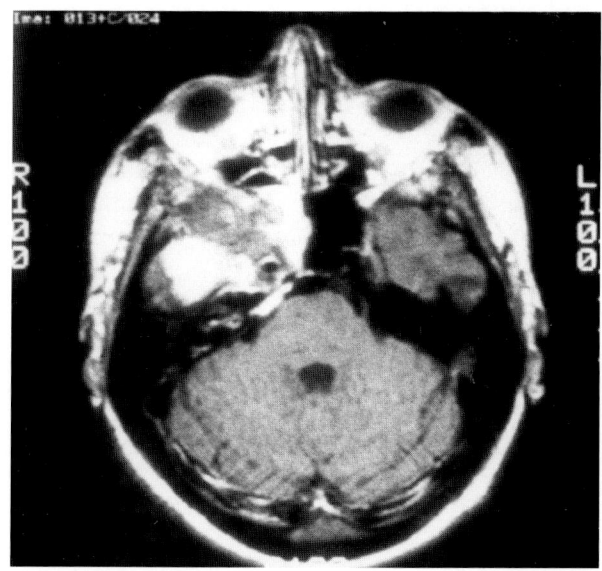 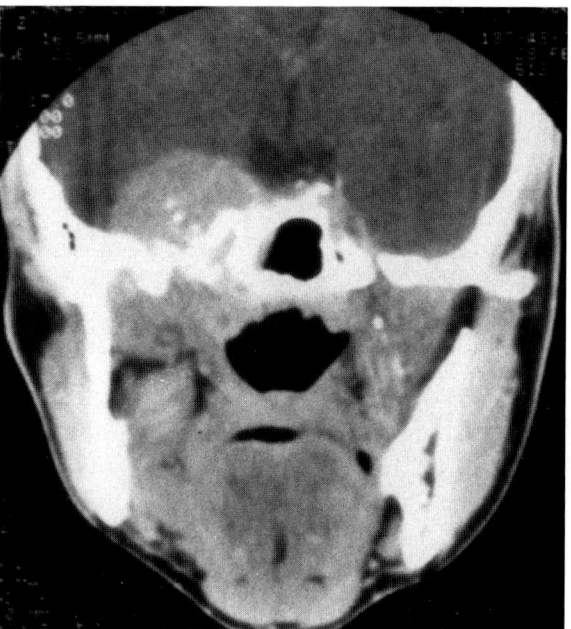

FIG. 4. A: Axial MRI showing a right-sided meningioma extensively involving the lateral wall of the sphenoid sinus. **B:** Coronal CT scan of the same patient showing the hyperostotic bony involvement by the tumor in the middle fossa and lateral wall of the sphenoid sinus.

Management

If the leak is small, a trial period of CSF drainage through a lumbar spinal drain is recommended. The amount of fluid drained must be closely regulated by volume (30–50 ml every 8 hr), in order to avoid development of pneumocephalus. This is continued for 4–5 days, after which the situation is reevaluated. Persistent leakage or a large leak is indication for surgical exploration.

The sphenoid sinus, because of its variable size and multiple extensions, has been the most common site of leakage in the present series. Transsphenoidal repair of the leak has been attempted on two occasions but has succeeded only once. The procedure of choice in our hands for leaks from the anterior fossa and the sphenoid sinus is through a bifrontal craniotomy, wide opening of the planum sphenoidale, and packing the frontal and sphenoid sinuses with fat, fascia lata, and fibrin glue and covering the entire floor with a large pericranial flap (Fig. 5). The obvious drawbacks of this operation are the need for a craniotomy and loss of smell but the advantage is the ability to address such a large area of the cranial base with the use of healthy vascularized tissue for reconstruc-

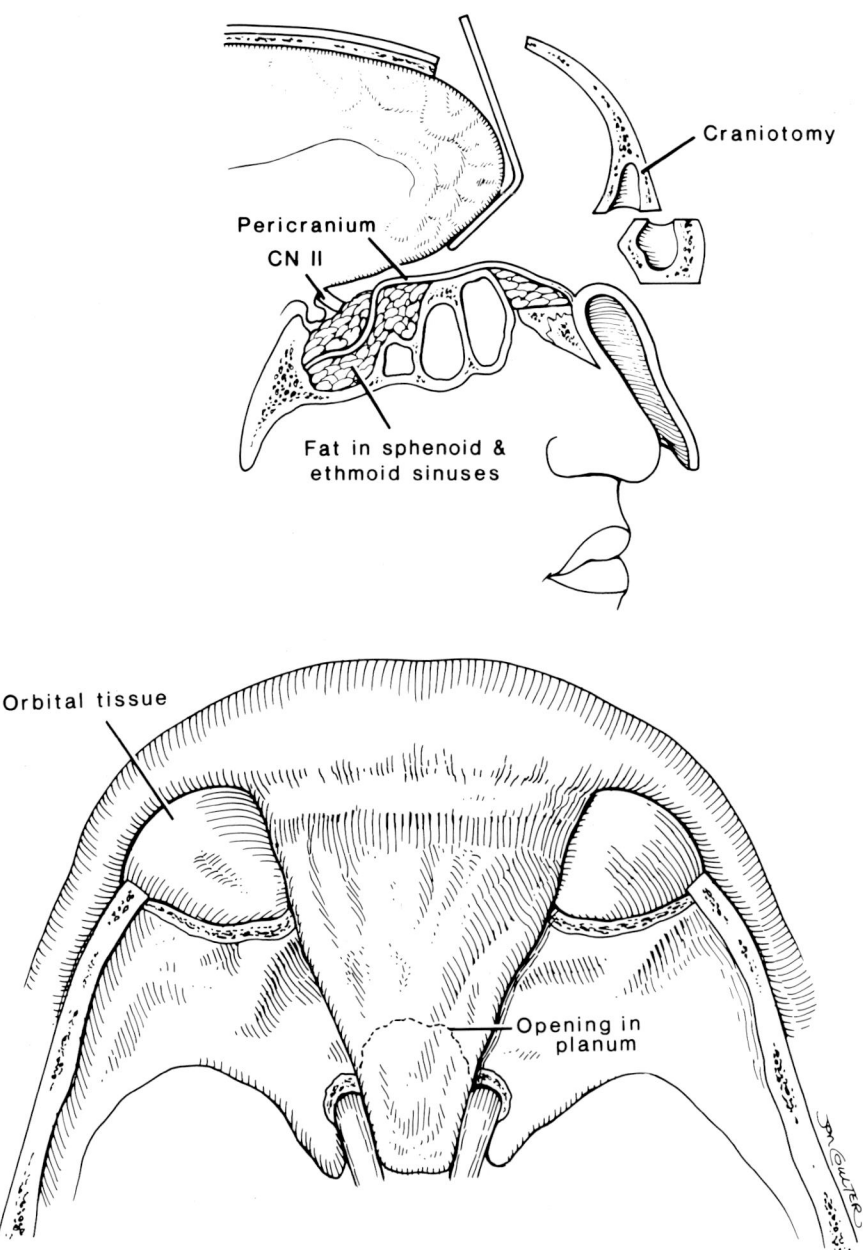

FIG. 5. Diagram showing reconstruction of the anterior cranial base with fat and pericranial flap, which covers the sphenoid, ethmoid, and frontal sinuses.

tion. Leaks from the eustachian tube (Fig. 6) have to be reexplored and the pharyngeal end of the tube has to be packed and resutured, while the middle ear leaks may require mastiodectomy and obliteration of the middle ear unless the site can be repaired directly. A point of major importance is to determine the presence of hydrocephalus, which must be confirmed by pressure measurements and treated appropriately since any repair performed will otherwise fail.

VASCULAR (ARTERIAL) PROBLEMS

Close proximity of the lesions to the carotid and vertebrobasilar system and also the fact that some of the operative approaches traverse the region of the ICA or the vertebral arteries make it imperative for the skull base surgeon to be prepared to manage injury to these vessels or their branches. Injury is manifested as intraoperative or postoperative hemorrhage or infarction in the territory of its supply.

Prevention

Evaluation

Adequate radiographic evaluation is the first step in anticipating problems with the arteries. While MRI is an excellent tool to define the length and circumference of involvement, the arteriogram reveals narrowing and vessel wall abnormalities. In general, vessels in the subarachnoid space are delineated by an arachnoid plane from the tumor, which is not available in the skull base and cavernous sinus. Hence complete encasement in these two areas indicates a different problem compared to similar encasement in the subarachnoid space. The histology of the tumor and history of prior operations will indicate the ease or difficulty of such dissection. When the potential problem has been identified, a balloon test occlusion of the involved ICA is carried out to assess the collateral circulation. This will dictate the further management for potential reconstruction or repair in the event of intraoperative injury. The balloon test occlusion with stable xenon CT cerebral blood flow has been very reliable for this purpose in relation to the carotid system; however, a similar reliable test for the vertebrobasilar system is not available. As far as possible, the collateral reserve of the cerebral circulation should be reconstituted and sacrifice of a major vessel should be avoided for benign lesions.

Surgical Technique

Generally, when dissecting around arteries, the surgeon must secure proximal and, if possible, distal control. Thus if the lesion is in the cavernous sinus, the petrous ICA must be controlled, and for the proximal vertebral artery, the vessel must be controlled extradurally. The path of dissection must be parallel to the direction of the artery and from a normal to abnormal area. Separation of tumors from the vessel should be carried out sharply to avoid irregular tears, which are much more difficult to repair. When a major vessel is exposed to the paranasal sinuses or the pharynx after completion of the tumor resection, it is imperative that meticulous reconstruction be carried out to maintain isolation of the vessel from the contaminated areas by the use of vascularized tissue to avoid subsequent infection and rupture of the vessel with fatal consequences. Such hemorrhage has occurred in two cases: from an ICA and a vertebral artery (Fig. 7) and in a third case a pseudoaneurysm developed in the ICA that was treated with permanent balloon occlusion.

Management

Lacerations can be repaired with simple sutures if the tears are clean and produced by sharp dissection techniques. If the laceration is irregular with loss of vessel wall (usually from blunt dissection), direct repair will compromise the lumen and it is recommended that an autologous vein patch be used for the purpose. If the vessel cannot be repaired, direct vein graft reconstruction of the ICA or some type of external to internal carotid revascularization should be carried out. During the period of temporary occlusion, adequate brain protec-

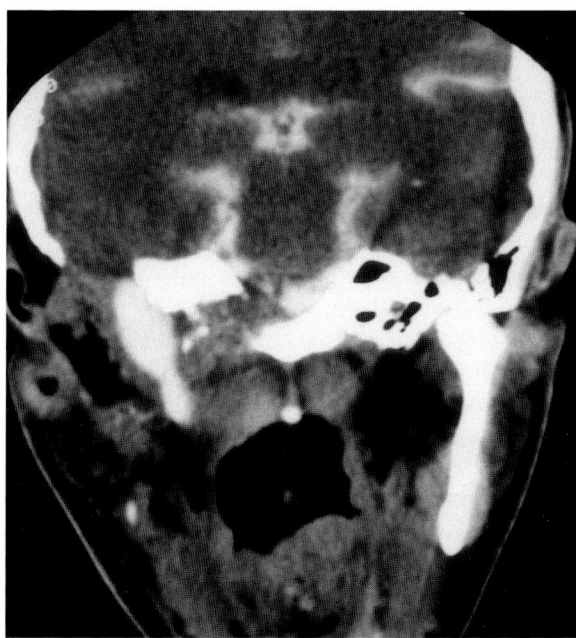

FIG. 6. Coronal CT cisternogram with intrathecal metrizamide in a patient after removal of a large glomus jugulare tumor showing extravasation of the dye into the eustachian tube. The patient was reexplored for closure.

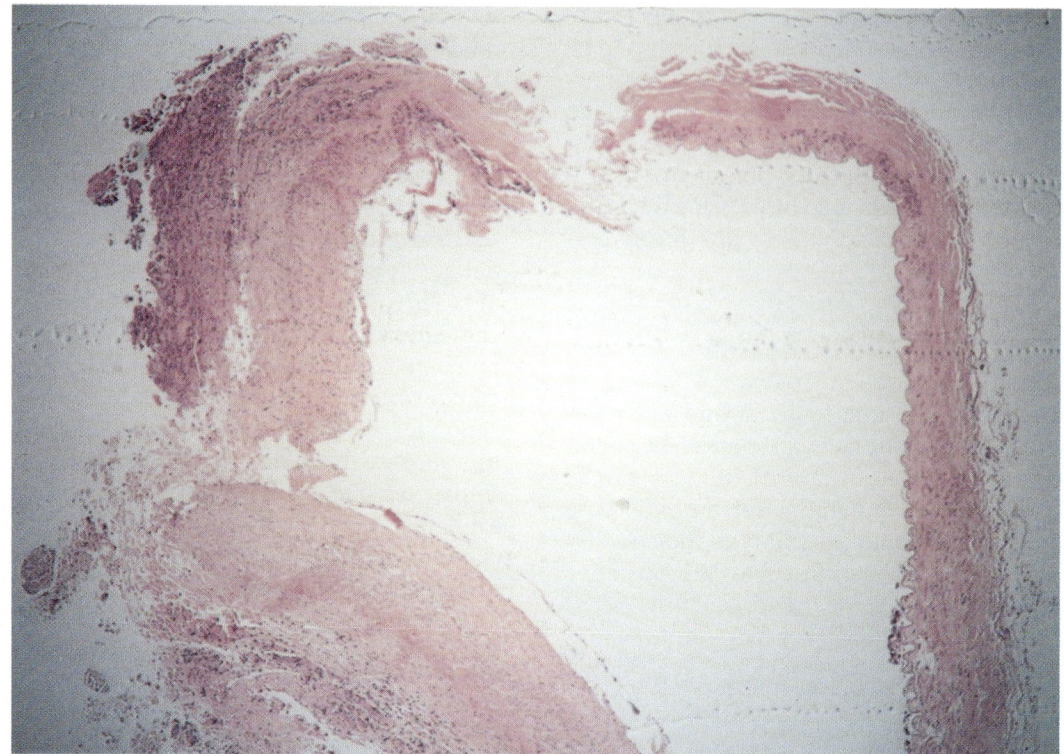

FIG. 7. Postmortem H&E stained section of a ruptured vertebral artery through a transoral exposure. Note the area of rupture in the upper left quadrant infiltrated with inflammatory cells.

tion using barbiturates or etomidate and hypothermia should be employed. Injury to smaller branches may be irreparable and the surgeon must exercise judgment about the feasibility of dissecting such vessels.

Special vigilance must be continued in the postoperative period when vessels have been manipulated or graft reconstruction has been carried out. If a new neurological deficit develops, an arteriogram must be performed to exclude vascular occlusion. In the event of acute vascular or graft occlusion, urgent revascularization must be considered provided there is no infarction seen on the xenon CT blood flow.

INFECTIONS

Despite the frequent communications established between the subarachnoid space and the contaminated passages of the upper aerodigestive system, infection is relatively uncommon. Infections may manifest themselves as an extradural abscess or meningitis, the presentation of which is quite classical unless the patient is obtunded.

Factors Influencing the Incidence of Infection

Length of the operation and staged procedures would seem to promote the occurrence of infection; however, this was not borne out in the present series. Surgical technique is of great importance in these lengthy operations and tissues must be handled properly so as to avoid devitalization and desiccation, which may later form a nidus for infection. Intraoperative antibiotics are routinely used and consist of either ceftriaxone or the combination of aminoglycoside and vancomycin given at the beginning of the operation and continued for 48 hr postoperatively or until the drains are removed. Drains must be removed as soon as their purpose is served. During the operation, the field is copiously irrigated with an antibiotic solution such as bacitracin or streptomycin. This is even more important when gross contamination from oropharyngeal or sinus secretions has occurred. Intradural and extradural portions of the operation may be performed at different times to limit the contamination but this is not always necessary.

An important factor is proper reconstruction of the barriers separating the intradural contents from the exterior and the aerodigestive system. Skin incisions must be carefully planned to preserve sufficient blood supply to the scalp and dead spaces must be obliterated with vital tissues to prevent hematoma formation. Reconstruction may be performed by using local flaps such as the galea, pericranium, temporalis muscle, or sternomastoid muscle, provided they appear viable at the end of the operation. In cases of large defects, vascularized free flaps of the rectus abdominis, latissimus dorsi, or the greater omentum may be necessary. Prior operations and irradiation are major predisposing factors for developing in-

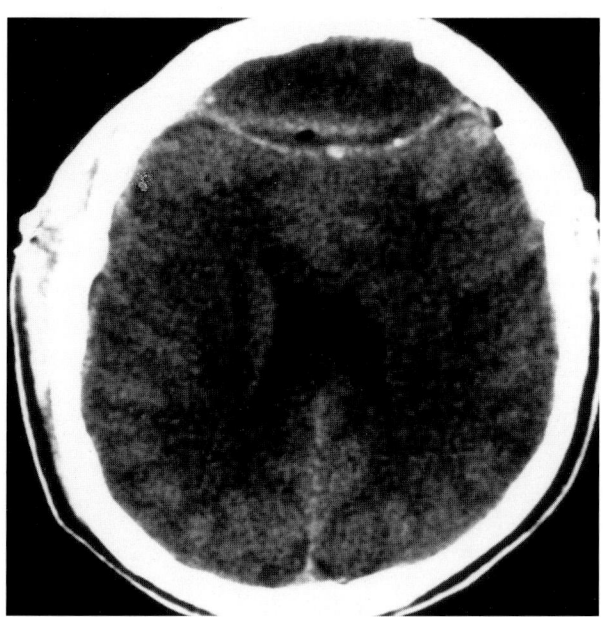

FIG. 8. Frontal epidural abscess following a bifrontal craniotomy and biorbital osteotomies. The patient was successfully treated by reexploration and bone flap removal, but the orbital rims were left in place.

fection. Cerebrospinal fluid leakage is usually the cause of meningitis and must be promptly addressed.

Treatment

Meningitis is treated with appropriate antibiotics as determined by the spinal fluid analysis. Cerebrospinal leaks, if present, must be repaired to eradicate the infection. Extradural abscesses need to be explored and thoroughly debrided of fat grafts and bone pieces (Fig. 8). The craniotomy bone flap is removed but facial osteotomy pieces such as the zygomatic arch or the supraorbital rim need not always be removed since they are thin cancellous bones that get revascularized early. Fistulous communication with the pharynx, if present, must be obliterated with vascularized tissues and parenteral antibiotics are continued for an extended period of time.

SYSTEMIC COMPLICATIONS

Complications involving other organ systems arise as a result of the length of the operation, loss of cranial nerve function, and cerebral hemispheric or brain stem dysfunction causing alteration of consciousness and hemiparesis. Modern neuroanesthetic techniques as well as monitoring have made significant improvements in this respect. Fluid and electrolyte imbalance and pulmonary atelectasis are greatly reduced despite a lengthy operation. Intraoperative use of sequential compression devices and avoidance of hypovolemia have reduced the incidence of lower extremity deep vein thrombosis (DVT). Postoperatively, the lower extremity compression stockings and subcutaneously administered minidose heparin are continued until the patient is ambulatory. Despite these precautions, patients do develop DVT and pulmonary embolism, which is further promoted by the hypercoagulable state produced by some tumors. Hence constant awareness and suspicion need to be maintained for early detection.

The respiratory system needs particular attention in obtunded patients as well as in those that have lower cranial nerve dysfunction and are prone to aspiration. Such patients are observed in an intensive care setting in close cooperation with an intensivist. Frequent suctioning, postural drainage, and intermittent positive pressure breathing performed regularly are excellent preventive measures. In patients with airway protection difficulties, a tracheostomy is better performed early since the morbidity of the procedure itself is so low.

Nutrition is very important and must be started as early as possible. In obtunded patients as well as those with swallowing difficulties, a temporary gastrostomy or jejunostomy is much better tolerated than a nasogastric feeding tube. This should be done early, when a protracted disability is anticipated, and is beneficial in the long run. Close monitoring of fluid and electrolyte balance is necessary to avoid abnormalities that may complicate the neurological problems. Anticonvulsant levels are maintained in the therapeutic range. Generally, patients with benign skull base lesions are young and otherwise healthy and with attention to the above factors the surgical results can be enhanced.

Successful outcome after skull base surgery is not only dependent on the performance of the operative procedure but a large share rests on the team providing postoperative care. Aside from the physicians involved, this consists of the nursing and rehabilitation staff and social workers. Extreme vigilance, anticipation, and prompt intervention are the key elements in avoiding disasters.

Subject Index

A

Abducens (abducent) nerve (cranial nerve VI)
  acoustic neuroma and, 690
  in cavernous sinus, 521, 523, 526, 527
    in lateral wall, 110
    reconstruction of, 548, 603
    after tumor resection, 602
    combined lateral suboccipital-infralabyrinthine approach and, 385
  exit zone of, 137, 139
  intracisternal course of, 139
  intraoperative monitoring of function of, 95
    during cavernous sinus surgery, 534
    otological approaches to acoustic neuromas and, 723
  risks to in skull base surgery, 833
Abscesses
  cerebral, and petroclival meningioma surgery, 658
  sellar, transsphenoidal approach for resection of, 349
Abulia minor, in craniopharyngioma, 789
  after surgery, 805
Accessory hypophyseal arteries, 108
Accessory nerve (spinal accessory nerve, cranial nerve XI), 117
  acoustic neuroma and, 690, 691
  combined lateral suboccipital-infralabyrinthine approach and, 385
  exit zone of, 138–139
  intracisternal course of, 141
  intraoperative monitoring of function of, 95
Accessory sinus, 134
Acinar cell carcinoma, parotid, 318
  adjuvant treatment for, 325
Acoustic meatus, internal, 144–146
Acoustic nerve, and otologic approaches to acoustic neuroma, 723
Acoustic neuromas. See also Acoustic tumors
  accessory nerve and, 690, 691
  arterial relationships and, 695–699
  brain stem relationships and, 689–695, 696
  central electroauditory prosthesis placement and, 826
  cerebellar-brain stem fissures and, 691–693
  choroid plexus and, 693–695, 696
  diagnosis of, 715
  flocculus and, 693–695, 696
  foramen of Luschka and, 693–695, 696
  giant, operative approaches for resection of, 663
  glossopharyngeal nerve and, 690, 691
  mastoid retrosigmoid approach for resection of, 720–722
  meatal relationships and, 687, 688, 689
  microsurgical anatomy of, 687–699
  middle fossa approach for resection of, 709–710, 710–712, 719–720, 721
  neural relationships and, 687
  operative technique for resection of, 701, 702–713
  otological approaches for resection of, 715–724
    anesthesia for, 715–716
    complications of, 722–723
    cranial nerve dysfunction and, 723
    diagnosis and, 715
    operative technique for, 716–722
    patient positioning for, 716
    patient selection for, 715
    postoperative management and, 722
  pontomedullary sulcus and, 689–691
  recurrence of, 712–713, 723
  retrosigmoid approach for resection of, 701, 702–710
    exposure for, 701, 702
    instrumentation for, 705, 708
    intraoperative monitoring and, 703, 706, 707
    mastoid, 720–722
    patient positioning for, 701, 702–703
    stereotactic radiosurgery for, 712
    translabyrinthine approach for resection of, 711, 712, 716–719, 720
    transtemporal and infratemporal approach for resection of, 286, 287
  vagus nerve and, 690, 691
  venous relationships and, 699
Acoustic tumors. See also Acoustic neuromas
  bilateral, internal auditory canal decompression for, 377
  middle fossa approach for resection of, 367–377
  petrous apex, 305
  translabyrinthine approach for resection of, 351–362
    anesthesia for, 351
    closure for, 361
    complete/simple mastoidectomy and, 353
    complications of, 361–362
    cortical mastoidectomy and, 352–353
    dural incision and, 356–357
    postoperative management and, 361
    tumor isolation and, 357–359
    tumor removal and completion of, 361
    partial, 357
    venous bleeding and, 356
  transtemporal and infratemporal approach for resection of, 286, 287
Acromegaly, pituitary adenoma in, transsphenoidal surgery and, 337, 349
ACTH. See Adrenocorticotropic hormone
Adenocarcinoma
  cranial base, site of origin of, 21
  petroclival, 219
Adenoid cystic carcinoma
  anterior cranio-orbital resection with free-flap reconstruction for, 500, 503–504
  cavernous sinus, 603
  facial translocation approach for resection of, 256
  imaging characteristics of, 26
  of lacrimal gland, en bloc orbitectomy for, 781, 783–784
  petroclival, 219
  site of origin of, 20, 21
  spread of, 26, 27
Adenomas, pituitary
  in cavernous sinus, 603
  surgical resection of
    case examples illustrating, 584, 585, 586
    indications for, 533
  imaging characteristics of, 26
  petroclival invasion by, 219
  recurrence of, 305
  site of origin of, 20
  transsphenoidal approach for resection of, 337–338, 342, 343, 346, 347–348, 349

Adjuvant therapy
  for paranasal/nasal sinus carcinoma, 500
  for petrous bone tumors, 325
Adrenocorticotropic hormone-secreting pituitary adenoma, intracavernous invasion and, 584, 585, 586
Aesculap bipolar, for cranial base surgery, 4, 5
Age
  and craniopharyngioma incidence, 787
  patient selection for glomus vagale tumor surgery and, 764
AICA. See Anterior inferior cerebellar artery
Air embolism, venous, 76–77
  and hypovolemia, 74
"Air lock", 76, 77
Airway
  management of in paranasal/nasal sinus carcinoma resection, 499
  postoperative care of, 79–80
    in transmaxillary approach, 240
    in transoral surgery, 232
Algorithms, signal processing, for Neuronet, 87, 88
Alloplastic materials in skull base reconstruction, 461–469
  anesthesia and, 462
  for anterior base of skull, 468
  antibiotics and, 464
  cases illustrating use of, 465–468
  complications of, 464–465
  for congenital fistula involving floor of sella turcica and sphenoid sinus, 465–468
  diagnostic considerations and, 461
  for ethmoid bone roof, 468
  for frontal sinus posterior wall, 468
  for frontobasal fracture, 464, 465
  for lateral skull base, 468–469
  for olfactory fissure, 468
  operative technique for, 462, 463
  patient positioning and, 462
  patient selection and, 461–462
  for petrosal bone fracture, 467, 468
  postoperative management and, 464
  for recurrent meningioma, 466, 468
  technical problems and, 462–464
Amenorrhea, in craniopharyngioma, 789
Ampicillin, for otological approaches to acoustic neurilemoma, 716
Amplifier bandpass, for intraoperative electromyography, 95
Analgesia, postoperative
  for transmaxillary approach, 240
  for transoral surgery, 232
Anastomoses, embolization and, 147
Anesthesia for cranial base surgery, 3–4, 69–81. See also specific procedure
  blood transfusion and, 77–78
  carotid artery cross-clamping and, 78
  for cavernous sinus tumor surgery, 534
  clinical management and, 71–76
  coagulopathy and, 77–78
  complications and, 76–80
  cranial nerve cardiovascular reflexes and, 76
  and effects of anesthetic agents on intracranial contents, 69–71
  for extreme lateral transcondylar and transjugular surgery, 390
  and facilitation of surgical exposure, 75–76
  fluid management and, 74–75
  for glomus jugulare tumor surgery, 749
  for glomus vagale tumor surgery, 765
  hypothermia and, 79

844 / SUBJECT INDEX

Anesthesia for cranial base surgery (contd.)
  induction of, 72–74
    for jugular foramen neurilemoma surgery, 732
    for juvenile angiofibroma surgery, 486
  maintenance of, 72–74
  monitoring and, 71–72, 89. See also Intraoperative neurophysiologic monitoring
    for olfactory groove meningioma surgery, 508
    for osseous lesion (anterior and middle base) surgery, 810
    for otologic approaches for acoustic neurilemoma, 715–716
    for paranasal/nasal sinus carcinoma surgery, 499
  patient positioning and, 75
    for petroclival meningioma surgery, 607
    for petrosal approach for clivus tumors, 308
    for petrous bone tumor surgery, 318–319
  postoperative airway management and, 79–80
  postoperative nausea and vomiting and, 80
  preoperative preparation and, 71
    for reconstruction with alloplastic materials, 462
    for revascularization, 46
  tension pneumocephalus and, 79
    for transcondyle approach for foramen magnum meningiomas, 672
    for translabyrinthine surgery, 351
    for transmaxillary surgery, 235–236
    for transoral surgery, 227
    for transsphenoidal surgery, 338
    for transtemporal and infratemporal surgery, 269
    for transzygomatic and transpalatal resection of juvenile nasopharyngeal angiofibroma, 477
    for tuberculum sella meningioma surgery, 508
  venous air embolism and, 76–77
Aneurysms. See also specific type
  imaging characteristics of, 26
  site of origin of, 20
Angiofibromas
  embolization of, 40–41, 43
  facial translocation approach for resection of, 245, 253, 255
  juvenile, 485–496
    cavernous sinus, 603
      indications for surgical resection of, 533
    combined extracranial-intracranial approach for resection of, 488–489, 492–495
    diagnosis of, 485–486
    differential diagnosis of, 485
    endonasal microendoscopic approach without external incision for resection of, 486, 491
    extracranial approach for resection of, 486–488
    imaging characteristics of, 21, 26
    with intracranial extension, 477–484, 485
    midfacial degloving technique for resection of, 487
    radiation therapy for, 486
    site of origin of, 21, 485
    spontaneous remission of, 486
    spread of, 485
    surgical resection of
      anesthesia for, 486
      cases illustrating, 489, 490, 491–495
      complications of, 489–491
      operative techniques for, 486–489
      patient positioning for, 486
      patient selection for, 486
      postoperative management after, 489
      preoperative planning for, 485–486
    symptoms of, 485, 486
    transfacial technique through an extended Moure incision for resection of, 487–488, 490–491, 491–492, 493
    transzygomatic and transpalatal excision of, 477–484
      anesthesia for, 477
      cases illustrating, 480–483
      complications of, 480
      operative technique for, 477–480
      patient positioning for, 478
      patient selection for, 477
      postoperative management of, 480
      preoperative preparation for, 477
      technical problems in, 480
      transpalatal stage of, 479–480
      transzygomatic stage of, 478–479
    vascularity of, 485
Angiography
  for evaluation of skull base masses
    cavernous sinus tumors, 533
    glomus jugulare tumors, 747–748
    glomus vagale tumors, 764
    jugular foramen tumors, 380, 381
      neurilemomas, 731
    juvenile angiofibroma, 485
    olfactory groove meningiomas, 507
    orbital lesions, 771
    osseous lesions, 809
    petroclival meningiomas, 607
    petrous bone tumors, 318
    trigeminal neurilemomas, 738
    tuberculum sella meningiomas, 507
  in extreme lateral transcondylar and transjugular approaches, 389–390
  in preoperative patient evaluation, 3
  superselective
    for embolization, 37
    for juvenile angiofibroma, 485
    for transmaxillary approach, 235
Annulus tympanicus, 113
Anosmia, after craniofacial resection for esthesioneuroblastoma, 476
Anterior approach, to orbit, 771, 772–773, 774
Anterior cerebral vein, 103
Anterior circulation bypass grafting, 64–65
Anterior clinoid process
  and cavernous meningioma resection, 541, 542
  space exposed by removal of, 521. See also Clinoid space
Anterior cranial fossa, 103
  anatomy of, 99–121
  blood vessels related to, 103
  brain structures related to, 103
  dura mater of, 103
Anterior craniofacial resection, 147–156
  bifrontal craniotomy in, 150, 154
  complications of, 155
  for ethmoid sinus carcinoma, 500, 501
  follow-up and, 155
  incisions for, 147, 150
  including brain tissue, 500, 502
  planning for, 147
  postoperative care for, 155
  preoperative care for, 155
  reconstruction after, 151, 152
  specific concerns related to, 154–155
  surgical steps in, 147–151, 152
Anterior cranio-orbital resection
  with free-flap reconstruction, for adenoid cystic carcinoma, 500, 503–504
  for orbital and paranasal sinus rhabdomyosarcoma, 500, 503
Anterior ethmoidal canal, 127
Anterior inferior cerebellar artery, 142–143
  acoustic neuromas and, 695–697, 698
Anterior orbitotomy, 771, 772–773, 774
  extraperiosteal approach in, 773, 774
  incision sites for, 772
  transconjunctival approach in, 772, 773
  transseptal approach in, 773
Anterior petroclinoid fold, 106
Anterior subtemporal/frontotemporal-transsylvian approach, with zygomatic osteotomy, for petroclival meningioma, 608
Anterolateral approach, for cavernous sinus surgery, 540
Anterolateral craniofacial resection, 147–156
  complications of, 155
  facial osteotomies in, 151, 153, 154
  follow-up and, 155
  incisions for, 151, 152
  planning for, 147
  postoperative care for, 155
  preoperative care for, 155
  reconstruction after, 151–154
  specific concerns related to, 154–155
  surgical steps in, 151–154
Antibiotics. See also specific agent
  for otological approaches to acoustic neurilemoma, 716
  for paranasal/nasal sinus carcinoma resection, 499
  after reconstruction with alloplastic materials, 464
  after transmandibular-transcervical surgery, 265
  after transmaxillary surgery, 240
  after transoral surgery, 227–228, 232
Antidiuretic hormone, inappropriate secretion of, after cavernous sinus tumor surgery, 602
Antiemetics
  after transmaxillary surgery, 240
  after transoral surgery, 232
Arachnoid cyst, transsphenoidal approach for resection of, 349
Arnold's nerve, 109, 131
Arterial complications, after skull base surgery, 837–838
  evaluation of, 837
  management of, 837–838
  prevention of, 837
  surgical technique and, 837
Arterial pressure. See also Blood pressure
  mean, anesthetic agents affecting, 70, 71
Arteriovenous malformation, sigmoid, operative approaches for, 663
Artery-to-artery microanastomosis, in cerebral revascularization, 48–49
Articular eminence, 113
Articular fossa, 113
Articular tubercle, 113, 114

Subject Index / 845

Ascending palatine artery, 118
Ascending pharyngeal artery, 118
  bone and dura of posterior cranial fossa supplied by, 132
Aspiration pneumonia, and petroclival meningioma surgery, 658
Aspiration
  after complex cranial nerve injury, 820–822
  after jugular foramen neurilemoma resection, 735
  after single cranial nerve injury, 819–820
  after transmandibular-transcervical surgery, 265
Aspiratory, Cavitron ultrasonic, for cranial base surgery, 8
Ataxia, gait and limb, in petroclival meningioma, 606
Atrial myxomas. *See also* Cardiac myxomas
  metastatic, surgical resection of, 329, 330, 331
Audiometry, in preoperative patient evaluation, 3
Auditory canal, internal
  decompression of for bilateral acoustic tumors, 377
  dissection of in translabyrinthine approach, 354–356
Auditory evoked potentials, monitoring during cranial base surgery, 84, 93–94. *See also* Evoked potential studies
Auditory meatus. *See* Acoustic meatus
Auditory pathway, stimulation of by cochlear implantation, 825–829. *See also* Central electroauditory prosthesis
Auricular nerve, greater
  course of, 437
  for reconstruction of facial nerve, 435, 441, 442–443
Autologous blood donation, 78
Autoregulation, cerebrovascular, anesthetic agents affecting, 70

B
Bacterial sinusitis, imaging characteristics of, 26
BAEPs. *See* Auditory evoked potentials
Balloon test occlusion
  of internal carotid artery, 33–36
    in assessing need for revascularization, 45
    before cavernous sinus surgery, 533
    for evaluation of petroclival meningiomas, 607
    for evaluation of petrous bone tumors, 318
    for evaluation of trigeminal neurilemomas, 738
    in preoperative patient evaluation, 3
  of vertebral artery, 46
Bandpass, for intraoperative electromyography, 95
Barbiturate coma in cranial base anesthetic management, 3
  for cavernous sinus surgery, 534
Barbiturates
  for cavernous sinus surgery, 534
  protective effects of, 78
Basal cell carcinoma, petroclival, 219
Basal frontal approach, for clival tumors, 171–175
  cases illustrating, 190–194, 200–201, 202–207

disadvantages of, 175
entry into sphenoid sinus in, 173, 174
orbito-fronto-ethmoidal osteotomy in, 172–173
reconstruction and, 175
subtemporal-infratemporal approach combined with, 175, 176, 177
tumor resection in, 173–174
Basal vein of Rosenthal, 103
Basilar artery, 142
  aneurysms of, transoral approach for repair of, 227
  and transmaxillary approach, 239–240
Bick procedure, in eye reanimation, 451, 458
Bicoronal incision
  for combined frontotemporal-orbitozygomatic approach for tumors of sphenoid wing and orbit, 775, 779
  for subtemporal and infratemporal approach for clival tumor resection, 162, 163
Bicoronal scalp flap
  for reconstruction after anterior craniofacial resection, 151, 152
  for subfrontal approach for craniopharyngiomas, 792, 793
Bifrontal approach, for clival chordomas, 679, 680
Bifrontal craniotomy
  in anterior craniofacial resection, 150, 154
  for olfactory groove meningiomas, 515–516
Bill's bar
  and identification of facial nerve, 359
  in internal auditory canal dissection, 356
Bill's island, in internal auditory canal dissection, 354
Bipolar cautery, for cranial base surgery, 4, 5
Bleeding. *See also* Hemorrhage
  with cavernous meningioma surgery, control of, 547
  with translabyrinthine approach, 356
  with transmaxillary approach, 239
  with transoral surgery, 232
Blepharoplasty, in eye reanimation, 451
Blindness, in esthesioneuroblastoma, 473
Blood pressure
  anesthetic agents affecting, 70, 71
  control of, and facilitating surgical exposure, 76
Blood transfusions, complications of, 77–78
Bone grafting, transoral, 232
Bovine bone chips, in skull base reconstruction, 461
Brain contusion, after skull base surgery, 832
Brain edema. *See* Brain swelling
Brain function impairment, after skull base surgery, 834
Brain retraction, 4, 14
  minimizing use of, 4
Brain stem
  acoustic neuromas and, 689, 690, 692, 695
  fissures of, acoustic neuromas and, 691–693
  injury of after transtemporal and infratemporal surgery, 275
  swelling of after otological approaches to acoustic neurilemomas, 722
Brain stem evoked response
  monitoring during cranial base surgery, 4, 84, 91–93
    cavernous sinus surgery and, 534

extreme lateral transcondylar and transjugular approaches and, 390
petroclival meningioma surgery and, 607
petrous bone tumor surgery and, 318–319
revascularization and, 46
trigeminal neurilemoma surgery and, 738
preoperative, for petrous bone tumor surgery, 318
Brain swelling. *See also* Cerebral edema
  after skull base surgery, 832
  after tuberculum sella and olfactory groove meningioma surgery, 516–517
Bridging veins, of tentorium, 131
Brow lift, in eye reanimation, 451
BSEPs (brain stem evoked potentials). *See* Brain stem evoked response
BSER. *See* Brain stem evoked response
BTO. *See* Balloon test occlusion
Burrs, for cranial base surgery, 4
Bypass thrombosis, and cerebral revascularization, 65–66

C
C1-occipital condyle, resection of tumors of, 273
Canaliculi, lacrimal, stenting, in facial translocation approach, 250, 251
Cancer chemotherapy
  for esthesioneuroblastoma, 473
  for juvenile angiofibroma, 486
  for petrous bone tumors, 325
Canthal incision, for facial translocation approach, 249–250
Canthoplasty, medial, in eye reanimation, 451
Capsular arteries, 108
  of McConell, 521
Carbon dioxide laser, for cranial base surgery, 4–8
Carbon dioxide responsiveness, anesthetic agents affecting, 70
Carcinoma. *See also specific type*
  facial translocation approach for resection of, 253
  transsphenoidal approach for resection of, 349
Cardiac myxomas, metastatic
  to petroclivus, 219
  surgical resection of, 329, 330, 331
Cardiovascular reflexes, cranial nerve, 76
Caroticocavernous arteries, 108
Caroticoclinoid foramen (carotid foramen), 106
Carotid angiography. *See also* Angiography
  for evaluation of glomus jugulare tumors, 747–748
  for evaluation of glomus vagale tumors, 764
Carotid artery
  dissection of
    in cavernous meningioma surgery, 545–547
    in tuberculum sella meningioma surgery, 511–512, 513
  internal. *See* Internal carotid artery
Carotid artery bypass grafts, imaging in assessment of patency of, 29, 30
Carotid artery cross-clamping, 78
Carotid canal, 115
Carotid foramen (caroticoclinoid foramen), 106

Carotid sinus, 118
Cartilage implantation, in lower lid
  in eye reanimation, 451
  and postoperative facial paralysis, 443
Catecholamine secretion, by glomus jugulare
  tumors, preoperative preparation
  and, 749
Cavernoma, giant, operative approaches for,
  663
Cavernous hemangiomas
  indications for surgical resection of, 533
  orbital, transconjunctival approach for, 773
Cavernous internal carotid artery, 521, 522,
  528
  bone and dura of posterior cranial fossa
    supplied by, 132
  meningioma resection and, 545–547
    with grafting, 534–535
    without grafting, 535
    reconstruction and, 547–548
Cavernous meningioma, 512, 515, 603, 604
  embolization of, 40
  surgical resection of, 540–549
    anterior clinoid process and, 541, 542
    carotid artery and, 545–547
    cases illustrating, 550–554, 555,
      570–583, 584, 585–601
    cranial base reconstruction after, 549
    cranial nerves and, 545, 546
      reconstruction of, 548–549
    with ICA grafting, 534–535
    without ICA grafting, 535
    incisions for, 534–535
    indications for, 533
    intracavernous dissection in, 545–547
    lateral wall dissection in, 543–545
    optic nerve and, 541, 542
    petroclival bone and, 548
    petrous apex and, 548
    pituitary gland and, 548
    reconstruction after, 548–549
    subdural tumor resection in, 541
    superior approach for, 543
    sylvian dissection in, 540
    temporal lobe resection in, 540
    vascular reconstruction and, 547–548
    venous bleeding and, 547
Cavernous sinus, 101, 106. *See also* Hypo-
    physeal area
  adenoid cystic carcinoma of, 604
  anatomy of, 521, 522–532
  anterolateral approach for resection of tu-
    mors of, 540
  benign tumors of, indications for surgical
    resection of, 533
  chondrosarcoma of, 604
    surgical resection of, 549–550
      incisions for, 535
      indications for, 533
  chordoma of, 604
    surgical resection of, 549–550
      incisions for, 535
      indications for, 533
  classification of tumors of, 532
  clinoid space in, 521, 526–531
  condylar resection in surgery for tumors of,
    538
  craniopharyngioma in, cases illustrating
    surgical resection of, 562–570
  craniotomy in resection of tumors of,
    535–537
  epidermoid in, cases illustrating surgical
    resection of, 584, 587–588
  extradural approach for resection of tu-
    mors of, 537–540
  hemangioma in, cases illustrating surgical
    resection of, 554–562, 563
  imaging of tumors of, 532–533
  inferior approach to, 525, 526
    for resection of tumors, 539
  intradural approach for resection of tu-
    mors of, 540–550
  juvenile angiofibroma in, 603
    indications for surgical resection of, 533
  lateral wall of
    nerves in, 109–110
    resection of for cavernous meningioma
      surgery, 543–545
  malignant tumors of, surgical resection of,
    550
    indications for, 533–534
  medial approach for resection of tumors
    of, 540
  meningioma of. *See* Cavernous
    meningioma
  neurilemoma of, 603
    indications for surgery of, 533
  orbitozygomatic osteotomy in resection of
    tumors of, 537–538
  paranasal/nasal sinus carcinoma in, 498
  petrous carotid artery exposure in resection
    of tumors of, 538–539
  pituitary adenoma in, 603
    surgical resection of
      cases illustrating, 584, 585, 586
      indications for, 533
  squamous cell carcinoma in, 604
    indications for surgical resection of,
      533–534
  superior approach to, 524
  supraclinoid internal carotid artery in, and
    petrosal artery bypass, 52–61
    results of, 62
  surgical anatomy of, 522–532
  surgical resection of tumors of, 533–550
    anesthesia for, 534
    cases illustrating, 550–601
    complications of, 601–602
    cranial nerve dysfunction and, 833
    craniotomy for, 535–537
    extradural approach for, 537–540
    follow-up examination and, 603–604
    incisions for, 534–535
    indications for, 533–534
    intradural approach for, 540–550
    monitoring during, 534
  in tuberculum sella meningioma surgery,
    512, 515
  venous plexus in, 521, 527, 531
Cavitron ultrasonic aspiratory, for cranial
  base surgery, 8
CBF. *See* Cerebral blood flow
Cefuroxime, for paranasal/nasal sinus carcinoma resection, 499
"Cell saver", for transfusion, 78
Central electroauditory prosthesis, 825–829
  anatomy and, 826
  operative technique for placement of,
    826–828
  patient selection for, 826
  postoperative management of, 828
  results of placement of, 828
Central venous pressure, and facilitating surgical exposure, 76
Central venous pressure catheter, air embolism controlled with, 77
CEP. *See* Central electroauditory prosthesis
Cephalosporin
  for transmaxillary approach, 236, 240
  for transoral surgery, 227–228, 232
Ceravital plates, in skull base reconstruction,
  461, 468
Cerebellar arteries
  anterior inferior, 142–143
    acoustic neuromas and, 695–697, 698
    replacement and, 144
  superior, 143–144
    acoustic neuromas and, 697–699
Cerebellar dysfunction, and otologic approaches to acoustic neuroma, 723
Cerebellar fissures, acoustic neuromas and,
  691–693
Cerebellar injury, after transtemporal and
  infratemporal surgery, 275
Cerebellar peduncle, middle, vein of, acoustic
  neuroma and, 699
Cerebellomedullary fissure
  acoustic neuromas and, 691–693
  vein of, acoustic neuromas and, 699
Cerebellopontine angle
  extreme lateral transcondylar and transju-
    gular approaches for tumors of, 400
  topography of, 144–146
  translabyrinthine approach to, 351
    hematoma after, 361
Cerebellopontine fissure
  acoustic neuromas and, 691–693
  vein of, acoustic neuromas and, 699
Cerebellum, acoustic neuromas and, 689,
  690, 692, 695
Cerebral abscess, and petroclival meningioma surgery, 658
Cerebral angiography. *See* Angiography
Cerebral arteries, damage to, after tuberculum sella and olfactory groove
  meningioma surgery, 516
Cerebral blood flow
  anesthetic agents affecting, 70
  xenon/CT technique for measurement of,
    33–36
    and assessing need for revascularization,
      45
    before cavernous sinus surgery, 533
Cerebral edema. *See also* Brain swelling
  fluid administration and, 74–75
  petroclival meningioma surgery and, 658
Cerebral hematoma, and petroclival meningioma surgery, 658
Cerebral hemispheric injury, after transtemporal and infratemporal surgery,
  275
Cerebral hemorrhage, and petroclival meningioma surgery, 658
Cerebral hypoperfusion, EEG patterns in, 90
Cerebral infarction, and petroclival meningioma surgery, 658
Cerebral ischemia
  and carotid cross-clamping, 78
  revascularization complicated by, 65
Cerebral metabolic oxygen consumption
  rate, anesthetic agents affecting, 70,
  71
Cerebral revascularization, 45–68
  anesthesia for, 46
  artery-to-artery microanastomosis in,
    48–49
  complications of, 65–66
  extracranial-to-distal middle cerebral ar-
    tery bypass in, 63–64

extracranial-internal carotid bypass grafting in, 63–65
extracranial-to-proximal anterior circulation artery bypass in, 64–65
long-term outcome with, 66
monitoring during, 46
need for, assessment of, 45–46
petrosal to supraclinoid internal carotid artery cavernous sinus bypass in, 52–61
results of, 62
petrosal to upper cervical internal carotid artery interposition grafting in, 50–52
posterior circulation bypass grafting in, 65
postoperative medical management and, 65
preparation for, 46–47
reimplantation in, 61
saphenous vein harvesting for, 46–47
vein-to-artery microanastomosis in, 49
vein graft results and, 61–62
venous patch grafting in, 50
vertebral artery interposition grafting in, 61
Cerebral veins
anterior, 103
great, 133
Cerebrospinal fluid
anesthetic agents affecting
production of, 70, 71
resistance to absorption of, 70
disturbances in circulation of, and otologic approaches to acoustic neuroma, 723
drainage of, in esthesioneuroblastoma resection, 473
intracranial confinement of, in anterior and anterolateral craniofacial resection, 154
leakage of. *See* Cerebrospinal fluid leak
withdrawal of, and facilitating surgical exposure, 76
Cerebrospinal fluid fistula, petrous apex, 305
Cerebrospinal fluid leak, 9, 31, 32, 834–837
after cavernous sinus tumor surgery, 602
after craniofacial resection for paranasal sinus tumors, 504
diagnosis of, 835
after extreme lateral transcondylar and transjugular surgery, 399–400
after facial translocation surgery, 253
after glomus jugulare surgery, 757
incidence of, 834–835
after juvenile angiofibroma surgery, 489
management of, 836–837
after osseous lesion (anterior and middle base) surgery, 816
after petroclival meningioma surgery, 658
after petrous bone tumor surgery, 325
after subtemporal and infratemporal approach for clival tumor resection, 171
after transsphenoidal surgery for invasive lesions, 344, 345
after transtemporal and infratemporal surgery, 276
after trigeminal neurilemoma surgery, 739
after tuberculum sella and olfactory groove meningioma surgery, 516
Cerebrovascular autoregulation, anesthetic agents affecting, 70
Cervical exposure, for jugular foramen tumors, 381

Cervical to petrous carotid graft revascularization, 62
results of, 62
Cheek swelling, in juvenile angiofibroma, 485, 486
Chemodectomas, jugular foramen, 379
Chemotherapy
for esthesioneuroblastoma, 473
for juvenile angiofibroma, 486
for petrous bone tumors, 325
Chest physiotherapy, after transoral surgery, 232
Cholesteatomas
imaging characteristics of, 26
petrous apex, 305
imaging characteristics of, 292
site of origin of, 20
Cholesterol granulomas
imaging characteristics of, 23, 26
petroclival, 219
petrous apex, imaging characteristics of, 292
site of origin of, 20
Chondroblastomas, petroclival, 219
Chondromas, middle fossa, surgical resection of, 810–811
Chondrosarcomas
cavernous sinus, 603
surgical resection of
incisions for, 535
indications for, 533
clival, subtemporal-infratemporal lateral and transethmoidal anterior approach for resection of, 198–199
extreme lateral transcondylar and transjugular approaches for resection of, 389, 398, 402–403, 404, 405
imaging characteristics of, 24, 25, 26
petroclival, 219
site of origin of, 20, 21
Chorda tympani, 119
Chordomas
cavernous sinus, 603
surgical resection of
incisions for, 535
indications for, 533
clival, 379, 679–685
basal frontal, subtemporal-infratemporal, and transcavernous approach for, cases illustrating, 188–194
diagnosis of, 679
extreme lateral transcondylar and transjugular approaches for resection of, 205, 208, 389, 398
standard surgical approaches for resection of, 679, 680
subtemporal-infratemporal approach for resection of, 211
and basal frontal approach, 202–207
transoral approach for resection of, 681–683, 684
transseptal transsphenoidal approach for resection of, 679–683, 684
exposure for, 680–681
patient positioning for, 680
postoperative care for, 681
preoperative preparation for, 680
steps in, 680–681
facial translocation approach for resection of, 245, 253, 254
imaging characteristics of, 26
middle fossa, surgical resection of, 810–811

petroclival, 219
operative approaches for, 663
recurrent, 28–29, 31
site of origin of, 20, 21
spinal, extreme lateral transcondylar and transjugular approaches for resection of, 399
transmaxillary approach for resection of, 242–243
transoral approach for resection of, 232–233
transsphenoidal approach for resection of, 345–346, 349
Choroid plexus
acoustic neuromas and, 693–695, 696
malignant papillomas and, 318
Cisternography, cerebrospinal fluid leak diagnosed with
computed tomographic, 835
radioisotope, 835
Clinoid process
anterior
and cavernous meningioma resection, 541, 542
space exposed by removal of, 521, 526–531
posterior, 105
Clinoid space, 521, 526–531
Clinoidal internal carotid artery, 526
Clival chordomas, 379, 679–685
basal frontal, subtemporal-infratemporal, and transcavernous approach for, cases illustrating, 188–194
diagnosis of, 679
extreme lateral transcondylar and transjugular approaches for resection of, 205, 208, 389, 398
standard surgical approaches for resection of, 679, 680
subtemporal-infratemporal approach for resection of, 211
and basal frontal approach, 202–207
transoral approach for resection of, 681–683, 684
transseptal transsphenoidal approach for resection of, 679–683, 684
exposure for, 680–681
patient positioning for, 680
postoperative care for, 681
preoperative preparation for, 680
steps in, 680–681
Clival meningiomas. *See also* Petroclival meningiomas
cavernous sinus involvement and, case illustrating surgical resection of, 580–583
Clivus, 132. *See also under* Petroclival
anatomy of, 246, 605–606
blood supply of, 132
combined anterior and lateral approach for tumors of, 175, 176, 177
cranial nerve dysfunction after surgery on, 834
extended frontal approach for tumors of, 171–175
disadvantages of, 175
entry into sphenoid sinus in, 173, 174
orbito-fronto-ethmoidal osteotomy in, 172–173
reconstruction and, 175
tumor resection in, 173–174
extradural tumors of, anterior/anterolateral/lateral approaches to, 157–223

Clivus, extradural tumors of (*contd.*)
  approach selection and, 157–159
  cases illustrating, 181–218
    combined anterior and lateral, 175, 176, 177
    extended frontal, 171–175
    extreme lateral/transcondyle/transjugular, 175–181
    subtemporal/infratemporal, 161–171
    subtemporal/transcavernous/transpetrous apex, 159–161
  extreme lateral transcondylar and jugular approaches to tumors of, 175–181, 389–411
    anesthesia for, 390
    cases illustrating, 400–405, 406–409
    cerebrospinal fluid leakage and, 399–400
    complications of, 399–400
    cranial nerve function and, 399
    disadvantages of, 181
    neurologic deficits and, 399
    operative procedure for, 390–394, 395–396
    operative technique for, 390–397
    patient positioning for, 390
    postoperative care and, 397
    preoperative evaluation for, 389–390
    reconstruction after, 180–181
    results of, 397–400
    stability and, 394–397, 399
    tumor resection extent and, 398–399
  facial translocation approach for tumors of, 245–259
    complications of, 253, 256
    craniofacial skeleton and, 251, 252
    facial incisions/scars and, 249, 251
    facial nerve and, 249, 250, 438, 440, 441
    follow-up and, 258
    indications for, 245–248, 253, 258
    infraorbital nerve and, 250–251, 252
    midfacial split approach and, 257–258
    nasal mucosa and, 251
    nasolacrimal duct and, 250, 251
    planning for, 245–248
    postoperative care for, 256
    preoperative care for, 253–256
    specific concerns in, 248–253
    surgical steps in, 247, 248
    temporalis muscle and, 253
    vascularity and, 248
  meningiomas of. *See* Petroclival meningiomas
  myeloma of, transmaxillary approach for resection of, 242–243
  petrosal approach for tumors of, 307–315
    anesthesia for, 308
    case studies illustrating, 313–314
    closure for, 312
    complications of, 312–313
    craniotomy flap in, 308–309
    diagnosis and, 307
    dural opening in, 309
    exposure for, 309
    monitoring during, 308
    operative technique for, 308–312
    patient position for, 308
    patient selection for, 307–308
    postoperative management for, 312
    temporal bone drilling for, 309
    tentorium sectioning in, 309
    tumor resection in, 309–312
  subtemporal/infratemporal approach for tumors of, 161–171

disadvantages of, 171
division of V_3 in, 167, 169, 170
reconstruction and, 167–171
subtemporal/transcavernous/transpetrous apex approach to, 159–161
  reconstruction and, 161
transmaxillary approach for tumors of, 235–244
  and accurate replacement of upper jaw, 240
  anesthesia for, 235–236
  basilar artery and, 239–240
  bleeding and, 239
  case studies illustrating, 242–243
  closure for, 239
  complications of, 240
  diagnosis and, 235
  exposure for, 236–239
  and extended maxillectomy, 240–241
    operative technique for, 241–242
  operative technique for, 235–239
  patient position for, 236
  patient selection for, 235
  postoperative management for, 240
  technical problems with, 239–240
  tumor access and, 239
transsphenoidal approach for invasive lesions of, 337–349
  anesthesia for, 338
  cases illustrating, 345–348
  complications of, 345
  diagnosis and, 337
  operating room arrangement for, 338
  operative technique for, 338–344
  patient position for, 338
  patient selection for, 337–338
  pernasal approach for, 339–340
  postoperative management and, 344
  sublabial incision for, 339
transtemporal and infratemporal approach for tumors of, 269
Closed eyelid spring implantation technique, for eye reanimation in paralyzed face without facial nerve, 454
Closure. *See also specific procedure*
  for clivus chordoma surgery, 680
  for petrosal approach to clival tumors, 312
  for transmandibular-transcervical approach, 265
  for transmaxillary approach, 239
  for transoral approach, 231–232
  for tuberculum sella meningioma surgery, 515
Clotting factor deficiencies, 77–78
CMRO$_2$. *See* Cerebral metabolic oxygen consumption rate
CNC. *See* Cochlear nucleus complex
Coagulopathy, transfusion-related, 77–78
Cochlear implantation, electrical stimulation of auditory pathway by, 825–829. *See also* Central electroauditory prosthesis
Cochlear nerve, and acoustic neuroma removal, 687, 688, 689
Cochlear nucleus
  anatomy of, 826
  stimulation of by implant, 825–829. *See also* Central electroauditory prosthesis
Cochlear nucleus complex, 826
Cochleovestibular nerve (cranial nerve VIII)
  and acoustic neuroma removal, 687
  exit zone of, 138
  intracisternal course of, 139

and petroclival meningioma, 606
total section of, 362
Colloid cyst, transsphenoidal approach for resection of, 349
Colloids, for blood replacement during cranial base surgery, 4, 74–75
Combined anterior and lateral approach, for clival tumors, 175, 176, 177
Combined extracranial-intracranial approach, for juvenile angiofibroma surgery, 488–489, 492–495
Combined frontotemporal-orbitozygomatic approach, 775–781
  for intraorbital tumors with and without intracranial extension, 781–784
  for sphenoid wing, orbit, and middle fossa tumors, 775–781
Combined lateral suboccipital-infralabyrinthine approach for jugular foramen tumors, 381–386
  advantages of, 385–386
  cranial nerve affected in, 384, 385
  patient positioning for, 381
  results of, 384–386
  steps in, 382–383
Combined middle-posterior fossa approach for petrous apex lesions, 300–301
  indications for, 299, 300
  surgical technique for, 300–301
Combined supra- and infraparapetrosal approach for petroclival lesions, 661–669
  cases illustrating, 667–669
  closure for, 667
  craniotomy for, 664, 665
  dural incision for, 664–667
  indications for, 663
  microsurgical instrumentation for, 663–664
  operative technique for, 663–667
  patient positioning for, 664
  scalp incision for, 664, 665
  tumor access with, 664–667
  tumor resection and, 667
Complete, simple mastoidectomy, in translabyrinthine approach, 353
Complications of cranial base surgery, 9, 831–839. *See also specific type and procedure*
  systemic, 839
Computed tomographic cisternogram, cerebrospinal fluid leak diagnosed with, 835
Computed tomography
  for cerebral blood flow measurements, xenon-enhancement and, 33–36
  and assessing need for revascularization, 45
  for evaluation of skull base masses, 3, 15–32
    avenues of spread and, 26–28
    cavernous sinus tumors, 532–533
    craniopharyngiomas, 789
    esthesioneuroblastomas, 471
    facial nerve neurilemomas, 725
    glomus jugulare tumors, 747–748
    glomus vagale tumors, 764
    as guide to surgical management, 28–29
    jugular foramen tumors, 379, 380
    neurilemomas, 731
    juvenile angiofibromas, 485
    orbital lesions, 771
    osseous lesions, 809

paranasal/nasal sinus carcinoma, 497–498
petroclival meningiomas, 607, 667–669
petrous apex lesions, 293
petrous bone tumors, 318
postoperative evaluation and, 29–32
problem areas in, 29
techniques for, 15–19
trigeminal neurilemomas, 738
tumor identification and, 19, 20–25, 26
in extreme lateral transcondylar and transjugular approaches, 389
in transmaxillary approach, 235
in transsphenoidal approach for invasive and sellar clival lesions, 337
xenon-enhanced, for cerebral blood flow measurement, 33–36
and assessing need for revascularization, 45
Computer network architecture, for NeuroNet, 85
Concha, nasal, middle, 123–124
Conductive hearing loss. *See also* Hearing loss
after transmandibular-transcervical surgery, 265
after transtemporal and infratemporal surgery, 276
Condylar emissary vein, 135
Condylar resection, in cavernous sinus surgery, 538
Conjunctival incision, for facial translocation approach, 249–250
Connective tissue, in orbit, 101–102
Contact lasers, for cranial base tumors, 4–8
Contact zone, 140–141
Contusion, brain, after skull base surgery, 832
Cortex, electrical activity of, monitoring during cranial base surgery, 84, 89–91
Cortical mastoidectomy, in translabyrinthine approach, 352–353
Corticosteroid replacement, for craniopharyngioma surgery, 791, 804
Cranial base (skull base)
anterior, alloplastic materials in reconstruction of, 468
divisions of, 1
inferior
anatomy of, 112–115
muscles of, 115–116
nerves of, 116–118
lateral, alloplastic materials in reconstruction of, 468–469
middle
anatomy of, 103–105
transmandibular-transcervical approach to, 261–265
reconstruction of. *See* Reconstruction
veins of, 119
Cranial base nurse coordinator, on skull base team, 3
Cranial base surgery. *See also specific procedure*
anesthesia for, 3–4
cerebral revascularization in, 45–68
complications of, 9, 831–839
systemic, 839
exposure for, 4
facilitating, 75–76
facial nerve management and reconstructive techniques in, 435–447
instrumentation for, 4–8, 13–14
and otolaryngologic/plastic surgery operative techniques and instrumentation, 11–14

patient evaluation and, 3
perioperative management for, 8
postoperative follow-up and, 9–10
reconstruction and, 8–9, 12–13
as team effort, 2–3
neurophysiologic monitoring and, 84–85
techniques in, 1–10
from otolaryngologic and plastic surgery, 11–14
and tumor resection plan, 8
Cranial base tumors. *See also specific type*
computed tomography in evaluation of, 3, 15–32
definition of, 1
devascularization of, by embolization, 37–44
imaging characteristics of, 19, 26
magnetic resonance imaging in evaluation of, 3, 15–32
operative techniques for, 1–10. *See also* Cranial base surgery
sites of origin of, 20–21
types of, 831
Cranial fossae. *See* Anterior cranial fossa; Middle cranial fossa; Posterior cranial fossa
Cranial nerve I. *See* Olfactory nerve
Cranial nerve II. *See* Optic nerve
Cranial nerve III. *See* Oculomotor nerve
Cranial nerve IV. *See* Trochlear nerve
Cranial nerve V. *See* Trigeminal nerve
Cranial nerve V_1. *See* Ophthalmic nerve
Cranial nerve V_2. *See* Maxillary nerve
Cranial nerve V_3. *See* Mandibular nerve
Cranial nerve VI. *See* Abducens (abducent) nerve
Cranial nerve VII. *See* Facial nerve
Cranial nerve VIII. *See* Cochleovestibular nerve
Cranial nerve IX. *See* Glossopharyngeal nerve
Cranial nerve X. *See* Vagus nerve
Cranial nerve XI. *See* Accessory nerve
Cranial nerve XII. *See* Hypoglossal nerve
Cranial nerve cardiovascular reflexes, 76
Cranial nerve deficits. *See also* Cranial nerve function; Cranial nerves
after glomus jugulare tumor surgery, 757
in jugular foramen neurilemoma resection, 735
in juvenile angiofibroma, 485, 486
after skull base surgery, 833–834
after transtemporal and infratemporal surgery, 275–276
Cranial nerve function. *See also* Cranial nerve deficits; Cranial nerves
after cavernous sinus tumor surgery, 602
and extreme lateral transcondylar and transjugular approaches, 389, 399
monitoring during cranial base surgery, 84, 95–96
cavernous sinus surgery and, 534
and otologic approaches to acoustic neuroma, 723
in petroclival meningioma, 606
Cranial nerves. *See also specific type*
in cavernous sinus, 521, 522, 526, 527, 530
meningioma resection and, 545, 546
reconstruction of, 548–549
tumor resection and, 602
in combined lateral suboccipital-infralabyrinthine approach, 385
exit zones of, 137–141
in extreme lateral transcondylar and transjugular approaches, 399

function of. *See* Cranial nerve function
intracisternal course of, 139–141
after otological approaches to acoustic neurilemomas, 723
swallowing dysfunction caused by injury to complex nerve injury, 820–822
single nerve injury, 819–820
Cranial roots, 138–139
Craniectomy
for middle fossa approach for petrous apex lesions, 296
in occipito-transmastoid-cervical approach, 303
for posterior fossa approach for petrous apex lesions, 299
Craniocervical junction, stability of, and extreme lateral transcondylar and transjugular approaches, 394–397, 399
Craniofacial osteotomy, in anterolateral craniofacial resection, 151, 153
Craniofacial resection
anterior and anterolateral, 147–156
complications of, 155
for ethmoid sinus carcinoma, 500, 501
follow-up and, 155
including brain tissue, 500, 502
planning for, 147
postoperative care for, 155
preoperative care for, 155
specific concerns related to, 154–155
surgical steps in, 147–155
for esthesioneuroblastoma, 473
patient positioning for, 473
technique for, 473–476
for paranasal/nasal sinus carcinoma, 409–505
adjuvant therapy and, 500
and anterior cranio-orbital resection, 500, 503
with free-flap reconstruction, 500, 503–504
including brain tissue, 500, 502
cases illustrating, 500, 501–504
cavernous sinus involvement and, 498
cerebrospinal fluid leak and, 504
complications of, 504–505
cribriform plate involvement and, 498
dural involvement and, 498
eye protection and, 499
functional and esthetic results of, 499–500
hard palate involvement and, 498–499
instrumentation for, 499
neuroanesthesia for, 499
ocular dystopia after, 505
operative procedure for, 499–500
orbital involvement and, 498
Craniofacial skeleton
disassembly and reconstruction of, 421–424
complications of, 425
follow-up care and, 425
postoperative care and, 425
preoperative preparation and, 425
in facial translocation approach, 251, 252
Craniofacial structures, and facial translocation approach, 245
Craniofacial surgery, 11
Cranio-orbital resection, anterior
with free-flap reconstruction, for adenoid cystic carcinoma, 500, 503–504
for orbital and paranasal sinus rhabdomyosarcoma, 500, 503

Craniopharyngiomas, 787–807
  calcification of, 788
  cavernous sinus, surgical resection of
    cases illustrating, 562–570
    indications for, 533
  clinical features of, 788–789
  cystic, 788
    treatment of, 791
  diagnosis of, radiologic, 789
  embryologic origin of, 787–788
  incidence of, 787
  location of, 788
  pathology of, 788
  recurrent, 805–806
  solid, 788
    biopsy and radiation of, 790
    stereotactic radiosurgery for, 791
    subtotal resection of, with postoperative radiation, 790
    total resection of, 790
    treatment of, 789–791
  subfrontal approach for resection of, 792–797, 798
  subfrontal-transsphenoidal approach for resection of, 799–802, 803
  surgical pathology of, 788
  surgical resection of
    approaches for, 792–804
    complications of, 804–805
    for cystic lesions, 791
    hydrocephalus and, 792
    patient selection for, 789–791
    postoperative follow-up for, 805
    preoperative care for, 791–792
    for solid lesions, 790
    staged procedures for, 802–804
  translamina terminalis approach for resection of, 797–799, 800
  transsphenoidal approach for resection of, 349
Craniospinal foramen magnum meningioma, transcondyle approach for resection of, 675, 676–677
Craniotomes, for cranial base surgery, 14
Craniotomy
  air bubbles introduced during, 76
  bifrontal
    in anterior craniofacial resection, 150, 154
    for olfactory groove meningiomas, 515–516
  in combined supra- and infraparapetrosal approach for petroclival lesions, 664
  frontal, in extended frontal approach for clival tumors, 172
  frontotemporal
    in cavernous sinus surgery, 535–537
    in frontotemporal transcavernous and transpetrous apex approach for petroclival meningiomas, 609
    in frontotemporal-transsylvanian/anterior subtemporal approach for petroclival meningiomas, 608
  pterional, 679
  sphenoidal, in en bloc orbitectomy, 783, 785
  in middle fossa approach for petrous apex lesions, 295–296
  in paranasal/nasal sinus carcinoma resection, 499
  rectosigmoid, in retrosigmoid approach for acoustic neurilemoma, 721
  subfrontal, for clival chordomas, 679
  in subtemporal/transcavernous/transpetrous apex approach, 159
  in transcondyle approach for foramen magnum meningiomas, 672
Craniotomy flap, in petrosal approach for clival tumors, 308–309
Crawford nasolacrimal stent, 250
Cribriform plate, paranasal/nasal sinus carcinoma and, 498
Crista alaris (Sylvi), 103
Crockard transoral instrumentation, 7
Crossbite deformity, after transtemporal and infratemporal surgery, 276
Cross-clamping, carotid artery, 78
Crusting, after juvenile angiofibroma surgery, 489
CSF. See Cerebrospinal fluid
CSF leak. See Cerebrospinal fluid leak
CT. See Computed tomography
CUSA. See Cavitron ultrasonic aspiratory
Cushing's disease, pituitary adenoma in, transsphenoidal surgery and, 337, 349
Cushing's method, for transsphenoidal surgery, 338
CVP. See Central venous pressure
Cyclophosphamide, for esthesioneuroblastoma, 473
Cysts
  neurenteric, transoral approach for resection of, 233–234
  transsphenoidal approach for resection of, 349

D

Dacryocystorhinotomy, endonasal microsurgical, for impaired lacrimal drainage after juvenile angiofibroma surgery, 489
DDAVP. See Desmopressin
Dementia, in petroclival meningioma, 606
Dermoids
  imaging characteristics of, 26
  orbital, extraperiosteal approach for resection of, 773
  site of origin of, 20
Derome's bifrontal approach, for clival chordomas, 679, 680
Derome's transbasal approach, extended frontal approach as modification of, 171
Desmopressin
  for diabetes insipidus after craniopharyngioma surgery, 804
  for excess urinary output after transsphenoidal surgery for invasive lesions, 344
Dexamethasone, for combined frontotemporal-orbitozygomatic approach for tumors of sphenoid wing and orbit, 775
Diabetes insipidus
  after cavernous sinus tumor surgery, 602
  in craniopharyngiomas, 789
    after surgery, 804
  after petroclival meningioma surgery, 658
  after transsphenoidal surgery for invasive lesions, 344, 345
  after tuberculum sella and olfactory groove meningioma surgery, 517
Diaphragma sellae, 106
  in transsphenoidal surgery for invasive tumors, 344
Diethylstilbestrol, before transzygomatic and transpalatal resection of juvenile nasopharyngeal angiofibroma, 477
Digastric sulcus, 113–115
Digital subtraction angiography, in jugular foramen neurilemomas, 731
Dilutional thrombocytopenia, 77
Diskless work stations, in NeuroNet, 86
Dissectors, for cranial base tumors, 6
Disseminated intravascular coagulation, after cranial base surgery, 77
Dorello's canal, 527
Dorsum sellae, 105, 132
Drills, for cranial base surgery, 4, 14
Droperidol, for otological approaches to acoustic neurilemoma, 715
DSA. See Digital subtraction angiography
Dura mater
  of anterior cranial fossa, 103
  of cavernous sinus, 521
  closure of, in transoral approach, 231–232
  in hypophyseal area, 106, 107
  opening
    in combined parapetrosal approach, 664
    in extreme lateral transcondylar and transjugular approaches, 392, 393
    in petrosal approach, 309
    in translabyrinthine approach, 356–357
  paranasal/nasal sinus carcinoma and, 498
  of posterior cranial fossa
    blood supply of, 132
    nerve supply of, 132–133
Dural defect, and osseous lesion (anterior and middle base) surgery, 812–813
Dural tail, in spread of meningioma, 26–28
Dysembryonic tumors, transsphenoidal approach for resection of, 349
Dysphagia. See also Swallowing
  complex cranial nerve injury and, 820–822
  after jugular foramen neurilemoma resection, 735
  single cranial nerve injury and, 819–820
  after transmandibular-transcervical surgery, 265
Dysplasia, fibrous
  imaging characteristics of, 26
  optic nerves affected by, surgical resection of, 811–812
Dystopia, ocular, after craniofacial resection for paranasal sinus tumors, 505

E

Echography, for orbital lesions, 771
Edema. See Brain swelling; Cerebral edema
EEG. See Electroencephalogram
Electroauditory prosthesis, central, 825–829
  anatomy and, 826
  operative technique for, 826–828
  patient selection for, 826
  postoperative management for, 828
  results of, 828
Electrodes, for intraoperative electromyography, 95
Electroencephalogram
  anesthetic agents affecting, 71
  monitoring during cranial base surgery, 4, 84, 89–91
    cavernous sinus surgery and, 534
    petroclival meningioma surgery and, 607
    petrous bone tumor surgery and, 319
    revascularization and, 46
  NeuroNet and, 86
  two-channel, 72

Electromyography, cranial nerve function monitored by, 95–96
  cavernous sinus surgery and, 534
  extreme lateral transcondylar and transjugular approaches and, 390
  NeuroNet and, 86
Electron microscopy, for evaluation of esthesioneuroblastoma, 471
Electrophysiologic monitoring, during cranial base surgery, 4. *See also* Intraoperative neurophysiologic monitoring
  petrosal approach for clival tumors and, 308
Embolism, venous air, 76–77
  and hypovolemia, 74
Embolization, by interventional neuroradiology, 37–44
  for glomus vagale tumors, 766
  for juvenile nasopharyngeal angiofibromas, 477, 485
  for orbital lesions, 771
  patient preparation and, 43
  technique considerations and, 43
Emissary foramen, mastoid, 135
Emissary veins. *See also specific type*
  in posterior cranial fossa, 135–136
En bloc orbitectomy, 781–784
"En plaque" hyperostosing meningioma, surgical resection of, 810–811
Encephalocele
  imaging characteristics of, 26
  site of origin of, 20, 21
Endonasal microendoscopic approach, without external incision, for juvenile angiofibroma surgery, 486, 491
Endonasal microsurgical dacryocystorhinotomy, for impaired lacrimal drainage after juvenile angiofibroma surgery, 489
Endosteum, in transsphenoidal approach for invasive tumors, 342–343
Enflurane, effects of, 70, 71
EOM. *See* Extraocular muscles
Epidermoids
  cavernous sinus, cases illustrating surgical resection of, 584, 587–588
  imaging characteristics of, 26
  jugular foramen, 379
  petroclival, 219
  site of origin of, 20
  supracavernous, cases illustrating surgical resection of, 584, 587–588
Epiphora, in esthesioneuroblastoma, 473
Epistaxis
  in esthesioneuroblastoma, 471, 473
  in juvenile angiofibroma, 485
Erb's point, and monitoring somatosensory system, 91
Esthesioneuroblastoma (olfactory neuroblastoma), 471–476
  biopsy of, 471
  clinical presentation of, 472–473
  diagnosis of, 471–472
  differential diagnosis of, 472
  imaging characteristics of, 22, 26
  pathogenesis of, 471
  prognosis for, 476
  site of origin of, 20, 21
  staging of, 472
  surgical removal of, 473–476
  transcranial, anterior craniofacial resection for, 500, 502

transsphenoidal approach for resection of, 349
  treatment of, 473
    complications of, 476
    technique for, 473–476
  ultrastructure of, 471–472
Ethernet, in NeuroNet configuration, 85
Ethmoid bone, roof of, alloplastic materials in reconstruction of, 468
Ethmoid mucocele, site of origin of, 20, 21
Ethmoid sinus carcinoma, anterior craniofacial resection for, 500, 501
Ethmoidal arteries, anterior cranial fossa supplied by, 103
Ethmoidal bulla, 124
Ethmoidal canals, 127
Ethmoidal infundibulum, 125
Ethmoidal recess, 129
Ethmoidosphenoidal osseous lesions, medial, surgical resection of, 811–812
Etomidate, effects of, 70
Eustachian tube, cerebrospinal fluid leak at, 835
EVD. *See* External ventricular drain
Evoked potential studies
  of auditory system, 93–94
  monitoring during cranial base surgery, 4, 84
    cavernous sinus surgery and, 534
    extreme lateral transcondylar and transjugular approaches and, 390
    petroclival meningioma surgery and, 607
    petrous bone tumor surgery and, 318–319
    revascularization and, 46
    trigeminal neurilemoma surgery and, 738
  NeuroNet and, 86
  in preoperative patient evaluation, 3
  for petrous bone tumor surgery, 318
  of somatosensory system, 91–93
  of visual system, 94–95
Exposure, for cranial base surgery, 4. *See also specific procedure*
  for cavernous sinus surgery, 534
  for clivus chordoma surgery, 680
  facilitation and, 75–76
  for glomus jugulare tumor surgery, 749, 750
  for jugular foramen neurilemoma surgery, 733
  for petrosal approach for clival tumor surgery, 309, 310, 311
  for petrous bone tumor surgery, 319–321
  for retrosigmoid approach for acoustic neuroma surgery, 701, 702
  for subfrontal approach for craniopharyngioma surgery, 792, 793
  for subtemporal and infratemporal approach for clival tumor surgery, 162
  for transcondyle approach for foramen magnum meningioma surgery, 672
  for transmandibular-transcervical approach, 262
  for transmaxillary approach, 236–239
  for transoral approach, 228–230
  for transtemporal and infratemporal approach, 269–270
Extended facial recess approach, for jugular foramen tumors, 384–385
Extended frontal approach for clival tumors, 171–175
  cases illustrating, 190–194, 200–201, 202–207

disadvantages of, 175
  entry into sphenoid sinus in, 173, 174
  orbito-fronto-ethmoidal osteotomy in, 171, 172–173
  reconstruction and, 175
  subtemporal-infratemporal approach combined with, 175, 176, 177
  tumor resection in, 173–174
Extended maxillectomy, 240–241
  operative technique for, 241–242
External otitis, malignant
  imaging characteristics of, 26
  site of origin of, 20, 21
External ventricular drain, for craniopharyngioma-induced hydrocephalus, 792
Extracranial approach, for juvenile angiofibroma surgery, 486–488
  endonasal microendoscopic without external incision, 486, 491
  with intracranial approach, 488–489, 492–495
  and midfacial degloving technique, 487
  transfacial, through extended Moure incision, 487–488, 490–491, 491–492, 493
Extracranial-to-distal middle cerebral artery bypass graft, 63–64
Extracranial-internal carotid bypass grafting, 63–65
Extracranial-to-proximal anterior circulation arteries, bypass grafting, 64–65
Extradural approach, for cavernous sinus surgery, 537–540
Extradural hematomas, after skull base surgery, 832–833
Extradural pneumatoceles, after osseous lesion (anterior and middle base) surgery, 816–817
Extradural tumors
  clival
    anterior/anterolateral/lateral approaches for resection of, 157–223
    cases illustrating, 181–218
    approach selection for, 157–159
    combined anterior and lateral approach for resection of, 175, 176, 177
    extended frontal approach for resection of, 171–175
      disadvantages of, 175
      entry into sphenoid sinus in, 173, 174
      orbito-fronto-ethmoidal osteotomy in, 172–173
      reconstruction and, 175
      tumor resection in, 173–174
    extreme lateral/transcondyle/transjugular approach for, resection of, 175–181
    subtemporal/infratemporal approach for resection of, 161–171
      disadvantages of, 171
      division of V_3 in, 167, 169, 170
      reconstruction and, 167–171
    subtemporal/transcavernous/transpetrous apex approach for resection of, 159–161
      reconstruction and, 161
  petroclival, anterior/anterolateral/lateral approaches for resection of, 219–223
    complications of, 219–223
    transmaxillary approach for resection of, 235, 236, 242–243

Extradural tumors (contd.)
  transoral approach for resection of, 225–234
    anesthesia for, 227
    bleeding and, 232
    bone grafting and, 232
    cases illustrating, 232–234
    closure in, 231–232
      of hard and soft palates, 232
    complications of, 232
    diagnosis and, 225–226
    dural closure in, 231–232
    exposure for, 228–230
    intradural surgery and, 231
    and lesions above foramen magnum, 230–231
    and lesions below foramen magnum, 228
    operative technique for, 227–231
    patient position for, 227–228
    patient selection for, 226–227
    postoperative management for, 232
    technical problems with, 232
Extraocular muscles, 100, 101
  after cavernous sinus tumor resection, 602
Extraperiosteal approach, in anterior orbitotomy, 773, 774
Extreme lateral transcondylar and transjugular approaches, 175–181, 389–411, 611
  anesthesia for, 390
  cases illustrating, 205, 208–210, 213–218, 400–405, 406–409
  cerebrospinal fluid leakage and, 399–400
  for clival tumors, 175–181
  complications of, 399–400
  cranial nerve function and, 399
  disadvantages of, 181
  neurologic deficits and, 399
  operative procedure for, 390–394, 395, 396
  operative technique for, 390–397
  patient positioning for, 390
  for petroclival meningiomas, 611, 657
    cases illustrating, 618–619, 620, 626–630, 631–635, 647, 648–653
  for posterior fossa lesions
    complications of surgery and, 399
    extent of tumor resection and, 398–399
  postoperative care and, 397
  preoperative evaluation for, 389–390
  reconstruction after, 180–181
  results of, 397–400
  for spinal lesions
    cases illustrating, 404–410
    complications of surgery and, 399–400
    extent of tumor resection and, 399
    stability and, 394–397, 399
    tumor resection extent and, 398–399
Eye
  displacement of, after juvenile angiofibroma surgery, 489
  protection of in paranasal/nasal sinus carcinoma resection, 499
  reanimation of, in paralyzed face without facial nerve, 449–450, 450–454
Eyeball, 101
Eyelid spring implantation technique, for eye reanimation in paralyzed face without facial nerve, 458–459
  adjunctive static procedures and, 451–454
  closed, 454
  open, 450–454

F

Face, paralyzed without facial nerve, reanimation of, 449–459
  adjunctive static techniques and, 455–459
  examples of results of, 458–459
  eye and, 449–450, 450–454
  gold weight implantation technique for, 450, 451
  lower face and, 454–455, 456–458
  mouth and, 454–455, 456–458
  open eyelid spring implantation technique in, 450–454
  temporalis muscle transposition technique in, 454–455, 456–458
Face-lift, and reanimation of paralyzed face without facial nerve, 455
Facial deformity, after juvenile angiofibroma surgery, 489
Facial-to-facial reconstruction, and translabyrinthine approach for petrous apex lesions, 294
Facial incisions, in facial translocation approach, 249–250, 251
Facial nerve (cranial nerve VII)
  acoustic neuroma removal and, 687, 688, 689, 690, 718
  anatomic course of, 436
  branches of, 436
  clinical assessment of function of, 443
  in combined lateral suboccipital-infralabyrinthine approach, 385
  decompression of
    middle fossa approach for, 376
    translabyrinthine approach for, 362
  exit zone of, 137–138
  facial translocation approach and, 249, 250, 438, 440, 441
  grafting, 435, 440–443, 444, 445
  identification of in patients previously operated on, 443
  in infratemporal fossa approach for glomus jugulare tumors, 752
  intracisternal course of, 141
  intraoperative monitoring of function of, 95, 96
    during cavernous sinus surgery, 534
    during transcochlear approach, 363
  isolation of, 436–437, 438
  in jugular foramen neurilemoma resection, 733–734
  management of in cranial base surgery, 435–447
    planning, 435, 436
  middle fossa approach for decompression and repair of, 376
  mobilization of, 437, 438, 440
  and otologic approaches to acoustic neuroma, 723
  peripheral branching of, 436, 438
  petroclival meningiomas and, 606
  postoperative loss of function of, 444–446
  protection of during surgery, 435, 436
  reanimation of face without, 449–459
    adjunctive static techniques and, 455–459
    examples of results of, 458–459
    eye and, 449–450, 450–454
    gold weight implantation technique for, 450, 451
    lower face and, 454–455, 456–458
    mouth and, 454–455, 456–458
    open eyelid spring implantation technique in, 450–454
    temporalis muscle transposition technique in, 454–455, 456–458
  reconstruction/repair of, 435–447, 726, 727
    complications of, 446
    concerns in, 443
    after facial nerve neurilemoma resection, 726, 727
    follow-up care and, 446
    graft for, 435, 440–443, 444, 445
    middle fossa approach for, 376
    neurorrhaphy for, 438–440
    planning, 436, 437
    postoperative care and, 444–446
    preoperative care and, 443–444
    primary, 438–440
    surgical steps in, 435–443
    translabyrinthine approach for, 362
  resection of during surgery, 435
  risks to in skull base surgery, 834
  target organs of, 436
  translabyrinthine approach and
    for acoustic neurilemoma resection, 718
    for decompression or repair, 362
    dissection in, 359–360
    identification and, 359
    for petrous apex lesions, 293–294
  vascularity of, protection of, 443
Facial nerve graft, 435, 440–443, 444, 445
Facial nerve neurilemomas, 725–730
  diagnosis of, 725
  location of, 725, 726
  surgical resection of
    cases illustrating, 727, 728, 729
    complications of, 728
    follow-up for, 728
    planning, 725
    postoperative care and, 727
    procedures for, 725–726
    recommendations for, 728–729
    statistical analyses related to, 728–729
Facial nerve neurinomas, 305
Facial nerve neuromas, and translabyrinthine approach for facial nerve decompression or repair, 362
Facial nerve trauma, 305
Facial neurorrhaphy, 438–440, 441
Facial osteotomy, in anterolateral craniofacial resection, 151, 153, 154
Facial paralysis, after facial nerve neurilemoma resection, 728
Facial scars, and facial translocation approach, 249–250, 251
Facial translocation approach, to nasopharynx/clivus/infratemporal fossa, 245–259
  complications of, 253, 256
  craniofacial skeleton and, 251, 252
  facial incisions/scars and, 249, 251, 438, 440
  facial nerve and, 249, 250, 438, 440, 441
  follow-up and, 258
  indications for, 245–248, 253, 258
  infraorbital nerve and, 250–251, 252
  and midfacial split approach, 257–258
  nasal mucosa and, 251
  nasolacrimal duct and, 250, 251
  planning for, 245–248
  postoperative care for, 256
  preoperative care for, 253–256
  specific concerns in, 248–253
  surgical steps in, 247, 248
  temporalis muscle and, 253
  vascularity and, 248

Facial weakness, after translabyrinthine approach, 362
Fascia lata graft, and transsphenoidal surgery for invasive lesions, 344, 345
Fascia lata slings, in facial nerve reconstruction, 443, 444
"Fat hernia", 113
Fentanyl
  for cranial base surgery, 73
  effects of, 70
  for otological approaches to acoustic neurilemoma, 715
Fiberoptic laryngoscopy, for transoral approach, 227
Fibrin glue, for cavernous sinus tumor surgery, 534
Fibrous dysplasia
  imaging characteristics of, 26
  surgical resection and, 810
    optic nerve involvement and, 811–812
File servers, for NeuroNet, 86
Fissures
  cerebellar-brain stem, acoustic neuromas and, 691–693, 699
  olfactory, alloplastic materials in reconstruction for, 468
  orbital
    inferior, 99, 100, 112
    superior, 99, 101, 103–104
  petrotympanic, 113
  sphenomaxillary, 113
Fixed orbital retractors, 772
Flaps. See also Grafts
  craniotomy, in petrosal approach for clival tumors, 308–309
  hemipalatal, in transmandibular-transcervical approach, 263, 264
  latissimus dorsi, 430–433
  pectoralis muscle (myocutaneous), 417, 420, 421
  pericranial, 414, 415, 416
  rectus abdominis, 427–430
  scalp, 417, 419–420
    bicoronal
      for reconstruction after anterior craniofacial resection, 151, 152
      for subfrontal approach for craniopharyngiomas, 792, 793
  soft tissue, for facial translocation approach, vascularity of, 248
  temporalis fascia, for middle fossa approach for petrous apex lesions, 295
  temporalis muscle, 415–417, 418, 419
  trapezius muscle (myocutaneous), 417–421
Flocculus, acoustic neuromas and, 693–695, 696
Fluid management, during cranial base surgery, 74–75
Fluothane, for glomus vagale tumor surgery, 765
Follicle-stimulating hormone deficiency, after craniopharyngioma surgery, 804
Follow-up care, 9–10. See also specific procedure
  after anterior and anterolateral craniofacial resection, 155
  after cavernous sinus tumor surgery, 603–604
  after craniofacial disassembly and reconstruction, 425
  after craniopharyngioma surgery, 805

  for facial nerve management and reconstruction, 444–446
  after facial translocation surgery, 258
  after juvenile angiofibroma surgery, 489–491
  after latissimus dorsi flap, 433
  after rectus abdominis flap, 430
  after regional flaps, 425
Foramen (foramina). See also specific type
  jugular, 135, 136
    condylar emissary vein and, 135
    nerves and vessels passing through, 135
    tumors of, 379–387
      cervical exposure for resection of, 381
      combined lateral suboccipital-infralabyrinthine approach for resection of, 381–386
      diagnosis of, 379–381
      distribution of types of, 379
      lateral suboccipital route for resection of, 381
      neurilemomas, 731–735
      neurinomas, 305
      occipito-transmastoid-cervical approach for resection of, 301–304
      surgical approach for resection of, 381–386
      transtemporal and infratemporal approach for resection of, 267–289
  of Luschka, acoustic neuromas and, 693–695, 696
  magnum
    blood supply of, 132
    cranial nerve dysfunction after surgery on, 834
    extreme lateral transcondylar and transjugular approaches to, 392, 400–404, 405, 406, 407
    transcondyle approach for meningiomas of, 671–678
      anesthesia for, 672
      cases illustrating, 674, 675–677
      complications of, 675
      craniospinal type, 675, 676–677
      craniotomy for, 672
      diagnosis and, 671
      laminectomy for, 672
      operative technique for, 671–674
      patient positioning for, 672
      postoperative management for, 675
      skin incision for, 672
      spinocranial type, 673, 674, 675–676
      surgical steps in, 672, 673
    transoral approach to
      for lesions above, 230–231
      for lesions below, 228
  mastoid emissary, 135
  ovale, 104, 115
  rotundum, 104, 115
  spinosum, 104
  of Vesalius, 104
Forceps, for cranial base tumors, 7
Fossa, cranial. See Cranial fossa
Four-vessel angiography, for transmaxillary approach, 533
Fourth segment of vertebral artery, 120
Free-fat graft, in temporal fossa after temporalis muscle transfer, 417, 419
Free-flap reconstruction, 427–433
  with anterior cranio-orbital resection, for adenoid cystic carcinoma, 500, 503–504

Frialit plates, in skull base reconstruction, 461
Frontal approach, extended (basal), for clival tumors, 171–175
  cases illustrating, 190–194, 200–201, 202–207
  disadvantages of, 175
  entry into sphenoid sinus in, 173, 174
  orbito-fronto-ethmoidal osteotomy in, 171, 172–173
  reconstruction and, 175
  subtemporal-infratemporal approach combined with, 175, 176, 177
  tumor resection in, 173–174
Frontal bone flap, for craniofacial resection for esthesioneuroblastoma, 473, 474
Frontal lobe, 103
Frontal mucocele, site of origin of, 20
Frontal nerve, 101
  in cavernous sinus, 530
Frontal ostium, 126–127
Frontal recess, 124
Frontal sinus, 126–127
  cerebrospinal fluid leak at, 835
  posterior wall of, alloplastic materials in reconstruction of, 468
Frontobasal artery, anterior cranial fossa supplied by, 103
Frontobasal fracture, reconstruction with alloplastic materials for, 464, 465
Frontonasal duct, 126–127
Frontonasal osteotomy, in anterior craniofacial resection, 150
Frontotemporal approach
  extended (basal), cases illustrating, 198–199
  and preauricular infratemporal approach, for petroclival meningiomas, cases illustrating, 630–635, 635–639
Frontotemporal craniotomy
  in cavernous sinus surgery, 535–537
  for clival chordomas, 679
  in frontotemporal transcavernous and transpetrous apex approach for petroclival meningioma resection, 609
  in frontotemporal-transsylvian/anterior subtemporal approach with zygomatic osteotomy, 608
Frontotemporal-orbitozygomatic approach combined, 775–781
  for intraorbital tumors with and without intracranial extension, 781–785
  for sphenoid wing, orbit, and middle fossa tumors, 775–781
  and transcavernous approach, for petroclival meningioma resection, 657
Frontotemporal sphenoidal craniotomy, in en bloc orbitectomy, 781, 783
Frontotemporal transcavernous and presigmoid and transsigmoid transpetrous approach, for petroclival meningiomas, cases illustrating, 639–647, 648
Frontotemporal transcavernous and transpetrous apex approach, for petroclival meningiomas, 608–611
  cases illustrating, 639–647, 648
Frontotemporal transsylvian approach
  and anterior subtemporal approach with zygomatic osteotomy, for petroclival meningioma resection, 608, 657
  and total petrosectomy, for petroclival meningioma resection, cases illustrating, 647–656

Fukushima modification of combined petrosal approach for petroclival lesions, 662
Fungal sinusitis, imaging characteristics of, 26
Furosemide
　for combined frontotemporal-orbitozygomatic approach for tumors of sphenoid wing and orbit, 775
　for petroclival meningioma surgery, 607

G

Gait ataxia, in petroclival meningioma, 606
Giant acoustic neuroma, operative approaches for, 663
Giant cavernoma, operative approaches for, 663
Gigli saw, for tuberculum sella and olfactory groove meningioma surgery, 509
Glass-ionomer cement, in skull base reconstruction, 461, 469
Glomus jugulare tumors, 747–762
　clinical presentation of, 747
　diagnosis of, 747–748
　extreme lateral transcondylar and transjugular approaches for resection of, 389, 398
　infratemporal fossa approach for resection of, 752–757
　　with intracranial extension, 756–757
　petroclival, 219
　surgical resection of
　　anesthesia for, 749
　　cases illustrating, 758–759, 760–761
　　complication prophylaxis and, 757
　　operative approaches for, 749
　　operative technique for, 749
　　patient positioning for, 749
　　patient selection for, 748
　　postoperative management and, 757
　　technical problems and, 749
　　transtemporal and infratemporal approach for resection of, 286–289
　　transtemporal skull base approach for resection of, 749–752
Glomus vagale tumors, 763–768
　bilateral, surgical intervention and, 765
　clinical presentation and, 763–764
　diagnosis of, 763–764
　paragangliomas and, 763
　surgical intervention and, 765
　patient age and, surgical intervention and, 764
　surgical resection of
　　anesthesia for, 765
　　complications of, 768
　　operative technique for, 765–768
　　patient positioning for, 766
　　patient selection for, 764–765
　　postoperative management for, 768
　　steps in, 766, 767
　　technical considerations for, 766–768
Glossopharyngeal nerve (cranial nerve IX), 116
　acoustic neuroma and, 690, 691
　in combined lateral suboccipital-infralabyrinthine approach, 385
　exit zone of, 138–139
　intracisternal course of, 141
　intraoperative monitoring of function of, 95
　and otologic approaches to acoustic neuroma, 723

in petroclival meningioma, 606
risks to in skull base surgery, 834
swallowing dysfunction caused by injury to
　complex nerve injury, 820–821
　single nerve injury, 820
Glottic closure, in swallowing dysfunction, 822
Gold weight implantation technique
　for eye reanimation in paralyzed face without facial nerve, 450, 451, 458
　adjunctive static procedures and, 451–454
　for postoperative facial paralysis, 443, 445
Gonadal failure, in craniopharyngioma, 789
Grafts. See also Flaps
　bone, transoral approach and, 232
　bypass
　　anterior circulation, 64–65
　　carotid artery, imaging in assessment of patency of, 29, 30
　　cervical to petrous carotid
　　　results of, 62
　　　revascularization and, 62
　　extracranial-to-distal middle cerebral artery, 63–64
　　extracranial-internal carotid, 63–65
　　extracranial-to-proximal anterior circulation arteries, 64–65
　　P-S, 52–61
　　　results of, 62
　　posterior circulation, 65
　facial nerve, 440–443, 444, 445
　fascia lata, and transsphenoidal surgery for invasive lesions, 344, 345
　free-fat, in temporal fossa after temporalis muscle transfer, 417, 419
　pericranial, for reconstruction after anterior craniofacial resection, 151
　petrosal to upper cervical ICA interposition, 50–52, 53–54
　vein, results of, 61–62
　venous patch, in cerebral revascularization, 50, 51, 52
　vertebral artery interposition, 61
Granulomas
　cholesterol
　　imaging characteristics of, 23, 26
　　petroclival, 219
　　site of origin of, 20
　　transsphenoidal approach for resection of, 349
Great cerebral vein, 133
Greater auricular nerve, course of, 437
Greater auricular nerve graft, for reconstruction of facial nerve, 435, 441, 442–443
Greater petrosal nerve, 104–105
Growth hormone replacement, after craniopharyngioma surgery, 804
Growth rate, after craniopharyngioma surgery, 804

H

Hakuba modification of combined petrosal approach for petroclival lesions, 662
Haller's cells, 125–126
Halothane, effects of, 70
Hard palate
　paranasal/nasal sinus carcinoma and, 498–499
　transoral approach and, 230–231
　closure of, 232

Headache
　in craniopharyngioma, 789
　in juvenile angiofibroma, 485, 486
　in petroclival meningioma, 606
Hearing loss
　and central electroauditory prosthesis, 825–829
　in glomus jugulare tumors, 747
　and petrous apex lesions, 291–292
　after transmandibular-transcervical surgery, 265
　after transtemporal and infratemporal surgery, 276
Heat loss, as intraoperative complication, 79
Hemangiomas, cavernous
　cavernous sinus, indications for surgical resection of, 533
　intracavernous, cases illustrating surgical resection of, 554–562, 563
　orbital, transconjunctival approach for, 773
Hemangiopericytomas
　petrous bone, 318
　transsphenoidal approach for resection of, 349
Hematoma
　after petroclival meningioma surgery, 658
　after skull base surgery, 832–833
　after transmandibular-transcervical surgery, 265
　after tuberculum sella and olfactory groove meningioma surgery, 516
Hemipalatal flap, in transmandibular-transcervical approach, 263, 264
Hemiparesis, and petroclival meningioma surgery, 658
Hemisensory loss, in petroclival meningioma, 606
Hemodynamics, systemic, anesthetic agents affecting, 70
Hemolytic transfusion reaction, 77
Hemorrhage. See also Bleeding
　and otological approaches to acoustic neurilemomas, 722
　and petroclival meningioma surgery, 658
　and transzygomatic and transpalatal resection of juvenile nasopharyngeal angiofibroma, 480
Heubner's recurrent artery, anterior cranial fossa supplied by, 103
Hitselberger-House modification of combined petrosal approach for petroclival lesions, 662
Hormone deficiencies, after craniopharyngioma surgery, 804
Hourglass trigeminal neurilemomas
　cases illustrating, 739–740, 740, 741, 742–743, 744
　diagnosis of, 737–738
　surgical approach for, 739
House Urban dissector
　for transcochlear approach, 364
　for translabyrinthine approach, 357, 358, 361
Hydrocephalus. See also Increased intracranial pressure
　in craniopharyngiomas, 789
　preoperative management of, 792
　after petroclival meningioma surgery, 658
　after tuberculum sella and olfactory groove meningioma surgery, 516–517
Hyperglycemia, outcome of ischemic injury affected by, 75
Hyperostosing meningioma "en plaque", surgical resection of, 810–811

Hyperperfusion hemorrhage and edema, and cerebral revascularization, 65–66
Hyperphagia, in craniopharyngioma, 789
Hyperventilation with anesthesia, 73
  facilitating surgical exposure and, 75–76
  intracranial pressure affected by, 70
  for petroclival meningioma surgery, 607
Hypoglossal canal, venous plexus of, 135
Hypoglossal-to-facial anastomosis, and translabyrinthine approach for petrous apex lesions, 294
Hypoglossal nerve (cranial nerve XII), 117–118
  and acoustic neuroma, 690
  in combined lateral suboccipital-infralabyrinthine approach, 385
  exit zone of, 139
  intracisternal course of, 141
  intraoperative monitoring of function of, 95
  in petroclival meningioma, 606
  risks to in skull base surgery, 834
  swallowing dysfunction caused by injury to
    complex nerve injury, 820–821
    single nerve injury, 820
Hypoglossal venous plexus, 135
Hypophyseal area, 105–120
  cavernous sinus in, 106
  dura mater of, 106, 107
  inferior skull base anatomy and, 112–114
  infratemporal fossa in, 118–120
  internal carotid artery supplying, 110, 111
  muscles of inferior cranial base and, 115–116
  nerves of inferior skull base and, 116–118
  nerves in lateral wall of cavernous sinus and, 109–110
  osteology of, 105–106
  pituitary cisterns in, 106–109
  portals for nerves and vessels and, 115
  variations of sella turcica and, 106
  vertebral artery and veins in, 120
  vessels of parapharyngeal space and, 118
Hypophyseal arteries
  accessory, 108
  superior, 106–108, 528
Hypophyseal fossa, 105
Hypophyseal veins, 109
Hypothalamic disturbances, after craniopharyngioma surgery, 805
Hypothalamus, dissection of, in tuberculum sella meningioma surgery, 512
Hypothermia
  cranial base anesthetic management and, 3
  as intraoperative complication, 79
  petroclival meningioma surgery and, 607
Hypovolemia, during cranial base surgery, 74

I

ICA. *See* Internal carotid artery
ICP. *See* Intracranial pressure
IGFs. *See* Insulin-like growth factors
Immunoperoxidase studies, for evaluation of esthesioneuroblastoma, 471
Impedance testing, and petrous apex lesions, 292
Inappropriate secretion of antidiuretic hormone, after cavernous sinus tumor surgery, 602
Incision, skin. *See* Exposure
Incisura Rivini, 113
Increased intracranial pressure. *See also* Hydrocephalus
  in craniopharyngioma, 789
  preoperative management of, 792
  after tuberculum sella and olfactory groove meningioma surgery, 517
Infections, after skull base surgery, 9, 838–839
  craniofacial resection for paranasal sinus tumors and, 505
  factors influencing incidence of, 838–839
  osseous lesion (anterior and middle base) surgery and, 817
  transmandibular-transcervical surgery and, 265
  treatment of, 839
Inferior approach, for cavernous sinus surgery, 539
Inferior cavernous sinus artery, 521
Inferior cerebellar artery
  anterior, 142–143
    acoustic neuromas and, 695–697, 698
  posterior, extreme lateral transcondylar and transjugular approaches for resection of, 398
Inferior head of lateral pterygoid muscle, 115
Inferior olive, 137
Inferior orbital fissure, 99, 100, 112
Inferior petrosal sinus, 134–135
  termination of, 135–136
Inferior skull base
  anatomy of, 112–115
  muscles of, 115–116
  nerves of, 116–118
  veins of, 119
Inferolateral recess, 130
Inferolateral trunk, 108
Infralabyrinthine approach
  for jugular foramen tumors, 384
  and lateral suboccipital approach, 381–386
    advantages of, 385–386
    cranial nerve affected in, 384, 385
    patient positioning for, 381
    results of, 384–386
    steps in, 382–383
Infraorbital artery, 102
Infraorbital nerve, in facial translocation approach, 250–251, 252
Infratemporal approach
  for benign tumors of jugular foramen and temporal bone, 267–289
    anesthesia for, 269
    case studies illustrating, 276–289
    choice of surgical approach and, 268–269
    complications of, 275–276
    incision for, 269–270
    infratemporal fossa exposure in, 270–271, 272
    for limited lesions, 273, 274, 275
    operative technique for, 269–275
    patient position for, 269
    planning for, 267
    posterior fossa tumor resection and, 273, 274
    preoperative evaluation for, 267–268
    reconstruction after, 273–275
    soft tissue dissection in, 270
    transtemporal dissection in, 271–273
    tumor isolation in, 273
  and frontotemporal approach, for petroclival meningiomas, cases illustrating, 630–635, 635–639
  for glomus jugulare tumors, 752–757
    with intracranial extension, 756–757
  and subtemporal approach
    for clival tumors, 161–171
      cases illustrating, 190–194, 195–197, 198–199, 200–201, 202–207, 211, 213–218
      disadvantages of, 171
      division of V_3 in, 167, 169, 170
      reconstruction after, 167–171
      skin incision for, 162
    for petroclival meningiomas, 612, 657
      cases illustrating, 620–626, 626–630
Infratemporal fossa, 113, 118–119
  anatomy of, 246
  exposure of, 270–271, 272
  facial translocation approach to, 245–259
    complications of, 253, 256
    craniofacial skeleton and, 251, 252
    facial incisions/scars and, 249, 251
    facial nerve and, 249, 250, 438, 440, 441
    follow-up and, 258
    indications for, 245–248, 253, 258
    infraorbital nerve and, 250–251, 252
    midfacial split approach and, 257–258
    nasal mucosa and, 251
    nasolacrimal duct and, 250, 251
    planning for, 245–248
    postoperative care for, 256
    preoperative care for, 253–256
    specific concerns in, 248–253
    surgical steps in, 247, 248
    temporalis muscle and, 253
    vascularity and, 248
Infratemporal fossa approach, for glomus jugulare tumors, 752–757
  with intracranial extension, 756–757
Infratemporal head, of lateral pterygoid muscle, 115
Infratemporal spine, 113
Instrumentation
  for cranial base surgery, 4–8, 13–14
    from otolaryngologic and plastic surgery, 13–14
  for NeuroNet, 86–87
  for orbital surgery, 772
  for paranasal/nasal sinus carcinoma resection, 499
  for retrosigmoid approach for acoustic neuromas, 705, 708
Insulin levels, after craniopharyngioma surgery, 804
Insulin-like growth factors, after craniopharyngioma surgery, 804–805
Intermastoid line, 113
Internal acoustic meatus, 144–146
Internal auditory canal
  decompression of for bilateral acoustic tumors, 377
  dissection of in translabyrinthine approach, 354–356
Internal carotid artery, 110, 111, 118
  anterior cranial fossa supplied by, 103
  balloon test occlusion of, 33–36
    in assessing need for revascularization, 45
    before cavernous sinus surgery, 533
    for evaluation of petroclival meningiomas, 607
    for evaluation of petrous bone tumors, 318
    for evaluation of trigeminal neurilemomas, 738
    in preoperative patient evaluation, 3
  cavernous, 521, 522, 528
    meningioma resection and, 545–547
      with grafting, 534–535
      without grafting, 535
      reconstruction and, 547–548

Internal carotid artery, cavernous (contd.)
  clinoidal, 526
  and glomus jugulare tumors, 747
  occlusion of, and revascularization, 45
  petrous
    in cavernous sinus, 525
      exposure of, 538–539
    meningioma encasing, case illustrating surgical resection of, 647–656
    reconstruction of, 322–323, 324, 325
    in subtemporal and infratemporal approach for clival tumor resection, 164–167, 168, 169
    transtemporal and infratemporal approach for tumors around, 269, 273, 276–278
  reconstruction of, after cavernous meningioma surgery, 547–548, 602
  supraclinoid cavernous sinus, and petrosal artery bypass, 52–61
    results of, 62
Internal jugular vein, 119
Interventional neuroradiology, 37–44
  in preoperative patient evaluation, 3
Intracranial approach, for juvenile angiofibroma surgery, with extracranial approach, 488–489, 492–495
Intracranial contents, anesthetic agents affecting, 69–71
Intracranial hemorrhage. See Hemorrhage
Intracranial pressure
  anesthetic agents affecting, 70, 71
  increased. See also Hydrocephalus
    in craniopharyngiomas, 789
      preoperative management of, 792
    after tuberculum sella and olfactory groove meningioma surgery, 517
Intradural approach
  for cavernous chondrosarcoma resection, 549–550
  for cavernous chordoma resection, 549–550
  for cavernous meningioma resection, 540–549
    anterior clinoid process and, 541, 542
    cranial base reconstruction after, 549
    cranial nerves and, 545, 546
      reconstruction of, 548–549
    internal carotid artery and, 545–547
    intracavernous dissection in, 545–547
    lateral wall dissection in, 543–545
    optic nerve and, 541, 542
    petroclival bone and, 548
    petrous apex and, 548
    pituitary gland and, 548
    reconstruction after, 548–549
    subdural tumor resection and, 541
    superior approach in, 543
    sylvian dissection in, 540
    temporal lobe resection in, 540
    vascular reconstruction and, 547–548
    venous bleeding and, 547
  transoral, 231
Intradural hematomas, after skull base surgery, 832–833
Intradural tumors
  transmaxillary approach for, 242–243
  transoral approach for, 225–234
    anesthesia for, 227
    bleeding and, 232
    bone grafting and, 232
    case studies illustrating, 232–234
    closure for, 231–232
      of hard and soft palates, 232
    complications of, 232
    diagnosis and, 225–226
    dural closure in, 231–232
    exposure for, 228–230
    intradural surgery and, 231
    and lesions above foramen magnum, 230–231
    and lesions below foramen magnum, 228
    operative technique for, 227–231
    patient position for, 227–228
    patient selection and, 226–227
    postoperative management for, 232
    technical problems with, 232
Intraoperative neurophysiologic monitoring, 83–98
  anesthesia and, 71–72, 89
  of auditory system, 93–94
  during cavernous sinus surgery, 534
  computer network architecture for, 85–86
  of cranial nerve function, electromyography for, 95–96
  of electroencephalogram, 89–91
  general procedures for, 88–89
  instrumentation for, 86–87
  measures used in, 88–96
  during petroclival meningioma surgery, 607–608
  during petrosal approach for clival tumors, 308
  during petrous bone tumor surgery, 318
  Pittsburgh approach for, 83–85
  during retrosigmoid approach to acoustic neuromas, 703, 706, 707
  signal processing algorithms for, 87
  of somatosensory system, 91–93
  system for, 85–87
  for trigeminal neurilemoma surgery, 738
  of visual system, 94–95
Intrapetrous aneurysm, site of origin of, 20
"Inverse steal" syndrome, 78
Ionos bone cement (glass-ionomer cement), in skull base reconstruction, 461, 469
Ischemia, cerebral
  and carotid cross-clamping, 78
  revascularization complicated by, 65
Isoflurane, for cranial base anesthetic management, 3, 71, 74
  effects of, 70
  neurophysiologic monitoring and, 89
  for otological approaches to acoustic neurilemoma, 715
  for petroclival meningioma surgery, 607

J
Jaw, upper, accurate replacement of after transmaxillary surgery, 240
JNA. See Juvenile nasopharyngeal angiofibroma
Jugular bulb
  tearing of, in translabyrinthine approach, 356
  transtemporal and infratemporal approach for tumors of, 268–269, 273, 274, 276–278
Jugular foramen, 135, 136
  condylar emissary vein and, 135
  nerves and vessels passing through, 135
  tumors of, 379–387
    cervical exposure for resection of, 381
    combined lateral suboccipital-infralabyrinthine approach for resection of, 381–386
      advantages of, 385–386
      cranial nerve affected in, 384, 385
      patient positioning for, 381
      results of, 384–386
      steps in, 382–383
    diagnosis of, 379–381
    distribution of types of, 379
    lateral suboccipital route for resection of, 381
    neurilemomas, 731–735
    neurinomas, 305
    occipito-transmastoid-cervical approach for resection of, 301–304
    surgical approach for resection of, 381–386
    transtemporal and infratemporal approach for resection of, 267–289
      anesthesia for, 269
      cases illustrating, 276–289
      choice of surgical approach and, 268–269
      complications of, 275–276
      operative technique for, 269–275
      patient position for, 269
      planning for, 267
      preoperative evaluation for, 267–268
Jugular foramen neurilemomas, 731–735
  classification of, 731
  clinical presentation of, 731
  diagnosis of, 731
  surgical resection of
    anesthesia for, 732
    exposure for, 733
    operative technique for, 732–735
    patient positioning for, 732
Jugular foramen neurinomas, 305
Jugular fossa, transtemporal and infratemporal approach for tumors of, 278, 279–282
Jugular paragangliomas, embolization of, 42, 43
Jugular vein, internal, 119
Juvenile angiofibroma. See Juvenile nasopharyngeal angiofibroma
Juvenile nasopharyngeal angiofibroma, 485–496
  cavernous sinus, 603
    indications for surgical resection of, 533
  combined extracranial-intracranial approach for resection of, 488–489, 492–495
  diagnosis of, 485–486
  differential diagnosis of, 485
  endonasal microendoscopic approach without external incision for resection of, 486, 491
  extracranial approach for resection of, 486–488
  imaging characteristics of, 21, 26
  with intracranial extension, 477–484, 485
  midfacial degloving technique for resection of, 487
  radiation therapy for, 486
  site of origin of, 21, 485
  spontaneous remission of, 486
  spread of, 485
  surgical resection of
    anesthesia for, 486
    cases illustrating, 489, 490, 491–495
    complications of, 489–491
    operative techniques for, 486–489
    patient positioning for, 486
    patient selection for, 486

postoperative management after, 489
preoperative planning for, 485–486
symptoms of, 485, 486
transfacial technique through an extended Moure incision for resection of, 487–488, 490–491, 491–492, 493
transzygomatic and transpalatal excision of, 477–484
anesthesia for, 477
cases illustrating, 480–483
complications of, 480
operative technique for, 477–480
patient positioning for, 478
patient selection for, 477
postoperative management of, 480
preoperative preparation for, 477
technical problems in, 480
transpalatal stage of, 479–480
transzygomatic stage of, 478–479
vascularity of, 485

K
Karnofsky scores, for petrous bone tumors, 334
Keratitis, neurotrophic, after cavernous sinus tumor surgery, 602
Ketamine, brain metabolic demand and, 71
"Key/keyhole" pattern of osteotomies, 421, 423
Kuhnt-Sztmanowsky procedure, in eye reanimation, 451

L
Labbe's vein, preservation of with middle fossa approach for petrous apex lesions, 297
Labyrinthectomy, in translabyrinthine approach, 353–354
Lacrimal artery, 102
Lacrimal canaliculi, stenting, in facial translocation approach, 250, 251
Lacrimal drainage, after juvenile angiofibroma surgery
impairment of, 489
preservation of, in transfacial technique through extended Moure incision, 488
Lacrimal gland, 102
tumors of, en bloc orbitectomy for, 781, 783–785
Lacrimal nerve, 101, 102
Lamina terminalis, in craniopharyngioma resection, 797–799
Laminae pterygospinosae, 113
Laminectomy, in transcondyle approach for foramen magnum meningiomas, 672
Laryngeal nerve
recurrent, swallowing dysfunction caused by injury to, 820
superior, swallowing dysfunction caused by injury to, 820
Laryngectomy, in swallowing dysfunction, 822
Laryngotracheal separation, in swallowing dysfunction, 821, 822
Laser surgery, for cranial base tumors, 4–8
Lateral approach
for glomus vagale tumors, 765–768
anesthesia for, 765
complications of, 768
patient positioning for, 766
postoperative management and, 768
steps in, 766, 767
technical considerations for, 766–768
to orbit, 771, 773–775, 776–778
Lateral canthal incision, for facial translocation approach, 249
Lateral cavernous sinus wall dissection, for cavernous meningioma resection, 543–545
Lateral frontobasal artery, anterior cranial fossa supplied by, 103
Lateral medullary vein, acoustic neuroma and, 699
Lateral orbital wall, 102
Lateral orbitotomy, 771, 773–775, 776–778
incision for, 773–774, 775
Lateral position, for transoral approach, 227
Lateral pterygoid muscle, 114, 115
Lateral recesses, superior and inferior, 129
Lateral rectus muscle, 102
Lateral suboccipital route, for jugular foramen tumors, 381
Lateral suboccipital-infralabyrinthine approach, for jugular foramen tumors, 381–386
advantages of, 385–386
cranial nerve affected in, 384, 385
patient positioning for, 381
results of, 384–386
steps in, 382–383
Lateral torus, 124
Lateral transcondylar and transjugular approaches, extreme, 175–181, 389–411, 611
anesthesia for, 390
cases illustrating, 205, 208–210, 213–218, 400–405, 406–409
cerebrospinal fluid leakage and, 399–400
for clival tumors, 175–181
complications of, 399–400
cranial nerve function and, 399
disadvantages of, 181
neurologic deficits and, 399
operative procedure for, 390–394, 395, 396
operative technique for, 390–397
patient positioning for, 390
for petroclival meningiomas, 611, 657
cases illustrating, 618–619, 620, 626–630, 631–635, 647, 648–653
for posterior fossa lesions
complications of surgery and, 399
extent of tumor resection and, 398–399
postoperative care and, 397
preoperative evaluation for, 389–390
reconstruction after, 180–181
results of, 397–400
for spinal lesions
cases illustrating, 404–410
complications of surgery and, 399–400
extent of tumor resection and, 399
stability and, 394–397, 399
tumor resection extent and, 398–399
Lateral venous sinus, and glomus jugulare tumor surgery, 750
Lateral wall dissection, for cavernous meningioma resection, 543–545
Latissimus dorsi flap, 430–433
follow-up care for, 433
planning for, 430–431
surgical steps for, 431–433
Laudanosine, brain metabolic demand and, 71
Lazy "S" incision, for lateral orbitotomy, 773–774, 775
Le Fort I osteotomy, in facial translocation approach, 251
Le Fort maxillectomy, extended maxillectomy and, 240–241
Lessor petrosal nerve, 104
Levator palpebrae superioris muscle, 100, 101
nerve to, preservation of during surgery, 101
Levator veli palatini muscle, 116
Liliequist membrane, in tuberculum sella meningioma surgery, 512
Limb ataxia, in petroclival meningioma, 606
Limbus sphenoidalis, 105
Locked in syndrome, and petroclival meningioma surgery, 658
Long tract deficits, and otologic approaches to acoustic neuroma, 723
Lower clivus, 157, 158, 606. *See also* Clivus
approach selection for tumors of, 157–159
Lower facial reanimation, 454–455, 456–458
Lumbar drain
after transmaxillary surgery, 240
after transoral surgery, 232
Luschka's foramen, acoustic neuromas and, 693–695, 696
Luteinizing hormone deficiency, after craniopharyngioma surgery, 804
LVS. *See* Lateral venous sinus
Lymphomas, cranial base, imaging characteristics of, 26

M
MacCarty's keyhole, for tuberculum sella and olfactory groove meningioma surgery, 509
McConnell's capsular artery, 521
Macroadenomas, pituitary, transsphenoidal approach for resection of, 342, 343, 346, 347–348
Magnetic resonance imaging
for evaluation of skull base masses, 3, 15–32
avenues of spread and, 26–28
cavernous sinus tumors, 532–533
classification and, 532
craniopharyngiomas, 789
esthesioneuroblastomas, 471
facial nerve neurilemomas, 725
glomus jugulare tumors, 747–748
glomus vagale tumors, 764
as guide to surgical management, 28–29
jugular foramen tumors, 379–380
neurilemomas, 731
juvenile angiofibroma, 485
orbital lesions, 771
osseous lesions, 809
paranasal/nasal sinus carcinoma, 497–498
petroclival meningiomas, 607, 667–669
petrous apex lesions, 293
petrous bone tumors, 318
postoperative evaluation and, 29–32
problem areas in, 29
techniques for, 19
trigeminal neurilemomas, 738
tumor identification and, 19, 20–25, 26
in extreme lateral transcondylar and transjugular approaches, 389
in transmaxillary approach, 235
in transsphenoidal approach for invasive and sellar clival lesions, 337
Malignant choroid plexus papilloma, 318

Malignant external otitis
  imaging characteristics of, 26
  site of origin of, 20, 21
Malis irrigation bipolar, for cranial base surgery, 4, 5
Malis modification of combined petrosal approach for petroclival lesions, 662
Malis subtemporal transtentorial approach, for clival chordomas, 679
Malocclusion
  after transmaxillary surgery, avoiding, 240
  after transtemporal and infratemporal surgery, 276
Mandibular fossa, 113
Mandibular nerve (cranial nerve V_3), 104, 119
  in cavernous sinus
    in lateral wall, 109
    tumor resection and, 602
Mandibulotomy, in transmandibular-transcervical approach, 262
Mannitol
  for combined frontotemporal-orbitozygomatic approach for tumors of sphenoid wing and orbit, 775
  and facilitating surgical exposure, 75
  for otological approaches to acoustic neurilemoma, 716
  for petroclival meningioma surgery, 607
MAP. See Mean arterial pressure
Masseter muscle, origin of, 115–116
Masticatory space, 118–119
Mastoid carcinoma, 379
Mastoid emissary foramen, 135
Mastoid process, 113–115
Mastoid retrosigmoid approach, for acoustic neurilemoma, 720–722
Mastoidectomy
  complete, simple, in translabyrinthine approach, 353
  cortical, in translabyrinthine approach, 352–353
  in extreme lateral transcondylar and transjugular approaches, 392
  in jugular foramen neurilemoma resection, 734
  in occipito-transmastoid-cervical approach, 303
  in retrosigmoid approach for acoustic neurilemoma, 720, 721
Matas test, of internal carotid artery, 33–36. See also Balloon test occlusion
Maxillary artery, 118–119
Maxillary nerve (cranial nerve V_2), 104
  in cavernous sinus
    in lateral wall, 109, 521
    tumor resection and, 602
  neurilemmoma of, 740–743, 745
Maxillary sinus, 125
Maxillary tuber, 112
Maxillectomy
  extended, 240–241
    operative technique for, 241–242
  Le Fort, extended maxillectomy and, 240–241
  in transmandibular-transcervical approach, 263–264
Mayfield headrest
  for transcondyle approach for foramen magnum meningiomas, 672
  for tuberculum sella and olfactory groove meningioma surgery, 508
Mean arterial pressure. See also Blood pressure
  anesthetic agents affecting, 70

Meckel's cave, 526, 532
Medial approach, for cavernous sinus surgery, 540
Medial canthal incision, for facial translocation approach, 249
Medial canthoplasty, in eye reanimation, 451
Medial ethmoidosphenoidal osseous lesions, surgical resection of, 811–812
Medial frontobasal artery, anterior cranial fossa supplied by, 103
Medial orbital vein, 103
Medial orbital wall, 99
Medial pterygoid muscle, 116
Median nerve somatosensory evoked potentials, monitoring during cranial base surgery, 91–93
Medulla, acoustic neuromas and, 689, 690, 692, 695
Medullary vein, lateral, acoustic neuroma and, 699
Memory deficits, in craniopharyngioma, 789
Meningeal artery, anterior cranial fossa supplied by, 103
Meningiomas
  calcified, imaging in evaluation of, 15
  cavernous, 512, 515, 603, 604
    embolization of, 40
    surgical resection of, 540–549
      anterior clinoid process and, 541, 542
      carotid artery and, 545–547
      cases illustrating, 550–554, 555, 570–583, 584, 585–601
      cranial base reconstruction after, 549
      cranial nerves and, 545, 546
        reconstruction of, 548–549
      with ICA grafting, 534–535
      without ICA grafting, 535
      incisions for, 534–535
      indications for, 533
      intracavernous dissection in, 545–547
      lateral wall dissection in, 543–545
      optic nerve and, 541, 542
      petroclival bone and, 548
      petrous apex and, 548
      pituitary gland and, 548
      reconstruction after, 548–549
      subdural tumor resection in, 541
      superior approach for, 543
      sylvian dissection in, 540
      temporal lobe resection in, 540
      vascular reconstruction and, 547–548
      venous bleeding and, 547
  craniocervical, 379
    embolization of, 38–39, 43
    extreme lateral transcondylar and transjugular approaches for, 389, 398, 400–402
    foramen magnum, transcondyle approach for resection of, 671–678
      anesthesia for, 672
      cases illustrating, 674, 675–677
      complications of, 675
      craniospinal type, 675, 676–677
      craniotomy for, 672
      diagnosis and, 671
      laminectomy for, 672
      operative technique for, 671–674
      patient positioning for, 672
      postoperative management for, 675
      skin incision for, 672

      spinocranial type, 673, 674, 675–676
      surgical steps in, 672, 673
    hyperostosing, "en plaque", surgical resection of, 810–811
    imaging characteristics of, 26
    intraosseous, 379
    jugular foramen, 379
    of olfactory groove, 507–519
      diagnosis of, 507
      surgical resection of
        anesthesia for, 508
        cases illustrating, 517, 518
        complications of, 516–517
        operative technique for, 515–516
        patient positioning for, 508
        patient selection for, 507–508
        postoperative management and, 516
    petroclival, 219, 299, 300, 379, 605–659. See also Petroclival tumors
      cavernous sinus involvement and, cases illustrating surgical resection of, 578–579, 580, 581, 585–601
      classification of, 605–606
      clinical presentation of, 606–607
      combined middle-posterior fossa approach for resection of, 300–301
      computed tomography in evaluation of, 667–669
      extreme lateral transcondylar approach for resection of, 611, 657
        cases illustrating, 618–619, 620, 626–630, 631–635, 647, 647–653
      frontotemporal and preauricular infratemporal approach for resection of, cases illustrating, 630–635, 635–639
      frontotemporal transcavernous and transpetrous apex approach for, 608–611
        cases illustrating, 639–647, 648
      frontotemporal-transsylvian/
        anterior subtemporal approach for, with zygomatic osteotomy, 608, 657
      magnetic resonance imaging in evaluation of, 667
      operative approaches for resection of, 663
      petrosal approach for resection of, 313, 314
      petrosectomy for, 613–617
        cases illustrating, 618–619, 619, 620, 620–624, 647–656
      posterior subtemporal/transzygomatic and presigmoid transpetrous approach for resection of, 612–613, 614–615, 657
      postoperative management and, 618
      radiologic evaluation of, 607
      rehabilitation and, 618
      retrosigmoid approach for resection of, 611, 657
        cases illustrating, 620–626, 626–630
      signs and symptoms of, 606–607
      subtemporal-preauricular infratemporal fossa approach for resection of, 612
        cases illustrating, 620–626, 626–630
      subtemporal transzygomatic approach for resection of, cases illustrating, 619, 620–624, 657
      and surgical anatomy of clivus, 605
      surgical resection of
        anesthesia for, 607–608
        approaches for, 608–616, 657
        cases illustrating, 618–656
        complications of, 657–658

general principles of, 608
monitoring during, 607–608
operative techniques for, 607–608
reconstruction after, 618
results of, 657
technical problems of, 617–618
total petrosectomy approach for, 613–617
cases illustrating, 618–619, 619, 620, 620–624, 647–656
petrous apex, 305
imaging characteristics of, 292
occipito-transmastoid-cervical approach for, 301
petrous bone, benign, 318, 326, 327, 328
surgical resection of, 326, 327, 328
postoperative scan of, 29
recurrent, and reconstruction with alloplastic materials, 466, 468
sphenocavernous, cases illustrating surgical resection of, 554–558
sphenocavernous-orbital, cases illustrating surgical resection of, 562, 564–567
sphenoid wing, planum, and suprasellar, cases illustrating surgical resection of, 584–585, 589–594
spinal, extreme lateral transcondylar and transjugular approaches for resection of, 399
spread of, 268
transsphenoidal approach for resection of, 349
transtemporal and infratemporal approach for resection of, 278–283
of tuberculum sella, 507–519
diagnosis of, 507
optic canal involvement and, 512, 514
optic nerve involvement and, 510–511
supraorbital approach for resection of, 508–509, 510
surgical resection of
anesthesia for, 508
arterial dissection during, 511–512, 513
cases illustrating, 517, 518
cavernous sinus involvement and, 512, 515
closure after, 515
complications of, 516–517
hypothalamus dissection in, 512, 513, 514
operative technique for, 508–515
patient positioning for, 508
patient selection for, 507–508
pituitary stalk dissection in, 512, 513, 514
postoperative management for, 516
tissue dissection for resection of, 510
tumor attachment and, 515
tumor resection and, 510
Meningitis
after osseous lesion (anterior and middle base) surgery, 817
after petroclival meningioma surgery, 658
after translabyrinthine approach, 362
after transsphenoidal surgery for invasive lesions, 345
Meningo-orbital foramina, posterior, 103
Metastatic disease, transsphenoidal approach for resection of, 349
Metoclopramide
for transmaxillary approach, 240
for transoral surgery, 232

Metronidazole
for transmaxillary approach, 236, 240
for transoral surgery, 228, 232
Microanastomosis
artery-to-artery, 48–49
vein-to-artery, 49
Microinstruments, for cranial base surgery, 4, 5
Microplates, vitallium, for craniofacial skeleton fixation, 423, 424
Microscope for cranial base surgery, 4
introduction of, 12
Microvascular anastomosis, in facial translocation approach, 248
Midas Rex drill, for tuberculum sella and olfactory groove meningioma surgery, 509
Middle cerebellar peduncle, vein of, acoustic neuroma and, 699
Middle clivus (midclivus), 157, 158, 606. See also Clivus
approach selection for tumors of, 157–159
Middle cranial base anatomy, 103–105
Middle cranial fossa, 103
anatomy of, 99–121
arteries of, 105
osseous lesions of, surgical resection of, 810–811
portals of, 103–105
Middle ear problems, in juvenile angiofibroma, 485, 486
Middle fossa approach
for acoustic tumor removal, 367–377, 709–710, 710–712, 719–720, 721
anesthesia for, 368
bone flap elevation and, 368–369
closure for, 376
complications of, 376
dura elevation and, 369–372
incision for, 368
indications for, 367–368
internal auditory canal exposure and, 372–374, 375
modifications of, 376–377
for neuromas, 709–710, 710–712, 719–720, 721
operative management for, 368–376
patient positioning for, 368
patient selection for, 367–368
tumor removal and, 374–376
for facial nerve decompression and repair, 376
for internal auditory canal decompression, 377
modifications of, 376–377
for petrous apex lesions, 294–297
indications for, 294–295, 296
posterior fossa approach and, 300–301
surgical technique for, 295–297
for vestibular nerve section, 376–377
Middle nasal concha, 123–124
Middle nasal meatus, 123–124
Middle-posterior fossa approach, combined, to petrous apex lesions, 300–301
indications for, 299, 300
surgical technique for, 300–301
Midfacial degloving technique, for juvenile angiofibroma surgery, 487
Midfacial split approach, 257–258
Miniplate fixation, 421–424
Miniplates, titanium, for craniofacial skeleton fixation, 423, 424
Mixed myoepithelial carcinoma, petrous bone, 318

Mobilization, after transoral surgery, 232
Morrison-King modification, of combined petrosal approach for petroclival lesions, 662
Motor weakness, in petroclival meningioma, 606
Moure incision, extended, for transfacial approach for juvenile angiofibroma surgery, 487–488, 490–491, 491–492, 493
Mouth
evaluation of, for transoral approach, 227
reanimation of, in paralyzed face without facial nerve, 454–455, 456–458
Mouth care, after transmaxillary surgery, 240
MRI. See Magnetic resonance imaging
MSPs. See Median nerve somatosensory evoked potentials
Mucoceles
cranial base
imaging characteristics of, 25, 26
site of origin of, 20
orbital, extraperiosteal approach for, 773
Musculoaponeurotic system, superficial, facial nerve access and, 437, 440
Myelomas, of clivus, transmaxillary approach for resection of, 242–243
Myoepithelial carcinoma, mixed, petrous bone, 318
Myxomas, cardiac, metastatic
to petroclivus, 219
surgical resection of, 329, 330, 331

N
Narcotic-based anesthesia, 73–74
Nasal bleeding. See Epistaxis
Nasal care, after transmaxillary surgery, 240
Nasal concha, middle, 123–124
Nasal dermoids
imaging characteristics of, 26
site of origin of, 20
Nasal fossae, wide opening of, and osseous lesion (anterior and middle base) surgery, 812–813
Nasal meatus, middle, 123–124
Nasal mucosa, in facial translocation approach, 251
Nasal obstruction
in esthesioneuroblastoma, 471, 473
in juvenile angiofibroma, 485, 486
Nasal packs, after transmaxillary surgery, 240
Nasal polyps, site of origin of, 20, 21
Nasal sinus carcinoma, 497–505
adjuvant therapy and, 500
anterior craniofacial resection for, 500, 501
including brain tissue, 500, 502
anterior cranio-orbital resection for, 500, 503
with free-flap reconstruction, 500, 503–504
biology of, 498
cavernous sinus involvement and, 498
cribriform plate involvement and, 498
diagnosis of, 497–498
dural involvement and, 498
extent of, determination of, 497–498
hard palate involvement and, 498–499
incidence of, 497
orbital involvement and, 498
surgical resection of
cases illustrating, 500, 501–504
cerebrospinal fluid leak after, 504
complications of, 504–505

Nasal sinus carcinoma, surgical resection of (*contd.*)
  eye protection in, 499
  functional and esthetic results of, 499–500
  infection after, 505
  instrumentation for, 499
  neuroanesthesia for, 499
  ocular dystopia after, 505
  operative procedure for, 499–500
  patient positioning for, 499
  perioperative antibiotics and, 499
  planning for, 498–499
  pneumocephalus after, 504
  preoperative preparation for, 499
  vision loss after, 504–505
  symptoms of, 497
  therapeutic options for, 498
  trigeminal nerve involvement and, 498
  tumor containment and, 499
  vascularity of, determination of, 498
Nasal speech, in juvenile angiofibroma, 485, 486
Nasal split, 257
Nasogastric intubation, for transoral approach, 227
Nasolacrimal duct, stenting, in facial translocation approach, 250, 251
Nasopharyngeal carcinoma, facial translocation approach for resection of, 245
Nasopharynx
  anatomy of, 246
  facial translocation approach to, 245–259
    complications of, 253, 256
    craniofacial skeleton and, 251, 252
    facial incisions/scars and, 249, 251
    facial nerve and, 249, 250, 438, 440, 441
    follow-up in, 258
    indications for, 245–248, 253, 258
    infraorbital nerve and, 250–251, 252
    midfacial split approach and, 257–258
    nasal mucosa and, 251
    nasolacrimal duct and, 250, 251
    planning for, 245–248
    postoperative care for, 256
    specific concerns in, 248–253
    surgical steps in, 247, 248
    temporalis muscle and, 253
    vascularity and, 248
Nasotracheal intubation, for transoral approach, 227
Nausea and vomiting, postoperative, 79–80
Nelson's syndrome, pituitary adenoma in, case illustrating, 584
Nerve sheath tumors
  imaging characteristics of, 26
  sites of origin of, 20, 21
  trigeminal, imaging in evaluation of, 17
Nervus intermedius
  exit zone of, 138
  intracisternal course of, 139
Neurenteric cyst, transoral approach for resection of, 233–234
Neurilemomas
  acoustic. *See* Neuromas, acoustic
  cavernous sinus, 603
    indications for surgery of, 533
  clival, subtemporal-infratemporal approach and basal frontal approaches for resection of, 200–201
  extracranial-intracranial V₂, cases illustrating, 740–743, 745
  extreme lateral transcondylar and transjugular approaches for resection of, 389

facial nerve, 725–730
  diagnosis of, 725
  location of, 725, 726
  surgical resection of
    cases illustrating, 727, 728, 729
    complications of, 728
    follow-up for, 728
    planning, 725
    postoperative care and, 727
    procedures for, 725–726
    recommendations for, 728–729
    statistical analyses related to, 728–729
jugular foramen, 731–735
  classification of, 731
  clinical presentation of, 731
  diagnosis of, 731
  surgical resection of, 732–735
    anesthesia for, 732
    exposure for, 733
    patient positioning for, 732
petroclival, 219
transtemporal and infratemporal approach for resection of, 283–286
trigeminal, 737–746
  clinical presentation of, 737
  diagnosis of, 737–738
  middle fossa involvement and, 810–811
  surgical resection of
    cases illustrating, 739–743, 744–745
    complications of, 749
    operative technique for, 738–739
    patient selection for, 738
    preoperative evaluation and, 738
Neurinomas
  acoustic, 305. *See also* Acoustic neuromas
  facial nerve, 305
  jugular foramen, 379
  petrous apex, occipito-transmastoid-cervical approach for, 301
  trigeminal, 669
    operative approaches to, 663
Neuroanesthesia. *See also* Anesthesia
  for paranasal/nasal sinus carcinoma resection, 499
Neuroblastomas, olfactory (esthesioneuroblastomas), 471–476
  biopsy of, 471
  clinical presentation of, 472–473
  diagnosis of, 471–472
  differential diagnosis of, 472
  imaging characteristics of, 22, 26
  pathogenesis of, 471
  prognosis for, 476
  site of origin of, 20, 21
  staging of, 472
  surgical removal of, 473–476
  transcranial, anterior craniofacial resection for, 500, 502
  transsphenoidal approach for resection of, 349
  treatment of, 473
    complications of, 476
    technique for, 473–476
  ultrastructure of, 471–472
Neuroendocrine carcinoma, olfactory. *See* Esthesioneuroblastoma
Neurofibromas, extreme lateral transcondylar and transjugular approaches for resection of, 389
  spinal, 399
Neurolept anesthesia, for reconstruction with alloplastic materials, 462
Neurologic complications, after skull base surgery, 832–833

Neurologic deficits
  and extreme lateral transcondylar and transjugular approaches, 399
  and transtemporal and infratemporal approach for benign tumors, 267
Neuromas
  acoustic. *See also* Acoustic tumors
    accessory nerve and, 690, 691
    arterial relationships and, 695–699
    brain stem relationships and, 689–695, 696
    central electroauditory prosthesis placement and, 826
    cerebellar-brain stem fissures and, 691–693
    choroid plexus and, 693–695, 696
    flocculus and, 693–695, 696
    foramen of Luschka and, 693–695, 696
    giant, operative approaches for resection of, 663
    glossopharyngeal nerve and, 690, 691
    mastoid retrosigmoid approach for resection of, 720–722
    meatal relationships and, 687, 688, 689
    microsurgical anatomy of, 687–699
    middle fossa approach for resection of, 709–710, 710–712, 719–720, 721
    neural relationships and, 687
    operative technique for resection of, 701, 702–713
    otological approaches for resection of, 715–724
      anesthesia for, 715–716
      complications of, 722–723
      cranial nerve dysfunction and, 723
      diagnosis and, 715
      operative technique for, 716–722
      patient positioning for, 716
      patient selection for, 715
      postoperative management and, 722
    pontomedullary sulcus and, 689–691
    recurrence of, 712–713, 723
    retrosigmoid approach for resection of, 701, 702–710
      exposure for, 701, 702
      instrumentation for, 705, 708
      intraoperative monitoring and, 703, 706, 707
      mastoid, 720–722
      patient positioning for, 701, 702–703
    stereotactic radiosurgery for, 712
    translabyrinthine approach for resection of, 711, 712, 716–719, 720
    transtemporal and infratemporal approach for resection of, 286, 287
    vagus nerve and, 690, 691
    venous relationships and, 699
  facial nerve, and translabyrinthine approach for facial nerve decompression or repair, 362
Neuromuscular blockers, for cranial base surgery, 74
NeuroNet
  instrumentation for, 86–87
  for neurophysiologic monitoring, 85–87, 88
  configuration of, 85–86
  signal processing algorithms for, 87, 88
Neurophysiologic monitoring, intraoperative, 83–98
  anesthesia and, 71–72, 89
  of auditory system, 93–94
  during cavernous sinus surgery, 534
  computer network architecture for, 85–86
  of cranial nerve function, electromyography for, 95–96

of electroencephalogram, 89–91
  during extreme lateral transcondylar and transjugular approaches, 390
  general procedures for, 88–89
  instrumentation for, 86–87
  measures used in, 88–96
  during petroclival meningioma surgery, 607–608
  during petrosal approach for clival tumors, 308
  during petrous bone tumor surgery, 318
  Pittsburgh approach for, 83–85
  during retrosigmoid approach to acoustic neuromas, 703, 706, 707
  signal processing algorithms for, 87
  of somatosensory system, 91–93
  system for, 85–87
  for trigeminal neurilemoma surgery, 738
  of visual system, 94–95
Neurorrhaphy, facial, 438–440, 441
Neurotrophic keratitis, after cavernous sinus tumor surgery, 602
Nitrous oxide
  for otological approaches to acoustic neurilemoma, 715
  for petroclival meningioma surgery, 607
  and tension pneumocephalus, 79
Nitrous oxide (N_2O)
  effects of, 70, 71
  and venous air embolism, 77
N_2O. *See* Nitrous oxide

O

Obesity, in craniopharyngioma, 789
Occipital artery, bone and dura of posterior cranial fossa supplied by, 132
Occipital artery bypass, artery-to-artery microanastomosis in, 48
Occipital bone, blood supply of, 132
Occipito-transmastoid-cervical approach, for petrous apex lesions, 301–304
  indications for, 301
  surgical techniques for, 302–304
Ocular dystopia, after craniofacial resection for paranasal sinus tumors, 505
Oculomotor nerve (cranial nerve III), 101
  in cavernous sinus, 109–110, 521, 523, 527, 530
    reconstruction of, 548, 603
    after tumor resection, 602
  entry portal of, 106
  intraoperative monitoring of function of, 95
    during cavernous sinus surgery, 534
  in lateral wall of cavernous sinus, 109–110
  risks to in skull base surgery, 833
Odontoid peg, and exposure for transoral approach, 228, 229
Olfactory fissure, alloplastic materials in reconstruction for, 468
Olfactory groove, meningiomas of, 507–519
  anesthesia for resection of, 508
  cases illustrating, 517, 518
  complications of surgery for, 516–517
  diagnosis of, 507
  operative technique for resection of, 515–516
  patient positioning for resection of, 508
  patient selection for resection of, 507–508
  postoperative management after surgery for, 516
Olfactory gyrus, vein of, 103
Olfactory nerve (cranial nerve I), after cavernous sinus tumor resection, 602

Olfactory neuroblastoma (olfactory neural neoplasm, esthesioneuroblastoma), 471–476
  biopsy of, 471
  clinical presentation of, 472–473
  diagnosis of, 471–472
  differential diagnosis of, 472
  imaging characteristics of, 22, 26
  pathogenesis of, 471
  prognosis for, 476
  site of origin of, 20, 21
  staging of, 472
  surgical removal of, 473–476
  transcranial, anterior craniofacial resection for, 500, 502
  transsphenoidal approach for resection of, 349
  treatment of, 473
    complications of, 476
    technique for, 473–476
  ultrastructure of, 471–472 craniofacial resection for, 500, 502
Olfactory sulcus, 103
Olfactory tract, 103
Open eyelid spring implantation technique, for eye reanimation in paralyzed face without facial nerve, 450–454
  adjunctive static procedures and, 451–454
Operating microscope for cranial base surgery, 4
  introduction of, 12
Operative techniques for cranial base surgery, 1–10. *See also specific procedure*
  from otolaryngologic and plastic surgery, 11–14
Ophthalmic artery, 99, 100
  and cavernous internal carotid artery, 521
Ophthalmic branch of facial nerve, and facial translocation approach, 249, 250
Ophthalmic nerve (cranial nerve V_1), 101
  in cavernous sinus, 109, 521, 523, 526
  reconstruction of, 549, 603
    after tumor resection, 602
Ophthalmic vein, 101
Optic canal, 99–100
  in neonates vs adults, 100
  in tuberculum sella meningioma surgery, 512, 514
Optic nerve (cranial nerve II)
  and cavernous meningioma resection, 541, 542
  fibrous dysplasia causing compression of, surgical resection and, 811–812
  removal of for tumor, 781, 782–784
  transconjunctival approach to, 772
  tuberculum sella meningioma and, 510–511
Orbit, 99–102
  anterior approach to, 771, 772–773, 774
  apex of, 101
    combined frontotemporal-orbitozygomatic approach for lesions of, 781–784
  combined frontotemporal-orbitozygomatic approach to, 775–784
  connective tissue in, 101–102
  contents of, 100–101
    displacement of in juvenile angiofibroma, 485, 486
    paranasal/nasal sinus carcinoma and, 498
  en bloc orbitectomy for malignancies of, 781–784
  extraperiosteal approach to, 773, 774
  lateral approach to, 771, 773–775, 776–778

medial wall of, 99
  optic canal in, 100
  portals of, 99
  rhabdomyosarcoma of, anterior cranio-orbital resection of, 500, 503
  superior approach to, 771
  superior wall of, 99
  surgical indications and approaches to, 769–786. *See also* Orbital surgery; Orbitectomy; Orbitotomy
  transconjunctival approach to, 772, 773
  transfrontal approach to, 771
  transseptal approach to, 773
Orbital fissures
  inferior, 99, 100, 112
  superior, 99, 101, 103–104
Orbital osteotomy, in anterior craniofacial resection, 150
Orbital retractors, fixed, 772
Orbital surgery, 769–786
  approaches for, 771–772
    anterior, 771, 772–773, 774
    combined frontotemporal-orbitozygomatic, 775–785
    extraperiosteal, 773, 774
    lateral, 771, 773–775, 776–778
    superior, 771
    transconjunctival, 772, 773
    transfrontal, 771
    transseptal, 773
  and distribution of orbital disease, 770
  en bloc, 781–785
  imaging and, 770–771
  indications for, 770
  instrumentation for, 772
  and presentation of orbital disease, 769
  and profile of orbital disease, 769–770
  techniques for, 772
Orbital vein, medial, 103
Orbitalis muscle, 100
Orbitectomy, en bloc, 781–785
Orbitocranial lesions, combined frontotemporal-orbitozygomatic approach for, 781–784
Orbito-fronto-ethmoidal osteotomy, in extended frontal approach for clival tumors, 171, 172–173
Orbitotomy
  anterior, 771, 772–773, 774
    extraperiosteal approach in, 773, 774
    incision sites for, 772
    transconjunctival approach in, 772, 773
    transseptal approach in, 773
  lateral, 771, 773–775, 776–778
    incision for, 773–774, 775
Orbitozygomatic osteotomy
  in cavernous sinus surgery, 536, 537–538
  in frontotemporal transcavernous and transpetrous apex approach for petroclival meningiomas, 609
Orotracheal tube, for transmaxillary approach, 235–236
Oscillating saw, for paranasal/nasal sinus carcinoma resection, 499
Osseous lesions, 809–817
  diagnosis of, 809
  lateral (middle fossa and pterional area), 810–811
  medial ethmoidosphenoidal, 811–812
  surgical resection of
    anesthesia for, 810
    cerebrospinal fluid leak and, 816
    complications of, 816–817
    dural defect and, 813, 814
    extradural pneumatoceles and, 816–817

862 / SUBJECT INDEX

Osseous lesions, surgical resection of (contd.)
  infection and, 817
  one-stage multiple approaches for, 814–816
  operative technique for, 810–816
  patient selection for, 809–810
  reconstruction materials for, 814
  technical problems in, 812–814
  visual deficits and, 817
  and wide opening of nasal fossae, 812–813
  transfacial approach for resection of, 815, 816
  transsphenoidal approach for resection of, 814–816
Osteogenic sarcomas
  petroclival, 219
  petrous bone, 318
  surgical resection of, 329–332, 333
Osteoplastic bone graft technique, and juvenile angiofibroma surgery, 489
Osteotomy, in cranial base surgery, 4
  in craniofacial disassembly, 421, 422, 423
  in craniofacial resection
    anterior, 150
    anterolateral, 151, 153, 154
  in facial translocation approach, 251
  lateral, in craniofacial resection for esthesioneuroblastoma, 474
  orbito-fronto-ethmoidal, in extended frontal approach for clival tumors, 171, 172–173
  orbitozygomatic
    in cavernous sinus surgery, 536, 537–538
    in frontotemporal transcavernous and transpetrous apex approach for petroclival meningiomas, 609
  zygomatic
    in cavernous sinus surgery, 537–538
    and frontotemporal-transsylvian/anterior subtemporal approach for petroclival meningiomas, 608
    in subtemporal/transcavernous/transpetrous apex approach, 159
Otitis, malignant external
  imaging characteristics of, 26
  site of origin of, 20, 21
Otolaryngologic surgery, techniques and instrumentation for in cranial base surgery, 11–14
Otological approaches, for acoustic neurilemoma, 715–724
  anesthetic considerations for, 715–716
  complications of, 722–723
  cranial nerve dysfunction and, 723
  diagnosis and, 715
  mastoid retrosigmoid, 720–722
  middle fossa, 719–720, 721
  operative technique for, 716–722
  patient positioning for, 716
  patient selection for, 715
  postoperative management and, 722
  translabyrinthine, 716–719, 720
Otoneurosurgical approach, for jugular foramen tumors, 381–386
  advantages of, 385–386
  cranial nerve affected in, 384, 385
  patient positioning for, 381
  results of, 384–386
  steps in, 382–383
Otoscopy, and petrous apex lesions, 292
Oxygen consumption, cerebral, anesthetic agents affecting, 70, 71

P-Q
P-S bypass graft, 52–61
  results of, 62
Pain, orbital, in esthesioneuroblastoma, 473
Palate
  hard
    paranasal/nasal sinus carcinoma and, 498–499
    in transoral approach, 230–231
      closure of, 232
  soft, in transoral approach, 228, 229
    closure of, 232
Palatine artery, ascending, 118
Palatine recess, 129
Papillomas, malignant choroid plexus, 318
Paragangliomas
  embolization of, 42, 43
  glomus vagale tumors and, 763
    surgical intervention and, 765
  imaging characteristics of, 26
  imaging in evaluation of, 16
  jugular foramen, 379
  multicentric characteristics of, 763, 764
  petrous apex, 305
    occipito-transmastoid-cervical approach for, 301
  site of origin of, 20, 21
Paramastoid crest, 113–115
Paranasal incision, for facial translocation approach, 249
Paranasal sinuses
  anatomy of, 123–130
  carcinoma of, 497–505
    adjuvant therapy and, 500
    anterior craniofacial resection for, 500, 501
      including brain tissue, 500, 502
    anterior cranio-orbital resection for, 500, 503
      with free-flap reconstruction, 500, 503–504
    biology of, 498
    cavernous sinus involvement and, 498
    cribriform plate involvement and, 498
    diagnosis of, 497–498
    dural involvement and, 498
    extent of, determination of, 497–498
    hard palate involvement and, 498–499
    incidence of, 497
    orbital involvement and, 498
    surgical resection of
      cases illustrating, 500, 501–504
      cerebrospinal fluid leak after, 504
      complications of, 504–505
      eye protection in, 499
      functional and esthetic results of, 499–500
      infection after, 505
      instrumentation for, 499
      neuroanesthesia for, 499
      ocular dystopia after, 505
      operative procedure for, 499–500
      patient positioning for, 499
      perioperative antibiotics and, 499
      planning for, 498–499
      pneumocephalus after, 504
      preoperative preparation for, 499
      vision loss after, 504–505
    symptoms of, 497
    therapeutic options for, 498
    trigeminal nerve involvement and, 498
    tumor containment and, 499
    vascularity of, determination of, 498
  ethmoidal bulla, 124
  frontal recess and, 124
  frontal sinus, 126–127
  Haller's cells and, 125–126
  maxillary sinus, 125
  middle nasal meatus and, 123–124
  rhabdomyosarcoma of, anterior cranio-orbital resection of, 500, 503
  semilunar hiatus and, 124
  sphenoid sinus, 127–130
Parapetrosal approach, combined, for petroclival lesions, 661–669
  cases illustrating, 667–669
  closure for, 667
  craniotomy for, 664, 665
  dural incision for, 664–667
  indications for, 663
  microsurgical instrumentation for, 663–664
  operative technique for, 663–667
  patient positioning for, 664
  scalp incision for, 664, 665
  tumor access with, 664–667
  tumor resection and, 667
Parapharyngeal space, vessels of, 118
Parasellar aneurysm, imaging in evaluation of, 18
Parkinson's triangle, 523, 529
Parolivary area, 137
Parotid acinar cell carcinoma, 318
  adjuvant treatment for, 325
Parotid salivary gland neoplasms, facial translocation approach for resection of, 245–248
Parotidectomy incision
  for glomus jugulare tumor surgery, 749, 750
  for subtemporal and infratemporal approach for clival tumor resection, 162, 163
Pars flaccida, 113
Pars oculomotoria, 101
Pars optica, 101
Pars tensa, of tympanic membrane, 113
Patient evaluation, 3–4
Patient positioning for cranial base surgery, 75. *See also specific procedure*
  for clivus chordoma surgery, 680
  for combined lateral suboccipital-infralabyrinthine approach, 381
  for combined supra- and infraparapetrosal approach for petroclival lesions, 664
  for craniofacial resection for esthesioneuroblastoma, 473
  for extreme lateral transcondylar and transjugular approaches, 175, 390
  for glomus jugulare tumor surgery, 749
  for glomus vagale tumor surgery, 765
  for jugular foramen neurilemoma resection, 732
  for juvenile angiofibroma surgery, 486
  for olfactory groove meningioma surgery, 508
  for otological approaches to acoustic neurilemoma, 716
  for paranasal/nasal sinus carcinoma resection, 499
  for petrosal approach for clival tumors, 308
  for posterior fossa approach for petrous apex lesions, 297–299
  for reconstruction with alloplastic materials, 462
  for retrosigmoid approach for acoustic neuromas, 701, 702–703

for transcondyle approach for foramen magnum meningiomas, 672
for translabyrinthine approach, 351–352
for transmaxillary approach, 236
for transoral approach, 227–228
for transsphenoidal surgery, 338
for transtemporal and infratemporal approach, 269
for transzygomatic and transpalatal resection of juvenile nasopharyngeal angiofibroma, 478
for tuberculum sella meningioma surgery, 508
Pectoralis muscle flap, 417, 420, 421
Pectoralis myocutaneous flap, 417, 420, 421
PEEP. *See* Positive-end-expiratory pressure
Pentothal, for cranial base surgery, 73–74
Pericranial flap, 414, 415, 416
Pericranial graft, for reconstruction after anterior craniofacial resection, 151
Perioperative management, 8
Pernasal paraseptal approach, 339–340
Petroclinoid folds, anterior and posterior, 106
Petroclival bone, and cavernous meningioma resection, 548
Petroclival meningiomas, 219, 299, 300, 379, 605–659. *See also* Petroclival tumors
   cavernous sinus involvement and, cases illustrating surgical resection of, 578–579, 580, 581, 585–601
   classification of, 605–606
   clinical presentation of, 606–607
   combined middle-posterior fossa approach for resection of, 300–301
   computed tomography in evaluation of, 667–669
   extreme lateral transcondylar approach for resection of, 611, 657
     cases illustrating, 618–619, 620, 626–630, 631–635, 647, 647–653
   frontotemporal and preauricular infratemporal approach for resection of, cases illustrating, 630–635, 635–639
   frontotemporal transcavernous and transpetrous apex approach for resection of, 608–611
     cases illustrating, 639–647, 648
   frontotemporal-transsylvian/anterior subtemporal approach for, with zygomatic osteotomy, 608, 657
   magnetic resonance imaging in evaluation of, 667
   operative approaches for resection of, 663
   petrosal approach for resection of, 313, 314
   petrosectomy for, 613–617
     cases illustrating, 618–619, 619, 620, 620–624, 647–656
   posterior subtemporal/transzygomatic and presigmoid transpetrous approach for resection of, 612–613, 614–615, 657
   postoperative management and, 618
   radiologic evaluation of, 607
   rehabilitation and, 618
   retrosigmoid approach for resection of, 611, 657
     cases illustrating, 620–626, 626–630
   signs and symptoms of, 606–607
   subtemporal-preauricular infratemporal fossa approach for resection of, 612
     cases illustrating, 620–626, 626–630
   subtemporal transzygomatic approach for resection of, cases illustrating, 619, 620–624, 657
   and surgical anatomy of clivus, 605
   surgical resection of
     anesthesia for, 607–608
     approaches for, 608–616, 657
       general principles of, 608
     cases illustrating, 618–656
     complications of, 657–658
     monitoring during, 607–608
     operative techniques for, 607–608
     reconstruction after, 618
     results of, 657
     technical problems of, 617–618
   total petrosectomy approach for resection of, 613–617
     cases illustrating, 618–619, 619, 620, 620–624, 647–656
Petroclival tumors. *See also* Petroclival meningiomas
   combined supra- and infraparapetrosal approach for resection of, 661–669
     cases illustrating, 667–669
     closure for, 667
     craniotomy for, 664, 665
     dural incision for, 664–667
     indications for, 663
     microsurgical instrumentation for, 663–664
     operative technique for, 663–667
     patient positioning for, 664
     scalp incision for, 664, 665
     tumor access with, 664–667
     tumor resection and, 667
   extradural, anterior/anterolateral/lateral approaches to, 219–223
     complications of, 219–223
   operative approaches to, 661
Petrosal approach
   for clival tumors, 307–315
     anesthesia for, 308
     cases illustrating, 313–314
     closure for, 312
     complications of, 312–313
     craniotomy flap in, 308–309
     diagnosis and, 307
     dural opening in, 309
     exposure for, 309
     monitoring during, 308
     operative technique for, 308–312
     patient position for, 308
     patient selection for, 307–308
     postoperative management for, 312
     temporal bone drilling for, 309
     tentorium sectioning in, 309
     tumor resection in, 309–312
   combined, for petroclival lesions, 662–663
Petrosal bone, fracture of, and reconstruction with alloplastic materials, 467, 468
Petrosal nerves, greater and lesser, 104–105
Petrosal sinus
   inferior, 134–135
     termination of, 135–136
   superior, 105
Petrosal to supraclinoid internal carotid artery cavernous sinus bypass, 52–61
   results of, 62
Petrosal to upper cervical internal carotid artery interposition grafting, 50–52, 53–54
Petrosal vein, and translabyrinthine approach, 357
Petrosectomy
   subtotal, for petroclival lesions, 662
   total, for petroclival lesions, 662
   for meningiomas, 613–617
     cases illustrating, 618–619, 619, 620, 620–624, 647–656
Petrosquamous sinus, 134
Petrotympanic fissure, 113
Petrous apex, and cavernous meningioma resection, 548
Petrous apex lesions. *See also* Petrous bone tumors
   combined middle-posterior fossa approach for, 299, 300–301
   middle fossa, 294–297
   surgical resection of, 291–305
     approaches for, 292–304
     contraindications to, 292
     cranial nerve dysfunction and, 833
     diagnosis and, 291–292
     difficulties in, 292
     occipito-transmastoid-cervical approach for, 301–304
     patient selection for, 292
     posterior fossa approach for, 297–299
     radiologic examination and, 292
     translabyrinthine approach for, 292–294
       with cavity obliteration, 292–294
       with marsupialization, 292, 293
   types of, 305
Petrous bone tumors. *See also* Petrous apex lesions
   benign, 321
     Karnofsky functional scores for, 334
   classification of spread of, 325–326
   malignant, 321–322
     Karnofsky functional scores for, 334
   low grade, 321
   surgical resection of, 317–335
     adjuvant treatment and, 325
     anesthesia for, 318–319
     cases illustrating, 326–332
     complications of, 325
     early treatment and, 334
     en bloc, 321–322
     exposure for, 319–321
     historical perspective of, 333
     incision for, 319–321
     indications for, 317–318
     monitoring for, 318–319
     outcome of, 325
     patient population and, 317–318
     patient positioning for, 318–319
     piecemeal, 321
     postoperative care and, 323–325
     preoperative evaluation and treatment and, 318
     reconstruction after, 322–323, 324, 325
     technical limitations of, 333–334
   transcochlear approach for resection of, 363–364
     indications for, 363
     operative technique for, 363–364
Petrous internal carotid artery
   in cavernous sinus, 525
   exposure of, 538–539
   meningioma encasing, case illustrating surgical resection of, 647–656
   reconstruction of, 322–323, 324, 325
   in subtemporal and infratemporal approach for clival tumor resection, 164–167, 168, 169
   transtemporal and infratemporal approach for tumors around, 269, 273, 276–278

Pharyngeal artery, ascending, 118
  bone and dura of posterior cranial fossa supplied by, 132
Pharyngogastric tube, for transmaxillary approach, 236
  postoperative care and, 240
Phonosurgery, for swallowing dysfunction associated with superior and recurrent laryngeal nerve injury, 820
Pituitary adenomas
  cavernous sinus, 603
    surgical resection of
      case illustrating, 584, 585, 586
      indications for, 533
  imaging characteristics of, 26
  petroclival invasion by, 219
  recurrence of, 305
  site of origin of, 20
  transsphenoidal approach for resection of, 337–338, 342, 343, 346, 347–348, 349
Pituitary capsule, 109
Pituitary cisterns, 106–109
Pituitary fossa, 105
  floor of, 106
Pituitary gland, and cavernous meningioma resection, 548
Pituitary macroadenomas, transsphenoidal approach for resection of, 342, 343, 346, 347–348
Pituitary stalk, dissection of, in tuberculum sella meningioma surgery, 512, 513, 514
Plain films, skull. *See* Skull x-ray
Planum meningioma, cases illustrating surgical resection of, 584–585, 589–594
Planum sphenoidale, 106
Plasmacytomas, extreme lateral transcondylar and transjugular approaches for resection of, 398
Plastic surgery, techniques and instrumentation for in cranial base surgery, 11–14
Pneumatoceles, extradural, after osseous lesion (anterior and middle base) surgery, 816–817
Pneumocephalus
  after anterior and anterolateral craniofacial resection, prevention of, 154
  after craniofacial resection for paranasal sinus tumors, 504
  tension, 79
Pneumonia, aspiration, and petroclival meningioma surgery, 658
Polyps
  imaging characteristics of, 26
  nasal, site of origin of, 20, 21
Pons, 136
  acoustic neuromas and, 689, 690, 692, 695
Pontomedullary sulcus
  acoustic neuromas and, 689–691
  vein of, acoustic neuroma and, 699
Positioning for cranial base surgery, 75. *See also specific procedure*
  for clivus chordoma surgery, 680
  for combined lateral suboccipital-infralabyrinthine approach, 381
  for combined supra- and infraparapetrosal approach for petroclival lesions, 664
  for craniofacial resection for esthesioneuroblastoma, 473
  for extreme lateral transcondylar and transjugular approaches, 175, 390
  for glomus jugulare tumor surgery, 749
  for glomus vagale tumor surgery, 765
  for jugular foramen neurilemoma resection, 732
  for juvenile angiofibroma surgery, 486
  for olfactory groove meningioma surgery, 508
  for otological approaches to acoustic neurilemoma, 716
  for paranasal/nasal sinus carcinoma resection, 499
  for petrosal approach for clival tumors, 308
  for posterior fossa approach for petrous apex lesions, 297–299
  for reconstruction with alloplastic materials, 462
  for retrosigmoid approach for acoustic neuromas, 701, 702–703
  for transcondyle approach for foramen magnum meningiomas, 672
  for translabyrinthine approach, 351–352
  for transmaxillary approach, 236
  for transoral approach, 227–228
  for transsphenoidal surgery, 338
  for transtemporal and infratemporal approach, 269
  for transzygomatic and transpalatal resection of juvenile nasopharyngeal angiofibroma, 478
  for tuberculum sella meningioma surgery, 508
Positive-end-expiratory pressure
  and facilitating surgical exposure, 76
  for venous air embolism, 77
Posterior circulation bypass grafting, 65
Posterior clinoid process, 105
Posterior cranial fossa, 131–146
  accessory sinus of, 134
  anatomy of, 131–146
  arteries supplying, 141–144
  blood supply of bone and dura of, 132
  cerebellar arteries in, replacement and, 144
  cerebellopontine angle of, 144–146
  cranial nerves in, 137–141
  emissary veins of, 135–136
  extreme lateral transcondylar and transjugular approaches to tumors of, 397
    complications and, 399
    extent of tumor resection and, 398–399
  great cerebral vein in, 133
  inferior petrosal sinus of, 134–135
    termination of, 135–136
  internal acoustic meatus and, 144–146
  nerve supply of dura mater of, 132–133
  petrosquamous sinus of, 134
  pons in, 136
  retro-olivary area of, 137–141
  roof of, 131–132
  sigmoid sinus of, 134
  squamopetrosal sinus of, 134
  straight sinus of, 134
  transtemporal and infratemporal approach for tumors of, 273, 274, 275, 276–278
  transverse sinus of, 134
Posterior ethmoidal canal, 127
Posterior fossa approach
  for petrous apex lesions, 297–298
    indications for, 297, 298
    middle fossa approach and, 300–301
    surgical techniques for, 297–298
  retrosigmoid, in jugular foramen neurilemoma resection, 734–735
Posterior inferior cerebellar artery, extreme lateral transcondylar and transjugular approaches for resection of, 398
Posterior meningo-orbital foramen, 103
Posterior petroclinoid fold, 106
Posterior subtemporal/transzygomatic and presigmoid transpetrous approach, for petroclival meningiomas, 612–613, 614–615, 657
Postoperative care, 9–12, 232. *See also specific procedure and* Follow-up care
  after anterior and anterolateral craniofacial resection, 232
  after central electroauditory prosthesis placement, 828
  after cerebral revascularization, 65
  computed tomography in, 29–32
  after craniofacial skeleton disassembly and reconstruction, 425
  after craniopharyngioma surgery, 804
  for facial nerve management and reconstruction, 444–446
  after facial nerve neurilemoma resection, 727
  after facial translocation surgery, 256
  imaging studies in, 29–32
  after juvenile angiofibroma surgery, 489
  after otological surgery for acoustic neurilemomas, 722
  after petroclival meningioma surgery, 618
  after petrosal surgery for clival tumors, 312
  after petrous bone tumor surgery, 323–325
  after regional flaps, 425
  after translabyrinthine surgery, 361
  after transmaxillary surgery, 240
  after transoral surgery, 232
  after transsphenoidal surgery for invasive lesions, 344
  after transzygomatic and transpalatal resection of juvenile nasopharyngeal angiofibroma, 480
  after tuberculum sella and olfactory groove meningioma surgery, 516
Preauricular infratemporal approach
  and frontotemporal approach, for petroclival meningiomas, cases illustrating, 630–635, 635–639
  and subtemporal approach
    for clival tumors, 161–171
      cases illustrating, 190–194, 195–197, 198–199, 200–201, 211, 213–218
      disadvantages of, 171
      division of V_3 in, 167, 169, 170
      extended frontal approach combined with, 175, 176, 177
      reconstruction after, 167–171
      skin incision for, 162
    for petroclival meningiomas, 612, 657
      cases illustrating, 620–626, 626–630
Preoperative preparation for cranial base surgery, 71. *See also specific procedure*
  for anterior and anterolateral craniofacial resection, 155
  for clivus chordoma surgery, 680
  for craniofacial skeleton disassembly and reconstruction, 424–425
  for craniopharyngioma surgery, 791–792
  for facial nerve management and reconstruction, 443–444
  for facial translocation surgery, 253–256
  for paranasal/nasal sinus carcinoma resection, 499

patient evaluation and, 3
  for petrous bone resection, 318
  for regional flaps, 424–425
  for transtemporal and infratemporal surgery, 267–268
  for trigeminal neurilemoma surgery, 738
Presigmoid-subtemporal approach, and extreme lateral transcondylar approach, for petroclival meningiomas, cases illustrating, 647, 648–653
Presigmoid transpetrous approach, and posterior subtemporal/transzygomatic approach, for petroclival meningiomas, 612–613, 614–615, 657
Presigmoid and transsigmoid transpetrous approach, and frontotemporal-transcavernous approach, for petroclival meningiomas, 639–647, 648
Prevertebral segment of vertebral artery, 120
Prolactinomas, transsphenoidal approach for resection of, 349
Proptosis, in esthesioneuroblastoma, 471, 473
Provocative testing, for embolization, 36
Pseudoprefixity, in craniopharyngiomas, 788, 793
Pterion, 103
  osseous lesions of, surgical resection of, 810–811
Pterional approach, for petroclival lesions, 661, 663
Pterional craniotomy, for clival chordomas, 679
Pterygoid canal, 104
Pterygoid lamina, spinous process of, 113
Pterygoid muscle
  lateral, 114, 115
  medial, 116
Pterygoid process, 113
Pterygoid recess, 130
Pterygopalatine fossa, 112, 113
Pterygospinal ligament, 113
Pulmonary embolism, after tuberculum sella and olfactory groove meningioma surgery, 517
Pyramid, 137

R
Radiation therapy
  for craniopharyngiomas
    with biopsy, 790
    intracavitary, 791
    with subtotal resection, 790
  for esthesioneuroblastomas, 473
  for juvenile angiofibromas, 486
  for paranasal/nasal sinus carcinoma, 500
  for petrous bone tumors, 325
Radioisotope cisternography, cerebrospinal fluid leak diagnosed with, 835
Radiosurgery, stereotactic
  for acoustic neuromas, 712
  for craniopharyngiomas, 791
Rami sinus carotici, 116
Rathke's pouch cysts, transsphenoidal approach for resection of, 349
Reanimation procedures, for paralyzed face without facial nerve, 449–459
  adjunctive static techniques and, 455–459
  examples of results of, 458–459
  eye and, 449–450, 450–454
  gold weight implantation technique for, 450, 451
  lower face and, 454–455, 456–458
  mouth and, 454–455, 456–458

open eyelid spring implantation technique in, 450–454
  temporalis muscle transposition technique in, 454–455, 456–458
Reciprocating saw, for cranial base surgery, 4
  for paranasal/nasal sinus carcinoma resection, 499
Reconstruction, 8–9, 12–13. *See also specific procedure*
  alloplastic materials in, 461–469
    anesthesia and, 462
    for anterior base of skull, 468
    antibiotics and, 464
    cases illustrating, 465–468
    complications of, 464–465
    for congenital fistula involving floor of sella turcica and sphenoid sinus, 465–468
    diagnosis and, 461
    for ethmoid bone roof, 468
    for frontal sinus posterior wall, 468
    for frontobasal fracture, 464, 465
    for lateral skull base, 468–469
    for olfactory fissure, 468
    operative technique and, 462, 463
    patient positioning and, 462
    patient selection and, 461–462
    for petrosal bone fracture, 467, 468
    postoperative management and, 464
    for recurrent meningioma, 466, 468
    technical problems and, 462–464
  after anterolateral and anterior craniofacial resection, 151, 152
  after cavernous meningioma surgery
    of cranial base, 549
    of cranial nerves, 548–549
    of internal carotid artery, 547–548
  of craniofacial skeleton, 421–424
    complications of, 425
    follow-up care and, 425
    postoperative care and, 425
    preoperative preparation and, 425
  after extended frontal approach for clival tumor resection, 175
  after extreme lateral transcondylar and transjugular approaches, 180–181
  facial-to-facial, and translabyrinthine approach for petrous apex lesions, 294
  of facial nerve, 435–447
    complications of, 446
    concerns in, 443
    follow-up care and, 446
    graft for, 435, 440–443, 444, 445
    middle fossa approach for, 376
    neurorrhaphy for, 438–440
    planning, 436, 437
    postoperative care and, 444–446
    preoperative care and, 443–444
    primary, 438–440
    surgical steps in, 435–443
    translabyrinthine approach for, 362
  free-flap, 427–433
    after anterior cranio-orbital resection for adenoid cystic carcinoma, 500, 503–504
  latissimus dorsi flap for, 430–433
  microvascular, 427–433
  after osseous lesion (anterior and middle base) surgery, materials for, 814
  pectoralis muscle (myocutaneous) flap for, 417, 420, 421
  pericranial flap for, 414, 415, 416
  pericranial graft for, 151
  after petroclival meningioma surgery, 618

after petrous bone tumor surgery, 322–323, 324, 325
  reanimation procedures in, 449–459
  rectus abdominis flap for, 427–430
  regional flaps for, 413–426
  scalp flaps for, 417, 419–420
    bicoronal, 151, 152, 792, 793
  after subtemporal and infratemporal approach for clival tumor resection, 167–171
  after subtemporal/transcavernous/transpetrous apex approach for clival tumor resection, 161
  temporalis muscle flap for, 415–417, 418, 419
  after transtemporal and infratemporal surgery, 273–275
  trapezius muscle (myocutaneous) flap for, 417–421
  vein graft, after cavernous sinus tumor surgery, 602
Rectosigmoid craniotomy, in retrosigmoid approach for acoustic neurilemoma, 721
Rectus abdominis flap, 427–430
  follow-up care and, 430
  surgical steps for, 427–430
Rectus muscles, 100, 101
  lateral, 102
Recurrent artery of Heubner, anterior cranial fossa supplied by, 103
Recurrent laryngeal nerve, swallowing dysfunction caused by injury to, 820
Regional flaps, 413–426. *See also specific type*
  complications of, 425
  follow-up care and, 425
  pectoralis muscle (myocutaneous), 417, 420, 421
  pericranial, 414, 415, 416
  planning and, 413–415
  postoperative care and, 425
  preoperative care and, 424–425
  scalp, 417, 419–420
  surgical steps for, 414, 415–424
  temporalis muscle, 415–417, 418, 419
  trapezius muscle (myocutaneous), 417–421
Reimplantation, of avulsed artery, 61
Repair. *See* Reconstruction
Retraction
  brain, 4, 14
    minimizing use of, 4
  in orbital surgery, 772
Retrolabyrinthine approach, for jugular foramen tumors, 385
Retromastoid approach, for petroclival lesions, 661, 663
Retro-olivary area, 137–141
Retrosigmoid approach
  for acoustic neuromas, 701, 702–710
    exposure for, 701, 702
    instrumentation for, 705, 708
    intraoperative monitoring and, 703, 706, 707
    mastoid, 720–722
    patient positioning for, 701, 702–703
  mastoid, 720–722
  for petroclival meningiomas, 611, 657
    cases illustrating, 620–626, 626–630
  posterior fossa, in jugular foramen neurilemoma resection, 734–735
Retrosigmoid craniectomy, in occipito-transmastoid-cervical approach, 303
Revascularization, cerebral, 45–68
  anesthesia for, 46

Revascularization, cerebral (contd.)
  artery-to-artery microanastomosis in, 48–49
  complications of, 65–66
  extracranial-to-distal middle cerebral artery bypass in, 63–64
  extracranial-internal carotid bypass grafting in, 63–65
  extracranial-to-proximal anterior circulation artery bypass in, 64–65
  long-term outcome with, 66
  monitoring during, 46
  need for, assessment of, 45–46
  petrosal to supraclinoid internal carotid artery cavernous sinus bypass in, 52–61
    results of, 62
  petrosal to upper cervical internal carotid artery interposition grafting in, 50–52
  posterior circulation bypass grafting in, 65
  postoperative medical management and, 65
  preparation for, 46–47
  reimplantation in, 61
  saphenous vein harvesting for, 46–47
  vein-to-artery microanastomosis in, 49
  vein graft results and, 61–62
  venous patch grafting in, 50
  vertebral artery interposition grafting in, 61
Rhabdomyosarcomas
  imaging in evaluation of, 18–19
  orbital and paranasal, anterior cranioorbital resection of, 500, 503
Rhinorrhea, after transsphenoidal surgery for invasive lesions, 345
Rhinotomy, in craniofacial resection for esthesioneuroblastoma, 474
Rhoton forceps, for cranial base tumors, 7
Rivini's incisura, 113
"Robin Hood" syndrome, 78
Rongeurs, for cranial base tumors, 6
Rosenthal's basal vein, 103

S

Saphenous vein, harvesting for revascularization, 46–47, 48
Sarcomas. *See also specific type*
  facial translocation approach for resection of, 245, 253
  imaging characteristics of, 26
  osteogenic
    petroclival, 219
    petrous bone, 318
      surgical resection of, 329–332, 333
Scalp flaps, 417, 419–420
  bicoronal
    after anterior craniofacial resection, 151, 152
    in subfrontal approach for craniopharyngiomas, 792, 793
Scars, facial, after anterior and anterolateral craniofacial resection, 154
Schirmer's test, and petrous apex lesions, 292
Schwannomas
  orbital, extraperiosteal approach for resection of, 774
  petroclival, petrosal approach for resection of, 313–314
Scissors, for cranial base tumors, 7
Seizures
  anesthetic agents affecting, 70
  and carotid cross-clamping, 78
  in petroclival meningioma, 606

Sella dura. *See* Endosteum
Sella turcica, 103, 105
  congenital fistula involving, reconstruction with alloplastic materials for, 465–468
  transsphenoidal approach for invasive lesions of, 337–349
    anesthesia for, 338
    cases illustrating, 345–348
    complications of, 345
    diagnosis and, 337
    operating room arrangement for, 338
    operative technique for, 338–344
    patient position for, 338
    patient selection for, 337–338
    pernasal approach for, 339–340
    postoperative management and, 344
    sublabial incision for, 339
  variations of, 106
Sellar abscess, transsphenoidal approach for resection of, 349
Sellar bridges, 106
Sellar spine, 106
Semilunar hiatus, 124
Sensory-neural hearing loss, and petrous apex lesions, 291
SEPs (somatosensory evoked potentials). *See* Somatosensory evoked response
Septum, of sphenoid sinus, 127–129
Short stature, in craniopharyngioma, 789
SIADH. *See* Inappropriate secretion of antidiuretic hormone
Sigmoid arteriovenous malformation, operative approaches for resection of, 663
Sigmoid sinus, 134
  tearing of, in translabyrinthine approach, 356
Signal processing algorithms, for NeuroNet, 87, 88
Simple mastoidectomy, complete, in translabyrinthine approach, 353
Sinonasal undifferentiated carcinoma, esthesioneuroblastoma differentiated from, 472
Sinusitis
  imaging characteristics of, 26
  site of origin of, 20, 21
Skin incision. *See* Exposure
Skull, and middle cranial base anatomy, 103
Skull base. *See* Cranial base
Skull base masses. *See* Cranial base tumors
Skull base surgery. *See* Cranial base surgery
Skull base team, 2–3
  and neurophysiologic monitoring, 84–85
  nurse coordinator on, 3
Skull x-ray
  for evaluation of craniopharyngioma, 789
  for evaluation of osseous lesions, 809
SMA. *See* Superficial musculoaponeurotic system
SNUC. *See* Sinonasal undifferentiated carcinoma
Sodium thiopental, for petroclival meningioma surgery, 607
Soft palate, and transoral approach, 228, 229, 230–231
  closure of, 232
Soft tissue dissection, for transtemporal and infratemporal approach, 270
Soft tissue flaps
  for facial translocation approach, vascularity of, 248
  regional, 413–426. *See also specific type and* Regional flaps

Somatosensory evoked response
  monitoring during cranial base surgery, 4, 84, 91–93
    cavernous sinus surgery and, 534
    extreme lateral transcondylar and transjugular approaches and, 390
    petroclival meningioma surgery and, 607
    petrous bone tumor surgery and, 318–319
    revascularization and, 46
    trigeminal neurilemoma surgery and, 738
  preoperative, for petrous bone tumor surgery, 318
Sphenocavernous meningioma, cases illustrating surgical resection of, 554–558
Sphenocavernous-orbital meningioma, cases illustrating surgical resection of, 562, 564–567
Sphenoid bone, 105
Sphenoid sinus, 127–130
  congenital fistula involving, reconstruction with alloplastic materials for, 465–468
  in extended frontal approach for clival tumors, 173, 174
  opening, for resection of invasive lesions, 342–343
  postoperative cerebrospinal fluid leak at, 835
  recesses of, 129–130
  septum of, 127–129
Sphenoid wing
  combined frontotemporal-orbitozygomatic approach for tumors of, 775–784
  meningioma of, cases illustrating surgical resection of, 584–585, 589–594
Sphenomaxillary crest, 113
Sphenomaxillary fissure, 113
Sphenopalatine foramen, 124
  juvenile nasopharyngeal angiofibroma originating in, 485
Sphenopetrosal ligament, superior (abducent bridge), 110
Spinal accessory nerve (accessory nerve, cranial nerve XI), 117
  acoustic neuroma and, 690, 691
  combined lateral suboccipital-infralabyrinthine approach and, 385
  exit zone of, 138–139
  intracisternal course of, 141
  intraoperative monitoring of function of, 95
Spinal drain, for subtemporal and infratemporal approach for clival tumor resection, 162
Spinal lesions, extreme lateral transcondylar and transjugular approaches for
  cases illustrating, 404–410
  complications of, 399–400
  extent of tumor resection and, 399
Spinocranial foramen magnum meningiomas, transcondyle approach for, 673, 674, 675–676
Squamopetrosal sinus, 134
Squamous cell carcinoma
  cavernous sinus, 604
    surgical resection of, indications for, 533–534
  imaging characteristics of, 26
  petroclival, 219

petrous bone, 318
  adjuvant treatment for, 325
  site of origin of, 20, 21
SSEP (somatosensory evoked potential). *See* Somatosensory evoked response
SSER. *See* Somatosensory evoked response
Stability, craniocervical junction, and extreme lateral transcondylar and transjugular approaches, 394–397
Stature, short, in craniopharyngioma, 789
Stereotactic radiosurgery
  for acoustic neuromas, 712
  for craniopharyngiomas, 791
Straight sinus, 134
Styloid process, 113
  muscle origin and, 116
Stylopharyngeal muscle, origin of, 116
Subdural hematoma
  and cerebral revascularization, 65–66
  and petroclival meningioma surgery, 658
Subdural hygroma, and petroclival meningioma surgery, 658
Subdural meningioma, cavernous sinus. *See also* Cavernous meningioma
  resection of, 541
Subfrontal approach, to craniopharyngioma, 792–797, 798
  incisions for, 792, 793
Subfrontal craniotomy, for clival chordomas, 679
Subfrontal-transsphenoidal approach, to craniopharyngiomas, 799–802, 803
Sublabial-paraseptal approach, 339
Suboccipital approach, lateral, for jugular foramen tumors, 381
  with infralabyrinthine approach, 381–386
    advantages of, 385–386
    cranial nerves affected in, 384, 385
    patient positioning for, 381
    results of, 384–386
    steps in, 382–383
Suboccipital transcondyle approach, for foramen magnum meningiomas, 671–678
  anesthesia for, 672
  cases illustrating, 674, 675–677
  complications of, 675
  craniospinal type, 675, 676–677
  craniotomy for, 672
  diagnosis and, 671
  laminectomy for, 672
  operative technique for, 671–674
  patient positioning for, 672
  postoperative management for, 675
  skin incision for, 672
  spinocranial type, 673, 674, 675–676
  surgical steps in, 672, 673
Subtemporal approach, anterior, or frontotemporal transsylvian approach, with zygomatic osteotomy, for petroclival meningiomas, 608
Subtemporal and infratemporal approach
  for clival tumors, 161–171
    cases illustrating, 190–194, 195–197, 198–199, 200–201, 202–207, 211, 213–218
    disadvantages of, 171
    division of V$_3$ in, 167, 169, 170
    extended frontal approach combined with, 175, 176, 177
    reconstruction after, 167–171
    skin incision for, 162
  for petroclival meningiomas, 612, 657
    cases illustrating, 620–626, 626–630

Subtemporal-presigmoid approach, and extreme lateral transcondylar approach, for petroclival meningiomas, cases illustrating, 647, 648–653
Subtemporal/transcavernous/transpetrous apex approach for clival tumors, 159–161
  cases illustrating, 190–194
  reconstruction and, 161
Subtemporal transtentorial approach
  Malis', for clival chordomas, 679
  for petroclival lesions, 661, 663
Subtemporal/transzygomatic approach
  for petroclival meningiomas, cases illustrating, 619, 620–624
  posterior, and presigmoid transpetrous approach, for petroclival meningiomas, 612–613, 614–615, 657
Sugita position, for extreme lateral transcondylar and transjugular approach for clival tumors, 175
Superficial musculoaponeurotic system, facial nerve access and, 437, 440
Superficial temporal artery bypass, artery-to-artery microanastomosis in, 48
Superior approach
  for cavernous meningioma resection, 543
  to orbit, 771
Superior cerebellar artery, 143–144
  acoustic neuromas and, 697–699
Superior hypophyseal arteries, 106–108
Superior laryngeal nerve, swallowing dysfunction caused by injury to, 820
Superior orbital fissure, 99, 101, 103–104
Superior orbital wall, 99
Superior petrosa sinus, 105
Superior sphenopetrosal ligament (abducent bridge), 110
Superior tentorial sinuses, 131
Superselective angiography
  for embolization, 37
  for juvenile angiofibroma, 485
Supracavernous epidermoid, cases illustrating surgical resection of, 584, 587–588
Supraclinoid internal carotid artery, cavernous sinus, and petrosal artery bypass, 52–61
  results of, 62
Supraglottic closure, in swallowing dysfunction, 822
Supraorbital approach, for tuberculum sella meningioma surgery, 508–509, 510
Suprasellar meningioma, cases illustrating surgical resection of, 584–585, 589–594
Sural nerve
  course of, 437
  for reconstruction of facial nerve, 435
Surgical closure. *See also specific procedure*
  for clivus chordoma surgery, 680
  for petrosal approach to clival tumors, 312
  for transmandibular-transcervical approach, 265
  for transmaxillary approach, 239
  for transoral approach, 231–232
  for tuberculum sella meningioma surgery, 515
Surgical exposure, for cranial base surgery, 4. *See also specific procedure*
  for cavernous sinus surgery, 534
  for clivus chordoma surgery, 680
  facilitation and, 75–76

  for glomus jugulare tumor surgery, 749, 750
  for jugular foramen neurilemoma surgery, 733
  for petrosal approach for clival tumor surgery, 309, 310, 311
  for petrous bone tumor surgery, 319–321
  for retrosigmoid approach for acoustic neuroma surgery, 701, 702
  for subfrontal approach for craniopharyngioma surgery, 792, 793
  for subtemporal and infratemporal approach for clival tumor surgery, 162
  for transcondyle approach for foramen magnum meningioma surgery, 672
  for transmandibular-transcervical approach, 262
  for transmaxillary approach, 236–239
  for transoral approach, 228–230
  for transtemporal and infratemporal approach, 269–270
Suspension procedures, for swallowing dysfunction, 820
Swallowing
  complex cranial nerve injury affecting, 820–822
  after jugular foramen neurilemoma resection, 735
  physiology of, 819
  rehabilitation of, 819–823
    laryngotracheal separation for, 822
  single cranial nerve injury affecting, 819–820
  after transmandibular-transcervical surgery, 265
Sylvian dissection, for cavernous meningioma resection, 540
Sympathetic nerve, in cavernous sinus, 521
Sympathetic trunk
  dura mater of posterior cranial fossa supplied by, 132–133
  inferior skull base supplied by, 116

T
Temporal bone
  anatomy of, 268
  benign tumors of, transtemporal and infratemporal approach for resection of, 267–289
    anesthesia for, 269
    case studies illustrating, 276–289
    and choice of surgical approach, 268–269
    complications of, 275–276
    operative technique for, 269–275
    patient position for, 269
    planning for, 267
    preoperative evaluation for, 267–268
  dissection of, 271–273
  postoperative cerebrospinal fluid leak at, 835
  tympanic part of, 113
Temporal bone drilling, in petrosal approach for clival tumors, 309
Temporal craniotomy, for subtemporal/transcavernous/transpetrous apex approach, 159
Temporal lobe resection, for cavernous meningioma surgery, 540
Temporal muscle, origin of, 115
Temporal petrous bone resection, 317–335. *See also* Petrous bone tumors, surgical resection of

Temporalis fascia flap, in middle fossa approach for petrous apex lesions, 295
Temporalis muscle, in facial translocation approach, 253
Temporalis muscle flap, 415–417, 418, 419
Temporalis muscle transposition
  adjunctive static techniques and, 455
  for eyelid reanimation, 450–451
  for mouth (lower facial) reanimation in paralyzed face without facial nerve, 454–455, 456–458, 459
  for swallowing dysfunction, 820
Temporomandibular joint, 113, 114
Tension pneumocephalus, 79
Tentorial arteries, 131, 132
Tentorial sinuses, superior, 131
Tentorium, sectioning, in petrosal approach for clival tumors, 309
Tentorium cerebelli, 131
  blood supply of, 132
Teratomas
  benign, petroclival, 219
  petrous apex, 305
  transsphenoidal approach for resection of, 349
Tertiary ethmoidal canal, 127
Thiopental, for cranial base anesthetic management, 3
  for cavernous sinus surgery, 534
  effects of, 70
Third segment of vertebral artery, 120
Three-dimensional imaging reconstructions, for transmaxillary approach, 235
Thrombocytopenia, dilutional, 77
Thyroid replacement, for craniopharyngioma surgery, 791, 804
L-Thyroxine, for craniopharyngioma surgery, 791, 804
Tinnitus, in glomus jugulare tumors, 747
Titanium miniplates, for craniofacial skeleton fixation, 423, 424
Torus, lateral, 124
Total cochleovestibular nerve section, 362
Total petrosectomy, for petroclival lesions, 662
  cases illustrating, 618–619, 619, 620, 620–624, 647–656
  for meningiomas, 613–617, 657
Total petrous temporal bone resection, 317–335. See also Petrous bone tumors, surgical resection of
Tracheobronchial-pulmonary dysfunction, after otological approaches to acoustic neurilemomas, 722
Tracheoesophageal diversion procedure, in swallowing dysfunction, 821
Tracheostomy
  for transmaxillary approach, 236
  for transoral approach, 227
Transbasal approach of Derome, extended frontal approach as modification of, 171
Transcavernous approach
  frontotemporal
    and presigmoid and transsigmoid transpetrous approach for petroclival meningiomas, 639–647, 648
    and transpetrous apex approach for petroclival meningiomas, 608–611
    and subtemporal and transpetrous apex approaches to clival tumors, 159–161
  cases illustrating, 190–194
  reconstruction and, 161

Transcervical-transmandibular approach to skull base, 261–265
  closure for, 265
  complications of, 265
  incision for, 262
  indications for, 261
  surgical technique for, 261–265
Transcochlear approach, 363–365
  complications of, 364
  indications for, 363
  for jugular foramen tumors, 384
  operative technique for, 363–364
  postoperative management of, 364
Transcondylar and transjugular approaches, extreme lateral, 175–181, 389–411
  anesthesia for, 390
  cases illustrating, 205, 208–210, 213–218, 400–405, 406–409
  cerebrospinal fluid leakage and, 399–400
  complications of, 399–400
  cranial nerve function and, 399
  disadvantages of, 181
  neurologic deficits and, 399
  operative procedure for, 390–394, 395, 396
  operative technique for, 390–397
  patient positioning for, 390
  to petroclival meningiomas, 611, 657
    cases illustrating, 618–619, 620, 626–630, 631–635, 647, 648–653
  posterior fossa lesions and
    complications of surgery for, 399
    extent of tumor resection and, 398–399
  postoperative care and, 397
  preoperative evaluation for, 389–390
  reconstruction after, 180–181
  results of, 397–400
  spinal lesions and
    cases illustrating, 404–410
    complications of surgery for, 399–400
    extent of tumor resection and, 399
  stability and, 394–397, 399
  tumor resection extent and, 398–399
Transcondyle approach for foramen magnum meningiomas, 671–678
  anesthesia for, 672
  cases illustrating, 674, 675–677
  complications of, 675
  craniospinal type, 675, 676–677
  craniotomy for, 672
  diagnosis and, 671
  laminectomy for, 672
  operative technique for, 671–674
  patient positioning for, 672
  postoperative management for, 675
  skin incision for, 672
  spinocranial type, 673, 674, 675–676
  surgical steps in, 672, 673
Transconjunctival approach, to orbit, 772, 773
Transcranial lesions, facial translocation approach for resection of, 245
Transethmoidal anterior approach, for clival tumors, cases illustrating, 198–199
Transfacial approach
  through extended Moure incision, for juvenile angiofibroma surgery, 487–488, 490–491, 491–492, 492
  for osseous lesions of anterior and middle base, 814–816
Transfrontal approach, to orbit, 771
Transfusions, blood, complications of, 77–78
Transjugular and transcondylar approaches, extreme lateral, 175–181, 389–411
  anesthesia for, 390
  cases illustrating, 205, 208–210, 213–218, 400–405, 406–409
  cerebrospinal fluid leakage and, 399–400
  to clival tumors, 175–181
  complications of, 399–400
  cranial nerve function and, 399
  disadvantages of, 181
  neurologic deficits and, 399
  operative procedure for, 390–394, 395, 396
  operative technique for, 390–397
  patient positioning for, 390
  to petroclival meningiomas, 611, 657
    cases illustrating, 618–619, 620, 626–630, 631–635, 647, 648–653
  posterior fossa lesions and
    complications of surgery for, 399
    extent of tumor resection and, 399
  postoperative care and, 397
  preoperative evaluation for, 389–390
  reconstruction after, 180–181
  results of, 397–400
  spinal lesions and
    cases illustrating, 404–410
    complications of surgery for, 399–400
    extent of tumor resection and, 399
  stability and, 394–397, 399
  tumor resection extent and, 398–399
Translabyrinthine approach
  for acoustic tumor resection, 351–362, 711, 712, 716–719, 720
  anesthesia for, 351
  closure for, 361
  complete/simple mastoidectomy and, 353
  complications of, 361–362
  cortical mastoidectomy and, 352–353
  dural incision and, 356–357
  facial nerve and
    dissection of, 359–360
    identification of, 359
  hemostasis for, 361
  indications for, 351
  internal auditory canal dissection and, 354–356
  labyrinthectomy and, 353–354
  limits of, 716
  modifications to, 362
  for neuromas, 711, 712, 716–719, 720
    preoperative preparation and, 716
  operating room arrangement for, 352
  operative technique for, 351–361
  patient positioning for, 351–352
  patient selection for, 351
  petrosal vein and, 357
  postoperative management and, 361
  tumor isolation and, 357–359
  tumor removal and
    completion of, 361
    partial, 357
  venous bleeding and, 356
  for central electroauditory prosthesis placement, 827
  for cochleovestibular nerve section, 362
  for facial nerve decompression or repair, 362
  for jugular foramen tumor surgery, 384
  for petrous apex lesion resection, 292–294
    with cavity obliteration, 292–294
      facial nerve management in, 293–294
      indications for, 292–293
      surgical techniques for, 293

with marsupialization, 292, 293
  indications for, 292, 293
  surgical technique for, 292
Translamina terminalis approach, for craniopharyngioma, 797–799, 800
Transmandibular-transcervical approach to skull base, 261–265
  closure for, 265
  complications of, 265
  incision for, 262
  indications for, 261
  surgical technique for, 261–265
Transmaxillary approach to clivus, 235–244
  and accurate replacement of upper jaw, 240
  anesthesia for, 235–236
  basilar artery and, 239–240
  bleeding and, 239
  cases illustrating, 242–243
  closure for, 239
  complications of, 240
  diagnosis and, 235
  exposure for, 236–239
  and extended maxillectomy, 240–241
    operative technique for, 241–242
  and middle fossa approach for petrous apex lesions, 295, 296
  operative technique for, 235–239
  patient position for, 236
  patient selection for, 235
  postoperative management for, 240
  technical problems with, 239–240
  tumor access and, 239
Transoral approach
  for clivus chordomas, 681–683
  instrumentation for, 4, 7
  for intra/extradural tumors, 225–234
    anesthesia for, 227
    bleeding and, 232
    bone grafting and, 232
    case studies illustrating, 232–234
    closure for, 231–232
      of hard and soft palates, 232
    complications of, 232
    diagnosis and, 225–226
    dural closure in, 231–232
    exposure for, 228–230
    intradural surgery and, 231
    and lesions above foramen magnum, 230–231
    and lesions below foramen magnum, 338
    operative technique for, 227–231
    patient position for, 227–228
    patient selection for, 226–227
    postoperative management for, 232
    technical problems with, 232
Transoral bone grafting, 232
Transpalatal stage, of transzygomatic and transpalatal excision of juvenile nasopharyngeal angiofibroma, 479–480
  patient positioning for, 478
Transpetrous apex approach
  and frontotemporal transcavernous approach, for petroclival meningiomas, 608–611
  and subtemporal and transcavernous approaches
    to clival tumors, 159–161
      cases illustrating, 190–194
      reconstruction and, 161
Transpetrous approach
  presigmoid, and posterior subtemporal approach, for petroclival meningiomas, 612–613, 614–615, 657

presigmoid and transsigmoid, and frontotemporal- transcavernous approach, for petroclival meningiomas, 639–647, 648
Transseptal approach
  in anterior orbitotomy, 773
  transsphenoidal, for clivus chordomas, 679–683, 684
    exposure for, 680–681
    patient positioning for, 680
    postoperative care for, 681
    preoperative preparation for, 680
    steps in, 680–681
Transsigmoid and presigmoid transpetrous approach, and frontotemporal-transcavernous approach, for petroclival meningiomas, 639–647, 648
Transsphenoidal approach
  for invasive sellar and clival lesions, 337–349
    anesthesia for, 338
    cases illustrating, 345–348
    complications of, 345
    diagnosis and, 337
    operating room arrangement for, 338
    operative technique for, 338–344
    patient position for, 338
    patient selection for, 337–338
    pernasal approach for, 339–340
    postoperative management and, 344
    sublabial incision for, 339
  for osseous lesions of anterior and middle base, 814–816
  transseptal, for clivus chordomas, 679–683, 684
    exposure for, 680–681
    patient positioning for, 680
    postoperative care for, 681
    preoperative care for, 680
    steps in, 680–681
Transsylvian approach, frontotemporal
  or anterior subtemporal approach with zygomatic osteotomy, to petroclival meningioma, 608
  and total petrosectomy, for petroclival meningiomas, cases illustrating, 647–656
Transtemporal approach
  for benign tumors of jugular foramen and temporal bone, 267–289
    anesthesia for, 269
    cases illustrating, 276–289
    and choice of surgical approach, 268–269
    complications of, 275–276
    incision for, 269–270
    infratemporal fossa exposure in, 270–271, 272
    for limited lesions, 273, 274, 275
    operative technique for, 269–275
    patient position for, 269
    planning for, 267
    posterior fossa tumor resection and, 273, 274
    preoperative evaluation for, 267–268
    reconstruction after, 273–275
    soft tissue dissection in, 270
    transtemporal dissection in, 271–273
    tumor isolation in, 273
  for glomus jugulare tumors, 749–752
    exposure for, 749–750
Transtemporal dissection, 271–273
Transtrigeminal approach, in intracavernous dissection in meningioma surgery, 545

Transverse segment of vertebral artery, 120
Transverse sinus, 134
Transzygomatic stage, of transzygomatic and transpalatal excision of juvenile nasopharyngeal angiofibroma, 478–479
  patient positioning for, 478
Transzygomatic/subtemporal approach
  for petroclival meningiomas, cases illustrating, 619, 620–624
  posterior, and presigmoid transpetrous approach, for petroclival meningiomas, 612–613, 614–615, 657
Transzygomatic and transpalatal excision, of juvenile nasopharyngeal angiofibroma with intracranial extension, 477–484
  anesthesia for, 477
  cases illustrating, 480–483
  complications of, 480
  operative technique for, 477–480
  patient positioning for, 478
  patient selection for, 477
  postoperative management of, 480
  preoperative preparation for, 477
  technical problems in, 480
  transpalatal stage of, 479–480
  transzygomatic stage of, 478–479
Trapezius muscle flap, 417–421
Trapezius myocutaneous flap, 417–421
Trigeminal ganglion, in lateral wall of cavernous sinus, 110
Trigeminal nerve (cranial nerve V)
  and cavernous meningioma resection, reconstruction of, 549
  in cavernous sinus, 521, 523
  in combined lateral suboccipital-infralabyrinthine approach, 385
  intracisternal course of, 139
  intraoperative monitoring of function of, 95
  neurinoma of, 669
    operative approaches for, 663
  in otological approaches to acoustic neuromas, 723
  paranasal/nasal sinus carcinoma and, 498
  petroclival meningiomas and, 606
  risks to in skull base surgery, 833, 834
  in subtemporal and infratemporal approach for clival tumor resection, 167, 169, 170
  swallowing dysfunction caused by injury to, 820
  topography of, 140
Trigeminal nerve sheath tumor, imaging in evaluation of, 17
Trigeminal neurilemomas, 737–746
  clinical presentation of, 737
  diagnosis and, 737–738
  middle fossa involvement and, 810–811
  surgical resection of
    cases illustrating, 739–743, 744–745
    complications of, 749
    operative technique for, 738–739
    patient selection for, 738
    preoperative evaluation and, 738
Trigeminal neurinomas, 305
Trigeminal portal, 139, 140
Trochlear nerve (cranial nerve IV), 101
  acoustic neuroma and, 690
  in cavernous sinus, 521, 523, 530
  reconstruction of, 548–549, 603
    after tumor resection, 602

Trochlear nerve (cranial nerve IV), in cavernous sinus, (contd.)
  intraoperative monitoring of function of, 95
  in lateral wall of cavernous sinus, 109
  risks to in skull base surgery, 833
Tubercle, and exposure for transoral approach, 228, 229
Tuberculum sella, 105
  meningiomas of, 507–519
    anesthesia for resection of, 508
    arterial dissection during resection of, 511–512, 513
    cases illustrating, 517, 518
    cavernous sinus involvement and, 512, 515
    closure after surgery for, 515
    complications of surgery for, 516–517
    diagnosis of, 507
    hypothalamus dissection in surgery for, 512, 513, 514
    operative technique for resection of, 508–515
    optic canal involvement and, 512, 514
    optic nerve involvement and, 510–511
    patient positioning for resection of, 508
    patient selection for resection of, 507–508
    pituitary stalk dissection in surgery for, 512, 513, 514
    postoperative management after surgery for, 516
    supraorbital approach for resection of, 508–509, 510
    tissue dissection for resection of, 510
    tumor attachment and, 515
    tumor resection and, 510
Tumor access, with transmaxillary approach, 239
Tumor excision, in cranial base surgery, 8
Tumor identification, imaging in, 19, 20–25, 26
Tumors, cranial base. *See* Cranial base tumors
Two-channel electroencephalography, for intraoperative monitoring, 72
Tympanic bone, 113
Tympanic nerve, 116
Tympanic part of temporal bone, 113

U

Ultrasonic aspiratory, Cavitron, for cranial base surgery, 8
Upper clivus, 157, 158, 606. *See also* Clivus
  approach selection for tumors of, 157–159
Upper jaw, accurate replacement of after transmaxillary surgery, 240
Urine output, after transsphenoidal surgery for invasive lesions, 344, 345
Uvular muscle, 116

V

Vagus nerve (cranial nerve X), 117
  acoustic neuroma and, 690, 691
  in combined lateral suboccipital-infralabyrinthine approach, 385
  exit zone of, 138–139
  intracisternal course of, 141
  intraoperative monitoring of function of, 95
  and otologic approaches to acoustic neuroma, 723
  in petroclival meningioma, 606
  risks to in skull base surgery, 834
  swallowing dysfunction caused by injury to
    complex nerve injury, 820–821
    single nerve injury, 820
Vagus nerve palsy, in glomus vagale tumor surgery, 768
Vascular complications after skull base surgery, 837–838
  evaluation of, 837
  management of, 837–838
  prevention of, 837
  surgical technique and, 837
Vascular reconstruction, after cavernous meningioma surgery, 547–548
Vascular tumors, in jugular foramen, 379
Vascularity
  and facial translocation approach, 248
  of paranasal/nasal sinus carcinomas, 498
Vasopressin, for transsphenoidal approach, 338
Vein-to-artery microanastomosis, 49
Vein grafts, results of, 61–62
Venography, for orbital lesions, 771
Venous air embolism, 76–77
  and hypovolemia, 74
Venous bleeding, in intracavernous dissection in meningioma surgery, 547
Venous patch grafting, in cerebral revascularization, 50, 51, 52
Venous pressure, reduction of, and facilitating surgical exposure, 76
VEPs. *See* Visual evoked potentials
Vertebral artery, 120, 141–142
  bone and dura of posterior cranial fossa supplied by, 132
  occlusion of, and assessing need for revascularization, 45
Vertebral artery interposition grafting, 61
Vertebral veins, 120
Vertigo, cochleovestibular nerve section for, 362
Vesalius, foramen of, 104
Vestibular nerve
  and acoustic neuroma removal, 687, 688
  resection of, 376–377
Vestibular nerves, inferior and superior, and acoustic neuroma removal, 687, 688
Vestibular testing, and petrous apex lesions, 292

Vestibulocochlear nerve (cranial nerve VIII)
  and acoustic neuroma, 687, 688, 690
  exit zone of, 138
  intracisternal course of, 139
  in petroclival meningioma, 606
  total section of, 362
Vincristine, for esthesioneuroblastoma, 473
Visual evoked potentials, monitoring during cranial base surgery, 84, 94–95. *See also* Evoked potential studies
Visual field testing, in preoperative patient evaluation, 3
Visual loss
  after craniofacial resection for paranasal sinus tumors, 504–505
  in craniopharyngiomas, 788, 789
    after surgery, 804
  after osseous lesion (anterior and middle base) surgery, 817
  and tuberculum sella meningiomas, 507–508
  after tuberculum sella and olfactory groove meningioma surgery, 517
Vitallium microplates, for craniofacial skeleton fixation, 423, 424
Vomiting
  in craniopharyngioma, 789
  postoperative, 79–80

W

Wharton's duct, in transmandibular-transcervical approach, 262
Work stations, diskless, in NeuroNet, 86
Wound closure
  and transmaxillary approach, 239
  and transoral approach, 231–232
Wound infection, after petroclival meningioma surgery, 658
Wrisberg nerve, and otologic approaches to acoustic neuroma, 723

X-Y

Xenon/CT/cerebral blood flow study, 33–36
  and assessing need for revascularization, 45

Z

Z-plasty, for swallowing dysfunction, 820
Zeiss-Contraves microscope, for cranial base surgery, 4
Zygomatic osteotomy
  in cavernous sinus surgery, 537–538
  in frontotemporal-transsylvian/anterior subtemporal approach for petroclival meningiomas, 608
  in subtemporal/transcavernous/transpetrous apex approach, 159